AMERICAN
HANDBOOK OF
CLINICAL
MEDICINE

Second Edition

Published and forthcoming Oxford American Handbooks

Oxford American Handbook of Clinical Medicine
Oxford American Handbook of Anesthesiology
Oxford American Handbook of Cardiology
Oxford American Handbook of Clinical Dentistry
Oxford American Handbook of Clinical Diagnosis
Oxford American Handbook of Clinical Pharmacy
Oxford American Handbook of Critical Care
Oxford American Handbook of Disaster Medicine
Oxford American Handbook of Emergency Medicine
Oxford American Handbook of Endocrinology and Diabetes
Oxford American Handbook of Geriatric Medicine
Oxford American Handbook of Hospice and Palliative Medicine
Oxford American Handbook of Infectious Diseases
Oxford American Handbook of Nephrology and Hypertension
Oxford American Handbook of Neurology
Oxford American Handbook of Obstetrics and Gynecology
Oxford American Handbook of Oncology
Oxford American Handbook of Otolaryngology
Oxford American Handbook of Pediatrics
Oxford American Handbook of Physical Medicine and Rehabilitation
Oxford American Handbook of Psychiatry
Oxford American Handbook of Pulmonary Medicine
Oxford American Handbook of Radiology
Oxford American Handbook of Reproductive Medicine
Oxford American Handbook of Rheumatology
Oxford American Handbook of Sports Medicine
Oxford American Handbook of Surgery
Oxford American Handbook of Urology

OXFORD AMERICAN HANDBOOK OF CLINICAL MEDICINE

Second Edition

EDITED BY

JOHN A. FLYNN, MD, MBA, MED
GENERAL INTERNAL MEDICINE
AND RHEUMATOLOGY
JOHNS HOPKINS UNIVERSITY

MICHAEL J. CHOI, MD
MEDICINE AND NEPHROLOGY
JOHNS HOPKINS UNIVERSITY

L. DWIGHT WOOSTER, MD
MEDICINE AND PULMONARY DISEASE
JOHNS HOPKINS UNIVERSITY

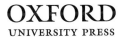

OXFORD
UNIVERSITY PRESS

OXFORD
UNIVERSITY PRESS

Oxford University Press is a department of the University of Oxford.
It furthers the University's objective of excellence in research, scholarship,
and education by publishing worldwide.

Oxford   New York
Auckland   Cape Town   Dar es Salaam   Hong Kong   Karachi
Kuala Lumpur   Madrid   Melbourne   Mexico City   Nairobi
New Delhi   Shanghai   Taipei   Toronto

With offices in
Argentina   Austria   Brazil   Chile   Czech Republic   France   Greece
Guatemala   Hungary   Italy   Japan   Poland   Portugal   Singapore
South Korea   Switzerland   Thailand   Turkey   Ukraine   Vietnam

Oxford is a registered trademark of Oxford University Press
in the UK and certain other countries.

Published in the United States of America by
Oxford University Press
198 Madison Avenue, New York, NY 10016

© Oxford University Press, 2013

Library of Congress Cataloging-in-Publication Data
Oxford American handbook of clinical medicine / edited by John A. Flynn, Michael
J. Choi, L. Dwight Wooster.— 2nd ed.
    p. ; cm.—(Oxford American handbooks)
Adapted from: Oxford handbook of clinical medicine / Murray Longmore,
Ian B. Wilkinson, Supraj R. Rajagopalan, 6th ed. 2004.
Includes bibliographical references and index.
ISBN 978-0-19-991494-4 (alk. paper)—ISBN 978-0-19-998515-9 (alk. paper)—
ISBN 978-0-19-998516-6 (alk. paper)
I. Flynn, John A., MD.   II. Choi, Michael J.   III. Wooster, L. Dwight (Lyman
Dwight)
IV. Oxford handbook of clinical medicine.   V. Series: Oxford American handbooks.
[DNLM: 1. Clinical Medicine—Handbooks. WB 39]
LC Classification not assigned
616—dc23   2012038115

9 8 7 6 5 4 3 2 1
Printed in the United States of America
on acid-free paper

Preface

The Hippocratic Oath is a pledge by all physicians to practice medicine ethically and honestly. As part of that oath, our beliefs hold a promise "to teach (our students) this art, if they desire to learn it, without fee or covenant; to give a share of precepts and oral instruction and all the other learning to … pupils who have signed the covenant and have taken an oath according to the medical law…". Clearly, as we were embarking on writing and editing this medical text, we were not dwelling on the magnitude of this late 5th-century Greek work. We were, nonetheless, thinking about and motivated by the long-standing tradition in medicine of sharing medical knowledge with colleagues, especially with our students of medicine. In contrast to the early days of medicine, this sharing of medical knowledge is distributed to all cultures and all countries and is incredibly more open to all who "desire to learn it."

The Oxford American Handbook of Clinical Medicine is particularly written for physicians-in-training; students in medical school and physicians in their residency. The tradition of teaching and sharing medical information had its beginnings at our hospital more than 120 years ago. It is here that Sir William Osler wrote and published, in 1892, The Principles and Practice of Medicine. This book was heralded as the most current work of clinical management of patients based on known scientific principles. In addition to his review of the science of medicine, Osler's text provided sage advice on the art of compassionate patient care. Unlike in the days of Osler, we now have access to current medical information at the speed of electrons with our various hand-held devices, search engines, and electronic medical records. As a result, now more than ever, our trainees must assiduously balance the science of medicine with the art of medicine. Although this handbook is replete with medical information, as authors and editors we also worked diligently to balance the art and compassionate delivery of medicine with the facts of clinical decisions. We are acutely aware of new health care policies, both local and national, of clinical cost containment, of the importance of quality medical outcomes with high efficiency, and with goals of professionalism. In this new edition, we have attempted to incorporate these aspects into medical decision-making processes and recommendations for accurate diagnosis and treatment.

This book aims to present both the science and the art of patient management. Our trainees are challenged in their clinical years to remember and assimilate an enormous volume of medical information; additionally, students of medicine are applying and synthesizing this material within the context of their care of patients in the hospital and the outpatient environment. The process of integrating medical knowledge with patient care is a repetitive one, in which learning will come in many forms and from numerous sources. This book is one of those sources. The Oxford American Handbook of Clinical Medicine is designed as a reference when contemplating symptoms and signs and medical conditions. Although relatively small and constructed to fit into pockets or backpacks, this text is formatted to accommodate the growth and development of your medical knowledge. The contributors of this manual have the understanding and experience to emphasize one of the grandest sources of medical knowledge—your patients. As you interact with each patient, questions will arise; use each clinical question and each patient experience to stimulate your quest for medical knowledge. Allow your patients to become the foundations of this knowledge; allow your patient's illnesses and their reactions to their illnesses and treatments to formulate your compassion and your art of medicine. Relish the journey; it will last a lifetime.

Acknowledgments

We, the three editors of the *Oxford American Handbook of Clinical Medicine*, express our most profound gratitude to all of the authors who have contributed to this book. These contributors are highly respected colleagues from the Johns Hopkins School of Medicine. They have been fastidious in their development of these chapters, incorporating the most recent evidence-based guidelines into clinical practice.

We also have the distinct privilege of participating in the care of our patients while teaching physicians-in-training within Johns Hopkins Medicine. The care of patients, the recognition of their ills, the definition of their clinical problems, and the provision of their care are the foundations of the practice of medicine. This privilege of caring, cemented by medical knowledge, is commonly a bilateral interaction shared mutually whether with our patients or with our students. Through these interactions we have learned as much as we have imparted.

The sharing of medical information with our colleagues, our students, and our patients is imperative for successful health care. The presentation of current, accurate, and dependable medical knowledge is essential for successful, evidence-based quality outcomes for our patients. Our participation in writing and editing this medical text was motivated by our indebtedness to our patients and our students.

We also wish to acknowledge all of the efforts provided by Oxford University Press, in particular Andrea Seils, Senior Editor of Clinical Medicine. She has served throughout this effort as a steadfast advocate for the excellence and clarity of this text. Her many hours of dedication and profound patience are greatly appreciated.

JF would like to thank his children, Emilee, John, Sarah, Jayne, Christian, Patrick, and W. Andrew for their constant support of one another as our family advances. He also wishes to thank Bill Baumgartner for his mentorship. Most importantly he must thank Monica—his wife, his life—for her infinite support and strength during the past 35 years of being together.

MC would like to thank his wife Mia, his son Chris, and his daughter Julia for their endless support and infinite patience. They have forgiven him far too many things. He would like to thank his parents for always doing their best for him. He would also like to thank his mentor Pedro Fernandez, on behalf of all of his mentees, for simply making us better doctors.

DW extends his appreciation to his fiancée, Tina Blasi, who has unequivocally supported his decision to work on this text; she has been his cornerstone and source of encouragement. Tina's love and devotion are his emotional foundations from which he changed professional paths and expanded his professional and personal horizons. Additionally, his children Ashley, Margaux, and Tyler are universally helpful in contributing to his energy and ideas, and to his wish for better health care for them and for their children. He also wishes to thank Mike Weisfeldt for giving him the opportunity to join the faculty of Johns Hopkins' Medicine.

Finally, we wish to dedicate this book to Dr. Frederick L. Brancati for being a constant source of strength, courage, and guidance to us, through not only his words but through his actions.

Contents

List of Contributors

Sumera Ali, M.D.
Johns Hopkins University
Radiology

Arjun S. Chanmugam, M.D.
Johns Hopkins University
Emergency Medicine

Colleen Christmas, M.D.
Johns Hopkins University
Geriatric Medicine

April Fitzgerald, M.D.
Johns Hopkins University
Signs and Symptoms

John A. Flynn, M.D., M.B.A., M.ED.
Johns Hopkins University
Rheumatology

Matthew Foy, M.D.
Louisiana State University
Renal Medicine

Susan L. Gearhart, M.D.
Johns Hopkins University
Surgery

Mark T. Hughes, M.D., M.A.
Johns Hopkins University
Thinking About Medicine

Joshua D. King, M.D.
University of Virginia
Biochemistry

Daniel Laheru, M.D.
Johns Hopkins University
Oncology

L. David Martin, M.D.
Johns Hopkins University
Signs and Symptoms

Alison R. Moliterno, M.D.
Johns Hopkins University
Hematology

Kendall F. Moseley, M.D.
Johns Hopkins University,
Endocrinology

Rodney Omron, M.D., M.P.H.
Johns Hopkins University
Emergency Medicine

Gregory P. Prokopowicz, M.D., M.P.H.
Johns Hopkins University
Epidemiology

Jason Rosenberg, M.D.
Johns Hopkins University
Neurology

Stuart Russell, M.D.
Johns Hopkins University
Cardiovascular Medicine

Paul E. Segal, D.O.
Johns Hopkins University
Biochemistry

Shmuel Shoham, M.D.
Johns Hopkins University
Infectious Disease

Lanaya W. Smith, M.D.
Johns Hopkins University
Rheumatology

Ellen M. Stein, M.D.
Johns Hopkins University
Gastroenterology

C. Matthew Stewart, M.D., PH.D.
Johns Hopkins University
Practical Procedures

Rosalyn W. Stewart, M.D., M.S.
Johns Hopkins University
Practical Procedures

Sumeska Thavarajah, M.D.
Johns Hopkins University
Renal Medicine

Clifford R. Weiss, M.D.
Johns Hopkins University Radiology

L. Dwight Wooster M.D.
Johns Hopkins University
Pulmonary Medicine

Symbols and abbreviations

1°	Primary
2°	Secondary
–ve; +ve	negative and positive, respectively
6-MP	thiopurine
A_2	aortic component of second heart sound
A_2A	angiotensin-2 receptor antagonist (AT-2, A2R, and AIIR)
Ab	antibody
ABC	airway, breathing, and circulation: basic life support
ABG	arterial blood gas measurement (PaO_2, $PaCO_2$, pH, HCO_3^-)
ABI	ankle brachial index
ABPA	allergic bronchopulmonary aspergillosis
ac	*ante cibum* (before food)
ACE	angiotensin-converting enzyme
ACS	acute coronary syndrome
ACTH	adrenocorticotropic hormone
AD	Alzheimer's disease
ADH	antidiuretic hormone
Ad lib	ad libitum; as much/as often as wanted (Latin for *at pleasure*)
ADL	activities of daily living
AF	atrial fibrillation
AFB	acid-fast bacillus
AFP	(and α-FP) α-fetoprotein
Ag	antigen
AIDS	acquired immunodeficiency syndrome
AIH	autoimmune hepatitis
AIN	acute interstitial nephritis
AKI	acute kidney injury
alk phos	alkaline phosphatase (also ALP)
ALL	acute lymphoblastic leukemia
AMA	antimitochondrial antibody
AML	acute myeloid leukemia
AMP	adenosine monophosphate
ANA	antinuclear antibody
ANCA	antineutrophil cytoplasmic antibody
APTT	activated partial thromboplastin time
AR	aortic regurgitation
ARB	angiotensin receptor blocker
ARDS	acute respiratory distress syndrome
ARF	acute renal failure
ART	antiretroviral therapy
AS	aortic stenosis
ASD	atrial septal defect
ASO(T)	antistreptolysin o (titer)
AST	aspartate transaminase

AT-2	angiotensin-2 receptor blocker (also AT-2, A2R, and AllR)
ATN	acute tubular necrosis
ATP	adenosine triphosphate
AV	atrioventricular
AVM	arteriovenous malformation(s)
AVNRT	AV nodal reentry tachycardia
AVRT	AV reentry tachycardia
AXR	abdominal x-ray (plain)
AZA	azathioprine
AZT	zidovudine
Ba	barium
BAL	bronchoalveolar lavage
BET	benign essential tremor
BHL	bilateral symmetrical hilar lymphadenopathy
BID	*bis die* (twice a day)
BKA	below-knee amputation
BMD	bone mineral density
BMI	body mass index
BNP	brain natriuretic peptide
BP	blood pressure
bpm	beats per minute (e.g., pulse)
BUN	blood urea nitrogen
ca	carcinoma
Ca	calcium
CABG	coronary artery bypass graft
CAD	coronary artery disease
cAMP	cyclic adenosine monophosphate (AMP)
CAP	community-acquired pneumonia
CAPD	continuous ambulatory peritoneal dialysis
CBC	complete blood count
CBD	common bile duct
CC	creatinine clearance
CCPD	continuous cyclic peritoneal dialysis
CCU	coronary care unit
CDC	Centers for Disease Control, U.S.
CEA	carcino-embryonic antigen
CF	cystic fibrosis
CGM	continuous glucose monitoring
CHB	complete heart block
CHD	coronary heart disease (related to ischaemia and atheroma)
CHF	congestive heart failure (i.e., left and right heart failure)
Chol	cholesterol
CI	contraindications
CIPD	chronic inflammatory demyelinating polyradiculoneuropathy
CK	creatine (phospho)kinase (also CPK)

CKD	chronic kidney disease
CLL	chronic lymphocytic leukemia
CML	chronic myeloid leukemia
CMV	cytomegalovirus
CNS	central nervous system
CONS	coagulase-negative *Staphylococcus*
COPD	chronic obstructive pulmonary disease
COX	cyclo-oxygenase
CPAP	continuous positive airways pressure
CPPD	calcium pyrophosphate dihydrate
CPR	cardiopulmonary resuscitation
CRC	colorectal cancer
CrCl	creatinine clearance
CRF	chronic renal failure
CRP	C-reactive protein
CRRT	continuous renal replacement therapy
CSF	cerebrospinal fluid
CT	computed tomography
CVD	cardiovascular disease
CVP	central venous pressure
CVS	cardiovascular system
CXR	chest x-ray
d	day(s) (also expressed as ×/7)
DC	direct current
DIC	disseminated intravascular coagulation
DIP	distal interphalangeal
dL	deciliter
DEXA	dual energy x-ray absorptiometry
DLCO	diffusing capacity of lung
DM	diabetes mellitus
DOT	directly observed therapy
DTPA	diethylenetriamine penta-acetic acid
DU	duodenal ulcer
D&V	diarrhea and vomiting
DVT	deep venous thrombosis
EAA	extrinsic allergic alveolitis
EBM	evidence-based medicine
EBV	Epstein–Barr virus
ECG	electrocardiogram
Echo	echocardiogram
EDTA	ethylene diamine tetraacetic acid (e.g., in a CBC bottle)
EEG	electroencephalogram
EKG	electrocardiogram; also ECG
EGD	esophagogastric-duodenoscopy
ELISA	enzyme linked immunosorbent assay

EM	electron microscope
EMG	electromyogram
ENT	ear, nose, and throat
ERCP	endoscopic retrograde cholangiopancreatography
ESR	erythrocyte sedimentation rate
ESRD	end-stage renal disease
EUA	examination under anesthesia
EUS	endoscopic ultrasonography
EVAR	endovascular aneurysm repair
FB	foreign body
FDA	U.S. Food and Drug Administration
FDP	fibrin degradation products
FEV_1	forced expiratory volume in first second
FFP	fresh frozen plasma
FGF	fibroblast growth factor
FH	family history
FHF	fulminant hepatic failure
F_IO_2	partial pressure of O2 in inspired air
FNA	fine needle aspiration
FROM	full range of movements
FSH	follicle-stimulating hormone
FUO	fever of unknown origin
FVC	forced vital capacity
g	gram
GA	general anesthetic
GB	gall bladder
GC	gonococcus
GCA	giant cell arteritis
GCS	Glasgow Coma Scale
GERD	gastroesophageal reflux disease
GFR	glomerular filtration rate
GGT	gamma glutamyl transpeptidase
GH	growth hormone
GI	gastrointestinal
G6PD	glucose-6-phosphate dehydrogenase
GN	glomerulonephritis
GPA	granulomatosis with polyangiitis
GTT	glucose tolerance test (also OGTT: oral GTT)
GU	genitourinary; also gastric ulcer
h	hour
HAART	highly active antiretroviral therapy
HAP	hospital-acquired pneumonia
HAV	hepatitis A virus
Hb	hemoglobin
HBsAg/HBV	hepatitis B surface antigen/hepatitis B virus

HBIG	hepatitis B immune globulin
HCAP	health care acquired pneumonia
HCC	hepatocellular cancer
Hct	hematocrit
HCV	hepatitis C virus
HD	hemodialysis
HDL	high-density lipoprotein
HDV	hepatitis D virus
HELLP	hemolysis, elevated liver enzymes, low platelet count syndrome
HH	hereditary hemochromatosis
HHS	hyperosmolar hyperglycemic state
HHT	hereditary hemorrhagic telangiectasia
HHV	human herpes virus
HIDA	hepatic iminodiacetic acid
HIT	heparin-induced thrombocytopenia
HIV	human immunodeficiency virus
HLA	human leukocyte antigen
HOCM	hypertrophic obstructive cardiomyopathy
HONK	hyperosmolar nonketotic (diabetic coma)
HPV	human papilloma virus
HRCT	high-resolution computed tomography
HRS	hepatorenal syndrome
HRT	hormone replacement therapy
HSV	Herpes simplex virus
HTN	hypertension
HUS	hemolytic uremic syndrome
IBD	inflammatory bowel disease
IBS	irritable bowel syndrome
ICP	intracranial pressure
ICS	intercostal space
ICU	intensive care unit
IDA	iron-deficiency anemia
IDDM	insulin-dependent diabetes mellitus
IFN-α	α interferon
IE	infective endocarditis
IFG	impaired fasting glucose
Ig	immunoglobulin
IGRA	interferon gamma release assay
IGT	impaired glucose tolerance
IHD	ischemic heart disease
IL	interleukin
IM	intramuscular
IMNM	immune-mediated necrotizing myopathy
IND	indinavir

INR	international normalized ratio (prothrombin ratio)
IPPV	intermittent positive pressure ventilation
ISH	isolate systolic hypertension
ITP	idiopathic thrombocytopenic purpura
iu	international unit
IVC	inferior vena cava
IVDU	intravenous drug user
IVIG	intravenous immunoglobulin
IVF	
IV(I)	intravenous (infusion)
IVU	intravenous urography
JVP	jugular venous pressure
K	potassium
kg	kilogram
L	liter
LA	left atrium of heart
LAD	left axis deviation on the ecg
LBBB	left bundle branch block
LDH	lactate dehydrogenase
LDL	low-density lipoprotein
LFT	liver function test
LH	luteinizing hormone
LLQ	left lower quadrant
LMN	lower motor neuron
LMWH	low-molecular-weight heparin
LMP	last menstrual period
LP	lumbar puncture
LR	lactated Ringer's
LRD	living related donor
LTOT	long term oxygen therapy
LUQ	left upper quadrant
LV	left ventricle of the heart
LVF	left ventricular failure
LVH	left ventricular hypertrophy
LVOT	left ventricular outflow tract
μg	microgram
MAI	*Mycobacterium avium intracellulare*
MAOI	monoamine oxidase inhibitors
MC & S	microscopy, culture, and sensitivity
MCP	metacarpophalangeal joints
MCV	mean cell volume
MDCT	multidetector computed tomography
MDMA	3,4-methylenedioxymethamphetamine
MDRD	Modification of Diet in Renal Disease
MELD	model for end-stage liver disease

OPD	outpatient department
ORh–	blood group O, Rh negative
OT	occupational therapist
P_2	pulmonary component of second heart sound
P_aCO_2	partial pressure of carbon dioxide in arterial blood
PAD	*peripheral artery disease*
PAN	polyarteritis nodosa
P_aO_2	partial pressure of oxygen in arterial blood
PAS	periodic acid-Schiff
PBC	primary biliary cirrhosis
PCN	penicillin
PCOS	polycystic ovary disease
PCR	polymerase chain reaction (DNA diagnosis)
PCV	packed cell volume
PD	peritoneal dialysis; also Parkinson's disease
PDGF	platelet-derive growth factor
PE	pulmonary embolism
PEEP	positive end-expiratory pressure
PERLA	pupils equal and reactive to light and accommodation
PEF(R)	peak expiratory flow (rate)
PET	positron emission tomography
PFT	pulmonary function tests
PI	protease inhibitor
PID	pelvic inflammatory disease
PIP	proximal interphalangeal (joint)
PMH	past medical history
PMR	polymyalgia rheumatica
PND	paroxysmal nocturnal dyspnea
PO	*per os* (by mouth)
POEM	peroral endoscopic myotomy
PPF	purified plasma fraction (albumin)
PPI	proton pump inhibitor; e.g., omeprazole, lansoprazole, etc.
PR	*per rectum* (by the rectum)
PRN	*pro re nata* (as required)
PSA	prostate specific antigen
PSC	primary sclerosing cholangitis
PTCA	percutaneous transluminal coronary angioplasty
PTH	parathyroid hormone
PTT	prothrombin time
PTU	propylthiouracil
PUD	peptic ulcer disease
qd	each day
qid	*quater in die* (4 times a day); qqh: *quarta quaque hora* (every 4h)
R	right
RA	rheumatoid arthritis; also right atrium of heart

RAD	right axis deviation on the ECG
RBBB	right bundle branch block
RBC	red blood cell
RCT	randomized controlled trial
RF	renal failure
R/O	rule out
RLQ	right lower quadrant
RUQ	right upper quadrant
RV	right ventricle of heart; also residual volume of lung
RVF	right ventricular failure
RVH	right ventricular hypertrophy
R_x	*recipe* (treat with)
s or sec	second(s)
S1, S2	first and second heart sounds
SARS	severe acute respiratory syndrome
SBE	subacute bacterial endocarditis (IE, *infective endocarditis*, is better)
SBP	spontaneous bacterial peritonitis
SC	subcutaneous
SCD	spontaneous compression device
SD	standard deviation
SE	side effect(s)
SEER	Surveillance Epidemiology and End Results program
SEM	systolic ejection murmur
SL	sublingual
SLE	systemic lupus erythematosus
SOB	short of breath
SPECT	single positron emission computed tomography
SQ	subcutaneous
SR	slow-release (also called modified-release)
SNRI	serotonin-norepinephrine reuptake inhibitor
SSRI	selective serotonin reuptake inhibitor
stat	*statim* (immediately; as initial dose)
STD/STI	sexually transmitted disease; sexually transmitted infection
SVC	superior vena cava
SVT	supraventricular tachycardia
sy(n)	syndrome
T°	temperature
$t_{1/2}$	biological half-life
T1DM	type 1 diabetes mellitus
T2DM	type 2 diabetes mellitus
T3	triiodothyronine
T4	thyroxine
TB	tuberculosis
TCC	transitional cell carcinoma
TFTs	thyroid function tests (e.g., tsh)

TIA	transient ischemic attack
TIBC	total iron binding capacity
Tid	*ter in die* (3 times a day)
TEE	trans-esophageal echocardiogram
TENS	transcutaneous electrical nerve stimulation
TGF	tumor growth factor
TLC	total lung capacity
TLS	tumor lysis syndrome
TMP/SMX	trimethoprim/sulfamethoxazole
TNF	tumor necrosis factor
TPR	temperature, pulse, and respirations count
TR	tricuspid regurgitation
TRH	thyroid-releasing hormone
Trig	triglycerides
TSH	thyroid-stimulating hormone
TSST	toxic shock syndrome toxin
TTE	trans-thoracic echocardiogram
TTP	thrombotic thrombocytopenic purpura
TUIP	transurethral incision of the prostate
TURP	transurethral resection of the prostate
U	units
UC	ulcerative colitis
U&E	urea & electrolytes & creatinine in plasma, unless stated otherwise
UDCA	ursodeoxycholic acid
UMN	upper motor neuron
URT	upper respiratory tract
URTI	upper respiratory tract infection
US(S)	ultrasound (scan)
UTI	urinary tract infection
VAP	ventilator-acquired pneumonia
VAT	video-assisted thorascopy
VDRL	Venereal Diseases Research Laboratory
VEGF	vascular endothelial growth factor
VISA/VRSA	vancomycin intermediate/resistant Staphylococcus aureus
VF	ventricular fibrillation
VLDL	very low density lipoprotein
VMA	vanillyl mandelic acid (HMMA)
V./Q.	ventilation/perfusion ratio
VSD	ventriculo-septal defect
VT	ventricular tachycardia
WBC	white blood cell
WCC	white cell count
wk(s)	week(s)
WPW	Wolff-Parkinson-White syndrome
WHO	World Health Organization

WR	Wassermann reaction
yr(s)	year(s)
ZN	Ziehl–Neelsen (stain for acid-fast bacilli; e.g., mycobacteria)

Other abbreviations are given on pages where they occur: consult the *index*.

Thinking about medicine

Mark T. Hughes, M.D., M.A.

Contents

Ideals

Decision and *intervention* are the essence of action. Reflection and conjecture are the essence of thought. The essence of medicine is combining these realms of decision and intervention in the service of others. We offer these ideals to stimulate both thought and action: Like the stars, these ideals are hard to reach—but they serve for navigation during the night.

- *Remember the goal of healing is to make the person whole:* This applies whether the aim is cure, relief of symptoms in an acute or chronic illness, prevention of complications in a chronic disease, or comfort in an incurable disease.
- *Do not blame the sick for being sick:* They come to you for help. You are there for them, not the other way around.
- *If the patient's wishes are known, comply with them.*
- *Work for your patients, not your attending.*
- *Use ward rounds to boost the patient's morale*, not your own.
- *Treat the whole patient*, not the disease.
- *Admit people*—not "strokes," "infarcts," "shooters," or "gomers."
- *Spend time with the bereaved*; you can help them shed their tears.
- *Question your conscience*—however strongly it tells you to act.
- *Respect the opinions of nurses;* they know the patient, spend the most time with the patient, and are usually right.
- *Work as a team member;* everyone on the interdisciplinary team has a valuable role in the patient's care.
- *Be kind to yourself*—you are not an inexhaustible resource.
- *Give the patient (and yourself) time:* Time to ask questions, time to reflect, time to allow healing to take place, and time to gain autonomy.
- *Give the patient the benefit of the doubt.* If you can, *be optimistic:* Patients want physicians to be realistic but also to instill hope.

While these ideals speak to our actions—*what we do*—we also have to be mindful of *who we are*. None of us is perfect and will never be perfect, but we can strive to reach asymptotically for perfection. This entails trying to develop habits of character that lead to virtues… and a virtuous life. The virtues especially important in medicine include honesty and integrity, courage and fortitude, *phronesis* (practical wisdom), temperance and equanimity, justice, self-effacement, compassion, and care.[1]

Ideal and less than ideal methods of care

The story of Ivan Ilyich illustrates the options: "Special foods were prepared for him on the doctor's orders, but these became more and more unpalatable, more and more revolting… Special arrangements, too, were made for his bowel movements. And this was a regular torture—a torture because of the filth, the unseemliness, the stench, and the knowledge that another person had to assist him… Yet it was precisely through this unseemly business that Ivan Ilyich derived some comfort. The pantry boy, Gerasim, always came to carry out the chamber pot. Gerasim was a clean, ruddy-faced young peasant who was thriving on town food. He was always bright and cheerful… 'Gerasim,' said Ivan Ilyich in a feeble voice… 'This must be very unpleasant for you. You must forgive me. I can't help it.'… 'Oh no, sir!' said Gerasim as he broke into a smile, his eyes and strong white teeth gleaming. 'Why shouldn't I help you? You're a sick man.' Gerasim did everything easily, willingly, simply, and with a goodness of heart that moved Ivan Ilyich. Health, strength, and vitality in other people offended Ivan Ilyich, whereas Gerasim's strength and vitality had a soothing effect on him."[2]

It was the pantry boy who was his true healthcare provider and caregiver, who took him on his own terms, cared for him, and gave him time and dignity. While Ivan Ilyich's physicians and others cooperated in the "lie" that he was ill but not dying, "Gerasim was the only one who understood and pitied him." Gerasim did not find his work burdensome, because he understood he was doing it for a dying man. As T. S. Eliot said, "*there is, at best, only a limited value in the knowledge derived from experience*" (e.g., the knowledge encompassed in this book). The pantry boy had the innate understanding and the natural compassion that we all too easily lose amid the science, the knowledge, and our stainless steel universe of organized healthcare.

The oft-quoted advice of Francis Peabody nearly a century ago still provides guidance: "for the secret of the care of the patient is in caring for the patient."[3]

Health and medical ethics

Medicine has its own internal morality. This derives from a patient's illness and his or her subsequent vulnerability, coupled with the physician's intent to help the patient improve. Each time a physician asks of the patient, "How can I help you?" there is an implicit understanding that the physician will use his or her expertise to serve the best interests of the patient.

As members of a profession, physicians declare publicly that they will put aside their self-interest in the service of others. Although society grants physicians certain privileges (e.g., prescribing medication, determining

1 Pellegrino ED, Thomasma DC. *The Virtues in Medical Practice*. New York: Oxford University Press; 1993.
2 Tolstoy L. *The Death of Ivan Ilyich*. New York: Bantam Books; 1981.
3 Peabody F. 1927, The care of the patient. *JAMA*. 1927;88(12):877–882.

disability), it also expects certain duties of the profession, namely that physicians be the stewards of valuable societal resources. Professionalism is our contract with society and entails certain commitments on the part of physicians.[4]

In the sphere of ethics, physicians are called upon to lead as often as to follow. To do this, we need to return to basic principles and put society's expectations temporarily to one side.

Our analysis starts with our aim: To do good by promoting people's health. *Health* entails being sound in body and mind, and having powers of growth, development, healing, and regeneration. *How many people have you made healthy (or at least healthier) today? Good* is the most general term of commendation and entails four chief duties:

- Not doing harm (nonmaleficence). We owe this duty to all people, not just our patients.
- Doing good by positive actions (beneficence). We particularly owe this to our patients. There are four ways by which the patient's good can be defined: (1) the ultimate good, that which has the highest meaning for the patient; (2) the biomedical good, obtained by treatment of the disease; (3) the patient's perception of the good based on his or her life plan; and (4) the good of the patient as a person, deserving respect and the freedom to make reasoned choices.[5]
- Respecting autonomy or respecting the person. Autonomy (self-determination) is not universally recognized; in some cultures, such as those facing starvation, it may be irrelevant or even subversive. But respecting persons and their inherent dignity is to be found across cultures. This is manifested in medicine by upholding patients' rights to be informed, to be offered all the options, to be told the truth, and to have their confidentiality protected.
- Promoting justice—distributing scarce resources fairly and treating people fairly, such as when we respect their legal rights.

The point of having these guiding principles is to provide a context for our negotiations with patients. If we want to be better doctors, a good starting point is trying to put these principles into action. Inevitably, when we try, there are times when the principles seem to conflict with each other. What should guide us when these principles conflict? It is not just a case of deciding off the top of one's head. It requires further inquiry, deliberation, and aspiring to a *synthesis*—if you have the time (time will so often be what you do *not* have; but, in retrospect, when things have gone wrong, you realize that they would not have done so if you had *made* time).

Synthesis When we must act in the face of two conflicting duties, one of the duties will take precedence. How do we tell which one? Trying to find out involves getting to know our patients and asking some questions:

- Are the patient's wishes being complied with?
- What do the patient's loved ones (family and/or friends) think? First, ask the patient's permission to speak to the loved ones. Do the patient's loved ones have his or her best interests at heart?
- What do colleagues think? Often having the input of other clinicians can help sort out the complexities of a difficult case.

4 ABIM Foundation. American Board of Internal Medicine; ACP-ASIM Foundation. American College of Physicians-American Society of Internal Medicine; European Federation of Internal Medicine. Medical professionalism in the new millennium: A physician charter. *Ann Intern Med.* 2002;136(3): 243-246.
5 Pellegrino ED, Thomasma DC. *For the Patient's Good: The Restoration of Beneficence in Healthcare.* New York: Oxford University Press; 1988.

- Is it desirable that the reason for an action be universalizable? (That is, if I say this person is too old for such-and-such an operation, am I happy to make this a general rule for everyone?—Kant's "law.")[6]
- What would the man on the street say? These opinions are valuable as they are readily available, and they can stop decision making from becoming dangerously medicalized. Seeking these opinions also prompts one to think about the "reasonable person" standard when getting informed consent.
- If an investigative journalist were to sit on a sulcus of mine, having full knowledge of my thoughts and actions, would she be bored or would she be composing vitriol for tomorrow's newspapers? If so, can I answer her, point for point? Am I happy with my answers? Or are they tactical cerebrations designed to outwit her?
- What would I do if nobody were watching? Would I act the same way if there were no consequences in terms of public scrutiny? Will I be able to face myself in the mirror the next morning?
- Do I need the input of the hospital ethics committee? In some cases, ethics consultants can help to facilitate discussion among interested parties, sort out the ethical issues at stake, and provide an opinion about ethically permissible options for resolution of the problem.

Good ethics starts with good facts. Understanding a situation completely, or as complete as possible, can go a long way in figuring out the most appropriate course of action. Four domains of knowledge need to be explored:

1 *Medical indications*—diagnosis, prognosis, goals of treatment, and probabilities of success;
2 *Patient preferences*—the values and perspective of the patient relative to the medical indications; is the patient competent to make decisions, and, if not, who will speak for him?;
3 *Quality of life*—the prospects for improving or restoring the patient's quality of life and what to do if there is treatment failure;
4 *Contextual features*—ranging from family or provider issues to legal, economic, or cultural factors.[7]

The bedside manner and communication skills

Our bedside manner matters because it indicates to patients whether they can *trust* us. Where there is no trust, there can be little healing. A good bedside manner is not static: It develops in coordination with the patients' needs, but it is grounded in the timeless clinical virtues of honesty, humor, and humility in the presence of human weakness and human suffering.

The following are examples from an endless variety of phenomena that arise whenever doctors meet patients. One of the great skills (and pleasures) in medicine is to learn how our actions and attitudes influence patients, and how to take this knowledge into account when assessing the validity and significance of the signs and symptoms we elicit. The information we

---

6 There are problems with universalizability: Sometimes only intuition can suggest how to resolve conflicts between competing universal principles. Universal principles work in the abstract but have drawbacks when applied to real-life situations. Also, there is a sense in which all ethical dilemmas are unique—they *cannot* be universal. This leads some ethicists to favor case-based reasoning (i.e., casuistry).
7 Jonsen AR, Siegler M, Winslade WJ. *Clinical Ethics: A Practical Approach to Ethical Decisions in Clinical Medicine*, 6th ed. New York: McGraw-Hill; 2006.

receive from our patients is not "hard evidence," but a much more plastic commodity, molded as much by the doctor's attitude and the hospital or consulting room environment as by the patient's own hopes and fears. It is our job to adjust our attitudes and environment, so that these hidden hopes and fears become manifest and the channels of communication are always open.

Anxiety reduction or intensification A simple explanation of what you are going to do often defuses what can be a highly charged affair. With children, try more subtle techniques, such as examining the abdomen using the child's own hands, or examining their teddy bear first.

Pain reduction or intensification Compare: "I'm going to press your stomach. If it hurts, cry out" with "I'm going to touch your stomach. Let me know what you feel." The examination can be made to sound frightening, neutral, or joyful, and the patient will relax or tense up accordingly.

The tactful or clumsy invasion of personal space The physical examination can involve close contact with the patient that is normally not acceptable as part of usual social interaction. Acknowledging this to the patient can set both parties at ease. For example, during ophthalmoscopy, simply explain "I need to get very close to your eyes for this."

The use of distraction to gather information Skillful practitioners palpating the painful abdomen will start away from the part that hurts. They will watch the patient's face while talking about a hobby or the patient's family while they press as hard as they need to. If the patient stops talking and frowns only when the doctor's hand is over the right lower quadrant, the doctor will already have found out something useful.

Awareness of the patient experience If you ask the patient to hold his breath while listening to the carotid artery, also hold your breath, so that you know when it might be getting uncomfortable for the patient as you intently listen for the tell-tale bruit.

Communication Your skills are useless unless you communicate well. Be simple, and direct. Avoid jargon: "Remission" and "growth" are frequently misunderstood. Give the most important details first. Be specific. "Drink 6 cups of water per day" is better than "Drink more fluids." Provide written information with easy readability. Aim for a sixth-grade reading level—more like the *Reader's Digest* than the *Wall Street Journal*. If possible, show videos for patient education. Do not assume your patient can read. Naming the pictures but not the words on our visual test chart helps find this out tactfully.

Inquire about your patient's views of what should be done. Patient-centered care improves provider–patient interactions and patient satisfaction. Find goals of care that can be mutually agreed upon. Learn more about the patient's values. We often talk of *compliance* with our regimens, when what we should talk of is *concordance*, for concordance recognizes the central role of patient participation in all good plans of care.

Asking questions

No class of questions is "correct." Sometimes you need to ask one type of question; sometimes another. The good clinician can shift from one kind to another, in order to use the most effective questions for each individual patient. The aim of asking questions is to *describe*, to find a shared world between the doctor and patient. Questions provide the means to offer practical help: Once the illness is described, a diagnosis can be made and a possible cure offered. If not curable, the experience can at least be shared, mitigated, and so partially overcome. Different kinds of questions either throw light on the experience or obscure it, as in the examples below.

Leading questions On seeing a bloodstained handkerchief you ask: "How long have you been coughing up blood?" "Six weeks, doctor," so you assume hemoptysis for 6 weeks. In fact, the stain could be due to an infected finger, or to epistaxis. On finding this out later (and perhaps after expensive and unpleasant investigations), you will be upset, but the patient was politely trying to give the sort of answer you were obviously expecting. With such leading questions as these, the patient is not given an opportunity to deny your assumptions.

Questions suggesting the answer "Was the vomit red, yellow, or black—like coffee grounds?"—the classic description of vomited blood. "Yes, like coffee grounds, doctor." The doctor's expectations and hurry to get the evidence into a pre-determined format have so tarnished the story as to make it useless.

Open-ended questions The most open is "How are you?" This suggests no particular answer, so the direction a patient chooses offers valuable information. Other examples are gentle imperatives such as "Tell me about the vomit." "It was dark." "How dark?" "Dark with little chunks in it." "Like…?" "Like bits of soil in it." This information is pure gold, although it is not cast in the form of "coffee grounds."

Close-ended questions Sometimes in obtaining the history, it is necessary to ask specific, close-ended questions to round out the information. These may only require a "Yes/No" answer or might prompt the patient to give more details. This line of questioning can aid in formulating the differential diagnosis and make sure you do not miss important clues. "Did you have a fever?" "Did you notice wheezing?" "Have you had swelling in your ankles?"

Patient-centered questions "What do you think is wrong?" "Are there any other aspects of this we might explore?" "Are there any questions you want to ask?" (a close-ended question). Better still, try "What are the other things on your mind? How is this affecting you? What is the worst thing? It makes you feel… (the doctor is silent)." Becoming patient-centered gives you a better chance of healing the whole person, and the patient may be more satisfied as a result.

Framing questions in the context of the family This is particularly useful in revealing if symptoms are caused or perpetuated by psychosocial factors. Family-oriented questions probe the network of causes and enabling conditions that allow nebulous symptoms to flourish in a person's life. "Who else is important in your life? Are they worried about you? Who really understands you?" Until this sort of question is asked, illness may be refractory to treatment. For example: "Who is present when your headache starts? Who notices it first—you or your wife? Who worries about it most (or least)? What does your wife do when (or before) you get it?" The spouse's view of the symptoms may be the best predictor of outcome for the patient.

Framing questions in the context of culture In medicine, we may encounter patients from diverse backgrounds, sometimes quite different from our own. The skillful clinician will be self-aware enough to recognize any biases he or she may have based on his or her own cultural identity. To be culturally competent, the clinician should be open to exploring the patient's health beliefs from the patient's cultural perspective. Admitting ignorance of the patient's culture in an inquiring, respectful manner may provide clues as to how best help the patient within his worldview. Curiosity can also fortify the relationship: "Help me understand what this means to you in light of your background."

Echoing Try repeating the last words said as a route to new intimacies, otherwise inaccessible, as you fade into the distance and the patient soliloquizes "I've always been suspicious of my wife." "Wife…" "My wife… and her boss working late at night together." "Together…" "I've never trusted them together." "Trusted them together…" "No, well, I've always felt I've known who my son's real father was… I can never trust those two together." Without any questions, you may unearth the unexpected, important clue that throws a new light on the history.

Empathic opportunities Remember that the purpose of the medical interview is not just to gain information, but to develop a relationship. Are you asking questions in a respectful way that validates the patient's emotional experience? After getting facts about the illness experience, ask the follow-up question, "How did you feel about that?" and acknowledge the emotions reported. Match body language to build rapport and make it more likely that the patient will be open to answering questions. Be attentive to nonverbal communication, which may shed light on the patient's underlying feelings and increase the yield of the information: Does the patient cross his arms in a defensive posture when talking about his wife? Maybe that's a clue as to why he is getting headaches.

The value of silence Sometimes not asking a question will give the patient the opportunity to share important information. There is value in the pregnant pause…

If you only ask questions, you will only receive answers in reply. If you interrogate a robin, he will fly away: Treelike silence may bring him to your hand.

What is the mechanism? Finding narrative answers

Like toddlers, we should always be asking *"Why?"*—not just to find ultimate causes, but to enable us to choose the simplest level for intervention. Some simple change early on in a chain of events may be sufficient to bring about a cure, whereas later on in the chain such opportunities may not arise.

For example, it is not enough for you to diagnose heart failure in your breathless patient. Ask: *"Why is there heart failure?"* If you do not, you will be satisfied with giving the patient an anti-failure drug, and any side effects from these, such as uremia or incontinence induced by diuretic-associated polyuria, will be attributed to an unavoidable consequence of necessary therapy. If only you had asked *"What is the mechanism of the heart failure?"* you might have found an underlying cause (e.g., anemia coupled with ischemic heart disease). You cannot cure the latter, but treating the anemia may be all that is required to cure the patient's breathlessness. But do not stop there. Ask: *"What is the mechanism of the anemia?"*

You find a low serum ferritin, and you might be tempted to say to yourself,"I have the root cause." Wrong! Put aside the idea of prime causes and go on asking *"What is the mechanism?"* Return to the patient (never think that the process of history-taking is over). Retaking the history reveals that the patient has a very poor diet. *"Why is the patient eating a poor diet?"* Is he ignorant or too poor to eat properly? You may find the patient's wife died a year ago, he is sinking into a depression, and cannot be bothered to eat. He would not care if he died tomorrow.

You now begin to realize that simply treating the patient's anemia may not be of much help to him—so go on asking *"Why?"*: "Why did you bother to go to the doctor at all if you are not interested in getting better?" It turns out that he only went to see the doctor to please his daughter. He is unlikely to take your treatment unless you really get to the bottom of what he cares about. His daughter is what matters, and, unless you can enlist her help, all your therapeutic initiatives will fail. Talk with his daughter, offer help for the depression, teach her about iron-rich foods, and, with luck, your patient's breathlessness may gradually begin to disappear. Even if it does not start to disappear, you may perhaps have forged a partnership with your patient that can be used to enable him to accept help in other ways—and this dialogue may help you to be a more humane and kinder doctor, particularly if you are feeling worn out and assaulted by long lists of technical tasks that you must somehow fit into impossibly overcrowded days and nights.

Constructing imaginative narratives yielding new meanings Doctors are often thought of as being reductionist and overmechanistic. The previous section shows that always asking "why" can sometimes enlarge the scope of our inquiries, rather than narrowing the focus. Another way to do this is to ask *"What does this symptom mean?"*—for this person, their family, and our world. For example, a limp might mean a neuropathy or inability to meet mortgage repayments (if you are a dancer)—or it may represent a medically unexplained symptom that subtly alters family hierarchies, both literally (during family walks through the country) and metaphorically. Science is about clarity, objectivity, and theory in modeling our external world. But there is another way of modeling the external world that involves subjectivity, emotion, ambiguity, and the seeking of arcane relationships between apparently unrelated phenomena. The medical humanities explore the latter—and have been burgeoning during the last two decades—leading to the existence of two camps—humanities and science. If, while reading this, you are getting impatient to get to the real nuts and bolts of technological medicine, you are in the latter camp. We are not suggesting that you leave it—only that you learn to operate out of both camps. If you do not, your professional life will be full of failures (which you may deny or of which you will remain ignorant). If you do straddle both camps, there will also be failures—but you will realize what these failures mean, and you will know how to transform them. With reflection comes growth.

Always remember that medicine is both an art and a science. In the *tekné iatrike* of medicine,[8] physicians are master craftsmen who must have the technical skill and knowledge to ply their craft, but also the artistry to practice it with compassion in the context of a patient's life. No matter his or her specialty, each physician should recognize that *every* contact with a patient in the practice of medicine has a technical dimension, to be sure, but also an artistic one.

Medicine, art, and the humanities

Let us start with an elementary observation: The most famous doctors are those immortalized in literature (e.g., Dr. Watson, Dr. Zhivago, Dr. Frankenstein, and Dr. Faustus).[9] Thus we demonstrate the power of the written word. And it *is* an extraordinary power. When we curl up in an armchair and read for pleasure, we open the portals of our minds because we are alone. While we are reading, there is no point in dissembling. We confront our subject matter with a steady eye because we believe that, while reading to ourselves, we cannot be judged. Then, suddenly, when we are at our most open and defenseless, literature takes us by the throat—and that eye which was so steady and confident a few minutes ago is now

---

8 Pellegrino ED, Thomasma DC. *A Philosophical Basis of Medical Practice: Toward a Philosophy and Ethic of the Healing Professions.* New York: Oxford University Press; 1981.

9 Of course, Dr. Faust, that famous charlatan, necromancer, and quack from medieval Germany, did have a real existence. In fact, there may have been two of them, who together gave rise to the myth of devil-dealing, debauchery, and the undisciplined pursuit of science, without the constraints of morality.

perhaps misting over, or our heart is missing a beat, or our skin is covered in a goose-flesh more papular than ever a Siberian winter produced. Once we have been on earth for a few decades, not much in our mundane world sends shivers down our spines, but the power of worlds of literature and art to do this continues to grow.

There are, of course, doctors who are quite well known as literary artists: Arthur Conan Doyle, William Carlos Williams, Somerset Maugham, and Anton Chekhov from the past and Michael Crichton, Oliver Sacks, Abraham Verghese, and Sherwin Nuland from more recent times. What about Sigmund Freud? Here is the exception that proves the rule—proves in the sense of testing, for he is not really an exception. We can accept him among the great only in so far as we view his collection of writings as an artistic oeuvre, rather than as a scientific one. Science has progressed for years without Freud, but, as art, his work and insights will survive: And survival, as Bernard Shaw pointed out, is the only test of greatness.

The reason for the ascendancy of art over science is simple. We scientists, in our humble way, are only interested in explaining reality. Artists are good at explaining reality, too: But they also *create* it. William Carlos Williams wrote in *Imaginations*, "... now works of art... must be real, not 'realism' but reality itself—they must give not the sense of frustration but a sense of completion, of actuality—It is not a matter of 'representation'—which may be represented actually, but of separate existence."[10]

Our most powerful impressions are produced in our minds not by simple sensations but by the association of ideas. It is a preeminent feature of the human mind that it revels in seeing something as, or through, something else: Life refracted through experience, light refracted through jewels, or a walk through the woods transmuted into a *Pastoral Symphony*. Ours is a world of metaphor, fantasy, and deceit.

William Carlos Williams noted, "There is neither beginning nor end to the imagination but it delights in its own seasons reversing the usual order at will. Of the air of the coldest room it will seem to build the hottest passions."[11] He poetically linked his imagination to his experiences as a physician doing house calls in New Jersey to capture the essence of humanity.

What has all this to do with the day-to-day practice of medicine? The answer lies in the word "defenseless." When we read alone and for pleasure, our defenses are down—and we hide nothing from the great characters of fiction. This openness to the story of another helps to keep us connected with our patients. So often, a professional detachment is all that is left after all those years inured to the foibles, fallacies, and frictions of our patients' tragic lives. It is at the point where art and medicine collide that doctors can reattach themselves to the human race and re-experience those emotions that motivate or terrify our patients. Art and literature can cultivate our empathy, so that, at some level, there can be truth to the statement, "I understand what you're going through," even though we ourselves may not have had to endure the illness experience of the patient.

We all have an Achilles heel: That part of our inner self that was not rendered forever invulnerable to mortal cares when we were dipped in the waters of the river Styx as it flowed down the wards of our first disillusion. Art and literature, among other things, may enable this Achilles heel to be the means of our survival as thinking, sentient beings, capable of maintaining a sympathetic sensibility to our patients.

10 Williams WC. *Imaginations*. New York: New Directions Publishing; 1970:116.
11 Williams WC. *Imaginations*. New York: New Directions Publishing; 1970:35.

Anton Chekhov wrote, "I feel more confident and more satisfied when I reflect that I have two professions and not one. Medicine is my lawful wife and literature is my mistress. When I get tired of one I spend the night with the other. Though it's disorderly it's not so dull, and besides, neither really loses anything, through my infidelity."[12]

Narrative medicine allows us to see *the patient as text*, and thereby foster speculation and curiosity about the patient's worldview of illness… and hone our ability make a diagnosis.

The art and science of diagnosing

The central processes of medicine are relieving symptoms, providing reassurance and prognostic information, and lending a sympathetic ear (see Table 1.1). But it is very difficult to do any of this without a working diagnosis. How is this achieved?

We diagnose, it is held, by a three-stage process: We take a history, we examine, and we do tests. We then collate this information, by a process which is never explained, and ultimately arrive at a diagnosis. So how *are* diagnoses made?

Diagnosing by recognition For students, this is the most irritating method. You spend an hour asking all the wrong questions, then in waltzes a doctor who names the disease and sorts it out before you have even finished taking the pulse. This doctor has simply recognized the illness like he recognizes an old friend (or enemy).

Diagnosing by probability theory Over the course of our clinical lives, we unconsciously build up a personal database of diagnoses and outcomes, and their associated pitfalls. We unconsciously run each new "case" through this personal and continuously developing fine-grained probabilistic algorithm.

Diagnosing by hypothesizing We formulate a hypothesis from the moment we hear the chief complaint. Our subsequent questions in history-taking, the focus of our physical exam, and/or our selection of tests provide the data to prove or disprove our original hypothesis, or to formulate a new one.

Diagnosing by reasoning Like Sherlock Holmes, we exclude each differential diagnosis; then, whatever is left must be the culprit. This process presupposes that our differential includes the culprit and that we have methods for *absolutely* excluding diseases. All tests are statistical, rather than absolute—which is why the Holmes technique is, at best, fictional.

Diagnosing by a "wait and see" approach Some doctors (and patients) need to know immediately and definitively what the diagnosis is, while others can tolerate more uncertainty. With practice, one can sense that the dangers and expense of exhaustive tests can be obviated by the skillful use of time. This cough *might* represent pneumonia, but I may choose not to get a chest x-ray or sputum culture. Rather, I may say "take this antibiotic if you get a fever—but you probably don't need it, and you'll get better on your own: Wait and see."

Diagnosing by selective doubting Traditionally, patients are "unreliable," signs are objective, and lab tests virtually perfect. When diagnosis is difficult, try inverting this hierarchy. The more you do so, the more you realize that there are no hard signs or perfect labs. But the game of medicine is unplayable if you doubt everything, so doubt selectively.

Table 1.1 Diagnosis by iteration and reiteration

A brief history suggests looking for a few signs, the assessment of which leads you to ask further questions and do a few tests. As this process reiterates, various diagnostic possibilities crop up and receive more or less confirmation. "I feel my heart racing"—and the doctor immediately puts his finger on the pulse, feels it to be irregularly irregular, and infers atrial fibrillation (AF; see p. 120). He wants to know *why* there is AF, so he asks about weight loss and heat intolerance. This suggests hyperthyroidism (p. 298) as the cause of the AF. While he takes the pulse, he notices clubbing of the fingers, so he makes a mental note to do a chest x-ray to see if there are signs of cancer (could this cause the AF?—yes). This reminds him to ask about smoking: While inquiring about habits, he asks about alcohol, and elicits excessive drinking. "Why now?" "Because I lost my job." In the time it takes to assess the pulse, the doctor has many promising leads to follow and is starting to formulate a diagnosis in three dimensions: Physical, psychological, and social. The patient's palms are clammy and the pulse is weak, so the doctor knows he must be prompt and decisive, and gently explains that admission for various tests is needed. Whereupon the patient, who has been holding back tears, now weeps. Now holding her hand, as well as continuing to take her pulse, the doctor becomes aware of a change in rhythm. Is this sinus rhythm, brought on by the Valsalva-like maneuver of weeping? So the doctor now says "Well... let's see how you do over the next hour—you'll feel better for crying." "Yes, you're right, I feel better already."

This is a microcosm of the intuitive world of medicine, which the solely systematic doctor never knows. He would come on to the pulse only after a "full history"—and would have missed everything. The doctor who can work on many different levels simultaneously will often be the first to know the diagnosis.

Diagnosing by computer Computing power is the only way of fully mapping the interrelatedness of diseases (e.g., hyponatremia with eosinophilia points to *Addison's disease*, and if there is oliguria, the computer "knows" that oliguria is a feature of shock, and shock is a complication of Addison's).

Prevention

Two mottos: "*The only good medicine is preventive medicine*" and "*If preventable...why not prevented?*" During life on the wards you will have many opportunities to practice preventive medicine, and, unconsciously, you will pass most of them over in favor of more glamorous tasks such as diagnosis and clever interventions, involving probes, scalpels, and imaging. But if we imagine a ward in which scalpels remain sheathed and the only thing being probed is our commitment to health, then preventive medicine comes to the forefront, and it is our contention that such a ward might produce more health than some entire hospitals.

Ways of thinking about prevention Preventing a disease (e.g., by vaccination) is *primary prevention*. Controlling disease in an early form (e.g., carcinoma *in situ*) is *secondary prevention*. Preventing complications in those already symptomatic is *tertiary prevention*.

The best way of thinking about prevention is to ask "*What can I do now with this patient in front of me?*" On the wards, this will often be secondary or tertiary prevention (e.g., blood pressure screening in diabetes, or colonoscopy in ulcerative colitis [looking for colon cancer], or endoscopic screening for esophageal cancer in Barrett's esophagus).

The first step in prevention is to motivate your patient to take steps to benefit his or her own health by asking Socratic questions. "Do you want to smoke?" "What does your family think about smoking" "Do you want your children to smoke?" "Would there be any advantages in giving up?" "Why is your health important to you?" "Is there anything more important we can help with?" "How would you spend the money you might save?" These types of questions, along with specific strategies in prevention (p. 87) are more likely to produce change than will withering looks and lectures on lung cancer. In summary: In any preventive activity, get the patient on your side—make her want to change. Once you have done this, preventive activities you might promote include:

Primary- and secondary disease prevention	General health	Cancer screening
Vaccination (e.g., flu shot if >65 yrs)	Healthy eating	Colon cancer screening
Aspirin if vascular disease	Regular exercise	Pap smears
Cardiovascular risk reduction	Advice on smoking and alcohol	Mammography and annual breast exam
Osteoporosis prevention if on steroids or postmenopausal (calcium, vitamin D, ± bisphosphonate)	House and car dangers: Seat belts, accidents, falls, gun safety	Genetic counseling (e.g., if family history positive in two 1st-degree relatives)

11

Sometimes referral to other agencies is needed (e.g., for genetic counseling, contraception, and preconception advice).

Concentrate on those preventive activities that are simple, cheap, and have a complication rate approaching zero. When considering a more complicated or "high-tech" preventive procedure, be on guard for unintended consequences, such as colon perforation in colonoscopy. When risk is involved with the preventive strategy, weigh the procedure in light of the patient's history and other medical problems. Get the patient's input about whether the preventive measure is right for him or her.

Individualized risk communication When counseling a patient about screening tests, communication should be based on a person's individual risk factors for a condition (e.g., age, family history, smoking status, cholesterol level). With some conditions, this can be achieved with decisional aids or using formulae. A Cochrane meta-analysis suggests this kind of individualized approach will "not necessarily" change behavior, although uptake of screening tests is improved. At least this technique promotes dialogue, and dialogue opens doors, minds, and possibilities for choice. *Informed participation* is the aim, not passive acceptance of advice. Improved knowledge, beliefs, and risk perceptions can be achieved with this approach. How clinical evidence is presented can make a difference in certain patient populations. Participatory decision-making is facilitated when the physician:

- Understands the patient's experience and expectations.
- Builds partnership.
- Provides evidence, including a balanced discussion of uncertainties.
- Checks for understanding and agreement.
- Presents recommendations informed by clinical judgment and patient preferences.

Prescribing drugs

Before prescribing any drug with which you are not thoroughly familiar, consult the *Physicians' Desk Reference* (PDR), your local equivalent, or a reliable online reference site like Micromedex:

<http://www.thomsonhc.com/micromedex2/librarian>

Before prescribing, ask if the patient is allergic to anything. The answer is often "Yes," but do not stop here. Find out what the reaction was, or else you run the risk of denying your patient a possibly life-saving and very safe drug, such as penicillin, because of a mild reaction like nausea. Is the reaction a *true allergy* (anaphylaxis, p. 748 or a rash?), a *toxic effect* (e.g., ataxia is inevitable if given large quantities of phenytoin), a *predictable adverse reaction* (e.g., GI bleeding from aspirin), or an *idiosyncratic reaction*?

Remember *primum non nocere*: First do no harm. The more minor the complaint, the more weight this dictum carries. The more serious the complaint, the more its antithesis comes into play: *Nothing ventured, nothing gained.*

Ten commandments These should be written on every tablet:

1 Explore any alternatives to a prescription. Prescriptions lead to doctor-dependency, which in turn frequently leads to bad medicine and drives up the expense of healthcare. There are three places to find alternatives:
   • *The kitchen*: Lemon and honey for sore throats, rather than penicillin.
   • *The blackboard:* For example, education about the self-inflicted causes of esophagitis. Rather than giving expensive drugs, advise against too many big meals, eating close to bedtime, smoking and alcohol excess, or wearing overly tight garments.
   • *Last, look to yourself.* Giving a piece of yourself, some real empathy, is worth more than all the drugs in your pharmacopoeia to patients who are frightened, bereaved, or weary of life.
2 Find out if the patient wants to take a drug. Are you prescribing for some minor ailment because you want to solve every problem? Patients may be happy just to know the ailment *is* minor. If they know what it is, they may be happy to live with it. Some people do not believe in drugs, and you must find this out.
3 Decide if the patient is responsible. If she swallows *all* the acetaminophen with codeine pills that you have prescribed for her acute pain at one time, death will be swift.
4 Know of other ways your prescription may be misused. Perhaps the patient whose "insomnia" you so kindly treated is actually grinding up your prescription for injection in order to get a fix. Will you be suspicious when he returns to say he has lost your prescription?
5 Address these questions when prescribing:
   • How many daily doses are there? 1–2 is much better than 4.
   • How many other drugs are to be taken? Can they be reduced?
   • Can the patient read the instructions on the bottle—and can he open it?
   • Is the patient agreeable to enlisting the help of a loved one or caretaker to ensure that she remembers to take the pills?
   • Is the patient taking the medication properly? Check by counting the remaining pills at the next visit.
   • How will the patient refill his prescription?
   • How will you know and what will you do if the patient does not come for a follow-up visit?
6 List the potential benefits of the drug for *this* patient.
7 List the risks (side-effects, contraindications, interactions, risk of allergy). Of any new problems, always ask yourself: *Is this a side-effect?*

8 Try to ensure there is true concordance between you and your patient on the risk–benefit ratio's favorability. Document your discussion.

9 Record how you will review the patient's need for each drug and quantify progress (or lack thereof) toward specified, agreed goals (e.g., pulse rate to mark degree of β-blockade or peak flow reading to guide steroid use in asthma).

10 Make a record of all drugs taken. Offer the patient a copy.

Is this new treatment any good? (Analysis and meta-analysis)

This question frequently arises when reading journals. Not only authors, but *all* clinicians have to decide what new treatments to recommend and which to ignore. Evidence-based medicine recognizes two fundamental principles: (1) the physician must assess the strength and validity of the evidence for the new treatment based on a hierarchy; (2) decision makers must consider the patient's values and trade off the benefits, risks, inconvenience, and costs of alternatives.

Users' Guides to the Medical Literature have been created to help the clinician decide whether the results of a research study will help in the care of his or her patients. In assessing the use of research, ask the following:

1 Are the results valid? Much must be taken on trust, since many statistical analyses depend on sophisticated computing. Few papers, unfortunately, present "raw" data. Look out for obvious faults by asking:

2 Were comparison groups (experimental and control groups) similar in terms of prognosis and clinical characteristics at the start of the study?

3 Were patients randomized to the comparison groups? Did randomization produce groups that were well matched? Were the treatments being compared carried out by practitioners equally skilled in each treatment?

4 Was the study placebo-controlled? Good research can go on outside the realm of double-blind, randomized trials, but you need to be more careful in drawing conclusions (e.g., for intermittent symptoms, a bad time [prompting a consultation] is followed by a good time, making any treatment given in the bad phase appear effective). *Regression toward the mean* occurs in many areas (e.g., repeated BP measurement: Because of transitory or random effects, most people having a high value today will have a less high value tomorrow—and most of those having a low value today will have a less extreme value tomorrow). This concept works at the bedside: If someone who is drowsy after a head injury has a high BP, and the next measurements are higher still (i.e., no regression to the mean), then this suggests a "real" effect, such as increased ICP.

5 Was the study blinded? In a double blind study, both patients and doctors are unaware of which treatment the patient is having. Could patients, doctors, or those assessing outcome have figured out which treatment was given (e.g., by the metabolic effects of the drug)?

6 Is the sample large enough to detect a clinically important difference, say a 20% drop in deaths from disease X? If the sample is small, the chance of missing such a difference is high. To reduce this chance to less than 5%, and if disease X has a mortality of 10%, more than 10,000 patients would need to be randomized. If a small trial that lacks power (the ability to detect true differences) does give "positive" results, the size of the difference between the groups is likely to be exaggerated. This is *type I error*; a *type II error* applies to results that indicate that there is no effect, when in fact there is one. So beware of quite big trials that

purport to show that a new drug is equally effective as an established treatment.

7 How large was the treatment effect, and how precisely was it measured?

8 Does the study give a clear, clinically significant answer, as well as a statistically significant answer in patients similar to those I treat? Are the likely treatment benefits worth the potential risks and costs if applied in the clinical setting?

9 Is the journal peer reviewed? Experts vet the paper before release (an imperfect process, as they have unknown axes to grind—as well as competing interests).

10 Has time been allowed for criticism of the research to appear in the correspondence columns of the journal in question?

11 If I were the patient, would I want the new treatment?

12 What have the Centers for Disease Control (CDC) or professional organizations said? Have clinical guidelines been developed as a result of the research findings?

Meta-analyses Systematic merging of similar trials can help resolve contentious issues and explain data inconsistencies. Meta-analysis is quicker and cheaper than doing new studies, and can establish generalizability of research. *Be cautious!* Bias can result from pharmaceutical funding or from the meta-analyst's own assumptions about the topic under study.

A well-planned large trial may be worth centuries of uncritical medical practice; but a week's experience on the wards may be more valuable than years reading journals. As William Osler said, "To study the phenomena of disease without books is to sail an uncharted sea, while to study books without patients is not to go to sea at all."[13]

This is the central paradox in medical education. How can we trust our own experiences, knowing they are all anecdotal; how can we be open to novel ideas but avoid being merely fashionable? A stance of wary open-mindedness may serve us best.

Resource allocation and distributive justice

Resource allocation: How to decide who gets what There is a perception in the United States that healthcare resources are scarce. When one looks at the availability of organ transplants, critical care beds, home care services, and other potentially beneficial treatments, this appears to be true. Resource allocation is about cutting the healthcare cake—the size of which is given based on how much society is willing to expend on healthcare relative to other societal priorities.

Making the cake Focusing on how to cut the cake diverts attention from the central issue: How large should the cake be? The answer may be that more needs to be spent on our healthcare services, not at the expense of some other health gain, but at the expense of something else. The percentage of gross domestic product (GDP) spent on healthcare differs from country to country, and economists debate how much is too much… or too little.

Slicing the cake In deciding how to slice the healthcare cake, methods have been developed to find a rational basis for allocating resources. One method used by health economists is the QALY.

What is a QALY? The essence of a QALY (Quality Adjusted Life Year) is that it takes a year of healthy life expectancy to be worth 1, but a year

---

13 Osler W. Books and men, in *Aequanimitas*, 2nd ed. Philadelphia: P. Blakiston's Son & Co.; 1925.

of unhealthy life expectancy is regarded as <1. Its exact value is lower the worse the quality of life of the unhealthy person. If a patient is likely to live for 8 yrs in perfect health on an old drug, he gains 8 QALYs; if a new drug would give him 16 yrs but at a quality of life rated by him at only 25% of the maximum, he would gain only 4 QALYs. The dream of health economists is to buy the most QALYs for his budget. QALYs *are* helpful in guiding rationing, but problems include accurate pricing, the invidiousness of choosing between the welfare of different patients—and the problem of QALYs not adding up: If a vase of flowers is beautiful, are 10 vases (or QALYs) 10 times as beautiful—or might the scent be overpowering?

Eating the cake In their daily practices, the majority of physicians will not have to contemplate the larger picture of how society spends its healthcare dollars. They will have to worry about whether the patient can afford the medication just prescribed, whether a proposed treatment will be covered by the insurance plan, where their patient is on the transplant waiting list, etc. How much the everyday clinician needs to factor allocation of resources into treatment recommendations (i.e., bedside rationing) is a controversial topic. The physician must resist the temptation to live by the dictum *primum non expendere*, and should stay focused on serving the best interests of the patient. Part of their responsibility in achieving the patient's best interests is in providing *cost-effective* medical care. Physicians and patients should be part of the societal discussion on cost-savings in the delivery of proven, effective treatments.

Distributive justice Distributive justice is that unyielding and perpetually problematic benchmark against which all civilizations must, sometime or other, come to measure themselves. Among the questions that must be asked about distributive justice are: *How are rights and responsibilities distributed in society? Is access to healthcare a fundamental right? Are the benefits and costs of healthcare being shared fairly across society?*

In the United Kingdom, even with the National Health Service, social and geographic inequalities in morbidity and mortality have been recognized for decades. This is called the *inverse care law*, in which the *"availability of good medical care tends to vary inversely with the need for it in the population served."*[14] The inverse care law seems to operate most when medical care is exposed to economic forces. The United States experiences this in its medical marketplace, with resulting variability in how healthcare is delivered across the country. One example is seen in the Dartmouth Atlas of Health Care: <http://www.dartmouthatlas.org/>

Whether new models of payment will enhance access, reduce overtreatment, curb spending, and improve quality remains to be seen. Calls for universal coverage of affordable healthcare are still hotly debated. The inverse care law is still in operation, and distributive justice remains elusive.

Quality and safety

Two reports from the Institute of Medicine—*To Err is Human: Building a Safer Healthcare System* (2000) and *Crossing the Quality Chasm: A New Health System for the 21st Century* (2001)—have helped to shape how we should think about the delivery of healthcare in the new millennium. It's a hard pill to swallow, but the reality is that patients can die as the result of medical errors. *Iatrogenesis* is illness at our hands. Knowing that physicians are human and humans make mistakes, our responsibility is to try to

14 Hart JT. The inverse care law. *Lancet*. 1971;1(7696):405–412.

minimize errors and maximize safety. Errors can occur either because of poor planning or poor execution of a treatment plan.[15]

Safety When the healthcare system focuses on safety, the aim is to reduce accidental injury to our patients. Establishing safe practices is a shared responsibility, and, when errors occur, we have to learn from them in order to prevent them for the next patient. For physicians to make considerations of safety part of their usual behavior, several elements need to be in place: Attitude (belief that safety behavior will protect patients); perceived control (feeling of self-efficacy and know-how about medical procedures); and subjective norms (perceived social pressure from the healthcare team or the patient to practice safe behavior). Another factor that can motivate us is the environment we work in, such as having checklists and standard operating procedures that remind us to think about safety.[16]

Quality Changing the healthcare working environment to focus on quality requires applying evidence to healthcare delivery (i.e., best practices), using information technology to automate patient information, influencing physician and patient behaviors through how healthcare is paid for, and preparing clinicians to work in new ways.[17]

Informatics has tremendous potential to reshape medical practice. The days of paper-based medical records are fading into the past. Using the Internet to store patient data (for clinical, research, and quality improvement purposes), prescribe medications or order tests, collaborate with distant colleagues, and share health information with patients provides physicians with an awesome tool. But a few caveats need to be in place for the busy house officer:

- Verify the information in an electronic record on your own. There is a temptation to "cut and paste" a documented history and physical (in part or in full) from someone else's, but what if they got something wrong (like a fatal allergy)?
- Do not just "data dump" (e.g., for purposes of billing or compliance). Still strive to make what is entered in the medical record coherent and readable.
- When entering medical orders, think about the end-user (e.g., the nurse who must institute the order). Have you provided sufficient detail to make the instructions understandable and logical?
- When electronically prescribing medications, use software to your advantage in calculating dosages, checking for drug-drug interactions, and monitoring for potential side effects. But double-check your work before finalizing the prescription (lest the nurse or pharmacist calls you later to alert you to a mistake in the order entry).
- Remember your obligations to protect patient privacy. Keep passwords for access into computerized records or ordering systems to yourself. Resist the urge to post patient-specific information on publicly available websites (however fascinating that x-ray looks or gruesome that wound appears).

15 Kohn LT, Corrigan JM, Donaldson MS, eds.; Committee on Quality of Health Care in America, Institute of Medicine. *To Err is Human: Building a Safer Healthcare System.* Washington, DC: National Academies Press; 2000.
16 Foy R et al. The role of theory in research to develop and evaluate the implementation of patient safety practices. *BMJ Qual Saf.* 2011;20(5):453–459.
17 Committee on Quality of Health Care in America, Institute of Medicine 2001. *Crossing the Quality Chasm: A New Health System for the 21st Century.* Washington, DC: National Academies Press; 2001.

Psychiatry on medical and surgical wards

Psychopathology is common in colleagues, patients, and relatives.

Current mental state Gently probe a patient's thoughts, as you might explore a new garden. What is in bloom now? Where do those paths lead? What is under that stone? *Focus on:* Appearance, speech (rate, content), affect (withdrawn? anxious? suspicious?), mood, beliefs, hallucinations, orientation, memory (recall of current events, president's name), concentration. Note the patient's insight and the degree of your rapport. Observe nonverbal behavior.

Depression This is common, and often ignored, at great cost to well-being. "I would be depressed in her situation…," you say to yourself, and so you do not think of offering treatment. The usual biological guides (early morning awakening, change in appetite, loss of weight, fatigue, and loss of energy) are common on general wards.

Screening questions for major depression are: "Are you depressed (or sad or blue)?" If so, the follow-up question, "*Have you found that you aren't enjoying activities that you normally enjoy doing, or that you have lost interest in doing much?*" If yes to both questions, there is a 95% chance the patient has depression. There may also be guilt and feelings of worthlessness. Do not neglect to ask the patient if he or she has thought about suicide or has passive death wishes. *Don't think it's not your job to recognize and treat depression.* It is as important as pain. Try to arrange activities to boost the patient's morale and confidence and encourage social interaction. Communicate your thoughts to other members of the team: Nurses, physical and occupational therapists—as well as the patient's loved ones (if the patient wishes). Among these, your patient may find a kindred spirit who can give insight and support. Counseling, psychotherapy, and/or antidepressants may be appropriate in some patients. Help guide your patient to the treatment that is right for him or her.

Alcohol This is a common cause of problems on the ward (both the results of abuse and the effects of withdrawal) (p. 229).

The violent patient Ensure your own and others' safety. Do not try to physically restrain violent patients until adequate help is available (e.g., hospital security guards). Prevent violence by being aware of its early signs (e.g., restlessness, earnest pacing, clenched fists, morose silences, chanting, or shouting). Try to keep your own intuitions alert to developing problems. Common causes: *Alcohol intoxication, drugs* (recreational or prescribed), *hypoglycemia, acute confusional states* (p. 353). Once help arrives, try to talk with the patient to calm him—and to gain an understanding of his mental state. Find a nurse who knows the patient. Assess for causes of delirium by measuring oxygen saturation level and blood glucose, or give IV dextrose stat (p. 782). If not hypoglycemic, before further investigation is possible, drugs may be needed (e.g., haloperidol ~2 mg IM; monitor vital signs closely).

If a rational adult refuses vital treatment, it may be as well to respect this decision, provided she is "competent" (i.e., she is able to understand the consequences of her actions and what you are telling her, she is able to retain this information, and she can form the belief that it is true). Decision-making capacity is rarely all or nothing, so don't hesitate to get the opinion of an attending physician or psychiatric consultant. Enlist the persuasive powers of someone the patient respects and trusts.

Physical restraints Familiarize yourself with hospital policies, local procedures, and laws pertaining to the use of physical restraints. Consider sitters and chemical restraints before resorting to physical restraints. A confused, violent patient may need to be physically restrained to prevent harm to himself or others. Reevaluate the need for restraints periodically.

Difficult patients

"Unless both the doctor and the patient become a problem to each other, no solution is found."

Great aphorisms, like this one from Jung, can both inspire and unsettle us, because they resonate with truth. But all great aphorisms also harbor some untruth. Jung's aphorism is untrue for half our waking lives: For an anesthesiologist, there is no need for the patient to become a problem in order for the anesthetic to work. Half our waking professional lives we spend as if asleep, on automatic pilot, following protocols or guidelines to some trite destination—or else we are dreaming of what we could do if we had more time, proper resources, and perhaps a different set of colleagues. Our settled and smug satisfaction at finishing a rotation without any problems is so often a sign of failure. We have kept the chaos at bay, but if we had Jung in our pockets, he would be shaking us awake, derailing our guidelines, and saluting our attempts to risk genuine interactions with our patients—however much of a mess we make of it, and however much pain we cause and receive. (Pain, after all, is the inevitable companion to lives led authentically.[18]) To the unreflective doctor, and to all average minds, this interaction is anathema, to be avoided at all costs, because it leads us away from anesthesia, to the unpredictable, and to destinations that are unknown.

So, every so often, try being pleased to have difficult patients: Those who become a problem to us, those who question us, those who do not respond to our treatments, or who complain when these treatments do work. Very often, it will seem that whatever you say, it is wrong: misunderstood, misquoted, and mangled by the mind you are confronting—perhaps because of fear, loneliness, or past experiences that you can only guess at. If this is happening, shut up—but don't give up. Stick with your patient. Listen to what he or she is saying… and not saying. And when you have understood your patient a bit more, then negotiate, cajole, and even argue—but don't bully or blackmail ("If you do not let your daughter have the operation she needs, I'll tell her just what sort of a mother you are…"). When you find yourself turning to walk away from your patient, turn back and say, "This is not going very well, is it? Can we start again?" Realize that the anger or disappointment that they hurl at you may not be directed at you at all—you may just be the closest target, the scapegoat, for their upset. Learn how to keep your emotional distance without becoming emotionally distant. And don't hesitate to call in your colleagues' help: Not to win by force of numbers, but to see if a different approach might bear fruit. By this process, you and your patient may grow in stature. You may even end up with a truly satisfied patient. And a satisfied patient is worth a thousand protocols.

Death: Diagnosis and management

Death is Nature's master stroke, albeit a cruel one, because it allows genotypes space and opportunity to try on new phenotypes. Our bodies and minds are these perishable phenotypes—the froth, on the wave of our genes. These genes are not really our genes. It is we who belong to them for a few decades. As our neurofibrils begin to tangle, and a neonate walks to a wisdom that eludes us, we are forced to give Nature credit for her daring idea.

---

18 "Some say that the world is a vale of tears. I say it is a place of soul making"—John Keats—the first medical student to formulate these ideas about pain. They did not do him much good, because he died shortly after expressing them. But his ideas can do us good—perhaps if, each day, we try at least once for authentic interactions with a patient, unencumbered by professional detachment, research interests, defensive medicine, a wish to show off to our peers, or to get though the day with the minimum of fuss.

Of course, Nature, in her haphazard way, can get it wrong: People often die in the wrong order (one of our chief roles is to prevent this misordering of deaths, not the phenomenon of death itself).

Death is not our enemy. A life well lived is the goal of every man, and our goal should be to help our patients achieve this as much as possible. As Osler said of the healing professions, "And, finally, remember what we are—useful supernumeraries in the battle, simply stage accessories in the drama, playing minor, but essential, parts at the exits and entrances, or picking up, here and there, a strutter, who may have tripped upon the stage."[19]

Causes of death Homicide, suicide, accident, or natural causes.

Diagnosing death The pronouncement of death is an important responsibility of the physician. The physical exam done to diagnose death is a key symbolic ritual that brings closure to the patient's life and closure for the physician, members of the healthcare team, and, most especially, the patient's family. Death is determined by the absence of pulse and respirations, no auscultated heart sounds, and fixed pupils.

If a patient is on a ventilator, brain death may be diagnosed even if the heart is still beating, via *brain death criteria* that entail the irreversible absence of brain function, particularly in the brainstem. Death of the brainstem is recognized by establishing the absence of cranial nerve and respiratory reflexes. The Uniform Determination of Death Act recognizes that death can be diagnosed by neurologic criteria. In addition to evidence of a catastrophic brain injury, the following prerequisite criteria must be met:

- Deep coma with absent respirations (hence on a ventilator).
- The absence of drug intoxication and hypothermia (<32°C).
- The absence of hypoglycemia, acidosis, hepatic failure, and electrolyte imbalance.

Tests: For determination of brain death, the following tests should be performed by qualified personnel. Repeat the tests after a suitable interval—at least 6 hrs, although sometimes 12-24 hrs is required to confirm irreversibility of the coma. It is often recommended that a neurologist perform the confirmatory tests.

- Tests to establish that brainstem reflexes are absent:
  - Unreactive pupils. Absent corneal response.
  - No oculocephalic reflex (Doll's eye test).
  - No vestibulo-ocular reflexes (i.e., no eye movement occurs after or during slow injection of 60 mL of ice-cold water into each ear canal in turn). Visualize the tympanic membrane first to eliminate false negative tests (e.g., due to wax).
  - No motor response within the cranial nerve distribution should be elicited by adequate stimulation (e.g., absent facial grimacing when pressing on supraorbital ridge).
  - No gag reflex or response to bronchial stimulation with a catheter to the level of the carina.
- Additional tests:
  - No spontaneous or reflex motor responses to noxious stimuli. There should also be no autonomic response to noxious stimuli or vagal stimulation. Spinal reflexes are not relevant to the diagnosis of brain death.
  - Positive apnea test: No respiratory effort in response to hypercarbia. A tube is inserted through the endotracheal tube to the level of the carina

19 Osler W. Doctor and Nurse, in *Aequanimitas*, 2nd ed. Philadelphia: P. Blakiston's Son & Co.; 1925.

in order to deliver continuous oxygen at a rate of 2–4 L/min. The ventilator is disconnected, allowing P_aCO_2 to rise to $\geq$60 mm Hg or more (for patients with COPD, a rise of 20 mm Hg above their baseline). P_aCO_2 typically rises at a rate of 3 mm Hg per minute. Patients should be monitored for any hemo-dynamic instability during the test, and the test should be stopped if SBP falls by $\geq$20%, cardiac arrhythmias emerge, or the patient becomes hypoxic.

Other considerations: Ancillary studies may be needed when the prerequisite criteria cannot be met (e.g., the patient is receiving sedative or anesthetic infusions). An electroencephalogram (EEG) recording is not a standard requirement, unless brain death is to be diagnosed within 6 h of apparent cessation of brain activity. Cerebral blood flow studies (e.g., with isotope angiography) are helpful when the patient is receiving treatments that suppress cerebral metabolic activity.

Organ donation: The point of diagnosing brain death is partly that this allows organs (kidney, liver, cornea, heart, or lungs) to be donated and removed with as little damage from hypoxia as possible. Do not avoid the topic with loved ones. Many are glad to give consent and to think that some good can come after the death of their relative, that some part of the relative will go on living, giving a new life to another person.

After death Inform the patient's attending and consultants. Meet with the patient's next of kin and offer emotional support. Ask if they want an autopsy. Autopsy permission may be granted (in order of priority) by spouse, adult child, parent, sibling. Sign death certificates promptly. If DOA or within 24 h of admission, or the cause is violence, trauma, accident, neglect, surgery, anesthesia, therapeutic mishap, drug/alcohol overdose, suicide, poisoning, or is unknown or suspicious, inform the Coroner/Medical Examiner.

Facing death

"People imagine that they are not afraid of death when they think of it while they are in good health" (Marcel Proust). So, to get into the mood, as a thought experiment, place a finger in your left supraclavicular fossa, and feel there the craggy node of Virchow, telling of some distant gastric malignancy, as if it were your death warrant. Perhaps you have just 4 months left. Live with this "knowledge" for the rest of the day, or rest of the week, and see how it changes your attitude to family and friends, on the one hand, and the million irrelevances that clutter our minds, on the other. As the week unfolds, you may experience thoughts and feelings that are new to you, but all too familiar to your patients. And as the months and years roll by, and you find yourself sitting opposite certain patients, put that finger once more on that metaphorical node and turn it over in your mind, and it will turn you, so you are sitting not opposite your patient but beside him. There is only so much comfort you can bring in this way, as, in the end, you cannot tame death.

Whenever you find yourself thinking *it is better for them not to know,* suspect that you mean: *It is easier for me not to tell.*

We find it hard to tell for many reasons: It distresses patients; it may hold up a ward round; we do not like acknowledging our impotence to alter the course of diseases; telling reminds us of our own mortality and may unlock our previous griefs. We use many tricks to minimize the pain: *rationalization* ("They would not want to know"); *intellectualization* ("Research shows that 37% of people at stage 3 survive 2 yrs…"); *brusque honesty* ("You are unlikely to survive 1 month" and, so saying, the doctor rushes off to more vital things); *inappropriate delegation* ("The nurse will explain it all to you when you are calmer").

Why it may help the patient to be told

- The patient already half knows but everyone shies away so he cannot discuss his fears (of pain, or that his family will not cope).
- There may be many affairs for the patient to put in order.
- To enable him to judge if unpleasant therapy is worthwhile and to set realistic goals.

Most patients are told less than they would like to know.

Breaking bad news Being able to deliver bad news compassionately and effectively is one of the most important skills of the physician. Although each discussion must be individualized to the particular patient, some general principles have been recommended. These have been encapsulated in the mnemonic SPIKES[20]:

- **S**etting the stage: Sit down. Arrange for privacy. Avoid interruptions.
- **P**atient's perceptions: What does the patient know about the situation?
- **I**nvitation for information: How does the patient want to be given information? Patients may either desire or shun information.
- **K**nowledge: Fire a warning shot before providing information, "*I'm sorry to tell you that …*" Use language that the patient can understand.
- **E**motions: Acknowledge emotions and offer empathetic statements, "*I can see that this is upsetting to you.*" Be authentic in your empathy.
- **S**ummary and strategy: Review discussion and set agenda based on goals of care. Address any lingering misunderstanding, uncertainty, or fears.

What are the patient's worries likely to be?

Put yourself in the patient's place.

- Give some information, and then the opportunity to ask for more.
- Be sensitive to hints that they may be ready to learn more. "I'm worried about my son." "What is worrying you most?" "Well, it will be a difficult time for him (pause) starting school next year." Silence, broken by the doctor "I get the impression there are other things worrying you." The patient now has the opportunity to proceed further, or to stop. Ensure that the patient's personal physician and the nurses know what you have and have not said. Also make sure that this is written in the notes.

Living wills/advance directives If a patient has the capacity to make her own decisions, then she should be asked directly what her treatment preferences are. If a patient lacks capacity and her views are known, comply with them. Some patients spell out their views in a written document. But these views change, are ambiguous, or are hard to interpret, even if a living will exists. Living wills only take effect when the patient is terminally ill. In many cases, there can be uncertainty or disagreement about whether to invoke the living will because it is not clear that the patient is "absolutely, hopelessly ill."

If a patient desires to complete an advance directive, it is often more preferable to have the patient designate a durable power of attorney for healthcare or a healthcare agent—a person who will speak for the patient if the patient is too ill to speak for himself. Designation of a healthcare agent can also be fraught with difficulties, especially if the named surrogate has not had a prior discussion with the patient about his wishes.

Perhaps the best strategy is to focus less on completion of the advance directive form and more on the discussion involved in advance care planning. This will be an ongoing process with the patient, reviewing the goals of care in light of the changing clinical situation and the patient's hopes, fears, prognosis, quality of life, loved ones' wishes, and underlying values.

Stages of acceptance Accepting death takes time, and may involve passing through "stages" on a path. It helps to know where your patient is on this path (but progress is rarely orderly and need not always be forward: The same ground often needs to be covered many times). At first, there may be *shock* and *numbness*, then *denial* (which reduces anxiety), then *anger* (which may lead you to dislike your patient, but anger can have positive attributes (e.g., in energizing people—and it can trump fear and pain; it is different from hostility), then *grief*, and then, perhaps, *acceptance*. Finally there may be intense longing for death as the patient moves beyond the reach of worldly cares.[21]

The physician can be a guide on the patient's journey. The physician is there to bid patients, in the words of T. S. Eliot, with the call, "Not fare well, but fare forward, voyagers."[22]

Palliative care

When the patient's journey finds him or her on the path of a life-limiting illness, it is time to start thinking about palliative care. The palliative care philosophy can be introduced at any point in a serious, debilitating illness and becomes more of the focus as the patient enters the terminal phases of his or her illness.

The National Consensus Project for Quality Palliative Care states: "The goal of palliative care is to prevent and relieve suffering and to support the best possible quality of life for patients and their families, regardless of the stage of the disease or the need for other therapies. Palliative care is both a philosophy of care and an organized, highly structured system for delivering care. Palliative care expands traditional disease-model medical treatments to include the goals of enhancing quality of life for patient and family, optimizing function, helping with decision making, and providing opportunities for personal growth. As such, it can be delivered concurrently with life-prolonging care or as the main focus of care."[23]

For conditions such as congestive heart failure, optimal symptom management and improved functional status are often achieved by prescribing the best evidence-based cardiac regimen.

Elements of palliative care (1) *Patient population,* anyone with a life-threatening illness, condition, or injury; (2) *patient- and family-centered care,* respecting the uniqueness of the patient and family as the unit of care; (3) *timing,* beginning at the diagnosis of the condition through cure, until death, or into the period of family bereavement; (4) *comprehensive care,* multidimensional care to identify and relieve suffering and distress; (5) *interdisciplinary team,* to utilize the skills of each discipline; (6) *attention to relief of suffering,* do not just think about pain, but other symptoms like dyspnea, anorexia, nausea, change in bowel habits, fatigue, insomnia, delirium, anxiety, depression (many of which can be assessed on a 0–10 scale to monitor treatment effect, as with pain); (7) *communication skills,* sharing information, listening, setting goals of care; (8) *skill in care of the dying and the bereaved,* with particular attention to prognostication (think especially of functional status, as with the Palliative Performance Scale,[24] which can be used across different diseases), preparation, and anticipatory guidance;

21 Bach JS. *Ich habe genug,* Cantata No. 82, composed for the Feast of the Purification, 1727.
22 Eliot TS. The dry salvages. In: *The Four Quartets.* New York: Mariner Books; 1968.
23 National Consensus Project for Quality Palliative Care. Clinical Practice Guidelines for Quality Palliative Care, 2nd ed. 2009. http://www.nationalconsensusproject.org. Accessed September 10, 2012.
24 Anderson F, Downing GM, Hill J. et al. Palliative performance scale (PPS): a new tool. *J Palliat Care.* 1996;12(1):5–11.

(9) *continuity of care across settings*, whether in hospital, home, long-term care facility, or inpatient hospice... or while transitioning from one to another; (10) *equitable access*, across all patient populations and settings; (11) *quality assessment and performance improvement*, consistent with the IOM aims for quality healthcare delivery.

In the words of Dame Cicely Saunders, the founder of the modern hospice movement: "You matter because you are you, and you matter to the end of your life. We will do all we can not only to help you die peacefully, but also to live until you die."[25]

Surviving residency

If some fool or visionary were to say that our aim should be to pro-duce the greatest health and happiness for the greatest number of our patients, we would not expect to hear cheering from the tattered ranks of midnight house staff: Rather, our ears are detecting a decimated groan—because these men and women know that there is something at stake in a house staff training program far more elemental than health or happiness: Namely, survival. Here, we are talking about our own survival, not that of our patients. It is hard to think of a greater peacetime challenge than the first few months on the wards. Within the first weeks, however brightly shone the intern's armor, it will now be smeared and splattered, if not with blood, then with the fallout from very many decisions that were taken with-out sufficient care and attention. It was not because the intern was lazy. All of us are stunned to realize at some point in our training that the forces of Nature (e.g., our need for sleep) and the exigencies of ward life teach us to be second-rate: For to insist on being first-rate in all areas at all times is to sign a kind of death warrant for many of our patients, and, more pertinently for this page, for ourselves.

Perfectionism cannot survive in our clinical world. The perfect is the enemy of the good. To cope with this fact, or, to put it less depressingly, to flour-ish in this new world, don't keep repolishing your armor (what are the 10 causes of atrial fibrillation—or are there 11?), rather furnish your mind—and nourish your body (regular food and drink make those midnight groans of yours less intrusive). Do not voluntarily deny yourself the restorative power of sleep. The move to an 80 hr work week is a recognition that our bodies (and minds) need time to rejuvenate.

We cannot prepare you for the adversity that you may encounter or the tests to your character that may ensue. Neither would we dream of impos-ing on you a set of standard regimens on how to survive. Finding out what can lead you through adversity is the art of living. Plan your free time and recreation in advance. What will you choose: physical fitness, martial arts, yoga, music, poetry, writing, culinary delights, the sermon on the mount, juggling, meditation, a love affair—or will you make an art form out of the ironic observation of your contemporaries?

Work–life balance does not necessarily mean that the time devoted to our professional and personal lives is evenly weighted. Our profession puts cer-tain demands on our time and energy that we cannot escape. Work–life bal-ance is about "figuring out what's really important and fulfilling to you, right now, and living intentionally, as best you can."[26] It's about remembering that patient care "ultimately depends on the soul of the doctor."[27]

25 Saunders C. *Nursing Times.* 1976; 72(26): 1003–1005.
26 Harrison R. Evolving trends in balancing work and family for future academic physicians: A role for personal stories. *Med Teacher.* 2008;30:316–318.
27 Gaufberg E. Time to care. *Health Affairs.* 2008;27(3):845–849.

Some physicians nourish their inner person through a religious belief and attend mosque, church, synagogue, or temple. Some find spirituality and meaning through other means. A multicultural society provides diversity and room for all branches of expression. Bear in mind not to compare yourself with your contemporaries. Those who make the most noise are often *not waving but drowning*. Find time to reflect on your experiences.

Residency can encompass tremendous up-and-down swings in energy, motivation, and mood, which can be precipitated by small incidents. If you are depressed for more than a day, speak to a sympathetic friend, partner, or counselor to help you put it in perspective. Seek help for your own problems. Find professional help if needed. You are not the best person to plan your assessment, treatment, and referral. When in doubt, communicate.

Think about your future career, and seek out an advisor and mentor in the specialty that you think you will pursue after your training. Such inquiries supply energy to get you through the long, though now limited, hours of residency, and may motivate you if the going gets tough. Not that this is any guarantee that the plans will work, but if your yoga, your sermons, and your fitness regimens turn to ashes in your mouth, then at least you will know the direction in which to spit.

Residency is not just a phase to get through and to enjoy where possible (there are frequently *many* such possibilities); it is also the anvil on which we are beaten into a new and perhaps rather uncomfortable shape. Luckily, not all of us are made of iron and steel, so there is a fair chance that, in due course, we will spring back into something resembling our normal shape, and, in so doing, we may come to realize that it was our weaknesses, not our strengths, which served us best. And, in the end, we will be better doctors (and our future patients will be better cared for) for our having endured the hardships.

On being busy: Corrigan's secret door

Unstoppable demands, increased expectations as to what medical care should bring, the rising number of elderly patients, coupled with the introduction of new and complex treatments all conspire, it might be thought, to make doctors ever busier. In fact, doctors have always been busy. In Great Britain, Sir Dominic Corrigan was so busy 150 yrs ago that he had to have a secret door made in his consulting room so that he could escape from the ever-growing waiting room of eager patients.

We are all familiar with the phenomenon of being hopelessly overstretched… and of needing Corrigan's secret door. Competing, urgent, and simultaneous demands make carrying out any task all but impossible: The resident is trying to put up an IV infusion on a hypotensive patient when his pager goes off. On his way to the phone, a patient is falling out of bed, being held in, apparently, only by his visibly lengthening catheter (which had taken the house officer an hour to insert). He knows he should stop to help but, instead, as he picks up the phone, he starts to tell the nurse about "this man dangling from his Foley" (knowing in his heart that the worst will have already happened). But he is interrupted by a thud coming from the bed of the lady who has just had her occluded left anterior descending artery attended to: However, it is not her, but her visiting husband who has collapsed and is now having a seizure. At this moment a Code Blue is called, summoning him to some other patient. In despair, he turns to the nurse and groans: "There must be some way out of here!" At times like this, we all need Corrigan to take us by the shadow of our hand and walk with us through his metaphorical secret door, into a calm inner world. To enable this to happen, make things as easy as possible for yourself.

First, however lonely you feel, you are not alone. Do not pride yourself on not asking for help. If a decision is a hard one, share it with a colleague. Second, take any chance you get to sit down and rest. Have a cup of coffee with other members of the staff, or with a friendly patient (patients are sources of renewal, not just devourers of your energies). Third, do not miss meals. If there is no time to go to the cafeteria, know where you can find food on the wards or ensure that food is put aside for you to eat when you can: Hard work and sleeplessness are twice as bad when you are hungry. Fourth, avoid making work for yourself. It is too easy for physicians in training, trapped in their image of excessive work and blackmailed by misplaced guilt, to remain on the wards following up on patients, rewriting notes, or rechecking lab results at an hour when the priority should be caring for themselves. Fifth, when a bad part of the rotation is looming, plan a good time for when you are off duty, to look forward to during the long nights.

Finally, remember that however busy the call day (and night), your period of duty will end. For you, as for Macbeth:

> Come what come may,
> Time and the hour runs through the roughest day.

Epidemiology

Gregory P. Prokopowicz, M.D., M.P.H.

Contents

Why epidemiology is relevant to the practicing physician

Epidemiology is the study of the distribution of clinical phenomena in human populations. Clinical epidemiology is the application of epidemiologic methods to the care of the patient. The fruits of clinical epidemiology include identification of the causes of disease, prediction of the development of disease and its clinical outcomes, rational use of clinical tests, assessment of the risks and benefits of therapies, and evaluation of screening technologies.

Identification of causes of disease Epidemiologic methods enable one to determine the *risk factors* responsible for disease. The association of smoking with lung cancer, dyslipidemia with coronary artery disease, and hypertension with stroke are examples of the valuable findings of epidemiology with relevance for the practitioner. Novel risk factors, such as C-reactive protein for coronary artery disease, continue to be identified. The up-to-date physician should have an awareness of how such associations are derived and whether they are likely to be important for clinical care.

Prediction of disease and its clinical outcomes By identifying risk factors, the physician can predict which of his or her patients is most likely to develop disease. Risk scores, such as the Framingham score for coronary artery disease or the CHADS2 score for thromboembolism in atrial fibrillation, can be used to estimate the risk of clinical outcomes in a given patient and thereby guide the choice of therapy.

Rational use of clinical tests Laboratory and radiographic tests are a daily part of clinical practice, but few tests provide totally unambiguous results. Quantification of test performance, using sensitivity, specificity, positive and negative predictive values, and likelihood ratios, facilitate appropriate selection and interpretation of tests.

Assessment of risks and benefits of therapy Quantitative measures of effect, such as the *number needed to treat,* enable the clinician to accurately weigh the benefits of therapy against any harms, and to compare the cost effectiveness of competing therapies.

Evaluation of screening technologies An increasing number of investigations may be performed on the healthy patient with the intent of detecting early disease. Emerging technologies, such as multislice spiral computed tomography and genetic testing with single nucleotide polymorphisms, will reveal new abnormalities of uncertain significance. Appropriate counseling of the patient with respect to such screening tests requires an understanding of the issues involved.

Evidence-based medicine

Evidence-based medicine (EBM) as been defined as the conscientious and judicious use of current best evidence from clinical research in the management of individual patients.

The problem Traditionally, the teaching and practice of medicine has relied largely on three sources of knowledge: Pathophysiology, expert opinion, and personal clinical experience. Important limitations have become apparent in these sources of information. Predictions from pathophysiology may not hold in clinical practice; for example, suppression of ventricular ectopy following myocardial infarction with encainide or flecainide led to a surprising increase in mortality. Expert opinion may be out of date or biased due to conflict of interest. And personal experience is likely to be unduly influenced by striking clinical outcomes, such as a rare but devastating side effect in a generally safe drug.

The solution EBM directs the physician to be aware of the quality of the information on which his or her practice is based, and to conscientiously choose the most reliable sources. This presupposes a *hierarchy of evidence* (i.e., a ranking of types of information according to susceptibility to bias and chance effects). Such hierarchies generally place randomized controlled trials (RCTs) at the highest tier, followed by observational studies, then unsystematic clinical observations, pathophysiologic reasoning, and expert opinion. *Meta-analyses* and *systematic reviews* are often given even greater credence than RCTs, although this depends on the quality of the review.

27

The four steps of EBM

Formulate the clinical question: The first step is to focus our sometimes vague uncertainty into a question that can be answered. The acronym PICO may be of help: What sort of *Patient* are we considering; what is the *Intervention* we are contemplating; to what alternative can we *Compare* the intervention; and what *Outcomes* are important for our patient?

Search the literature: The practice of EBM optimally requires access to computerized literature sources such as PubMed. Time spent learning appropriate search techniques (e.g., by using the tutorials) will pay off with better results.

Appraise the literature that you have found: Here, we are interested in the validity of the study, the results of the study, and the applicability to our patient.

Apply the findings to the individual patient: In applying the findings to our particular patient, we must consider our patient's unique clinical characteristics and values.

Criticisms of EBM Searching the primary literature and assessing its validity in the context of a busy clinical practice is difficult. In response, proponents of EBM have suggested the use of *pre-appraised literature sources*, such as ACP PIER, Clinical Evidence, Up-To-Date, and the journals *Evidence-Based Medicine* and *ACP Journal Club*. These resources provide clinically relevant summaries of the primary literature and obviate the laborious critical appraisal of individual papers by the clinician. In addition, tools for winnowing out the clinically useful articles from the morass of medical literature have been developed; these including literature filters and selective e-mail notification services.

The suggestion has been made that EBM is primarily a means of controlling costs by denying what would otherwise be considered appropriate care. While certain techniques of EBM may be used to this end, the principles of EBM do not require that the least expensive alternative be chosen, and evidence-based practice guidelines have not invariably resulted in lower costs.

Perhaps the most significant criticism of EBM is that it has never itself been subject to the sort of rigorous evaluation that it espouses for other therapies. Specifically, we do not know if physicians who adhere closely to the principles of EBM have better patient outcomes than those who do not. Proponents of EBM point to studies showing that expert opinions voiced in traditional review articles may lag behind evidence from the latest studies, and that patients receiving therapies for which there is good evidence do better than those who do not. But these are indirect measures of the effectiveness of EBM; direct comparisons of EBM practitioners with non-EBM practitioners, either in the form of RCTs or observational studies, are lacking.

Associations and causality

Association Epidemiological research is concerned with comparing rates of disease in populations with different exposures (e.g., rates of lung cancer in a population of men who smoke, compared with men who do not). A difference in rates suggests an *association* between the disease and the exposure (in this case, smoking). The search for meaningful associations may be complicated by the presence of *confounders*, or factors that are related to both the exposure and the disease. For example, an apparent association between alcohol use and lung cancer may simply reflect the fact that both are related to tobacco use. Associations may also be due simply to chance. The strength of an association is expressed as the *risk ratio*—the risk of developing the disease among those with the exposure, divided by the risk of developing the disease among those without the exposure, or the *odds ratio,* a similar but not identical measure.

Prevalence and incidence To compare rates of disease between groups, standard measures of disease occurrence are used. *Prevalence* is the number of cases of disease present in a defined population divided by the total number of people in that population. Since it is not usually practical to count an entire population at once, the *period prevalence* is often given, indicating that the measurement took place over a period of time. For example, the prevalence of obesity (body mass index [BMI] >30) in the United States during the 2009–10 National Health and Nutrition Examination Survey (NHANES) survey period was 35.7%. *Lifetime prevalence* is the proportion of a population that has *ever* experienced the condition of interest, and *point prevalence* is the proportion with the condition at a given point in time. For example, the lifetime prevalence of headache in women has been reported at 99%, and the point prevalence at 22%.

Incidence is the number of new cases occurring in a defined population that is initially free of the disease, over a specified time period (e.g., the incidence of breast cancer among U.S. women from 2008 was 127 per 100,000 [Surveillance Epidemiology and End Results (SEER) cancer statistics review]).

Observational studies Associations are often discovered using *observational studies*. Such studies are distinguished from experimental studies or *clinical trials* in that the investigator does not control the exposure; she or he merely observes the subjects who are exposed and those who are not and records the outcomes occurring in each group. Observational studies usually take one of three forms:

1 *Cohort studies:* The group, or cohort, consisting of subjects exposed to the suspected causal factor (e.g., smoking) is followed alongside a control group consisting of subjects not exposed. The incidence of the disease is compared between the groups over the duration of the study. Because the exposure information is recorded as it occurs, prospective cohort studies do not

have recall bias. However, they can be very expensive and time-consuming, particularly for diseases with low incidence rates.

2 *Case–control studies:* The study group consists of those with the disease (e.g., lung cancer); the control group consists of those without the disease. The previous occurrence of the exposure (e.g., smoking) is compared between each group. Case–control studies are particularly useful for the investigation of rare diseases, but they suffer from recall bias: inaccuracy in the subjects' reporting of the exposure (e.g., smoking).

3 *Cross-sectional studies:* The population of interest is surveyed for the presence of both the exposure and the disease at the same time. This design is usually quick and inexpensive, and provides prevalence data, but it may not enable the investigator to determine whether the exposure preceded development of the disease, since both are measured at the same time.

Establishing causality The finding of an association between an exposure and a disease does not prove that the exposure causes the disease. Reports abound in the media of supposed links between various foods and worsened or improved health; which will turn out to be valid? Sir Austin Bradford Hill, a British epidemiologist, recognized this problem in the context of evaluating occupational hazards, and proposed nine criteria for establishing causality:

1 *Strength of the association:* Does the disease occur *much* more frequently among the exposed than among the unexposed, such as with lung cancer, or is it only slightly more common?

2 *Consistency:* Does the relation hold across different studies in different populations?

3 *Specificity:* Is the exposure the only potential cause of the disease, or vice versa? This is not required for causality, but when present it strengthens the argument.

4 *Temporality:* Does the cause precede the effect?

5 *Dose response:* Does a greater exposure lead to a greater risk of disease?

6 *Plausibility:* Is there a plausible biologic mechanism to explain the causality?

7 *Coherence:* Does the cause-and-effect relation fit with histopathology and other information about the disease?

8 *Experiment:* Does alteration of the exposure, if possible, result in a change in frequency of outcome?

9 *Analogy:* Is there a similar disease known to be caused by a similar exposure?

Risk of disease and its outcomes

As physicians, we are frequently called on to prognosticate. Our patients want to know: Should I be worried about this cough? Is my cholesterol low enough? How long am I going to be in the hospital? Application of epidemiologic principles can help answer these questions.

Which is more likely: An uncommon manifestation of a common disease or a common manifestation of an uncommon disease? When we consider the significance of a new symptom reported by a patient, we are engaging in a process of risk stratification. Is the sudden, stabbing mid-back pain reported by this 65-yr-old diabetic with hypertension likely to be from muscle strain? Myocardial infarction? Aortic dissection? In formulating a diagnosis, we estimate the likelihood of various diseases in our patient and also consider how commonly each disease would present with the symptoms we see in front of us. Proper use of epidemiology can guide our application of this information to the patient. Consider the development of angioedema in a person taking an angiotensin-converting enzyme (ACE) inhibitor. Angioedema is a rare symptom with ACE inhibitor use (seen in 0.1–0.2% of patients), but is commonly seen in patients with C1 inhibitor deficiency (perhaps 90% of such patients). C1 inhibitor deficiency itself is rare, occurring in only about 1 in 50,000 in the general population. If a patient on an ACE-inhibitor develops angioedema, should we check for C1 inhibitor deficiency? We may intuitively feel that it is a reasonable part of a comprehensive evaluation of angioedema. However, the probability of our patient having ACE inhibitor-induced angioedema is 0.1–0.2%, whereas the probability that he or she has C1 inhibitor is 0.9 × 1/50,000 or 0.0018%. It is thus 50–100 times more likely that our patient's angioedema is due to the ACE inhibitor.

Medical decision-making as a type of gambling A busy physician might see 20 patients in an afternoon session. How should she or he decide which symptoms to monitor expectantly and which to investigate until a cause is found? Some patients may offer five separate symptom groups in the course of a single visit. Full elucidation of these symptoms might reveal additional complaints, leading to a potentially endless cycle of investigation. Certainly, some of these complaints might not seem too serious ("this pain in my toe…"). But on reflection, even toe pain might be dangerous if caused by emboli or osteomyelitis. Similarly, fingernail problems with a slight rash might mean arsenic poisoning, lethargy may mean cancer, and so on. Since almost any symptom can be seen as a manifestation of some fatal illness, an attitude of excessive pessimism is to be avoided, as it would lead to many sleepless nights for the doctor and much excessive testing for the patient. On the other hand, an attitude of complacency or blind optimism would be no better and might be worse, resulting in missed diagnoses.

Table 2.1 Calculation of the risk of disease outcomes

Epidemiologic investigations have enabled the practitioner to calculate a patient's overall risk based on the presence or absence of several individual risk factors. For example, the **Framingham Risk Calculator** permits an assessment of cardiac risk. It uses age, total cholesterol, high-density lipoprotein (HDL) cholesterol, blood pressure, diabetes, and smoking status to calculate the 10-yr risk of coronary heart disease.

Patient: 62-yr-old male smoker with total cholesterol of 242, HDL cholesterol of 41, blood pressure (BP) 148/90, not diabetic, on no medications.

Age: 60–64
↓
Total cholesterol: 240–279
↓
HDL cholesterol: 35–44
↓
BP: 140–159/90–99
↓
Diabetes: **No**
↓
Smoking: **Yes**
↓
↓
10-yr CHD risk
23%

This patient thus has a 23% chance of myocardial infarction in the next 10 yrs.

http://hp2010.nhlbihin.net/atpiii/calculator.asp

Rather, *the physician should be a shrewd gambler,* able to use subtle clues to change his or her outlook from pessimism to optimism and vice versa. Sometimes the approach is scientific, relying on quantitative estimates of the probability of disease, just as the poker player calculates the probability of filling an inside straight. But sometimes it is intuitive, as when the gambler reads the face of his opponent, or the physician relies on her gut sense that something is "not right" about the appearance of a patient, a sense that may be invaluable even if it cannot be expressed in words or numbers.

Evaluation of diagnostic tests

Only rarely does a single test provide a definitive diagnosis. More often, tests alter our assessment of the likelihood of a condition being present. When taking a history and examining patients, we estimate (consciously or unconsciously) how likely various diagnoses are. The results of testing modify those estimates. A test is worthwhile if it alters the post-test probability (i.e., the likelihood that a patient has disease, given the test results) and if the results affect our management of the patient.

Basic test statistics All tests have false positives and false negatives, as summarized below:

	Patient has the condition	Patient does not have the condition
Test result is positive	True positive (a)	False positive (b)
Test result is negative	False negative (c)	True negative (d)

For tests with a dichotomous outcome (i.e., positive or negative), the following statistics are commonly used:

- *Sensitivity:* The proportion of people with disease who test positive: ($a/a + c$).
- *Specificity:* The proportion of people without disease who test negative: ($d/d + b$).
- *Positive predictive value:* The proportion of people testing positive who have the disease: ($a/a + b$).
- *Negative predictive value:* The proportion of people testing negative who do not have the disease: ($c/c + d$).

Likelihood ratio In addition to the above, the *likelihood ratio* (LR) is quite useful, because it does not require that the test have a dichotomous outcome (i.e., be limited to one of two values).

The LR is calculated as the probability of having the given test result if the patient *has* disease, divided by the probability of having the same result if the patient *does not have* disease. The mnemonic WOWO (With Over WithOut) may be helpful. For example, the LR for iron deficiency anemia with a serum ferritin in the range of 15–24 is 8.8. This means that the likelihood of seeing a ferritin level in the range of 15–24 is 8.8 times greater in patients with iron deficiency than in those without. Furthermore, the LR for a ferritin level of 45–99 is 0.54. This means that it is almost 50% *less* common to obtain a ferritin level of 45–99 in a patient with iron deficiency than in a patient without iron deficiency.

Advantages of the likelihood ratio: There are two major advantages to using LRs. The first is that they enable us to take into account the exact value of a test result, rather than simply classifying it as positive or negative. This is in accord with how we practice medicine. For example, a patient with chest pain and a troponin I level of 20 ng/mL will certainly get our attention more than one with a troponin of 0.6 ng/mL, despite the fact that both would be reported as "positive" in a lab that uses a cutoff value of 0.5. In this case, the

LR for myocardial infarction associated with a troponin of 20 ng/mL would be much higher than the LR for a troponin of 0.5 ng/mL. The traditional test statistics (sensitivity, specificity, and positive and negative predictive values) treat all tests as either positive or negative and lose the important information carried by extreme values.

The second advantage to LRs is that they can be used to calculate a post-test probability, even when multiple tests are used in sequence. This uses the formula:

$$\text{Pre-test odds} \times \text{LR(test result)} = \text{post-test odds}$$

To use this formula, one must convert between probability and odds using the formulas:

$$\text{Odds} = \text{probability}/(1-\text{probability})$$
$$\text{Probability} = \text{odds}/(1+\text{odds})$$

Handy pocket-card nomograms are available to apply these formulas without having to do the actual calculations.

Using likelihood ratios: Assume you are faced with a patient with ascites and abdominal discomfort. You are considering the diagnosis of spontaneous bacterial peritonitis (SBP). After examining the patient, you estimate the chance that she has SBP to be low, about 20%. You perform a paracentesis, and find 600 polymorphonuclear leukocytes (PMNs)/μL. How does this affect the likelihood that she has SBP?

Number of PMNs in ascitic fluid	Likelihood ratio
>1,000	22.3
501–1,000	2.78
251–500	1.14
0–250	0.08

Pre-test odds = 0.2/(1 – 0.2) = 0.25
Post-test odds = 0.25 × 2.78 = 0.695
Post-test probability = 0.695/(1 + 0.695) = 0.41

Thus, our new estimate is that she has about a 40% probability of SBP. Had the fluid shown >1,000 PMNs, the post-test probability would have been 85%.

The effectiveness of therapy

While some therapies have gained general acceptance through dramatic uncontrolled demonstrations (e.g., insulin for diabetes or penicillin for streptococcal infection), most modern therapies require a comparison with a control group to demonstrate safety and effectiveness. This can sometimes be accomplished using an observational study, such as a cohort study. However, to minimize bias, *controlled clinical trials* are preferred.

Experimental studies In contrast to observational studies, *experimental studies* or *clinical trials* involve active assignment by the investigator of subjects to the treatment under consideration.

Randomized controlled trials: Assignment to the treatment and control groups is performed randomly to avoid selection bias and help ensure that the two groups do not differ with respect to confounding factors. This is generally felt to be the optimal design for assessing the effect of therapeutic interventions.

Comparability of groups: In both cohort studies and RCTs, it is desirable that the two groups be similar to one another with respect to all factors that could affect the outcome, except for the intervention being studied. In large RCTs, random assignment makes this likely to occur, but the reader should still check to see that the two groups are comparable. If they are not, adjustment procedures, such as multivariate analysis, may be used.

Allocation concealment: In RCTs, assignment to treatment or control is done without advance knowledge by the investigator or the subject.

Blinding: Following randomization, it is often desirable to prevent the subjects and members of the study team from knowing who is receiving treatment and who is receiving placebo. This helps minimize bias in the measurement of the outcome, and it equalizes the placebo effect between the two groups.

Outcome measures: If the risk of dying from an myocardial infarction (MI) after "standard treatment" is 10%, and a new treatment reduces this to 8%, then the relative risk is 0.8 (i.e., 8/10) and the relative risk reduction is 20% [(10 – 8/10) × 100%]. While this may sound impressive, it is important to also consider the absolute risk reduction (ARR), which is 10% – 8% = 2%. Thus, if 100 people with MI receive the drug, only ~2 would be expected to derive benefit. This may also be expressed as the number needed to treat, which is calculated as (1/ARR), with ARR expressed as a fraction rather than a percent. In this example the number needed to treat (NNT) would be 1/0.02 = 50; thus, one would need to treat 50 people to prevent one death from MI.

If the outcome being studied is rare, the NNT may be quite high. For example, in some preventive studies of mild hypertension in the young, ~800 people may need to be treated to prevent one stroke. Furthermore, if one were to compare a new antihypertensive regimen to an older one, with the NNT for the older treatment being 800 and the new treatment only marginally better, the NNT to prevent one death or stroke by adopting the new regimen in place of the old might be *several thousand*. The implication is that adoption of the new treatment, if it is more expensive than the old, is not likely to be cost-effective.

Intention-to-treat analysis: Despite the best efforts of the investigators, some subjects inevitably fail to follow the study protocol. What should be done with patients assigned to the control group who wind up taking the treatment, and vice versa? One option is to analyze the subjects according to what they actually did in the study (i.e., if a subject did not adhere to the treatment plan, he or she should be lumped in with the control group). Similarly, if a subject who was assigned to control opted to use the therapy, he or she should be analyzed as part of the treatment group. This is called *on-treatment analysis*, and it has a certain plausibility. However, it is now common practice to analyze subjects according to the group to which they were randomized, regardless of whether they stuck with the study plan. This is known as *intention-to-treat analysis*, and offers the following advantages:

• The initial comparability of groups produced by randomization is preserved.
• The results reflect imperfect adherence and are therefore more similar to what will happen when the intervention is used in actual practice.
• Outcomes such as death, which may or may not be due to the therapy or control, will not be overlooked.

Table 2.2 Examples of NNTs

Study	Outcome	NNT
Statins for 1° prevention	Death (MI)	931 (78) for 5 yrs
Statins for 2° prevention	Death (MI)	30 (15) for 5.4 yrs
Mild hypertension	Stroke	850 for 1 yr
Systolic hypertension in elderly	Stroke	43 for 4.5 yrs
Aspirin in acute MI	Death	40
ACE-inhibitor for CHF (NYHA class IV)	Death	6 for 1 yr

Screening

Screening is defined as the application of a test to detect a potential disease or condition in a person who has no known signs or symptoms of that disease, so that treatment might be more effective, less expensive, or both; or with the aim of identifying and modifying risk factors to prevent disease.[1]

Because screening is applied to a generally healthy population, most of whom will not benefit from the screening (because they would not have developed the disease regardless), extra care must be taken to ensure that the screening is worthwhile.

Wilson and Jungner criteria for screening[2]

1 The condition being sought should be an important health problem, for the individual and the community.
2 There should be an acceptable form of treatment for patients with identified disease.
3 The natural history of the condition, including its development from latent to declared disease, should be adequately understood.
4 There should be a recognizable latent or early symptomatic stage.
5 There should be a suitable screening test or examination for detecting the disease at the latent or early symptomatic stage, and this test should be acceptable to the population.
6 The facilities required for diagnosis and treatment of patients revealed by the screening program should be available.
7 There should be an agreed policy on whom to treat as patients.
8 Treatment at the presymptomatic, borderline stage of a disease should favorably influence its course and prognosis.
9 The cost of case-finding (which would include the cost of diagnosis and treatment) needs to be economically balanced in relation to possible expenditure on medical care as a whole.
10 Case-finding should be a continuing process, not a "once and for all" project.

Biases Assessment of screening programs may reveal the following problems:

• *Lead-time bias:* Patients who are screened for asymptomatic disease may simply find that they are being diagnosed earlier, even if the early diagnosis does nothing to improve their ultimate prognosis. If the success of the screening program is measured in 5-yr survival from the time of diagnosis,

1 Modified from Eddy D. How to think about screening. In D. Eddy, ed., *Screening for Diseases: Prevention in Primary Care.* acp Press, 1991.
2 Wilson JMG, Jungner G. *Principles and Practice of Screening for Disease.* Geneva: World Health Organisation, 1968.

Table 2.3 Screening effectiveness

Examples of effective screening	Unproven/ineffective screening
Papanicolaou smears for cervical cancer	Chest radiography for lung cancer
Mammography for breast cancer	CA-125 for ovarian cancer
Colonoscopy for colorectal adenomas	Digital rectal exam and PSA for prostate cancer
Blood pressure for hypertension	Total body CT scanning

NB: Screenings for cervical cancer and mammography (p. 425) are far from perfect—both are susceptible to false negatives, and a negative result might lead that patient to take risks or be inattentive to signs of disease occurring between screenings.

one may get the incorrect impression that screening is helping patients when it is not.

- *Length bias:* Cases of indolent disease, such as slow-growing prostate cancers, are more likely to be discovered on routine screening because they remain in the population for a longer time. Because such cases have a generally better prognosis, studies that use survival from time of diagnosis as the outcome will find benefit among patients who are screened over those who are not.

- *Overdiagnosis bias:* In the extreme case, some patients may harbor cancers (e.g., of the prostate, kidney, or thyroid) that would never have caused symptoms during their natural life. Identification and removal of such "cancers" is not helpful to the patient and may cause harm, yet inclusion of such cases in survival statistics may give the false impression of improved survival among those undergoing screening.

Clinical skills

L. David Martin, M.D.

Contents

Clinicians who are skilled at the bedside clinical evaluation make better use of diagnostic tests and order fewer unnecessary tests. The way to learn physical signs is at the bedside, with guidance from an experienced colleague. This chapter is not intended as a substitute for this process: It is simply an aid and an introduction to the important science behind the art of clinical examination.*

We ask questions to get information to help with the differential diagnosis. But we also ask questions to find out about the inner life and past exploits of our patients so that we can respect them as individuals and understand them as a whole. In the words of Sir William Osler, "The good physician treats the disease; the great physician treats the patient who has the disease." Knowing our patients as individuals helps build the mutual respect and trust that are the foundation of effective doctor-patient relationships. Optimal patient care requires understanding patients' preferences, abilities, resources, and family and social circumstances. Beyond the mechanics of delivering medical care lies the art of healing. See Table 3.1.

---

* Principal sources for this chapter are Talley NJ, O'Connor S. *Clinical Examination: A Systematic Guide to Physical Diagnosis*, 5th ed. London: Elsevier, 2005; Burton JL, Burton JBL. *Aids to Undergraduate Medicine*, 6th ed. New York: Churchill Livingstone, 1997; McGee SR. *Evidence-Based Physical Diagnosis*. New York: Elsevier, 2007; Simel DL, Rennie D (eds.). *The Rational Clinical Examination: Evidence-Based Clinical Diagnosis*. New York: McGraw-Hill, 2007; and The Stanford 25: An initiative to revive the culture of bedside medicine. http://stanford25.wordpress.com.

Table 3.1 The patient now waiting for you in room 9...1

The first news of your next patient will often be via a phone call: "There's an MI on the way in," or "There's someone delirious in room 9," or "Can you take the overdose in room 12?" On hearing such dehumanized descriptions, our minds will start painting pictures, colored by the tone of these messages. So, when we arrive at the bedside, our mind is far from a *tabula rasa* or blank canvas on which the patient can paint his woes.

The mind is always painting pictures, filling in gaps—and falling into traps. Perception is an active process, for, as Marcel Proust, that life-long all-knowing patient, observed[1]:

> We never see the people who are dear to us save in the animated system, the perpetual motion of our incessant love for them, which before allowing the images that their faces present to reach us catches them in its vortex, flings them back upon the idea that we have always had of them, makes them adhere to it, coincide with it.

So, if you want to know your patient, take snapshots of him from various angles and briefly contemplate him in the round before Proust's vortex whisks you off track. You can prepare for these snapshots in the blink of an eye, saying to yourself: "When I open my eyes, I'm going to see my patient face to face" and in that clinical blink, divest yourself of those prejudices and expectations that all good diagnosticians somehow ignore. When you open your eyes, you will be all set for a Gestalt recognition of incipient myxedema (the cause of the delirium in room 9), jaundice, anemia, or, perhaps more important, the recognition that the person in front of you is frightened, failing, or dying.

1 Proust M. The Guermantes Way, trans. Scott Moncrieff.

Taking a history

Taking histories is what most of us spend much of our professional life doing: It is worth doing it well. An accurate history is the biggest step in making the correct diagnosis. History-taking, examination, and treatment of a patient begin the moment one reaches the bedside. (The divisions imposed by our page titles are somewhat misleading.) Try to put the patient at ease: A good rapport may relieve distress on its own. Always introduce yourself and explain your role (student, resident, attending, etc.). It often helps to shake hands. Please do so gently, for if they have an underlying arthritis, a "normal" grasp may be quite uncomfortable. Check whether the patient is comfortable and ask permission to minimize distractions (such as a loud television). Be conversational rather than interrogative in tone. General questions ("Before we get into the story of your symptoms, can you tell me about yourself?") help break the ice and help assess mental functions.

Chief complaint (CC) "What has been the trouble recently?" Record the patient's own words rather than medical shorthand (e.g., short of breath rather than "dyspnea").

Set the agenda Elicit the patient's additional presenting concerns, if any, beyond the chief complaint.

Style of questioning At first, questions should be open-ended. Once a differential diagnosis begins to crystallize, ask specific directed questions about the diagnoses you have in mind and associated risk factors (e.g., travel history; p. 546).

History of presenting illness (HPI) "Tell me more about your symptoms/illness." Establish chronology. When did it start? What was the first thing noticed? Progress since then. "Ever had it before?"

PQRST Questions: Provocative/palliative factors, Quality of pain (sharp/burning/deep/aching), Region/radiation, Severity (scale of 1–10, 10 being most severe), Timing (duration and sequence with other symptoms).

Appreciate the patient's perspective What does the patient think is going on? What are the patient's worries or fears about his or her symptoms/health? How is this illness affecting his or her life?

Past medical history (PMH) Ever hospitalized? Illnesses? Operations? Ask specifically about common conditions such as diabetes, asthma, hypertension, heart disease, cancer.

Allergies Ask the features of allergies; often patients report significant medication side effects that are not true allergies.

Medications Prescribed medications? Any "over-the-counter" drugs, including aspirin? Herbal remedies, oral contraceptives, insulin or other injections?

Family history (FH) Age, health, and cause of death, if known, of parents, siblings, and children; ask about common conditions and conditions relevant to the patient's illness. Areas of the FH may need detailed questioning (e.g., to determine if there is a significant FH of heart disease, you need to specify the age at which an affected first-degree relative had his or her first heart attack or stroke [prior to age 50 in men, prior to age 60 in women is considered significant]). See Table 3.2 and Figure 3.1.

Social history (SH) Probe without prying. "Who else is there at home?" Include elements of education, language, and health literacy; relationships, marital status, family, and support (including faith/religion); important life events, job, lifestyle, and home situation; sexual history; dietary habits, substance use and abuse (see below), and other risk behaviors.

Alcohol, illicit drugs, tobacco How much? How long? When stopped? There are several ways to screen for unhealthy alcohol use, including the CAGE questionnaire (p. 69). Ever injected drugs? Shared needles? Quantify smoking in terms of *pack-years*: 20 cigarettes smoked per day for 1 yr equals 1 pack-year. Don't make assumptions about substance use based on age or other demographic information: All patients should be screened.

Review of systems (ROS) To uncover undeclared symptoms. Some of this may already have been incorporated into the history.

Don't hesitate to retake the history after a few days: Recollections change.

Table 3.2 Drawing family trees to reveal dominantly inherited disease

Advances in genetics touch all branches of medicine. It is increasingly important for doctors to identify patients at high risk of genetic disease and to make appropriate referrals. The key skill is drawing a family tree to help you structure a family history as follows:

1 *Start with your patient:* Draw a square for a male and a circle for a female. Add a small arrow (see below) to show that this person is the *propositus* (the person through whom the family tree is ascertained).
2 *Add your patient's parents, brothers, and sisters:* Record basic information only (e.g., age, and if alive and well [a&w]). If dead, note age and cause of death, and pass a diagonal line through that person's symbol.

(Continued)

Table 3.2 (*Continued*)

3 *Ask the key question* "Has anybody else in your family had a similar problem as yourself?" (e.g., heart attack/angina/stroke/cancer). Ask only about the family of diseases that relate to your patient's main problem. Do not record a full medical history for each family member: Time is too short.

4 *Extend the family tree upward to include grandparents:* If you haven't revealed a problem by now, go no further—you are unlikely to miss important familial disease. If your patient is elderly, it may be impossible to obtain good information about grandparents. If so, fill out the family tree with your patient's uncles and aunts on both the mother's and father's sides.

5 *Shade those in the family tree affected by the disease:* • = an affected female; ■ = an affected male. This helps to show any genetic problem and, if there is one, will help demonstrate the pattern of inheritance.

6 *Extend the tree:* If you have identified a familial susceptibility, or your patient has a recognized genetic disease, extend the family tree down to include children, to identify others who may be at risk and who may benefit from screening. You must find out who is pregnant in the family, or may soon be, and arrange appropriate genetic counseling.

The family tree in Figure 3.1 shows these ideas at work and indicates that there is evidence for genetic risk of colon cancer.

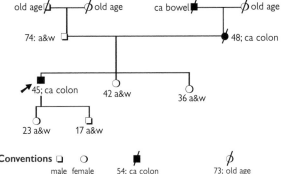

Conventions ☐ ○ ■ ∅
           male female   54; ca colon   73; old age
                           (=male died aged 54yrs   (female died aged 73yrs
a&w = alive and well   and had colon cancer)   from old age)

"This section owes much to Dr. Helen Firth, whom we thank."

Review of systems

The review of systems is a compendium of medical symptoms, grouped by body system. It is an important safety net to identify issues the clinician may have forgotten to ask about or the patient forgot to mention. It is typically presented as a series of closed yes-or-no questions, heralded by a transition statement such as, "Now I'd like to ask you a series of questions about whether you've *recently* experienced different types of medical symptoms, and you can simply answer yes or no." Obtain enough detail about positive responses to determine whether positive symptoms are significant or trivial (the more severe and chronic the symptom, the more likely it is to be important). With increasing experience, the review of systems can often be parsed down and greatly expedited. Some experienced clinicians systematically review systems as they are performing the physical examination.

Elements of selected system reviews are illustrated below.

General questions may be the most significant (e.g., in identifying cancer, endocrine problems, or tuberculosis [TB]):

- Weight loss
- Night sweats
- Any lumps
- Fatigue
- Sleeping pattern
- Appetite
- Fevers
- Itching
- Recent trauma

Cardiorespiratory symptoms Chest pain. Palpitations (awareness of heartbeats). Exertional dyspnea (= breathlessness; quantify exercise tolerance *and how it has changed*: E.g., stairs climbed or distance walked before onset of breathlessness). Paroxysmal nocturnal dyspnea (sensation of shortness of breath, often with coughing/choking, that awakens the patient). Orthopnea (breathlessness on lying flat: Quantify the number of pillows the patient must sleep on to prevent dyspnea). Edema. Intermittent claudication (reproducible leg pain that occurs with exercise and is relieved by rest). Cough. Sputum. Hemoptysis (coughing up blood). Wheezing.

GI symptoms Think of symptoms throughout the GI tract, from mouth to anus:

- Swallowing
- Indigestion
- Nausea/vomiting
- Abdominal pain
- Bowel habit

Tenesmus is a feeling of incomplete defecation (e.g., due to rectal inflammation or tumor). Hematemesis is vomiting blood. Melena refers to black, tarry, foul-smelling stools, and hematochezia refers to passage of red blood per rectum, usually in or with stools.

Genitourinary symptoms

- Incontinence (stress or urge)
- Dysuria (painful micturition)
- Hematuria (bloody urine)

- Nocturia (needing to urinate at night)
- Frequency (frequent urination) or polyuria (passing excessive amounts of urine)
- Hesitancy (difficulty starting urination)
- Terminal dribbling
- Vaginal discharge
- Menses: Frequency, regularity, heavy or light, duration, painful
- First day of last menstrual period (LMP)
- Number of pregnancies
- Menarche
- Menopause
- Any chance of pregnancy now?

Neurological symptoms

- *Special senses:* Sight, hearing, smell, and taste
- Seizures, fainting
- Headache
- "Pins and needles" (paresthesias) or numbness
- Weakness ("Do your arms and legs work?"), poor balance
- Speech problems
- Sphincter disturbance
- Higher mental function and psychiatric symptoms

The important thing is to assess function: What the patient can and cannot do at home, work, etc.

Musculoskeletal symptoms

- Pain, stiffness, swelling of joints
- Trauma
- Functional deficit

Thyroid symptoms

- *Hyperthyroidism:* Prefers cold weather, ill-tempered, sweaty, diarrhea, oligomenorrhea, weight loss (although often ↑ appetite), tremor, palpitations, visual problems
- *Hypothyroidism:* Depressed, slow, tired, thin hair, hoarseness, heavy periods, constipation, dry skin, prefers warm weather

History-taking may seem deceptively easy, as if the patient knew the hard facts and the only problem was extracting them; but what a patient says is a mixture of hearsay ("she said I looked very pale"), innuendo ("you know, doctor: down below"), legend ("I suppose I bit my tongue; it was a real seizure, you know"), exaggeration ("I haven't slept for 2 weeks"), and improbabilities ("the Pope put a transmitter in my brain"). The great skill (and pleasure) in taking a history lies not in ignoring these garbled messages, but in making sense of them. Collateral history taken from family members and other caregivers can also be very important in developing the story of a patient's illness.

Physical examination

The physical examination is performed to make diagnoses (in most of dermatology and much of neurology, for instance) and as a tool to generate hypotheses. Patients often expect to be examined, and, as such, the physical exam is also a ritual that helps affirm the physician's connection and commitment to the patient and helps build trust. We must act respectfully and professionally and recognize the vulnerability of patients, who are disrobing and allowing touch by a physician who they may have just met.

With a few exceptions (e.g., blood pressure [BP]), the physical examination is not a good screening test for detecting unsuspected disease. Although you will generally be expected to examine all four major systems (cardiovascular, respiratory, abdominal, and neurological), plan your examination to emphasize those areas that the history suggests may be abnormal. A few well-directed, problem-oriented minutes can save hours of fruitless, but very thorough, physical examination. It is also very important to communicate well with patients as you examine them, letting them know what you are doing and commenting on findings. Practice is the key; the physical exam must be explored at the bedside!

Look at your patient as a whole to decide how sick he or she seems to be. Does he or she appear well or *in extremis*? Try to decide *why* you think so. Is he in pain, and does it make him lie still (e.g., peritonitis) or writhe about (e.g., colic)? Is breathing labored and rapid? Is she obese or cachectic? Is behavior appropriate? Can you detect any unusual **smell** (e.g., hepatic fetor, ketosis, cigarettes, alcohol)?

Specific diagnoses can often be made from **the face and body habitus,** and these may be missed unless you stop and consider them: E.g., acromegaly, thyrotoxicosis, myxedema, Cushing's syndrome, or hypopituitarism. Is there an abnormal distribution of body hair (e.g., bearded ♀ or hairless ♂) suggestive of endocrine disease? Is there anything to trigger thoughts about Paget's disease, Marfan's syndrome, or Parkinson's disease? Look at the skin (e.g., the spider telangiectasia, palmar erythema, dilated abdominal veins of liver disease, and the butterfly facial rash of lupus).

Assess the degree of **hydration** by examining the skin turgor (reliable in pediatric populations), the axillae, and mucus membranes. Check peripheral perfusion. Compare lying and standing BP to identify postural hypotension, a sign of volume depletion. The hands and fingernails hold a wealth of clues; see Table 3.3.

Check for **cyanosis** (central and peripheral, p. 72). Is the patient **jaundiced** (usually first noticed in the conjunctiva of the eyes)? **Pallor** is a nonspecific sign and depends in part on the patient's natural skin pigments. **Anemia** is assessed from the palmar skin creases and conjunctivae—usually pale if Hb is <9 g/dL. No physical sign convincingly argues *against* a diagnosis of anemia. Pathological **hyperpigmentation** is seen in Addison's disease, hemochromatosis, and amiodarone, gold, and minocycline therapy.

Check **vital signs**, which can provide an early indication that a patient is ill. **Weight** (and input/output charts) may be helpful in monitoring patients who are volume-overloaded. The average oral **temperature** is 36.8°C (98.2°F), and temperature is usually lowest at 6 am and highest at 4–6 pm ("diurnal variation"). Rectal temperatures are on average 0.4° to 0.5°C (0.7°–1.0°F) higher than oral measurements, which in turn are 0.4° to 0.7°C (0.7°–1.3°F) higher than axillary temperatures and 0.4°C (0.7°F) higher than tympanic membrane measurements. An oral temperature >37.7°C (99.9°F) constitutes a *fever* (defined as the 99th percentile of maximum temperatures in healthy persons). Do not always believe the temperature chart—if the patient feels warm and you suspect fever, take the temperature yourself. **Pulse** (rate, contour, rhythm), **BP**, and **respiratory rate** and breathing pattern are discussed in the next sections.

Table 3.3 The hands

A wealth of information can be gained from gently shaking hands and then inspecting the hands of the patient. Are they warm and well-perfused? Warm, sweaty hands may signal hyperthyroidism, whereas cold, moist hands may be due to anxiety. Are the rings tight with edema? Are there any nicotine stains? Does the patient have difficulty shaking your hand (rheumatoid arthritis, p. 413)? Inability to let go of your hand suggests myotonia.

Nails Koilonychia (spoon-shaped nails) suggests iron deficiency (also fungal infection or Raynaud's). Onycholysis (detachment of the nail from the nail bed) is seen with fungal nail infection, psoriasis, and hyperthyroidism. Beau's lines are transverse furrows that signify temporary arrest of nail growth and occur with periods of severe illness. As nails grow at a rate of about 1 mm/week, by measuring distance from the cuticle it may be possible to date the stress. Mees' lines are single, white, transverse bands that are also seen in acute illness (including arsenic poisoning) and grow out during recovery. Muehrcke's lines are paired, white, transverse bands sometimes seen in hypoalbuminemia. Terry's nails: Proximal portion of nail is white/pink, nail tip is red/brown (nonspecific, seen in cirrhosis, chronic renal failure, heart failure, others). Pitting is seen in psoriasis and alopecia areata.

Splinter hemorrhages are fine longitudinal hemorrhagic streaks (under nails), which in the febrile patient may suggest infective endocarditis. They are also associated with trauma, scleroderma, and other conditions.

Nail-fold infarcts are characteristically seen in vasculitic disorders.

Digital clubbing occurs with many disorders (p. 72) and is characterized by enlargement of the terminal segments of the fingers or toes that results from the proliferation of the connective tissue between the nail matrix and the distal phalanx. There is loss of the angle between the nail and the nail-fold (i.e., no dip), and the nail feels "boggy." Exact pathogenesis is unknown.

Chronic paronychia is a chronic infection of the nail folds and presents as a painful swollen nail with intermittent discharge. Predisposing factors include diabetes mellitus, nail biting, and frequent immersion of the hands in water.

Changes occur in **the hands** in many diseases. Palmar erythema is associated with cirrhosis, pregnancy, and polycythemia. Pallor of the palmar creases suggests anemia. Pigmentation of the palmar creases is normal in Asians and blacks but is also seen in Addison's disease. A symmetrical red, scaly eruption on the knuckles (Gottron's sign) with abnormal capillary nail bed loops suggests dermatomyositis (p. 404). Dupuytren's contracture (fibrosis and contracture of palmar fascia) increases with age and is associated with repetitive hand use and vibratory trauma, diabetes mellitus, complex regional pain syndrome, the presence of other localized fibrosing conditions, and cigarette smoking and alcohol consumption. Swollen proximal interphalangeal (PIP) and metacarpophalangeal (MCP) joints with sparing of the distal (DIP) joints suggest rheumatoid arthritis; swollen DIP joints suggest osteoarthritis, gout, or psoriatic arthritis. Look for Heberden's (bony DIP joint enlargements) and Bouchard's (PIP joint enlargements) "nodes" in osteoarthritis.

The cardiovascular system

History Ask about age, occupation, exercise tolerance, and risk factors. "Typical" angina is exertional chest pain relieved by rest.

Presenting symptoms	Risk factors for coronary artery disease (CAD)
Chest pain	Smoking
Dyspnea—exertional? orthopnea? Paroxysmal nocturnal dyspnea (PND)?	Hypertension Diabetes mellitus
Ankle swelling	Hyperlipidemia
Palpitations; dizziness; blackouts	Family history of premature CAD[a]
Intermittent claudication	

Past history	Past tests and procedures:	
Angina or myocardial infarction (MI)	Electrocardiogram (ECG)	Echocardiography
Rheumatic fever	Angiograms	Stress tests
	Angioplasty/stents	CABG (coronary artery bypass grafts)

a First-degree relative <50 yrs (men) or <60 yrs (women)

Appearance Ill or well? In pain? Dyspneic? Is the patient pale, cold, and clammy? Is there corneal arcus or xanthelasma (hyperlipidemia)? Are there signs of Graves' disease (bulging eyes, goiter; p. 298)? Are there dysmorphic body features suggestive of a genetic disease (e.g., Down's, Marfan's, or Turner's syndromes, etc.)? Can you hear the click of a prosthetic valve?

Hands Digital clubbing occurs in congenital cyanotic heart disease and endocarditis (also seen in lung cancer, pus in the lung, and others). Splinter hemorrhages, Osler's nodes (tender nodules in finger pulps), and Janeway lesions (red nonpainful macules on palms and soles) are signs of infective endocarditis, as are Roth spots (hemorrhagic lesions of the retina).

Pulse See p. 48.

Blood pressure See Table 3.7 for review of measurement technique. The *systolic* BP is the pressure at which repetitive sounds are first heard (Korotkoff phase 1) as the cuff is deflated; the *diastolic* is when the heart sounds disappear (phase 5) or become muffled (phase 4; used in children, and when sounds are heard nearly to a level of 0 mm Hg). The *pulse pressure* is defined as the difference between systolic and diastolic. It is narrow in aortic stenosis and wide in aortic regurgitation. Examine the fundi for hypertensive changes. *Shock* may occur if systolic BP is <100 mm Hg.

Postural hypotension is defined as a drop in systolic BP of >20 mm Hg or diastolic BP >10 mm Hg on standing. When checking postural vital signs, wait 2 min before measuring the supine vitals and at least 1 min after standing before measuring the upright vitals.

Jugular venous pressure see p. 48.

Precordium Inspect for *scars*: Median sternotomy (CABG or valve replacement). Inspect for any implanted device (e.g., pacemaker, defibrillator). Palpate the *apical impulse*. Normal position: Fifth intercostal space in the mid-clavicular line. Is it displaced laterally (cardiomegaly, depressed ejection fraction)? Is the diameter ≥4 cm (dilated heart)? Is it sustained (left ventricular pressure and/or volume overload due to aortic valvular disease or ventriculo-septal defect (VSD), cardiomyopathy, or ventricular aneurysm)? Feel for *left parasternal heave* (right ventricle [RV] enlargement; e.g., in pulmonary stenosis, cor pulmonale, atrial septal defect [ASD]) or *thrills* (transmitted murmurs).

Auscultating the heart see Figure 3.2.

Lungs Examine the lung bases for crackles and pleural effusions (can detect high left heart pressure in patients with known heart disease).

Edema Examine the ankles, legs, and sacrum for pitting edema (in the context of elevated central venous pressure [CVP]; e.g., abnormally distended neck veins; indicates cardiac disease or pulmonary hypertension).

Abdomen Hepatomegaly and ascites may occur in right-sided heart failure. Pulsatile liver occurs with tricuspid regurgitation. *Aortic aneurysm* may be palpable in the epigastrium (physical exam is highly sensitive for detecting aneurysms >5 cm in diameter; the diameter usually indicating surgical repair).

Peripheral pulses Palpate radial, brachial, carotid, femoral, dorsalis pedis, and posterior tibial pulses. The dorsalis pedis pulse is not palpable in up to 14% of healthy persons, and the posterior tibial is not palpable in up to 10% of healthy persons (although distal pulses are rarely *both* missing in the absence of disease). See Table 3.4 for review of diagnosing peripheral vascular disease. Diminished or delayed femoral pulses are also a classic finding in coarctation of the aorta. Auscultate for carotid *bruits* in patients with stroke or transient ischemic attack (TIA) symptoms (increases the likelihood of an important stenotic lesion, but the absence of a bruit does not rule out carotid stenosis). A continuous femoral bruit following femoral artery puncture (e.g., for cardiac catheterization) is diagnostic for arteriovenous fistula.

Figure 3.2 Auscultating the heart

- The bell is used to detect low-frequency sounds and the diaphragm detects high-frequency sounds. When using the bell, apply it lightly to the body wall with only enough force to create an air seal (excessive pressure with the bell turns it into a diaphragm). The room should be quiet. Close the door to the examination room and turn off the television.

- Listen with diaphragm and bell at the apex (mitral area). Identify first and second *heart sounds*: Are they normal? Listen for *added sounds* (p. 51) and *murmurs* (Figure 3.6, p. 52) during systole and then during diastole. Repeat at lower left sternal edge and in aortic and pulmonary areas (right and left of manubrium)—and, in patients with systolic murmurs, listen in both the left axilla (radiation of mitral regurgitation) and over the carotids and right clavicle (radiation of aortic stenosis).

- Listen with the patient in three positions: Supine, left lateral decubitus, and seated upright. The lateral decubitus position is best for detection of S3 and S4 and the diastolic rumble of mitral stenosis. Upright positioning is necessary to detect some pericardial rubs and the blowing diastolic murmur of aortic regurgitation.

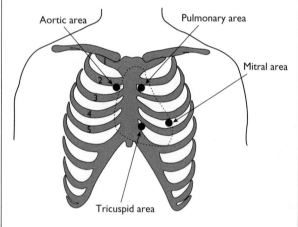

Locations for auscultating heart valve murmurs. After N Talley, S O'Connor. *Clinical Examination* 4th ed. Blackwell Science, 2002.

Table 3.4 Diagnosis of peripheral vascular disease

The *ankle brachial index* (ABI) is the diagnostic standard for detecting peripheral arterial disease (PAD). The ABI has also been shown to predict mortality and adverse cardiovascular events independent of traditional risk factors.

Technique and interpretation:

- Position patient supine.
- Measure the highest systolic BP at each ankle (dorsalis pedis and posterior tibial arteries) with a hand-held Doppler device and divide these by the highest BP in the brachial artery to get the ABI for each leg.
- Normal ABI ranges from 1.0 to 1.2; <0.9 is diagnostic of PAD, and <0.5 indicates severe disease.

Other signs *helpful* in detecting peripheral vascular disease in the symptomatic leg (although classic intermittent claudication occurs only in the minority of patients with PAD) include the absence of both pedal pulses or the femoral pulse, and the presence of wounds or sores on the foot or an asymmetrically cool foot. Findings that are *unhelpful* include atrophic skin, hairless lower limbs, and a prolonged capillary refill time.

Jugular venous pressure

The jugular veins (either the external or internal jugular veins may be used, optimally on the right side of the patient's neck) act as a manometer of right atrial pressure (e.g., CVP). Observe two features: The *height* (jugular venous pressure, JVP) and the *waveform* of the pulse. JVP observations are often difficult, especially in obese patients. Do not be downhearted if the skill seems to elude you. Keep on watching necks and the patterns you see will slowly start to make sense. See Table 3.5 for differentiating between arterial and venous pulses.

The height First assess JVP with the patient reclined to 45 degrees, with his head turned slightly to the left. The patient should be repositioned as needed, to whichever angle between the supine and upright position best reveals the top of the neck veins. The top of the neck veins is indicated by the point above which the subcutaneous conduit of the external jugular vein disappears or above which the pulsating waveforms of the internal jugular wave become imperceptible. The JVP is the vertical height of the pulse above the sternal angle. It is raised if >3 cm. Pressing firmly over the patient's midabdomen often produces a transient rise in the JVP. If a rise in JVP of ≥4 cm persists throughout a 10 sec compression, it is a *positive abdominojugular reflux sign* (also called hepatojugular reflux). Many clinicians recognize a positive test by observing the neck veins at the moment the abdominal pressure is released, regarding a fall >4 cm as positive. This is an accurate sign of elevated left atrial pressure (e.g., in patients with dyspnea, it indicates that at least some of the dyspnea is due to disease in the left side of the heart).

The jugular venous waveform See Figure 3.3. To identify individual waveforms, listen to the heart sounds as you look at the neck veins. The x descent ends just *before* S_2, and the y descent begins just *after* S_2. The normal venous waveform has a prominent x descent and a small or absent y descent.

Abnormalities of the jvp

Raised jvp with normal waveform: Fluid overload, heart failure (due to heart or lung disease)

Raised jvp with absent pulsation: Superior vena cava (SVC) obstruction

Large a wave: Pulmonary hypertension, pulmonic or tricuspid stenosis

Cannon a wave: When the right atrium contracts against a closed tricuspid valve, large "cannon" *a* waves result. *Causes:* Atrioventricular dissociation, ventricular tachycardia, other arrhythmias

Absent a wave: Atrial fibrillation

Large systolic v waves: Coincide with the carotid pulsation and collapse after S_2 (prominent y descent); seen in tricuspid regurgitation

Constrictive pericarditis: High plateau of JVP (which rises on inspiration—Kussmaul's sign) with deep x and y descents

Pulses

Assess the radial pulse to determine *rate* and *rhythm*. *Contour* may be best assessed at the brachials or carotids.

Rate Count the pulse for 30 sec and double the result. Is the pulse tachycardic (>100 bpm) or bradycardic (<50 bpm)?

Rhythm An irregularly irregular pulse occurs in AF or multiple ectopics. A regularly irregular pulse occurs in second-degree heart block and ventricular bigeminy.

Volume and contour

Normal carotid volume is easily felt with light palpation, whereas reduced carotid volume is difficult to feel even with firm palpation.

Normal carotid upstroke feels like a sharp tap, whereas reduced/delayed carotid upstroke feels like a nudge.

Pulsus parvus et tardus (carotid pulse with small volume and reduced/delayed upstroke) is a finding of aortic stenosis.

Palpable femoral pulse indicates a systolic BP of >60 mm Hg (presence or absence of femoral pulse can help determine severity of shock).

Collapsing pulses (also called *water hammer pulses*; felt at the radial artery when the patient's wrist is elevated above the heart) occur most commonly in chronic aortic regurgitation but are seen in many conditions associated with increased stroke volume.

Pulsus bisferiens (two beats per cardiac cycle, both in systole) can occur in hemodynamically significant aortic regurgitation (also in combined aortic stenosis and regurgitation). See Figure 3.4.

Dicrotic pulses (two beats per cardiac cycle, one in systole and one in diastole) occur in younger patients with severe myocardial dysfunction, low stroke volumes, and high systemic resistance.

Pulsus alternans (alternating strong and weak beats) indicates severe left ventricular dysfunction.

Pulsus paradoxus (inspiratory fall in systolic BP of >10–12 mm Hg) is a common finding in cardiac tamponade and acute asthma. See Table 3.5 for review of technique.

Table 3.5 Distinguishing arterial and venous pulses

In distinguishing venous from arterial pulses in the neck, note that the venous pulse:

- Has a prominent *descending* movement, versus arterial pulsations that have a prominent *ascending* or *outward* movement.
- Is not usually palpable.
- Is obliterated by finger pressure on the vein.
- Rises transiently following pressure on the abdomen (*abdominojugular reflux*).
- Drops lower in the neck as the patient sits up (and becomes more prominent when you lower the head of the bed).
- Becomes more prominent during inspiration (but also drops lower in the neck).
- Usually has a double pulse for every arterial pulse (flicking like a snake's tongue).

Figure 3.3 The jugular venous pressure wave

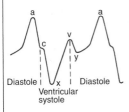

• a wave:	atrial systole
• c wave:	closure of tricuspid valve, not normally visible
• x descent:	fall in atrial pressure during ventricular systole
• v wave:	atrial filling against a closed tricuspid valve
• y descent:	opening of tricuspid valve

The jugular venous pressure wave. After Macleod, ed., Clinical Examination, 4th ed. New York: Churchill Livingstone.

Table 3.6 Pulsus paradoxus

- Have the patient breathe normally (vigorous respirations can induce a pulsus paradoxus).
- Begin checking the BP in the usual way. As you slowly deflate the cuff, note the BP at which you first hear Korotkoff sounds. Sounds will disappear during inspiration and then reappear, corresponding to the higher systemic BP occurring during expiration.
- Keep slowly deflating the cuff until you hear Korotkoff sounds with every heartbeat. Note the BP at this point.
- The difference between the two BP recordings is the pulsus paradoxus. It is considered significant if it is >10–12 mm Hg.

Figure 3.4 Arterial pulse waveforms

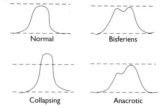

Normal

Bisferiens

Collapsing

Anacrotic

Typical arterial pulse waveforms. After J Burton. *Aids to Undergraduate Medicine*, 6th ed. New York: Churchill Livingstone.

Table 3.7 Measuring blood pressure

- Patients should be seated quietly for 5 min in a chair, with their feet on the floor and the arm supported at heart level.
- Use the correct size cuff (a too small cuff will overestimate BP). The blood pressure cuff's bladder should encircle at least 80% of the arm. The bladder should be centered over the brachial artery, and the cuff applied snugly.
- Inflate the cuff while palpating the brachial artery until the pulse disappears. This provides an estimate of systolic pressure.
- Inflate the cuff until 20–30 mm Hg above systolic pressure, then place stethoscope over the brachial artery. Deflate the cuff at 2 mm Hg/sec.
- *Systolic pressure:* The appearance of repetitive sounds (Korotkoff phase 1).
- *Diastolic pressure:* Usually the disappearance of sounds (phase 5). However, in some individuals (e.g., pregnant women), sounds are present until the zero point. In this case, the muffling of sounds, Korotkoff phase 4, should be used.
- Record pressure, patient position (e.g., seated), arm, and cuff size. Obtain two readings, separated by at least 30 sec, and average them.

Heart sounds

Listen systematically: Sounds then murmurs. While listening, palpate the carotid artery: S_1 is synchronous with the upstroke.

The heart sounds The first and second sounds are usually clear. Confident pronouncements about other sounds and soft murmurs may be difficult. Even senior colleagues disagree with one another about the more difficult sounds and murmurs.

The first heart sound (S_1) is usually loudest at the apex and represents closure of mitral and tricuspid valves. See Figure 3.5.

Abnormally loud S_1 can occur because of delayed closure of the mitral valve (as in mitral stenosis) or due to vigorous ventricular contractions (as in fever, thyrotoxicosis). *Faint or absent S_1* occurs due to weak ventricular contractions (MI, left bundle branch block [LBBB]) or due to early closure of the mitral valve (when PR interval is >0.20 sec or in acute aortic regurgitation). *Varying intensity of S_1* (assuming the rhythm is *regular*) indicates atrioventricular dissociation. *Prominent splitting of S*$_1$ can occur in patients with RBBB or paced beats.

The second heart sound (S$_2$*)* represents aortic (A$_2$) and pulmonary valve (P$_2$) closure. The most important diagnostic feature of S$_2$ is the "splitting" of its A$_2$ and P$_2$ components; intensity of S$_2$ has less diagnostic importance (despite traditional teachings, no evidence supports a loud P$_2$ as a sign of pulmonary hypertension).

Splitting in inspiration is normal and is mainly due to the variation with respiration of right heart venous return, causing P$_2$ to be further delayed. Splitting is usually heard only in the pulmonary area (second left interspace; see p. 46), because P$_2$ is too faint elsewhere. *Wide physiologic splitting* (A$_2$P$_2$ interval widens further during inspiration) occurs most commonly in right bundle branch block (RBBB). *Wide fixed splitting* (A$_2$P$_2$ interval remains constant during inspiration and expiration) occurs in ASD. *Paradoxic ("reversed") splitting* (i.e., splitting ↑ on expiration) occurs in LBBB, RV pacing, aortic stenosis, and ischemic heart disease.

A *third heart sound (S*$_3$*)* may occur just after S$_2$ and represents exaggerated early diastolic filling. It is low-pitched and best heard with the bell of the stethoscope. S$_3$ can be physiologic in individuals younger than 40 yrs. An S$_3$ is an important finding indicating depressed ejection fraction and elevated left atrial pressures (associated with heart failure, aortic valve disease).

A *fourth heart sound (S*$_4$*)* occurs just before S$_1$ and represents atrial contraction against a ventricle made stiff by any cause; for example, due to hypertension, other cardiomyopathy, or aortic stenosis. S$_4$ has less diagnostic value (does not predict ejection fraction, left heart filling pressures, or severity of aortic stenosis).

"Gallop" rhythms: Third and fourth heart sounds are also called *gallops*, as they can give the impression of galloping hooves. An S$_3$ gallop sounds like "Ken-tucky," whereas an S$_4$ gallop sounds like "Tenne-ssee." When S$_3$ and S$_4$ occur during tachycardia, they may appear together as a single loud sound, a *summation gallop*.

An *aortic ejection sound* is heard early in systole with bicuspid aortic valves, aortic stenosis, or a dilated aortic root. The right heart equivalent lesions may also cause clicks (e.g., pulmonary ejection sound).

Mid-systolic clicks occur in mitral valve prolapse.

An *opening snap* precedes the mid-diastolic murmur of mitral stenosis.

A *pericardial knock* is a loud early diastolic sound that can occur in constrictive pericarditis (higher frequency than S$_3$ and heard over a wider area).

Prosthetic sounds are caused by mechanical valves. Prosthetic mitral valve clicks occur in time with S$_1$, and aortic valve clicks are timed with S$_2$.

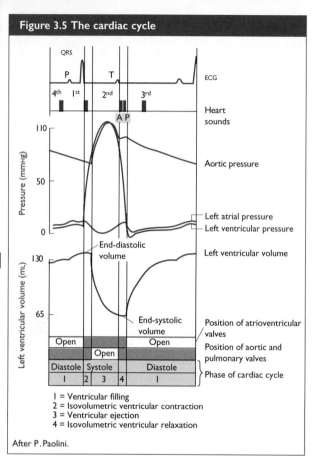

Figure 3.5 The cardiac cycle

QRS

P   T

ECG

4th 1st   2nd   3rd

Heart sounds

A P

110

50

0

Pressure (mmHg)

Aortic pressure

Left atrial pressure
Left ventricular pressure

End-diastolic volume

Left ventricular volume

130

65

Left ventricular volume (mL)

End-systolic volume

Position of atrioventricular valves

| Open | | Open |

Position of aortic and pulmonary valves

| | Open | |

| Diastole | Systole | Diastole |
| 1 | 2 | 3 | 4 | 1 |

Phase of cardiac cycle

1 = Ventricular filling
2 = Isovolumetric ventricular contraction
3 = Ventricular ejection
4 = Isovolumetric ventricular relaxation

After P. Paolini.

Heart murmurs

Always consider other symptoms and signs before auscultation and think: What do I expect to hear? However, don't let your expectations determine what you hear.

Use the stethoscope correctly. Remember that the bell is used to detect low-pitched sounds (e.g., mitral stenosis) and should be applied gently to the skin (a bell applied tightly to the skin becomes a diaphragm). The diaphragm is used to detect higher-pitched sounds (e.g., aortic regurgitation).

Consider any murmur in terms of *timing* (systolic, diastolic, or continuous), *intensity* (see Table 3.8 and Figure 3.6), *pitch*, and *location* (where the murmur is loudest and where it radiates).

An *innocent systolic murmur* (also called *functional murmur*) is soft (grade 1 or 2), early in systole, and heard along the left sternal border. Anything beyond this description (including all diastolic murmurs) could indicate underlying structural heart disease and may need an echocardiogram to further evaluate.

Timing and quality A *systolic-ejection murmur* (SEM, crescendo–decrescendo) usually originates from abnormal flow over an outflow tract and waxes and wanes with the intraventricular pressures. SEMs may be innocent and are common in children and high-output states (e.g., tachycardia, pregnancy). Pathologic causes include aortic stenosis and sclerosis, pulmonary stenosis, and hypertrophic obstructive cardiomyopathy (HOCM).

A *holosystolic murmur* (HSM) is of uniform intensity and obscures both S_1 and S_2. It occurs due to regurgitation from a ventricle into a low-pressure chamber (e.g., mitral or tricuspid regurgitation, VSD). Mitral valve prolapse may produce a late systolic murmur and a midsystolic click.

Early diastolic murmurs are high-pitched, blowing, and decrescendo. These occur in aortic and, although rare, pulmonary regurgitation.

Mid-diastolic murmurs are low-pitched and rumbling. They occur in mitral stenosis (often accentuated presystolically also) and are easily missed: Listen for the "absence of silence" in diastole. Also often seen in moderate or severe aortic regurgitation (Austin Flint murmur).

Continuous murmurs begin in systole and continue into diastole and may occur with a patent ductus arteriosus, arteriovenous fistula, or coarctation of the aorta.

Intensity Intensity is generally a poor guide to the severity of a lesion (exceptions include aortic and mitral regurgitation, where murmurs of grade ≥ 3 indicate more severe disease). Many patients with right-sided valvular lesions (such as tricuspid regurgitation), and many with *mild* mitral or aortic regurgitation, do not have audible murmurs. To help distinguish the etiology of a systolic murmur, observe how its intensity changes with changing cardiac cycle lengths (as in atrial fibrillation): Mitral regurgitation does not change in intensity, but aortic stenosis becomes louder after a longer duration diastole (HOCM responds unpredictably to changing cycle lengths). See Table 3.8.

Area where loudest The location (and timing) of a systolic murmur does not reliably distinguish aortic stenosis from mitral regurgitation. However, highest intensity of murmur at second right intercostal space (among systolic murmurs radiating to the right clavicle) can help determine likelihood of severe aortic stenosis.

Radiation The SEM of aortic stenosis classically radiates to the right clavicle and carotids (if the murmur over the right clavicle is absent, then aortic stenosis is considerably less likely), in contrast to the HSM of mitral regurgitation, which classically radiates to the axilla.

Accentuating maneuvers Movements that bring the relevant part of the heart closer to the stethoscope accentuate murmurs (e.g., leaning forward for aortic regurgitation, left lateral decubitus position for mitral stenosis).

Right-sided murmurs characteristically intensify during normal *inspiration* (inspiration increases venous return to the right side of the heart and decreases it to the left side of the heart). The *Valsalva maneuver* (forced expiration against a closed glottis) decreases systemic venous return, accentuating the systolic murmur of HOCM. Squatting-to-standing also decreases venous return and may also intensify mitral valve prolapse.

Increasing afterload (via isometric handgrip exercise or transient arterial occlusion) will intensify murmurs of mitral regurgitation and VSD.

Nonvalvular murmurs A *pericardial friction rub* may be heard in pericarditis. It is a superficial scratching sound, not confined to systole or diastole.

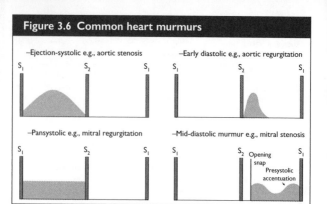

Figure 3.6 Common heart murmurs

-Ejection-systolic e.g., aortic stenosis

-Early diastolic e.g., aortic regurgitation

-Pansystolic e.g., mitral regurgitation

-Mid-diastolic murmur e.g., mitral stenosis

Opening snap

Presystolic accentuation

Table 3.8 Grading intensity of heart murmurs

The intensity of murmurs is graded on a 1–6 scale:

Grade 1/6:	Very soft, only heard after listening for a while
Grade 2/6:	Soft, but detectable immediately
Grade 3/6:	Clearly audible, but no thrill palpable
Grade 4/6:	Clearly audible, palpable thrill
Grade 5/6:	Audible with stethoscope partially touching chest
Grade 6/6:	Can be heard without placing stethoscope on chest

The respiratory system

Presenting symptoms

- *Cough*

  Duration (see Table 3.9)? Character (e.g., dry vs. productive; bloody)? Nocturnal (asthma)? Exacerbating factors (cold air, dust, fumes, fragrances)? Associated symptoms (including constitutional symptoms, wheezing, dyspnea, rhinorrhea, heartburn, hoarseness, etc.)?

- *Dyspnea*

  Duration? Steps climbed/distance walked before onset? Associated symptoms (cough, wheezing, chest pain, orthopnea, leg swelling, etc.)?

- *Hoarseness*

  Duration? Acute laryngitis is usually a viral infection; chronic laryngitis is due to an irritant such as acid reflux or inhaled toxins. Risk factors for cancer (e.g., tobacco, alcohol use)? Differential diagnosis includes benign vocal fold lesions, malignancy, neurologic disease, and many others.

- *Fever/ night sweats (p. 76)*   • *Chest pain (p. 90)*   • *Wheeze (p. 57)*   • *Stridor (pp. 56,82)*

Past history Previous history with presenting symptoms? History of heart, lung, or neuromuscular disease? Immunocompromised (e.g., due to HIV infection, malignancy, chemotherapy or other immunosuppressive medications)? Atopy (asthma/eczema/hay fever)? Previous chest x-ray (CXR) abnormalities (e.g., lung nodule, or hilar adenopathy as in sarcoidosis)?

Family history Atopy? chronic obstructive pulmonary disease (COPD)/ emphysema? Pulmonary embolism? TB? Other lung or neuromuscular disease?

Social history Quantify smoking in terms of pack-years (20 cigarettes/day for 1 yr = 1 pack-year). Occupational and other exposures (farming, mining, asbestos, secondhand smoke exposure)? Animals at home (e.g., birds)? Recent travel/TB contacts? Illicit drugs?

Medications Review all, with particular attention to inhaled or nebulized respiratory medications and those with respiratory side effects (e.g., ACE inhibitors, cytotoxics, β-blockers, amiodarone)?

Examining the chest See Figure 3.7 for review of anatomy. See next section for review of inspection, palpation, percussion, and auscultation.

Other relevant examination:

Review vital signs including pulse oximetry.

Examine the hands for *clubbing* (p. 72), peripheral cyanosis, nicotine staining, and wasting/weakness of the intrinsic muscles (e.g., Pancoast's tumor; also accompanied by Horner's syndrome). Pain on palpation of the hands, wrists, ankles, or other joints may indicate hypertrophic pulmonary osteoarthropathy (often associated with lung cancer).

Inspect the face Check for the ptosis and miosis of Horner's syndrome (e.g., Pancoast's tumor). Are the tongue and lips bluish (central cyanosis)?

Examine the heart Including assessment of JVP (p. 47) and for signs of *cor pulmonale* (p. 198).

Table 3.9 Differential diagnosis of cough

Cough is a relatively nonspecific symptom, resulting from mechanical or chemical irritation of cough receptors anywhere from the pharynx to the lungs (and also located in the pericardium, esophagus, diaphragm, and stomach). Duration of cough helps inform the differential diagnosis:

Acute cough (<3 wks) is usually due to acute respiratory tract infection; also consider COPD exacerbation, pneumonia, pulmonary embolism.

Subacute cough (3–8 wks) is often postinfectious; also consider Pertussis infection.

Chronic cough (>8 wks) is most commonly due to postnasal drip, asthma, gastroesophageal reflux disease (GERD), angiotensin-converting enzyme (ACE)-inhibitor therapy, and chronic bronchitis (also lung infections, bronchiectasis, pulmonary fibrosis, neoplasm, and many others).

Do not ignore a change in character of a chronic cough; it may signify a new problem, such as infection or malignancy.

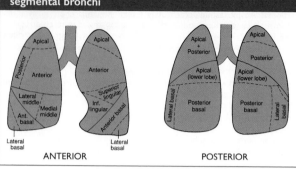

Figure 3.7 The respiratory segments supplied by the segmental bronchi

ANTERIOR

POSTERIOR

This diagram reminds us that we must auscultate anteriorly in order to examine the right middle lobe.

Examining the chest

Inspection Look for deformities of the spine (kyphoscoliosis) or chest wall (e.g., barrel chest, p. 71) or scars from surgery. Count *respiratory rate* (usually done while pretending to count the radial pulse, as the respiratory rate may change if attention is drawn to it), note *breathing pattern* (e.g., Is the expiratory phase prolonged? Lips pursed? Periods of apnea? Cheyne-Stokes breathing? p. 71) and note use of accessory muscles of respiration (sternocleidomastoid and scalene muscles).

Palpation *Lymphadenopathy:* Check for cervical, supraclavicular, and axillary lymphadenopathy. *Tracheal position:* Is it central or displaced to one side (toward an area of collapse, away from a large pleural effusion or tension pneumothorax; slight deviation to the right is normal). *Expansion (or "excursion"):* Stand behind the patient, touch the lateral thorax bilaterally, and assess for any visible difference in excursion between the two sides of the chest. Unilaterally reduced chest expansion suggests pleural effusion or consolidation, and bilateral reduction is seen in chronic airflow obstruction. Classically, <5 cm change in chest circumference between maximum inspiration and expiration (using a tape measure at the level of the fourth ICS) is considered abnormal, although this overlaps with the lower limit seen in normal persons (2–3 cm). Test *tactile fremitus* (the palpation of low-frequency vibrations transmitted by a patient's voice through the chest) by asking the patient to repeat "ninety-nine" while firmly palpating the chest wall over symmetric respiratory segments bilaterally. Absence of tactile fremitus can be a normal finding; focus on *asymmetry* as being abnormal (asymmetrically diminished fremitus seen in unilateral pneumothorax, pleural effusion, pleural thickening, or neoplasm; increased fremitus suggests consolidation, as in unilateral pneumonia).

Percussion Percuss symmetrical areas of the anterior, posterior, and axillary regions of the chest wall. A normal chest should sound equally resonant on both sides. However, patients with significant lung disease also often have normal percussion findings. It is important to know the upper border of liver dullness on the right side: In the fifth space in the mid-clavicular line, the seventh space in the mid-axillary line, and the ninth space in the scapular line ("579 rule"). *Causes of a dull percussion note:* Pleural effusion, consolidation, pleural thickening, atelectasis, or elevated hemidiaphragm. *Causes of a hyperresonant percussion note:* Pneumothorax or hyperinflation (COPD).

Auscultation Ask the patient to breathe normally in and out of the mouth. Listen with the diaphragm over symmetrical areas of the anterior, posterior, and axillary regions of the chest wall, focusing on *quality* and *intensity* of breath sounds, the *transmission of spoken words*, and the presence of *adventitious sounds*.

Quality and intensity Normal breath sounds (as heard over the posterior chest) have a soft, rustling quality and are described as *vesicular*. *Bronchial breath sounds* (normally heard over the trachea and right apex; abnormal elsewhere) have a prominent expiratory component and much harsher quality, as if air was blown forcibly through a hollow tube. Bronchial breath sounds occur when lung tissue that has become solid, collapsed, or consolidated is contiguous with the chest wall (usually due to pneumonia or pleural effusion). *Diminished breath sounds* occur with pleural effusions, pleural thickening, pneumothorax, bronchial obstruction, asthma, or COPD. *The silent chest* occurs in life-threatening asthma and is due to severe bronchospasm that prevents adequate air entry into the chest.

Transmission of spoken words (to a stethoscope placed on the patient's chest) is called "vocal resonance" and is usually muffled, weak, and unintelligible. Abnormalities include *bronchophony* (patient's voice sounds much louder than normal), *whispered pectoriloquy* (patient's whispered words are intelligible), and *egophony* (patient's "E" vocalization changes into a loud nasal "A" or "AH", also called "E-to-A" change). *Asymmetry* of findings is again key in detecting abnormality. Abnormal vocal resonance has the same significance as bronchial breath sounds.

Adventitious sounds Wheezes are caused by air passing through narrowed airways. They are classically heard in COPD and asthma, although decompensated left ventricular failure ("cardiac asthma") is always important to consider in the dyspneic patient (remember to examine the neck veins for elevated jugular venous pressure). Longer and high-pitched wheezes indicate worse obstruction than shorter and low-pitched ones. *Crackles (rales)* are caused by the reopening, during inspiration, of the small distal airways that collapsed during expiration. The sound resembles pulling apart strips of Velcro. Coarse crackles are thought to originate in larger, more proximal airways than are fine crackles. The timing of crackles is important; early inspiratory crackles suggest small airways disease (e.g., COPD), whereas late inspiratory fine crackles are typical of interstitial fibrosis. The crackles of heart failure and pneumonia are either coarse or fine and can be pan inspiratory. *Rhonchus* is an ambiguous term that should be avoided. That said, *rhonchi* most often refers to coarse discontinuous sounds heard in patients with airway secretions; we suggest simply labeling these "coarse breath sounds" (these often clear with cough). *Stridor* is a loud, high-pitched musical sound confined to inspiration that indicates upper airway obstruction. *Pleural rubs* are caused by movement of the visceral pleura over the parietal pleura, when both surfaces are roughened (e.g., by an inflammatory exudate). Causes include adjacent pneumonia, pulmonary infarction.

GI history

Presenting symptoms

Abdominal pain
Nausea and vomiting (p. 207)
Dysphagia (p. 206)
Upper GI bleeding (hematemesis, melena p. 217)

Indigestion (dyspepsia, GERD p. 208)
Recent change in bowel habit
Diarrhea (p. 210) or constipation (p. 213)
Rectal bleeding (p. 82)
Appetite, weight change
Jaundice (p. 202)
Pruritus; dark urine, pale stools

Past history

Peptic ulcer
Cancer
Jaundice, hepatitis
Blood transfusions
Previous operations
Last menstrual period, LMP

Medications

GI drugs
NSAIDs
Antibiotics
Metformin
Steroids
Oral contraceptives

Social history

Smoking, alcohol
Intranasal cocaine, injection drugs (risk factors for hepatitis C [HCV] infection)
High-risk sexual activity (risk for HBV infection)
Overseas travel, tropical illnesses
Contact with jaundiced persons
Occupational exposures,
dietary history, recent changes

Family history

Irritable bowel disease
Inflammatory bowel disease
Peptic ulcer
Polyps, cancer

Examining the GI system

Signs of chronic liver disease

- Fetor hepaticus (sign of severe portosystemic shunting; breath is a mix of rotten eggs and garlic)

- Drowsiness, confusion

- Parotid (and lacrimal) gland enlargement

- Spider telangiectasia (spider angiomas; also seen in pregnancy and malnutrition)

- Jaundice

- Diminished axillary hair

- Male gynecomastia

- Asterixis (an irregular hand and finger "flap" seen when patient holds arms outstretched with wrists fully extended and fingers spread apart; not specific to liver disease, but one of the earliest findings of encephalopathy)

- Palmar erythema (pale hand with islands of redness over thenar and hypothenar eminence)

- Clubbing (rare; only in biliary cirrhosis)

- Terry's nails (p. 43)

- Scratch marks

- Edema

- Testicular atrophy

- Dilated abdominal veins (e.g., caput medusae; in contrast, dilated abdominal veins due to SVC or IVC syndrome tend to appear on the lateral aspects of the abdominal wall)

- Splenomegaly, ascites (see Table 3.10)

Genitourinary history

Presenting symptoms

Fever, groin pain, dysuria, urinary frequency, hematuria, incontinence

Urethral/vaginal discharge
Sex: Any problems? Painful intercourse (dyspareunia)

Menses: Menarche, menopause, length of periods, amount, pain? Irregular bleeding? Last period (LMP)?

Past history

Urinary tract infection (UTI), Sexually transmitted disease (STD)
Kidney disease, stones
Prostate disease

Diabetes mellitus (DM), hypertension (HTN), NSAID use
Irregular menses, endometriosis
Pregnancy
Previous operations

Medications

Anticholinergics
Diuretics
Prostate drugs

Social history

Smoking
Sexual history
Contraception

Lower urinary tract symptoms (e.g., from benign prostatic enlargement causing bladder outlet obstruction, or overactive bladder). Ask:

- Any pain or burning on urination? (*Dysuria*)
- On feeling an urge to urinate, do you have to go at once? (*Urgency*)
- Do you urinate often at night? (*Nocturia*)
- Too often during the day? (*Frequency*)
- When you want to urinate, is it hard to get the stream started? (*Hesitancy*)
- Is your stream getting weaker? (*Weak stream*)
- Does the flow stop and start? Do you go on dribbling when you think you've stopped? (*Terminal dribbling*)
- Do you ever leak urine? (*Incontinence*)
- Do you feel the bladder is not empty after urinating? (*Sense of incomplete emptying*)

Important note on physical examination

Remember to have a chaperone present when performing intimate examinations (breast, genitourinary, rectal).

Table 3.10 Examining the abdomen

Adjust the patient so that he or she is lying flat, with his or her head resting on only one pillow and arms at the sides. The examiner is positioned on the patient's right side. Ask permission to expose the patient's abdomen and open a drape (flat sheet) to first cover patient's legs and pelvic area prior to the patient raising his or her gown.

Inspection Inspect abdomen for contour (distention, bulging flanks, hernia), scars, ecchymoses (may indicate intraperitoneal or retroperitoneal hemorrhage), dilated veins, striae, masses (e.g., Sister Mary Joseph's nodule; i.e., metastatic carcinoma of the umbilicus), pulsations, peristalsis.

Auscultation Listen with the diaphragm of the stethoscope for *bowel sounds* for 10–15 sec just below and to the right of the umbilicus. Do this before percussing or palpating (which may stimulate bowel sounds and alter the exam findings). In patients with small bowel obstruction, about 40% have hyperactive bowel sounds (>34/min) and about 25% have hypoactive (<5/min) or absent (none heard for 2 min) bowel sounds. Listen for *abdominal bruits* (may be general markers of vascular disease or indicate renovascular hypertension), although they occur in 4–20% of healthy persons.

Percussion and palpation Clinicians' hands should be warm and expected tender areas should be examined last. If the abdominal wall is tense, it can be further relaxed by asking the patient to bend her knees. Observe the patient's face for signs of discomfort during the exam.

Briefly percuss in all four quadrants, listening for tympany and dullness. Then systematically perform light palpation followed by deep palpation. Note *tenderness* and *guarding* (involuntary tensing of abdominal muscles because of pain or fear of it). If the patient has abdominal pain, test for *rebound tenderness* (a sign of peritoneal inflammation) by releasing your hand quickly from the abdomen.

- *Examining the liver:* A practical approach involves starting with palpation. Beginning deep in the right lower quadrant, place right hand on patient's abdomen just lateral to the rectus abdominis; ask patient to take a deep breath and try to feel the liver edge as it descends. Note liver texture (soft, firm, nodular) as it passes under your fingers. If liver edge is not felt below the costal margin, do not proceed with percussion. If liver edge is palpated, then percuss for the upper border (>15 cm = enlargement by percussion in mid-clavicular line). Percussed liver span correlates modestly with the actual span, but underestimates it. As percussed liver span is also dependent on technique, you will develop your sense of "normal" vs. "abnormal" based on using your individual technique to examine many patients. Evidence does not support using the "scratch test" to measure liver span. Two important points in assessing for hepatomegaly:
- Palpating the liver edge below the costal margin is an unreliable sign of hepatomegaly, as half of all palpable livers are not enlarged.
- About half of all livers that extend below the costal margin are not palpable (consistency seems to be important, and diseased/firm livers are much more likely to be palpable).

(Continued)

Table 3.10 (Continued)

Examining the spleen: The physical exam is best used when ruling in a diagnosis of splenomegaly in a patient for whom suspicion is moderately high (the exam is more specific than sensitive). Start by percussing in the lower left rib spaces in the mid-axillary line. If dull (instead of tympanic), proceed with supine, one-handed palpation (many other methods of palpation are also acceptable). Start in the right lower quadrant with gentle pressure and feel for a descending spleen as patient takes a long, deep breath. Reposition and repeat palpation at 2 cm increments heading through the umbilical area to the left upper quadrant. *To confidently rule out splenomegaly, imaging (e.g., ultrasound) is required.*

Assessing for ascites: Fluid wave and edema are the most helpful findings in diagnosing ascites. To elicit a *fluid wave*, the examiner places one hand firmly against the lateral abdominal wall and uses the other hand to tap firmly on the opposite lateral wall (unless there is "tense" ascites, the patient or an assistant must also apply firm pressure against the anterior abdominal wall during the exam to restrict waves from travelling through the subcutaneous tissue). *Shifting dullness* (flank dullness whose position shifts as the patient rolls on to one side) also increases the probability of ascites. *To confidently rule out ascites, imaging (e.g., ultrasound) is required.*

The neurological system

History This should be taken from the patient and, if possible, from a close friend or relative as well. The patient's memory, perception, or speech may be affected by the disorder, making the history difficult to obtain. Note the progression of the symptoms and signs: Gradual deterioration (e.g., tumor) versus intermittent exacerbations (e.g., multiple sclerosis) versus rapid onset (e.g., stroke). Ask about age, occupation, right- or left-handed? See Table 3.11.

Presenting symptoms

- *Headache:* (p. 345) Different from usual headaches? Acute/chronic? Speed of onset? Intensity (worst headache of your life?). Course (recurrent, progressive)? Unilateral or bilateral? Associated aura (migraine, p. 349)? Any meningismus? Other associated symptoms (e.g., fever, visual disturbance, nausea, etc.)?
- *Weakness:* Speed of onset? Muscle groups affected (e.g., symmetric proximal weakness is usually due to muscle disease)? Sensory loss? Pain? Varies during the day? Associated ptosis or dysphagia?
- *Visual disturbance:* E.g., blurring, double vision (diplopia), photophobia, visual loss, red eye, eye pain. Speed of onset? Any preceding or associated symptoms? Trauma?
- *Special senses:* Hearing, smell, taste.
- *Dizziness:* (p. 355) Clarify vertigo (illusion of surroundings moving, spinning) versus light-headedness (feeling faint) versus dysequilibrium? Hearing loss or tinnitus? Any loss of consciousness? New medications?
- *Speech disturbance:* Difficulty in expression, articulation, or comprehension? Sudden onset or gradual? Other focal symptoms?
- *Dysphagia:* Solids and/or liquids? Intermittent or constant/progressive? Temporal progression of symptoms? Associated symptoms (e.g., weight loss, heartburn)? Painful (odynophagia)?

- *Seizures:* (p. 378) Context/circumstances? Preceding aura? Describe ictal events. Loss of consciousness? Tongue biting? Incontinence? Any residual weakness/confusion? Family history? Alcohol or benzodiazepine withdrawal?
- *Sensory disturbance:* E.g., numbness, "pins and needles" (paresthesias), pain, odd sensations? Distribution? Speed of onset? Associated weakness?
- *Tremor:* (p. 384) Amplitude? Appears with rest, posture, or activity? Taking β-agonists? Metoclopramide? Neuroleptics? Suspicion for hyperthyroidism? Any family history?

Cognitive state If there is any doubt about the patient's cognition, an objective measure is performance on a cognitive test such as the Mini-Mental State Examination (MMSE, p. 67).

Past medical history Ask about cancer, HIV infection, mental illness; meningitis/encephalitis, head/spine trauma, seizures, previous operations, risk factors for stroke (atrial fibrillation [AF], HTN, hyperlipidemia, DM, smoking). Is there any chance that the patient is pregnant (preeclampsia)?

Medications Any anticonvulsant/antipsychotic/antidepressant medication? Any medication with neurological side effects (e.g., isoniazid)?

Social and family history Functional status (activities of daily living [ADLs], etc.) and limitations? Tobacco, alcohol, illicit drugs? Caffeine intake, dietary history? Recent travel? Any neurological or psychiatric disease in the family?

Table 3.11 Examining the neurological system

Along with the history, the neurologic exam is performed to help precisely localize the site of pathology within the nervous system (p. 329). The neurological system is usually the most daunting examination to learn, but the most satisfying once perfected. Learn at the bedside from a senior colleague, preferably a neurologist. There is no substitute for practice. Be aware that books present ideal situations: Often one or more signs are equivocal or even contrary to expectation. Don't be put off; consider the whole picture, and consider retaking the history.

Level of consciousness Can say awake, drowsy, stuporous, or comatose; but be sure to more precisely describe the patient's level of arousal (e.g., "Patient is very drowsy; falls asleep between questions").

General inspection During history, note speech quality (assess for dysarthria, fluency, coherence). On looking at the patient, do you notice any *asymmetry* (facial, extremities, movements)? Reduced muscle bulk or tone? Are movements and walking fluid and coordinated? Any tremor or muscle twitching?

Mental status examination See p. 69.

Cranial nerves See p. 63.

Motor exam Test muscles individually by asking the patient to contract the muscle strongly while you try to resist any movement. Grade muscle strength (p. 332); note any asymmetry. Identify whether the pattern of motor weakness is consistent with lower or upper motor neuron dysfunction (lower or upper motor neurons [LMN or UMN], p. 332).
Pronator drift: Detects subtle weakness. Ask the patient to extend both arms straight out in front of himself with palms up, as if he is holding a tray, for 10 sec. Does one arm pronate and drift downward (positive pronator drift)?

(Continued)

Table 3.11 (Continued)

Tone: Look for *hypotonia* (flaccidity; a sign of LMN disease), *spasticity* (increased muscle tone with associated weakness, and flexor and extensor tone differ; a sign of UMN disease), or *rigidity* (increased tone with no associated weakness, and flexor and extensor tone are the same; a sign of extrapyramidal disease, e.g., Parkinson's).

Coordination: Look for ataxic movements that lack the speed, smoothness, and accuracy seen in normal persons (a sign of cerebellar disease). Tests include *finger-to-nose* (must be done at full arm's extension), *heel-to-shin,* and *rapid alternating movements* (if abnormal, this is called dysdiadochokinesia).

Gait: Observe patient walking normally, then on the toes, heels, and using tandem steps (heel-to-toe). Note whether any gait disturbance is symmetric or asymmetric. A positive *Romberg's sign* is inability to stand for 60 sec with feet together and eyes closed (signals a disturbance of proprioception, either from neuropathy or posterior column disease; *not* a sign of cerebellar disease).

Reflexes Proper patient positioning and good technique are required to elicit muscle stretch reflexes. Grade as *absent* (0), 1+ (present with reinforcement; e.g., when patient hooks fingers of both hands and pulls them apart as strongly as possible), *normal* (2+), *brisk* (3+), or *hyperactive* (4+ including *clonus;* i.e., rhythmic oscillations that continue as long as tension is applied to a hyperreflexic muscle). Enhanced reflexes are a sign of UMN disease, and reduced/absent reflexes are a sign of LMN disease (although these findings are nonspecific and may be seen in persons without neurologic disease). Associated nerve roots to memorize include C6 (biceps and brachioradialis), C7 (triceps), L3–4 (patellar), and S1 (ankle). Also assess the *Babinski reflex* bilaterally (use a key or handle of reflex hammer to slowly scratch a J-shaped stroke beginning at the lateral plantar surface up to the ball of the foot). A normal response (i.e., Babinski is "absent" or "normal") is flexion of all toes, and a positive response is an upgoing (extension) of the great toe (with a fanning of the other four toes).

Sensory exam Extent of testing depends on the clinical setting but may include all four simple sensations: Light touch (cotton wool), pain (pin-prick), vibration (128 Hz tuning fork), and temperature (cold stem of tuning fork). Compare patient's perceptions to the contralateral side; note distribution and symmetry of abnormality. Also assess *proprioception* (sensation of movement of great toe up or down); proprioceptive loss is common in peripheral neuropathy, spinal cord disease, and severe hemispheric disease.

Cranial nerve examination

Approach to examining the cranial nerves In patients without neurologic complaints, a quick screening exam can include testing pupillary responses to light, eye movements, visual field testing (in one eye), and facial strength. For clinical correlations, see Table 3.12.

I: *Smell:* Test ability of each nostril to differentiate familiar smells (rarely performed).

II: *Acuity:* Test in each eye separately using a pocket Snellen card; have patients wear usual corrective lenses. *Visual fields:* Compare during confrontation with your own fields. *Pupils:* (p. 81) Assess responses to the "swinging flashlight test" (in relative afferent papillary defect, pupils constrict with light into the normal eye and dilate with light into the abnormal eye). *Funduscopic exam:* Darken the room. Starting 12–18 inches away from the patient's eye, look through the scope to find the red reflex. Slowly move in and bring a retinal vessel into focus; trace vessels medially toward the nose to find the optic disc, inspecting its shape, color, and clarity.

III, IV, and VI: Assess for *ptosis* and test *eye movements*. *III palsy*: Ptosis, eye down and out, +/– dilated pupil. May cause both vertical and horizontal diplopia. *IV palsy*: Vertical diplopia (often noticed on descending stairs). Tilting the head toward the affected side aggravates the diplopia; many patients compensate by tilting their head away from the side of the lesion. *VI nerve palsy*: Esotropia (inward deviation) and an inability to abduct the affected eye. Patient complains of horizontal diplopia on looking out at a distance. *Nystagmus* is involuntary, often jerky, eye oscillations. Nystagmus lasting two beats or less is normal, as is brief nystagmus at the extremes of gaze. Horizontal nystagmus is often due to cerebellar disease or peripheral vestibular disease (but may be due to other central nervous system disorders). Vertical nystagmus is often from a central etiology.

V: *Motor palsy*: "Open your mouth": Jaw deviates to side of lesion. *Sensory*: Corneal reflex lost first; check light touch in all three divisions on the face.

VII: *Facial nerve lesions* cause facial asymmetry (droop) and weakness of ipsilateral facial movements (except for lid movements). As the forehead has bilateral representation in the brain, only the lower two-thirds is affected in UMN lesions, but all of one side of the face in LMN lesions. Ask patient to "raise your eyebrows" and "show me your teeth."

VIII: *Hearing*: Rub your fingers together softly while holding them a few inches away from the patient's ear. An alternative is the "whispered voice test" (whisper a combination of three letters or numbers while standing 2 feet behind the patient; the examiner must occlude and rub the external auditory canal of the untested ear). The Weber and Rinne tests are not recommended for routine screening.

IX and X: *Ipsilateral palate elevation*: Ask the patient to say "aaah" and observe whether the two sides of the palate move fully and symmetrically. Can also use a swab to assess pharyngeal sensation and gag reflex, although the gag reflex is often absent in normal persons, especially the elderly.

XI: *Trapezius*: "Shrug your shoulders" against resistance. *Sternocleidomastoid*: "Turn your head to the left/right" against resistance.

XII: *Tongue protrusion*: Deviates to the side of the lesion.

Table 3.12 Causes of cranial nerve lesions

Any cranial nerve may be affected by diabetes mellitus, stroke, multiple sclerosis (MS), tumors, sarcoidosis, vasculitis (e.g., polyarteritis nodosa [p. 416]), lupus, syphilis. Chronic meningitis (malignant, TB, or fungal) tends to pick off the lower cranial nerves one-by-one.

I: Trauma, respiratory tract infection, frontal lobe tumor, meningitis

II: *Field defects* may start as small areas of visual loss (*scotomas*; e.g., in glaucoma).

Monocular blindness: Lesions of one eye or optic nerve (e.g., MS, giant cell arteritis, trauma)

Bilateral blindness: Diabetes, glaucoma, infection, methanol

Field defects: Bitemporal hemianopsia: Optic chiasm compression (e.g., pituitary adenoma, craniopharyngioma, internal carotid artery aneurysm)

Homonymous hemianopsia: Affects half the visual field contralateral to the lesion in each eye. Lesions lie beyond the chiasm in the tracts, radiation, or occipital cortex (e.g., stroke, abscess, tumor).

(Continued)

Table 3.12 (Continued)

Papilledema (swollen discs): (1) ↑ Intracranial pressure (ICP) (tumor, abscess, encephalitis, hydrocephalus, benign intracranial hypertension); (2) retro-orbital lesion (e.g., cavernous sinus thrombosis, p. 368)
Optic atrophy (pale optic discs and reduced acuity): MS, frontal tumors, Friedreich's ataxia, retinitis pigmentosa, syphilis, glaucoma, Leber's optic atrophy, optic nerve compression
III alone: Diabetes, giant cell arteritis, syphilis, posterior communicating artery aneurysm, idiopathic, ↑ ICP (if uncal herniation through the tentorium compresses the nerve); third nerve palsies without a dilated pupil are typically "medical" (e.g., diabetes; ↑BP). Early dilatation of a pupil implies a compressive lesion, from a "surgical" cause (tumor, aneurysm).
IV alone: Rare and usually due to trauma to the orbit.
VI alone: MS, Wernicke's encephalopathy, false localizing sign in ↑ICP, pontine stroke (presents with fixed small pupils ± quadriparesis).
V: *Sensory:* Trigeminal neuralgia (pain but no sensory loss), herpes zoster, nasopharyngeal cancer, acoustic neuroma (p. 356) *Motor:* Rare
VII: *LMN:* Bell's palsy (p. 389), polio, otitis media, skull fracture, cerebello-pontine angle tumors (e.g., acoustic neuroma, parotid tumors, herpes zoster [Ramsay Hunt syndrome]). *UMN:* (spares the forehead—bilateral innervation) stroke, tumor
VIII: Noise, Paget's disease, Ménière's disease, herpes zoster, acoustic neuroma, brainstem CVA, drugs (e.g., aminoglycosides)
IX, X, XII: Trauma, brainstem lesions, neck tumors
XI: Rare; polio, syringomyelia, tumors near jugular foramen, stroke, bulbar palsy, trauma, TB
Groups of cranial nerves VIII, then V ± VI: Cerebellopontine angle tumors; e.g., acoustic neuroma (p. 356; facial weakness is, surprisingly, not a prominent sign). V, VI: Gradenigo's syndrome: Lesions within the petrous temporal bone III, IV, VI: Stroke, tumors, Wernicke's encephalopathy, aneurysms, MS III, IV, V$_a$, VI: Cavernous sinus thrombosis, superior orbital fissure lesions (Tolosa–Hunt syndrome) IX, X, XI: Jugular foramen lesion *Other differential diagnoses:* Myasthenia gravis, muscular dystrophy, myotonic dystrophy, mononeuritis multiplex (p. 385)

Speech and higher mental function

Aphasia (Impairment of language caused by brain damage)
Assessment:

1 If speech is fluent, grammatical, and meaningful, aphasia is unlikely.
2 *Comprehension:* Can the patient follow one, two, and multistep commands ("Touch your ear, stand up, then close the door")?
3 *Repetition:* Can the patient repeat a sentence?
4 *Naming:* Can the patient name common and uncommon things (e.g., parts of a watch)?
5 *Reading and writing:* Normal? They can be affected like speech in dysphasia. (See Table 3.13.)

Classification: Broca's (expressive) aphasia: Nonfluent speech produced with effort and frustration with malformed words 356 (e.g., "spoot" for "spoon," or "that thing"). Reading and writing are impaired but comprehension is relatively intact. Patients understand questions and attempt to convey meaningful answers. *Site of lesion:* Inferolateral dominant frontal lobe

Wernicke's (receptive) aphasia: Empty, fluent speech, like talking ragtime with phonemic (*flush* for *brush*) and semantic (*comb* for *brush*) paraphasias/neologisms (may be mistaken for psychotic speech). The patient is oblivious of errors. Reading, writing, *and* comprehension are impaired (replies are inappropriate). *Site of lesion:* Posterior superior temporal lobe (dominant)

Conduction aphasia: Traffic between Broca's and Wernicke's area is interrupted. Fluent aphasia with impaired repetition and frequent paraphasic errors but relatively preserved comprehension.

Anomic aphasias: Naming is affected in all aphasias, but in anomic aphasia, objects cannot be named but other aspects of speech are normal. This occurs with dominant posterior temporoparietal lesions.

Mixed aphasias are common. Discriminating features take time to emerge after an acute brain injury. Consider speech therapy (of variable use).

Dysarthria Difficulty with articulation due to incoordination or weakness of the musculature of speech. Language is normal (see above).

Assessment: Ask to repeat "baby hippopotamus."

Cerebellar disease: Ataxic speech muscles cause slurring (as if drunk) and speech that is irregular in volume and rhythm.

Extrapyramidal disease: Soft, indistinct, and monotonous speech.

Pseudobulbar palsy: Spastic dysarthria (*upper motor neuron*; speech is slow, indistinct, and effortful ("Donald Duck" or "hot potato" voice) from bilateral hemispheric lesions or severe MS.

Bulbar palsy: Lower motor neuron (e.g., facial nerve palsy, Guillain–Barré)—any associated palatal paralysis gives speech a nasal character.

Dysphonia Difficulty with speech volume due to weakness of respiratory muscles or vocal cords (myasthenia, p. 390; Guillain–Barré syndrome, p. 387). Parkinson's disease gives a mixed picture of dysarthria and dysphonia.

Apraxia Loss of the ability to perform complex movements despite ability to perform each individual component. Test by asking the patient to copy unfamiliar hand positions or mime an object's use (e.g., a comb). Can they make familiar gestures (e.g., a salute)? The term "apraxia" is used in three other ways:

• *Dressing apraxia:* The patient is unsure of the orientation of clothes on his body. Test by pulling one sleeve of a sweater inside out before asking the patient to put it back on (mostly nondominant hemisphere lesions).

• *Constructional apraxia:* Difficulty in assembling objects or drawing a 5-pointed star (nondominant hemisphere lesions, hepatic encephalopathy).

• *Gait apraxia:* Inability to initiate the process of walking; the gait is broad-based with short steps, with a tendency to fall backward. Seen with bilateral frontal lesions, lesions in the posterior temporal region, and hydrocephalus.

Table 3.13 The Mini-Mental Status Examination (MMSE)

(*Kafka's law:* "In youth we take examinations to get into institutions. In old age to keep out of them.") The MMSE is a quick screening test for dementia (although it is sometimes used to serially examine hospitalized patients with delirium). On longitudinal follow-up, only changes of ≥4 points indicate a significant change of cognition. An important limitation of the MMSE is that performance is affected by the patient's level of education.

Orientation
- *What is the year? Season? Date? Day? Month?* [1 point for each correct answer]
- *Where are we now?* (e.g., specific hospital, doctor's office) *State? County? City? Floor?* [1 point each]

Registration
- *I am going to name three objects. After I have finished saying all three, I want you to repeat them. Remember what they are because I am going to ask you to name them again in a few minutes.* The first repetition determines the score [1 point each, e.g., APPLE, PENNY, AIRPLANE]; repeat until all are learned.

Attention and Calculation
- *Begin with the number 100 and count backward by 7s (so you're subtracting 7 each time).* [1 point for each correct; stop after 5 answers] Alternative: *Spell "world" backward.* [1 point for each letter in correct order]

Recall
- *What were the three objects I asked you to remember a little while ago?* [1 point each]

Language
- *Show and ask patient to name a pencil and wristwatch.* [1 point each]
- *Please repeat this sentence:* "No ifs, ands, or buts." [1 point if exactly correct; 1 trial only]
- *I am going to give you a piece of paper. When I do, take the paper in your right hand. Fold the paper in half. Put the paper on the floor.* ["3-stage command"; 1 point for each correct task]
- *Please read what is written here and do what it says.* Show card with "CLOSE YOUR EYES" written on it. [1 point]
- *Please write a complete sentence on this sheet of paper.* [1 point if sentence contains a noun and verb and makes sense]

Here is a drawing. Please copy the drawing. (See Figure 3.8) Give 1 point if the two figures intersect to form a four-sided figure and if all angles are preserved.

Interpreting the score The maximum is 30; assuming there is no evidence of delirium, scores of 23 or lower strongly suggest dementia (and scores of 26–30 rule it out).

Figure 3.8

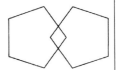

Close your eyes

Psychiatric assessment

Introduce yourself, ask a few factual questions (full name, age, marital status, job, and who is at home). These will help your patient to relax.

Presenting problem Ask for the main problems that led to this consultation. Sit back and listen for 3–5 min. Don't worry whether the information is in a convenient form or not—this is an opportunity for the patient to come out with his or her worries unsullied by your expectations.

History of presenting problem For each problem, obtain details, both current state and history of onset, precipitating factors, and effects on life. Ask what treatments have already been tried, including prescriptions and over-the-counter meds.

Check of major psychiatric symptoms Check those that have not yet been covered: *Depression* (low mood), anhedonia (inability to feel pleasure), thoughts of worthlessness/hopelessness, sleep and appetite disturbance. Ask specifically about *suicidal ideation* (and plans, if positive response) "Have you ever been so low that you thought of harming yourself?", "Do you feel you'd be better off dead?"(*passive death wish*); *mania* (periods of excessive energy and activity, euphoria, little need for sleep, reckless behavior); *hallucinations* ("Have you ever heard voices when there hasn't been anyone there, or seen visions?"); *delusions* ("Have you ever had any thoughts or beliefs that have struck you afterward as bizarre?", "Do you believe you are being monitored or that others want to harm you?"); *anxiety* and *avoidance behavior* (e.g., avoiding shopping because of anxiety or phobias); *obsessive thoughts* and *compulsive behavior* (e.g., handwashing); and *eating disorders*.

Past psychiatric history Note prior hospitalizations and outpatient treatment (e.g., from therapists, psychiatrists, and primary docs). "Do you know what you were diagnosed with?" History of response to medications and side effects.

Alcohol and illicit drug use See Table 3.14. Ask how often they use or ever used (e.g., alcohol, cocaine, marijuana, amphetamines, heroin, pain pills, benzodiazepines, etc.). Ask about past and current drug treatment.

Social History Housing, finance, work, relationship status, sexual orientation, children, friends, religion, education level, who raised them and where.

Family history Note psychiatric and substance abuse history in parents, sibs, grandparents, aunts/uncles.

Abuse history Ask about past and present sexual, physical, and verbal abuse.

Mental status examination This is the state *now*, at the time of interview.

- *Nonverbal behavior:* Dress and grooming, eye contact, affect, tears, laughter, pauses (while listening to voices?), attitude (e.g., withdrawn), psychomotor slowing or agitation, and abnormal movements (e.g., lip smacking, hand tremor)
- *Speech:* Include rate of speech (e.g., pressured) and organization (e.g., circumstantial)
- *Mood:* Sad, euthymic, anxious, irritable, euphoric? Note thoughts about harming self or others.
- *Beliefs:* E.g., about one's self, one's own body, about other people, and the future; note persecutory, grandiose, or bizarre ideas.
- *Hallucinations:* Visual, auditory, tactile
- *Orientation:* In time, place, and person

- *Memory:* Ask patient if she has concerns about her memory. Give examples. Test short-term (see MMSE p. 67) and remote memory (e.g., "Where did you get married?").
- *Attention/Concentration:* Ask patient to recite days of the week, then ask for them *backward*.
- Note the patient's *insight* and the degree of your *rapport*.

Table 3.14 Screening for unhealthy alcohol use

There is more than one way to screen for unhealthy alcohol use. The National Institute on Alcohol Abuse and Alcoholism (NIAAA) recommends a single-item screening test for people who drink alcoholic beverages at least sometimes. The question is: "How many times in the past year have you had five or more drinks in a day *(for men)* or four or more drinks in a day *(for women)*?" The test is positive if the answer is one or more times. Note that one "standard drink" is equivalent to 12 ounces of beer, 5 ounces of wine, or 1.5 ounces of 80-proof spirits. It is also a good idea to define alcohol as beer, wine, or liquor. Other screening tests are available, but a practical approach is to ask directly about "risky drinking"[1] amounts (amounts associated with adverse consequences; for men, >14 drinks/week or >4/occasion; for women, >7/week or >3/occasion), plus the familiar CAGE questionnaire:

- Have you ever felt you should *Cut down* on your drinking?
- Have people *Annoyed* you by criticizing your drinking?
- Have you ever felt bad or *Guilty* about your drinking?
- Have you ever taken a drink first thing in the morning (*Eye-opener*) to steady your nerves or get rid of a hangover?

The CAGE questionnaire alone, using one affirmative response as a positive test, is about 80–90% sensitive and specific for an alcohol use disorder (using two as a cutoff is less sensitive). These questions can be asked verbatim as part of the routine medical history, or can be asked only when patients report drinking risky amounts. Asking everyone will identify more patients with past problems or patients with current heavy drinking who did not understand the prior questions or accurately report their drinking amounts.

1 Risky drinking is much more common than alcohol dependence (also referred to as alcoholism or addiction): Almost one-third of drinkers in the United States drink risky amounts, and nearly one in four of these individuals have alcohol dependence.

Symptoms and signs

April S. Fitzgerald, M.D.

Symptoms are the features of a disease that a patient reports. **Signs** are the objective findings elicited by a physician, often at the bedside. Together, **symptoms and signs** constitute the features of a disease. Their evolution over time, and interaction with the physical, psychological, and social setting, comprise the natural history of a patient's disease.

In this chapter, we discuss symptoms and signs in isolation. Although this is an artificial construct, it is the necessary step in learning the art of diagnosis.

Abdominal distension

Causes: The famous five "**F**'s" are **F**at, **F**luid, **F**eces, **F**etus, or **F**latus. Also **F**ood (e.g., in malabsorption) can cause distension. Specific groups include:

Air	Ascites	Solid masses	Pelvic masses
Gastrointestinal obstruction (incl. fecal)	Malignancy	Malignancy	Bladder: Full or cancer
	Hypoproteinemia (e.g., nephrotic)	Lymph nodes	Fibroids; fetus
		Aortic aneurysm	Ovarian cyst
Aerophagia (air swallowing)	Right heart failure	*Cysts*: Renal, pancreatic	Ovarian cancer
	Portal hypertension		Uterine cancer

Air is resonant on percussion.

Ascites (free fluid in peritoneal cavity): Signs: Shifting dullness (p. 61); fluid wave (place patient's hand firmly on his abdomen in sagittal plane and tap one flank with your finger while your other hand feels on the other flank for a fluid wave).

The characteristic feature of *pelvic masses* is that you cannot palpate below them (i.e., their lower border cannot be defined). Causes of *right iliac fossa masses:* Appendix mass or abscess (p. 467), kidney mass, cecal cancer, a Crohn's or tubercular (TB) mass, intussusception, amoebic abscess or any pelvic mass (above).

Causes of *ascites with portal hypertension* (p. 220): See causes of *hepatomegaly* (p. 77), *splenomegaly*.

Abdominal pain

varies greatly depending on the underlying cause. Examples include irritation of the mucosa (acute gastritis), smooth muscle spasm (acute enterocolitis), capsular stretching (liver congestion in congestive heart failure [CHF]), peritoneal inflammation (acute appendicitis), and direct splanchnic nerve stimulation (retroperitoneal extension of tumor). The *character (constant or intermittent, sharp or dull)*, *duration*, and *frequency* depend on the mechanism of production. The *location* and *distribution* of referred pain depend on the anatomical site. *Time of occurrence* and *aggravating or relieving factors*, such as meals, defecation, and sleep, also have special significance related to the underlying disease process. The site of the pain may provide a clue as to its cause.

Amaurosis fugax (see p. 363)

Anemia

may be assessed from the skin creases and conjunctivae (pale if Hb is <9 g/dL). Koilonychia and stomatitis (p.) suggest iron deficiency. Anemia with jaundice suggests malignancy or hemolysis (p. 609).

Apex beat (aka apical impulse or point of maximum impulse [PMI]). This is the point furthest from the manubrium where the heart can be felt beating—normally the fifth intercostal space in the mid-clavicular line (fifth ICS MCL). Lateral displacement may be from cardiomegaly or mediastinal shift. Assess character using your palm or fingertips: A *pressure loaded* apex is a forceful, sustained undisplaced impulse (blood pressure (BP) ↑ or aortic stenosis causing LV hypertrophy with unenlarged cavity). A *volume over-loaded* (hyperdynamic) apex is forceful, nonsustained, and displaced down and laterally (e.g., cavity enlargement from aortic or mitral regurgitation). It is *tapping* in mitral *Apex beat–Chvostek's sign* stenosis (palpable 1st heart sound), *dyskinetic* after anterior myocardial infarction (MI) or with left ventricular (LV) aneurysm, *double* or *triple impulse* in hypertrophic obstructive cardiomyopathy (HOCM) (p. 53).

Athetosis is due to a lesion in the putamen, which causes slow sinuous writhing movements in the hands, which are present at rest. *Pseudoathetosis* refers to athetoid movements in patients with severe proprioceptive loss.

Backache (p. 401)

Breathlessness (dyspnea) (p. 74)

Breast pain Most common cause is hormonal fluctuations' effect on breast tissue (*cyclical mastalgia,* but patients sometimes worry that breast cancer is causing the symptom. Perform a careful examination (p. 497) and refer for ultrasound or mammography as appropriate. If there is no sign of breast pathology, and it is not cyclical, think of:

- Tietze's syndrome
- Gallstones
- Angina
- Estrogens (hormone replacement therapy [HRT])
- Bornholm's disease
- Pulmonary embolus
- Cervical radiculopathy

If none of the above, *wearing a supportive bra* may help, as may *NSAIDs.*

Cachexia Severe generalized muscle wasting implying malnutrition, neoplasia, CHF, Alzheimer's disease, hyperthyroidism, prolonged inanition, or infection (e.g., TB, AIDS, intestinal parasites, such as from *Cryptosporidium,* p. 545).

Carotid bruits indicate atheroma. A bruit is a poor predictor of carotid stenosis or stroke risk but is a predictor of ischemic cardiac disease; consider risk factor management. The key question for carotid disease is whether the patient is symptomatic. Stroke or transient ischemic attack (TIA) from carotid stenosis are considered symptomatic and often benefit from carotid revascularization. Asymptomatic patients usually benefit from medical management without surgery, but a select subset may also benefit from endarterectomy.

Chest deformity *Barrel chest:* ↑AP diameter, tracheal descent and expansion reduced; seen in chronic hyperinflation (e.g., asthma/chronic obstructive pulmonary disease [COPD]). *Pigeon chest (pectus carinatum):* Prominent sternum with a flat chest, seen in chronic childhood asthma and rickets. *Funnel chest (pectus excavatum)* (PLATE 10): Developmental defect involving local sternum depression (lower end). *Kyphosis:* "Humpback" from increased thoracic spine curvature. *Scoliosis:* Lateral curvature; both may cause restrictive ventilatory defect.

Chest pains (see p. 90)

Cheyne–Stokes respiration Breathing becomes progressively deeper and then shallower (± episodic apnea) in cycles. *Causes:* Brainstem lesions or compression (stroke, ↑ intracerebral pressure [ICP]); if the cycle is long (e.g., 3 min), the cause may be a long lung-to-brain circulation time (e.g., in chronic pulmonary edema, poor cardiac output). It is enhanced by narcotics.

Chorea means dance—a continuous flow of jerky movements, flitting from one limb or part to another. Each movement looks like a fragment of a normal movement. *Cause:* Basal ganglia lesion: Huntington's, Sydenham's (p. 137), systemic lupus erythematosus (SLE) (p. 410), Wilson's (p. 233), kernicterus, polycythemia vera (p. 633), neuroacanthocytosis (a familial association of acanthocytes in peripheral blood with chorea, orofacial dyskinesia, and axonal neuropathy), thyrotoxicosis (p. 298), drugs (L-dopa, contraceptive steroids). Early stages of chorea may be detected by feeling fluctuations in muscle tension while the patient grips your finger. Treat the underlying cause; reserve drugs (i.e., dopamine receptor blockers) for severe cases. Ask a neurologist for help.

Chvostek's sign Tapping on the facial nerve causes a facial twitch in hypocalcemia; caused by nerve hyperexcitability.

Clubbing Fingernails have exaggerated longitudinal curvature with loss of angle between nail and nail-fold, and the nail-fold feels boggy.

Thoracic causes	*GI causes*	*Cardiac causes*
• Bronchial carcinoma (usually *not* small cell)	• Inflammatory bowel (especially Crohn's disease)	• Cyanotic congenital heart disease
• Chronic lung suppuration		• Endocarditis
• Empyema, abscess	• Cirrhosis	• Atrial myxoma
• Bronchiectasis	• GI lymphoma	
• Cystic fibrosis	• Malabsorption, e.g., celiac	
• Fibrosing alveolitis	*Rare:*	
• Mesothelioma	• Familial	
	• Thyroid acropathy	
	• Unilateral clubbing, from:	
	• axillary artery aneurysm	
	• brachial arteriovenous malformations	

Constipation (see p. 213)

Cough p. 54; see also **Hemoptysis** (p. 76)

Cramp (painful muscle spasm) Cramp in the legs is common, especially at night. It may also occur after exercise. It only occasionally indicates a disease, in particular salt depletion, muscle ischemia, or myopathy. Forearm cramps suggest motor neuron disease. Quinine is no longer recommended for leg cramps due to potential for serious side effects. Writer's cramp is a focal dystonia causing difficulty with the motor act of writing. The pen is gripped firmly, with excessive flexion of the thumb and index finger (± tremor). There is normally no CNS deficit. Oral drugs or psychotherapy rarely help, but botulinum toxin can help—sometimes dramatically—but it has side effects. Similar specific dystonias may apply to other tasks.

Cyanosis Dusky blue skin (*peripheral*, e.g., of the fingers) or mucosa (*central*, e.g., of the tongue; occurs more readily in polycythemia than anemia). *Causes:*

1 Lung disease resulting in inadequate oxygen transfer (e.g., COPD, severe pneumonia); often correctable by increasing inspired O_2.
2 Shunting from pulmonary to systemic circulation (e.g., R–L shunting VSD, patent ductus arteriosus, transposition of the great arteries); cyanosis is *not* reversed by increasing inspired O_2.
3 Inadequate oxygen uptake (e.g., met-, or sulf-hemoglobinemia).

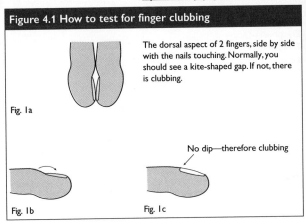

Figure 4.1 How to test for finger clubbing

The dorsal aspect of 2 fingers, side by side with the nails touching. Normally, you should see a kite-shaped gap. If not, there is clubbing.

Fig. 1a

No dip—therefore clubbing

Fig. 1b

Fig. 1c

Acute cyanosis is a sign of impending emergency. Is there asthma, an inhaled foreign body, a pneumothorax (X-RAY PLATE 6), or left ventricular failure (LVF) (p. 128)?

Peripheral cyanosis will occur in causes of central cyanosis, but may also be induced by changes in the peripheral and cutaneous vascular systems in patients with normal oxygen saturations. It occurs in the cold, in hypovolemia, and in arterial disease and is therefore not a specific sign.

Deafness (p. 357)

Dehydration (p. 458)

Diarrhea (p. 210)

Dizziness is a trinity: (1) *Vertigo* (p. 355) is the illusion of rotation, as if one just stepped off a merry-go-round. (2) *Imbalance* (i.e., difficulty in walking straight) e.g., from peripheral nerve, posterior column, cerebellum, or other central pathway failure. (3) *Faintness* (sense of collapse) e.g., seen in anemia, ↓BP, hypoglycemia, carotid sinus hypersensitivity, and epilepsy. 1–3 may coexist.

Dysarthria (p. 66)

Dyspepsia and **indigestion** These are broad terms, used by patients to signify epigastric or retrosternal pain (or discomfort) that is usually related to meals. Find out exactly what your patient means. Thirty percent have no real abnormality on endoscopy. Of positive findings:

Esophagitis alone	24%	Gastritis	9%	≥2 lesions	23%
Duodenal ulcer (DU)	17%	Duodenitis	6%	Bile reflux	0.7%
Hiatal hernia	15%	Gastric ulcer	5%	Gastric cancer	0.2%

Endoscopic or nonendoscopic testing can be used to diagnose *Helicobacter pylori* infection. Noninvasive tests include the ^{13}C-urea breath test, serological tests, and stool antigen tests. Antibody testing identifies an immunologic reaction to the disease, whereas the breath test and stool antigen test detect the presence of active infection. Prior to performing a urea breath test, patients must be off antibiotics for 4 wks and off proton pump inhibitors for 2 wks to avoid false negatives. Do endoscopy if there are "alarm"

73

symptoms (>45 yrs, ↓weight, vomiting, hematemesis, anemia, dysphagia, family history of upper GI malignancy).

Dysphasia (p. 84)

Dysphonia (p. 66)

Dyspnea (p. 90) is the subjective sensation of shortness of breath, often exacerbated by exertion. Try to quantify exercise tolerance (e.g., dressing, distance walked, climbing stairs, New York Heart Association [NYHA] classification [p. 129]). Causes:

- *Cardiac*: E.g., mitral stenosis or left ventricular failure of any cause; LVF is associated with *orthopnea* (dyspnea worse on lying; "how many pillows?") and *paroxysmal nocturnal dyspnea* (PND; dyspnea waking with the sensation of air hunger). There may also be ankle edema. Any patient who is in shock may also be dyspneic: This may be shock's presenting feature.
- *Lung*: Both airway and interstitial disease. May be hard to separate from cardiac causes; asthma may wake the patient as well as cause early morning dyspnea and wheeze. Focus on the circumstances in which dyspnea occurs (e.g., on exposure to an occupational allergen).
- *Anatomical*: I.e., diseases of the chest wall, muscles, or pleura.
- *Others*: Thyrotoxicosis, ketoacidosis, aspirin poisoning, anemia, psychogenic. Look for other clues: Dyspnea at rest, *not associated with exertion* may be psychogenic; look for respiratory alkalemia (peripheral ± perioral paresthesia ± carpopedal spasm). Speed of onset helps diagnosis:

Acute	*Subacute*	*Chronic*
Foreign body	Asthma	COPD and chronic
Pneumothorax (PLATE 6)	Parenchymal disease (e.g., alveolitis)	parenchymal diseases
Acute asthma		Nonrespiratory causes (e.g., cardiac failure)
Pulmonary embolus	Effusions	
Acute pulmonary edema	Pneumonia	Anemia

74

Dyspraxia (p. 358)

Dysuria is painful micturition (from urethral or bladder inflammation, typically from infection; also urethral syndrome [p.257]).

Edema *Causes:* ↑*Venous pressure* (e.g., DVT or right-heart failure) or *lowered intravascular oncotic pressure* (↓plasma proteins; e.g., cirrhosis, nephrosis, malnutrition, or protein-losing enteropathy; here, water moves down the osmotic gradient into the interstitium to dilute the solutes there). On standing, venous pressure at the ankle rises due to the height of blood from the heart (~100 mm Hg). This is short-lived if leg movement pumps blood through valved veins; but if venous pressure rises or valves fail, capillary pressure rises, fluid is forced out (edema), PCV rises locally, and microvascular stasis occurs. *Pitting edema, nonpitting* (i.e., nonindentible)edema; caused by poor lymph drainage (lymphedema), either primary (Milroy's syndrome) or secondary (radiotherapy, malignant infiltration, infection, filariasis). The mechanism is complex.

Epigastric pain *Acute causes:* Peritonitis, pancreatitis, GI obstruction, gall bladder disease, peptic ulcer, ruptured aortic aneurysm, irritable bowel syndrome. Referred pain: Myocardial infarct, pleural pathology; psychological causes are also important. *Chronic causes:* Peptic ulcer, gastric cancer, chronic pancreatitis, aortic aneurysm, nerve root pain.

Facial pain This can be neurological (e.g., trigeminal neuralgia) or from any other pain-sensitive structure in the head or neck (see Table 4.1). *Postherpetic neuralgia:* This nasty burning-and-stabbing pain (e.g., ophthalmic division of V) all too often becomes chronic and intractable. Skin previously affected

Table 4.1 Non-neurological causes of facial pain

Neck	Cervical disc pathology
Sinuses	Sinusitis, neoplasia
Eye	Glaucoma, iritis, eye strain
Temporomandibular joint	Arthritis
Teeth	Caries, abscess, malocclusion
Ear	Otitis media, otitis externa
Vascular	Giant cell arteritis

When all causes are excluded, a group that is mostly young and female remains ("atypical facial pain") who complain of unilateral pain deep in the face or at the angle of cheek and nose, which is constant, severe, and unresponsive to analgesia. Do not dismiss this as psychological. Do not expose these patients to the risks of destructive surgery; few meet the criteria of depression. Although many are prescribed antidepressants, some neurologists advocate no treatment.

by zoster is exquisitely sensitive. Treatment is difficult. Give strong psychological support, whatever else is tried. Transcutaneous nerve stimulation, capsaicin ointment, and infiltration of local anesthetic may be tried. Amitriptyline (e.g., 10–25 mg at bedtime) may help, as may carbamazepine (number needed to treat [NNT] ≈ 4). **NB**: Meta-analyses indicate that famciclovir and valacyclovir given in the acute stage may decrease duration of neuralgia.

Fecal incontinence Common in the elderly; be sure to find out who bathes the patient as they may be under particular stress and benefit from assistance at home. The cause may disappear if constipation (p. 213) is treated ("overflow incontinence"/diarrhea). A rectal exam will help identify overflow incontinence from retained hard stool. *Other GI causes:* Rectal prolapse, sphincter laxity, severe hemorrhoids. Others: See Table 4.2.

Fatigue This feeling is so common that it is a variant of normality. Only 1 in 400 episodes leads to a consultation with a doctor. Do not miss depression, which often presents in this way. Even if the patient is depressed, a screening history and examination is important to rule out chronic disease. *Tests* should ##include CBC, erythrocyte sedimentation rate (ESR), chemistry panel, thyroid function tests (TFTs) ± chest x-ray (CXR). Arrange follow-up to see what develops and to address any emotional problems that develop.

Table 4.2 Nongastrointestinal causes of fecal incontinence

Neurological	Spinal cord compression, Parkinson's disease, stroke, epilepsy
Endocrinological	Diabetes mellitus (autonomic neuropathy), myxedema
Obstetric	Damage to puborectalis (or nerve roots) at childbirth

Treatment is directed to the cause if possible. Avoid dehydration. If all sensible measures fail, try the brake-and-accelerator approach: Enemas to empty the rectum (e.g., twice weekly) and codeine phosphate (e.g., 15 mg/12 h PO) on nonenema days to constipate. This is not a cure, but makes the incontinence predictable.

Fever and night sweats Although moderate night sweating is common in anxiety states, drenching sweats requiring several changes of night-clothing is a more ominous symptom associated with infection (e.g., TB), lymphoproliferative disease, or mesothelioma. Patterns of fever may be relevant (p. 542). *Rigors* are uncontrolled, sometimes violent episodes of shivering that occur with some causes of fever (often acute pyogenic infections ± bacteremia).

Flank pain *Causes:* Pyelonephritis, hydronephrosis, renal calculus, renal tumor, perinephric abscess, pain referred from vertebral column.

Flatulence 400–1,300 mL of gas are expelled PR per day, and if this, coupled with belching (eructation) and abdominal distension, seems excessive to the patient, the patient may complain of flatulence. Eructation may occur in those with hiatal hernia. Most patients complaining of flatulence have no GI disease. The most likely cause is air-swallowing (aerophagia).

Frequency (urinary) means increased frequency of micturition. It is important to differentiate increased urine production (e.g., diabetes insipidus [p. 325], diabetes mellitus, polydipsia, diuretics, renal tubular disease, adrenal insufficiency, and alcohol) from frequent passage of small amounts of urine (e.g., cystitis, urethritis, neurogenic bladder, extrinsic bladder compression [e.g., pregnancy], bladder tumor, enlarged prostate).

Guarding Reflex contraction of abdominal muscles occurring as you press (gently!) on the abdomen; signifies local or general peritoneal inflammation. It is an imperfect sign of peritonitis, but is one of the best we have; e.g., if you decide not to operate on someone with right lower quadrant guarding, the risk of missing appendicitis is about 25%. If you *do* operate, the chance of finding appendicitis is 50%.

Gynecomastia (p. 319)

Hematemesis (p. 204)

Hematuria (p. 251)

Halitosis (bad breath; see Table 4.3) results from gingivitis (Vincent's angina), metabolic activity of bacteria in plaque, or sulfide-yielding food putrefaction. *Contributory factors:* Smoking, alcohol, drugs (disulfiram, isosorbide), lung disease. Delusional halitosis is quite common. *Treatment:* Try to eliminate anaerobes:

• Use the toothbrush more frequently
• Use dental floss
• 0.2% aqueous chlorhexidine gluconate

Headache (see p. 345)

Heartburn An intermittent, gripping, retrosternal pain usually worsened by stooping/lying, large meals, and pregnancy. See **Esophagitis** (p. 209).

Hemiballismus This refers to the uncontrolled unilateral movements of proximal limb joints caused by subthalamic lesions.

Hemoptysis See Table 4.4. The blood is *coughed up* (e.g., frothy, alkaline, and bright red, often in a context of known chest disease). Always think of TB ± malignancy. Don't confuse with hematemesis: The vomiting of blood—acidic and dark "coffee grounds." **NB**: Melena occurs if enough blood is swallowed. Blood not mixed with sputum suggests infarction or trauma. Consider upper airway source: Epistaxis, gum bleeding. Hemoptysis rarely needs treating in its own right, but if massive (e.g., trauma, TB, echinococcus, cancer, arteriovenous [AV] malformation), call a chest physician/surgeon (the danger is drowning; lobe resection, endobronchial tamponade, or artery embolization may be needed); set up IVF, do CXR, blood gases, CBC, International Normalization Ratio/activated partial thromboplastin time (INR/aPTT), cross-match. If distressing, consider *prompt* IV morphine (e.g., if inoperable malignancy).

Table 4.3 The science of halitosis

Locally retained bacteria metabolize sulfur-containing amino acids to yield volatile hydrogen sulfide and methylmercaptan. Not only do these stink, but they also damage surrounding tissue, thereby perpetuating bacterial retention and periodontal disease.

At night and between meals, conditions are optimal for odor production. To supplement conventional oral hygienic measures some people advise brushing of the tongue. Oral care products containing metal ions, especially zinc (Zn), inhibit odor formation, possibly by affinity between the metal ion and sulfur.

Table 4.4 Causes of hemoptysis

1 *Respiratory causes of hemoptysis*	
Traumatic	Wounds, postintubation, foreign body
Infective	Acute bronchitis, pneumonia, lung abscess, bronchiectasis, TB, fungi, paragonimiasis
Neoplastic	Primary or secondary
Vascular	Lung infarction, vasculitis (Wegener's, rheumatoid arthritis [RA], SLE, Osler–Weber–Rendu), AV fistula, malformations
Parenchymal	Diffuse interstitial fibrosis, sarcoidosis, hemosiderosis, Goodpasture's syndrome, cystic fibrosis
2 *Cardiovascular (pulmo-nary hypertension)*	Pulmonary edema, mitral stenosis, aortic aneurysm, Eisenmenger's syndrome
3 *Bleeding diatheses*	

Hepatomegaly *Causes: Hepatic congestion:* Right heart failure—may be pulsatile in tricuspid incompetence, hepatic vein thrombosis. *Infection:* Mononucleosis, hepatitis viruses, malaria, amoebic abscess, hydatid cyst. *Malignancy:* Metastatic or primary (usually hard ± nodular hepatomegaly), myeloma, leukemia, lymphoma. *Others:* Sickle-cell disease, other hemolytic anemias, porphyria, myeloproliferative disorders (e.g., myelofibrosis), storage disorders (e.g., amyloidosis, Gaucher's disease), early cirrhosis, or fatty infiltration.

Hoarseness (p. 54)

Hyperpigmentation See **Skin discoloration** (p. 82).

Hyperventilation is overbreathing that may be either fast (tachypnea; i.e., >20 breaths/min) or deep (hyperpnea; i.e., ↑tidal volume). Hyperpnea may not be perceived by the patient (unlike dyspnea) and is usually "excessive" in that it produces a respiratory alkalosis. This may be appropriate (Kussmaul respiration) or inappropriate; the latter results in palpitations, dizziness, faintness, tinnitus, chest pains, perioral, and peripheral tingling (↓plasma Ca^{2+}). The most common cause for hyperventilation is anxiety; others include fever and brainstem lesions.

- *Kussmaul respiration* is deep, sighing breathing that is principally seen in metabolic acidoses, such as diabetic ketoacidosis and uremia.
- *Neurogenic hyperventilation* is produced by pontine lesions.

Insomnia When we are sleeping well this is a trivial and irritating complaint, but if we suffer a few sleepless nights, sleep becomes the most desirable thing imaginable and the ability to bestow sleep the best thing we can do for a patient, second only to relieving pain.

Do not resort to drugs without asking: "What is the cause? Can it be treated?"

Self-limiting causes		*Psychological*	*Some typical organic causes*	
Travel	Jet lag	Depression	Drugs	Nocturia	Alcoholism
Stress	Shift work	Anxiety	Pain/itch	Asthma	Dystonias
Arousal	In hospital	Mania, grief	Tinnitus	Sleep apnea (p. 189)

Management: "Sleep hygiene"

- Avoid daytime naps. Establish regular bedtime and waking time with an alarm clock set for morning even if the patient reports spontaneously awaking at the correct time.
- Bedroom should be completely dark and quiet for sleeping, without background music or noise.
- Do not read, eat, or watch TV in the bedroom. Upon waking in the middle of the night, do not eat or get out of bed.
- Avoid caffeine, nicotine, and alcohol. Avoid exercise within 2 hours of bedtime (sexual activity may be the exception).
- Encourage daytime aerobic exercise to fatigue muscles.
- Do not prescribe benzodiazepines or alcohol at bedtime due to their addictive nature and interference with quality of sleep.
- Consider sedating antihistamine as a sleep aid.
- Consider sleep study to evaluate for restless legs or sleep apnea.
- Trazodone at bedtime is helpful for nightmares from posttraumatic stress disorder

Internuclear ophthalmoplegia A failure of eye adduction (on the affected side) with nystagmus in the other, abducting, eye. It is due to a lesion in the medial longitudinal fasciculus (e.g., caused by multiple sclerosis [MS] or stroke).

Itching (pruritus) is common and can be as debilitating as pain.

Local causes	*Systemic* (perform CBC, ESR, ferritin, liver function tests [LFT], urinalysis, TFTs)	
Eczema, atopy, urticaria	Liver disease (bile salts)	Old age, pregnancy
Scabies	Chronic renal failure	Drug reactions
Lichen planus	Lymphomas	Iron deficiency
Dermatitis herpetiformis	Polycythemia	Thyroid disease

Questions: Are there wheals (urticaria)? Is itching worse at night, and are others affected (scabies)? What provokes it? After a bath, look for polycythemia or aquagenic urticaria. Exposure (e.g., to animals [?atopy] or fiberglass [irritant eczema])? *Look for local causes:* Scabies burrows in the finger webs, lice on hair shafts, knee and elbow blisters (dermatitis herpetiformis). *Systemic:* Splenomegaly, nodes, jaundice, or flushed face or thyroid signs? *Treat* primary diseases; try moisturizing creams, ± emollient bath oils and H1-antihistamines at night (e.g., hydroxyzine or diphenhydramine).

Jaundice (p. 215)

Jugular venous pulse and pressure (p. 47)

Left iliac fossa pain *Acute:* Gastroenteritis, ureteric colic, urinary tract infection (UTI), diverticulitis, ovarian torsion, salpingitis, ectopic, volvulus, pelvic abscess, cancer in undescended testis. *Chronic/subacute:* Constipation, irritable bowel syndrome, colon cancer, inflammatory bowel disease, hip pathology.

Left upper quadrant pain *Causes:* Large kidney or spleen, gastric or colonic (splenic flexure) cancer, pneumonia, subphrenic or perinephric abscess, renal colic, pyelonephritis, splenic rupture.

Lid lag is lagging behind of the lid as the eye looks down. **Lid retraction** is the static state of the upper eyelid traversing the eye *above* the iris, rather than over it. *Causes* (both): Thyrotoxicosis and anxiety.

Lymphadenopathy Causes may be divided into:

Reactive: Infective: Bacterial (pyogenic, TB, brucella, syphilis), fungal (coccidiomycosis), viral (Epstein-Barr virus [EBV], cytomegalovirus [CMV], HIV), toxoplasmosis, trypanosomiasis. *Noninfective:* Sarcoid, connective tissue disease (rheumatoid), dermatopathic (eczema, psoriasis), drugs (phenytoin), berylliosis.

Infiltrative: Benign: Histiocytosis, lipoidoses. *Malignant:* Lymphoma, metastases.

Musculoskeletal symptoms Chiefly *pain, deformity, reduced function*. *Pain: Degenerative arthritis* generally produces an aching pain worse with exercise and relieved by rest. Discomfort may be increased in certain positions or with certain motions. Cervical or lumbar spine degeneration may also produce subjective changes in sensation not following dermatome distribution. Both inflammatory and degenerative joint disease produce *morning stiffness* in the affected joints but, in the former, this generally improves during the day, whereas in the latter, the pain is worse at the end of the day. The pain of *bone erosion* due to tumor or aneurysm tends to be deep, boring, and constant. The pain of *fracture* or *infection* of the bone is severe and throbbing and is increased by any motion of the part. *Acute nerve compression* causes a sharp, severe pain radiating along the distribution of the nerve. Joint pain may be referred (e.g., that from a hip disorder to anterior and lateral aspect of the thigh or to knee; shoulder to the lateral aspect of the humerus; cervical spine to the interscapular area, medial border of scapulae or tips of shoulders + lateral side of arms). (See *back pain* [p. 402].)

Reduced function: Causes: Pain, bone or joint instability, or restriction of joint movement (e.g., due to muscle weakness, contractures, bony fusion or mechanical block by intracapsular bony fragments or cartilage).

Nodules *(subcutaneous)* Rheumatoid nodules, polyarteritis nodosa (PAN), xanthomata, tuberous sclerosis, neurofibromata, sarcoid, granuloma annulare, rheumatic fever.

Oliguria is defined as a urine output of <400 mL/24 h. This occurs in extreme dehydration, severe cardiac failure, urethral or bilateral ureteral obstruction, acute and chronic renal failure.

Orthopnea (p. 40).

Pallor is a nonspecific sign and may be racial or familial. Pathology suggested by pallor includes anemia, shock, Stokes–Adams attack, vasovagal syncope, myxedema, hypopituitarism, and albinism.

Palmar erythema *Causes:* Pregnancy, polycythemia, cirrhosis (e.g., via reduced inactivation of vasoactive endotoxins by the liver).

Palpitations represent to the patient the sensation of feeling his own heart beat; the symptom is notoriously elusive. Have the patient tap out the rate and regularity of the palpitations.

Palpitations–Ptosis

- Irregular fast palpitations are likely to be paroxysmal atrial fibrillation (AF), or flutter with variable block.
- Dropped or missed beats related to rest, recumbency, or eating are likely to be atrial or ventricular ectopic beats.
- Regular pounding is likely to be due to anxiety.
- Slow palpitations are likely to be due to drugs, such as β-blockers, or to bigeminy. Ask about associated pain, dyspnea, and syncope (fainting), suggesting hemodynamic compromise. Ask *when* symptoms occur: People often feel their (normal) heart beat in the anxious nocturnal silence of the bedroom.

Consider checking electrocardiogram (ECG), thyroid stimulating hormone (TSH), and hematocrit (Hct). Event monitors allow event capturing and are more likely to capture an event than 48 hour Holter monitoring. If a diagnosis of "normal" ectopy is made, reassurance is essential.

Paraphimosis occurs when a tight foreskin is retracted and then becomes nonreplaceable as the glans swells. It can occur when a doctor/nurse fails to replace the patient's foreskin after catheterization. The general principle is to start with the least invasive techniques (manual manipulation) and progress to more invasive techniques (needle puncture or incision) if initial efforts are unsuccessful. If significant glans penis ischemia with necrosis is present, emergent involvement by urologist is warranted—these patients warrant sedation and immediate reduction by invasive techniques.

Pelvic pain *Causes:* UTI, urine retention, bladder stones, menses, labor, pregnancy, endometriosis, salpingitis, endometritis, ovarian cyst. Cancer of rectum, colon, ovary, cervix, bladder.

Percussive pain Pain on percussion of the abdomen is a sign of peritonitis and is often less painful for the patient than testing rebound abdominal pain (p. 467).

Phimosis The foreskin occludes the meatus, obstructing urine. Time (± trials of gentle retraction) usually obviates the need for circumcision.

Polyuria (e.g., urine >3.5 L/24 h). *Causes:* Diabetes mellitus (DM), over-enthusiastic IVF treatment, diabetes insipidus (p. 325), ↑Ca^{2+}, polydipsia, chronic renal failure.

Postural hypotension is defined as a drop in systolic or diastolic of >15 mm Hg on standing for 3 min, compared with lying down. *Causes:* Hypovolemia, Addison's disease (p. 312), hypopituitarism, autonomic neuropathy (e.g., diabetes, multisystem atrophy), idiopathic orthostatic hypotension, drugs (e.g., vasodilators, diuretics).

Prostatism (p. 681) Symptoms of prostate enlargement are often termed "prostatism," but it is better to use the terms *cystitis* symptoms or *obstructive* bladder symptoms. Don't assume the cause is prostatic. (1) *Irritative bladder symptoms*: Urgency, dysuria, frequency, nocturia (the last two are also caused by UTI, polydipsia, detrusor instability, hypercalcemia, or uremia); (2) *obstructive symptoms* (e.g., reduced size and force of urinary stream, hesitancy, and interruption of stream during voiding) may also be produced by strictures, tumors, urethral valves, or bladder neck contracture. Maximum flow rate of urine is normally ~18–30 mL/sec.

Pruritus See **Itching** (p. 78)

Ptosis is drooping of the upper eyelid. It is best observed with the patient sitting up with head held by the examiner. The third cranial nerve (CN III) innervates the levator palpebrae superioris, but nerves from the cervical sympathetic chain innervate the adjoining smooth muscle of the superior tarsal. A lesion of these nerves will cause a mild ptosis that can be overcome on looking up.

Causes: (1) Third-nerve lesions usually causing unilateral complete ptosis. Look for other evidence of third-nerve lesion (ophthalmoplegia with outward deviation of the eye, pupil dilated and unreactive to light, and accommodation). (2) Sympathetic paralysis usually causes unilateral partial ptosis. Look for other evidence of sympathetic lesion (constricted pupil, lack of sweating on same side of the face [Horner's syndrome]). (3) Myopathy (dystrophia myotonica, myasthenia gravis); these usually cause bilateral partial ptosis. (4) Congenital (present since birth); may be unilateral or bilateral, is usually partial and is not associated with other neurological signs. (5) Syphilis.

Pulses (p. 48)

Pupillary abnormalities The key questions are:

• Are the pupils equal, central, circular, dilated, or constricted?
• Do they react to light, directly and consensually?
• Do they constrict normally on convergence/accommodation?

Irregular pupils are caused by iritis, syphilis, or globe rupture. *Dilated pupils Causes:* Third cranial nerve lesions and mydriatic drugs. But always ask: "Is this pupil dilated, or is it the other which is constricted?" *Constricted pupils* are associated with old age, sympathetic nerve damage (Horner's syndrome; and see **Ptosis** [p. 80]), opiates, miotics (e.g., pilocarpine eye-drops for glaucoma), and pontine damage. *Unequal pupils (anisocoria)* may be due to a unilateral lesion, eyedrops, eye surgery, syphilis, or be a Holmes–Adie pupil (below). Some inequality is normal.

Reaction to light: Test by covering one eye and shining light into the other obliquely. Both pupils should constrict (one by the direct, the other by the consensual or indirect light reflex). Lesion site may be deduced by knowing the pathway: From the retina, the message passes up the optic nerve to the superior colliculus (midbrain) and thence to the third-nerve nuclei bilaterally. The third nerve causes pupillary constriction. If a light in one eye causes only contralateral constriction, the defect is "efferent," as the afferent pathways from the retina being stimulated must be intact. Test for a *relative afferent pupillary defect* by moving the light quickly from pupil to pupil. If an eye has severely reduced acuity (e.g., due to optic atrophy), the affected pupil will paradoxically dilate when the light is moved from the normal eye to the abnormal eye. This is because, in the face of reduced afferent input from the affected eye, the consensual pupillary relaxation response from the normal eye predominates. This phenomenon is also known as the *Marcus Gunn sign.*

Reaction to accommodation/convergence: If the patient first looks at a distant object and then at the examiner's finger held a few inches away, the eyes will converge and the pupils constrict. The neural pathway involves a projection from the cortex to the nucleus of the third nerve.

Holmes-Adie (myotonic) pupil: This is a benign condition, which occurs usually in women and is unilateral in about 80% of cases. The affected pupil is normally moderately dilated and is poorly reactive to light, if at all. It is slowly reactive to accommodation; wait and watch carefully: It may eventually constrict more than a normal pupil. It is often associated with diminished or absent ankle and knee reflexes, in which case, the *Holmes-Adie syndrome* is present.

Argyll Robertson pupil: This occurs in neurosyphilis, but a similar phenomenon may occur in diabetes mellitus. The pupil is constricted. It is unreactive to light, but reacts to accommodation. The iris is usually patchily atrophied and depigmented.

Hutchinson pupil: This is the sequence of events resulting from rapidly rising unilateral intracranial pressure (e.g., in intracerebral hemorrhage). The pupil on the side of the lesion first constricts then widely dilates. The other pupil then goes through the same sequence.

Rebound abdominal pain is present if, on the sudden removal of pressure from the examiner's hand, the patient feels a *momentary increase* in pain. It signifies local peritoneal inflammation, manifest as pain as the peritoneum rebounds after being gently displaced.

Rectal bleeding Ascertain details about
• Pain on defecation?
• Is blood mixed with stool, or just on surface?
• Is blood just on toilet paper, or also in the toilet bowl?

Causes and classical features: Diverticulosis (painless, large volumes of blood in bowl), colorectal cancer (blood mixed with stool), hemorrhoids (bright red blood on paper and in bowl), anal fissure (painful, bright red blood on paper and surface of stool), inflammatory bowel disease (blood and mucus mixed with loose stool), trauma, polyps, vascular malformation, ischemic colitis, iatrogenic (radiation proctitis, postpolypectomy bleeding, aortoenteric fistula after aortic surgery).

Regurgitation Gastric and esophageal contents are regurgitated effortlessly into the mouth, without contraction of abdominal muscles and diaphragm (so distinguishing it from true vomiting). Regurgitation is rarely preceded by nausea, and when due to gastroesophageal reflux, it is often associated with heartburn. An esophageal pouch may cause regurgitation. Very high GI obstructions (e.g., gastric volvulus) cause nonproductive retching rather than true regurgitation.

Right iliac fossa pain *Causes:* All causes of left iliac fossa pain (p. 79) plus appendicitis, but usually excluding diverticulitis.

Right upper quadrant pain *Causes:* Gallstones, hepatitis, appendicitis (e.g., if pregnant), colonic cancer at the hepatic flexure, right kidney pathology (e.g., renal colic, pyelonephritis), intrathoracic conditions (e.g., pneumonia), subphrenic or perinephric abscess.

Rigors are uncontrolled, sometimes violent episodes of shivering that occur as a patient's temperature rises quickly from normal. See FUO (p. 542).

Skin discoloration Generalized hyperpigmentation due at least in part to melanin may be genetic, or due to radiation, Addison's (p. 312), chronic renal failure, pregnancy, oral contraceptive pill, any chronic wasting (e.g., TB, carcinoma), malabsorption, biliary cirrhosis, hemochromatosis, or medications such as antipsychotics (chlorpromazine), alkylating agents (busulfan), antibiotics (tetracyclines). Hyperpigmentation due to other causes occurs in jaundice, carotenemia, and gold therapy.

Splenomegaly means an abnormally large spleen. If massive, think of leishmaniasis, malaria, myelofibrosis, chronic myeloid leukemia.

Sputum (p. 155)

Stridor is an inspiratory sound caused by partial obstruction of the upper airways. An obstruction may be due to something within the lumen (e.g., foreign body, tumor, bilateral vocal cord palsy), within the wall (e.g., edema from anaphylaxis, laryngospasm, tumor, croup, acute epiglottitis), or extrinsic (e.g., goiter, lymphadenopathy). It is a medical (or surgical) emergency if the airway is compromised.

Subcutaneous emphysema is a crackling sensation felt on palpating the skin over the chest or neck, caused by air tracking from the lungs (e.g., due to a pneumothorax). It may rarely occur due to a pneumomediastinum (e.g., following esophageal rupture).

Tactile vocal fremitus (p. 56)

Tenesmus is a sensation felt in the rectum of incomplete emptying following defecation, as if there was something else left behind that cannot be passed. It is very common in irritable bowel syndrome but can be caused by a tumor.

Terminal dribbling Dribbling at the end of urination, often seen in conjunction with incontinence following incomplete urination; it is commonly associated with outlet obstruction. See **prostatism** (p. 79).

Tinnitus (p. 357)

Tiredness See **Fatigue** (p. 75)

Tremor is rhythmic oscillation of limbs, trunk, head, or tongue. Three types:

1 *Resting tremor.* Worst at rest; feature of parkinsonism, but the tremor is more resistant to treatment than bradykinesia or rigidity. This is usually a slow tremor (frequency: 3–5 Hz)

2 *Postural tremor.* Made worse with certain positions (e.g., arms outstretched). Typically, a rapid tremor (frequency: 8–12 Hz). May be exaggerated physiological tremor (e.g., anxiety, thyrotoxicosis, alcohol, drugs), metabolic (e.g., hepatic encephalopathy, CO_2 retention), due to brain damage (e.g., Wilson's disease, syphilis), or *benign essential tremor* (BET). This last is usually a familial (autosomal dominant) tremor of arms and head presenting at any age. It is suppressed by alcohol and is rarely progressive. Propranolol (40–80 mg/8–12 h PO) helps ~30%.

3 *Intention tremor.* Made worse with movement; occurs in cerebellar disease (e.g., in MS). No effective drug has been found.

Trousseau's sign is elicited by inflating a BP cuff on an arm/leg to above systolic pressure. The hands and feet go into spasm (carpopedal spasm) in hypocalcemia. The metacarpophalangeal joints become flexed and the interphalangeal joints are extended. See **Chvostek's sign** (p. 72).

83

Urinary changes *Cloudy urine* suggests pus (infection, UTI) but is often normal phosphate precipitation in an alkaline urine. *Pneumaturia* (bubbles in urine as it is passed) occurs with UTI due to gas-forming organisms or may signal an enterovesical (bowel-bladder) fistula from diverticulitis or neoplastic diseases of the gut. *Nocturia* is caused by bladder outlet obstruction (prostate enlargement), uncontrolled diabetes mellitus, UTI, and absorption of peripheral edema. *Hematuria* (red blood cells [RBCs] in urine) is due to neoplasia or glomerulonephritis until proven otherwise.

Visual loss Get ophthalmic help. *If sudden, ask:*

• Is the eye painful/red (glaucoma; iritis)? Optic neuritis may be painful.
• What is each eye's acuity? Is there a contact lens problem (e.g., infection)?
• History of trauma, migraine, TIA, MS, or diabetes; what is the blood sugar?
• Any flashes/floaters (TIA, migraine, retinal artery occlusion, detachment)?
• Is the cornea cloudy (corneal ulcer; glaucoma)?
• Is there a visual field problem/hemianopsia (stroke, space-occupying lesion, glaucoma)? Formal field testing requires ophthalmic help.
• Any heart disease/bruits (emboli)? Hyperlipidemia (xanthoma)?
• Is the BP raised or lowered? Measure it lying and standing.
• Are there focal central nervous system (CNS) signs? Is there an afferent pupillary defect (p. 81)?
• Tender temporal arteries ± ↑ESR points to giant cell arteritis: Urgent steroids (p. 418).
• Any distant signs, such as HIV (causes retinitis), SLE, sarcoid, Behçet's disease, etc.?

Voice and disturbance of speech (p. 66) may be noted by the patient or the doctor. Assess if difficulty is with articulation (dysarthria, e.g., from muscle problems), or of word command (dysphasia; always central).

Vomiting Causes of nausea/vomiting include:

Gastrointestinal	CNS	Metabolic/endocrine
Gastroenteritis	Meningitis/encephalitis	Uremia
Peptic ulceration	Migraine	Hypercalcemia
Pyloric stenosis	↑Intracranial pressure	Hyponatremia
Intestinal obstruction	Brainstem lesions	Pregnancy
Paralytic ileus	Motion sickness	Diabetic ketoacidosis
Acute cholecystitis	Ménière's disease	Addison's disease
Acute pancreatitis	Labyrinthitis	Drugs:
	Psychiatric disorder:	• Alcohol
Other	• Self-induced	• Antibiotics
Myocardial infarction	• Psychogenic	• Cytotoxics
Autonomic neuropathy	• Bulimia nervosa	• Digoxin
UTI		• Opiates

The history is very important: Ask about timing, relationship to meals, amount, and content (liquid, solid, bile, blood, "coffee grounds"). Associated symptoms and previous medical history often indicate the cause. *Signs:* Look for signs of dehydration. Examine the abdomen for distension, tenderness, an abdominal mass, a succussion splash (pyloric stenosis), or tinkling bowel sounds (intestinal obstruction). See Table 4.5 for non-GI causes of vomiting.

Walking difficulty In the elderly, this is a common and nonspecific presentation: The reason may be *local* (typically osteo- or rheumatoid arthritis, but remember fractured neck of femur), *systemic* (e.g., pneumonia, UTI, anemia, drugs, hypothyroidism, renal failure, hypothermia), or even a manifestation of depression or bereavement. *It is only rarely a manipulative strategy.*

More specific causes to consider are Parkinson's disease (p. 382), polymyalgia rheumatica (very treatable, p. 417), and various neuropathies/myopathies. One of the key questions is "Is there pain?" Another issue to address is whether there is muscle wasting and, if so, is it symmetrical?

If there is also ataxia, the cause is not always alcohol: Other chemicals may be involved (cannabis, arsenic, thallium, mercury, or prescribed

---

Table 4.5 Non-GI causes of vomiting

Never forget these, as they can be a sign of serious disease. The following mnemonic covers the most important nongastrointestinal causes of vomiting: **ABCDEFGHI**

• **A**cute renal failure/**A**ddison's disease
• **B**rain (e.g., ↑ICP [p. 722])
• **C**ardiac (myocardial infarct)
• **D**iabetic ketoacidosis
• **E**ars (e.g., labyrinthitis, Ménière's disease)
• **F**oreign substances (alcohol, drugs [e.g., opiates])
• **G**ravidity (e.g., hyperemesis gravidarum)
• **H**ypercalcemia/**H**yponatremia
• **I**nfection (e.g., UTI, meningitis)

sedatives), or there may be a metastatic or nonmetastatic manifestation of malignancy—or a CNS primary or vascular lesion.

Remember also treatable conditions, such as pellagra (p. 245), ↓B12, and beriberi, and infections such as encephalitis, myelitis, Lyme disease, brucellosis, or rarities such as botulism (p. 581).

Bilateral weak legs in an otherwise fit person suggests a cord lesion (p. 333). If there is associated incontinence ± saddle anesthesia, prompt treatment for cord compression may be needed.

Water brash refers to the excessive secretion of saliva, which suddenly fills the mouth. It typically occurs after meals and may denote gastroesophageal reflux disease. It is suggested that this is an exaggeration of the esophagosalivary reflex. It should not be confused with **regurgitation** (p. 209).

Weight loss is a feature of chronic disease and depression and also of malnutrition, chronic infections, and infestations (e.g., TB, HIV/AIDS), malignancy, diabetes mellitus, and hyperthyroidism (typically in the presence of increased appetite). Severe generalized muscle wasting is also seen as part of a number of degenerative neurological and muscle diseases and in cardiac failure (cardiac cachexia), although in the latter, right heart failure may not

---

Table 4.6 Unexplained signs and symptoms: How to refer a patient for an opinion

▶ *When you don't know: Ask.*
▶ *If you find yourself wondering if you should ask: Ask.*

Frequently, you may require the help of a consultant. If so, during ward rounds, agree who should be asked for an opinion. You will be left with the job of making the arrangements. This can be a daunting task, if you are very junior and have been asked to contact an intimidating consultant. Don't be intimidated: Perhaps this may be an opportunity to learn something new. A few simple points can help the process go smoothly.

• Have the patient's notes, observations, and drug charts at hand.
• Be familiar with the history: You may be interrogated.
• Ask if it is a convenient time to talk.
• At the outset, state if you are just looking for advice or if you are asking if the patient could be seen. Make it clear exactly what the question is that you want addressed, "We wonder why Mr. Smith's legs have become weak today…" This helps the listener to focus his or her thoughts while you describe the story and will save you wasting time if the page operator has put you through to the wrong specialist.
• Give the patient's age and occupation, to give a snapshot of the person.
• Run through a brief history. Do not present the case as if you are in formal rounds—it will take ages to get to the point and the listener will get irritated.
• If you would like the patient to be seen, give warning if you know that the patient will be going off the ward for a test at a particular time.
• If you are on the ward when the consultant arrives, offer to introduce him or her to the patient.

We thank Martin Zeidler for providing the first draft of this page.

make weight loss a major complaint. Do not forget anorexia nervosa as a possible underlying cause of weight loss.

Focus on treatable causes (e.g., diabetes is easy to diagnose; TB can be very hard). For example, the CXR may look like cancer, so you may forget to send bronchoscopy samples for acid-fast bacillus (AFB) stain and TB culture (to the detriment not just of the patient, but the entire ward).

Wheeze (p. 57)

Whispered pectoriloquy refers to the increased transmission of a patient's whispers heard when auscultating over consolidated lung. It is a manifestation of increased vocal resonance. (*Vocal resonance* is sound vibration of the patient's spoken or whispered voice transmitted to the stethoscope.) *Tactile fremitus* is the sound vibration of the spoken or whispered voice transmitted via the lung fields and detected by palpation over the back.

Xanthomata are localized deposits of fat under the skin surface, commonly occurring over joints, tendons, hands, and feet. They are a sign of hyperlipidemia (p. 109). *Xanthelasma palpebra* is a xanthoma on the eyelid.

Knowing when to refer a patient for an expert opinion is equally important as making the diagnosis yourself. See Table 4.6 for guidelines.

Cardiovascular medicine

Stuart D. Russell, M.D.

Contents

Cardiovascular health

Maintaining good cardiovascular health is important to all patients. Table 5.1 discusses the most important parameters of heart health.

Table 5.1 Cardiovascular health

Ischemic heart disease (IHD), even though decreasing in incidence, is still the most common cause of death worldwide. Encouraging cardiovascular health is not *only* about preventing IHD. The activities associated with improving cardiovascular health have many beneficial side effects as well. Exercise will improve cardiovascular health (blood pressure [BP]↓, high-density lipoprotein [HDL]↑) but can also prevent osteoporosis, improve glucose tolerance, and promote weight loss. People who improve *and maintain* their fitness live longer: *Age-adjusted mortality from all causes is reduced by >40%.* Avoiding obesity helps too, but there is no evidence that losing weight will lengthen life. However, the risk of diabetes (DM) *will* diminish if weight loss can be achieved.

Smoking is the major modifiable risk factor for cardiovascular mortality. You *can* help people quit, and quitting *does* undo much of the harm of smoking. *Simple advice works.* Most smokers want to give up. Just because smoking advice does not *always* work, do not stop giving it. Ask about smoking during every visit—especially those concerned with smoking-related diseases.

- Ensure advice is congruent with the patient's beliefs about smoking.
- Concentrate on the benefits of giving up.
- Invite the patient to choose a date (when there will be few stressors) on which he or she will become a nonsmoker. You may suggest the birthday of a loved one or an anniversary so that they stop as a "gift."
- Suggest throwing away all accessories (cigarettes, pipes, ashtrays, lighters, matches) in advance; inform friends of the new change; practice saying "no" to their offers of "just one cigarette."
- *Nicotine gum,* chewed intermittently to limit nicotine release: Ten 2 mg sticks may be needed/day. *Transdermal nicotine patches* may be easier. Written advice offers no added benefit to advice from nurses. Always offer follow-up.
- *Bupropion* may improve the success rate in those who want to quit to 30% at 1 yr vs. 16% with patches and 15.6% for placebo (patches + bupropion: 35.5%): Consider if the above fails. *Dose:* 150 mg/d PO (while still smoking; quit within 2 wks); dose may be twice daily from day 7; stop after 7 wks. *Warn of side effects (se):* Seizures (risk <1:1,000), insomnia, headache. Contraindicated (CI) in epilepsy, cirrhosis, pregnancy/lactation, bipolar depression, eating disorders, central nervous system (CNS) tumors, on antimalarials etc., alcohol or benzodiazepine withdrawal.

Lipids and BP (pp. 108, 132) are the other major modifiable risk factors. Nonmodifiable risk factors include sex and family history.

Apply preventive measures such as healthy eating (see p. 203) *early* in life to maximize impact, when there are more years to save and before bad habits get ingrained.

For more on risk factors and their impact, see the American Heart Association *Heart Disease and Stroke Statistics* 2012 update.

Cardiovascular symptoms

Chest pain Cardiac-sounding chest pain may have no serious cause, but always think "Could this be an myocardial infarction (MI), dissecting aortic aneurysm, pericarditis, or pulmonary embolism?"

Nature of pain: Constricting suggests angina, esophageal spasm, or anxiety; a *sharp* pain may be from the pleura or pericardium, especially if exacerbated by inspiration. A prolonged (>0.5 h), dull, central crushing pain or pressure suggests MI. Stabbing, short lasting (<30 sec), or pain in continually varying location is less likely to be cardiac.

Radiation: To shoulder, either or both arms, or neck/jaw suggests cardiac ischemia. The pain of aortic dissection is classically instantaneous, tearing, and interscapular, but may be retrosternal. Epigastric pain may be cardiac.

Precipitants: Pain associated with cold, exercise, palpitations, or emotion suggest cardiac pain or anxiety; if brought on by food, lying flat, hot drinks, or alcohol, consider esophageal spasm (but meals *can* cause angina).

Relieving factors: If pain is relieved *within minutes* by rest or nitroglycerin, suspect angina. Nitroglycerin can relieve esophageal spasm, but usually more slowly. If antacids help, suspect GI causes. Pericarditis pain improves on leaning forward.

Associations: Dyspnea occurs with cardiac pain, pulmonary embolism, pleurisy, or anxiety. MI may cause nausea, vomiting, or sweating. In addition to coronary artery disease, angina may be caused by aortic stenosis (AS), hypertrophic obstructive cardiomyopathy (HOCM), or paroxysmal supraventricular tachycardia (SVT) and be exacerbated by anemia. Chest pain with *tenderness* suggests self-limiting costochondritis (Tietze's syndrome). See Table 5.2 for tips on how to decipher a patient's description of cardiac sensations.

Differential diagnosis of chest pain: Pleuritic pain (i.e., exacerbated by inspiration) implies inflammation of the pleura secondary to pulmonary infection, inflammation, or infarction. The patient may "catch his breath." *Musculoskeletal pain:* Exacerbated by pressure on the affected area. *Fractured rib:* Pain on respiration, exacerbated by gentle pressure on the sternum. *Subdiaphragmatic pathology* may also mimic cardiac pain.

Acutely ill patients:

- Admit to hospital.
- Check pulse, BP in both arms, jugular venous pressure (JVP), heart sounds, and examine the legs for deep vein thrombosis (DVT).
- Give O_2 by face mask.
- Insert an IV line.
- Relieve pain (e.g., morphine 5–10 mg IV slowly + an antiemetic).
- Place on cardiac monitor; do 12-lead electrocardiogram (ECG).
- Obtain chest x-ray (CXR).
- Obtain Arterial blood gas (ABG).

Famous traps: Aortic dissection (a tearing or ripping sensation, often midscapular). Make sure you check all pulses and bilateral BP; herpes zoster (p. 557), ruptured esophagus, cardiac tamponade (shock with JVP↑), opiate addiction.

Dyspnea may be from left ventricular failure (LVF), pulmonary embolism, any respiratory cause, or anxiety. Severity: Emergency presentations. Ask about shortness of breath at rest or on exertion, orthopnea, paroxysmal nocturnal dyspnea (PND), exercise tolerance, and coping with daily tasks. Associations: Specific symptoms associated with heart failure are orthopnea (ask about number of pillows used at night or if sitting in a recliner), paroxysmal nocturnal dyspnea (waking up at night gasping for breath), and peripheral edema. Pulmonary embolism is associated with acute onset of dyspnea and pleuritic chest pain; ask about risk factors for DVT.

Palpitation(s) may be due to premature ventricular contractions, atrial fibrillation (AF), SVT and ventricular tachycardia (VT), thyrotoxicosis, anxiety, and rarely pheochromocytoma. History: Ask about previous episodes, precipitating/relieving factors, duration of symptoms, associated chest pain, dyspnea, or dizziness. *Did the patient check her pulse?*

Syncope may reflect cardiac or CNS events. Vasovagal "faints" are common (pulse↓, pupils dilated). The history from an observer is invaluable in diagnosis. *Prodromal symptoms:* Chest pain, palpitations, or dyspnea point to a cardiac cause (e.g., arrhythmia). Aura, headache, dysarthria, limb weakness indicate CNS causes. *During the episode:* Was there a pulse? Was there limb jerking, tongue biting, or urinary incontinence? **NB**: Hypoxia from lack of cerebral perfusion may cause seizures. *Recovery:* Was this rapid (arrhythmia) or prolonged and associated with postictal drowsiness (seizure)?

Table 5.2 How patients communicate ischemic cardiac sensations

In emergency departments, we are always hearing questions such as "Is your pain sharp or dull?" followed by an equivocal answer. The doctor goes on "Sharp like a knife—or dull and crushing?" The doctor is getting irritated because the patient must know the answer, but is not saying it. Instead of asking the questions that we relate to cardiac chest pain (chest heaviness associated with dyspnea and radiation to the jaw and left arm), allow the patient to tell his story. Patients often avoid using the word "pain" to describe ischemia: "Heaviness," "tightening," "pressure," "burning," or "a lump in the throat" (angina means to choke) may be used. They may say "sharp" to communicate severity and not character. So be as vague in your questioning as your patient is in his answers. "Tell me some more about what you are feeling (long pause)... as if someone was doing *what* to you?" "Sitting on me," or "like a hotness" might be the response (suggesting cardiac ischemia). Do not ask "Does it go into your left arm." Try "Is there anything else about it?" (pause)... "Does it go anywhere?" Note your patient's exact words.

Note also nonverbal clues: The clenched fist placed over the sternum is a telling feature of cardiac pain (Levine sign positive).

A good history, taking account of these features, is the best way to stratify patients likely to have cardiac pain. If the history is nonspecific, there are no risk factors for cardiovascular diseases, and ECG and plasma troponin T (p. 114) are normal (<0.2 mcg/L) 6–12 h after the onset of pain, discharge will probably be OK. But when in doubt, get help.

Features making cardiac pain unlikely:
- Stabbing, shooting pain
- Pain lasting <30 sec, however intense
- Well-localized, left submammary pain ("In my heart, doctor")
- Pains of continually varying location
- Youth

Do not feel that you must diagnose every pain. *Chest pain with no cause* is common. Extensive testing, including cardiac catheterization and ruling out depression, may not find the cause. Do not reject these patients: Explain your findings to them. Some have a "chronic pain syndrome" that responds to a tricyclic (e.g., imipramine 50 mg at night[1]; this dose does not imply any depression). It is similar to postherpetic neuralgia.

1 Cannon RO, Quyyumi AA, Mincemoyer R, *et al.* Imipramine in patients with chest pain despite normal coronary angiograms. *N Engl J Med.* 1994 May 19;330(20):1411–1147.

ECG: A methodical approach

First confirm the patient's name and age, and the ECG date. Then:

- *Rate:* At usual speed (25 mm/sec) each "big square" is 0.2 sec; each "small square" is 0.04 sec. To calculate the rate, divide 300 by the number of big squares per R–R interval (p. 93).
- *Rhythm:* If the cycles are not clearly regular, use the "card method": Lay a card along the ECG, marking positions of three successive R waves. Slide the card to and fro to check that all intervals are equal. If not, note if different rates are multiples of each other (i.e., varying block) or if it is 100% irregular (AF or ventricular fibrillation [VF]). *Sinus rhythm* is characterized by a P wave (upright in II, III, and aVF; inverted in aVR) followed by a QRS complex. AF has no discernible P waves, and the QRS complexes are irregularly irregular. *Atrial flutter* usually has a "sawtooth" baseline of atrial depolarization (~300/min) and regular QRS complexes. *Nodal rhythm* has a normal QRS complex, but P waves are absent or occur just before or within the QRS complex. *Ventricular rhythm* has QRS complexes of >0.12 sec with P waves following them.

Axis: The mean frontal axis is the sum of all the ventricular forces during ventricular depolarization. The axis lies at 90 degrees to the isoelectric complex (i.e., the one in which positive and negative deflections are equal). *Normal axis* is between –30° and +90°. As a simple rule of thumb, if the complexes in leads I and II are both "positive," the axis is normal. *Left axis deviation* (LAD) is –30° to –90°. *Causes:* Left anterior hemiblock, inferior MI, VT from LV focus, Wolff–Parkinson–White (WPW) syndrome (some types). *Right axis deviation* (RAD) is +90° to +180°. *Causes:* Right ventricular hypertrophy (RVH), PE, anterolateral MI, left posterior hemiblock (rare), WPW syndrome (some types).

- *P wave:* Normally precedes each QRS complex. *Absent p wave:* AF, sinoatrial block, junctional (AV nodal) rhythm. Dissociation between P waves and QRS complexes indicates complete heart block. *p mitrale:* Bifid P wave in lead II and biphasic P wave in lead V_1 indicate left atrial hypertrophy. *p pulmonale:* Peaked P wave (>2.5 mm in lead II) indicates right atrial hypertrophy. Pseudo-P-pulmonale is seen in K⁺↓.
- *P-R interval:* Measure from start of P wave to start of QRS. *Normal range:* 0.12–0.2 sec (3–5 small squares). A *prolonged P-R interval* implies delayed atrioventricular (AV) conduction (first-degree heart block). A *short P-R interval* implies unusually fast AV conduction down an accessory pathway (e.g., WPW [ECG, p. 124]). In second-degree block, some P waves aren't followed by a QRS. If the PR interval increases with each cycle until there is a P wave not followed by a QRS, this is Mobitz type I (Wenckebach) AV block. If the PR interval is constant and a P wave is not followed by a QRS, this is Mobitz type II AV block. In third-degree block, the P waves and QRS waves are independent of each other.
- *QRS complex: Normal duration:* <0.12 sec. If ≥0.12 sec, suggests ventricular conduction defects (e.g., a bundle branch block [p. 95]). Large QRS complexes suggest *ventricular hypertrophy* (p. 96). *Normal Q wave* is <0.04 sec wide and <2 mm deep. *Pathological q waves* may occur within a few hours of an acute MI.
- *QT interval:* Measure from start of QRS to *end* of T wave. It varies with rate. Calculate *corrected QT interval (QT^c)* by dividing the measured QT interval by the square root of the cycle length, i.e., $QT^c = (QT)/(\sqrt{R-R})$. Normal QT^c: 0.38–0.43 sec. *Prolonged qt interval:* Acute myocardial ischemia, myocarditis, bradycardia (e.g., AV block), head injury, hypothermia, electrolyte imbalance (K⁺↓, Ca²⁺↓, Mg²⁺↓), congenital (Romano–Ward and Jervell–Lange–Nielson syndromes), sotalol, quinidine, antihistamines, macrolides (e.g., erythromycin), amiodarone, phenothiazines, tricyclics.

- *ST segment:* Usually isoelectric. Planar elevation (>1 mm) or depression (>0.5 mm) usually implies infarction (p. 97) or ischemia (p. 100), respectively.
- *T wave:* Abnormal if inverted in I, II, and V_4–V_6. It is peaked in hyperkalemia (ECG 13 [p. 672]) and flattened in hypokalemia.
- *U wave:* May be prominent in hypokalemia but can also be normal
- *J wave:* Associated with hypothermia

Figure 5.1 ECG nomenclature (ventricular activation time, VAT)

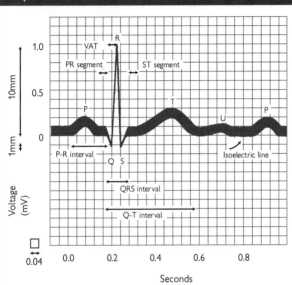

Seconds

Calculating the R–R interval To calculate the rate, divide 300 by the number of big squares per R–R interval if the standard ECG speed of 25 mm/sec is used (elsewhere, 50 mm/sec may be used: Don't be confused!)

R–R duration(s)	Big squares	Rate (per min)
0.2	1	300
0.4	2	150
0.6	3	100
0.8	4	75
1.0	5	60
1.2	6	50
1.4	7	43

Figure 5.2 Determining the ecg axis

- The axis lies at 90° to the isoelectric complex (the one in which positive and negative deflections are equal in size).
- If the complexes in I and II are both predominantly positive, the axis is normal.

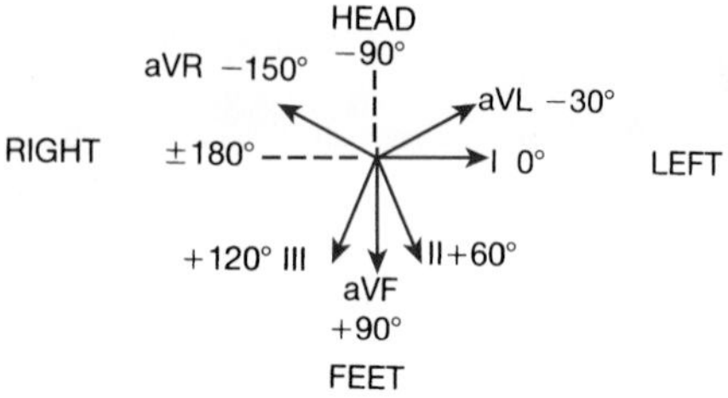

Causes of lad
Left anterior hemiblock
Inferior MI
VT from LV focus
WPW syndrome (some); p. 124
Left ventricular hypertrophy

Causes of rad
RVH
Pulmonary embolism
Anterolateral MI
Left posterior hemiblock (rare)
WPW syndrome (some)

ECG:Abnormalities

Sinus tachycardia: Rate >100. Anxiety, exercise, pain, fever, sepsis, hypovolemia, heart failure, pulmonary embolism, pregnancy, thyrotoxicosis, beriberi, CO_2 retention, autonomic neuropathy, sympathomimetics; e.g., caffeine, adrenaline, and nicotine (may produce abrupt changes in sinus rate, and other arrhythmias).

Sinus bradycardia: Rate <60. Physical fitness, vasovagal attacks, sick sinus syndrome, acute MI (esp. inferior), drugs (β-blockers, digoxin, amiodarone, verapamil), hypothyroidism, hypothermia, intracranial pressure (ICP) ↑, cholestasis.

AF (ECG p. 120): *Common causes:* IHD thyrotoxicosis, hypertension.

First- and second-degree heart block: Normal variant, athletes, sick sinus syndrome, IHD, acute carditis, drugs (digoxin, β-blockers).

Complete heart block: Idiopathic (fibrosis), congenital, IHD, aortic valve calcification, cardiac surgery/trauma, digoxin toxicity, infiltration (abscesses, granulomas, tumors, parasites).

ST elevation: Normal variant (high take-off), acute MI, Prinzmetal's angina, acute pericarditis (saddle-shaped), left ventricular aneurysm.

ST depression: Normal variant (upward sloping), digoxin (downward sloping), ischemic (horizontal): Angina, acute posterior MI.

T inversion: In V_1-V_3: Normal (African Americans and children), right bundle branch block (RBBB), pulmonary embolism. In V_2-V_5: Subendocardial MI, HOCM, subarachnoid hemorrhage, lithium. In V_4-V_6 and *AVL*: Ischemia, left ventricular hypertrophy (LVH), associated with left bundle branch block (LBBB).

NB: ST and T wave changes are often nonspecific, and must be interpreted in the light of the clinical context.

MI (ECG p. 97):

- Within hours, the T wave may become peaked and the ST segment may begin to rise.
- Within 24 h, the T wave inverts as ST segment elevation begins to resolve. ST elevation rarely persists, unless a left ventricular aneurysm develops. T wave inversion may or may not persist.
- Within a few days, pathological Q waves begin to form. Q waves usually persist, but may resolve in 10%.

The leads affected reflect the site of the infarct: Inferior (II, III, a VF), anteroseptal (V_{1-4}), anterolateral (V_{4-6}, I, aVL), posterior (tall R and ST↓ in V_{1-2}).

"Non-Q wave infarcts" (formerly called subendocardial infarcts) may have ST and T changes without Q waves.

Pulmonary embolism: Sinus tachycardia is most common. There may be RAD, RBBB (p. 97), right ventricular strain pattern V_{1-3}, or AF. Rarely, the classic "$S_I Q_{III} T_{III}$" pattern occurs: Deep S waves in I, pathological Q waves in III, inverted T waves in III.

Metabolic abnormalities: Digoxin effect: ST depression and inverted T wave in V_{5-6}. In *digoxin toxicity,* any arrhythmia may occur (ventricular ectopy and nodal bradycardia are common). *Hyperkalemia:* Tall, tented T wave, widened QRS, absent P waves, "sine wave" appearance (ECG 13, p. 672). *Hypokalemia:* Small T waves, prominent U waves. *Hypercalcemia:* Short QT interval. *Hypocalcemia:* Long QT interval, small T waves.

95

ECG: Additional points

Figure 5.3 Where to place the chest leads

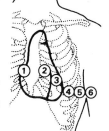

V_1: Right sternal edge, fourth intercostal space
V_2: Left sternal edge, fourth intercostal space
V_3: Half-way between V_2 and V_4
V_4: The patient's apex beat
All subsequent leads are in the same horizontal plane as V_4
V_5: Anterior axillary line
V_6: Mid-axillary line (V_7: Posterior axillary line)
Finish 12-lead ECGs with a long rhythm strip in lead II.

Disorders of ventricular conduction

Bundle branch block (see ECGs 1 and 2) Delayed conduction is evidenced by prolongation of QRS >0.12 sec. Abnormal conduction patterns lasting <0.12 sec are incomplete blocks. The area that would have been reached by the blocked bundle depolarizes slowly and late. Taking V_1 as an example, right ventricular depolarization is normally +ve and left ventricular depolarization is normally −ve.

In RBBB, the following pattern is seen: QRS >0.12 sec, "RSR" pattern in V_1, dominant R in V_1, inverted T waves in V_1–V_3 or V_4, deep wide S wave in V_6. *Causes:* Normal variant (isolated RBBB), pulmonary embolism, cor pulmonale.

In LBBB, the following pattern is seen: QRS >0.12 sec, "M" pattern in V_5, no septal Q waves, inverted T waves in I, aVL, V_5–V_6. *Causes:* IHD, hypertension, cardio-myopathy, idiopathic fibrosis. **NB:** If there is LBBB, no comment can be made on the ST segment or T wave.

Bifascicular block is the combination of RBBB and left bundle hemi-block, manifest as an axis deviation (e.g., LAD in the case of left anterior hemiblock).

Trifascicular block is the combination of bifascicular block and first-degree heart block.

Ventricular hypertrophy There is no single marker of ventricular hypertrophy: Electrical axis, voltage, and ST wave changes should all be taken into consideration. Relying on a single marker such as voltage may be unreliable as a thin chest wall may result in large voltage, whereas a thick chest wall may mask it.

Suspect *LVH* if the R wave in V_6 >25 mm or the sum of the S wave in V_1 and the R wave in V_6 is >35 mm (ECG 8, p. 136).

Suspect *RVH* if dominant R wave in V_1, T wave inversion in V_1–V_3 or V_4, deep S wave in V_6, RAD.

Other causes of *dominant r wave in V1*: RBBB, posterior MI, some types of WPW syndrome (p. 124).

Causes of low-voltage QRS complex: QRS <5 mm in all limb leads. Hypothyroidism, chronic obstructive pulmonary disease (COPD), hematocrit↑ (intra-cardiac blood resistivity is related to hematocrit), changes in chest wall impedance (e.g., in renal failure, subcutaneous emphysema but *not* obesity), pulmonary embolism, bundle branch block, carcinoid heart disease, myocarditis, cardiac amyloid, Adriamycin cardiotoxicity, and other heart muscle diseases, pericardial effusion, pericarditis.

Figure 5.4   ECG 1: Left bundle branch block. Note the W pattern in V_1 and the M pattern in V_6

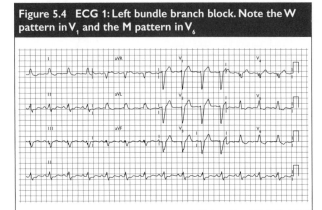

Figure 5.5 ECG 2: Right bundle branch block. Note the M pattern in V_1 and the W pattern in V_5

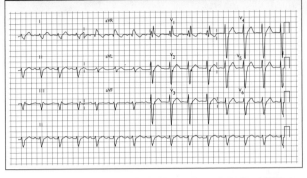

Figure 5.6 ECG 3: Acute inferolateral myocardial infarction. Note the marked ST elevation in the inferior leads (II, III, aVF), but also in V_5 and V_6, indicating lateral involvement as well. There is also "reciprocal change"; i.e., ST-segment depression in leads I and aVL. The latter is often seen with a large myocardial infarction.

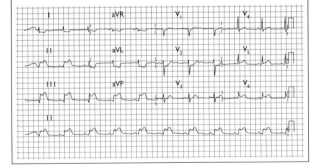

Figure 5.7 ECG 4: Acute anterior myocardial infarction. Note the marked ST segment elevation and evolving Q waves in leads V_1–V_4.

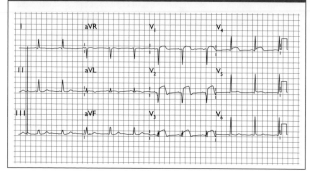

Figure 5.8 ECG 5: Complete heart block. Note the dissociation between the P waves and the QRS complexes. QRS complexes are relatively narrow, indicating that there is a ventricular rhythm originating from the conducting pathway.

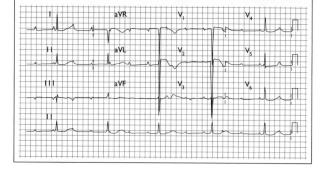

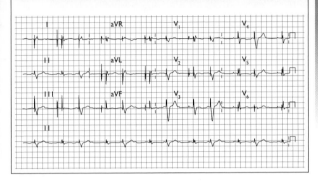

Figure 5.9 ECG 6: Ventricular tachycardia. Note the broad complexes.

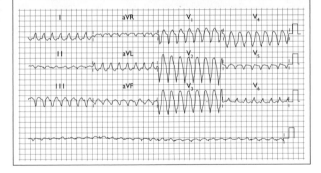

Figure 5.10 ECG 7: Dual-chamber pacemaker. Note the pacing spikes that occur before some of the P waves, and the QRS complexes.

Exercise ECG testing

The patient undergoes a graduated treadmill exercise test with continuous 12-lead ECG and BP monitoring. There are numerous treadmill protocols; the "Bruce protocol" is the most widely used.

Indications:

- To help confirm a suspected diagnosis of IHD
- To assess cardiac function and exercise tolerance
- To develop prognosis following MI; often done predischarge (if +ve, worse outcome)

- To evaluate response to treatment (drugs, angioplasty, coronary artery bypass grafting [CABG])
- To assess exercise-induced arrhythmias

Contraindications:

- Unstable angina
- Recent Q wave MI (<5 d)
- Severe AS
- Uncontrolled arrhythmia, hypertension (systemic or pulmonary), or heart failure

Be cautious about arranging tests that will be hard to perform or interpret. These patients should have some type of imaging in addition to a stress test:

- Complete heart block, LBBB
- Pacemaker patients
- Osteoarthritis, COPD, stroke, or other limitations to exercise

Stop the test if:

- Chest pain or dyspnea occurs. You want to make sure that the patient has a maximal test and would consider not stopping for minor chest pain without ECG changes.
- The patient feels faint, exhausted, or is in danger of falling.
- ST segment elevation/depression >2 mm is present(with or without chest pain).
- Atrial or ventricular arrhythmia (not just ectopy) is present.
- Fall in BP or excessive rise in BP (systolic >230 mm Hg)occurs.
- AV block or LBBB develops.
- Maximal or 90% maximal heart rate for age is achieved.

Interpreting the test: A +ve test only allows one to assess the *probability* that the patient has IHD. 75% of patients with significant coronary artery disease have a +ve test, but so do 5% of people with normal arteries (the false-positive rate is even higher in middle-aged women, e.g., 20%). The more +ve the result, the higher the predictive accuracy. Down-sloping ST depression is much more significant than up-sloping; e.g., 1 mm J-point depression with down-sloping ST segment is 99% predictive of 2–3 vessel disease.

Morbidity: 24 in 100,000. *Mortality:* 10 in 100,000.

Ambulatory ECG monitoring

Continuous ECG monitoring for 24 h may be used to evaluate for paroxysmal arrhythmias. However, >70% of patients will not have symptoms during the period of monitoring. ~20% will have a normal ECG during symptoms and only up to 10% will have an arrhythmia coinciding with symptoms. Give these patients an event recorder they can activate themselves during a symptomatic episode. These episodes can then be transmitted via a telephone for evaluation. Recorders may also be programmed to detect ST segment depression, either symptomatic (to prove angina), or to reveal "silent" ischemia (predictive of reinfarction or death soon after MI).

Figure 5.11

(a)

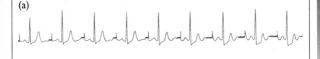

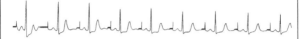

Each complex is taken from sample ECGs (lead V_5) recorded at 1-min intervals during exercise (*top line*) and recovery (*bottom line*). At maximum ST depression, the ST segment is almost horizontal. This is a positive exercise test.

(b)

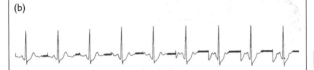

This is an exercise ECG in the same format. It is negative because although the J point is depressed, the ensuing ST segment is steeply up sloping.

Cardiac catheterization

This involves the insertion of a catheter into the heart via the femoral (or radial/brachial) artery or vein. The catheter is manipulated within the heart and great vessels to measure pressures. (See Tables 5.3 and 5.4.) Catheterization can also be used to:

• Sample blood to assess oxygen saturation
• Inject radiopaque contrast medium to image the anatomy of the heart and flow in blood vessels
• Perform angioplasty (± stenting), valvuloplasty, and cardiac biopsies
• Perform intravascular ultrasound to quantify arterial narrowing

During the procedure, ECG and arterial pressures are monitored continuously.

Indications:

• *Coronary artery disease:* Diagnostic (assessment of coronary vessels and graft patency); therapeutic (angioplasty, stent insertion)
• *Valve disease:* Diagnostic (to assess severity); therapeutic valvuloplasty
• *Congenital heart disease:* Diagnostic (assessment of severity of lesions); therapeutic (balloon dilatation or septostomy)
• *Other:* Cardiomyopathy; pericardial disease; endomyocardial biopsy

Preprocedure checks:

- Brief history/examination (**NB:** Peripheral pulses, bruits, aneurysms)
- Investigations: Electrolytes, blood urea nitrogen (BUN)/creatinine, CBC, prothrombin time (PT)/partial thromboplastin time (PTT), type and screen, ECG
- Obtain consent for angiogram ± angioplasty ± stent depending on the indication of the procedure; explain reason for procedure and possible complications (below).
- Obtain IV access.
- Patient should be nothing by mouth (NPO) for at least 6 h before the procedure.
- Patients should take all their morning drugs (and premedication if needed). Withhold oral hypoglycemics and only give half dose of insulin.

Postprocedure checks:

- Pulse, BP, arterial puncture site (for bruising or swelling; false aneurysm), peripheral pulses
- Investigations: CBC and PT/PTT (if suspected blood loss), ECG

Complications:

- *Hemorrhage.* Apply firm pressure for a long period of time (>10 min) over puncture site. If you suspect a false aneurysm, diagnostic ultrasound is required. Some require ultrasound-guided or surgical repair.
- *Contrast reaction.* This is usually mild with modern contrast agents.
- *Loss of peripheral pulse.* May be due to dissection, thrombosis, distal embolus, or arterial spasm; occurs in <1% of brachial catheterizations, rare with femoral catheterization.
- *Angina.* May occur during or after cardiac catheterization; usually responds to sublingual nitroglycerin (NTG); if not, give analgesia and IV nitrates.
- *Arrhythmias.* Usually transient; manage along standard lines and remove all catheters from the heart.
- *Pericardial tamponade.* Rare, but should be suspected if the patient becomes hypotensive and/or anuric.
- *Infection.* Postcatheter fever is usually due to a contrast reaction. If it persists for >24 h, take blood cultures before giving antibiotics.

Mortality: <1 in 1,000 patients, in most centers.

Intracardiac electrophysiology This catheter technique can determine types and origins of arrhythmias and locate (and ablate) aberrant pathways (e.g., causing atrial flutter or VT). Arrhythmias may be induced and the effectiveness of control by drugs assessed.

Table 5.3 Normal values for intracardiac pressures and saturations

Location	Pressure (mm Hg) Mean	Range	Saturation (%)
Inferior vena cava			76
Superior vena cava			70
Right atrium	4	0–8	74
Right ventricle			74
Systolic	25	15–30	
End-diastolic	4	0–8	
Pulmonary artery			74
Systolic	25	15–30	
Diastolic	10	5–15	
Mean	15	10–20	
Pulmonary artery	a	3–12	74
Wedge pressure	v	3–15	
Left ventricle			
Systolic	110	80–140	98
End-diastolic	8	5–12	
Aorta			
Systolic	110	80–140	98
Diastolic	70	60–90	
Mean	85	70–105	
Brachial			
Systolic	120	90–140	98
Diastolic	72	60–90	
Mean	83	70–105	

Table 5.4 Gradients across stenotic valves

Valve	Normal gradient (mm Hg)	Stenotic gradient (mm Hg) Mild	Moderate	Severe
Aortic	0	<30	30–50	>50
Mitral	0	<5	5–15	>15
Prosthetic	5–10			

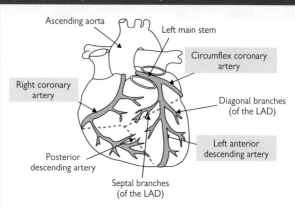

Figure 5.12 Diagram of coronary circulation

Ascending aorta

Left main stem

Circumflex coronary artery

Right coronary artery

Diagonal branches (of the LAD)

Posterior descending artery

Left anterior descending artery

Septal branches (of the LAD)

Reproduced from Myerson SG, Choudhury RP, Mitchell ARJ (eds.). *Emergencies in Cardiology*. New York: Oxford University Press, 2006. By permission of the publisher.

Echocardiography

This noninvasive technique uses the differing ability of various structures within the heart to reflect ultrasound waves. It not only demonstrates anatomy but also provides a continuous display of the functioning heart throughout its cycle. There are various types of scans:

M-mode (motion mode): Scans are displayed to produce a permanent single-dimension (time) image.

Two-dimensional (real-time): A 2-D, fan-shaped image of a segment of the heart is produced on the screen, which may be "frozen" and hard-copied. Several views are possible; the four most common are: Long axis, short axis, four-chamber, and subcostal. 2-D echocardiography is good for visualizing ventricular function, congenital heart disease, LV aneurysm, mural thrombus, left atrial (LA) myxoma, and septal defects.

Doppler and color-flow echocardiography: Different colored jets illustrate flow and gradients across valves and septal defects (p. 148).

Transesophageal echocardiography (tee) can be more sensitive than transthoracic echocardiography (TTE) because the transducer is nearer to the heart and the images are not limited by lung or fat interference. Indications: Diagnosis of aortic dissections; assessment of prosthetic valves; finding of cardiac source of emboli and endocarditis. Contraindicated in esophageal disease or cervical spine instability.

Stress echocardiography: Used to evaluate ventricular function, ejection fraction, myocardial thickening, and regional wall motion pre- and postexercise. Dobutamine may be used if the patient cannot exercise. Inexpensive and as sensitive and specific as a thallium scan (p. 107).

Uses of echocardiography

Quantification of global rv and lv function: Echo is useful for detecting focal and global wall motion abnormalities, LV aneurysm, mural thrombus, and LVH (echo is 5–10 times more sensitive than the ECG in detecting this). The size of the ventricle can also be assessed.

Estimating right-heart hemodynamics: Doppler studies of pulmonary artery flow allow evaluation of RV function and pressures.

Valve disease: Measurement of pressure gradients and valve orifice areas in stenotic lesions. Detecting valvular regurgitation. Evaluating function of prosthetic valves is another role.

Congenital heart disease: Establishing the presence of lesions and determining their functional significance.

Endocarditis: Vegetations may not be seen if <2 mm in size. TTE with color Doppler is best for aortic regurgitation (AR). TTE is useful for visualizing mitral valve vegetations, leaflet perforation, or looking for an aortic root abscess.

Pericardial effusion is best diagnosed by echo. Fluid may first accumulate between the posterior pericardium and the left ventricle, then anterior to both ventricles and anterior and lateral to the right atrium. There may be paradoxical septal motion.

HOCM (p. 144): Echo features include asymmetrical septal hypertrophy, small LV cavity, dilated left atrium, and systolic anterior motion of the mitral valve.

Figure 5.13

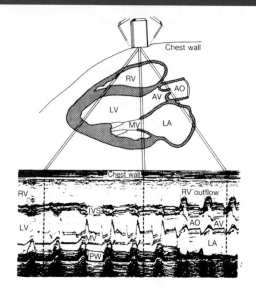

Chest wall

RV
AO
AV
LV
MV
LA

Chest wall

RV
RV outflow
IVS
LV
AO   AV
MV
LA
PW

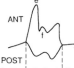

e
ANT
f

POST
1. Normal mitral valve

CLOSED | OPEN | CLOSED

2. Mitral stenosis
• reduced e–f slope

3. Aortic regurgitation
• fluttering of ant. leaflet

a

b

4. (a) Systolic anterior leaflet movement (SAM) in HOCM
   (b) Mitral valve prolapse (late systole)

Normal M-mode echocardiogram (RV, right ventricle; LV, left ventricle; AO, aorta; AV, aortic valve; LA, left atrium; MV, mitral valve; PW, posterior wall of LV; IVS, interventricular septum). After Hall R. *Med International* **17** 774.

Nuclear cardiology and other cardiac scans

Myocardial perfusion imaging

A noninvasive method of assessing regional myocardial blood flow and the cellular integrity of myocytes. The technique uses radionuclide tracers, which cross the myocyte membrane and are trapped intracellularly.

Thallium-201, a K^+ analog, is the most widely used agent. It is distributed via regional myocardial blood flow and requires cellular integrity for uptake. Newer *technetium-99*-based agents are similar to thallium-201 but have improved imaging characteristics and can also be used to assess myocardial perfusion and LV performance in the same study.

Myocardial territories supplied by unobstructed coronary vessels have normal perfusion, whereas regions supplied by stenosed coronary vessels have poorer relative perfusion, a difference that is accentuated by exercise. For this reason, exercise tests are used in conjunction with radionuclide imaging to identify areas at risk of ischemia/infarction. Exercise scans are compared with resting views. *Reperfusion* (ischemia) or *fixed defects* (infarct) can be seen, and the coronary artery involved is reliably predicted. Drugs (e.g., adenosine and dipyridamole) can also be used to induce perfusion differences between normal and underperfused tissues in patients who can't exercise.

Myocardial perfusion imaging has also been used in patients presenting with acute MI (to determine the amount of myocardium salvaged by thrombolysis) and in diagnosing acute chest pain in those without classical ECG changes (to define the presence of significant perfusion defects).

Positron emission tomography (PET)

Severely underperfused tissues, such as those supplied by a critically stenotic coronary artery, switch from fatty acid metabolism to glycolytic metabolism. Such altered cellular biochemistry may be imaged by PET using ^{18}F-labelled deoxyglucose (FDG), which identifies glycolytically active tissue that is viable. This phenomenon, called *hibernating myocardium*, occurs in up to 40% of fixed defects seen on thallium-201 scans.

Computed tomography (CT) allows only limited assessment of cardiac structures. It can help evaluate cardiac disease (e.g., constrictive pericarditis). CT is also part of first-line assessment for abnormalities of the ascending and descending aorta, especially in aortic dissection, and for detecting pulmonary emboli. Ultra-fast CT is now shown to reliably evaluate for lesions of coronary arteries and assist with evaluating congenital anomalies.

Magnetic resonance imaging (MRI) is used in assessing congenital heart disease, infiltrating disease of the myocardium, intracardiac structures, and the great vessels. Its advantages over CT are the lack of exposure to radiation, the wide field of view and high-image resolution, the ability to orient images in multiple planes, and the ability to gate or trigger the MRI scanner, according to the cardiac cycle, thus allowing stop-frame imaging of the heart and great vessels. Spin-echo MRI has a high sensitivity for detecting false lumina and intra-mural flaps in aortic dissection compared with CT. Its main limitation, compared with TEE (p. 105) and CT, is its inability to image significantly unstable patients. Additionally, significant artifact occurs in patients who have implantable devices, and some patients' devices will be altered by the magnet.

New uses of MRI include myocardial phosphorus-31 NMR spectroscopy (^{31}P-NMR), which may demonstrate ischemia in the not-uncommon problem of women with chest pain but normal coronary angiograms. ("Syndrome X" denotes this type of uncertain chest pain.) ^{31}P-NMR may suggest abnormal dilator responses of the microvasculature to stress.

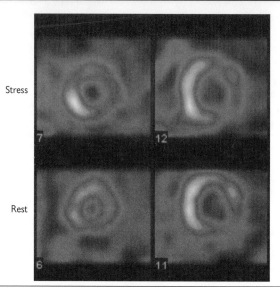

Figure 5.14 Technetium perfusion scan showing perfusion defect in the left ventricle anterior and lateral walls at stress which is reversible (difference between stress and rest images).

Stress

Rest

Hyperlipidemia

Cholesterol is a major risk factor for coronary heart disease (CHD) and, due to the efficacy of current medications, is very treatable. The decision to treat hypercholesterolemia should be based on multiple factors. The Adult Treatment Panel III (ATP III) has established clinical guidelines for cholesterol testing and management (http://www.nhlbi.nih.gov/guidelines/cholesterol/atp3_rpt.htm). See Table 5.5 for a list of primary hyperlipidemias.

- First, determine if the patient has CHD or its equivalent (DM, symptomatic carotid artery disease, peripheral vascular disease, or an abdominal aortic aneurysm).
- Second, determine if the patient has other risk factors for CHD (smoking, BP↑, family history, HDL <40 mg/dL, or age: Male >45, female >55).
- Third, decide to treat based on LDL level and their risk for CHD using the Framingham risk calculator (http://hin.nhlbi.nih.gov/atpiii/calculator.asp?usertype=prof).

Trial evidence that treating hypercholesterolemia is worthwhile

- *"4S" study.* Secondary prevention trial (patients with IHD) using simvastatin ≥20 mg/d PO in 4,444 men aged 35–70 (cholesterol 212–309 mg/dL). Number needed to treat (NNT) to prevent 1 fatal MI was 25 (over 6 yrs) and 14 for nonfatal events.

- *WOSCOPS.* Primary prevention trial in Scotland with more than 6,500 men (cholesterol >155 mg/dL), pravastatin 40 mg/24 h PO. NNT to prevent 1 fatal MI was 142 (over 5 yrs) and for all cardiac events was 55.
- *CARE study.* Secondary prevention trial with pravastatin 40 mg/24 h PO in 4,159 people, post-MI, with "normal" cholesterol (average 209 mg/dL). NNT for fatalities was 91 (over 5 yrs), and for nonfatal MI was 38.
- *HEART PROTECTION STUDY.* Secondary prevention trial with 40 mg simvastatin to patients irrespective of cholesterol. NNT for death was 55. No evidence of "threshold of cholesterol" for benefit. 33% of the patients had an LDL <113 mg/dL and still demonstrated reduction in mortality and cardiovascular events.

Who to screen

- CHD or elevated risk (e.g., DM, BP↑)
- Family history of hyperlipidemia or CHD before 65 yrs
- Xanthoma or xanthelasma
- Corneal arcus before 50 yrs old

Management

- Exclude familial or second-degree hyperlipidemias; treat as appropriate.
- Lifestyle advice. Aim for BMI of 20–25. Diet with <10% of calories from saturated fats and plenty of fiber. Exercise.
- Treat those with known CHD.
- If *0 or 1 risk factors*, treat at LDL >160. If ≥2 risk factors and MI risk <20%, treat at LDL >130 mg/dL. If CHD or >20% MI risk, treat at LDL >100 mg/dL.
- Statins are first choice; they decrease cholesterol synthesis in the liver (e.g., simvastatin 10–40 mg PO at night). CI: Porphyria, LFT↑. se: Myositis (stop if CK↑ by ≥10-fold. If any muscle aches, check CK; risk is 1/100,000 treatment yrs); abdominal pain; LFT↑ (stop if AST ≥100U/L).
- Second-line therapy: Fibrates, such as bezafibrate (useful in familial mixed hyperlipidemias); cholesterol absorption inhibitors of ezetimibe (useful in combination with a statin to enhance cholesterol reduction); anion exchange resins, such as cholestyramine; and nicotinic acid (HDL↑; LDL↓; SE: Severe flushes; aspirin 325 mg half-hour pre-dose helps this).
- Hypertriglyceridemia responds best to fibrates, nicotinic acid, or fish oil.

Familial or primary hyperlipidemias Increased risk of CHD. Lipids travel in blood packaged with proteins as lipoproteins. There are four classes: Chylomicrons (mainly triglyceride); LDL (mainly cholesterol, the lipid correlating most strongly with CHD); very-low-density lipoprotein (VLDL; mainly triglyceride); HDL (mainly phospholipid, correlating *inversely* with CHD). See Table 5.5.

Secondary hyperlipidemias A result of DM, alcohol abuse, T4↓; renal failure, nephrosis, and cholestasis.

Xanthomata These yellowish lipid deposits may be eruptive (itchy nodules in crops in hypertriglyceridemia), tuberous (yellow plaques on elbows and knees), planar (also called palmar; orange-colored streaks in palmar creases that are virtually diagnostic of remnant hyperlipidemia), or deposits in tendons, eyelids (xanthelasmata), or cornea (arcus).

Table 5.5 Primary hyperlipidemias

	Chol = plasma cholesterol (mg/dL)	Lipoprotein	
Familial hyperchylomicronemia (lipoprotein lipase deficiency or apoCII deficiency)[I]	Chol <250, Trig 900–1,300 Chylomicrons	↑	Eruptive xanthomata, lipemia retinalis, hepatosplenomegaly (HSM)
Familial hypercholesterolemia[ii] (LDL receptor defects)	Chol 300–600 Trig <200	LDL↑	Tendon xanthoma, corneal arcus, xanthelasma
Familial defective apoprotein B-100[IIa]	Chol 300–600 Trig <200	LDL↑	Tendon xanthoma, arcus, xanthelasma
Polygenic hyper-cholesterolemia[IIa]	Chol >300 Trig <200	LDL↑	*The most common 1°lipidemia* xanthelasma; corneal arcus
Familial combined hyperlipidemia[IIb, IV or V]	Chol 250–400 Trig 200–1,000	LDL↑, VLDL↑ HDL↑	*Next most common 1°lipidemia* xanthelasma; arcus
Dysbetalipoproteine-mia (remnant particle disease)[III]	Chol 350–550 Trig 800–1,200	IDL↑+HDL↓ LDL↓	Palmar striae; tubero-eruptive xanthoma
Familial hypertriglyceridemia[IV]	Chol 290–450 Trig 250–550	VLDL↑	
Type V hyperlipoproteinemia	Trig 850–2,500; chylomicrons		Eruptive xanthoma; lipemia retinalis; HSM

1° HDL abnormalities:
Hyperalphalipoproteinemia: HDL↑ chol >80
Hypoalphalipoproteinemia (Tangier's disease): HDL↓ chol <35

1° Primary LDL abnormalities:
Abetalipoproteinemia: Trig <30, Chol <50, missing LDL, VLDL and chylomicrons, and fat malabsorption, retinopathy, and acanthocytosis
Hypobetalipoproteinemia: Chol <60, LDL↓, HDL↓; longevity↑

Trig = plasma triglyceride (mg/dL); Chol = plasma cholesterol (mg/dL); colored numerals = **WHO** phenotype

Atherosclerosis and statins

Think of atheroma as the slow accumulation of snow on a mountain. Nothing much happens until one day an avalanche devastates the community below. The snow is lipid and lipid-laden macrophages; the mountain is an arterial wall; the avalanche is plaque rupture; and the community below is, all too often, myocardium or CNS neurons. The devastation is infarction. In assessing risk of thrombi, remember Rudolph Virchow's (1821–1902) triad of *changes in the vessel wall, changes in blood flow,* and *changes to the blood constituents.*

Plaque biology Atheroma is the result of cycles of vascular wall injury and repair, leading to the accumulation of T lymphocytes, which produce growth factors, cytokines, and chemoattractants. LDL gains access by a process called *transcytosis,* where it undergoes modification by macrophage-derived oxidative free radicals—a process enhanced by smoking tobacco and hypertension. Rupture of atheromatous plaque triggers most acute coronary events. These plaques have a core of lipid-laden macrophages and a fibrous cap. Many factors predispose to plaque formation; e.g., genetics, sex (σ), BP, smoking, and DM. Plaques are not static. They can regress or accumulate, or become inflamed (e.g., in unstable angina). The balance between LDL efflux and influx is alterable (e.g., by diet or antilipid drugs). Neither is the vessel wall a nonparticipatory audience to these great events. A sclerotic arterial wall comprises areas of chronic inflammation, with monocytes, macrophages, and T lymphocytes—with smooth muscle proliferation and elaboration of extracellular matrix. These macrophages make cholesterol and also produce enzymes (e.g., interstitial collagenase, gelatinase, and stromelysin), which have been implicated in digesting the plaque cap. The thinner the cap, and the fewer smooth muscle cells involved, the more unstable the plaque and the more likely it is to rupture. Endothelial cells also release a number of anti- and proatherogenic molecules, including nitric oxide and endothelin-1. Normal endothelial function is lost early in the process of atherosclerosis with a shift to the production of proatherogenic molecules.

After plaque rupture, what happens to fibrinogen and passing platelets partly determines the extent of the impending catastrophe. Hypercholesterolemia (if present) is associated with hypercoagulable blood and enhanced platelet reactivity at sites of vascular damage.

Disease prevention What can we do about plaques? First, try to prevent them: Eat a healthy diet (p. 203), encourage *some* exercise, discourage smoking; treat high BP and DM. Once a plaque is there, it can be bypassed, ablated (physically removed or compressed), or stented (with a metal stent). Angioplasty splits the plaque, causing an injury response: Elastic recoil → thrombus formation → inflammation → smooth muscle proliferation → arterial remodeling. An alternative to this drastic change is to give a statin, even if the cholesterol is "normal" since the whole process described above is favorably influenced by statins. Statins inhibit the enzyme HMG-COA reductase, which is responsible for the *de novo* synthesis of cholesterol in the liver. This leads to an increase in LDL receptor expression by hepatocytes and, ultimately, reduced circulating LDL cholesterol. In the past, reducing LDL to <100 was the goal but recent data suggest that even lower levels may be beneficial. Besides this, statins have other favorable effects:

- Thrombotic state↓
- Suppress inflammation (c-reactive protein [CRP]↓)
- Plaque stabilization
- Restoration of normal endothelial function
- Reduction in cholesterol synthesis by within-vessel macrophages
- Reduction of within-vessel macrophage proliferation and migration

Other cardiovascular drugs

Antiplatelet drugs Aspirin irreversibly acetylates cyclo-oxygenase, preventing production of thromboxane A$_2$, thereby inhibiting platelet aggregation. It is commonly used in low doses (e.g., 81 mg) for secondary prevention following MI, transient ischemic attack (TIA)/stroke, and for patients with angina or peripheral vascular disease. May have a role in primary prevention. ADP receptor antagonists (e.g., clopidogrel) also block platelet aggregation, but may cause less gastric irritation. They have a role in patients intolerant of aspirin and in post-coronary stent insertion.

β-blockers Block β-adrenoceptors, thus antagonizing the sympathetic nervous system. Blocking β$_1$-receptors is negatively inotropic and chronotropic and delays AV conduction, and blocking β$_2$-receptors induces peripheral vasoconstriction and bronchoconstriction. Drugs vary in their β$_1$/β$_2$ selectivity (e.g., propranolol is nonselective, and bisoprolol relatively β$_1$ selective), but this does not seem to alter their clinical efficacy. *Uses:* Angina, hypertension, antidysrhythmic, post MI (mortality↓), heart failure (with caution). *CI:* Asthma/COPD, heart block. Caution: Peripheral vascular disease, heart failure, DM. *SE:* Lethargy, impotence, *depression*, nightmares, headache.

Diuretics Loop diuretics (e.g., *furosemide*) used in heart failure and hypertension to inhibit the Na/K/2Cl co-transporter. Thiazides are used in hypertension to inhibit Na/Cl co-transporter. *SE: Loop* dehydration, K$^+$↓, Ca^{2+}↓, ototoxic; *thiazides:* K$^+$↓, Ca^{2+}↑, Mg^{2+}↓,urate↑ (+/− gout), impotence.

Vasodilators are used in heart failure, IHD, and hypertension. Nitrates preferentially dilate veins and the large arteries, reducing filling pressure (preload), while hydralazine primarily dilates the resistance vessels thus lowering BP (afterload). Prazosin (an α-blocker) dilates arteries and veins.

Calcium antagonists These reduce cell entry of Ca^{2+} via voltage-sensitive channels on smooth muscle cells, thereby promoting coronary and peripheral vasodilatation and reducing myocardial oxygen consumption.

Pharmacology: Effects of specific Ca^{2+} antagonists vary because they have different effects on the L-Ca^{2+}-type channels. The *dihydropyridines* (e.g., nifedipine and amlodipine) are mainly peripheral vasodilators (they also dilate coronary arteries) and can cause a reflex tachycardia, so are often used with a β-blocker. They are used mainly in hypertension and angina. Verapamil and diltiazem (*nondihydropyridines*) also slow conduction at the atrioventricular and sinoatrial nodes and may be used to treat hypertension, angina, and dysrhythmias. Don't give verapamil with β-blockers (risk of bradycardia ± LVF). *SE:* Flushes, headache, edema (diuretic unresponsive), LV↓ function, gingival hypertrophy. *CI:* Heart block.

Digoxin Blocks the Na$^+$/K$^+$ pump. It is used to slow the pulse in fast AF (p. 123; aim for <100). As it is a weak +ve inotrope, its role in heart failure in sinus rhythm may be best reserved if the patient is symptomatic despite optimal ACE-inhibitor and β-blocker therapy. For HF there is no benefit with mortality (but admissions for worsening CHF are decreased by ~25%). Elderly people and people with renal insufficiency are at increased risk of toxicity: Use lower doses. Check plasma levels >6 h post-dose. *Typical dose:* 0.25 mg/d, 0.125 mg (or renal function↓). Toxicity risk is increased if K$^+$↓, Mg^{2+}↓, or Ca^{2+}↑. t½ approximately 36 h. If on digoxin, use less energy in cardioversion (start with 5J). *SE:* Any arrhythmia (supraventricular tachycardia SVT with AV block is suggestive), nausea, reduced appetite, yellow vision, confusion, gynecomastia. In toxicity, stop digoxin, check K$^+$, treat arrhythmias, consider Digibind® by IVI (p. 789). *CI:* HOCM, WPW syndrome (p. 124).

ACE-inhibitors (p. 131), **nitrates** (p. 117), **antihypertensives** (p. 134).

Acute coronary syndrome

Definitions Acute coronary syndrome (ACS) includes unstable angina and evolving MI, which share a common underlying pathology—plaque rupture, thrombosis, and inflammation. However, ACS may rarely be due to emboli or coronary spasm in normal coronary arteries or vasculitis (p. 416). Usually divided into *ACS with ST-segment elevation* or new-onset LBBB—what most of us mean by acute MI—and *ACS without ST-segment elevation*—the ECG may show ST-depression, T-wave inversion, nonspecific changes, or be normal (includes non-Q wave or subendocardial MI). The degree of irreversible myocyte death varies, and significant necrosis can occur without ST-elevation. Cardiac troponins (T and I) are the most sensitive and specific markers of myocardial necrosis and have become the test of choice in patients with ACS (see below).

Risk factors Nonmodifiable: Age, ♂ sex, family history of IHD (MI in first-degree relative <55 yrs). *Modifiable:* Smoking, hypertension, DM, hyperlipidemia, obesity, sedentary lifestyle. *Controversial* risk factors include stress, type A personality, LVH, apoprotein A↑, fibrinogen↑, hyperinsulinemia, homocysteine levels↑, ACE genotype, and cocaine use.

Diagnosis is based on the presence of at least two out of three of: Typical history, ECG changes, and cardiac enzyme rise (World Health Organization [WHO] criteria).

Symptoms Acute central chest pain, lasting >20 min, often associated with nausea, diaphoresis, dyspnea, palpitations. May present without chest pain ("silent" infarct) or with atypical chest pain (e.g., in elderly or diabetic patients). In such patients, presentations may include syncope, pulmonary edema, epigastric pain and vomiting, postoperative hypotension or oliguria, acute confusional state, stroke, diabetic hyperglycemic states.

Signs Distress, anxiety, pallor, sweatiness, pulse↓ or ↑, BP↑ or ↓, fourth heart sound. There may be signs of heart failure (JVP↑, third heart sound, and bibasilar crackles) or a pansystolic murmur (papillary muscle dysfunction/rupture; ventral septal defect [VSD]). A low-grade fever may be present. Later, a pericardial friction rub or peripheral edema may develop.

Tests *ECG:* Classically, hyperacute (tall) T waves, ST elevation or new LBBB occur within hours of acute Q wave (transmural infarction). T wave inversion and the development of pathological Q waves follow over hours to days (p. 95). *In other ACS:* ST-depression, T-wave inversion, nonspecific changes, or normal. *In 20% of MIS, the ECG may be normal initially.*

CXR: Look for cardiomegaly, pulmonary edema, or a widened mediastinum (?aortic dissection). Don't routinely delay treatment while waiting for a CXR.

Blood: CBC, electrolytes, renal function, glucose↑, lipids↓, cardiac enzymes↑ (CK, troponin); CK is found in myocardial and skeletal muscle. It is raised in MI, after trauma (falls, seizures) or prolonged exercise, and in myositis, hypothermia, and hypothyroidism. Check CK-MB isoenzyme levels if there is doubt as to the source (normal CK-MB/CK ratio <5%). Troponin T better reflects myocardial damage (peaks at 12–24 h; elevated for >1 wk). If normal ≥6 h after onset of pain, and ECG normal, risk of missing MI is tiny (0.3%). Peak post-MI levels also help risk stratification.

Differential diagnosis (p. 90) Angina, pericarditis, myocarditis, aortic dissection, pulmonary embolism, and esophageal reflux/spasm

Management See *emergencies* (p. 749). The management of ACS with and without ST-segment elevation varies. Likewise, if there is no ST-elevation, and symptoms settle without a rise in cardiac troponin, then no myocardial damage has occurred, the prognosis is good, and patients can be discharged.

Therefore, the two key questions are: Is there ST-segment elevation? And, is there a rise in troponin?

Mortality 50% of deaths occur within 2 h of onset of symptom.

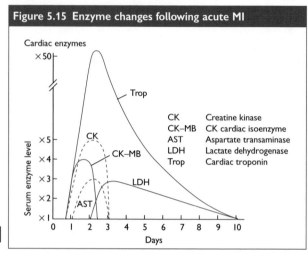

Figure 5.15 Enzyme changes following acute MI

CK	Creatine kinase
CK–MB	CK cardiac isoenzyme
AST	Aspartate transaminase
LDH	Lactate dehydrogenase
Trop	Cardiac troponin

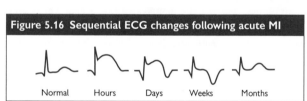

Figure 5.16 Sequential ECG changes following acute MI

Normal   Hours   Days   Weeks   Months

Management of ACS

Prehospital Arrange emergency ambulance. Aspirin 325 mg chewed (if no *absolute* CI) and NTG sublingual. Analgesia, such as morphine 5–10 mg IV (not IM because of risk of bleeding with thrombolysis). Ask if the patient took a PDE 5 inhibitor (sildenafil, vardenafil, tadalafil) since nitrates are contraindicated in that situation.

In the hospital O_2, morphine, aspirin (p. 751).

Then the key question for subsequent management of ACS is whether there is ST-segment elevation (includes new-onset LBBB or a true posterior MI).

ST-segment elevation

• *Primary* angioplasty or thrombolysis, if no contraindication
• *β-blocker*, e.g. atenolol 5 mg iv, unless contraindicated
• *ACE-inhibitor*: Consider starting ace-inhibitor (e.g., lisinopril 2.5 mg) in all normotensive patients within 24 h of acute MI, especially if there is clinical evidence of heart failure or echo evidence of LV dysfunction.

ACS without st-segment elevation

- β-*blocker*, e.g., atenolol 5 mg iv, unless contraindicated
- *Low-molecular-weight heparin (LMWH)* (e.g., enoxaparin)
- *Nitrates*, unless contraindication (usually given IV)
- High-risk patients (persistent or recurrent ischemia, ST-depression, DM, troponin↑) require infusion of a GPIIb/IIIa antagonist (e.g., tirofiban), and, ideally, urgent angiography. Clopidogrel may be useful in addition to aspirin.
- Low-risk patients (no further pain, flat or inverted T waves, or normal ECG, **and** negative troponin) can be discharged if a repeat troponin is negative. Treat medically and arrange further investigation (e.g., stress test, angiogram).

Subsequent management *Bed rest for 48 h; continuous ECG monitoring.*

- Daily examination of heart, lungs, and legs for complications (p. 116)
- Daily 12-lead ECG, electrolytes and renal function, cardiac enzymes for 2–3 d
- The length of time to give anticoagulant therapy and the type of anticoagulant therapy (heparin or LMWH, direct thrombin inhibitors, IIb/IIIa antagonists) is an area of active research.
- *Prophylaxis against thromboembolism:* E.g., LMWH SC until fully mobile. If large anterior MI, consider warfarin anticoagulation for 3 months as prophylaxis against systemic embolism from LV mural thrombus. Continue daily *low-dose aspirin* (e.g., 81 mg) indefinitely. Aspirin reduces vascular events (MI, stroke, or vascular death) by 29%.
- *Start oral* β-*blocker* (e.g., metoprolol ~50 mg/6 h, enough to lower the pulse to ~60; continue for at least 1 yr). Long-term β-blockade reduces mortality from all causes by ~25% in patients who have had a previous MI. If contraindicated, consider verapamil or diltiazem as an alternative.
- *Continue ACE-inhibitor in all patients:* ACE-inhibitor in those with evidence of heart failure reduces 2-yr mortality by 25–30%.
- *Start a statin:* Cholesterol reduction post-MI has been shown to be of benefit in patients with both elevated and normal cholesterol levels. Some treat all patients, others only if total cholesterol >200 mg/dL or LDL >130 mg/dL.
- *Address modifiable risk factors:* Discourage smoking (p. 89). Encourage exercise. Identify and treat DM, hypertension, and hyperlipidemia.
- *Exercise ECG:* May be useful in risk stratification post-MI and in subjects without ST-segment elevation or a troponin rise. Not necessary in patients who received a cardiac cath and appropriate intervention.
- *General advice:* If uncomplicated, discharge after 5–7 d. *Work:* Return to work after 4–12 wks. A few occupations should not be restarted post-MI: airline pilots, air traffic controllers, divers. Drivers of public service or heavy goods vehicles may be permitted to return to work if they meet certain criteria. Patients undertaking heavy manual labor should be advised to seek a lighter job. *Diet:* A diet high in fish, fruit, vegetables, and fiber, and low in saturated fats should be encouraged. *Exercise:* Encourage regular daily exercise. *Sex:* Intercourse is best avoided for 1 month. *Travel:* Avoid air travel for 2 months.

Review symptoms at 5 wks post-MI: Angina? Dyspnea? Palpitations?

- If angina recurs, treat conventionally, and consider coronary angiography.

Review at 3 months

- *Check fasting lipids:* Does the dose of statin need to be raised to reach goal levels?

Figure 5.17 Acute posterolateral MI

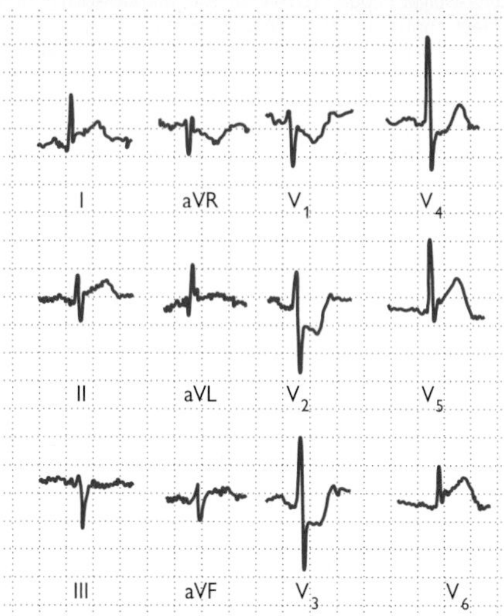

I aVR V₁ V₄

II aVL V₂ V₅

III aVF V₃ V₆

Complications of MI

- *Cardiac arrest* (p. 736); *cardiogenic shock* (p. 757)
- *Unstable angina:* Manage along standard lines (p. 752) and refer to a cardiologist for urgent investigation.
- *Bradycardias or heart block: Sinus bradycardia:* Treat with atropine 0.6–1.2 mg IV. Consider temporary cardiac pacing if no response, or poorly tolerated by the patient. *First-degree AV block:* Observe closely as approximately 40% develop higher degrees of AV block. *Wenckebach (Mobitz type I) block:* Does not require pacing unless poorly tolerated. *Mobitz type II block:* Carries a high risk of developing complete AV block; should be paced. *Complete AV block:* Insert pacemaker; may not be necessary after inferior MI if narrow QRS and reasonably stable pulse ≥40–50. *Bundle branch block:* MI complicated by trifascicular block or nonadjacent bifascicular disease should be paced.
- *Tachyarrhythmias:* **NB:** K⁺↓, hypoxia, and acidosis all predispose to arrhythmias and should be corrected. Regular wide complex tachycardia after MI is almost always VT. If hemodynamically stable, give lidocaine or amiodarone. If this fails, can repeat at a lower dose. Would review ACLS protocols. Consider maintenance antidysrhythmic therapy. *Early VT (<24 h):* Give lidocaine by infusion for 12–24 h or amiodarone. *Late VT (>24 h)* amiodarone and start oral therapy (amiodarone or sotalol). *SVT. AF or flutter:* If compromised, DC cardioversion. Otherwise, control rate with digoxin, β-blockers, or calcium channel blockers. In atrial flutter or intermittent AF, try amiodarone or sotalol.
- *Left ventricular failure (LVF)* (p. 754)
- *Right ventricular failure (RVF)/infarction:* Presents with low cardiac output and JVP↑. Insert a Swan–Ganz catheter to measure right-sided pressures

and guide fluid replacement. If BP remains low after fluid replacement, give inotropes.

- *Pericarditis:* Central chest pain, relieved by sitting forwards. *ECG:* Saddle-shaped ST elevation. *Treatment:* NSAIDs. Echo to check for effusion.
- *DVT and PE:* Patients are at risk of developing DVT and PE and should be prophylactically heparinized until fully mobile.
- *Systemic embolism:* May arise from an LV mural thrombus. After large anterior MIs, consider anticoagulation with warfarin for 3 months.
- *Cardiac tamponade* (p. 755): Presents with low cardiac output, pulsus paradoxus, JVP↑, muffled heart sounds. *Diagnosis:* Echo. *Treatment:* Pericardial aspiration (provides temporary relief [p. 730]), surgery
- *Mitral regurgitation:* May be mild (minor papillary muscle dysfunction) or severe (chordal or papillary muscle rupture or ischemia). *Presentation:* Pulmonary edema. *Diagnosis:* Echo. Treat LVF (p. 754) and consider valve replacement.
- *Ventricular septal defect:* Presents with pansystolic murmur, JVP↑, cardiac failure. *Diagnosis:* Echo. *Treatment:* Surgery. 50% mortality in first week
- *Late malignant ventricular arrhythmias:* Occur 1–3 wks post-MI and are the cardiologist's nightmare. Avoid hypokalemia, the most easily avoidable cause.
- *Dressler's syndrome:* Recurrent pericarditis, pleural effusions, fever, anemia and ESR↑ 1–3 wks post-MI. *Treatment:* NSAIDs; steroids if severe
- *Left ventricular aneurysm:* This occurs late (4–6 wks post-MI) and presents with LVF, angina, recurrent VT, or systemic embolism. *ECG:* Persistent ST segment elevation. *Treatment:* Anticoagulate, consider excision.

Angina pectoris

This is due to myocardial ischemia and presents as a central chest tightness or heaviness that is brought on by exertion and relieved by rest. It may radiate to one or both arms, the neck, jaw, or teeth. *Other precipitants:* Exercise, emotion, cold weather, and heavy meals. *Associated symptoms:* Dyspnea, nausea, diaphoresis, lightheadedness.

Causes Mostly atheroma; rarely, anemia, AS, tachyarrhythmias, HOCM, arteritis/small vessel disease.

Types of angina *Stable angina:* Induced by effort, relieved by rest. *Unstable (crescendo) angina:* Angina of increasing frequency or severity; occurs on minimal exertion or at rest; associated with highly increased risk of MI. *Decubitus angina:* Precipitated by lying flat. *Variant (Prinzmetal's) angina:* Caused by coronary artery spasm (rare; may coexist with fixed stenoses).

Tests *ECG:* Usually normal, but may show ST depression; flat or inverted T waves; signs of past MI. If resting ECG normal, consider exercise ECG (p. 99), thallium scan (p. 107), or coronary angiography.

Management *Alteration of lifestyle:* Stop smoking, encourage exercise, weight loss. *Modify risk factors:* Hypertension, DM, etc. (p. 89).
- Aspirin (81 mg/24 h) reduces mortality by 34%.
- β-*blockers:* E.g., atenolol 50–100 mg/24 h PO, unless contraindications (asthma, COPD, LVF, bradycardia, coronary artery spasm).
- *Nitrates:* For symptoms, give NTG spray or sublingual tabs, up to every half hour. Prophylaxis: Give regular oral nitrate, e.g., isosorbide mononitrate 10–30 mg PO (e.g., bid; an 8 h nitrate-free period to prevent tolerance) or slow-release nitrate (e.g., Imdur® 60 mg/24 h). *Alternatives:* Adhesive nitrate skin patches. *SE:* Headaches, BP↓.
- *Calcium antagonists:* Amlodipine 5–10 mg/24 h; diltiazem 90–180 mg/12 h PO.

- If total cholesterol >200 mg/dL, give a statin (p. 111).
- Unstable angina requires admission and urgent treatment: See *Emergencies* (p. 752).

Indications for referral Diagnostic uncertainty; new angina of sudden onset; recurrent angina if past MI or CABG; angina uncontrolled by drugs; unstable angina.

Percutaneous transluminal coronary angioplasty (PTCA) involves balloon dilatation of the stenotic vessel(s). *Indications:* Poor response or intolerance to medical therapy; refractory angina in patients not suitable for CABG; previous CABG; post-thrombolysis in patients with severe stenoses, symptoms, or positive stress tests. Comparisons of PTCA versus drugs alone show that PTCA may control symptoms better but with more frequent cardiac events (e.g., MI and need for CABG) and little effect on overall mortality. *Complications:* Restenosis (20–30% within 6 months); emergency CABG (<3%); MI (<2%); death (<0.5%). Stenting reduces restenosis rates and the need for bail-out CABG. NICE recommends that >70% of angioplasties should be accompanied by stenting. Drug-coated stents reduce restenosis. Antiplatelet agents (e.g., clopidogrel) reduce the risk of stent thrombosis. IV platelet glycoprotein IIb/IIIa-inhibitors (e.g., eptifibatide) can reduce procedure-related ischemic events.

CABG: Indications: Left main disease, multivessel disease, multiple severe stenoses, distal vessel disease, patient unsuitable for angioplasty, failed angioplasty, refractory angina, MI, pre-operatively (valve or vascular surgery). Comparisons of CABG versus PTCA have found that CABG results in better symptom control and lower re-intervention rate but longer recovery time and length of inpatient stay. Studies also show that CABG improves long-term survival compared to medical therapy.

118

Arrhythmias

Disturbances of cardiac rhythm or arrhythmias are:

- Common
- Often benign (but may reflect underlying heart disease)
- Often intermittent, causing diagnostic difficulty
- Occasionally severe, causing cardiac compromise

Causes *Cardiac*: MI, coronary artery disease, LV aneurysm, mitral valve disease, cardiomyopathy, pericarditis, myocarditis, aberrant conduction pathways. *Noncardiac*: Caffeine, smoking, alcohol, pneumonia, drugs (β_2-agonists, digoxin, tricyclics, Adriamycin, doxorubicin), metabolic imbalance (K^+, Ca^{2+}, Mg^{2+}, hypoxia, hypercapnia, metabolic acidosis, thyroid disease, pheochromocytoma). Presentation is with palpitation, chest pain, presyncope/syncope, hypotension, or pulmonary edema. Some arrhythmias may be asymptomatic and incidental (e.g., AF).

History Take a detailed history of palpitations. Ask about precipitating factors, onset, nature (fast or slow, regular or irregular) duration, associated symptoms (chest pain, dyspnea, light headedness). Review drug history. Ask about past medical history or family history of cardiac disease.

Tests CBC, electrolytes, glucose, Ca^{2+}, Mg^{2+}, thyroid-stimulating hormone (TSH). *ECG*: Look for signs of IHD, AF, short P–R interval (WPW syndrome), long QT interval (metabolic imbalance, drugs, congenital), U waves (hypokalemia). Undertake 24 h ECG monitoring; several recordings may be needed. May need a continuous monitor. *Echo*: To look for structural heart disease (e.g., mitral stenosis). *Provocation tests*: Exercise ECG, cardiac catheterization, and electrophysiological studies may be required.

Treatment If the ECG is normal during palpitations, reassure the patient. Otherwise, treatment depends on the type of arrhythmia.

Bradycardia (p. 120): If asymptomatic and rate is >40 bpm, no treatment is required. Look for a cause (drugs, sick sinus syndrome, hypothyroidism) and stop any drugs that may be contributing (β-blocker, digoxin). If rate is <40 bpm or patient is symptomatic, give atropine 0.5–1.0 mg IV (up to maximum of 3 mg). If no response, insert a temporary pacing wire (p. 732). If necessary, start an isoproterenol infusion or use external cardiac pacing.

Sick sinus syndrome: Sinus node dysfunction causes bradycardia ± arrest, sinoatrial block or SVT alternating with bradycardia/asystole (tachy–brady syndrome). AF and thromboembolism may occur. Pace if symptomatic.

SVT (p. 121): Narrow complex tachycardia (rate >100 bpm, QRS width <120 ms). *Acute management:* Vagotonic maneuvers followed by IV adenosine or verapamil (if not on β-blocker); DC shock if compromised. *Maintenance therapy:* β-blockers or verapamil.

af/flutter (p. 123): May be incidental finding. Control ventricular rate with β-blockers, calcium channel blockers, or digoxin. Use flecainide for preexcited AF. DC shock if compromised (p. 731).

VT (p. 125): Broad complex tachycardia (rate >100 bpm, QRS duration >120 ms). *Acute management:* IV lidocaine or amiodarone, if no response or if compromised DC shock. *Oral therapy:* Amiodarone loading dose (400 mg/8 h PO for 7 d, then 400 mg/12h for 7 d) followed by maintenance therapy (200–400 mg/24 h). *SE:* Corneal deposits, photosensitivity, hepatitis, pneumonitis, lung fibrosis, nightmares, INR↑ (warfarin potentiation), T4↑, T3↓. Monitor LFT and thyroid function tests (TFT).

Finally, pacing may be used to overdrive tachyarrhythmias, to treat bradyarrhythmias, or prophylactically in conduction disturbances (p. 127). Implanted automatic defibrillators can save lives and are indicated for patients with an ejection fraction <35% and New York Heart Association (NYHA) class II–III heart failure symptoms.

Figure 5.18 Diagnosis of bradycardias and AV block

(a)

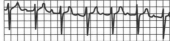

First degree AV block. P–R interval = 0.28s

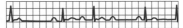

Möbitz type I (Wenckebach) AV block. With each succesive QRS, the P–R interval increases—until there is a non-conducted P wave.

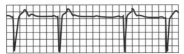

Möbitz type II AV block. Ratio of AV conduction varies from 2:1 to 3:1

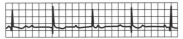

Complete AV block with narrow ventricular complexes. There is no relation between atrial and the slower ventricular activity.

(b)

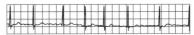

Atrial fibrillation

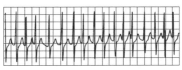

Atrial fibrillation with a rapid ventricular response. Diagnosis is based on the totally irregular ventricular rhythm.

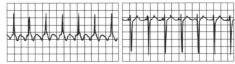

Atrial flutter with 2:1 AV block. Lead avF (on left) shows the characteristic saw-tooth baseline whereas lead V_1 (on right) shows discrete atrial activity, alternate 'F' waves being superimposed on ventricular T waves.

Narrow complex tachycardia

ECG shows rate of >100 bpm and QRS complex duration of <120 ms.

Differential diagnosis

- *Sinus tachycardia* Normal P wave followed by normal QRS
- *SVT:* P wave absent or inverted after QRS
- *AF:* Absent P wave, irregular QRS complexes
- *Atrial flutter:* Atrial rate usually 300 bpm giving "flutter waves" or "sawtooth" baseline (p. 120), ventricular rate often 150 bpm (2:1 block). See Table 5.6.
- *Atrial tachycardia* Abnormally shaped P waves, may outnumber QRS
- *Multifocal atrial tachycardia* Three or more P wave morphologies, irregular QRS complexes
- *Junctional tachycardia* Rate 150–250 bpm, P wave either buried in QRS complex or occurring after QRS complex

Principles of management See algorithm (Figure 5.19).

- If the patient is compromised, use DC cardioversion (p. 731).
- Otherwise, identify the underlying rhythm and treat accordingly.
- Vagal maneuvers (carotid sinus massage, Valsalva maneuver) transiently increase AV block, and may unmask an underlying atrial rhythm.
- If unsuccessful, give adenosine, which causes transient AV block. It has a short half-life (10–15 sec) and works in two ways: By transiently slowing ventricles to show the underlying atrial rhythm and by cardioverting a junctional tachycardia to sinus rhythm.

Give 6 mg IV bolus into a large vein; follow by saline flush, while recording a rhythm strip; if unsuccessful, give 12 mg, then 12 mg again at 2 min intervals, unless on dipyridamole or post cardiac transplantation. *Warn of SE:* Transient chest tightness, dyspnea, headache, flushing. *CI:* Asthma, second-/third-degree AV block, or sinoatrial disease (unless pacemaker). Drug interactions: Potentiated by dipyridamole, antagonized by theophylline.

Specific management Sinus tachycardia Identify and treat the cause.

SVT: If adenosine fails, use verapamil 5–10 mg IV over 2 min, or over 3 min if elderly (not if already on β-blocker). If no response, give further dose of 5 mg IV after 5–10 min. *Alternatives:* Atenolol 2.5 mg IV at 1 mg/min repeated at 5 min intervals to a maximum of 10 mg or sotalol. If no good, use DC cardioversion.

AF/flutter: Manage along standard lines (p. 123).

Atrial tachycardia: Rare. If due to digoxin toxicity, stop digoxin; consider digoxin-specific antibody fragments (p. 789). Maintain K^+ at 4–5 mmol/L.

Multifocal atrial tachycardia: Most commonly occurs in COPD. Correct hypoxia and hypercapnia. Consider verapamil if rate remains >110 bpm.

Junctional tachycardia: There are three types of junctional tachycardia: AV nodal reentry tachycardia (AVNRT), AV reentry tachycardia (AVRT), and His bundle tachycardia. Where anterograde conduction through the AV node occurs, vagal maneuvers are worth trying. Adenosine will usually cardiovert a junctional rhythm to sinus rhythm. If it recurs, treat with a β-blocker or amiodarone. Radiofrequency ablation is increasingly being used in AVRT and in some patients with AVNRT.

WPW syndrome (ECG, p. 124) Caused by congenital accessory conduction pathway between atria and ventricles. Resting ECG shows short P-R interval and widened QRS complex due to slurred upstroke or "delta wave." Two types: WPW type A (+ve δ wave in V_1), WPW type B (–ve δ wave in V_1). Patients present with SVT, which may be due to an AVRT, preexcited AF, or preexcited atrial flutter. Refer to cardiologist for electrophysiology and ablation of the accessory pathway.

Figure 5.19

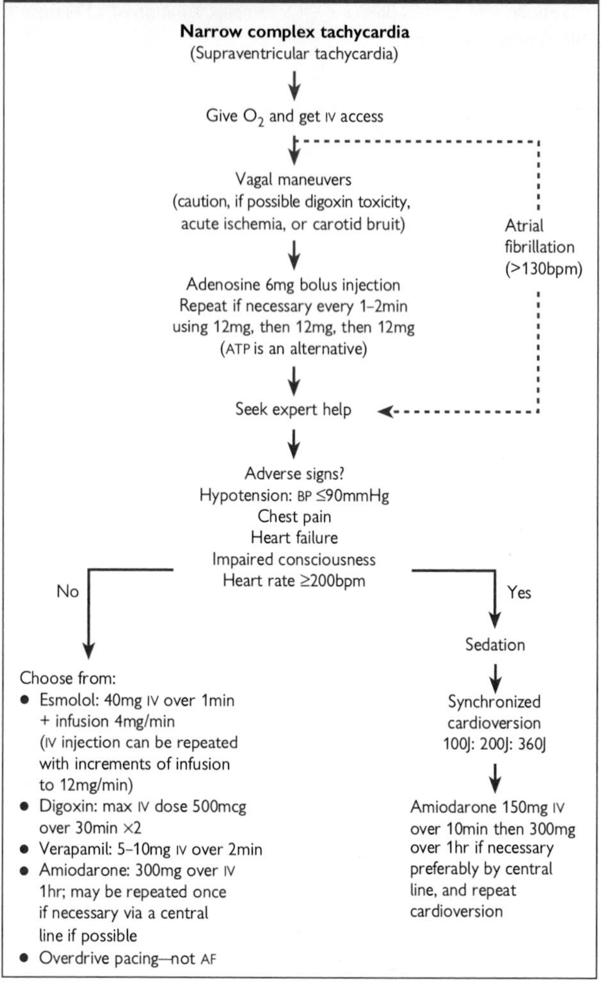

Narrow complex tachycardia
(Supraventricular tachycardia)

↓

Give O$_2$ and get IV access

↓

Vagal maneuvers
(caution, if possible digoxin toxicity,
acute ischemia, or carotid bruit)

↓

Adenosine 6mg bolus injection
Repeat if necessary every 1–2min
using 12mg, then 12mg, then 12mg
(ATP is an alternative)

↓

Seek expert help ←----------

Atrial
fibrillation
(>130bpm)

↓

Adverse signs?
Hypotension: BP ≤90mmHg
Chest pain
Heart failure
Impaired consciousness
Heart rate ≥200bpm

No ←

Yes →

Sedation

↓

Synchronized
cardioversion
100J: 200J: 360J

↓

Amiodarone 150mg IV
over 10min then 300mg
over 1hr if necessary
preferably by central
line, and repeat
cardioversion

Choose from:
- Esmolol: 40mg IV over 1min
  + infusion 4mg/min
  (IV injection can be repeated
  with increments of infusion
  to 12mg/min)
- Digoxin: max IV dose 500mcg
  over 30min ×2
- Verapamil: 5–10mg IV over 2min
- Amiodarone: 300mg over IV
  1hr; may be repeated once
  if necessary via a central
  line if possible
- Overdrive pacing—not AF

Atrial fibrillation and flutter

AF is a chaotic, irregular atrial rhythm at 300–600 bpm. The AV node responds intermittently, hence the irregular ventricular rate. It is common in the elderly (≤9%). The main risk is of embolic stroke, which is preventable by warfarin (reducible to 1%/yr from 4%; higher risk if old, poor LV function, DM, past TIA or stroke, or large left atrium on echocardiogram).

Common causes: Heart failure, hypertension, cardiac ischemia, MI (seen in 22%), mitral valve disease, pneumonia, hyperthyroidism, alcohol.

Rare causes: Cardiomyopathy, constrictive pericarditis, sick sinus syndrome, bronchial carcinoma, atrial myxoma, endocarditis, hemochromatosis, sarcoidosis, or other causes of atrial dilatation. "Lone" AF means none of the above causes.

Signs and symptoms: It may be asymptomatic (found incidentally) or present with chest pain, palpitations, dyspnea, or presyncope. On examination, the pulse is *irregularly irregular*, the apical pulse rate is greater than the radial rate, and the first heart sound is of variable intensity. Look for signs of mitral valve disease or hyperthyroidism.

Tests: ECG shows absent P waves, irregular QRS complexes. *Blood tests:* Electrolytes, cardiac enzymes, thyroid function tests. Echo to look for LA enlargement, mitral valve disease, poor LV function, and other structural abnormalities.

Acute af (e.g., ≤72 h):
- Treat any associated acute illness (e.g., MI, pneumonia).
- Control ventricular rate with either a β-blocker or a calcium channel blocker—intravenously if necessary. Digoxin can also be used but is not considered a first-line agent. If AF does not resolve, consider drug or electrical cardioversion.
- Drug cardioversion: Amiodarone IVI (5 mg/kg over 1 h then ~900 mg over 24 h via a central line max 1.2 g in 24 h) or PO (200 mg/8 h for 1 wk, 200 mg/12 h for 1 wk, 100–200 mg/24 h maintenance). Alternative (if hemodynamically stable and no known IHD): Flecainide 2 mg/kg IV over >25 min (max 150 mg) with ECG monitoring. 300 mg stat PO may also work.
- DC cardioversion is indicated: (1) electively, following a first attack of AF with an identifiable cause; (2) as an emergency, if the patient is compromised. *Protocol:* 200 J → 300 J → 360 J (100 J may be tried first, but is successful in <20%).
- Anticoagulation is not required if AF is of recent onset (<48 h) with a structurally normal heart on echo, but aspirin may be given. Otherwise, anticoagulate with warfarin for at least 3 wks before and 4 wks after DC cardioversion or perform TEE to look for left atrial thrombus.

Chronic AF:
- Control rate with β-blockers or calcium channel blockers. If the rate is not controlled on high doses of one, consider adding a second agent. Digoxin can be used but will not control the rate during exercise. *Alternative:* amiodarone PO.
- Anticoagulate with warfarin if >60 unless contraindication. Aim for an INR of 2.0–3.0. For those with no other risk factors (CHADS2 score: Heart failure, hypertension, age >75, DM, previous stroke, TIA, or thromboembolism), or those in whom warfarin is contraindicated, aspirin (325 mg PO) can be used.

Paroxysmal af:
- Many antiarrhythmic agents can be used to try to maintain sinus rhythm. Be cautious to not use an agent contraindicated in a certain patient population (e.g., flecainide in ischemic heart disease). Anticoagulate with warfarin.

Figure 5.20 Summary of treatment of AF

- Treat any reversible cause.
- Control ventricular rate.
- Consider cardioversion to sinus rhythm, if onset within last 12 months (do echo first; is heart structurally normal?).
- Prevent emboli: Warfarin (or aspirin).

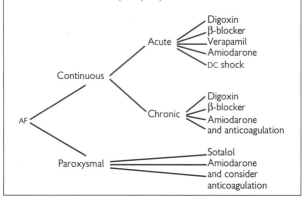

```
                                          ┌─ Digoxin
                                          ├─ β-blocker
                              Acute ──────┼─ Verapamil
                             /            ├─ Amiodarone
                            /             └─ DC shock
                 Continuous
                /           \             ┌─ Digoxin
               /             \            ├─ β-blocker
        AF                    Chronic ────┼─ Amiodarone
               \                          └─ and anticoagulation
                \
                 Paroxysmal ──────────────┌─ Sotalol
                                          ├─ Amiodarone
                                          └─ and consider
                                             anticoagulation
```

Table 5.6 Note on atrial flutter

- ECG: Continuous atrial depolarization (e.g., ~300/min, but very variable) produces a sawtooth baseline with variable block 2:1 or 3:1 usually.
- Carotid sinus massage or IV adenosine transiently blocks the AV node and may unmask flutter waves.
- Treatment: Same as AF. Consider cavotricuspid isthmus ablation (this "flutter isthmus" is low in the right atrium).

Figure 5.21 Wolff–Parkinson–White syndrome

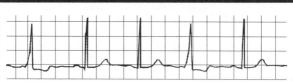

ECG of WPW syndrome (p. 121) in first and fourth beats; compared with the other beats, it can be seen how the delta wave both broadens the ventricular complex and shortens the PR interval.

Wide complex tachycardia

ECG shows rate of >100 and QRS complexes >120 ms (>3 small squares [p. 93]). If no clear QRS complexes, it is VF or asystole (p. 126).

Principles of management

- Identify the underlying rhythm and treat accordingly.
- If in doubt, treat as VT (the commonest cause).

Differential diagnosis

- VT; includes Torsade de pointes (see below)
- SVT with aberrant conduction (e.g., AF, atrial flutter)

(**NB:** Premature ventricular beats should not cause confusion when occurring singly; but if >3 together at rate of >120, this constitutes VT.)

Identification of the underlying rhythm (see Figure 5.22) may be difficult; seek expert help. Diagnosis is based on the history (IHD↑ the likelihood of a ventricular arrhythmia), a 12-lead ECG, and the lack of response to IV adenosine (p. 140). ECG findings in favor of VT:

- +ve QRS concordance in chest leads
- Marked LAD
- AV dissociation (occurs in 25%) or 2:1 or 3:1 AV block
- Fusion beats or capture beats
- RSR complex in V_1 (with +ve QRS in V_1)
- QS complex in V_6 (with -ve QRS in V_1)

Concordance means QRS complexes are all +ve or -ve. A *fusion beat* is when a "normal beat" fuses with a VT complex to create an unusual complex, and a *capture beat* is a normal QRS between abnormal beats (see Figure 5.22).

125

Management Connect to a cardiac monitor; have a defibrillator at hand.

- Give high-flow oxygen by face mask.
- Obtain IV access and take blood for electrolytes, cardiac enzymes, Ca^{2+}, Mg^{2+}.
- Obtain 12-lead ECG.
- Obtain ABG (if evidence of pulmonary edema, reduced conscious level, sepsis).

VT: Hemodynamically stable.

- Correct hypokalemia and hypomagnesemia.
- Amiodarone 150 mg IV over 10 min, then 1 mg/min IV × 6 h.
- *OR* lidocaine 1–1.5 mg/kg over 2 min, repeated every 5 min to 300 mg max.
- If this fails, or cardiac arrest occurs, use DC shock.
- After correction of VT, establish the cause from history/investigations.
- Maintenance antiarrhythmic therapy may be required. If VT occurs <24 h after MI, give IV lidocaine or amiodarone IVI for 12–24 h. If VT occurs >24 h after MI, give IV lidocaine or amiodarone infusion and start oral antiarrhythmic (e.g., amiodarone).
- Prevention of recurrent VT: Surgical isolation of the arrhythmogenic area or implantation of an automatic defibrillator may help.

VF: ECG (see Figure 5.23): Use asynchronized DC shock (p. 731). See also the *American Heart Association ACLS Guidelines* (p. 737).

Ventricular extrasystoles (PVCS) are the most common post-MI arrhythmia but they are also seen in healthy people (≥10/h). Post-MI, they suggest electrical instability, and there is a risk of VF if the "R on T" pattern (i.e., no gap before the T wave) is seen. Specific therapies to decrease PVCs have been shown to increase mortality so only treat with β-blockers. Otherwise, just observe patient and replace electrolytes.

Torsade de pointes: Looks like VF but is VT with varying axis (ECG, see Figure 5.23). It is due to ↑QT interval (congenital, drug-induced, or biochemical) and also occurs post MI. *Treatment:* Mg sulfate ± overdrive pacing.

Figure 5.22 Fusion and capture beats

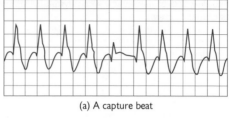

(a) A capture beat

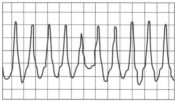

(b) A fusion beat

Figure 5.23 Specimen rhythm strips

(a)
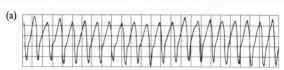

VT with a rate of 235/min.

(b)
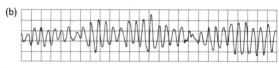

VF.

(c)
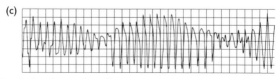

Torsade de pointes tachycardia.

Pacemakers

Pacemakers supply electrical initiation to myocardial contraction. The pacemaker lies subcutaneously, where it may be programed through the skin as necessary. Pacemakers usually last 7–15 yrs. See Table 5.7 for pacemaker terminology.

Indications for temporary cardiac pacing

• Symptomatic bradycardia, unresponsive to atropine
• Acute conduction disturbances following MI:
  • After acute *anterior* MI, prophylactic pacing is required in:
    – Complete AV block
    – Mobitz type II AV block
    – Nonadjacent bifascicular or trifascicular block (p. 95)
    – After *inferior* MI, pacing may not be needed in complete AV block if reasonably stable, rate is >40–50, and QRS complexes are narrow.
• Suppression of drug-resistant tachyarrhythmias (e.g., SVT, VT)
• Special situations: During general anesthesia, during cardiac surgery, during electrophysiological studies, drug overdose (e.g., digoxin, β-blockers, verapamil).

Indications for a permanent pacemaker

• Complete AV block (Stokes–Adams attacks, asymptomatic, congenital) or Mobitz type II AV block (p. 120) with symptoms or HR <40 or >3 sec asystole
• Persistent AV block after anterior MI
• Symptomatic bradycardias (e.g., sick sinus syndrome [p. 118])
• Drug-resistant tachyarrhythmias

Some say persistent bifascicular block after MI requires a permanent system: This remains controversial.

Preoperative assessment: CBC, PT/PTT. Insert IV cannula. Obtain consent for procedure under local anesthetic. Consider premedication. Give antibiotic coverage 20 min before, and 1 and 6 h after.

Postprocedure assessment: Prior to discharge, check wound for bleeding or hematoma, check position on CXR, check pacemaker function. During first week, inspect for wound dehiscence, or muscle twitching. Count apical rate (p. 71): If this is ≥6 bpm less than the rate quoted for the pacemaker, suspect malfunction. Other problems: Lead fracture, pacemaker interference (e.g., from patient's muscles).

Types of pacemakers: Three-letter pacemaker codes enable the identification of the pacemaker: The first letter indicates the chamber paced (A = atria, V = ventricles, D = dual chamber); the second letter identifies the chamber sensed (A = atria, V = ventricles, D = dual chamber, 0 = none), and the third letter indicates the pacemaker response (T = triggered, I = inhibited, D = dual, R = reverse). DDD pacemakers are the only pacemakers that sense and pace both chambers. The fourth letter (if present) is for rate responsiveness during motion.

ECG of paced rhythm (ECG 7 [p. 99] and Figure 5.24 for rhythm strip): If the system is on "demand" of 60 bpm, a pacing spike will only be seen if the intrinsic heart rate is <60 bpm. If it is cutting in at a higher rate, its sensing mode is malfunctioning. If it is failing to cut in at slower rates, its pacing mode is malfunctioning(i.e., the lead may be dislodged, the pacing threshold is too high, or the lead [or insulation] is faulty). If you see spikes but no capture (i.e., no systole), suspect dislodgment.

Figure 5.24 ECG of paced rhythm.

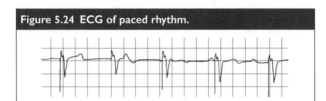

Heart failure: Basic concepts

Definition Heart failure occurs when the heart fails to maintain the cardiac output and BP to meet the body's requirements. Prognosis is poor, with >50% of patients dying within 5 yrs of diagnosis.

Classification *LVF* and *RVF* may occur independently, or together as *congestive heart failure (CHF)*. *Low-output cardiac failure:* The heart's output is inadequate (e.g., ejection fraction <0.35) or is only adequate with high filling pressures. *Causes:* Usually ischemia, hypertension, valve disorders, or idiopathic. See Table 5.8 for the New York Heart Association (NYHA) classification of heart failure.

- *Pump failure due to:*
  - *Heart muscle disease:* IHD, cardiomyopathy (p. 144).
  - *Restricted filling:* Constrictive pericarditis, tamponade, restrictive cardiomyopathy. This may be the mechanism of action of fluid overload: For constriction or tamponade, an expanding right heart impinges on the LV, so filling is restricted by the ungiving pericardium. For restriction, the heart is unable to expand properly because of intrinsic myocardial disease.
  - *Inadequate heart rate:* β-blockers, heart block, post MI
  - *Negative inotropic drugs:* E.g., most antiarrhythmic agents
- *Excessive preload:* E.g., mitral regurgitation or fluid overload; fluid overload may cause LVF in a normal heart if renal excretion is impaired or big volumes are involved (e.g., IVI running too fast). More common if there is simultaneous compromise of cardiac function and in the elderly.
- *Chronic excessive afterload:* E.g., AS, hypertension

NB: High-output failure is rare. Here, output is normal or increased in the face of much increased needs. Failure occurs when cardiac output fails to meet needs. It will occur with a normal heart, but even earlier if there is heart disease. *Causes:* Heart disease with anemia or pregnancy, hyperthyroidism, Paget's disease, arteriovenous malformation or fistulas, beriberi. *Consequences:* Initially features of RVF; later LVF becomes evident.

Symptoms depend on which ventricle is more affected. *LVF:* Dyspnea, poor exercise tolerance, fatigue, orthopnea, paroxysmal nocturnal dyspnea (PND), nocturnal cough (± pink frothy sputum), wheeze (cardiac "asthma"), nocturia, cool peripheries, weight loss, muscle wasting. *RVF:* Peripheral edema (up to thighs, sacrum, abdominal wall), abdominal distension (ascites), nausea, anorexia, facial engorgement, pulsation in neck and face (tricuspid regurgitation), epistaxis. In addition, patients may be depressed or complain of drug-related side effects.

Signs The patient may look ill and exhausted, with cool peripheries and peripheral cyanosis. *Pulse:* Resting tachycardia, pulsus alternans. Systolic BP↓, narrow pulse pressure, JVP↑. *Precordium:* Displaced apex (LV dilatation), RV heave (pulmonary hypertension). *Auscultation:* S₃ gallop (p. 51), murmurs of mitral or aortic valve disease. *Chest:* Tachypnea, bibasal end-inspiratory crackles, wheeze ("cardiac asthma"), pleural effusions. *Abdomen:* Hepatomegaly (pulsatile in tricuspid regurgitation), ascites, peripheral edema.

Investigations

Blood tests: CBC, electrolytes, brain natriuretic peptide (BNP), TSH, iron studies. *CXR:* Cardiomegaly (cardiothoracic ratio >50%), prominent upper lobe veins (upper lobe diversion), peribronchial cuffing, diffuse interstitial or alveolar shadowing, classical perihilar "bat's wing" shadowing, fluid in the fissures, pleural effusions, Kerley B lines (variously attributed to interstitial edema and engorged peripheral lymphatics). *ECG* may indicate cause (look for evidence of ischemia, MI, or ventricular hypertrophy). It is rare to get a completely normal ECG in chronic heart failure. *Echocardiography* is the key investigation. It may indicate the cause (MI, valvular heart disease) and can confirm the presence or absence of LV dysfunction. *Endomyocardial biopsy* is rarely needed but is occasionally helpful to diagnose the cause of restrictive cardiomyopathies.

129

Table 5.8 New York classification of heart failure: Summary

I	Heart disease present, but no dyspnea with ordinary activity
II	Comfortable at rest; dyspnea with ordinary activities
III	Dyspnea present with mild activity
IV	Dyspnea present at rest or with minimal activity

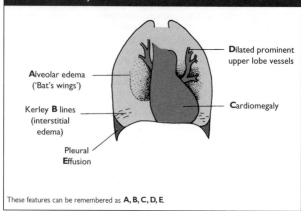

Figure 5.25 The cxr in left ventricular failure (see also X-RAY PLATE 2)

Dilated prominent upper lobe vessels

Alveolar edema ('Bat's wings')

Kerley **B** lines (interstitial edema)

Cardiomegaly

Pleural **E**ffusion

These features can be remembered as **A, B, C, D, E**.

Heart failure: Management

Acute heart failure is a medical emergency (p. 754).

Chronic heart failure Treat the cause (e.g., if arrhythmias; valve disease).

• Treat exacerbating factors (anemia, thyroid disease, infection, BP↑).
• Avoid exacerbating factors, such as NSAIDs (cause fluid retention, increase in afterload, and ↓ the effectiveness of ACE-inhibitors).
• Stop smoking. Eat less salt. Maintain optimal weight and nutrition.
• Drugs: The following are used:

  1 *Diuretics:* Loop diuretics routinely used to relieve symptoms (e.g., furosemide; increase dose and frequency as necessary. *SE:* Mg ↓, K⁺↓, renal impairment. Monitor electrolytes and add K⁺-sparing diuretic (e.g., *spironolactone*) if K⁺ <3.2 mEq/L, predisposition to arrhythmias, concurrent digoxin therapy (K⁺↓ increases risk of digoxin toxicity), or preexisting K⁺-losing conditions. If refractory fluid, consider adding *metolazone* 5 mg/24 h PO prior to the furosemide dose.

  2 *ace-inhibitor:* Consider in all patients with left ventricular systolic dysfunction; improves symptoms and prolongs life (see Table 5.9). If cough is a problem, an angiotensin receptor antagonist may be substituted (e.g., valsartan 40–160 mg/bid).

  3 *β-blockers* (e.g., carvedilol, metoprolol XL). Recent randomized trials show that β-blockers decrease mortality in heart failure. These benefits appear to be additive to those of ACE-inhibitor in patients with heart failure due to LV dysfunction. Should be initiated after diuretic and ACE-inhibitor only if the patient is euvolemic. *Use with caution*: "Start low and go slow"; if in doubt seek specialist advice first.

  4 *Aldosterone antagonists:* The RALES and EMPHASIS-HF trials have shown aldosterone antagonists) reduce mortality when added to conventional therapy. It should be initiated in NYHA I-IV patients. It improves endothelial dysfunction (↑nitric oxide bioactivity) and inhibits vascular angiotensin I/angiotensin II conversion. Spironolactone is K⁺-sparing, and hyperkalemia should be monitored closely in the elderly or those with renal insufficiency.

5 *Digoxin* improves symptoms even in those with sinus rhythm (data from the RADIANCE and other trials). Use it if diuretics, ACE-inhibitor, and β-blocker do not control symptoms, or in patients with AF. *Dose:* 0.125–0.25 mg/24 h PO. Monitor K^+ and maintain at 4–5 mEq/L. Other inotropes are unhelpful in terms of outcome.

6 *Vasodilators:* Long-acting nitrates reduce preload by causing venodilation (e.g., isosorbide mononitrate 60 mg/24 h PO). Second-line agents include arterial vasodilators, which reduce afterload (e.g., hydralazine, SE: Drug-induced lupus) or α-blockers, which are combined arterial and venous vasodilators (e.g., prazosin). Vasodilators improve arterial hemodynamics and reduce mortality (so especially valuable if ACE-inhibitor is contraindicated).

Intractable heart failure Reassess the cause. Is the patient taking his drugs? At maximum dose? Is he compliant with diet? Admit to hospital for:

- Bed rest
- IV furosemide ± metolazone
- IV opiates and nitrates may relieve symptoms—rarely used
- Daily weight and frequent electrolytes ($K^+\downarrow$)
- DVT prophylaxis: Heparin 5,000 U/12 h SC and TED stockings
- *In extremis,* IV inotropes (p. 757) may be needed but will not prolong life (it may be difficult to wean patients off them).
- Consider "*tailoring therapy*" with a right-heart catheterization.
- Finally, consider a heart transplant or left ventricular assist device.

How to start ACE-inhibitors

See Table 5.9.

Table 5.9 How to start ACE-inhibitor

Check that there are no contraindications/cautions:

- Renal failure (serum creatinine >2.5 mg/dL; but not an absolute CI)
- Hyperkalemia: K^+ >5.0 mEq/L
- Hyponatremia: Caution if <130 mEq/L (relates to a poorer prognosis)
- Hypovolemia
- Hypotension (systolic BP <90 mm Hg)
- AS or LV outflow tract obstruction
- Pregnancy or lactation
- Severe COPD or cor pulmonale (not an absolute CI)
- Renal artery stenosis.[2] (Suspect if arteriopathic, e.g., cerebrovascular disease, IHD, peripheral vascular disease. ACE-inhibitors reduce glomerular filtration rate (GFR) and may precipitate acute renal failure.)

Warn the patient about possible SE:

- Hypotension
- Dry cough (1:10)
- Taste disturbance
- Hyperkalemia
- Renal impairment
- Urticaria and angioedema (<1:1,000)
- Rarely: Proteinuria, leukopenia, fatigue

2 If renovascular disease precludes the use of ACE-inhibitors, and furosemide is providing no answer, consider maximal vasodilatation with nitrates and hydralazine: seek expert advice.

(Continued)

Table 5.9 (*Continued*)

Starting ACE-inhibitors:

Hypertensive patients can be safely started on ACE-inhibitors as outpatients. Warn them about postural hypotension and advise them to take the first dose on going to bed. Use a long-acting ACE-inhibitor at low doses.

Patients with CHF are best started on ACE-inhibitors under close medical supervision. Start with small dose and increase every 2 wks until at target dose (equivalent of 40 mg lisinopril a day) or side effects supervene (↓BP, ↑creatinine). Review in ~1 wk for assessment; monitor CHEM 7 regularly. Patients on high doses of diuretics (>80 mg furosemide a day) may need a reduction in their diuretic dose first—seek expert help.

Hypertension

Hypertension is a major risk factor for stroke and MI. It is usually asymptomatic, so screening is vital.

Defining hypertension BP has a skewed normal distribution within the population and risk is continuously related to BP. Therefore, it is impossible to define "hypertension." We choose to select a value above which risk is significantly elevated and the benefit of treatment is clear cut (see below). BP should be assessed over a period of time (don't rely on a single reading). The "observation" period depends on the BP and the presence of other risk factors or end-organ damage. See Tables 5.10 and 5.11.

Who to treat All patients with malignant hypertension or a sustained pressure ≥140/90 mm Hg should be treated (p. 133). For those >140/90, the decision depends on the risk of coronary events, presence of DM or end-organ damage (see the *Joint National Committee Guidelines*, *[JNC VII]*). See also Table 5.12.

Systolic or diastolic pressure? For many years, diastolic pressure was considered to be more important than systolic pressure. However, evidence from the Framingham and the MrFIT studies indicates that systolic pressure is the most important determinant of cardiovascular risk in the over 50s.

Systolic hypertension in the elderly: The age-related rise in systolic BP was considered part of the "normal" aging process, and isolated systolic hypertension (ISH) in the elderly was largely ignored. But evidence from major studies indicates, beyond doubt, that benefits of treating are even greater than treating moderate hypertension in middle-aged patients.

"Malignant" hypertension: This refers to severe hypertension (e.g., systolic >200, diastolic >130mmHg) in conjunction with bilateral retinal hemorrhages and exudates; papilledema may or may not be present. Symptoms are common (e.g., headache ± visual disturbance). Alone, it requires urgent treatment. However, it may precipitate acute renal failure, heart failure, or encephalopathy, which are hypertensive emergencies. Untreated, 90% die in 1 yr; treated, 70% survive 5 yrs. Pathological hallmark is fibrinoid necrosis. It is more common in younger patients and in black people. Look hard for any underlying cause.

Causes

Essential hypertension (primary, cause unknown: ~95% of cases.

Secondary *hypertension:* ~5% of cases. Causes include:

- *Renal disease:* The most common secondary cause. 75% are from *intrinsic renal disease:* Glomerulonephritis, polyarteritis nodosa (PAN), systemic sclerosis, chronic pyelonephritis, or polycystic kidneys. 25% are due to *renovascular disease,* most frequently atheromatous (elderly male cigarette smokers, associated peripheral vascular disease) or rarely fibromuscular dysplasia (young females)(p. 279).
- *Endocrine disease:* Cushing's (p. 309) and Conn's syndromes (p. 313), pheochromocytoma (p. 315), acromegaly, hyperparathyroidism
- *Others:* Coarctation, pregnancy, steroids, MAOI

Signs and symptoms Usually asymptomatic (except malignant hypertension, above). Always examine the CVS system fully and check for retinopathy. Are there features of an underlying cause (pheochromocytoma [p. 315]), signs of renal disease, radiofemoral delay, or weak femoral pulses (coarctation), renal bruits, palpable kidneys, or Cushing's syndrome? Look for end-organ damage: LVH, retinopathy (Table 5.10) and proteinuria—indicates severity and duration of hypertension and associated with a poorer prognosis.

Investigations *Basic:* Electrolytes, creatinine, cholesterol, glucose, ECG, urine analysis (for protein, blood). *Specific* (exclude a secondary cause): Renal ultrasound, renal arteriography, 24 h urinary VMA and metanephrines, urinary free cortisol, renin, and aldosterone. ECHO and 24 h ambulatory BP monitoring may be helpful in some cases (e.g., white coat or borderline hypertension).

Table 5.10 Hypertensive retinopathy

Grade
I	Tortuous arteries with thick shiny walls (silver or copper wiring)
II	A-V nicking (narrowing where arteries cross veins)
III	Flame hemorrhages and cotton wool spots
IV	Papilledema

Figure 5.26 Seventh Report of the Joint National Committee on Prevention, Detection, Evaluation, and Treatment of High Bp (jnc 7)[3]

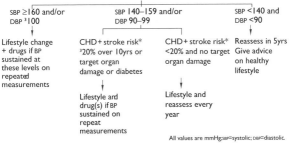

Algorithm for Treatment of Hypertension

Measure BP and other risk factors (plasma lipids, glucose)

SBP ≥160 and/or DBP ³100	SBP 140–159 and/or DBP 90–99		SBP <140 and DBP <90
Lifestyle change + drugs if BP sustained at these levels on repeated measurements	CHD+ stroke risk* ³20% over 10yrs or target organ damage or diabetes	CHD+ stroke risk* <20% and no target organ damage	Reassess in 5yrs Give advice on healthy lifestyle
	Lifestyle and drug(s) if BP sustained on repeat measurements	Lifestyle and reassess every year	

All values are mmHg; SBP=systolic; DBP=diastolic.

3 www.nhlbi.nih.gov/guidelines/hypertension/phycard.pdf

Table 5.11 Classification of BP

Category	SBP mm Hg		DBP mm Hg
Normal	<120	and	<80
Prehypertension	120–139	or	80–89
Hypertension, Stage 1	140–159	or	90–99
Hypertension, Stage 2	≥160	or	≥100

SBP, systolic BP; DBP, diastolic BP

Table 5.12 Compelling indications for Individual Drug Classes

Compelling indication	Initial therapy options
• Heart failure	THIAZ, BB, ACEI, ARB, ALDO ANT
• Post myocardial infarction	BB, ACEI, ALDO ANT
• High CVD risk	THIAZ, BB, ACEI, CCB
• Diabetes	THIAZ, BB, ACEI, ARB, CCB
• Chronic kidney disease	ACEI, ARB
• Recurrent stroke prevention	THIAZ, ACEI

THIAZ, thiazide diuretic; ACEI, angiotensin converting enzyme inhibitor; ARB, angiotensin receptor blocker; BB, β-blocker; CCB, calcium channel blocker; ALDO ANT, aldosterone antagonist

Hypertension: Management

Look for and treat underlying causes (e.g., renal disease, acute pain).

Treatment goal For most patients, aim for BP <140/90, but 130/80 in patients with DM and renal disease. Reduce BP gradually; a rapid reduction can be fatal, especially in the context of stroke.

Lifestyle changes Reduce concomitant risk factors: Stop smoking; low-fat diet. Reduce alcohol and salt intake; increase exercise; reduce weight if obese. (See DASH diet; http://www.nhlbi.nih.gov/health/public/heart/hbp/dash/new_dash.pdf.)

Drugs Explain the need for long-term treatment. Essential hypertension is not "curable." The recent ALLHAT study suggests that adequate BP reduction is more important than the specific drug used. However, ACE-inhibitor may provide additional renal benefit if coexisting DM is present.

- *Thiazide diuretics* are first choice, increasing the dose brings no benefit and produces more *SE:* Hypokalemia, hyponatremia, postural hypotension, impotence.
- *β-blockers:* E.g., atenolol 50 mg/24 h PO. Higher doses provide little additional benefit. *SE:* Bronchospasm, heart failure, lethargy, impotence. *CI:* Asthma; caution in heart failure.
- *ACE-inhibitor:* E.g., lisinopril 2.5–20 mg/24 h PO (max 40 mg/d) or enalapril. ACE-inhibitor may be first choice if coexisting LVF, or in diabetics with microalbuminuria or proteinuria. *SE:* Cough, K⁺↑, renal failure, angioedema. *CI:* Renal artery stenosis, AS.
- *Ca2⁺-channel antagonist:* E.g., nifedipine SR 30–90 mg/24 h PO. *SE:* Flushing, fatigue, gum hyperplasia, ankle edema. Avoid short-acting drugs.

- *Others:* Angiotensin receptor antagonists (e.g., losartan), methyldopa (used in pregnancy), and doxazosin (an α-blocker). For refractory cases: Clonidine, minoxidil, or hydralazine (causes a reflex tachycardia unless given with a β-blocker and may cause an SLE-like syndrome).

The four main classes of agent happen to start with ABCD. There is some evidence that in monotherapy A&B are more effective in younger people and C&D in older individuals (and African Americans). This may guide initial therapy, and if one drug fails, switch between groups. When adding drugs, it makes sense to combine A or B with C or D (e.g., a thiazide and ACE-inhibitor, or β-blocker and Ca^{2+}—channel antagonist)—the "ABCD rule." Remember that most drugs take 4–8 wks to produce their maximum effect, so don't assess efficacy on the basis of a single clinic BP measurement.

Malignant hypertension Most patients can be managed with oral therapy, except for those with encephalopathy. The aim is for a controlled reduction in BP over days, not hours. Avoid sudden drops in BP as cerebral autoregulation is poor (so stroke risk↑).

- Bed rest; start a loop diuretic (e.g., furosemide 40–80 mg daily ± a thiazide). There is no ideal antihypertensive therapy, but labetalol, atenolol, or long-acting calcium blockers may be used orally.
- Encephalopathy (headache, focal CNS signs, seizures, coma): Aim to reduce BP to ~110 mm Hg diastolic over 4 h. Admit to monitored area. Insert intra-arterial line for pressure monitoring. Furosemide 40–80 mg IV; then either IV labetalol (e.g., 50 mg IV over 1 min, repeated every 5 min, max 200 mg) or sodium nitroprusside infusion (0.5 mcg/kg/min IVI titrated up to 8 mcg/kg/min, e.g., 50 mg in 1L dextrose 5%; expect to give 100–200 mL/h for a few days at most to avoid cyanide risk). Labetalol or hydralazine can also be used intravenously. Avoid hydralazine if CAD.

Never use sublingual (SL) nifedipine to reduce BP (it can cause an uncontrollable drop in BP and stroke).

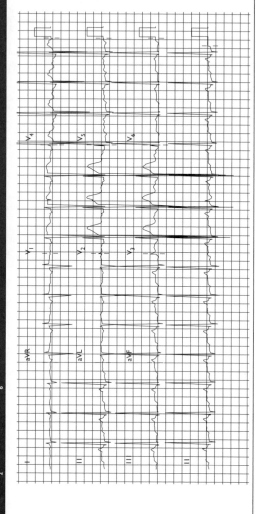

Figure 5.27 ECG 8: Left ventricular hypertrophy—this is from a patient with malignant hypertension—note the sum of the S-wave in V_2 and R-wave in V_6 is >35 mm.

136

Rheumatic fever

This systemic infection is still common in the Third World, although increasingly rare in the West. *Peak incidence:* 5–15 yrs. Tends to recur unless prevented. Pharyngeal infection with Lancefield Group A β-hemolytic strep-tococci triggers rheumatic fever 2–4 wks later, in the susceptible 2% of the population. An antibody to the carbohydrate cell wall of the streptococcus cross-reacts with valve tissue (antigenic mimicry) and may cause permanent damage to the heart valves.

Diagnosis Use the *revised Jones criteria.* There must be evidence of recent strep infection plus two major criteria, or one major + two minor.

Evidence of streptococcal infection:

• Recent streptococcal infection
• History of scarlet fever
• +ve throat swab
• Elevated in antistreptolysin O titer ASOT >200 U/mL
• Elevated in DNase B titer

Major criteria:

• *Carditis:* Tachycardia, murmurs (mitral or AR, mid diastolic murmur [mid diastolic, p. 53]), pericardial rub, CCF, cardiomegaly, conduction defects (45–70%). An apical systolic murmur may be the only sign.
• *Arthritis:* A migratory arthritis; usually affects the larger joints (75%)
• *Subcutaneous nodules:* Small, mobile painless nodules on extensor surfaces of joints and spine (2–20%)
• *Erythema marginatum:* Geographical-type rash with red, raised edges and clear center; occurs mainly on trunk, thighs, arms in 2–10%
• *Sydenham's chorea* (St. Vitus' dance): Occurs late in 10%. Unilateral or bilateral involuntary semipurposeful movements; may be preceded by emotional lability and uncharacteristic behavior

Minor criteria:

• Fever
• Raised ESR or CRP
• Arthralgia (but not if arthritis is one of the major criteria)
• Prolonged P–R interval (but not if carditis is major criterion)
• Previous rheumatic fever

Management

• Penicillin G 0.6–1.2 million units IM stat then penicillin V 250 mg/6 h PO
• *Analgesia for carditis/arthritis:* Aspirin 100 mg/kg/d PO in divided doses (maximum 8 g/d) for 2 d, then 70 mg/kg/d for 6 wks. Monitor salicylate level. Toxicity causes tinnitus, hyperventilation, metabolic acidosis. *Alternative:* NSAIDS.
• Steroids are thought not to have a major impact on sequelae, but they may improve symptoms.
• Immobilize joints in severe arthritis.
• Diazepam for the chorea

Prognosis 60% with carditis develop chronic rheumatic heart disease. This correlates with the severity of the carditis. Acute attacks last an average of 3 months. Recurrence may be precipitated by further streptococcal infections, pregnancy, or use of oral contraceptives. Cardiac sequelae affect mitral (70%), aortic (40%), tricuspid (10%), and pulmonary (2%) valves. Incompetent lesions develop during the attack, stenoses years later.

Secondary prophylaxis Penicillin V 250 mg/12 h PO until no longer at risk (>30 yrs). Thereafter, give antibiotic prophylaxis for dental or other surgery (p. 143). Erythromycin can be used if penicillin allergic.

Mitral valve disease

Mitral stenosis *Causes:* Rheumatic; congenital, mucopolysaccharidoses, endocardial fibroelastosis, malignant carcinoid, prosthetic valve.

Presentation: Dyspnea, fatigue, palpitations, chest pain, systemic emboli, hemoptysis, chronic bronchitis-like picture ± complications (below).

Signs: Malar (i.e., cheek) flush; low-volume pulse; AF common; tapping, undisplaced, apex beat (palpable S_1). *On auscultation:* Loud S_1; opening snap (pliable valve); rumbling mid-diastolic murmur (heard best in expiration, as the patient lies on their left side). Graham Steell murmur (early diastolic, p. 53) may occur. *Severity:* The more severe the stenosis, the longer the diastolic murmur, and the closer the opening snap is to S_2.

Tests: ECG: AF; P-mitrale if in sinus rhythm; RVH; progressive RAD. *CXR:* Left atrial enlargement; pulmonary edema; mitral valve calcification. *Echocardiography* is diagnostic. Significant stenosis exists if the valve orifice is <1 cm²/m² body surface area. Indications for *cardiac catheterization:* Previous valvotomy, signs of other valve disease, angina, severe pulmonary hypertension, calcified mitral valve.

Management: If in AF, *rate control is crucial* (add a β-blocker or calcium channel blocker if needed to keep the pulse rate <90); anticoagulate with warfarin. Diuretics reduce preload and pulmonary venous congestion. If this fails to control symptoms, balloon valvuloplasty (if pliable, noncalcified valve), open mitral valvotomy, or valve replacement. SBE/IE, prophylaxis for dental or surgical procedures (p. 143). Oral penicillin as prophylaxis against recurrent rheumatic fever if <30 yrs old.

Complications: Pulmonary hypertension; emboli, pressure from large LA on local structures; e.g., hoarseness (recurrent laryngeal nerve), dysphagia (esophagus), bronchial obstruction, infective endocarditis (rare).

Mitral regurgitation *Causes:* Functional (LV dilatation); annular calcification (elderly); rheumatic fever, infective endocarditis, mitral valve prolapse, ruptured chordae tendinea; papillary muscle dysfunction/rupture; connective tissue disorders (Ehlers–Danlos, Marfan's); cardiomyopathy; congenital (may be associated with other defects, e.g., atrial septal defect [ASD], AV canal); appetite suppressants (e.g., fenfluramine, phentermine).

Symptoms: Dyspnea, fatigue, palpitations, infective endocarditis. *Signs:* AF; displaced, hyperdynamic apex; RV heave; soft S_1; split S_2; loud P_2 (pulmonary hypertension) pansystolic murmur at apex radiating to axilla. *Severity:* The more severe, the larger the left ventricle.

Tests: ECG: AF ± P-mitrale if in sinus rhythm (may mean left atrial size↑, LVH. *CXR:* Big LA and LV, mitral valve calcification, pulmonary edema.

Echocardiogram to assess LV function (trans-esophageal to assess severity and suitability for repair rather than replacement). *Doppler* echo to assess size and site of regurgitant jet. *Cardiac catheterization* to confirm diagnosis, exclude other valve disease, assess coronary artery disease.

Management: Digoxin for fast AF. Anticoagulate if AF, history of embolism, prosthetic valve, additional mitral stenosis. Diuretics improve symptoms. Surgery for deteriorating symptoms; aim to repair or replace the valve before LV irreversibly impaired. Antibiotics to prevent endocarditis.

Mitral valve prolapse *Prevalence:* ~5%. Occurs alone or with: ASD, patent ductus arteriosus, cardiomyopathy, Turner's syndrome, Marfan's syndrome, osteogenesis imperfecta, pseudoxanthoma elasticum, WPW (p. 121). *Symptoms:* Asymptomatic—or atypical chest pain and palpitations. *Signs:* Mid-systolic click and/or a late systolic murmur. *Complications:* Mitral regurgitation, cerebral emboli, arrhythmias, sudden death. *Tests:* *Echocardiography* is diagnostic. *ECG* may show inferior T wave inversion. *Treatment:* β-blockers may help palpitations and chest pain. Give endocarditis prophylaxis (p. 143) if coexisting mitral regurgitation.

Aortic valve disease

Aortic stenosis (AS) *Causes:* Senile calcification is the commonest. Also congenital bicuspid valve.

Presentation: Angina, dyspnea, dizziness, syncope, systemic emboli if infective endocarditis, CCF, sudden death. *Signs:* Slow rising pulse with narrow pulse pressure (feel for diminished and delayed carotid upstroke—"parvus et tardus"); heaving, undisplaced apex beat; LV heave; aortic thrill; ejection systolic murmur (heard at the base, left sternal edge and the aortic area; radiates to the carotids). As stenosis worsens, A_2 is increasingly delayed, giving first a single S_2 and then reversed splitting. But this sign is rare. More common is a quiet A_2. In severe AS, A_2 may be inaudible (calcified valve). There may be an ejection click (pliable valve) or an audible S_4 (said to occur more commonly with bicuspid valves, but not in all populations).

Tests: ECG: P-mitrale, LVH with strain pattern; LAD (left anterior hemiblock); poor R wave progression; LBBB or complete AV block (calcified ring). *CXR:* LVH; calcified aortic valve; poststenotic dilatation of ascending aorta. *Echo* is diagnostic (p. 104). *Doppler echo* can estimate the gradient across valves: Severe stenosis if gradient >50 mm Hg and valve area <0.5 cm^2. If the aortic jet velocity is >4 m/sec (or is ↑ by >0.3 m/sec per year) risk of complications is increased. *Cardiac catheter* can assess valve gradient, LV function, coronary artery disease, the aortic root.

Differential diagnosis: HOCM.

Management: Symptomatic patients have a poor prognosis: 2–3-yr survival if angina/syncope; 1–2-yr survival with cardiac failure. Prompt valve replacement (p. 140) is recommended. In asymptomatic patients with severe AS and a deteriorating ECG, valve replacement is also recommended. If the patient is not medically fit for surgery, percutaneous valvuloplasty may be attempted. Endocarditis prophylaxis (p. 143). Percutaneous valve replacement is still experimental but may be approved soon.

Aortic sclerosis is senile degeneration of the valve. There is an ejection systolic murmur, no carotid radiation, and a normal pulse and S_2.

Aortic regurgitation (ar) *Causes:* *Congenital valve disease:* Rheumatic fever, infective endocarditis, rheumatoid arthritis, SLE, pseudoxanthoma elasticum, appetite suppressants (e.g., fenfluramine, phentermine). *Aortic root disease:* Hypertension, trauma, aortic dissection, seronegative spondyloarthritis (ankylosing spondylitis, reactive arthritis, psoriatic arthritis), Marfan's syndrome, osteogenesis imperfecta, syphilitic aortitis.

Symptoms: Dyspnea, palpitations, cardiac failure. *Signs:* Collapsing (water-hammer) pulse, wide pulse pressure, displaced, hyperdynamic apex beat, high-pitched early diastolic murmur (heard best in expiration, with patient sitting forward). Associated signs: Corrigan's sign (carotid pulsation), Quincke's sign (capillary pulsations in nail beds), Duroziez's sign (femoral diastolic murmur as blood flows backwards in diastole), Traube's sign ("pistol shot" sound over femoral arteries). In severe AR, an Austin Flint murmur may be heard (p. 53).

Investigations: ECG: LVH. *CXR:* Cardiomegaly, dilated ascending aorta, pulmonary edema. *Echocardiography* is diagnostic. *Cardiac catheterization* to assess severity of lesion, anatomy of aortic root, LV function, coronary artery disease, other valve disease.

Management: Indications for surgery: ↑ Symptoms, enlarging heart on CXR/echo, ECG deterioration (T wave inversion in lateral leads), infective endocarditis refractory to medical therapy. Aim to replace the valve before significant LV dysfunction occurs. Endocarditis prophylaxis (p. 143).

Right-heart valve disease

Tricuspid regurgitation *Causes*: Pulmonary hypertension, rheumatic fever, infective endocarditis (IV drug abusers), carcinoid syndrome, congenital (e.g., ASD, AV canal, Ebstein's anomaly).

Symptoms: Fatigue, hepatic pain on exertion, ascites; edema. *Signs*: Giant *v* waves and prominent *y* descent in JVP (p. 49); RV heave; pansystolic murmur, heard best at lower sternal edge in inspiration; pulsatile hepatomegaly; jaundice; ascites. *Management*: Treat underlying cause. *Drugs*: Diuretics, digoxin, ACE-inhibitors. Valve replacement (20% operative mortality).

Tricuspid stenosis *Causes*: Rheumatic fever; almost always occurs with mitral or aortic valve disease. *Symptoms*: Fatigue, ascites, edema. *Signs*: Giant *a* wave and slow *y* descent in JVP (p. 49); opening snap, early diastolic murmur heard at the left sternal edge in inspiration. *Diagnosis*: Doppler echo. *Treatment*: Diuretics; surgical repair.

Pulmonary stenosis *Causes*: Usually congenital (Turner's syndrome, Noonan's syndrome, William's syndrome, Fallot's tetralogy, rubella). *Acquired causes*: Rheumatic fever, carcinoid syndrome. *Symptoms*: Dyspnea, fatigue, edema, ascites. *Signs*: Dysmorphic facies (congenital causes); prominent *a* wave in JVP; RV heave. In mild stenosis, there is an ejection click, ejection systolic murmur (which radiates to the left shoulder); widely split S_2. In severe stenosis, the murmur becomes longer and obscures A_2. P_2 becomes softer and may be inaudible. *Tests*: ECG: RAD, P-pulmonale, RVH, RBBB. *CXR*: Poststenotic dilatation of pulmonary artery; RV hypertrophy; right atrial hypertrophy. Cardiac catheterization is diagnostic. *Treatment*: Pulmonary valvuloplasty or valvotomy.

Pulmonary regurgitation is caused by any cause of pulmonary hypertension (p. 195). A decrescendo murmur is heard in early diastole at the left sternal edge (the Graham Steell murmur).

Cardiac surgery

Valvuloplasty can be used in mitral or pulmonary stenosis (pliable, non-calcified valve, no regurgitation). A balloon catheter is inserted across the valve and inflated.

Valvotomy Closed valvotomy is rarely performed now. Open valvotomy is performed under cardiopulmonary bypass through a median sternotomy.

Valve replacements *Mechanical valves* may be of the ball-cage (Starr–Edwards), tilting disc (Björk–Shiley), or double tilting disc (St. Jude) type. These valves are very durable but the risk of thromboembolism is high; patients require lifelong anticoagulation. *Xenografts* are made from porcine valves or pericardium. These valves are less durable and may require replacement at 8–10 yrs. Anticoagulation is not required unless there is AF. *Homografts* are cadaveric valves. They are particularly useful in young patients and in the replacement of infected valves. *Complications of prosthetic valves*: Systemic embolism, infective endocarditis, hemolysis, structural valve failure, arrhythmias.

CABG see Table 5.13.

Cardiac transplantation Consider this when cardiac disease is *severely* curtailing quality of life and survival is not expected beyond 6–12 months. Refer to a specialty center. Main contraindications: Malignancy, age >70, significant peripheral or cerebrovascular disease, DM with end-organ dysfunction, noncompliance.

Table 5.13 Coronary artery bypass grafts

Indications for cabg: To improve survival

- Left main disease
- Triple vessel disease involving proximal part of the left anterior descending, especially with LV dysfunction

To relieve symptoms

- Angina unresponsive to drugs
- Unstable angina (sometimes)
- If angioplasty is unsuccessful

Procedure: Surgery is planned based on the result of angiograms. Not all stenoses are bypassable. The heart is stopped and blood is oxygenated and pumped artificially by a machine outside the body (cardiac bypass). The patient's own veins (saphenous) or arteries (internal mammary or radial)are used as the graft. Several grafts may be placed.
>50% of vein grafts close in 10 yrs (low-dose aspirin helps prevent this). Arterial grafts last longer.

After CABG: If angina persists or recurs (from poor run-off from the graft, distal disease, new atheroma, or graft occlusion), restart antianginal drugs and consider angioplasty (repeat surgery has increased risk). Mood, sex, and intellectual problems are common early. Cardiac rehabilitation improves survival:

- Exercise: Walk → cycle → swim → jog
- Drive at 4–8 wks: No need to tell DMV
- Get back to work (e.g., at 3 months)
- Address smoking cessation, BP, lipids
- Aspirin, statin for life

Infective endocarditis

Fever + new murmur = endocarditis until proven otherwise.

Classification

- 50% of all endocarditis occurs on *normal valves.* It follows an *acute course* and presents with acute heart failure.
- Endocarditis on *abnormal valves* tends to run a *subacute course.* Predisposing cardiac lesions: Aortic or mitral valve disease, tricuspid valves in IV drug users, coarctation, patent ductus arteriosus, VSD, prosthetic valves. Endocarditis on prosthetic valves may be "early" (acquired at the time of surgery, poor prognosis) or "late" (acquired hematogenously).

Causes *Bacteria:* Any cause of bacteremia exposes valves to the risk of bacterial colonization (e.g., dental work, UTI, urinary catheterization, cystoscopy, respiratory infection, endoscopy (controversial), colonic carcinoma, gall bladder disease, skin disease, IV cannulation, surgery, abortion, fractures). Quite often, no cause is found. *Streptococcus viridans* is the commonest (35–50%). Others: Enterococci, *Staphylococcus aureus/epidermidis*, diphtheroids and microaerophilic streptococci. *Rarely:* HACEK group of Gram –ve bacteria (*Haemophilus–Actinobacillus–Cardiobacterium–Eikenella–Kingella*), *Coxiella burnetii, Chlamydia. Fungi:* These include *Candida, Aspergillus,* and *Histoplasma. Other causes:* SLE (Libman–Sacks endocarditis), malignancy.

Clinical features The patient may present with any of the following: *Signs of infection:* Fever, rigors, night sweats, malaise, weight loss, anemia, splenomegaly, and clubbing. *Cardiac lesions:* Any new murmur or a change in the nature of a preexisting murmur should raise the suspicion of endocarditis. Vegetations may cause valve destruction and severe regurgitation or valve obstruction. An aortic root abscess causes prolongation of the P–R interval and may lead to complete AV block. LVF is a common cause of death. *Immune complex deposition:* Vasculitis (p. 416) may affect any vessel. Microscopic hematuria is common; glomerulonephritis and acute renal failure may occur. Roth spots (boat-shaped retinal hemorrhage with pale center), splinter hemorrhages (on finger or toe nails), Osler's nodes (painful pulp infarcts in fingers or toes) and Janeway lesions (painless palmar or plantar macules) are pathognomonic. *Embolic phenomena:* Emboli may cause abscesses in the relevant organ, e.g., brain, heart, kidney, spleen, GI tract. In right-sided endocarditis, pulmonary abscesses may occur.

Diagnosis The *Duke* criteria for definitive diagnosis of endocarditis are given. *Blood cultures:* Take three sets at different times and from different sites at peak fever. 85–90% are diagnosed from the first two sets; 10% is culture-negative. *Blood tests:* Normochromic, normocytic anemia, neutrophil leukocytosis, high ESR/CRP. Also check electrolytes, Mg^{2+}, LFTs. *Urinalysis* for microscopic hematuria. *CXR* (cardiomegaly) and ECG (prolonged P–R interval) at regular intervals. *Echocardiography* TTE may show vegetations, but only if >2 mm. TEE is more sensitive, and better for visualizing mitral lesions and possible development of aortic root abscess. See Table 5.14.

Management Consultation with Infectious Disease and Cardiology should be considered.
• Antibiotics (see Table 5.15)
• Consider surgery if: Heart failure, progressive heart block, valvular obstruction; repeated emboli or cerebral emboli; fungal endocarditis; persistent bacteremia; myocardial abscess; unstable infected prosthetic valve.

Prognosis 30% mortality with staphylococci; 14% with bowel organisms; 6% with sensitive streptococci.

142

Table 5.14 Duke criteria for infective endocarditis

Major criteria:
• Positive blood culture:
  • Typical organism in two separate cultures or
  • Persistently +ve blood cultures, e.g., three, >12 h apart (or majority if ≥4)
• Endocardium involved:
  • +ve echocardiogram (vegetation, abscess, dehiscence of prosthetic valve) or
  • New valvular regurgitation (change in murmur not sufficient)

Minor criteria:
• Predisposition (cardiac lesion; IV drug abuse)
• Fever >38°C
• Vascular/immunological signs
• +ve blood cultures that do not meet major criteria
• +ve echocardiogram that does not meet major criteria

How to diagnose: Definite infective endocarditis: Two major **or** one major and three minor **or** all five minor criteria (if no major criterion is met).

Table 5.15 Antibiotic therapy for infective endocarditis

- Consult Infectious Disease for the appropriate regimen based on bacterial sensitivities in your hospital. The following are guidelines only:
- *Empirical therapy:* Nafcillin or oxacillin 2 g/4 h IV + gentamicin or tobramycin 1 mg/kg q12h IV.
- *Streptococci:* Penicillin (PCN) G 20–30 million U/d IV for 4–6 wks; then amoxicillin 1 g/8 h PO for 2 wks. Monitor minimum inhibitory concentration (MIC) and add gentamicin 1 mg/kg q8–12h IV for the first 2 wks. Monitor gentamicin levels.
- *Enterococci:* Ampicillin[a] 1 g/6 h IV + gentamicin 1 mg/kg q8–12h IV for 4 wks. Monitor gentamicin levels.
- *Staphylococci:* Oxacillin or nafcillin 2 g/4 h IV + gentamicin 1 mg/kg q12h IV. Treat for 6–8 wks; stop gentamicin after 1 wk.
- *Coxiella:* Doxycycline 100 mg/12 h PO indefinitely + co-trimoxazole, rifampin, or ciprofloxacin.
- *Fungi:* Flucytosine 3 g/6 h IVI over 30 mins followed by fluconazole 50 mg/24 h PO (a higher dose may be needed). Amphotericin if flucytosine resistance or *Aspergillus*. Miconazole if renal function is poor.

[a] For penicillin allergy, use vancomycin 1 g/12 h IV

Prevention of endocarditis

Anyone with congenital heart disease, acquired valve disease, or prosthetic valves is at risk of infective endocarditis and should take prophylactic antibiotics before procedures that may result in bacteremia. The recommendations of the American Heart Association are:

Which conditions?
Prophylaxis recommended
- Prosthetic valve(s)
- Previous endocarditis
- Septal defects
- Mitral prolapse with regurgitation
- Acquired valve disease
- Surgical shunts

Prophylaxis not recommended
- Mitral prolapse (no regurgitation)
- Functional/innocent murmur

Which procedures?
Prophylaxis recommended
- Dental procedures
- Upper respiratory tract surgery
- Esophageal dilatation
- Sclerotherapy of varices
- Surgery/instrumentation of lower bowel, gall bladder, or GU tract

Prophylaxis not recommended
- Flexible bronchoscopy
- Diagnostic upper GI endoscopy
- TEE (p. 104)
- Cesarean or normal delivery
- Cardiac catheterization (unless high-risk patient)

Which regimen?

- *Dental procedures*
  - *Local or no anesthetic:* Amoxicillin 2 g PO, 1 h before the procedure. Alternative (if penicillin allergy or >1 dose of penicillin in previous month): Clindamycin 600 mg PO or cephalexin 2 g PO or azithromycin/clarithromycin 500 mg 1 h pre procedure.
  - *Intolerant of oral meds:* Ampicillin 2 g IV 30 min preprocedure.
- *Upper respiratory tract procedures*
  - As for dental procedures.
- *Gastrointestinal and genitourinary procedures*
  - *High risk* (prosthetic valve, prior endocarditis, surgical shunt): Ampicillin 2 g IM/IV + gentamicin 1.5 mg/kg IV/IM 30 min preprocedure. Vancomycin 1 g IV + gentamicin if penicillin allergy.
  - *Moderate risk:* Amoxicillin 2 g PO 1 h preprocedure. Vancomycin 1 g IV if penicillin allergy.

Diseases of heart muscle

Acute myocarditis *Causes:* Inflamed myocardium from viruses (coxsackie, enterovirus, adenovirus, HIV, and others); bacteria (*Clostridia*, diphtheria, *Meningococcus*, *Mycoplasma*, psittacosis); spirochetes (*Leptospirosis*, syphilis, Lyme disease); protozoa (Chagas' disease); drugs; toxins; vasculitis (p. 416).

Signs and symptoms: Fatigue, dyspnea, chest pain, palpitations, tachycardia, soft S_1, S_4 gallop.

Tests: ECG: ST segment elevation/depression, T wave inversion, atrial arrhythmias, transient AV block. Serology is rarely helpful for acute management.

Management: Treat the underlying cause. Supportive measures. Patients may recover or develop intractable heart failure (p. 128).

Dilated cardiomyopathy A dilated, poorly contractile heart of unknown cause. Associations: Alcohol, BP↑, hemochromatosis, viral infection, autoimmune, peri- or postpartum, thyrotoxicosis, congenital (X-linked). *Prevalence:* 0.2%.

Presentation: Fatigue, dyspnea, pulmonary edema, RVF, emboli, AF, VT. *Signs:* ↑Pulse, ↓BP, ↑JVP, displaced, diffuse apex, S_3 gallop, mitral or tricuspid regurgitation (MR/TR), pleural effusion, edema, jaundice, hepatomegaly, ascites.

Tests: CXR: Cardiomegaly, pulmonary edema. *ECG:* Tachycardia, nonspecific T wave changes, poor R wave progression. *Echo:* Globally dilated hypokinetic heart with low ejection fraction. Look for MR, TR, LV mural thrombus.

Management: Bed rest, diuretics, digoxin, ACE-inhibitor, β-blockers, anticoagulation. Consider cardiac transplantation. *Mortality:* Variable depending on severity of symptoms.

Hypertrophic cardiomyopathy *HOCM from LV* outflow tract (LVOT) obstruction from asymmetric septal hypertrophy.

Prevalence: 0.2%. Autosomal dominant inheritance, but 50% are sporadic. 70% have mutations in genes encoding β-myosin, α-tropomyosin, and troponin T. May present at any age. Ask about family history of sudden death.

The patient: Angina, dyspnea, palpitation, syncope, sudden death (VF is amenable to implantable defibrillators). Pulse with rapid upstroke, *a* wave in JVP, double apex beat, systolic thrill at lower left sternal edge, harsh ejection systolic murmur.

Tests: ECG: LVH, progressive T wave inversion, deep Q waves (inferior + lateral leads), AF, WPW syndrome (p. 121), ventricular ectopy, VT. *Echo:* Asymmetrical septal hypertrophy, small LV cavity with hypercontractile posterior wall, midsystolic closure of aortic valve, systolic anterior movement of mitral valve. *Cardiac catheterization* may provoke VT. It helps assess severity of gradient, coronary artery disease or mitral regurgitation. Electrophysiological studies may be needed if arrhythmias. Exercise test, Holter monitor, and echo to risk stratify yearly for increased risk of sudden death.

Management: β-blockers or verapamil for symptoms (p. 112). Amiodarone 100–200 mg/d for arrhythmias (AF, VT). Anticoagulate for paroxysmal AF or systemic emboli. Septal myectomy (surgical, or chemical, with alcohol, to reduce LV outflow tract gradient) is reserved for those with severe symptoms. Consider implantable defibrillator if patient has risk factors for sudden death (VT on Holter, family history of sudden death, syncope, drop in BP pressure with exercise, wall thickness >3 cm).

Mortality: 5.9%/yr if <14 yrs; 2.5%/yr if >14 yrs. *Poor prognostic factors:* Age < 14yrs or syncope at presentation; family history of HOCM/sudden death.

Restrictive cardiomyopathy *Causes:* Amyloidosis, hemochromatosis, sarcoidosis, scleroderma, Löffler's eosinophilic endocarditis, endomyocardial fibrosis. *Presentation* is like constrictive pericarditis (p. 147). Features of RVF predominate: ↑JVP, with prominent x and y descents, hepatomegaly, edema, ascites. *Diagnosis:* Echo, cardiac catheterization, +/- endomyocardial biopsy, MRI.

Cardiac myxoma Rare benign cardiac tumor. Prevalence ≤5/10,000, ♀:♂ ≈ 2:1. Usually sporadic, may be familial (autosomal dominant). It may mimic infective endocarditis (fever, weight loss, clubbing, ↑ESR), or mitral stenosis (left atrial obstruction, systemic emboli, AF). A "tumor plop" may be heard, and signs may vary according to posture. *Tests:* Echocardiography, CT or MRI. *Treatment:* Excision.

145

The heart in various, mostly rare, systemic diseases

See Table 5.16.

Table 5.16 The heart in various, mostly rare, systemic diseases

This list reminds us to look at the heart *and* the whole patient, not just in exams (where those with odd syndromes congregate), but always.

Acromegaly (p. 324): BP↑, LVH, hypertrophic cardiomyopathy, high-output cardiac failure, coronary artery disease
Amyloidosis (p. 635): Restrictive cardiomyopathy
Ankylosing spondylitis (p. 402): Conduction defects, AV block, AR
Behçet's disease (p. 416): AR, arterial ± venous thrombi
Cushing's syndrome (p. 309): Hypertension
Down's syndrome: ASD, VSD, mitral regurgitation
Ehlers-Danlos syndrome: Mitral valve prolapse + hyperelastic skin ± aneurysms and GI bleeds. Joints are loose and hypermobile; mutations exist, e.g., in genes for procollagen (COL3A1); there are six types.
Friedreich's ataxia: Hypertrophic cardiomyopathy
Hemochromatosis (p. 216): AF, cardiomyopathy

(Continued)

Table 5.16 (Continued)

Holt-Oram syndrome: ASD or VSD with upper limb defects

Human immunodeficiency virus (p. 566): Myocarditis, dilated cardiomyopathy, effusion, ventricular arrhythmias, SBE/IE, noninfective thrombotic (murantic) endocarditis, RVF (pulmonary hypertension), metastatic Kaposi's sarcoma

Hypothyroidism (p. 301): Sinus bradycardia, low pulse pressure, pericardial effusion, coronary artery disease, low-voltage ECG

Kawasaki disease: Coronary arteritis similar to PAN; more common than *rheumatic fever* as a cause of acquired heart disease.

Klinefelter's syndrome: Male; ASD. Psychopathy, learning difficulties, libido↓, gynecomastia, sparse facial hair and small firm testes; XXY

Marfan's syndrome: Mitral valve prolapse, AR, aortic dissection. Look for long fingers and a high-arched palate.

Noonan's syndrome: ASD, pulmonary stenosis ± low-set ears

PAN (p. 416): Small and medium vessel vasculitis + angina, MI, arrhythmias, CHF, pericarditis and conduction defects

Rheumatoid nodules: Conduction defects, pericarditis, LV dysfunction, AR, coronary arteritis. Look for arthritis signs (p. 399).

Sarcoidosis (p. 192): Infiltrating granulomas may cause complete AV block, ventricular or supraventricular tachycardia, myocarditis, CHF, restrictive cardiomyopathy; ECG may show Q waves.

Syphilis (p. 587): Myocarditis, ascending aortic aneurysm

Systemic lupus erythematosus (p. 410): Pericarditis/effusion, myocarditis, Libman–Sacks endocarditis, mitral valve prolapse, coronary arteritis

Systemic sclerosis (p. 410): Pericarditis, pericardial effusion, myocardial fibrosis, myocardial ischemia, conduction defects, cardiomyopathy

Thyrotoxicosis (p. 298): Pulse↑, AF ± emboli, wide pulse pressure, hyperdynamic apex, loud heart sounds, ejection systolic murmur, pleuropericardial rub, angina, high output cardiac failure

Turner's syndrome: Female; coarctation of aorta. Look for webbed neck; XO.

William's syndrome: Supravalvular aortic stenosis (visuospatial IQ↓)

Pericardial diseases

Acute pericarditis Inflammation of the pericardium that may be primary or secondary to systemic disease.

Causes:

- Viruses (coxsackie, flu, Epstein–Barr, mumps, varicella, HIV)
- Bacteria (pneumonia, rheumatic fever, TB)
- Fungi
- Myocardial infarct
- Dressler's syndrome
- Uremia
- Rheumatoid arthritis
- SLE
- Myxedema
- Trauma
- Surgery
- Malignancy
- Radiotherapy
- Procainamide; hydralazine

Clinical features: Central chest pain worse on inspiration or lying flat ± relief by sitting forward. A pericardial friction rub may be heard. Look for evidence of a pericardial effusion or cardiac tamponade (see below).

Tests: ECG classically shows concave (saddle-shaped) ST segment elevation, but may be normal or nonspecific (10%). Can also see PR depression. *Blood tests:* CBC, ESR, electrolytes, cardiac enzymes, viral serology, blood cultures, and, if indicated, autoantibodies, fungal cultures, thyroid function tests. Cardiomegaly on *cxr* may indicate a pericardial effusion. *Echo* to evaluate cardiac function and evaluate for effusions.

Treatment: Analgesia, e.g., ibuprofen 400 mg/8 h PO with food. Treat the cause. Consider colchicine before steroids/immunosuppressants if relapse or continuing symptoms occur. 15–40% DO recur.

Pericardial effusion Accumulation of fluid in the pericardial space.

Causes: Any cause of pericarditis (see above).

Clinical features: Dyspnea, ↑JVP (with prominent x descent [p. 49]), bronchial breathing at left base (Ewart's sign: Large effusion compressing left lower lobe). Look for signs of cardiac tamponade (see below).

Diagnosis: CXR shows an enlarged, globular heart. ECG shows low-voltage QRS complexes and alternating QRS morphologies (electrical alternans). *Echocardiography* shows an echo-free zone surrounding the heart.

Management: Treat the cause. Pericardiocentesis may be *diagnostic* (suspected bacterial pericarditis) or *therapeutic* (cardiac tamponade). Send pericardial fluid for culture, TB culture, and cytology.

Constrictive pericarditis The heart is encased in a rigid pericardium.

Causes: Often unknown; also TB or after *any* pericarditis.

Clinical features: These are mainly of right-heart failure with ↑JVP (with prominent x and y descents [p. 49]); Kussmaul's sign (JVP rising paradoxically with inspiration); soft, diffuse apex beat; quiet heart sounds; S₃; diastolic pericardial knock, hepatosplenomegaly, ascites, and edema.

Tests: CXR: Small heart ± pericardial calcification (if none, CT/MRI helps distinguish from other cardiomyopathies). *Echo:* Cardiac catheterization.

Management: Surgical excision.

Cardiac tamponade Accumulation of pericardial fluid raises intrapericardial pressure, hence poor ventricular filling and fall in cardiac output.

Causes: Any pericarditis (above), aortic dissection, hemodialysis, warfarin, trans-septal puncture at cardiac catheterization, post cardiac biopsy.

Signs: Pulse↑, BP↓, pulsus paradoxus, JVP↑, Kussmaul's sign, muffled S₁ and S₂.

Diagnosis: Beck's triad: Falling BP; rising JVP; small, quiet heart. *cxr:* Big globular heart (if >250 mL fluid). *ecg:* Low-voltage QRS ± electrical alternans. *Echo is diagnostic:* Echo-free zone (> 2 cm or >1 cm if acute) around the heart ± diastolic collapse of right atrium and right ventricle.

Management: Seek expert help. The pericardial effusion needs urgent drainage. Send fluid for culture, ZN stain/TB culture and cytology.

Figure 5.28 Pericarditis

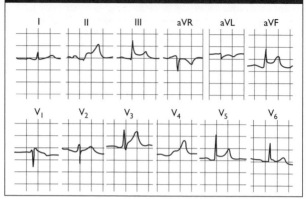

Congenital heart disease

The spectrum of congenital heart disease in adults is considerably different from that in infants and children; adults are unlikely to have complex lesions. The commonest lesions, in descending order of frequency, are:

Bicuspid aortic valve These function well at birth and go undetected. Most eventually develop AS (requiring valve replacement) and/or AR (predisposing to IE/SBE)(p. 141).

Atrial septal defect A hole connects the atria. *Ostium secundum* defects (high in the septum) are most common; *ostium primum* defects (opposing the endocardial cushions) are associated with AV valve anomalies. Primum ASDs present early. Secundum ASDs are often asymptomatic until adulthood, as the L → R shunt depends on compliance of the right and left ventricles. The latter decreases with age (esp. if BP↑). This augments L → R shunting, causing dyspnea and heart failure, usually by age 40–60. There may be pulmonary hypertension, cyanosis, arrhythmia, hemoptysis, and chest pain.

Signs: AF; ↑JVP; wide, fixed split S₂; pulmonary ejection systolic murmur. Pulmonary hypertension may cause pulmonary or tricuspid regurgitation.

Complications: Paradoxical embolism (rare). Reversal of left to right shunt (**Eisenmenger complex**). Eisenmenger complex is a congenital heart defect at first associated with a left-to-right shunt, which may lead to pulmonary hypertension and shunt reversal. If so, cyanosis develops (± heart failure and respiratory infections) and Eisenmenger's syndrome is present.

Tests: ECG: RBBB with LAD and prolonged P–R interval (primum defect) or RAD (secundum defect). *CXR:* Small aortic knuckle, pulmonary plethora, progressive atrial enlargement. Echocardiography is diagnostic. Cardiac catheterization shows step up in O₂ saturation in the right atrium.

Treatment: In children, surgical closure is recommended before age 10 yrs. In adults, closure is recommended if symptomatic, or if asymptomatic but having pulmonary to systemic blood flow ratios of ≥1.5:1.

Ventricular septal defect A hole connecting the two ventricles.

Causes: Congenital (prevalence 2:1,000 births); acquired (post-MI).

Symptoms: May present with severe heart failure in infancy or remain asymptomatic and be detected incidentally in later life.

Signs: These depend upon the size and site of the *VSD:* Smaller holes, which are hemodynamically less significant, give louder murmurs. Classically, a harsh pansystolic murmur is heard at the left sternal edge, accompanied by a systolic thrill, ± left parasternal heave. Larger holes are associated with signs of pulmonary hypertension.

Complications: AR, infundibular stenosis, infective endocarditis, pulmonary hypertension, Eisenmenger complex.

Tests: ECG: Normal (small VSD), LAD + LVH (moderate VSD) or LVH + RVH (large VSD). *CXR:* Normal heart size ± mild pulmonary plethora (small VSD) or cardiomegaly, large pulmonary arteries and marked pulmonary plethora (large VSD). *Cardiac catheter:* Step up in O_2 saturation in right ventricle.

Treatment: This is medical, at first, as many VSDs close spontaneously. Indications for surgical closure are failed medical therapy, symptomatic VSD, shunt >3:1, SBE/IE. Give SBE/IE prophylaxis for untreated defects (p. 143).

Coarctation of the aorta Congenital narrowing of the descending aorta; usually occurs just distal to the origin of the left subclavian artery. More common in boys. *Associations:* Bicuspid aortic valve, Turner's syndrome. *Signs:* Radiofemoral delay, weak femoral pulse, BP↑, scapular bruit, systolic murmur (best heard over the left scapula). *Complications:* Heart failure, infective endocarditis. *Tests:* CXR shows rib notching. *Treatment:* Surgery.

Pulmonary stenosis may occur alone or with other lesions (p. 140).

Driving and the heart

The rules on driving with heart conditions vary from state to state, and you should become familiar with the laws in your state before discussing driving with your patients. In general, it is the responsibility of the driver, but you should guide your patients appropriately.

Pulmonary medicine

L. Dwight Wooster, M.D., F.C.C.P.

Introduction

The respiratory system consists of the central nervous system, the peripheral nervous system, the nose and sinuses, the mouth and upper airways, the lungs, chest wall, and diaphragm and the pulmonary circulation. The functions of the respiratory system include filtering and humidification of air, oxygenating of blood and elimination of carbon dioxide, and the protection of each respiratory system component. Pulmonary disorders or those disorders affecting the lungs cause dysfunction of these respiratory functions, resulting in a variety of symptoms, the most common of which is dyspnea, difficulty in breathing. Other forms of breathlessness are orthopnea (shortness of breath when lying down), dyspnea on exertion, paroxysmal dyspnea and nocturnal paroxysmal dyspnea (sudden paroxysms of dyspnea), and platypnea, or shortness of breath when standing up. Cough, chest tightness or discomfort, wheezing, and hemoptysis are other frequent symptoms suggestive of respiratory system disorders.

Outline of pulmonary diseases

Airway diseases-predominately obstructive
- Acute bronchitis and upper respiratory tract infections
- Emphysema
- Chronic bronchitis/bronchiectasis
- Asthma
- Chronic obstructive pulmonary disease
- Bronchiolitis

Lung parenchyma disease-predominately restrictive
- Pulmonary fibrosis
- Sarcoidosis
- Lung abscess
- Pneumonia
- Malignancy: Primary or metastatic

Chest wall diseases-restrictive
- Skeletal: Pectus deformities, kyphoscoliosis, ankylosing spondylitis
- Extraskeletal: Obesity
- Neurological: Multiple sclerosis, amyotrophic lateral sclerosis, Guillain-Barré syndrome, paralyzed diaphragm

Vascular disease-neither obstructive nor restrictive
- Pulmonary emboli (PE)
- Pulmonary hypertension

History and physical exam

Refer to pp. 36–39; in addition to the clinical points in the chapter of Clinical Skills, a few other points;

Smoking history Ask the patient: "Have you ever smoked? How long? Number of cigarettes per day? Filtered or unfiltered? Generic versus brand-named cigarettes? Menthol or nonmenthol?" Did the patient's parents smoke?

If one has stopped smoking, how long?

Ask about other tobacco products; question about snuff or chew, frequency of use, history of previous dental or mouth examinations.

Ask about other inhalants, such as THC/cocaine.

Ask about occupational history; nature of the patient's work; exposure to fumes, chemicals dyes; e.g., if taking a history from a fire-fighter, is there a history of smoke inhalation?

Is there a modification of symptoms when away from work environment compared to symptoms at work? Ask about construction projects at work or at home. Question the patient about exposure to variations in temperature or humidity.

Physical exam of the chest In addition to examination of the chest discussed in Clinical Skills (p. 36):
- Listen to chest sound during quiet breathing and with deep breathing.
- With the stethoscope over the upper and anterior portion of the chest, have the patient perform a forced expiration—listen for wheezes or rhonchus.

Chest radiographs The routine chest radiograph (p. 691) is the first radiographic step in diagnosing pulmonary disease. Although chest computed tomography (ct) scans have greater lung and mediastinum resolution and are commonly ordered, the routine chest x-ray (cxr) is lower in cost and has less radiation exposure. The noncontrast ct has a radiation exposure of

7.00 millisieverts, whereas a routine cxr has an exposure of 0.02; concerning cost, national data from commercial insurance and Medicare show a cost range of $620-$386 for chest ct; the cost range for a cxr is $77-$51. Detailed analysis of chest radiographs are reviewed in the Radiology chapter.

The replications of chest radiographs in Figure 6.1 show characteristic changes of infiltrates or lung lesions in all five lobes.

Other chest imaging *Chest CT* is modality of choice for evaluating lung or thoracic abnormalities detected on a routine cxr; excellent for lung parenchyma, mediastinum, and chest wall abnormalities.

High-resolution CT (HRCT) produces cross-section images of 1–2 mm, in contrast to usual ct cross-sections of 7–10 mm; excellent for delineation of lung parenchyma and small airways, especially in interstitial lung disease.

Helical CT produces quicker ct scans with single-breath imaging, contrast images with collection of continuous data, and may develop three-dimensional (3-D) images. In 2010, the National Cancer Institute (NCI) reported on a lung cancer screening study that included participants who were between 55 and 74 years of age and who were smokers of at least 30 pack-years. The participants were randomized to low-dose helical ct or to screening routine chest radiographs. The findings indicated that screening with low-dose helical ct was beneficial in reducing mortality from lung cancer. Nonetheless, the nci recommended further lung cancer screening studies and advocated cost-effective review of low-dose helical ct for lung cancer screening.

Magnetic resonance imaging (MRI) is less sensitive than chest ct in the evaluation of lung parenchyma; effective for study of chest wall, breast, and mediastinum.

Nuclear medicine techniques Ventilation and perfusion nuclear scans were previously used to diagnose PE; ct angiography is now the radiographic tool of choice to evaluate for PE. Ventilation/perfusion ($\dot{V}/\dot{Q}$) scans are helpful in preoperative analysis of lung resection candidates, for regional blood flow and ventilation functional analysis of the proposed lung to be removed, and in calculating its contribution or noncontribution to overall lung function in comparison to the uninvolved lung.

Positron emission tomography (PET) scans utilize a radiolabeled glucose compound, fluoro-2-deoxyglucose, which is absorbed by metabolically active cells. 18-F decays and is detected by the PET camera. PET is useful for evaluation of solitary pulmonary nodules and for the inclusion or exclusion of metastatic lung disease. False negatives occur with neoplastic processes of low metabolic activity, such as carcinoid tumors and bronchioloalveolar carcinoma. False-positive results are detected in inflammatory processes having a high metabolic activity, such as pneumonias and inflammatory, granulomatous disorders.

Pulmonary angiography uses the direct injection of radiographic contrast dye into the pulmonary artery for evaluation of the pulmonary vasculature; it can be used to rule out PE or evaluate for arteriovenous malformations or congenital abnormalities of the pulmonary circulation.

CT angiography is presently the technique of choice for diagnosing PE; used instead of pulmonary angiography. ct angioradiography is ideal for the assessment of aortic aneurysms, aortic dissection, and of posttraumatic aortic arch injury. ct angiography uses less contrast material and is less risky than pulmonary angiography.

Ultrasound (US) of the chest uses echo images differentiate among tissue, air, and fluid, due to their differing acoustic properties. US is used for the detection and localization of pleural effusions, of an empyema, and for adjunct diagnosis of pneumothoraces. US is additive in percutaneous-guided thoracentesis or for biopsy of pleural/chest wall lesions and for guidance in placement of chest tubes. Portable US is useful in intensive care units for these applications and for evaluation of diaphragmatic movement.

Virtual bronchoscopy produces 3-D generated images from the multidetector ct (mdct); utilizes multiple sensors along the scanning axis; e.g., the mdct, 64-slice technique. Computers then generate a compilation of images to form a virtual bronchoscope image; there is high radiation exposure, but extraordinary images with significant airway specificity.

Figure 6.1

Left upper lobe collapse

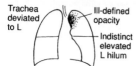

Trachea deviated to L

Ill-defined opacity

Indistinct elevated L hilum

Sharply defined posterior border due to anterior displacement of oblique fissure

Left lower lobe collapse

Triangular opacity visible through the heart with loss of medial end of diaphragm

Oblique fissure displaced posteriorly

Lingular consolidation

Indistinct L heart border

Right upper lobe collapse

Trachea deviated to R

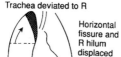

Horizontal fissure and R hilum displaced upwards

Triangular opacity with well-defined margins

Right middle lobe collapse

Horizontal fissure displaced down
Ill-defined opacity adjacent to R heart border
Loss of R heart border

Well-defined triangular opacity running from hilum

Right lower lobe collapse

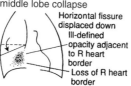

Horizontal fissure displaced downwards

Oblique fissure and hilum displaced posteriorly
Well-defined posterior opacity

Well-defined opacity adjacent to R heart border (R heart border still visible)

Clinical studies in pulmonary medicine

Sputum examination Collect a good sample; deep cough expectoration. Observe the appearance: Clear and colorless (chronic bronchitis), yellow/green (pulmonary infection), blood-streaked or grossly bloody (hemoptysis), black (smoke, coal), or frothy white/pink (pulmonary edema). Send the sample to the laboratory for microscopic examination: Gram stain for bacteria, special stains for fungi and mycobacterium, and for culture or cytology if indicated.

Peak expiratory flow (PEF) is measured by a maximal forced expiration through a peak flow meter or during routine pulmonary function studies (Figure 6.2).

PEF correlates well with the forced expiratory volume in 1 second (FEV_1) and is used as an estimate of airway caliber. PEF may be measured regularly in asthmatics to monitor response to therapy, disease control, and in the early detection of acute asthmatic exacerbations. See Figure 6.3.

Pulse oximetry is a noninvasive determination of peripheral O_2 saturation. Pulse oximetry is a valuable tool in clinical circumstances for the assessment of criticality of a patient's illness. It is also helpful in stable outpatient settings in determining the need and/or effectiveness of home or portable oxygen utilization. Normal O_2 saturation is between 96–98%. Oxygen saturation readings are useful in chronic obstructive pulmonary disease (COPD), as well as in acute or chronic congestive heart failure. Evaluating oxygen saturation during light exercise and during sleep are additive in judging severity of a pulmonary illness. Erroneous readings may occur with poor peripheral perfusion such as in Raynaud's phenomena and in instances of finger motion, presence of nail polish or rings, and in carbon monoxide intoxication. If pulse oximetry yields variable results then arterial blood gases (ABGs) are indicated (p. 177).

155

Arterial blood gas (ABG) analysis Heparinized blood is taken from the radial, brachial, or femoral artery, and pH, P_aO_2, and P_aCO_2 are measured using an automated analyzer. Remember to indicate the FiO_2 (fraction/percentage of inspired oxygen) on the requisition form.

- *Acid-base balance:* Normal pH is 7.35–7.45. A pH <7.35 indicates *acidosis* and a pH >7.45 indicates *alkalosis*.
- *Oxygenation:* Normal P_aO_2 is 85–100 mm Hg. Hypoxia is caused by one or more of ventilation/perfusion (V/Q) mismatch, hypoventilation, abnormal diffusion, right-to-left cardiac shunts. Of these, V/Q mismatch is the most common cause. Severe hypoxia is defined as a P_aO_2 <60 mm Hg.
- *Ventilation efficiency:* Normal P_aCO_2 is 35–45 mm Hg. P_aCO_2 is directly related to alveolar ventilation. A P_aCO_2 <35 mm Hg indicates *hyperventilation* and a P_aCO_2 >45 mm Hg indicates *hypoventilation*. Type I respiratory failure, or insufficient oxygenation, is defined as P_aO_2 <60 mm Hg and P_aCO_2 <45 mm Hg; Type II respiratory failure, or failure of alveolar ventilation, is defined as P_aO_2 <60 mm Hg and P_aCO_2 >45 mm Hg.

Alveolar–arterial O_2 concentration gradient may be calculated from the FiO_2, P_aO_2, and P_aCO_2. See Alveolar-arterial oxygen gradient calculation in Table 6.1.

Spirometry is a measurement of air flow and is used to evaluate the degree of obstruction in asthma, COPD, and bronchiectasis. FEV_1 and forced vital capacity (FVC) are measured from a full deep inspiration to a forced expiration into spirometer; exhalation continues until no more breath can be exhaled. Both FVC and FEV_1 are effort-dependent, yet FEV_1 is less effort-dependent than PEF. The FEV_1/FVC ratio gives a good estimate of severity of airflow obstruction; normal FEV_1/FVC ratio is 75–80%. See Figure 6.4.

Table 6.1 (Aa)po$_2$: The alveolar–arterial (Aa) oxygen gradient

The Aa oxygen gradient is the difference in the partial pressures of oxygen between the alveolar air and arterial blood. The normal Aa gradient for individuals ≤25 yrs is 2–12 mm Hg; however, aging influences the Aa gradient as normal for a 75-year-old is 12–25 mm Hg.

The partial pressure of oxygen in arterial blood is determined with ABG analysis. The partial pressure in alveolar air is calculated using the alveolar gas equation. This calculation is based on the body's oxygen consumption, which in turn is related to oxygen uptake and metabolic carbon dioxide production; the ratio of O_2 uptake/CO_2 production is called **R**, the respiratory quotient (≈0.85); this respiratory quotient depends on diet and on particular foods being metabolized. The partial pressure of alveolar oxygen calculation uses barometric pressure (**P^B** ≈ 760 mm Hg at sea level) and **P$_{H_2O}$**, the water saturation of airway gas (P_{H_2O} ≈ 47 mm Hg, as inspired air is usually fully saturated by the time it gets to the carina). P_AO_2 clearly depends on F_iO_2, the fractional concentration of O_2 in inspired air; e.g., F_iO_2 is 0.5 if breathing 50% O_2 and 0.21 if breathing room air). So:

$$P_AO_2 = (P_B + P_{H_2O}) \times F_iO_2 - P_aCO_2/R$$
$$= (760 + 47) \times F_iO_2 - P_aCO_2/0.8 \text{ (at sea level)}$$
$$= 713 \times F_iO_2 - 1.25 \times P_aCO_2$$

Once alveolar oxygen is determined, the difference between alveolar oxygen and arterial oxygen represents the Aa gradient. This calculation is especially useful in clinical instances of hypoventilation when the pCO$_2$ is high and one is determining the degree of hypoxemia related to hypoventilation; it is also useful in determining the degree/severity of hypoxemia with normal or low pCO$_2$.

- *Obstructive defect* (e.g., asthma, COPD): FEV$_1$ is reduced more than the FVC and the FEV$_1$/FVC ratio is <70%.
- *Restrictive defect* (e.g., interstitial fibrosis, or chest wall disorder): FVC is reduced and the FEV$_1$/FVC ratio is normal or raised. Other causes: Sarcoidosis; pneumoconiosis; interstitial pneumonias; connective tissue diseases; obesity; kyphoscoliosis; neuromuscular problems.

Pulmonary function tests PEF, FEV$_1$, FVC (p. 154). *Total lung capacity* (TLC) and *residual volume* (RV) are useful in distinguishing obstructive and restrictive diseases. TLC and RV are ↑ in obstructive airways disease and ↓ in restrictive lung diseases and musculoskeletal, chest wall limiting abnormalities. The *diffusing capacity* (DLCO) measuring gas exchange across the alveolar membrane is calculated by measuring carbon monoxide uptake from a single inspiration in a standard time (usually 10 sec). The diffusion capacity is reduced in emphysema and interstitial lung disease; it is high in alveolar hemorrhage. DLCO can be corrected for alveolar volume in appropriate circumstances.[1] *Flow volume loop* measures flow at various lung volumes. Characteristic flow-volume patterns are seen with intra-thoracic airways obstruction (asthma, emphysema) and extrathoracic airways obstruction (vocal cord paralysis, large goiter).

1 Johnson D. Importance of Adjusting Carbon Monoxide Diffusion Capacity and Carbon Monoxide Transfer Co-Efficient for Alveolar Volume. *Respir Med.* 2000;94:28–37.

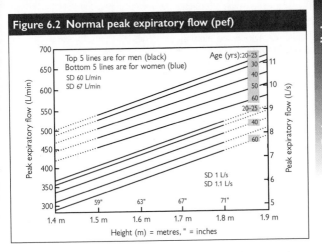

Figure 6.2 Normal peak expiratory flow (pef)

Top 5 lines are for men (black)
Bottom 5 lines are for women (blue)
SD 60 L/min
SD 67 L/min

Age (yrs):20–25
30
40
50
60
20–25
40
60

SD 1 L/s
SD 1.1 L/s

Peak expiratory flow (L/min)

Peak expiratory flow (L/s)

59"   63"   67"   71"

1.4 m   1.5 m   1.6 m   1.7 m   1.8 m   1.9 m

Height (m) = metres, " = inches

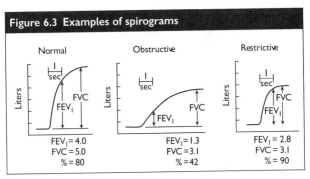

Figure 6.3 Examples of spirograms

Normal

Obstructive

Restrictive

FEV₁ = 4.0
FVC = 5.0
% = 80

FEV₁ = 1.3
FVC = 3.1
% = 42

FEV₁ = 2.8
FVC = 3.1
% = 90

157

Radiology For techniques, refer to Radiology chapter.

Fiberoptic bronchoscopy is performed under conscious sedation and local anesthetic via the nose or mouth. *Diagnostic indications:* Suspected lung malignancy, slowly resolving pneumonia, pneumonia in the immunosuppressed, interstitial lung disease. Bronchial lavage fluid may be sent to the lab for microscopy, culture, and cytology. Mucosal abnormalities may be brushed (cytology) and biopsied (histopathology). *Therapeutic indications:* Aspiration of mucus plugs causing lobar collapse or removal of foreign bodies. *Preprocedure investigations:* CBC, CXR, spirometry, pulse oximetry and ABG (if indicated); coagulation studies, especially in clinical circumstances of recent anticoagulation treatment and/or probable use of endobronchial lung biopsy. *Complications:* Respiratory depression, bleeding, pneumothorax (X-RAY PLATE 6).

Bronchoalveolar lavage (BAL) is performed at the time of bronchoscopy by instilling and aspirating a known volume of warmed buffered 0.9% saline into the distal airway. *Diagnostic indications:* Suspected malignancy, pneumonia in the immunosuppressed (especially HIV), suspected tuberculosis (TB; If sputum negative), interstitial lung diseases (e.g., sarcoidosis, extrinsic allergic alveolitis, histiocytosis X). *Therapeutic indications:* Alveolar proteinosis. *Complications:* Hypoxia, transient fever, transient CXR shadow, and procedure-related infection.

Lung biopsy may be performed in several ways. *Percutaneous needle biopsy* is performed under radiological guidance and is useful for peripheral lung and pleural lesions. *Transbronchial biopsy* performed during bronchoscopy may help in diagnosing diffuse lung diseases (e.g., sarcoidosis or diagnosing lung nodules, masses). If these biopsies are unsuccessful, an *open lung biopsy* may be performed under general anesthesia.

Surgical procedures are performed under general anesthesia. *Rigid bronchoscopy* provides a wider bronchoscope lumen, enables larger mucosal biopsies and control of bleeding, and allows the removal of foreign bodies. *Mediastinoscopy and mediastinotomy* enables examination and biopsy of the mediastinum lymph nodes/lesions.

Video-assisted-thoracoscopy (VAT) uses video technology and involves the insertion of VAT tubing through intercostal incisions. This procedure enables the operator to visualize the pleural space and to biopsy not only lesions in the pleural space but also lesions in the periphery of the lung. VAT has supplanted the use of open thoracotomy, yet the latter may be use in specific clinical circumstances.

Thoracoscopy allows examination and biopsy of pleural lesions, drainage of pleural effusions, and various pleurodesis.

Figure 6.4 Lung volumes: Physiological and pathological

(a)

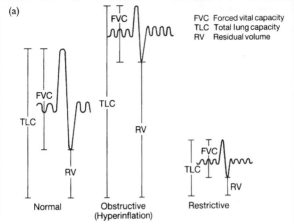

FVC Forced vital capacity
TLC Total lung capacity
RV Residual volume

Normal

Obstructive
(Hyperinflation)

Restrictive

Flow volume loops

(b)

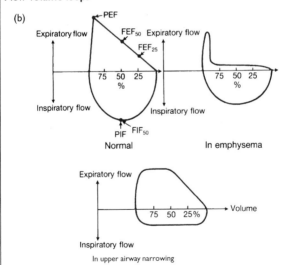

Normal

In emphysema

In upper airway narrowing

PEF, peak expiratory flow; FEF_{50}, forced expiratory flow at 50% TLC; FEF_{25}, forced expiratory flow at 25% TLC; PIF, peak inspiratory flow; FIF_{50}, forced inspiratory flow at 50% TLC.

Pneumonia

Pneumonia is an infection of the lung parenchyma and commonly presents with symptoms of fever, chest pain, cough and shortness of breath along with other systemic symptoms. Pneumonia may be categorized into three major pathognomonic groups: Community-acquired pneumonia (CAP); health care-acquired pneumonia (HCAP); this group includes hospital-acquired pneumonia (HAP) and ventilator-associated pneumonia (VAP), in addition to pneumonia acquired in institutions such as nursing homes and chronic care institutions. The last category of lung infections is *pneumonia in immunocompromised individuals*. One of the most critical problems in treating pneumonia is the evolution of multiple drug-resistant bacteria occurring not only in HCAP but also in CAP.

Classification and causes

1 CAP may be primary or secondary to underlying disease: *Streptococcus pneumoniae* is the most common, followed by *Haemophilus influenza, Mycoplasma pneumonia, Staphylococcus aureus, Legionella* species, and *Chlamydia*. Gram-negative bacilli, *Coxiella burnetii*, and anaerobes are rare. Viruses may account for up to 15–18% of CAP.

2 *HCAP(nosocomial and other health care institutions)* (>48 h after admission): Most common organisms in this group of pneumonia include enterobacteria or *Staphylococcus aureus*-methicillin resistant, *Streptococcus pneumonia*; *Pseudomonas, Klebsiella, Bacteroides, Clostridia, Haemophilus influenza*, and *Acinetobacter*.

3 *Aspiration pneumonia:* These pneumonias commonly occur in persons with impaired upper airway defence mechanisms, such as in patients with cerebral vascular events, myasthenia gravis, bulbar palsies, and those with altered level of consciousness (e.g., postseizure, or alcohol intoxication; other clinical instances predisposing to aspiration pneumonia include esophageal disease (achalasia, reflux) and persons with poor dental hygiene (a risk for aspirating oropharyngeal anaerobes).

Pneumonia in immunocompromised patients is related to the type and location of the neoplasm and to competency of the patient's bone marrow; i.e., the presence or absence of neutropenia or of lymphocyte depletion. *S. pneumoniae, H. influenza, S. aureus, Enterobacter*, other gram-negative bacilli, and *Pneumocystis*; fungi, viruses (cytomegalovirus [CMV], herpes simplex virus [HSV]), and mycobacteria.

4 *VAP:* The occurrence of VAP is related to the duration of artificial ventilation and to the colonization of the oropharynx with pathogenic organisms. VAP is associated with multiple drug-resistant organisms, with excessive sedation, and with aspiration of secretions from above the endotracheal or tracheal cuff; also, these pneumonias are associated with altered normal defense mechanisms such as in anemia, hyperglycemia, and malnutrition.

Clinical features of pneumonia *Symptoms:* Fever, rigors, malaise, anorexia, dyspnea, cough, and purulent sputum, hemoptysis, and pleuritic chest pain. *Signs:* Fever, cyanosis, confusion (may be the only sign in the elderly), tachypnea, tachycardia, hypotension, signs of consolidation (diminished expansion, dull percussion note, ↑ tactile vocal fremitus/vocal resonance, bronchial breathing), and a pleural rub.

Clinical studies are aimed to establish diagnosis, identify pathogen, and assess severity (see below). *CXR* (X-RAY PLATES 5 and 8): Lobar or multilobar infiltrates, cavitation, or pleural effusion. *Assess oxygenation:* Oxygen saturation (ABGs if s_aO_2 <92% or severe pneumonia). *Blood tests:* CBC, electrolytes, liver function tests (LFT), c-reactive protein (CRP), blood cultures. *Sputum:* For microscopy and culture; in severe cases, check for *Legionella* (sputum culture, urine antigen), atypical organism/viral serology (complement fixation tests acute/chronic-paired serology); may check for pneumococcal, legionella antigen in urine, sputum, or blood. *Pleural fluid* may be aspirated for culture. Consider *bronchoscopy* and BAL if patient is immunocompromised or if with multilobar, critical pneumonia.

Management (p. 708): *Antibiotics* (see Table 6.2, p. 162) may be administered orally if the pneumonia in uncomplicated and if the patient's oral intake is adequate. *Oxygen:* Keep P_aO_2 >60 and/or saturation ≥92%. *IV fluids:* Treatment of dehydration, shock. In severe pneumonia, treatment should consist of IV antibiotics; critical care utilization may be necessary if the patient does not improve quickly or if hypotension, hypercapnia, or uncorrected hypoxia evolve.

Complications of pneumonia (p. 161): Pleural effusion, empyema, lung abscess, respiratory failure, septicemia, brain abscess, pericarditis, myocarditis, cholestatic jaundice. Repeat CRP and CXR in patients not progressing satisfactorily.

Preventing pneumococcal infection Pneumococcal vaccine (23-valent Pneumovax II® 0.5 mL SC) indicated in:

- Chronic heart or lung conditions
- Cirrhosis
- Nephrosis
- Diabetes mellitus (DM)
- Immunosuppression (e.g., splenectomy, AIDS, or on chemotherapy).

CI: Pregnancy, lactation, fever. If high risk of fatal pneumococcal infection (asplenia, sickle-cell disease, nephrosis, post-transplant), revaccinate after 5 yrs.

Influenza prevention: Both inactivated and live attenuated vaccines are available for influenza A and B; inactivated vaccines are effective in 50–80% of persons in offering protection with a low incidence of adverse effects. Live attenuated vaccines may be administered in children with a 90% incidence of protection. Usually given by intranasal method; approved for use in nonpregnant healthy individuals 2–49 yrs. For inactivated vaccinations, the U.S. Public Health Service recommends vaccination of all persons >6 months.

Antiviral chemoprophylaxis is effective yet the evolution of viral resistance has limited the use of antiviral medications. *Recommended:* Zanamivir and oseltamivir have been >80% effective, yet amantadine and rimantadine are no longer recommended due to viral resistance to these drugs.

Table 6.2 Antibiotic treatment of pneumonia

Clinical setting	Organisms	Antibiotic
Community acquired		
Healthy w/o antibiotics in past 3 months	*Streptococcus pneumoniae, Haemophilus influenzae*	Azithromycin 500 mg PO once, then 250 mg/d for 4 days or clarithromycin 500 mg PO bid for 10 days
Antibiotics In past 3 months with comorbid diseases	*Streptococcus pneumoniae, Haemophilus influenzae, Mycoplasma pneumoniae*	Doxycycline 100 mg PO bid for 10 days Amoxicillin 1 g PO tid; or Augmentin 2 g bid or Cephitraxone 1–2 g IV qd or
Multilobar pneumonia w/o ICU care-hospitalized patient	Similar plus *Staph*, possible anaerobes	Cefuroxime 500 mg PO bid along with a macrolide Moxifloxacin 400 mg PO qd or Levofloxacin 750 mg PO qd Moxifloxacin 400 mg PO/IV qd or levofloxacin 750 mg PO/IV qd
Multilobar pneumonia-severe-ICU care	As above, plus gram-negative immunosuppressed patient	Cefotaxime 1–2 g IV q8h Ceftriaxone 1–2 g IV q8h Ertapenem 1 g IV qd Plus: Macrolide IV-clarithromycin, azithromycin Cefotaxime 1–2 g IV q8h Ceftriaxone 2 g IV qd Plus: Azithromycin IV or fluoroquinolone IV

Atypical	Legionella pneumophila	Clarithromycin 500 mg/12 h PO/IV ± rifampin
	Chlamydia sp.	Tetracycline
	Pneumocystis jiroveci	High-dose co-trimoxazole (p. 570)
Health care-associated pneumonias	Gram-negative bacilli, Pseudomonas, Anaerobes	Aminoglycoside IV + antipseudomonal penicillin IV or third-generation cephalosporin IV (p. 530)
Aspiration	Streptococcus pneumoniae, Anaerobe	Third-generation cephalosporin IV + clindamycin 600 mg/6 h IV
Immunocompromised patients	Gram-positive cocci, Gram-negative bacilli Fungi (p. 169)	Aminoglycoside IV + antipseudomonal penicillin IV or third-generation cephalosporin IV
		Consider antifungals after 48 h

Third-generation, e.g., cefotaxime (p. 530); gentamicin is an example of an aminoglycoside (p. 532).

Specific pneumonias

Pneumococcal pneumonia is the most common bacterial pneumonia, affecting all ages, yet is more common in the elderly, alcoholics, post-splenectomy patients, immunosuppressed patients, and patients with chronic heart failure or pre-existing lung disease. *Clinical features*: Fever, pleurisy, malaise, shortness of breath. CXR shows lobar consolidation. *Treatment*: Refer to Antibiotic Treatment Chart/Infectious disease chapter.

Staphylococcal pneumonia may complicate an influenza infection and may occur in the young, elderly, or in IV drug users, or in patients with underlying lung disease, such as cystic fibrosis (CF), or in immunosuppressed patients; frequently isolated in intubated patients in ICU, and a frequently causative agent in HAP. CAP secondary to Staph is usually associated with previous viral, influenza infection. *Treatment*: Refer to Antibiotic Treatment Chart/Infectious disease chapter.

Klebsiella pneumonia commonly occurs in individuals with comorbid diseases, COPD, DM, or alcoholism; frequent pathogen in HAP, with high incidence in hospitals and long-term care facilities; usually related to colonization of oropharynx; also seen in VAP; associated with pneumonia-related complications such as abscess formation, pulmonary necrosis, empyema. *Treatment*: Refer to Antibiotic Treatment Chart/Infectious disease chapter.

Pseudomonas is a common pathogen in bronchiectasis and CF. In CF, *Pseudomonas* infections are usually chronic and may never be completely eradicated; treatment in CF involves IV as well as inhalational therapy with aminoglycosides. *Pseudomonas* is commonly found in HAP most specifically in VAP; also causes hospital acquired infections, particularly in the ICU or postoperative surgery units. *Treatment*: Refer to Antibiotic Treatment Chart/ID chapter.

Mycoplasma pneumoniae occurs in sporadic epidemics about every 4–7 yrs. A frequent cause of community acquired respiratory illnesses in children and adults. Common presentations are flu-like symptoms, headache, myalgias, and, most commonly, a dry cough. Wheezes and crackles are detected in a large percentage of patients with *Mycoplasma* pneumonia. Treatment with penicillin and cephalosporins are ineffectual, whereas treatment with macrolides and others definitely shorten the duration of illness. *Diagnosis*: Polymerase chain reaction detection of *Mycoplasma* in upper respiratory secretions, tracheal secretions; IgM and IgG antibodies; enzyme-linked immune assay (primarily recommended). Cold agglutinins may cause an autoimmune hemolytic anemia; extrapulmonary complications include septic arthritis, Guillain-Barré syndrome, erythema multiforme, aseptic meningitis. *Treatment*: Azithromycin, clarithromycin, doxycycline, moxifloxacin and levofloxacin.

Legionella pneumophila colonizes water containers kept at <60°C (hotel air-conditioning and hot water systems); inhalation or aspiration of contaminated water results in outbreaks of Legionnaire's disease. Incubation period is usually 2–10 d; flu-like symptoms with especially high fever, malaise, precede a dry cough and dyspnea.

Chest discomfort and shortness of breath occur in 30–50% of patients. Extrapulmonary features include anorexia, diarrhea, vomiting, hepatitis, renal failure, confusion, and coma. CXR shows bibasal consolidation. Laboratory studies may show lymphopenia, hyponatremia. *Diagnosis*: Legionella serology/urine antigen. *Treatment*: Macrolides ± rifampin, or fluoroquinolone. 10% mortality.

Chlamydia pneumoniae is the most common chlamydial infection and may account for about 10% of CAP; person-to-person spread occurs, causing pharyngitis, hoarseness, otitis, followed by pneumonia. *Diagnosis*: Serology polymerase chain reaction (PCR) and culture. *Treatment*: Erythromycin, azithromycin, tetracycline, clarithromycin, fluoroquinolones.

Chlamydia psittaci causes psittacosis, an ornithosis acquired from infected birds, parrots, parakeets, turkeys, and ducks; greatest exposure to bird owners and poultry workers. Symptoms include headache, fever, dry cough, lethargy, arthralgia, anorexia, and diarrhea. CXR shows patchy consolidation. Diagnosis: *Chlamydia* serology. *Treatment*: Tetracycline 250 mg qid for at least 3 wks to avoid relapse; also erythromycin 500 mg qid.

Viral pneumonia: The development of viral diagnostic studies, PCR, tissue cultures, and immunofluorescence, have improved the detection of viruses; viral analyses have discovered viruses as a more frequent causative agent in both CAP and in HAP, with an incidence of 15–18%. In CAP, the most common viruses are influenza A/B and respiratory syncytial virus, as well as adenovirus, parainfluenza virus, rhinovirus, coronavirus, and the SARS virus; in HAP, the causative viruses are herpes simplex and cytomegalovirus.

Pneumocystis pneumonia: *Pneumocystis* is a world -wide distributed fungus that commonly colonizes immunosuppressed patients and persons with COPD. This opportunistic organism is a frequent cause of pneumonia in immunocompromised patients. Combination of cellular and humoral deficiencies predispose to *Pneumocystis* infection. Clinical presentation is relatively nonspecific; CXR may be normal or show bilateral perihilar interstitial infiltrates. *Diagnosis*: Visualization of the organism in induced sputum, BAL, or in lung biopsy specimens. *Treatment*: First choice is trimethoprim-sulfamethoxazole, 14 d treatment for non-HIV; 21 d therapy for HIV patients. Alternative treatments include trimethoprim with dapsone, clindamycin plus primaquine, pentamidine. *Prophylaxis for Pneumocystis*: First choice is trimethoprim-sulfamethoxazole, in patients with and without HIV, recovering from *Pneumocystis* pneumonia.

Complications of pneumonia

Respiratory failure (p. 176): Hypoxemia, respiratory failure (P_aO_2 <60 mm Hg) is relatively common. Treatment is with high-flow (60%) oxygen. *Transfer the patient to icu if hypoxia does not improve with O_2 therapy or P_aCO_2 rises to >45 mm Hg. Careful O_2 administration is required in COPD patients; check ABG frequently and consider elective mechanical ventilation if rising P_aCO_2 or worsening acidosis and hypoxemia.

Hypotension may be due to a combination of dehydration and vasodilatation due to bacteremia/ sepsis. If systolic blood pressure (BP) is <90 mm Hg, give an IV fluid challenge of 250 mL colloid/crystalloid over 15 min. If BP does not rise, insert a central line and infuse IV fluids to maintain the systolic BP >90 mm Hg. If systolic BP remains <90 mm Hg despite fluid therapy, asses for vasopressive support.

Atrial fibrillation (p. 120) is a quite common arrhythmia, particularly in the elderly; usually resolves with treatment of the pneumonia. Digoxin, calcium-channel blockers, or β-blockers may be required to slow the ventricular response rate.

Pleural effusion Inflammation of the pleura by adjacent pneumonia may cause fluid exudation into the pleural space. If fluid accumulates in the pleural space faster than reabsorption, a pleural effusion develops. If the effusion is small, <10% of the hemithorax area, then it may be of little consequence. If it becomes larger and symptomatic, or infected (empyema), drainage is required (pp. 180, 661).

Empyema is pus within the pleural space; clinically suspected if a patient with pneumonia and a pleural effusion does not respond to antibiotic therapy or if a patient with a resolving pneumonia develops a recurrent fever. Diagnosed by clinical features and a CXR indicating a pleural effusion. The aspirated pleural fluid is typically yellow and turbid, or with frank pus, with a pH <7.1, glucose↓, and lactate dehydrogenase(LDH)↑. The empyema should be drained using a chest drain, preferably inserted under sonographic guidance.

Lung abscess is a cavitating area of localized, suppurative infection within the lung.

Causes:

- Inadequately treated pneumonia
- Aspiration (e.g., alcoholism, esophageal obstruction, bulbar palsy)
- Bronchial obstruction (tumor, foreign body)
- Pulmonary infarction
- Septic emboli (septicemia, right-heart endocarditis, IV drug use)
- Subphrenic or hepatic abscess.

Clinical features: Cyclical fever; cough; purulent, foul-smelling sputum; pleuritic chest pain; hemoptysis; malaise; weight loss. Look for finger clubbing, anemia. Empyema develops in 20–30% of lung abscesses.

Tests: Blood: CBC (anemia, neutrophilia), erythrocyte sedimentation rate (ESR), CRP, blood cultures. *Sputum:* Microscopy, culture, and cytology. *CXR:* Walled cavity, often with a fluid level. Consider CT scan to exclude obstruction, and bronchoscopy to obtain diagnostic specimens.

Treatment: Antibiotics as indicated by sensitivities; continue until healed (4–6 wks). Postural drainage. Repeated aspiration, antibiotic instillation, or surgical excision may be required.

Septicemia may occur as a result of bacterial spread from the lung parenchyma into the bloodstream. Bacteremia may cause physiologic changes of hypotension, tachycardia, renal insufficiency, and metastatic infection (e.g., infective endocarditis, meningitis). Treatment is with IV antibiotic according to sensitivities.

Pericarditis and myocarditis may also complicate pneumonia.

Jaundice This is usually cholestatic, and may be due to sepsis or secondary to antibiotic therapy (particularly penicillin or erythromycin derivatives).

Cystic fibrosis

Cystic fibrosis (CF) is an autosomal recessive disease that is classically detected in childhood, yet 5% of patients are diagnosed with CF as adults. The primary mutations occur in CFTR gene found on chromosome 7; at least, 1,400 mutations have been documented. CF manifests ethnic variability with 1 in 3,000 Caucasian births 1 in 17,000 births in African Americans and 1 in 90,000 in Asian populations. Although in previous decades the life expectancy of a CF patient was short, today's median survival is >40 yrs. The genetic defect in the CFTR gene causes abnormalities in sodium absorption and in chloride secretion; this dysfunction of electrolyte movement affects normal hydration of the pulmonary airways, pancreatic ducts, sweat glands, and sex glands. This genetically induced dehydration within the airways impairs ciliary movement and airway clearance, both primary defense mechanisms, thus leading to susceptibility to infections. See Table 6.3.

Clinical manifestations

Neonates and early childhood: Common presentation in neonates; one-fifth of neonates present within 24 hours of birth with GI obstruction, meconium ileus, emesis, inability to pass stool; within the first 2 yrs of life, respiratory tract infections are prominent, along with recurrent sinusitis.

Children and young adults: As with early childhood, respiratory manifestation are major; however, with older ages the evolution of pancreatic insufficiency and insulin deficiency are common. *Respiratory:* Cough, wheeze, recurrent infections, bronchiectasis, pneumothorax, common in 10% of CF patients, hemoptysis, respiratory failure, cor pulmonale. *Gastrointestinal:* Pancreatic insufficiency (DM, steatorrhea), distal intestinal obstruction syndrome ("meconium ileus equivalent"), gallstones, cirrhosis. *Other:* Male infertility, osteoporosis, arthritis, vasculitis, nasal polyps, sinusitis, and hypertrophic pulmonary osteoarthropathy (HPOA). *Signs:* Cyanosis, finger clubbing, bilateral coarse crackles.

Diagnosis The diagnosis of CF is usually apparent especially at younger ages; nonetheless, the combination of clinical presentation and an abnormal sweat chloride or an abnormal nasal potential differential (PD) measurements complete the diagnosis: An elevated sweat chloride is pathognomonic for CF. Furthermore, *CFTR* analysis is available. In the 5% of the adult population who have CF, the diagnosis may be more insidious; 1–2% of CF patients have a normal sweat chloride study yet their nasal PD measurements are abnormal. *Sweat test:* Sweat sodium and chloride >60 mmol/L; chloride usually > sodium. *Genetics:* cftr mutation analysis; DNA testing identifies CF mutations in over 90% of patients with CF.

Tests *Blood:* CBC, electrolytes, LFTs; clotting; vitamin A, D, E levels; annual glucose tolerance test. *Bacteriology:* Cough swab, sputum culture. *Radiology:* CXR: Hyperinflation, bronchiectasis. *Abdominal US:* Fatty liver, cirrhosis, chronic pancreatitis. *Spirometry:* Obstructive defect. *Aspergillus serology/skin test* (20% develop allergic bronchopulmonary aspergillosis [ABPA; p. 164]). *Biochemistry:* Fecal fat analysis.

Table 6.3 Management of cystic fibrosis

The cornerstones of treatment are the control of infections with antibiotics, the movement of secretions with inhalational treatments and mucous-modifying agents, the use of chest physiotherapy, and the creation of a multidisciplinary plan involving parents, nurses, respiratory therapists, dieticians, and psychologists. Although 95% of CF patients expire as a consequence of pulmonary infections, the use of antibiotics in acute events, as well as their use in preventative therapy, have dramatically improved survival. The most common organisms are *Pseudomonas*, and *S. aureus, H. influenza*. Antibiotics in acute circumstances are administered IV; in subacute or chronic situations, antibiotics may be given orally and in inhalational solutions/therapy. With mild exacerbations, oral penicillin, cephalosporin, or ciprofloxacin, along with inhaled tobramycin or Colistin and chest physiotherapy are effective. In moderately severe or severe infections, antibiotic coverage is broadened to include cephalosporins and aminoglycosides IV, along with hospitalization and aggressive chest physiotherapy and antibiotic inhalational treatment.

Therapies to diminish the viscosity of the chronically infected sputum are mucolytic agents, hypertonic saline, and recombinant DNA. Breathing exercises, chest percussion, postural drainage, and mechanisms to improve mucociliary clearance are instrumental along with antibiotics in preserving lung function and modifying the progression of CF.

Gastrointestinal: Pancreatic enzyme replacement; fat soluble vitamin supplements (A, D, E, K); ursodeoxycholic acid for impaired liver function.

Other: Treatment of CF-related DM; screening for and treatment of osteoporosis; treatment of arthritis, sinusitis, and vasculitis; fertility and genetic counseling.

Advanced lung disease: Oxygen, diuretics (cor pulmonale); noninvasive ventilation; lung or heart/lung transplantation.

Prognosis: Median survival is >37.4 yrs.

Bronchiectasis

Bronchiectasis is a chronic infection of primarily the medium-sized airways, which results in irreversible dilation and destruction of the normal airway architecture. Bronchiectasis may be localized to one lobe or may be diffuse, involving all lobes of the lung; the extent of disease has a significant impact on clinical outcome. Classically, infections with *Bordetella pertussis* (whooping cough) in childhood have been associated with the development of bronchiectasis. Pulmonary infections with *Staph, Klebsiella, Pseudomonas, Haemophilus*, and anaerobes, as well as with adenovirus and influenza virus may be responsible for the evolution of bronchiectasis.

Tuberculosis is the major cause of bronchiectasis worldwide; atypical *Mycobacterium* infections may be a primary causative bacterium or more usually is a secondary infection. CF, with its thickened secretions and poor mucociliary clearance, is notoriously associated with bronchiectasis. Other predisposing causes of bronchiectasis include primary ciliary dyskinesis, hypogammaglobulinemia, HIV infections, endobronchial obstruction by a foreign body, and α_1-antitrypsin deficiency, as well as allergic bronchopulmonary aspergillosis, rheumatic diseases, and inhalation of toxic fumes.

Clinical features *Symptoms:* Constant or recurrent coughing of purulent sputum associated with recurrent respiratory tract infection is common in bronchiectasis; hemoptysis is common, occurring in 50–70% of patients. Historically, patients may recall an episode of pneumonia after which their symptoms of chronic cough started. On physical exam, auscultation of the chest may disclose a variety of sounds (crackles, rhonchi, wheezes), along with clubbing of digits, peripheral cyanosis, and signs of cor pulmonale. *Complications:* Pneumonia, pleural effusion; pneumothorax; hemoptysis; cerebral abscess.

Investigations *Sputum culture. CXR:* Cystic shadows, thickened bronchial walls (tram-tracking and ring shadows) Routine CXRs are the usual initial study, yet the most definitive radiographic study is CT and, especially, HRCT of the chest; it assesses the extent and distribution of disease. The findings are specific to the airways, with dilated thickened airways, cystic changes within the lung parenchyma with or without fluid levels, and saccular and peribronchial inflammatory changes of the airways. *Spirometry* often shows an obstructive airway pattern; reversibility with bronchodilators should be assessed. *Bronchoscopy:* Used to locate site of hemoptysis or exclude obstruction. *Other tests:* Serum immunoglobulins, CF sweat chloride test, *Aspergillus* precipitins.

Management/Treatment Treatment is fourfold: Treat infection, improve tracheobronchial clearance, diminish airway inflammation, and diagnose and/or reverse predisposing factors. Antibiotic selection is based on the clinical findings of acuity and on Gram stain and cultures; most commonly *Pseudomonas* and other gram-negative organisms, as well as *Staph*, are the offending bacteria; treatment with aminoglycosides and third-generation cephalosporins (e.g., carbapenem) is based on antibiotic sensitivity; in general, bronchiectasis requires a longer duration of treatment than other pulmonary infections, usually 14–21 d.

Medicated aerosol therapy with bronchodilators and normal saline diminish bronchial obstruction and promote bronchial dilation and thus airway clearance, especially in individuals with bronchiectasis with airway hyperactivity. Mucolytic agents and hydration of airways with IV fluid replacement or oral intake may thin secretions. Chest percussion and postural drainage may also facilitate secretion removal/expectoration. Fiberoptic bronchoscopy may be beneficial in instances of mucous plugging and airway obstruction. Decreasing generalized inflammation in airways is addressed with antibiotic treatment and purulent secretion removal; anti-inflammatory agents, such as leukotriene receptor antagonists and inhaled glucocorticosteroids, may be additive in reducing airway inflammation. In instances of localized bronchiectasis, surgery in the form of lobectomy is a reasonable approach to eliminating recurrent infections or hemoptysis; in cases of massive hemoptysis emanating from a specific lobe, surgical resection is relevant. A new approach in massive hemoptysis is bronchial artery embolization, most effectively used in cases of diffuse bronchiectasis where a single lobectomy is not indicated.

Lung abscess

Lung abscess is defined as an infectious process associated with necrosis of the lung parenchyma. Lung abscess are categorized as acute and chronic, and primary versus secondary. Acute lung abscesses occur with an immediate illness, whereas chronic lung abscesses are detected symptomatically or radiographically over 4–6 wks. Secondary lung abscesses occur with CF or in HIV infection, with lung neoplasms, in contrast to a primary lung abscess that develops in the absence of underlying pulmonary disorders (e.g., alcoholic-related aspiration). Common symptoms are fever, cough, fatigue, weight loss; lung abscesses are usually found in individuals with poor dental hygiene, pyorrhea, or gingivitis.

Physical examination is typically unrevealing; chest radiographs and chest CT are the primary methods for detecting and defining a lung abscess.

Routine sputum analysis is usually unreliable due to contamination of the specimen by upper airway organisms. Bronchoscopy with bronchial lavage should be helpful in establishing a diagnosis; CT-guided percutaneous drainage of a lung abscess may provide more specific identification of the cause and thus may facilitate more accurate antibiotic treatment.

Anaerobic bacteria are the most common finding in a primary lung abscess; other causes may include *Mycobacterium tuberculosis, Blastomycosis, Histoplasmosis, Coccidioidomycosis*, and atypical mycobacterium. In immunocompromised patients, causes of lung abscess are aspergillosis, *Nocardia, Legionella*, and *Klebsiella pneumonia*, in addition to the more common causes. In previously healthy individuals, S. *aureus, Streptococcus*, and *Klebsiella* and *Actinomyces* are causative considerations.

Treatment is based on identification of the causative organism; if an empyema is present, then pleural drainage is important; surgical resection is a consideration in cases of nonresponsiveness to antibiotics, yet lung resection is utilized in <10% of patients with lung abscess.

Fungal infection of the lung

Aspergillus This group of fungi affects the lung in five ways:

1 *Asthma:* This group includes those patients with severe asthma who may not meet clinical criteria of allergic bronchopulmonary aspergillosis, yet have considerable reactivity to the fungus; *Aspergillus fumigates* is a common fungus, thus commonly may be associated with asthma.
2 *Allergic bronchopulmonary aspergillosis:* The syndrome of ABPA consists of active asthma, whole blood eosinophilia, increased IgE level, pulmonary infiltrates and bronchial obstruction, bronchiectasis, and skin tests sensitivity to *A. fumigatus*. ABPA represent a hypersensitivity reaction to the fungus and is found in 1% of asthmatics and in up to 15% of CF patients. *Symptoms:* Wheeze, cough, sputum (plugs of mucus containing fungal hyphae), dyspnea, and "recurrent pneumonia." *Investigations:* CXR; transient segmental collapse or consolidation, central bronchiectasis, fleeting infiltrates; *Aspergillus* in sputum; positive *Aspergillus* skin test and/

or *Aspergillus*-specific IgE RAST; positive serum precipitins; eosinophilia; raised serum IgE. *Treatment:* Corticosteroids/Itraconazole.

3 *Aspergilloma:* A "fungus ball" within a pre-existing pulmonary cavity >2.5 cm in dimension; cavity often caused by TB, sarcoidosis; usually asymptomatic yet may cause cough, hemoptysis, lethargy ± weight loss (see Figure 6.5). Most common complication is life-threatening hemoptysis; may spontaneously resolve; however, the cavity is persistently infected. *Investigations:* CXR: Round opacity within a cavity, usually apical; sputum culture; strongly positive serum precipitins; *Aspergillus* skin test (30% +ve). *Treatment:* Surgery.

4 *Invasive aspergillosis is a true opportunistic organism in that primary risk factors for infection with this fungus are neutropenia and glucocorticosteroid use;* other risk factors: HIV, leukemia, underlying pulmonary disease, Wegener's granulomatosis, and systemic lupus erythematosus (SLE); treatment with antitumor necrosis factor may predispose to *Aspergillus* infection. Opportunistic infections are predominantly pulmonary and/or sinuses. *Investigations:* Sputum culture; serum precipitins; antigen detection; CXR findings include infiltrates, consolidation, or abscess; serum measurements of galactomannan (*Aspergillus* antigen) may be helpful. *Diagnosis:* Positive culture and confirmatory histology in affected tissue/ organ. In less than half of patients with invasive aspergillosis, the diagnosis is made postmortem. *Treatment:* IV itraconazole, caspofungin, micafungin, voriconazole, and Amphotericin B; voriconazole is preferred in invasive aspergillosis.

5 *Hypersensitivity pneumonitis:* Hypersensitivity to *A. clavatus/fumigatus* results in interstitial pneumonitis, eosinophilia associated with frequent expose to the fungus ("malt worker's lung"). Clinical features and treatment are as for other causes of EAA (p. 184). Diagnosis is based on a history of exposure and the presence of serum precipitins to *A. Clavatus/ fumigatus*. Pulmonary fibrosis may occur if untreated.

Histoplasmosis Infection with *Histoplasmosis capsulatum* is by inhalation of the microconidia; infections may vary from an asymptomatic presentation to a life-threatening illness; severity of illness depends on the extent of exposure, the health status of lungs, and cellular and humoral competence. In normal individuals residing in endemic areas, 50–80% may have chest radiograph or skin test evidence of prior exposure. In the United States, most common endemic areas are the Mississippi and Ohio River valleys. Most common presentations are in patients who seek medical attention with flu-like illnesses with chest radiographic changes of infiltrates associated with mediastinum lymphadenopathy and with a course of spontaneous resolution. The enlargement and subsequent calcification of chest lymph nodes is the most common finding in endemic areas, representing prior infection and usually requiring minimal evaluation or medical follow-up care.

In contrast, a most severe form of histoplasmosis is a progressive disseminated form that is most often found in immunocompromised individuals with HIV having a low T-cell count and in patients on immunosuppressive medications, such as prednisone and anti-tumor necrosis factor (TNF).

A chronic form of histoplasmosis is found in patients with emphysema and persistent smokers; usually associated with progressive chest radiographic changes of advancing infiltrates with or without cavitations.

Treatment is recommended in the chronic progressive form and in progressive disseminated histoplasmosis; preferred medications are lipid-formulations of Amphotericin B or Itraconazole; because acute histoplasmosis is self-limiting and is without clinical injury, treatment is not recommended.

Coccidioidomycosis is a fungal infection endemic to south-central Arizona, the southwestern United States, and the southern portion of the San Joaquin Valley of California, commonly described as "Valley Fever." The fungus exists in the soil as a filament yet subunits, *arthroconidia*, become airborne and cause disease through inhalation, predominately involving the lungs. Similar to histoplasmosis, coccidioidomycosis may be an asymptomatic subclinical infection, may present as a CAP, or rarely may present in a disseminated form. Along with the pulmonary infection, several skin manifestations of coccidioidomycosis occur and include erythema nodosum, erythema multiforme, and toxic erythema.

Usually, acute coccidioidomycosis infections resolve within weeks and do not require treatment; however, postinfection pulmonary nodules and cavities are notable. In immunosuppressed patients, the fungal pneumonia may progress to a diffuse pneumonia and rarely progress to a disseminated disease, not uncommonly including meningitis.

The diagnosis is usually based on travel and/or living within the endemic areas, presenting as a CAP. *Diagnostic findings*: Pulmonary infiltrates and positive serologic studies, including tube precipitin, complement fixation assays, immunodiffusion, and enzyme immunoassays to detect IgM and IgG antibodies. Coccidioidomycosis may be easily grown on culture and thus direct cultures are useful.

Treatment: Most cases of coccidioidomycosis do not need treatment; therapy is indicated in patients with a prolonged clinical course or who have extensive disease or in patients who are immunocompromised. Use fluconazole and itraconazole; Amphotericin in disseminated and meningitis cases.

Blastomycosis is primarily a pulmonary infection, yet skin manifestations of ulceration and verrucous lesions, as well as osteomyelitis, are common extrapulmonary conditions. Blastomycosis is found in the southeastern and south-central United States, and, similar to histoplasmosis, along the Ohio and Mississippi River basins. Acute blastomycosis presents with symptoms and signs of a community-acquired infection; it is frequently associated with epidemiological outbreaks. However, although spontaneous resolution is reported, progression is more usual. Most blastomycosis patients have a chronic pneumonia associated with fever, weight loss, and systemic symptoms. Blastomycosis has a high mortality rate in immunosuppressed patients. Diagnosis depends on the growth of the organism and *Blastomyces* antigen detection in serum and in urinary assays.

Treatment: Because prediction of those patients who may spontaneously resolve versus those patients who may progress/disseminate is impossible, almost all patients with blastomycosis require treatment with itraconazole, Amphotericin, or voriconazole.

Cryptococcosis is a rare fungal infection in individuals with normal humeral and cellular immune systems; infections commonly occur in patients with hematologic malignancies, HIV, with organ transplants, and in patients with high-dose glucocorticosteroids use. *Cryptococcus* infections are usually present as pneumonia or meningitis. *Cryptococcus* is usually inhaled as aerosolized particulate matter, and, depending on the immunologic status of the host, the organism is eliminated from the body or assumes a latent phase. A common presentation is chronic meningoencephalitis associated with headache, fever, and neurologic symptoms usually of several weeks duration. Pulmonary manifestations are less obvious with cough and possible fever, as numerous cases are discovered during an evaluation of an abnormal chest radiograph in an immunosuppressed patient. With India ink preparation, *Cryptococcus* may be found in the cerebrospinal fluid (CSF), along with positive cultures in the CSF and blood; diagnosis is also made with the *Cryptococcus* antigen in CSF/blood. Treatment is with fluconazole for pulmonary *Cryptococcus* in an immunocompetent individual; for extrapulmonary manifestations, Amphotericin B; for immunosuppressed patients, combination therapy with fluconazole, Amphotericin B, and flucytosine. Morbidity and mortality with and without treatment is high.

Figure 6.5

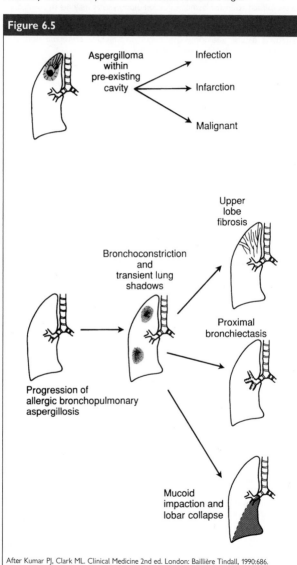

Aspergilloma within pre-existing cavity → Infection

→ Infarction

→ Malignant

Progression of allergic bronchopulmonary aspergillosis → Bronchoconstriction and transient lung shadows →

Upper lobe fibrosis

Proximal bronchiectasis

Mucoid impaction and lobar collapse

After Kumar PJ, Clark ML. Clinical Medicine 2nd ed. London: Baillière Tindall, 1990:686.

Neoplasms of the lung

Lung cancer is the leading cause of death in men and women; more patients die yearly from lung cancer than from breast, prostate, and colon cancers combined. Bronchogenic carcinoma accounts for about 30% of all cancer deaths/year. More women expire from lung neoplasm than from breast carcinoma; the 5-yr survival rate is now 15%; this survival improvement from previous decades is related to early detection and treatment regimens of surgery, radiation therapy, and chemotherapy. 85% of lung neoplasms are caused by cigarette smoking, found in both current smokers and former smokers. Conversely, 10–15% of lung neoplasms are discovered in individuals who have never smoked; a majority of these non-cigarette related tumors are found in women.

The major cell types are squamous cell carcinoma, adenocarcinoma, large cell carcinoma, and bronchoalveolar cell carcinoma. Although the distinction of cell types is important due to the differing cell type responses to treatment and clinical courses, the categorization into small cell carcinoma and non-small cell carcinoma is ultimately beneficial in consideration of treatment and outcomes. See Table 6.4.

Carcinoma of the bronchus Incidence is increasing in women. *Risk factors:* Cigarette smoking is the major risk factor. *Others:* Asbestos, chromium, arsenic, iron oxides, and radiation (radon gas). *Histology:* Squamous (30%), adenocarcinoma (30%), small cell (25%), large cell (15%), alveolar cell carcinoma (<1%). *Symptoms:* Cough (80%), hemoptysis (70%), dyspnea (60%), chest pain (40%), recurrent or slowly resolving pneumonia, anorexia, weight loss.

Signs: Cachexia, anemia, clubbing, hypertrophic pulmonary osteoarthropathy causing joint pain; supraclavicular or axillary lymphadenopathy. *Chest signs:* Chest exam may be normal yet may have auscultation/percussion findings of consolidation, collapse, pleural effusion. *Metastases:* Bone tenderness, hepatomegaly, confusion, seizures, myopathy, peripheral neuropathy. Lung neoplasms are uniquely associated with specific syndromes.

173

Pancoast syndrome Neoplastic growth from the apex of the lung into the eighth cervical and first/second thoracic nerves resulting in pain radiating into the arm and shoulder; often involving the first and second ribs.

Horner's syndrome Enophthalmos (an eye recessed into the orbit); ptosis (failure of eyelid opening); miosis (pupillary constriction), and, on the same side of the body, loss of sweating; the latter is related to sympathetic nerve invasion by tumor.

Superior vena cava syndrome Engorgement of the veins of the head, arms, and neck with facial edema associated with the obstruction of the superior vena cava by lung neoplasm; most instances of superior vena cava syndrome are medical emergencies. Treatment is aimed at alleviating elevated central venous pressure; usually represents a poor prognosis.

Endocrine syndromes

Hypercalcemia and hypophosphatemia associated with the production of PTH by a squamous cell carcinoma.

Antidiuretic hormone (adh) secretion by a small cell carcinoma results in inappropriately low serum sodium levels.

Adrenocorticotropic hormone(acth): Ectopic secretion by a tumor causing clinical findings of cortisone excess.

Eaton Lambert syndrome is usually associated with a small cell carcinoma of the lung; presentation of myasthenia gravis-like symptoms with proximal muscle and trunk weakness, with sparing of ocular dysfunction. Usually associated with increased muscle strength with repetitive contractions, in contrast to myasthenia gravis, in which muscle strength decreases with repetitive contractions; minimal response to edrophonium.

Trousseau's syndrome presents with migratory venous thrombophlebitis, especially with thrombosis in unusual areas of body.

Tests

Cytology: Sputum and pleural fluid. *CXR*: Peripheral abnormality or opacity; hilar enlargement; consolidation; lung collapse (X-RAY PLATE 4); pleural effusion; bony metastases. Peripheral lesions and superficial lymph nodes may be amenable to *percutaneous fine-needle aspiration/biopsy*. *Bronchoscopy*: To yield a histological diagnosis and to begin staging. *CT*: To stage the tumor. *Radionuclide bone scan*: For suspected metastases. *Lung function tests*: To asses physiologic staging.

Staging of a lung neoplasm requires a tissue diagnosis with lung or bronchial biopsies or biopsies of areas of obvious neoplastic disease. Once the diagnosis is established, then staging should be undertaken in two paths-one is anatomic staging and the other is physiologic staging.

Anatomic staging utilizes CT scans of the chest, brain, and abdomen; PET scans to search for yet-undetected metastatic disease; bone scans to search for osseous lesions. Refer to the anatomic staging Table 6.5 (p. 167).

Physiologic staging is aimed at assessing the overall ability of a patient to withstand surgery, radiation therapy, or chemotherapy; this staging includes laboratory studies, pulmonary function studies, cardiovascular assessment, and psychological appraisal.

Treatment: Non-small cell tumors: Excision is the treatment of choice for peripheral tumors, with no metastatic spread (~25%). *Curative radiotherapy* is an alternative in patients with inadequate respiratory reserve. *Small cell tumors* are almost always disseminated at presentation. They may respond to *chemotherapy*. *Palliation: Radiotherapy* is used for bronchial obstruction, superior vena cava obstruction, hemoptysis, bone pain, and cerebral metastases. *Endobronchial therapy* includes tracheal stenting, cryotherapy, laser therapy, and brachytherapy (a radioactive source is placed close to the tumor). *Pleural drainage/pleurodesis* for symptomatic pleural effusions. *Drug therapy*: Analgesia, corticosteroids, antiemetic, codeine, bronchodilators, antidepressants.

Prognosis: Non-small cell: 50% 2-yr survival without spread; 10% with spread. *Small cell:* Median survival is 3 months if untreated; 1–1.5 yrs if treated.

Prevention: Actively discourage smoking. Prevent occupational exposure to carcinogens.

Other lung tumors *Bronchial adenoma:* Rare, slow-growing tumor. 90% are carcinoid tumors; 10% are cylindromas. *Treatment:* Surgery. *Hamartoma:* Rare, benign tumor. *ct scan:* Lobulated mass with flecks of calcification. Often excised to exclude malignancy. *Mesothelioma* (p. 186).

Table 6.4 Coin lesions of the lung

• Malignancy (1° or 2°)	• Arteriovenous malformation
• Abscess	• Encysted effusion (fluid, blood, pus)
• Granulomata	• Cyst
• Carcinoid tumor	• Foreign body
• Pulmonary hamartoma	• Lung parenchyma scar

Table 6.5 TNM Staging for lung neoplasms

Primary tumor (T)	TX	Malignant cells in bronchial secretions, no other evidence of tumor
	Tis	Carcinoma *in situ*
	T0	None evident
	T1	≤3 cm, in lobar or more distal airway
	T2	>3 cm and >2 cm distal to carina *or* any size if pleural involvement *or* obstructive pneumonitis extending to hilum, but not all the lung
	T3	Involves the chest wall, diaphragm, mediastinal pleura, pericardium, or <2 cm from, but not at, carina
	T4	Involves the mediastinum, heart, great vessels, trachea, esophagus, vertebral body, carina, *or* a malignant effusion is present
Regional nodes (N)	N0	None involved (after mediastinoscopy)
	N1	Peribronchial and/or ipsilateral hilum
	N2	Ipsilateral mediastinum or subcarinal
	N3	Contralateral mediastinum or hilum, scalene, or supraclavicular
Distant metastasis (M)	M0	None
	M1	Distant metastases present

Stage	Tumor	Lymph nodes	Metastasis
Occult	TX	N0	M0
I	Tis, T1, or T2	N0	M0
II	T1 or T2	N1	M0
	T3	N0	M0
III a	T3	N1	M0
	T1–T3	N2	M0
III b	T1–T4	N3	M0
	T4	N0–N2	M0
IV	T1–T4	N0–N3	M1

Asthma

Asthma affects 10–12% of adults and 15% of children. Asthma is a syndrome complex characterized by variable airflow obstruction. Three factors are involved in airway obstruction: bronchial muscle hyperreactivity, inflammation in the airways, and bronchial mucous production. Factors contributing to the evolution and persistence of asthma are atopy (allergic rhinitis and atopic dermatitis, eczema), nonallergic influences, respiratory infections, genetic predisposition, and environmental elements including allergens, air pollution, and occupational exposure.

Symptoms Intermittent dyspnea, wheezing, cough (often nocturnal) and sputum production.

- *Precipitants:* Cold air, exercise, emotion, allergens (house dust, mites, pollen, animal fur), infection, drugs (e.g., aspirin, NSAIDs, β-blockers).
- *Diurnal variation* in symptoms or peak flow. Marked morning dipping of peak flow is common and can tip the patient over into a serious attack, despite having normal peak flow at other times.
- *Exercise:* Quantify the exercise tolerance.
- *Disturbed sleep:* Quantify as nights per week (a sign of serious asthma).
- *Acid reflux:* Individuals with asthma have an increased prevalence of gastroesophageal reflux disease; esophageal reflux of acid or acidic fumes may stimulate bronchospasm/laryngospasm.
- *Other atopic disease:* Eczema, hay fever, allergy, or family history?
- *The home (especially the bedroom):* Pets? Carpet? Feather pillows? Floor cushions and other "soft furnishings"?
- *Occupation:* If symptoms remit at weekends or holidays, something at work may be a trigger. Ask the patient to measure his or her peak flow at work and at home (at the same time of day) to confirm this.
- *Days per week off work or school.*

Signs Tachypnea, audible wheeze, hyperinflated chest, hyperresonant percussion, diminished air entry, widespread, polyphonic wheeze. *Severe attack:* Inability to complete sentences; pulse >110 bpm; respiratory rate >25/min; PEF 33–50% of predicted. *Life-threatening attack:* Silent chest, cyanosis, bradycardia, exhaustion, PEF <33% of predicted, confusion, feeble respiratory effort.

Tests *Peak expiratory flow:* PEF monitoring (p. 154): A diurnal variation of >20% on ≥ 3 d a week for 2 wks. Spirometry: Obstructive defect ($\downarrow FEV_1/FVC$, $\uparrow RV$); usually ≥15% improvement in FEV_1 following $\dot{O}_2$ agonists or steroid trial. CXR: Hyperinflation. Skin-prick tests may help to identify allergens. Histamine or methacholine challenge. *Aspergillus* serology. *Acute attack:* PEF, sputum culture, CBC, electrolytes, CRP, blood cultures. ABG analysis usually shows a normal or slightly reduced P_aO_2 and low P_aCO_2 (hyperventilation). If P_aO_2 is normal but the patient is hyperventilating, watch carefully and repeat the ABG a little later. *If P_aCO_2 is raised, transfer to a step-down unit or icu for mechanical ventilation.* CXR (to exclude infection or pneumothorax).

Treatment Refractory asthma, asthmatic bronchitis (p. 170). Emergency treatment (p. 702).

Differential diagnosis Pulmonary edema ("cardiac asthma"), COPD (often coexists), large airway obstruction (e.g., foreign body, tumor), superior vena cava (SVC) obstruction (wheeze/dyspnea not episodic), pneumothorax, PE, bronchiectasis, obliterative bronchiolitis (suspect in elderly).

Exercise-induced asthma Commonly misdiagnosed as wheezing during exercise; more accurately, exercise-induced asthma occurs after exertion has ended. It is usually self-limiting; may be pretreated with pre-exercise $\dot{O}_2$-agonist and antileukotriene.

Associated diseases Acid reflux; polyarteritis nodosa (PAN); Churg–Strauss syndrome; ABPA.

Natural history Most childhood asthmatics either grow out of asthma in adolescence or suffer much less as adults. A significant number of people develop chronic asthma late in life, adult-onset asthma, or asthmatic bronchitis.

Asthmatic bronchitis/Refractory asthma

Lifestyle education Stop smoking; avoid precipitants. Check inhaler technique. Teach patients to use a peak flow meter to monitor PEF twice a day. Educate patients to manage their disease by altering their medication in response to changes in symptoms or PEF. Give specific advice about what to do in an emergency; provide a written action plan.

National Asthma Education and Prevention Program (NAEPP) Guidelines Start treatment at the step most appropriate to severity. Review treatment every 1–6 months. A gradual stepwise reduction in treatment may be possible; alternatively, consider step-up if control is not maintained. A short course of prednisone may be used to gain control as quickly as possible.

Step 1 Mild intermittent asthma: Occasional short-acting inhaled β_2-agonist as required for symptom relief. If daytime symptoms occur >2 days per week (but not every day), or if nocturnal symptoms occur >2 nights per month, go to Step 2.

Step 2 Mild persistent asthma: Add low-dose inhaled steroid: beclomethasone 40–120 mcg/12 h, budesonide 100–200 mcg/12 h, or fluticasone 44–132 mcg/12 h. If symptoms occur daily or >1 night per week, go to Step 3.

Step 3 **Moderate persistent asthma**: Add long-acting β_2-agonist (e.g., salmeterol 50 mcg/12 h or formoterol 12 mcg/12 h). If benefit—but still inadequate control—continue and increase dose of inhaled steroid to medium-dose (beclomethasone 120–240 mcg/12 h, budesonide 200–600 mcg/12 h, or fluticasone 132–330 mcg/12 h). If symptoms are continual or occur frequently at night, go to Step 4.

Step 4 Severe persistent asthma: Continue long-acting β_2-agonist and increase dose of inhaled steroid to high-dose (beclomethasone up to 320 mcg/12 h, budesonide up to 800 mcg/12 h, or fluticasone up to 440 mcg/12 h).

Drugs β_2*-adrenoreceptor agonists* relax bronchial smooth muscle, acting within minutes. Albuterol is best given by inhalation (aerosol, powder, nebulizer), but may also be given PO (see Table 6.6). Side effects (*SE*): Tachyarrhythmia, ↓K$^+$, tremor, anxiety. *Long-acting inhaled β_2-agonist* (e.g., salmeterol, formoterol) can help nocturnal symptoms and reduce morning symptoms. They should never be used as mono-therapy for asthma, and should only be added when symptoms are inadequately controlled on inhaled corticosteroids. *SE*: Same as albuterol: Tolerance, arrhythmias, paradoxical bronchospasm (salmeterol),? ↑risk of death.

Corticosteroids are best inhaled (e.g., beclomethasone via spacer [or powder]), but may be given PO or IV. They act over days to reduce bronchial mucosal inflammation. Rinse mouth after inhaled steroids to prevent oral candidiasis. Oral steroids are used acutely (high-dose, short courses; e.g., prednisone 30–40 mg/24 h PO for 7 d) and longer term in lower dose (e.g., 5–10 mg/24 h) if control is not optimal on inhalers. Warn about SE.

Aminophylline (metabolized to theophylline) may act by inhibiting phospho-diesterase, thus reducing bronchoconstriction by increasing cyclic adenosine monophosphate (cAMP) levels. Stick with one brand name (bio-availability is variable). It may be useful as "add-on" treatment if inhaled therapy is inadequate. In acute severe asthma, it may be given IVI. It has a narrow therapeutic ratio, causing arrhythmias, GI upset, and seizures in the toxic range. Check theophylline levels, then do electrocardiogram (ECG) monitoring and check plasma levels after 24 h if IV therapy is used.

Anticholinergics (e.g., ipratropium) may reduce muscle spasm synergistically with β_2-agonists. They may be of more benefit in COPD than in asthma. Try each alone and then together; assess with spirometry.

Cromolyn May be used as prophylaxis in mild and exercise-induced asthma (always inhaled), especially in children. As an adverse effect, cromolyn may precipitate asthma.

Leukotriene receptor antagonists (e.g., montelukast, zafirlukast) block the effects of cysteinyl leukotrienes in the airways. May be used as "add-on" therapy to recommended inhaler regimens.

Table 6.6 Doses of inhaled medications used in asthma

	Inhaled aerosol	Inhaled powder	Nebulized (*supervised*)
Albuterol			
Dose example:	90–180 mcg/ 4–6 h		2.5–5 mg/6 h
(The same for **cfc** and **cfc**-free devices; Proventil HFA® is an example of a **cfc**-free inhaler)			
Salmeterol			
Dose/puff	—	50 mcg	—
Recommended regimen	—	50 mcg/12 h	—
Ipratropium bromide			
Dose/puff	17 mcg	—	500 mcg/ mL
Recommended regimen	20–80 mcg/6 h	—	500 mcg/6 h
Steroids			
Fluticasone (Flovent HFA®)			
Doses available/puff (CFC-free)	44, 110, & 220 mcg	—	—
Recommended regimen	88–440 mcg/12 h	—	—
Beclomethasone (Qvar®)			
Doses available/puff (CFC-free)	40 & 80 mcg	—	—
Recommended regimen	40–320 mcg/12 h		
Budesonide (Pulmicort®)			
Doses available/puff (CFC-free)	—	200 mcg	—
Recommended regimen	—	200–800 mcg/12 h	—

Any puff/dose ≤250 mcg produces significant steroid absorption.
Complications: Cataracts, easy bruisability, osteoporosis.

Chronic obstructive pulmonary disease

Definitions *COPD* is defined as a progressive disorder of airway obstruction ($\downarrow$FEV$_1$, $\downarrow$FEV$_1$/FVC) with little or no reversibility. COPD includes *chronic bronchitis* (chronic cough with sputum production), *emphysema* (destruction and expansion of alveolar air spaces), and *small airways disease* (narrowing of the small bronchioles). Although airway hyperresponsiveness is characteristic of asthma, a percentage of individuals with COPD have airway hyperresponsiveness to external stimuli, infections, and, in some cases, to allergens. COPD is favored by:

- Age of onset >35 yrs
- Smoking
- Chronic dyspnea
- Sputum production
- No marked diurnal or day-to-day FEV$_1$ variation. *Chronic bronchitis* is defined *clinically* as cough and sputum production on most days for 3 months in 2 successive years. There is no increase in mortality if lung function is normal. Symptoms improve in 90% of patients if they stop smoking. *Emphysema* is defined *histologically* as enlargement of the air spaces distal to the terminal bronchioles, with destruction of the alveolar walls.

Prevalence ~14 million in the United States. *COPD mortality:* 126,000 deaths/yr in the United States.

Pink puffers and blue bloaters *Pink puffers* have increased alveolar ventilation, a near normal P_aO_2, and a normal or low P_aCO_2. Patients have shortness of breath, yet maintain adequate ventilation without cyanosis. *Blue bloaters* have decreased alveolar ventilation, with a low P_aO_2 and a high P_aCO_2. They can be cyanotic but usually are not breathless; may go on to develop cor pulmonale. Their respiratory centers are relatively insensitive to CO_2, and they rely on their hypoxic drive to maintain respiratory effort—*supplemental oxygen should be given with care.* Although the traditional differentiation of pink puffers versus blue bloaters suggests that pink puffers have emphysema and blue bloaters have chronic bronchitis, more recent clinical studies show elements of both are present in COPD, and physiological/physical differentiation is no longer relevant.

Clinical features *Symptoms:* Cough, sputum, dyspnea, and wheeze. *Signs:* Tachypnea, use of accessory muscles of respiration, hyperinflation, $\downarrow$cricosternal distance (<3 cm), $\downarrow$expansion, resonant or hyperresonant percussion, quiet breath sounds (e.g., over bullae), wheeze, cyanosis, cor pulmonale. *Complications:* Acute exacerbations ± infection, polycythemia, respiratory failure, cor pulmonale (edema, JVP$\uparrow$), pneumothorax (ruptured bullae), lung cancer.

Tests *CBC:* PCV$\uparrow$. *CXR:* Hyperinflation (>6 anterior ribs seen above diaphragm in mid-clavicular line), flat hemidiaphragms, large central pulmonary arteries, $\downarrow$peripheral vascular markings, bullae. *ECG:* Right atrial and ventricular hypertrophy (cor pulmonale). *ABG:* $P_aO_2\downarrow$ ± hypercapnia. *Lung function* (p. 154): Obstructive + air trapping (FEV$_1$ <80% of predicted—see below, FEV$_1$/FVC ratio <70%, TLC$\uparrow$, RV$\uparrow$, DLCO$\downarrow$ in emphysema).

Treatment *Chronic stable:* See Table 6.7. *Emergency treatment* (p. 704). Smoking cessation advice. Body mass index (BMI) is often low: Diet advice ± dietary supplements may help. Mucolytic agents may help chronic productive cough. Disabilities may cause serious, treatable depression. Respiratory failure (p. 176). *Preventative treatment:* Flu and pneumococcal vaccinations.

Long-term O_2 therapy (ltot): An MRC trial showed that if P_aO_2 was maintained $\geq$60 mm Hg for 15 h a day, 3-yr survival improved by 50%. LTOT should be given for (1) clinically stable nonsmokers with P_aO_2 <55 mm Hg despite maximal treatment. These values should be stable on two occasions >3 wks apart; and (2) if P_aO_2 55–60 *and* pulmonary hypertension (e.g., right ventricular hypertrophy [RVH]; loud S_2) + cor pulmonale. O_2 can also be prescribed for terminally ill patients. For additional treatment guidelines, see Table 6.8.

Table 6.7 Predicted FEV_1

Caucasian males; ↓level in other races[a]

Height (cm) Age(yr) ♂	150	155	160	165	170	175	180	185	190	195
10	2.5	2.8	3.0	3.2	3.5	3.7	3.9	4.1	4.4	4.6
25	2.9	3.2	3.4	3.7	4.0	4.2	4.3	4.7	5.0	5.3
30	2.8	3.1	3.3	3.6	3.8	4.1	4.3	4.6	4.9	5.1
40	2.5	2.8	3.0	3.3	3.6	3.8	4.1	4.3	4.6	4.9
50	2.2	2.5	2.8	3.0	3.3	3.5	3.8	4.0	4.3	4.6
60	2.0	2.2	2.5	2.8	3.0	3.3	3.5	3.8	4.0	4.3
70	1.7	2.0	2.2	2.5	2.7	3.0	3.3	3.5	3.8	4.0
80	1.4	1.7	2.0	2.2	2.5	2.7	3.0	3.3	3.5	3.8

Caucasian females

Height (cm) Age(yr)	145	150	155	160	165	170	175	180	185	190
10	2.1	2.2	2.3	2.5	2.6	2.7	2.9	3.0	3.1	3.3
25	2.6	2.7	2.9	3.0	3.1	3.3	3.4	3.5	3.7	3.8
30	2.5	2.6	2.8	2.9	3.0	3.2	3.3	3.4	3.6	3.7
40	2.3	2.4	2.5	2.7	2.8	3.0	3.0	3.2	3.3	3.5
50	2.1	2.2	2.3	2.5	2.6	2.7	2.9	3.0	3.1	3.3
60	1.7	2.0	2.1	2.3	2.4	2.5	2.7	2.8	2.9	3.1
70	1.6	1.8	1.9	2.1	2.2	2.3	2.5	2.6	2.7	2.9
80	1.4	1.6	1.7	1.9	2.0	2.1	2.2	2.4	2.5	2.7

[a]African FEV_1 is 10–15% lower; Chinese: 20% lower; Indian: 10% lower. PEF varies little between groups.

www.nationalasthma.org.au/publications/spiro/appc.html# Mean

Table 6.8 Global Initiative for Chronic Obstructive Lung Disease (GOLD) 2003 Guidelines

Assessment of COPD	Spirometry (FEV_1/FVC <70%) Bronchodilator response Trial of oral steroids is a poor predictor of response to inhaled steroids. CXR?Bullae?Other pathology ABG?Hypoxia?Hypercapnia	
Severity of COPD (Stage)	At risk (0)	Normal spirometry
	Mild (I)	FEV_1 ≥80% predicted
	Moderate (II)	FEV_1 50–79% predicted
	Severe (III)	FEV_1 30–49% predicted
	Very-severe (IV)	FEV_1 <30% predicted

Treating stable COPD

NB: Patients who fly should be able to maintain an in-flight P_aO_2 of ≥50 mm Hg.

Nonpharmacological	Stop smoking, encourage exercise, treat poor nutrition or obesity, influenza and pneumococcal vaccination, pulmonary rehabilitation/palliative care
Pharmacological: Mild	Add PRN short-acting bronchodilator (inhaled ipratropium, albuterol, or combination of two)
Moderate	Add long-acting inhaled β_2 agonist (salmeterol or formoterol) or inhaled anticholinergic (tiotropium)
Severe	Add inhaled steroids if repeated exacerbations (Advair® combines salmeterol and fluticasone.)

More advanced COPD

- Pulmonary rehabilitation in patients with moderate or worse COPD
- Long-term oxygen therapy if P_aO_2 <55 mm Hg and/or oxygen saturation ≤85%.
- Indications for surgery: Recurrent pneumothoraces; isolated bullous disease; lung volume reduction surgery or lung transplantation in selected patients. In select COPD patients, lung volume reduction surgery improves lung function exercise tolerance, improves survival, and results in a better quality of life.
- Assess home set-up and support needed. Treat depression.

(Continued)

Table 6.8 (Continued)

Indications for specialist referral
- Uncertain diagnosis
- Suspected severe COPD or a rapid decline in FEV_1
- Onset of cor pulmonale
- Assessment for oral corticosteroids, nebulizer therapy, or LTOT
- Bullous lung disease (to assess for surgery)
- <10 pack-years smoking (PYS; equals the number of packs/day times the number of years of smoking). Smokers have an excess loss of FEV_1 of 7.4–12.6 mL per pack year for men and 4.4–7.2 mL per pack year for women.
- Symptoms disproportionate to pulmonary function tests
- Frequent infections (to exclude bronchiectasis)
- COPD in patient <40 yrs (exclude α_1-antitrypsin deficiency?)

Interstitial lung diseases

Interstitial lung disease is group of disorders that, in contrast to COPD, do not involve the airways but involve the interstitial region of lung parenchyma. The anatomy of the lung parenchyma primarily affected by these disorders are the alveoli, alveolar epithelium, the capillary endothelium, and the interstitial space surrounding those structures. Interstitial lung disease is characterized by progressive shortness of breath usually associated with a chronic nonproductive cough. Within this group of interstitial lung diseases, historical presentation, physical examination, and radiographic appearance do not help in differentiating among the various types of lung parenchyma diseases.

Histopathology may demonstrate alveolitis, fibrosis, and interstitial inflammatory changes or may indicate a granulomatous interstitial process.

A major portion of interstitial lung disease, 40%, is idiopathic, without a known cause, and with the histopathology revealing fibrosis, bronchiolitis, and/or pneumonia. A second common presentation of interstitial lung disease is related to inhalational exposures, such as in hypersensitivity pneumonitides, asbestosis, or fumes or gas exposure. Sarcoidosis, a granulomatous process of unknown cause, may present as interstitial lung disease, with histologic findings of granulomata present within the spaces between alveoli and pulmonary capillaries. Connective tissue diseases, such as SLE, rheumatoid arthritis, and systemic sclerosis, may be associated with interstitial fibrosis and inflammatory changes. Last, medications may initiate an inflammatory interstitial process and result in fibrosis; these drugs include amiodarone, gold, radiation therapy, and chemotherapy medications.

Dyspnea is the most common symptom; interstitial lung disease characteristics are a chronic presentation of illness, shortness of breath, and a nonproductive cough, especially prevalent in persons >60 yrs, with a family history of interstitial lung disease, a history of smoking, and a history of occupational or environmental exposures.

Physical exam, especially early in the disease process, is nonspecific, yet crackles heard bilaterally in the lung bases are a common finding. Laboratory studies are also nonspecific; however, excluding underlying connective tissue diseases with antibasement membrane antibodies, rheumatoid factor, and antinuclear antibody titer is important; serum precipitins aid in ruling out hypersensitivity pneumonitis; an elevation in angiotensin-converting enzyme may be present in sarcoidosis; an elevation in LDH is common yet also nonspecific. Depending on the phase of interstitial lung disease, an echocardiogram is helpful in excluding or including pulmonary hypertension with right ventricular hypertrophy or dilation.

Chest radiographs show a reticular, possibly nodular, pattern in both lung bases, usually in a clinical setting with associated symptoms/signs of an acute infection. HRCT is the best radiographic study, with clearer definition of an interstitial process and with the exclusion of other mediastinal or parenchyma disorders. Pulmonary function studies classically identify restrictive lung disease, demonstrating decreased total lung volumes, with decreased diffusion capacity and some reduction of expiratory flow; however, the ratio of FEV_1/FVC is usually normal or, in fact, increased due to the loss of lung compliance and increased elasticity secondary to fibrosis.

The most effective method of diagnosis is lung biopsy; fiberoptic bronchoscopy with BAL and with multiple lung biopsies may be useful, but a generous tissue biopsy is more helpful in defining the overall histology of an interstitial process and thus may necessitate surgical lung biopsy with video-assisted thoracic surgery or open surgical lung biopsy.

Treatment of interstitial lung disease is not effective; most cases have a progressive, advancing fibrosis terminating in hypoxemia, cor pulmonale, and respiratory failure. Glucocorticosteroids therapy may counteract the inflammatory phase (e.g., in alveolitis); however, with fibrosis, corticosteroids are not beneficial; in fact, although glucocorticosteroids may transiently improve symptoms, these drugs do not have an impact on morbidity and mortality. Other medications for interstitial lung disease are cyclophosphamide, azathioprine, colchicine, methotrexate, and penicillamine; all may have some positive effect in the short term, yet their long-term benefit is doubtful.

Idiopathic pulmonary fibrosis Most common; usual interstitial pneumonitis has a mixture of inflammation, fibroblasts interspersed between normal lung tissue, and dense fibrosis and honeycomb changes on hrct.

Nonspecific interstitial pneumonia is usually seen with clinical-serological evidence of connective tissue disease; more common in younger patients, especially women; uniform histologic involvement with fibrosis and cellular alterations.

Hamman-Rich syndrome High mortality; sudden onset, rapidly progressive (as in acute respiratory distress syndrome [ARDS]); deteriorating hypoxemia associated with histologic evidence of extreme alveolar damage. Most deaths occur within 6 months.

Interstitial lung disease associated with connective tissue diseases Typical interstitial lung disease presentation within clinical circumstances of SLE, rheumatoid arthritis, Sjögren's syndrome, dermatomyositis-polymyositis, progressive systemic sclerosis. Pulmonary involvement in these disorders portend a poor prognosis.

Interstitial lung disease associated with medications Chemotherapeutic agents, amiodarone, gold, antibiotics (nitrofurantoin); inflammatory lung changes usually resolve with discontinuation of medication.

Pulmonary alveolar proteinosis Presentation is similar to interstitial lung disease; lung biopsy reveals an abundance of lipoprotein in distal airspaces; common in men; elevated titer of anti-granulocyte-macrophage colony stimulating factor. Treatment consists of whole lung lavage.

Pulmonary lymphangioleiomyomatosis Rare; in premenopausal women; emphysema, recurrent pneumothorax and chylous pleural effusions; pulmonary function studies are mixed, with restrictive and obstructive patterns; survival of 8–10 yrs from time of diagnosis. No effective treatment.

Diffuse alveolar hemorrhage Primary example is Goodpasture's syndrome; alveolar hemorrhage with hypoxemia characterized by autoantibodies to renal glomerular and lung basement membranes; histologic finding of damage to the pulmonary capillary basement membrane. Treatment, especially when associated with connective tissue disease, is glucocorticosteroids; plasmapheresis is additive therapy.

Interstitial lung disease associated with cigarette smoking Diagnoses include desquamative interstitial pneumonia, respiratory bronchiolitis, pulmonary histiocytosis, all in smokers, mostly males; progressive hypoxemia; restrictive pulmonary function patterns with decrease diffusion capacity. Clinical improvement with smoking cessation.

Acute respiratory distress syndrome

The acute lung injury of ARDS may be caused by direct lung injury or occur secondary to severe systemic illness. Lung damage and release of inflammatory mediators cause increased capillary permeability and noncardiogenic pulmonary edema, often accompanied by failure in other organs systems.

Causes *Pulmonary:* Pneumonia, gastric aspiration, inhalation, injury, vasculitis, contusion. *Other causes:* Shock, septicemia, hemorrhage, multiple transfusions, disseminated intravascular coagulation (DIC; p. 577), pancreatitis, acute liver failure, trauma, head injury, fat embolism, burns, obstetric events (eclampsia, amniotic fluid embolus), drugs/toxins (aspirin overdose, heroin, paraquat). See Table 6.9.

Clinical features Cyanosis, tachypnea, tachycardia, peripheral vasodilatation, bilateral fine inspiratory crackles on lung auscultation.

Investigations CBC, electrolytes, LFT, amylase, clotting, CRP, blood cultures, ABG. CXR shows bilateral pulmonary infiltrates. Pulmonary artery catheter to measure pulmonary capillary wedge pressure (PCWP).

185

Diagnostic criteria One consensus requires these four to exist: (1) Acute onset. (2) CXR: Bilateral infiltrates. (3) PCWP <19 mm Hg or a lack of clinical congestive heart failure. (4) Refractory hypoxemia.

Management Admit to ICU, provide supportive therapy, and treat the under-lying cause; artificial ventilator support is common.

- *Respiratory support:* In early ARDS, continuous positive airway pressure (CPAP) with 40–60% oxygen may be adequate to maintain oxygenation; most patients need mechanical ventilation. Indications for ventilation: P_aO_2: <60 mm Hg despite 60% O_2; P_aCO_2: >45 mm Hg. The large tidal volumes (10–15 mL/kg) produced by conventional ventilation plus reduced lung compliance in ARDS may lead to high peak airway pressures ± pneumothorax. Positive end-expiratory pressure (PEEP) may improve oxygenation, but may reduce venous return, cardiac output, and perfusion of the kidneys and liver. Other approaches include inverse ratio ventilation (inspiration > expiration), permissive hypercapnia, high-frequency jet ventilation, and other low-tidal-volume techniques.
- *Circulatory support:* Invasive hemodynamic monitoring with an arterial line and Swan–Ganz catheter aids the diagnosis and may be helpful in monitoring PCWP and cardiac output. Maintain cardiac output and O_2 delivery with inotropes (e.g., dobutamine 2.5–10 mcg/kg/min IV), vasodilators, and blood transfusion. Consider treating pulmonary hypertension with low-dose (20–120 parts per million) nitric oxide, a selective pulmonary vasodilator. Hemodialysis may be needed in renal failure and to achieve a negative fluid balance.
- *Sepsis:* Identify organism(s) and treat accordingly. If clinically septic, but no organisms cultured, use empirical broad-spectrum antibiotics (p. 159). Avoid nephrotoxic antibiotics.

- *Other:* Nutritional support: Enteral nutrition is best. Steroids do not decrease mortality in the acute phase, but may help later on (>7 d), particularly if eosinophilia in blood or in fluid from BAL.

Prognosis Overall mortality is 50–75%. Prognosis varies with age of patient, cause of ARDS (pneumonia 86%, trauma 38%), and number of organs involved (three organs involved for >1 wk is invariably fatal).

Table 6.9 Risk factors for ARDS	
• Sepsis	• Massive transfusion
• Hypovolemic shock	• Burns
• Trauma	• Smoke inhalation
• Pneumonia	• Near drowning
• Diabetic ketoacidosis	• Acute pancreatitis
• Gastric aspiration	• DIC
• Pregnancy	• Head injury
• Eclampsia	• Intracranial pressure ↑
• Amniotic fluid embolus	• Fat embolus
• Drugs/toxins	• Heart/lung bypass
• Paraquat, heroin, aspirin overdose	• Tumor lysis syndrome
• Pulmonary contusion	• Malaria

Respiratory failure

Respiratory failure occurs when gas exchange is impaired, resulting in hypoxemia and/or impairment in CO_2 elimination. See Table 6.10.

Type I respiratory failure is defined as hypoxia (P_aO_2 <60 mm Hg) with a normal or low P_aCO_2. Type I respiratory failure is caused primarily by ventilation/perfusion (V/Q) mismatch. Causes include:

- Pneumonia
- Pulmonary edema
- PE
- Asthma
- Emphysema
- Pulmonary fibrosis
- ARDS (P. 174)

Type II respiratory failure is defined as hypoxia (P_aO_2 <60 mm Hg) with hypercapnia (P_aCO^2 is >45 mm Hg). Respiratory failure type II is caused by alveolar hypoventilation, with or without (V/Q) abnormalities. Causes include:

- *Pulmonary disease:* Asthma, COPD, pneumonia, pulmonary fibrosis, obstructive sleep apnea (OSA; p. 189)
- *Reduced respiratory drive:* Sedative drugs, CNS tumor, or trauma
- *Neuromuscular disease:* Cervical cord lesion, diaphragmatic paralysis, poliomyelitis, myasthenia gravis, Guillain–Barré syndrome
- *Thoracic wall disease:* Flail chest, kyphoscoliosis

Clinical features are those of the underlying cause, together with symptoms and signs of hypoxia, with or without hypercapnia.

Hypoxia: Dyspnea, restlessness, agitation, confusion, central cyanosis. If long-standing hypoxia: Polycythemia, pulmonary hypertension, cor pulmonale.

Hypercapnia: Headache, peripheral vasodilatation, tachycardia, bounding pulse, tremor/flap, papilledema, confusion, drowsiness, coma.

Investigations are aimed at determining the underlying cause:

• Blood tests: CBC, electrolytes, CRP, ABG
• Radiology: CXR
• Microbiology: Sputum and blood cultures (if febrile)
• Spirometry (COPD, neuromuscular disease, Guillain–Barré syndrome).

Management depends on the cause:

Type I respiratory failure:

• Treat underlying cause.
• Give oxygen (35–60%) by face mask to correct hypoxia.
• Assisted ventilation if P_aO_2 <60 mm Hg despite 60% O_2.

Type II respiratory failure: In type II respiratory failure, the respiratory center within the brainstem is relatively insensitive to CO_2; breathing may be driven by hypoxia. *Oxygen therapy should be administered with caution and with gradual increases in O_2.* Treatment of hypoxemia is crucial in prevention and modification of pulmonary hypertension caused by hypoxemia.

• Treat underlying cause.
• Controlled oxygen therapy: Start at 24% O_2.
• Recheck ABG after 20 min. If P_aCO_2 is steady or lower, ↑ O_2 concentration to 28%, If P_aCO_2 has risen >12 mm Hg and the patient is still hypoxic, consider assisted ventilation (i.e., noninvasive positive pressure ventilation).
• If type II respiratory failure progresses, consider intubation and ventilation.

Table 6.10 When to consider arterial blood gas (ABG) measurement

In these clinical scenarios:
Any unexpected deterioration in an ill patient
Anyone with an acute exacerbation of a chronic chest condition
Anyone with impaired level of consciousness
Anyone with impaired respiratory effort
Or if any of these signs or symptoms are present:
Bounding pulse, drowsiness, tremor (flapping), headache, pink palms, papilledema
Cyanosis, confusion, visual hallucinations (signs of hypoxia)
Or to monitor the progress of a critically ill patient:
Monitoring the treatment of known respiratory failure
Anyone ventilated in the ICU
After major surgery
After major trauma
To validate measurements from pulse oximetry:
Pulse oximetry (p. 154) effective for monitoring oxygen saturation; accurate readings are dependent on appropriate placement of monitor, on normal arterial perfusion, and on correlation with arterial pO_2.

Pulmonary embolism

PE and venous thromboembolism are the most common and preventable causes of death, especially in hospitalized patients. In addition to myocardial infarctions (MIs) and cerebral vascular accidents, venous thromboembolism is a major cause of death in nonhospitalized individuals. See Table 6.11.

Causes PE usually arise from a venous thrombosis in the pelvis or legs. Thrombus may dislodge and pass through the venous system to the right side of the heart before occluding an artery in the pulmonary circulation. Rare causes include right ventricular thrombus (post-MI); septic emboli (right-sided endocarditis); fat, air, or amniotic fluid embolism; neoplastic cells; parasites. *Risk factors:* Any cause of immobility or hypercoagulability:

• Prolonged travel in automobiles or planes without leg exercise and stretching.

• Recent surgery

• Recent stroke or MI
• Disseminated malignancy

• Thrombophilia/antiphospholipid syndrome (p. 590)
• Prolonged bed rest
• Pregnancy; postpartum; oral contraceptives/hormone replacement therapy

Clinical features depend on the number, size, and distribution of the emboli; small emboli may be asymptomatic whereas large, saddle emboli are critical/fatal. *Symptoms:* Acute breathlessness, pleuritic chest pain, hemoptysis; dizziness; syncope. Review risk factors (above), past history or family history of thromboembolism. *Signs:* Pyrexia; cyanosis; tachypnea; tachycardia; hypotension; ↑JVP, pleural rub; pleural effusion. Examine for signs of a cause; e.g., deep vein thrombosis (DVT); scar from recent surgery.

Prognosis of PE is related to comorbidities and to the presence or absence of hypotension and to the function of the right ventricle. PE in normotensive patients has an encouraging prognosis and usually requires anticoagulation only. In PE patients with hypotension or with normal BP, yet with evidence of right ventricular dysfunction, the prognosis is guarded; these PE patients may need thrombolysis and/or embolectomy in addition to anticoagulation.

Tests

• *CXR* may be normal or may show dilated pulmonary artery, linear atelectasis, small pleural effusion, wedge-shaped opacities; cavitations may occur with pulmonary infarction.
• *ECG* may be normal or show tachycardia, right bundle branch block, right ventricular strain (inverted T in V_1 to V_4). The classical $S_iQ_{iii}T_{iii}$ pattern is rare.
• *Echocardiogram* assessment of right ventricular function is important for prognosis; right ventricular heart failure is the cause of death in most patients with PE; evidence of right ventricular enlargement or dysfunction suggests significant physiologic impairment and thus a poor prognosis.
• *ABG* may show a low P_aO_2 and a low P_aCO_2.
• *Radiographic studies* Ultrasonography is crucial in evaluation of the lower extremities for thrombosis; pelvic US is difficult to assess for venous thrombosis.
• CT of the chest (spiral CT with contrast) is the radiographic study of choice for detecting PE; also may be useful in assessment of the right ventricle; right ventricular enlargement is associated with a poor prognosis.

Treatment (p. 710) Initiate anticoagulation with low-molecular-weight heparin (e.g., enoxaparin 1 mg/kg/12 h SC); start oral warfarin 10 mg

(p. 574). Stop heparin when International Normalized Ratio (INR) is >2 and continue warfarin for a minimum of 3 months; aim for an INR of 2–3. Consider placement of a *vena cava filter* in patients who develop emboli despite adequate anticoagulation, or in critically ill patients in whom another PE might be fatal. (NB ↑ risk of recurrence if placed without concomitant anticoagulation).

Prevention Give heparin (7,500 U/12 h or 5,000 U/8 h) to all immobile patients. Prescribe TED stockings and encourage early mobilization. Women should stop hormone replacement therapy (HRT) and oral contraceptives preoperatively. Patients with a past or family history of thromboembolism should be investigated for coagulation disorders associated with enhanced thrombus formation.

Pneumothorax

Management on p. 706 and X-RAY PLATE 6

Causes A pneumothorax is the presence of air/gas within the pleural space. Spontaneous pneumatothoraces occur (especially in young thin men) due to rupture of a subpleural bulla. *Other causes*: Asthma, COPD, TB, pneumonia, lung abscess, carcinoma, CF, lung fibrosis, sarcoidosis, connective tissue disorders (Marfan's syndrome, Ehlers–Danlos syndrome), trauma, iatrogenic (subclavian central venous pressure [CVP] line insertion, pleural aspiration or biopsy, percutaneous liver biopsy, positive pressure ventilation).

Table 6.11 Investigation of suspected PE

- First assess the likely probability of a PE.
- Numerous scoring systems are available.
- One simple system is the presence of clinical features of a PE (shortness of breath (SOB) and tachypnea, with or without pleuritic chest pain and hemoptysis) and either (a) the absence of another reasonable explanation or (b) the presence of a major risk factor. If a and b coexist, the probability is high; if only one exists, intermediate; if neither exist, the probability for PE is low.
- *D-dimer:* This study is useful as a screening test, especially in those patients *without* a high probability of a PE. A negative D-dimer test excludes a PE in patients with a low clinical probability, and imaging may not be required. A positive D-dimer test does not prove a diagnosis of a PE, and follow-up radiographic studies are crucial.
- *Imaging:* The recommended first-line imaging modality is a spiral CT scan, which show clots down to fifth-order pulmonary arteries. This may be useful in subjects with indeterminate isotope scans. Bilateral leg US (or rarely venograms) may confirm a DVT in patients with a coexisting clinical PE. Ventilation-perfusion nuclear lung scans are a secondary choice for diagnosing PE; may be useful in patients who have an allergy to radiographic dye.

Major risk factors for PE

Surgery
- Major abdominal/pelvic
- Hip/knee replacement
- Obstetrics
  - Late pregnancy; postpartum
  - Cesarean section

- Lower limb problems
- Fracture
- Varicose veins
- Malignancy
- Reduced mobility
- Previous PE
- Estrogen therapy

Clinical features *Symptoms:* Asymptomatic in well-conditioned younger individuals; pneumothorax may present as a sudden onset of dyspnea and/or pleuritic chest pain. Patients with asthma or COPD may present with emergent respiratory deterioration. Mechanically ventilated patients may develop hypoxia or an increase in ventilation pressures. *Signs:* Reduced expansion, hyperresonance to percussion, and diminished breath sounds on the affected side. *With a tension pneumothorax, the trachea will be deviated away from the affected side.*

Management of tension pneumothorax See p. 706, and placing a chest drain (p. 662).

Pleural effusion

Definitions A pleural effusion is excessive fluid in the pleural space. Effusions can be divided, by their protein and LDH concentrations, into *transudates* and *exudates* (see pleural fluid analysis, Table 6.12).

Blood in the pleural space is a *hemothorax,* pus in the pleural space is an *empyema,* and chyle in the pleural space (lymph with fat) is a *chylothorax.* Both blood and air in the pleural space is termed a *hemopneumothorax.*

Causes *Transudates* may be due to increased venous pressure (cardiac failure, constrictive pericarditis, fluid overload) or hypoproteinemia (cirrhosis, nephrotic syndrome, malabsorption). Transudative pleural fluid occurs in hypothyroidism and Meigs' syndrome (right pleural effusion and ovarian fibroma).

Exudates are mostly due to increased permeability of pleural capillaries secondary to infection, inflammation, or malignancy. *Causes:* Pneumonia, TB, pulmonary infarction, rheumatoid arthritis, SLE, bronchogenic carcinoma, malignant metastases, lymphoma, mesothelioma, lymphangitic carcinomatosis.

Symptoms Asymptomatic or symptoms of dyspnea, pleuritic chest pain, shortness of breath.

Signs Decreased chest *expansion with inspiration; dull percussion noted; diminished breath sounds* occur on the affected side. Tactile vocal fremitus and vocal resonance are ↓ (inconstant and unreliable). Above the effusion, where lung is compressed, there may be *bronchial breathing* and *egophony* (vocal resonance). With large effusions, there may be *tracheal deviation* away from the effusion. Look for aspiration marks and signs of associated disease: Malignancy (cachexia, clubbing, lymphadenopathy, radiation marks, and mastectomy scar), stigmata of chronic liver disease, cardiac failure, hypothyroidism, rheumatoid arthritis, butterfly rash of SLE.

Tests *CXR* Small effusions blunt the costophrenic angles, larger ones are seen as water-dense shadows with concave upper borders. A completely horizontal upper border implies that there is also a pneumothorax; an effusion-side-down chest radiograph may be helpful in detecting an effusion and determining whether it is free flowing or loculated.

US is useful in identifying the presence of pleural fluid and in guiding diagnostic or therapeutic aspiration.

Diagnostic aspiration Percuss the upper border of the pleural effusion and choose a site 1–2 intercostal spaces below it. Infiltrate down to the pleura with 5–10 mL of 1% lidocaine. Attach a 21 French (F) needle to a syringe and insert it just above the upper border of an appropriate rib (avoids neurovascular bundle). Draw off 10–30 mL of pleural fluid and send it to the lab for *clinical chemistry* (protein, glucose, pH, LDH, amylase), *bacteriology* (Gram and AFB staining, bacterial and TB culture), and *cytology.*

Pleural biopsy If pleural fluid analysis is inconclusive, consider parietal pleural biopsy. Video-assisted thoracoscopy or CT-guided pleural biopsy will increase diagnostic yield (by enabling direct visualization of the pleural cavity and biopsy of suspicious areas).

Management is of the underlying cause.

- *Drainage:* If the effusion is symptomatic, drain it, repeatedly if necessary. Fluid is best removed slowly (≤2 L/24 h). It may be aspirated in the same way as a diagnostic tap or using an intercostal drain (p. 661).
- *Pleurodesis* with tetracycline, bleomycin, or talc may be helpful for recurrent effusions. Thoracoscopic talc pleurodesis is most effective for malignant effusions. Empyemas (p. 161) are best drained using a chest tube drain, inserted under US or CT guidance.
- *Intrapleural streptokinase:* Doubtful benefit.
- *Surgery:* Persistent collections and increased pleural thickening may require video-assisted thoracoscopy or open thoracotomy.

Table 6.12 Pleural fluid analysis

Gross appearance	*Cause*
Clear, straw-coloured	Transudate, exudate
Turbid, yellow	Empyema, parapneumonic effusion
Hemorrhagic	Trauma, malignancy, pulmonary infarction
Cytology	
Neutrophils ++	Parapneumonic effusion, PE
Lymphocytes ++	Malignancy, TB, rheumatoid arthritis (RA), SLE, sarcoidosis
Mesothelial cells ++	Pulmonary infarction
Abnormal mesothelial cells	Mesothelioma
Multinucleated giant cells	RA
Lupus erythematosus cells	SLE
Clinical chemistry	
Pleural fluid/serum protein <0.5 *and*	If all 3 criteria are met, effusion is a transudate. Otherwise, it is an exudate
Pleural fluid/serum LDH <0.6 *and*	
Pleural fluid LDH <2/3 top normal serum LDH	
Glucose <60 mg/dL	Empyema, malignancy, TB, RA, SLE
pH <7.2	Empyema, malignancy, TB, RA, SLE
LDH↑(pleural: Serum >0.6)	Empyema, malignancy, TB, RA, SLE
Amylase↑	Pancreatitis, carcinoma, bacterial pneumonia, esophageal rupture

Sarcoidosis

Sarcoidosis is a multisystem noncaseating granulomatous disorder of unknown cause. Prevalence in the United States is $5/10^5$ of the population among Caucasians, $40/10^5$ among African Americans. It commonly affects adults aged 20–40 yrs. African Americans are affected more severely than Caucasians, particularly by extrathoracic disease.

Clinical features *Asymptomatic:* In 20–40%, the disease is discovered incidentally, after a routine CXR. *Acute sarcoidosis* often presents with erythema nodosum (PLATE 18) ± polyarthralgia; acute sarcoidosis usually resolves spontaneously.

Pulmonary disease: 90% have abnormal CXRs with *bilateral, symmetrical, hilar lymphadenopathy* (BHL) ± pulmonary infiltrates or fibrosis. *Symptoms:* Dry cough, progressive dyspnea, exercise intolerance and chest pain. In 10–20%, symptoms progress, with concurrent deterioration in lung function.

Nonpulmonary manifestations: Lymphadenopathy, hepatomegaly, splenomegaly, uveitis, conjunctivitis, keratoconjunctivitis, glaucoma, terminal phalangeal bone cysts, enlargement of lacrimal and parotid glands, Bell's palsy, neuropathy, meningitis, brainstem and spinal syndromes, space-occupying lesion, erythema nodosum (PLATE 18), lupus pernio, subcutaneous nodules, cardiomyopathy, arrhythmias, hypercalcemia, hypercalciuria, renal stones, pituitary dysfunction.

Investigations *Blood tests:* ↑ESR, lymphopenia, abnormal LFTS, ↑serum angiotensin-converting enzyme ↑immunoglobulins. *24 h urine:* Ca^{2+} ↑; hypercalciuria. *Tuberculin skin test* is –ve in two-thirds. *CXR* is abnormal 90%. *Stage 0:* Normal. *Stage 1:* BHL. *Stage 2:* BHL + peripheral pulmonary infiltrates. *Stage 3:* Peripheral pulmonary infiltrates alone. *Stage 4:* Progressive pulmonary fibrosis; bulla formation (honeycombing); pleural involvement. See Table 6.13.

ECG may show arrhythmias or bundle branch block. *Lung function tests* may be normal or show reduced lung volumes, impaired gas transfer, and a restrictive lung disorder. *Tissue biopsy* (lung, liver, lymph nodes, skin nodules, or lacrimal glands) is diagnostic and shows noncaseating granulomata.

BAL shows ↑lymphocytes in active disease; ↑neutrophils with pulmonary fibrosis.

US may show nephrocalcinosis or hepatosplenomegaly.

Bone x-rays show "punched out" lesions in terminal phalanges.

CT/MRI may be useful in assessing severity of pulmonary disease or diagnosing neuro-sarcoidosis. *Ophthalmology assessment* (slit lamp examination, fluorescein angiography) is indicated in ocular disease. *Kveim tests* are obsolete.

Management Patients with BHL alone do not require treatment since the majority resolve spontaneously. *Acute sarcoidosis:* Bed rest, NSAIDs. *Indications for corticosteroid therapy:*

• Parenchymal lung disease (symptomatic, static, or progressive)
• Uveitis
• Hypercalcemia
• Neurological or cardiac involvement.

Prednisone (40 mg/24 h) PO for 4–6 wks, then reduce dose over 1 yr according to clinical status. A few patients relapse and may need a further course or long-term therapy. In severe illness, IV methylprednisolone or immunosuppressants (methotrexate, cyclosporin, azathioprine, cyclophosphamide) may be needed.

Prognosis 60% of patients with thoracic sarcoidosis show spontaneous resolution within 2 yrs. 20% of patients respond to steroid therapy. In the remainder, improvement is unlikely despite therapy. For differential diagnoses, see Table 6.14.

Table 6.13 Causes of bilateral hilar lymphadenopathy (BHL)

Infection	TB
	Mycoplasma
Malignancy	Lymphoma
	Carcinoma
	Mediastinal tumors
Industrial dust disease	Silicosis
	Berylliosis
Extrinsic allergic alveolitis	

Table 6.14 Differential diagnosis of granulomatous diseases

Infections	Bacteria	TB
		Leprosy
		Syphilis
		Cat scratch fever
	Fungi	*Cryptococcus neoformans*
		Histoplasma capsulatumCoccidioides immitis
	Protozoa	Schistosomiasis
Autoimmune	Primary biliary cirrhosis	
	Granulomatous orchitis	
Vasculitis	Giant cell arteritis	
	Polyarteritis nodosa	
	Takayasu's arteritis	
	Wegener's granulomatosis	
Industrial dust disease	Silicosis	
	Berylliosis	
Idiopathic	Crohn's disease	
	de Quervain's thyroiditis	
	Sarcoidosis	
Extrinsic allergic alveolitis		
Histiocytosis X		

Hypersensitivity pneumonitis/Extrinsic allergic alveolitis (EAA)

In sensitized individuals, inhalation of allergens, fungal spores, or proteins provoke a hypersensitivity reaction. In the acute phase, the alveoli are infiltrated with acute inflammatory cells. With chronic exposure, granulomatous formation and obliterative bronchiolitis occur. Eosinophilia is specifically absent.

Causes (representative examples)

- *Bird fancier's and pigeon fancier's lung:* Proteins in bird droppings of pigeon, chicken, parakeet, turkey
- *Farmer's lung:* Thermophilic actinomycetes
- *Malt worker's lung:* Aspergillus fumigates or A. clavatus
- *Bagassosis:* Thermophilic actinomyces
- *Cheese washer's lung:* Penicillium casei
- *Familial hypersensitivity pneumonia:* Bacillus subtilis
- *Furrier's lung:* Animal fur particles
- *Mushroom worker's lung:* Thermophilic actinomycetes
- *Suberosis:* Cork dust, Penicillium glabrum
- *Wood worker's lung:* Oak, cedar, pine, mahogany dusts

Clinical features *4-6 h postexposure, Acute:* Fever, rigors, myalgias, dry cough, dyspnea, crackles (no wheeze). *Subacute:* Usually occurs over a 2-wk interval with cough and shortness of breath. *Chronic:* ↑ Dyspnea, weight↓, exertional dyspnea, progressive hypoxemia.

Tests *Acute:* Blood: CBC (neutrophilia); ESR↑; ABGs; eosinophilia is not present; positive serum precipitins (indicate exposure only). *CXR:* Mid-zone mottling/consolidation; hilar lymphadenopathy (rare).

HRCT yields greater definition of lung parenchymal changes, specifically, ground-glass infiltrates, reticulonodular or alveolar consolidation patterns. *Lung function tests:* Restrictive pulmonary disease findings; reduced diffusion capacity during acute attacks.

Chronic: Blood: Positive serum precipitins. *CXR:* Upper-zone fibrosis; honeycomb lung. *Lung function tests:* Persistent changes (see above). BAL fluid shows ↑ lymphocytes and mast cells.

Management *Acute attack:* Remove allergen and give O$_2$ (35–60%), then:

- Hydrocortisone 200 mg IV
- Prednisone (40 mg/24 h PO), followed by reducing dose

Chronic: Avoid exposure to allergens or wear a face masks. Long-term steroids often achieve radiographic and physiological improvement.

Hypersensitivity pneumonitis with eosinophilia

In contrast to hypersensitivity pneumonitis related to fungi, proteins, allergens, and the lack of eosinophilia, this group of disorder is associated with serum and pulmonary eosinophilia. The original description by Loeffler was a presentation of a benign migratory pneumonitis associated with eosinophilia; the clinical course was usually self-limiting, and most cases were subsequently attributed to a parasitic infection or to an adverse reaction to medications. The latter includes the classic culprits, nitrofurantoin, sulfonamides, penicillin, thiazide diuretics, gold salts, hydralazine, isoniazid, and chlorpropamide.

Other pulmonary syndromes with eosinophilia are allergic bronchopulmonary aspergillosis, acute eosinophilic pneumonia, allergic granulomatosis of Churg-Strauss, and chronic eosinophilic pneumonia. In most instances, the clinical presentation is one of a mild pneumonia with peripheral eosinophilia and with transient, peripheral infiltrates on CXR. BAL in these patients will usually yield a high percentage of eosinophils (>25%). However, in chronic eosinophilic pneumonia and in the hypereosinophilia syndrome, systemic symptoms of fever with constitutional symptoms exist; multiorgan involvement, especially cardiac involvement, is discovered in hypereosinophilia syndrome.

In hypersensitivity pneumonitis with eosinophilia, treatment with glucocorticosteroids most often produces immediate resolution of clinical symptoms and radiographic findings. Nonetheless, in chronic eosinophilic pneumonia, recurrence is common; in the hypereosinophilia syndrome, because of the cardiac complications, and in contrast to the benignity of other eosinophilic syndromes, a high morbidity and mortality occurs.

Pulmonary hypertension

Pulmonary hypertension is defined by an increase in pulmonary artery pressure and secondary changes of the right ventricular anatomy or function. A normal mean arterial pulmonary artery pressure is 8–20 mm Hg; determined by cardiac catheterization or by echocardiography, pulmonary artery hypertension is present when the mean pulmonary artery pressure is >25 mm Hg, with a pulmonary capillary wedge pressure of <15 mm Hg. Furthermore, if, during exercise, the mean pulmonary artery pressure is >30 mm Hg, then pulmonary artery hypertension is present. Pulmonary hypertension should be considered as primary or secondary and is best categorized in five groups:

- *Idiopathic pulmonary hypertension* is a rare group, 20% of which may be familial; may be related to medications/drug use and to collagen vascular diseases. Usually more common in women; pulmonary capillary wedge pressure is normal. Histological findings include vasoconstriction, inflammatory changes, and vascular proliferation in small pulmonary arterioles.
- *Pulmonary hypertension with left-heart disease:* Valvular heart disease or left ventricular failure; increases in mean pulmonary capillary wedge pressure
- *Pulmonary hypertension associated with primary lung disease and/or hypoxemia:* Associated with copd, interstitial fibrosis, restrictive lung diseases
- *Pulmonary hypertension caused by chronic thromboembolism disease/ PE*
- *Miscellaneous causes of pulmonary hypertension:* Sarcoidosis, chronic anemia

The most important component of treatment of pulmonary hypertension is the establishment of the diagnosis and the inclusion or exclusion of causative disease; e.g., anticoagulation in recurrent PE or modification of chronic hypoxemia from COPD or interstitial lung disease with supplemental oxygen.

Other forms of therapy include calcium-channel blockers causing vasodilatation and decrease in pulmonary artery pressure; endothelial receptor antagonists, which may improve exercise tolerance; phosphodiesterase inhibitors, which modify microvascular growth and enhance vasodilatation; and prostacyclins, which inhibit vascular smooth muscle growth, dilate the microvasculature, and result in platelet inhibition.

Once pulmonary hypertension is physiologically entrenched, the mean survival is 2–3 yrs; if patients have a functional cardiac classification of VI, then their mean survival is <6 months; death is usually secondary to right-heart failure, progressive hypoxemia, and hypotension.

Industrial dust diseases

Coal worker's pneumoconiosis (CWP) results from inhalation of coal dust particles (1–3 mcm in diameter) over 15–20 yrs; these microparticles are ingested by macrophages that degenerate, release their enzymes and cause an inflammatory reaction resulting in fibrosis.

Clinical features: Asymptomatic, but coexisting chronic bronchitis is common. A high incidence of cigarette smoking is common in coal workers.
CXR: Many round opacities (1–10 mm), especially upper zone.
Management: Avoid exposure to coal dust; treat coexisting chronic bronchitis.

Progressive massive fibrosis (PMF) is due to progression of CWP, which causes progressive dyspnea, fibrosis, and eventually, cor pulmonale.
CXR: Upper-zone fibrotic masses (1–10 cm).
Management: Avoid exposure to coal dust.

Caplan's syndrome is the association between rheumatoid arthritis, pneumoconiosis, and pulmonary rheumatoid nodules.

Silicosis is caused by inhalation of silica particles, which cause an intense fibrotic reaction. A number of jobs may be associated with exposure, e.g., metal mining, stone quarry exposure, sandblasting, and pottery/ceramic manufacture.

Clinical features: Progressive dyspnea, ↑incidence of TB, CXR shows diffuse miliary or nodular pattern in upper and mid-zones and egg-shell calcification of hilar nodes. PMF may occur. *Spirometry:* Restrictive ventilatory defect.
Management: Avoid exposure to silica.

Asbestosis is caused by inhalation of asbestos fibers. Chrysotile (white asbestos) is the least fibrogenic; crocidolite (blue asbestos) is the most fibrogenic. Amosite (brown asbestos) is the least common and has intermediate fibrogenicity. Asbestos was commonly used in the construction industry for fire-proofing, pipe wrapping, electrical wire insulation, and roofing tile.

Clinical features: Similar to other fibrotic lung diseases with progressive dyspnea, clubbing, and fine end-inspiratory crackles. Also causes pleural plaques, ↑risk of bronchial adenocarcinoma and mesothelioma.
Management: Symptomatic. Patients are often eligible for workers compensation.

Byssinosis is an asthmatic, obstructive airways-type pulmonary-occupational disorder characterized by chest tightness and a decreased FEV_1 when exposed to cotton dust, flax, and hemp in the production of yarns and textiles. Classically, employees describe symptoms on the first day of work, with lessening of their frequency and intensity throughout the work week. A chronic form of byssinosis may evolve over a period of years, resulting in COPD; especially found in cotton worker who are cigarette smokers.

Current environmental control measures have reduced cotton dust exposure and thus reduced the incidence of byssinosis; the Occupational and Safety and Health Administration has specific cotton dust exposure guidelines and requires pulmonary function surveillance in cotton/textile workers.

Beryllium is a lightweight, high-tensile-strength metal with solid electrical conduction, commonly used in manufacturing of alloys, ceramics, and high-technology electronics. The importance of beryllium exposure is primarily in the chronic form and in the patient's genetic makeup, which predisposes to a hypersensitive response to beryllium exposure.

Patient's sensitivity is associated with a genetic risk factor—the presence of HLA-DPB$_1$ alleles that are positive for glutamate at position 69. Although beryllium exposure has an acute form, chronic beryllium disease is similar to sarcoidosis and other granulomatous diseases. Clinical presentation and radiographic findings resemble sarcoidosis; pulmonary function studies are a mix of restrictive and obstructive patterns.

Toxic occupational exposure Exposure to toxic substances usually causes tracheobronchitis, a noxious airway reaction or, in severe instances, may cause destructive alveolar injury. Toxic chemicals affecting the lung include acid fumes, ammonia, formaldehyde, hydrogen sulfide, isocyanides, ozone and sulphur dioxide, and nitrogen dioxide.

The severity of toxic exposure may vary from a mixing of volatile cleaning agents in a closed bathroom to a massive chemical spill involving large populations. Ozone exposure results in a sterile inflammatory reaction associated with pulmonary macrophages releasing cytokines and pro-inflammatory mediators. Paraquat, a herbicide, induces acute lung injury; chlorine gas initiates an inflammatory reaction in the airways and alveoli and is associated with an oxidative lung injury secondary to reactive chlorinated by-products; nickel fumes cause a diffuse alveolitis/pneumonitis; sulphur mustard may cause an acute respiratory distress syndrome, acute bronchitis, bronchiolitis obliterans, or chronically evolving tracheobronchial stenosis.

Smoke inhalation is commonly encountered in fire-fighters; smoke inhalation and direct thermal injury to the airways are responsible for more deaths in fire victims and fire-fighters than are burn injuries. The toxicity of smoke inhalation to the lungs is related to the materials combusted in a fire; e.g., burning plastics may produce cyanide and hydrochloric acid.

The World Trade Center attack and the collapse of the buildings produced pulverized cement with a high alkalinity, resulting in acute respiratory symptoms and chronic lung disease. Follow-up studies of fire-fighters and victims with concentrated exposure from the New York catastrophe have defined a significant percentage of lung disease associated with long-term reduction in lung function. For more causes of interstitial lung disease, see Table 6.15.

Malignant mesothelioma is a neoplasm from mesothelial cells that usually occurs in the pleura and rarely in the peritoneum or other organs. Mesothelioma are associated with occupational exposure to asbestos; asbestos exists as fibers, either amphiboles or chrysotile. Because the risk of mesothelioma is more likely with amphibole exposure, the risk of mesothelioma is related to accumulative or total dose of exposure. >80% of patients report previous exposure to asbestos; only 20% of patients have pulmonary asbestosis. The latent period between exposure and development of a mesothelioma is 30–40 yrs, with rare occurrences at <20 years from exposure. Cigarette smoking does not affect the risk of developing mesothelioma.

Incidence in the United States 3–7 cases/million; with 2,200 new cases per year.

Clinical features include chest pain, dyspnea, weight loss, finger clubbing, recurrent pleural effusions. If the tumor has metastasized, there may be lymphadenopathy, hepatomegaly, bone pain/tenderness, abdominal pain/obstruction (peritoneal malignant mesothelioma). 50% of malignant mesothelioma metastases are usually local within the thorax or to the mediastinum or pericardium.

Tests: CXR/CT: Pleural thickening/effusion, decreased size of the hemithorax, bloody pleural fluid. Calcified pleural plaques are characteristic of asbestos exposure, especially when calcified pleural plaques are along the diaphragms.

Table 6.15 Causes of interstitial lung disease

Granulomatous diseases	Tuberculosis
	Sarcoidosis
Drugs	Amiodarone
	Bleomycin
	Busulfan
	Nitrofurantoin
	Sulfasalazine
Connective tissue diseases	Ankylosing spondylitis
	Rheumatoid arthritis
	SLE
	Systemic sclerosis
Extrinsic allergic alveolitis/Hyper-Sensitivity pneumonia (EAA) (p. 184)	Bird fancier's lung
	Farmer's lung
	Malt worker's lung
	Mushroom picker's lung
	Pigeon fancier's lung
Industrial dust diseases	Asbestosis
	Berylliosis
	Pneumoconiosis
	Silicosis
Radiation	
Chronic pulmonary edema (mitral stenosis)	
Bronchiolitis obliterans/ organizing pneumonia	
Idiopathic pulmonary fibrosis	

Individuals without evidence of mesothelioma yet with a history of asbestos exposure, with calcified or noncalcified pleural plaques, should be followed regularly; a routine asbestos evaluation includes a history and physical exam and pulmonary function studies, along with CXR and, if necessary, chest CT for detection of pleural or lung parenchyma neoplastic type changes and for detection of functional lung changes.

Diagnosis: Histology of tissue, following a pleural biopsy, video-assisted thoracic surgery, or limited thoracotomy. Often the diagnosis is made postmortem.

Management/Treatment: Symptomatic care; no effective radiation therapy or chemotherapy.

Prognosis is very poor (<2 yrs, produces 2,400 deaths/yr in the United States).

Cor pulmonale

Cor pulmonale is defined as secondary right-sided cardiac modifications and right ventricular dilation and/or hypertrophy in response to primary lung disease, either pulmonary vascular or lung parenchymal disorders. Causes include COPD, interstitial fibrosis, pulmonary vascular disorders, and neuromuscular and skeletal diseases (see Table 6.16). Although cor pulmonale or right-heart failure results from primary lung conditions, the most common cause of cor pulmonale is left-heart failure.

Clinical features Symptoms include dyspnea, fatigue, or syncope. *Signs*: Cyanosis, tachycardia, raised JVP with prominent *a* and *v* waves, right ventricular heave, loud P_2, pan-systolic murmur (tricuspid regurgitation), early diastolic Graham Steell murmur, hepatomegaly and edema.

Investigations *CBC*: Hemoglobin and hematocrit↑ (secondary polycythemia). *ABG*: Hypoxia, with or without hypercapnia and/or presence of respiratory acidosis. *CXR*: Enlarged right atrium and ventricle, prominent pulmonary arteries. *ECG*: Right axis deviation; right ventricular hypertrophy/strain; enlargement of P waves, P pulmonale.

Pulmonary function studies assist in differentiating between obstructive airways disease and restrictive pulmonary disease and in defining severity. Echocardiography reveals pulmonary hypertension, right ventricular function, right ventricular size, thickness, and paradoxical intraventricular septum motion and gives an assessment of left ventricular function and mitral/aortic valve functions.

Management
- *Treat underlying cause* (e.g., COPD, pulmonary infections, or treatment of left ventricular failure).
- *Treat respiratory failure*: In the acute situation, give 24% oxygen if P_aO_2 <60 mm Hg. Monitor ABG and gradually increase oxygen concentration if P_aCO_2 is stable. In COPD patients, LTOT for 18 h/d improves survival. Patients with chronic hypoxia, when clinically stable, should be assessed for LTOT.
- *Treat cardiac failure* with diuretics such as furosemide (e.g., 40–160 mg/24 h PO). Monitor electrolytes; treat with potassium supplements if necessary. *Alternative*: Spironolactone.

Table 6.16 Causes of cor pulmonale

- *Lung disease*
  Asthma (severe, chronic)
  COPD
  Bronchiectasis
  Pulmonary fibrosis
  Lung resection
- *Pulmonary vascular disease*
  PE
  Pulmonary vasculitis
  Primary pulmonary hypertension
  Pulmonary hypertension secondary to left-heart failure
  Sickle-cell disease
  Parasite infestation
- *Thoracic cage abnormality*
  Kyphosis
  Scoliosis
  Thoracoplasty
- *Neuromuscular disease*
  Myasthenia gravis
  Poliomyelitis
  Motor neuron disease
- *Hypoventilation*
  Sleep apnea/hypopnea syndrome
  Obesity
  Cerebral vascular disease

- Consider *phlebotomy* if the hematocrit is >55%.
- Consider *heart-lung transplantation* in young patients.

Prognosis Poor; once symptoms and signs of cor pulmonale develop, 50% of patients die within 5 yrs.

Obstructive sleep apnea/hypopnea syndrome

Obstructive sleep apnea/hypopnea syndrome is defined as daytime sleepiness associated with a minimum of five obstructive-type breathing events per hour of sleep; the events are *apnea,* defined as pauses of breathing lasting >10 sec, and *hypopnea,* defined as reduced ventilation by at least 50% for >10 sec during continuous breathing.

The cause of sleep apnea/hypopnea syndrome is related to relaxation of upper airway musculature and resultant inward movement of the upper airway soft tissue in inspiration during sleep. Predisposing factors include excessive weight, BMI of >30; male sex; shortened jaw and/or mandible; and age 40–65 yrs. The syndrome may occur in children with enlarged tonsils and adenoids.

Clinical points important in completion of the diagnosis include daytime sleepiness, reduced cognitive performance, depression, disturbed sleep, hypertension, morning headaches, decreased libido, increased incidence of auto accidents.

Clinical factors related to the sleep apnea/hypopnea syndrome are a greater risk of cardiovascular and cerebral vascular events; an association with DM related to increased insulin resistance; an elevation of liver function studies, unrelated to obesity; and, last, a higher risk of anesthesia and surgical procedures.

Diagnosis
- Detailed history from patient and patient's partner
- Sleep questionnaire
- Physical examination; BP readings; jaw and oral pharynx exams

Investigations Simple studies (pulse oximetry, video recordings) may be all that are required for diagnosis. Polysomnography (which monitors oxygen saturation, airflow at the nose and mouth, ecg, and electromyogram [emg] of chest and abdominal wall movement during sleep) is diagnostic. The occurrence of ≥15 episodes of apnea or hypopnea during 1 h of sleep indicates significant sleep apnea. The comparison of home- versus hospital-/office-based sleep studies reveals the home studies (especially in screening scenarios) are more cost effective, with similar clinical outcomes.

Management
- Weight reduction
- Avoidance of tobacco and alcohol
- CPAP Continuous positive airway pressure during sleep is effective.
- Surgical procedures to relieve pharyngeal obstruction (tonsillectomy, uvulopalatopharyngoplasty, or tracheostomy) are occasionally necessary.

Treatment/Outcomes
- Reduces sleepiness and improves quality of life
- Improves cognition
- Diminishes driving risk
- Hypertension resolves or is more easily controlled
- Betterment of work performance

Without daytime sleepiness and other daytime performance aberrations, patients with obstructive sleep apnea/hypopnea syndrome have doubtful clinical outcomes.

Lung transplantation

Lung transplantation is performed at a frequency of approximately 2,200 cases per year. The underlying pulmonary diseases for which lung transplantation is a treatment option are COPD, 30%; interstitial lung disease, 30%; CF, 15%; α_1-antitrypsin deficiency, 3%; and primary pulmonary artery hypertension, 2%.

Recipients of donor lungs basically do not have therapeutic options; their predictive transplant survival should be substantially greater than their native lung disease prognosis. Additionally, the recipient's quality of life should be predictably better with lung transplantation than with their predicted life quality with their present lung disease. Contraindications for lung transplantation include HIV infection, chronic hepatitis B and C infection, active smoking, malignancy (without remission or without cure), and alcohol or drug dependency. The upper age limit of lung transplant is about 65–70 yrs. Resistant bacterial infections, noncompliant persons, and ventilator-dependent individuals are other contraindications for lung transplant.

Organ procurement and timing of lung transplantation are based on a priority algorithm of risk of death on the waiting list versus probability of survival after transplantation. Candidates are matched for blood type and for lung size. The usual waiting time for transplantation is 6 months; deaths on the waiting list are about 50%.

Bilateral lung transplantation is the surgery of choice, performed in 65% of cases in the United States; bilateral lung transplants are necessary in CF and in diffuse bronchiectasis, in order to prevent the spread of infection, as may occur in a unilateral transplant scenario. Heart/lung transplants are utilized in patients with congenital heart-lung disease; single-lung transplants may be appropriate in other terminal lung diseases.

Post-transplant therapy consists of immunosuppressive regimens and prophylaxis for *Pneumocystis*-CMV-fungi. Within 3–6 months after transplantation, stability of lung function occurs; all patients have established follow-up for assessment of quality of life and for screening of complications and signs of rejection. The most common complication is a primary graft versus host dysfunction, as well as airway complications of bronchiolitis obliterans, acute and chronic rejections, and infections.

The cost of single-lung transplantation averages $450,000, whereas the expense of bilateral lung transplants is $657,000. Positive outcomes include restoration of lung function and an improvement in quality of life; the survival half-life for lung transplantation is 4–6 yrs.

Gastroenterology

Ellen M. Stein, M.D.

Contents

Oral manifestations of GI diseases

The oropharynx can provide diagnostic clues to a variety of GI diseases. Some examples are noted below.

Leukoplakia A potentially premalignant white thickening of the tongue or oral mucosa. When in doubt, refer all intraoral white lesions. *Causes:* Poor dental hygiene, smoking, sepsis, aphthous stomatitis, squamous papilloma, verruca vulgaris, secondary syphilis. Oral hairy leukoplakia is a painless, shaggy, whitish, streaky patch on the side of the tongue due to Epstein-Barr virus (EBV) that is often seen in patients with AIDS.

Necrotizing stomatitis Severe periodontal disease characterized by inflammation and necrosis of gingiva to adjacent soft tissue and nonalveolar bone. Often seen in patients with AIDS.

Aphthous ulcers Minute, painful, shallow white ulcers distributed along mucous membranes. Affects 20% of the population. *Causes:* Associated conditions include oral dental appliances (due to recurrent trauma), inflammatory bowel disease, Behçet disease, trauma, celiac sprue, erythema multiforme (see PLATE 17), lichen planus, pemphigus, pemphigoid, infections (herpes simplex, syphilis). Can be seen in otherwise healthy individuals. *Treatment* can be difficult: Steroid creams, treatment of underlying condition.

Candidiasis (thrush) White patches or erythema of the buccal mucosa. Patches may be hard to remove and bleed if scraped. *Risk factors*: Extremes of age, diabetes mellitus (DM), antibiotics, immunosuppression (long-term corticosteroids, including inhalers; cytotoxics; malignancy; HIV). Oropharyngeal candidiasis in an apparently healthy patient suggests underlying HIV infection *Treatment:* Nystatin swish-and-swallow suspension, fluconazole.

Angular cheilitis Fissuring at the angles of the mouth. Commonly associated with vitamin B deficiencies (riboflavin, niacin, and pyridoxine). Infectious causes include *Staphylococcus* and *Candida*.

Gingivitis Gum inflammation ± hypertrophy occurs with poor oral hygiene, drugs (phenytoin, cyclosporin, and nifedipine), pregnancy, vitamin C deficiency (scurvy), acute myeloid leukemia (p. 627), or Vincent's angina.

Microstomia The mouth is too small due to thickening and tightening of the perioral skin after burns or in epidermolysis bullosa (destructive skin and mucous membrane blisters ± ankyloglossia) or systemic sclerosis (p. 412); look for facial telangiectasia, sclerodactyly, Raynaud's, calcinosis.

Oral pigmentation Perioral melanin spots characterize Peutz–Jeghers' syndrome. Multiple telangiectasias of the buccal cavity suggest Osler–Weber–Rendu syndrome. Blue rubber bleb nevi syndrome can present with a mound-like venous anomaly on mucous membranes. Can be a cause of clinically overt or occult GI bleeding

Teeth A blue line at the gum–tooth margin suggests lead poisoning. Prenatal or childhood tetracycline exposure causes yellowish-brown discoloration.

Tongue *Ulcerated tongue:* May be seen in patients with graft-versus-host disease. Associated with tetrad of painful oral mucositis, enteritis, dermatitis, and hepatic dysfunction.

Glossitis A smooth, red, sore tongue is often caused by iron, folate, or B_{12} deficiency. If *local* loss of papillae leads to ulcer-like lesions that change in color and size, use the term *geographic tongue* (harmless migratory glossitis).

Macroglossia Diffusely enlarged tongue. Look for evidence of repeated tongue biting. *Causes:* myxedema, acromegaly, amyloid.

Healthy, enjoyable eating

There are no good or bad foods, and no universally good or bad diets. We must not consider diet out of context with a desired lifestyle, nor should we assume that everyone wants to be thin, healthy, and live forever. Excess body weight has been shown to increase the risk of progression of diseases like DM, osteoarthritis, and coronary disease. Providing sound nutritional advice to patients from many backgrounds requires sensitivity to cultural differences in diet (see Figure 7.1).

Current recommendations are based on three facts

- Obesity is an escalating epidemic, with as much as one-third of the U.S. population now estimated to be obese and estimated costs exceeding $147 billion annually in the United States alone.
- DM is burgeoning: The Centers for Disease Control (CDC) estimated the U.S. incidence of obesity at 9.1% in 2009 [http://www.cdc.gov/diabetes/statistics/incidence/fig2.html].
- Past advice has not changed eating habits in large sections of the population.

2010 U.S. Preventive Services Task Force (USPSTF) guidelines recommend screening children >6 for obesity and offer intervention and referral. Screening of adults continues to be recommended as well.

Advice is likely to focus on:

1 *Understand and use body mass index (BMI):* Weight in kilogram/(height in meters); aim for 18.5–25; i.e., *eat less, move more.* Controlling quantity may be more important than quality. In hypertension, eating the "right" things lowered blood pressure (BP) by 0.6 mm Hg, but controlling weight caused a 3.7 mm Hg reduction in 6 months in one randomized trial. BMI 25 to 30, overweight; BMI >30, obese. Consider referral to bariatric surgery if diet and exercise fail to improve BMI, and if BMI is >35 with a comorbidity or BMI >40 alone. (See Surgery.)

2 *Consider fish oil:* Eat fish rich in omega-3 fatty acid (e.g., mackerel, herring, salmon). This helps those with hyperlipidemia. If canned fish, avoid those in unspecified oils. Nuts are also valuable: Walnuts lower total cholesterol and have one of the highest ratios of polyunsaturates to saturates (7:1). Soya protein lowers cholesterol, low-density lipoproteins (LDL), and triglycerides.

3 *Use less refined sugar:* See Figure 7.1 for its deleterious effects. Use fruit to add sweetness. Have low-sugar drinks. Don't add sugar to drinks or cereals.

4 *Eat enough fruit and fiber:* See Figure 7.1.

5 *Reduce salt.*

Avoid this diet if:

- <5 yrs old
- Need for low residue (Crohn's, ulcerative colitis [UC, p. 238]) or special diet (celiac [p. 248])
- If weight *loss* is expected (e.g., HIV +ve).

Emphasis may be different in dyslipidemia (p. 108), DM, obesity, constipation, liver failure, chronic pancreatitis, renal failure (less protein), BP↑.

Figure 7.1 Traditional low-fat nutritional advice: The balance of good health

Fruits and vegetables

Bread, other cereals, and potatoes

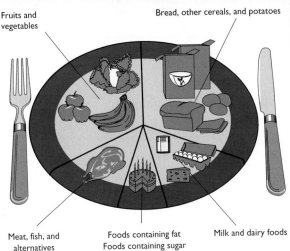

Meat, fish, and alternatives

Foods containing fat
Foods containing sugar

Milk and dairy foods

This shows rough proportions of food types that make up the putatively ideal meal. It is a model against which other diets are compared

Starchy foods: Bread, rice, pasta, potatoes, etc. form the main energy source (especially wholemeal). Increase fluid intake with a diet high in nonstarch polysaccharide (NSP)(e.g., 8 cups [1–2½ pints] daily). Warn about bulky stools. NSP ↓ calcium and iron absorption, so restrict main intake to one meal a day.

Fruit, vegetables: E.g., >6 different pieces of fruit (ideally with skins) or portions of pulses, beans, or lightly cooked greens per day. This may reduce cardiovascular and cancer mortality.

Meat and alternatives: Meat should be cooked without additional fat. Lower fat alternatives, such as white meat (poultry, without skin), white fish, and vegetable protein sources (e.g., pulses, soya) are encouraged.

Dairy foods: Low-fat skim milk/yogurt; cottage cheese.

Fat and sugary foods: Avoiding extra fat in cooking is advised ("grill, boil, roast, steam, or bake, but don't fry"). Fatty spreads (e.g., butter) are kept to a minimum and snack foods (potato chips, candies, cookies, or cake) are avoided.

Avoiding obesity: Excess sugar causes caries, DM, and obesity (this contributes to osteoarthritis, cancer, and hypertension, and raises oxidative stress, thus raising cardiovascular mortality).

Diets for obesity? Recent studies have shown a greater benefit for Mediterranean diets than for low-fat diets at inducing clinically relevant long-term changes in cardiovascular risk and inflammatory markers. The Mediterranean diet has been associated with lower all-cause mortality. The Mediterranean diet refers to a primarily plant-based diet originating from the habits of the peoples of Greece and southern Italy. The diet features high intake of fruits, vegetables, legumes, nuts, cereals, and whole-grains; use of olive oil rather than other fat sources; moderate consumption of fish and poultry and overall low consumption of red meat; moderate use of wine with meals is permitted.

(Continued)

Figure 7.1 (Continued)

Drugs for obesity? Indicated for a BMI of ≥30 or BMI ≥27 with obesity-related condition: high blood pressure (BP), type 2 DM, or dyslipidemia. Orlistat lowers fat absorption (hence SE of oily fecal incontinence).

Previous drugs were withdrawn from the market: Sibutramine (voluntarily withdrawn in 2010) and fenfluramine/dexfenfluramine (withdrawn 1997).

Dysphagia or odynophagia

Dysphagia is difficulty in swallowing, and odynophagia is pain with swallowing. Progressive or new-onset dysphagia lasting >3 wks deserves detailed investigation.

Causes May be classified as oropharyngeal or esophageal:

Mechanical block
Malignant stricture
Esophageal cancer
Metastatic cancer
Benign strictures
Esophageal web or ring
Peptic stricture
Extrinsic pressure
Lung cancer
Mediastinal lymph nodes
Retrosternal goiter
Aortic aneurysm
Left atrial enlargement

Pharyngeal pouch

Motility disorders
Achalasia
Diffuse esophageal spasm
Systemic sclerosis
Myasthenia gravis
Bulbar palsy
Pseudobulbar palsy
Syringobulbia
Bulbar poliomyelitis
Chagas disease

Others
Esophagitis
Eosinophilic esophagitis
Infection (*Candida*, herpes simplex virus [HSV])
Reflux esophagitis
Globus hystericus

Clinical features A careful history can establish whether dysphagia or odynophagia is oropharyngeal or esophageal in location and whether it is neuromuscular or structural in origin. Some discerning questions to ask include:

• Does dysphagia occur within 1 sec of swallowing? This implicates the oropharyngeal location.
• Is the dysphagia localized to the retrosternal or subxiphoid region? Often implicates an esophageal source.
• Was there difficulty in swallowing liquids and solids from the onset? If yes, then likely a motility disorder (achalasia, neurological dysfunction) is present; if no, likely a structural abnormality exists (stricture, ring, or web).
• Is it painful to swallow? Implicates mucosal disease (e.g., esophageal ulcerations due to malignancy, infections, or esophagitis).

- Is the dysphagia intermittent or progressive? Intermittent implies esophageal spasm.
- Does the neck bulge or gurgle on drinking? Suspect a pharyngeal pouch (e.g., Zenker diverticulum).

Investigations The first question is whether to obtain a barium swallow study prior to upper endoscopy. Patients with suspected oropharyngeal dysphagia or cervical esophageal dysphagia may benefit from a cine-esophagram first. When an endoscopy is performed, the endoscope is often passed quickly through the upper cervical esophagus. Guiding images can be safer for patients with strong suspicion of high strictures. In practice, a structural abnormality is often adequately treated with upper endoscopy. Findings suggestive of esophageal dysmotility or spasm should be further evaluated with esophageal manometry ± pH-impedance probe. Treatment is based on diagnosis.

Specific conditions *Diffuse esophageal spasm (DES)* is a disease characterized by rapid, nonperistaltic wave progression through the esophagus. Symptoms include intermittent dysphagia (30–60%) ± chest pain (80–90%). *Barium swallow:* Abnormal, nonperistaltic contractions; corkscrew esophagus. *Manometry:* >20% premature (e.g., contractions or nonperistaltic rapid contractions occurring during wet swallows). Medical therapy includes adequate acid control, smooth muscle relaxants, or tricyclic antidepressants. *Achalasia* is the most recognized motor disorder of the esophagus, and is characterized by incomplete relaxation of the lower esophageal sphincter (LES) (due to degeneration of the myenteric plexus). Secondary achalasia can result from Chagas' disease and pseudoachalasia. Symptoms include dysphagia, regurgitation, substernal cramps, and weight loss. *Barium swallow:* Dilated tapering esophagus (bird's beak), delay of clearance of barium, and usually without peristalsis. Diagnosis made with manometry reveals nonpropagating, low-amplitude aperistalic contractions of the esophagus and incomplete LES relaxation. *Treatment:* Chosen depending on age and comorbidities. *Surgery:* Laparoscopic Heller myotomy often done with partial fundoplication. *Endoscopy:* Pneumatic balloon dilatation, injection of Botox, peroral endoscopic myotomy (POEM; available at specialized academic centers). *Medication:* Smooth muscle relaxants, acid suppression. *Benign esophageal stricture:* Caused by gastroesophageal reflux disease (GERD) (p. 209), corrosives, surgery, or radiotherapy. Treatment is with endoscopic dilatation. *Esophageal cancer: Associations:* GERD, tobacco, alcohol, Barrett esophagus, achalasia. *Paterson-Brown-Kelly (Plummer-Vinson) syndrome:* Postcricoid web + iron-deficiency anemia.

Nausea and vomiting

Nausea is the subjective sensation of an impending urge to vomit, and vomiting is the forceful evacuation of gastric contents via the mouth. Causes of nausea and vomiting are protean and may originate from different body systems. Gross classifications include medications, central nervous system (CNS) disorders, GI and peritoneal disorders, endocrine and metabolic abnormalities, and infectious and miscellaneous causes (such as pregnancy).

Tests *Blood tests* including comprehensive metabolic panel. A metabolic alkalosis (pH >7.45, HCO_3^- ↑) suggests severe vomiting. A plain upright AXR may suggest a suspected bowel obstruction. Consider upper GI *endoscopy* if vomiting persists. Identify and *treat the underlying cause.*

Treatment *Fluids:* Give IV fluids for rehydration. *Drugs:* Various antiemetics may be chosen and administered IV or per rectum, if not tolerated orally. Avoid those antiemetics with prokinetic properties until bowel obstruction is ruled out. Metoclopramide 10 mg IV for GI causes (except intestinal obstruction). Avoid drugs in pregnancy.

207

Dyspepsia and peptic ulceration

Dyspepsia (indigestion) is a nonspecific group of symptoms (abdominal pain, bloating, and nausea) related to the upper GI tract. Causes of dyspeptic symptoms may include peptic ulcer disease (duodenal and gastric ulcers), gastritis, esophagitis, GERD, malignancy, or nonulcer dyspepsia (diagnosis of exclusion).

Symptoms and signs Physical examination, often normal, may reveal epigastric tenderness, tympanic percussion due to bloating, etc. These physical examination signs are non-specific.

Management of dyspepsia The initial management of patients with uninvestigated dyspepsia remains controversial. Clinical suspicion and economics often dictate when to test and perform invasive procedures on patients. For patients ≥50 yrs with long-standing symptoms or with alarm signs, upper endoscopy is indicated as part of the initial diagnostic workup. A reasonable approach for all patients without alarm symptoms or age <50 is to prescribe an empiric trial of a proton-pump inhibitor for 4–8 wks. American College of Gastroenterology (ACG) Guidelines advise treatment based on *Helicobacter pylori* prevalence within a community. If *H. pylori* prevalence is >10%, then dyspepsia patients should be tested and treated for *H. pylori* first; then, if symptoms persist, try proton pump inhibitor (PPI).[1]

Peptic ulcer disease

Abdominal pain occurs in 94% of patients with peptic ulcer disease (PUD). Typically described as burning, nonradiating epigastric pain that is often relieved with food or antacids. The pain may awaken patients in the middle of the night. Two-thirds of duodenal ulcer patients and one-third of gastric ulcer patients present with symptoms. Symptomatic pain is nonspecific, however, since one-third of patients with nonulcer dyspepsia also have similar pain. *Warning signs* of complicated PUD include signs of perforation, penetration, or hemorrhage. Ask for acute exacerbations in frequency, location, or severity of symptoms. Question patients for melena (90% of melena is due to upper GI hemorrhage), hematemesis, and radiating pain.

Duodenal ulcers (DU) are 4× more common than GU. *Risk factors*: *H. pylori* (~90%), drugs (aspirin, NSAIDs, steroids). Diseases associated with DU include Zollinger–Ellison syndrome, systemic mastocytosis, multiple endocrine neoplasia type I, chronic pulmonary disease, chronic renal failure, cirrhosis, nephrolithiasis, and α_1-antitrypsin deficiency.

Diagnosis: Upper GI endoscopy. Test for *H. pylori* (see p. 73). Gastrin concentrations should be measured if Zollinger–Ellison syndrome is suspected.

Gastric ulcers (GU) occur primarily in the elderly, on the lesser curve of the stomach. Ulcers elsewhere are more likely to be malignant. *Risk factors*: *H. pylori* (~70%), smoking, NSAIDs, stress-related ulcers (Cushing or Curling ulcers). *Diagnosis:* Upper GI endoscopy must be performed to exclude malignancy; take multiple biopsies from the rim and base of the ulcer (histology, *H. pylori*) and brushings (cytology).

Treatment of peptic ulcers *Lifestyle:* Avoid food that worsens symptoms. Stop smoking (slows healing in GU; hastens relapse rates in DU). Medical therapy includes antacids, H₂ receptor antagonists, proton-pump inhibitors, and cytoprotective agents (sucralfate, misoprostol). Misoprostol is contraindicated in women of childbearing age, and dose-related diarrhea is often the limiting factor in patient compliance. *H. pylori eradication:* Triple[2] or quadruple therapy. *NSAID-associated ulcers:* Stop NSAID if possible

---

1 Talley N, Vakil N. Guidelines for the management of dyspepsia. *Am J Gastroenterol.* 2005; 100:2324–2337.
2 Triple therapy for 7–14d: (1) PPI (e.g., lansoprazole 30 mg bid),(2) amoxicillin 1 g bid, (3) clarithromycin 500 mg bid.

(if not, use H_2-receptor antagonist, PPI, or misoprostol for prevention). If symptoms persist, re-endoscope, recheck for *H. pylori*, and reconsider the differential diagnosis. *Surgery* (p. 495): May be indicated for complications of PUD.

Gastroesophageal reflux disease

The development of signs, symptoms, or complications related to the retrograde passage of gastric contents into the esophagus is termed GERD. GERD is extremely common, with equal prevalence among genders; however, there is a male predominance for complications. Factors associated with GERD include the acidity of the refluxate, antireflux barriers, luminal acid clearance mechanisms, esophageal tissue resistance, and gastric emptying. Dysfunction of the lower esophageal sphincter predisposes to the gastroesophageal reflux. If reflux is prolonged or excessive, it may cause inflammation of the esophagus (esophagitis), benign esophageal stricture, Barrett's esophagus, and esophageal adenocarcinoma.

Associations Smoking, alcohol, hiatal hernia, pregnancy, obesity, large meals, myotomy of the lower esophageal sphincter for achalasia, drugs (tricyclics, anticholinergics, nitrates), systemic sclerosis. GERD may have a correlation with pulmonary or other extraintestinal manifestations.

Symptoms Heartburn (burning, retrosternal discomfort related to meals, lying down, and straining, relieved by antacids), belching, acid brash (acid or bile regurgitation), water brash (excessive salivation), odynophagia (painful swallowing (e.g., from esophagitis or stricture), nocturnal asthma (cough/ wheeze with apparently minimal inhalation of gastric contents).

Complications: Esophagitis, ulcers, iron deficiency anemia, benign strictures, Barrett esophagus, eosinophilic esophagitis, and esophageal adenocarcinoma.

Tests Isolated symptoms do not require investigation. *Indications for upper GI endoscopy*: Age >50 yrs, longer symptom duration (>4 wks), dysphagia, persistent symptoms despite treatment, relapsing symptoms, weight loss or other alarm signs/symptoms. Barium swallow may show hiatus hernia. 24 h esophageal pH monitoring ± esophageal manometry may be needed to distinguish refractory or hard to treat GERD from other causes, such as achalasia.

The Los Angeles (LA) classification: Minor diffuse changes (erythema, edema, friability) are not included and the term *mucosal break* is used to encompass the old terms "erosion" and "ulceration." There are four grades.

A One or more mucosal breaks <5 mm long, not extending beyond two mucosal fold tops. A mucosal break is a well-demarcated area of slough/ erythema.

B Mucosal break >5 mm long limited to the space between two mucosal fold tops.

C Mucosal break continuous between the tops of two or more mucosal folds but which involves <75% of the esophageal circumference.

D Mucosal break involving ≥75% of the esophageal circumference.

Treatment

- *Lifestyle:* Encourage weight loss; raise bed head; small, regular meals. Avoid hot drinks, alcohol, and eating <3 h before bed. Avoid drugs affecting esophageal motility (nitrates, anticholinergics, tricyclic antidepressants) or that damage the mucosa (NSAIDs, K^+ salts, alendronate).
- *Drugs: Antacids* to relieve symptoms. If symptoms persist for >4 wks (or weight↓; dysphagia; excessive vomiting; GI bleeding), *refer for GI endoscopy*. If esophagitis confirmed, try a *PPI* (the most effective option). *Prokinetic drugs:* These help gastric emptying (e.g., metoclopramide;

dystonias and tardive dyskinesia can be a serious side effect [see FDA Black Box warning]).

• *Surgery:* Endoscopic options such as Stretta or EndoCinch (endoscopic plication methods) have fallen out of use. Laparoscopic fundoplication performed by an experienced surgeon is a reliable therapeutic option for patients with proven reflux disease to achieve prolonged symptom relief.

Diarrhea

The normal daily stool weight is 100–200 g, and, in the United States, a daily stool weight >200 g is abnormal. *Diarrhea* means increased stool water (hence increased stool volume, e.g., >200 mL daily), and thus increased stool frequency and the passage of liquid stool. If it is the stool's fat content that is increased, the diarrhea is termed *steatorrhea.* Distinguish both from *fecal urgency* (may be caused by cancers or UC).

Conditions that cause diarrhea are broadly classified into *osmotic diarrhea* (stool output diminishes with reduced oral intake), *secretory diarrhea* (stool output persists despite reduction in oral intake), and *mucosal injury* categories. In reality, high-output diarrhea is usually a combination of these mechanisms. Normal-output diarrhea (stool volume <200 g/d) is typically related to anorectal dysfunction. Foul-smelling, greasy stools are characteristic of steatorrhea. See Table 7.1.

Clinical features It is important to take a detailed and accurate history:

Is it acute (<3 wks duration) or chronic (>3 wks duration)? Acute: Usually infectious or drug-induced. Ask about recent travel, sexual practices, ingestion of well water or inadequately cooked food and shellfish. Question for exposure to ill contacts

Chronic: Usually requires extensive history and further testing. Ask about prior bowel surgery and a family history. Additional testing should include stool studies for lactoferrin (fecal leukocytes), ova and parasites, cultures, and *Clostridium difficile* toxin. Check for signs of labs of malabsorption, including vitamins, and evaluate stool for steatorrhea (sudan stain). Often, radiographic and endoscopic evaluation with biopsies is required if above testing is normal.

• *Is the large or small bowel the source? Large bowel symptoms:* Watery stool ± blood or mucus, pelvic pain relieved by defecation, tenesmus,

Table 7.1 Common causes of diarrhea

Common causes	Uncommon	Rare
Gastroenteritis	Microscopic colitis	Autonomic neuropathy
Viral	Celiac disease	Addison's disease
Bacterial	Chronic pancreatitis	Ischemic colitis
Parasites/protozoa	Thyrotoxicosis	Amyloidosis
Irritable bowel	Laxative abuse; food allergy	Tropical enteropathy
Drugs (below)	Lactose intolerance	Gastrinoma, VIPoma
Colorectal cancer	Ileal/gastric resection	Carcinoid syndrome
Ulcerative colitis (UC)	Bacterial overgrowth	Medullary thyroid ca
Crohn disease	Pseudomembranous colitis	Pellagra

urgency. Small bowel symptoms: Periumbilical (or right iliac fossa [RIF]) right lower quadrant (RLQ) pain, not relieved by defecation; watery stool or steatorrhea.

- *Is there blood, mucus, or pus?* Bloody diarrhea: Campylobacter, Shigella, Salmonella, E. coli, amebiasis, inflammatory bowel disease, malignancy, pseudomembranous colitis, ischemic colitis. *Mucus* occurs in irritable bowel syndrome (IBS), colonic adenocarcinoma, polyps. *Pus* suggests inflammatory bowel disease or diverticulitis.
- *Could there be a non-gi cause?* Think of drugs (antibiotics, PPIs, cimetidine, propranolol, cytotoxics, NSAIDs, digoxin, alcohol, laxative abuse) and medical conditions (thyrotoxicosis, autonomic neuropathy, Addison's disease).

Examination *Look for* weight loss, anemia, dehydration, oral ulcers, clubbing, rashes, and abdominal scars. *Feel for:* Enlarged thyroid or an abdominal mass. *Do a rectal examination:* Any rectal mass (rectal carcinoma) or impacted feces (overflow diarrhea)? Test stools for fecal occult blood.

Tests *Blood:* In addition to above tests, look for evidence of iron deficiency or celiac sprue.

Stool: For pathogens and *C. difficile* toxin (pseudomembranous colitis). Fecal fat excretion or ^{13}C-hiolein breath test if symptoms of chronic pancreatitis, malabsorption, or steatorrhea are present.

Colonoscopy/barium enema: In colitis, and to exclude malignancy. If normal, consider small bowel radiology or capsule endoscopy (Crohn's) ± endoscopic ultrasound or endoscopic retrograde cholangiopancreatography (ERCP) (p. 222, e.g., chronic pancreatitis).

Management Treat causes. Oral rehydration is preferable to IV rehydration. If severely dehydrated, give 0.9% saline + 20 mmol K$^+$/L IVI. Codeine phosphate 30 mg/6 h PO reduces stool frequency. Avoid antibiotics unless the patient has infective diarrhea and is systemically unwell. See Figure 7.2.

Figure 7.2 Management of infective diarrhea

```
                              Diarrhoea
            ┌────────────────────┼────────────────────┐
No systemic signs      Systemic illness        Special circumstances:
                       • Fever> 39°C           • Food poisoning outbreak
                       • Bloody diarrhoea      • Travel (p556 & 558)
                         lasting>2 weeks       • Recent antibiotic use
                       • Dehydration           • Rectal intercourse
                                               • Immunocompromised host
Symptomic                                      • Raw sea food ingested
treatment
                        Consider noninfectious
                           causes (see text)
                        Admit to hospital
                        Give oral fluids
                        Consider presumptive
                        antimicrobial therapy*

Stool culture          Prompt, direct faecal       Routine stool culture
not needed             smear (then culture)         and microscopy

                                                          Confer with
                                                          microbiologist
              ┌───────────────────┼───────────────────┐
        Polymorphs seen      No Polymorphs         Parasites seen

        Likely culture:      Likely culture:       Specific therapy
        Shigella**           Salmonella**          (p616—p620)
        Campylobacter        E coli
        E coli               (C difficile*)
        (Yersinia—rare)
        (Samonella—rare)
        (C difficile*)
```

NB: Alternatively, classify into *secretory* (e.g., infections, UC/Crohn's, etc.) or *osmotic* causes (if water drawn into the gut, as in laxative use).

Constipation

Constipation is defined as the symptomatic reduction in stool frequency to fewer than three bowel movements per week or difficulty in defecation, with straining or discomfort.

Causes of constipation are numerous and relate either to colonic transit impairment or to structure or functional obstruction to fecal evacuation (see Table 7.2).

Clinical features Ask about frequency, nature, and consistency of the stool, and in comparison to their past habits. Is there blood or mucus in/on the stools? Is there diarrhea alternating with constipation? Has there been a recent change in bowel habit? Ask about diet and drugs. Rectal examination is essential.

Tests Most constipation does not need investigation, especially in young, mildly affected patients. Indications for investigation: Age >40 yrs, recent change in bowel habit, associated symptoms (weight loss, rectal bleeding, mucous discharge, or tenesmus). *Blood tests:* TSH. *Colonoscopy* and biopsy of abnormal mucosa if testing is abnormal. Special investigations (e.g., transit studies; anorectal physiology) are rarely indicated for constipation that responds to basic medical management.

Treatment Treat the cause (see Figure 7.2). Advise exercise and adequate fluid intake (a high-fiber diet is often advised, but this may cause bloating without helping the constipation). Consider drugs only if these measures fail and try to use them for short periods only. Often, a stimulant such as senna ± a bulking agent is cheaper than agents such as polyethylene glycol solutions. Both methods are effective.

Bulking agents increase fecal mass and thus stimulate peristalsis. *Contraindications* (*CI*): Difficulty in swallowing, intestinal obstruction, colonic atony, fecal impaction. *Stimulant laxatives* increase intestinal motility and should be avoided in intestinal obstruction. Prolonged use may rarely cause colonic atony and hypokalemia. Pure stimulant laxatives include *bisacodyl* tablets (5–10 mg at night) or suppositories (10 mg in the mornings) and *senna* (2–4 tablets at night). *Glycerol suppositories* act as a rectal stimulant.

Stool softeners: Docusate sodium acts as a stool softener. *Liquid paraffin* should not be used for a prolonged period. Side effects (*SE*): Anal seepage, lipoid pneumonia, malabsorption of fat-soluble vitamins.

Osmotic laxatives retain fluid in the bowel. *Lactulose*, a semisynthetic disaccharide, produces an osmotic diarrhea of low fecal pH that discourages growth of ammonia-producing organisms. It is useful in hepatic encephalopathy and is used frequently for constipation. A major SE is bloating that can often worsen the abdominal pain in constipated patients. A better alternative is polyethylene glycol (MiraLax®), which is an osmotic laxative. *Magnesium salts* (e.g., magnesium hydroxide and magnesium sulfate) are useful when rapid bowel evacuation is required. *Sodium salts* (e.g., Microlette® and Micralax® enemas) should be avoided as they may cause sodium and water retention. *Phosphate enemas* were useful for rapid bowel evacuation prior to procedures. Phosphate preparations have largely been removed from U.S. markets over concerns about renal failure and phosphate nephropathy when used without sufficient hydration techniques.

Chloride-channel(ClC-2) activators, such as lubiprostone (Amitiza®), have been demonstrated to be effective in treating chronic constipation.

Selective μ-opioid receptor antagonist, such as methylnaltrexone (Relistor®), when used as a subcutaneous injectable product has been shown to relieve constipation in opioid-induced constipation.

Agonist of guanylate cyclase C, such as linaclotide (Linzess®)is now FDA approved for control of constipation and IBS with constipation predominant symptoms.

What if laxatives don't help? A multidisciplinary approach with behavior therapy, psychological support, habit training ± sphincter-action biofeedback may help. Clinical trials are under way to evaluate prucalopride (selective 5HT-4 agonist) on safety and efficacy. This agent is under FDA review.

Table 7.2 Causes of constipation

Poor diet
Inadequate fluid intake or dehydration
Immobility (or lack of exercise)
Irritable bowel syndrome
Elderly
Postoperative pain
Anorectal disease
  Anal fissure
  Anal stricture
  Rectal prolapse
Intestinal obstruction
  Colorectal carcinoma
  Strictures (e.g., Crohn's disease)
  Pelvic mass (e.g., fibroids)
  Diverticular disease (stricture formation)
  Congenital abnormalities
  Pseudo-obstruction
Metabolic/endocrine
  Hypothyroidism
  Hypercalcemia
  Hypokalemia
  Porphyria
  Lead poisoning
Drugs
  Opiate analgesics (e.g., morphine, codeine)
  Anticholinergics (tricyclics, phenothiazines)
  Iron
Neuromuscular (slow transit with reduced propulsive activity)
  Spinal or pelvic nerve injury
  Aganglionosis (Chagas' disease, Hirschsprung's disease)
  Systemic sclerosis
  Diabetic neuropathy
Other causes
  Chronic laxative abuse (rare; diarrhea is more common)
  Idiopathic slow transit
  Idiopathic megarectum/colon
  Psychological (e.g., associated with depression or abuse as a child)

Jaundice

Jaundice (icterus) refers to a yellow pigmentation of skin, sclera, and mucosa due to an elevated plasma bilirubin level (visible at >3 mg/dL). Jaundice may be classified by the type of circulating bilirubin (conjugated or unconjugated) or by the site of the problem (prehepatic, hepatocellular, or cholestatic/obstructive). *Bilirubin metabolism:* Bilirubin is formed from the breakdown of hemoglobin. It is conjugated with glucuronic acid by hepatocytes, making it water soluble. Conjugated bilirubin is secreted into bile and passes into the duodenum. In the small intestine, bile is converted to urobilinogen by the gut flora. Most (>90%) of the urobilinogen is actively reabsorbed in the ileum and transported via the portal circulation to the liver. Some of the portal urobilinogen is retaken by the hepatocytes and resecreted into the bile (*enterohepatic circulation*). A portion of the bile bypasses the liver and is excreted by the kidneys into the urine. The remainder of urobilinogen that is not reabsorbed in the ileum is converted to stercobilin in the distal small intestine or proximal colon, giving feces its characteristic brown color.

Prehepatic jaundice If there is excess bilirubin production (hemolysis, inadequate liver uptake, or deficient hepatic conjugation), unconjugated bilirubin enters the blood. Because unconjugated bilirubin is water insoluble, it is not excreted in urine, resulting in an *unconjugated (indirect) hyperbilirubinemia*. *Causes:* Physiological (neonatal), hemolysis, ineffective erythropoiesis, glucuronyl transferase deficiency (e.g., Gilbert's syndrome, Crigler–Najjar's syndrome).

Hepatocellular jaundice occurs with hepatocyte damage ± cholestasis. *Causes:* Viruses Hepatitis (p. 564, e.g., A, B, C, etc.), cytomegalovirus (CMV), EBV (p. 559); drugs (see Table 7.3); alcoholic hepatitis; cirrhosis; liver metastases/abscess; hemochromatosis; autoimmune hepatitis (AIH); sepsis; leptospirosis; α_1-antitrypsin deficiency; Budd–Chiari syndrome; Wilson's disease (p. 233); failure to excrete conjugated bilirubin (Dubin–Johnson and Rotor's syndromes); right-heart failure, causing sinusoidal congestion; toxins, e.g., carbon tetrachloride; fungi (*Amanita phalloides*).

Cholestatic (obstructive) jaundice Blockage or obstruction of the common bile duct results in *conjugated hyperbilirubinemia*. Conjugated bilirubin is water soluble and thus easily excreted into the urine. Jaundiced patients complain of dark, tea-colored urine. The lack of conjugated bilirubin reaching the gut (due to bile duct obstruction) prevents adequate urobilinogen formation. This causes the feces to become clay-colored. *Causes:* Choledocholithiasis, pancreatic cancer, lymph nodes at the porta hepatis, drugs (see Table 7.3), cholangiocarcinoma, sclerosing cholangitis, primary biliary cirrhosis (PBC) (see Table 7.4), choledochal cyst, biliary atresia.

Clinical features Ask about clues to a possible viral hepatitis such as blood transfusions before 1990, IV drug use, body piercing, tattoos, sexual activity, travel abroad, jaundiced contacts, etc. Also, query family history, alcohol consumption, and *all* medications (e.g., old drug charts and records). *Examine* for signs of chronic liver disease, hepatic encephalopathy, lymphadenopathy, hepatomegaly, splenomegaly, palpable gallbladder, and ascites. Pale stools and dark urine suggest obstructive jaundice.

Tests *Urine:* Bilirubin is absent in prehepatic causes; urobilinogen is absent in obstructive jaundice. *Hematology:* Signs of hemolysis (anemia, elevated lactate dehydrogenase (LDH), low haptoglobin, elevated reticulocyte count, positive Coombs' test). *Biochemistry: Liver function tests* (LFT; bilirubin—direct and indirect, aspartate aminotransferase/alanine aminotransferase (AST/ALT), alk phos, total protein, albumin). *Virology:* EBV, CMV, hepatitis virus A, B, C (HVA, HVB, HVC) serologies. *Other specific tests*, e.g., for hemochromatosis (elevated ferritin and iron-to-total iron binding capacity (TIBC) ratio, causing a high serum % iron saturation (>55–60%); α_1-antitrypsin deficiency (serum for genetic analysis), Wilson's disease (e.g., low serum and high urine copper levels, low serum ceruloplasmin [p. 233]); PBC (high antimitochondrial antibody titers, AMA), and AIH (high antinuclear and anti-smooth muscle antibodies). *Ultrasound:* Are the bile ducts dilated (obstruction)? Are there gallstones, hepatic metastases, or pancreatic masses? Request magnetic resonance cholangiopancreatography (MRCP) (p. 223), *endoscopic ultrasound (EUS),* or ERCP if bile ducts are dilated. Consider performing a *liver biopsy* (p. 222) if the bile ducts are normal. Consider abdominal computed tomography *(CT) or magnetic resonance imaging (MRI) scan.*

Table 7.3 Drug-induced jaundice

Hepatitis	Phenytoin, carbamazepine, valproic acid
	Anti-tuberculosis (TB) meds (isoniazid, rifampin, pyrazinamide), nitrofurantoin, antifungals (ketoconazole, fluconazole, itraconazole), antivirals (DDI, AZT)
	Statins
	Angiotensin-converting enzyme (ACE)-inhibitors, methyldopa, calcium channel blockers
	Monoamine oxidase inhibitors (MAOIs), amitriptyline, imipramine
	Halothane (general anesthetic); NSAIDs (ibuprofen, sulindac, diclofenac, indomethacin)
Cholestasis	Antibiotics (erythromycin, nitrofurantoin, rifampin)
	Anabolic steroids
	Oral contraceptives
	Chlorpromazine
	Prochlorperazine,
	Sulfonylureas, chlorpropamide
	Gold salts, cyclosporin

Table 7.4 Causes of jaundice in a previously stable patient with cirrhosis

- Sepsis
- Alcohol
- Drugs
- Malignancy (e.g., hepatocellular carcinoma)
- GI bleeding

Upper GI bleeding 1

Hematemesis is vomiting of blood. It may be bright or resemble coffee grounds. *Melena* is black, tarry stool (signifies altered blood) with a characteristic odor. Both can indicate upper GI bleeding.

Causes

Common	Rare
Peptic ulcers	Bleeding disorders
Gastritis/gastric erosions	Portal hypertensive gastropathy
Mallory–Weiss tear	Aortoenteric fistula; angiodysplasia
Duodenitis	Hemobilia (bleeding from biliary tree)
Esophageal varicesEsophagitis	Dieulafoy lesion (rupture of a submucosal arteriole)
	Meckel's diverticulum
Malignancy	Peutz–Jeghers' syndrome
Drugs (NSAIDs, steroids thrombolytics, anticoagulants)	Osler–Weber–Rendu syndrome

Assessment Brief history and examination to assess severity.

History: Elicit a focused history evaluating for risk factors or conditions that are associated with severe GI bleeding. Assess for prior history of GI bleeding, history of PUD, known bleeding diathesis, underlying cirrhosis and portal hypertension, dysphagia, vomiting, weight loss, NSAID use, alcohol consumption. *Examination:* Look for stigmata of chronic liver disease and perform a digital rectal examination to check for melena. Assess for signs of vascular shock:

- Peripheral vasoconstriction (cool and clammy)
- Tachycardic (pulse >100 bpm, and jugular venous pressure (JVP) not elevated)
- Hypotensive (systolic BP <100 mm Hg)
- Postural drop in BP (orthostatic)
- Poor urine output, e.g., <30 mL/h

Calculating the *Rockall risk score* (see Table 7.5) may help to risk-stratify the patient.

Acute management (p. 769) Critical to management is early resuscitation of a bleeding patient (Table 7.6). In summary:

- Protect airway and give high-flow oxygen.
- Insert two large-bore (14–16 G) IV cannula and draw blood for hemoglobin levels, clotting assessment, and type and cross for 4–6 U packed red blood cells (PRBCs) (1 U/g/dL <14 g/dL).
- Give IV colloid while waiting for blood to be cross-matched. In an emergency, give group O Rh–ve blood.
- Transfuse until hemodynamically stable.
- Correct clotting abnormalities (vitamin K, frozen fresh plasma [FFP], platelets).
- Monitor pulse, BP, and central venous pressure (CVP) at least hourly until stable.
- Consider insertion of a urinary catheter and monitor hourly urine output.
- Consider a CVP line to monitor CVP and guide fluid replacement. Remember that standard CVP catheters infuse more slowly than peripheral large-bore IV.

- Obtain a chest x-ray (CXR), electrocardiogram (ECG), and arterial blood gas (ABG) in high-risk patients.
- Consult gastroenterologist and arrange for an urgent endoscopy (p. 221).
- Begin PPI therapy. May wish to notify surgery team of all severe bleeds on admission.
- If liver disease present, consider octreotide infusion.

Further management

- Reexamine after 4 h and give FFP if >4 U transfused.
- Monitor pulse, BP, CVP, and urine output hourly; decrease frequency to 4 h if hemodynamically stable.
- Check CBC, CMP, LFT, and clotting daily.
- Transfuse to goal Hb based on comorbidities; always keep 2 units of blood in reserve.
- Keep "NPO" for 24 h. Allow clear fluids after 24 h and light diet after 48 h if no evidence of rebleeding. Discuss with consulting gastroenterologist, if needed.
- Start IV or oral PPI pending clinical status.

Table 7.5 Rockall risk-scoring system for gi bleeds

Score	0	1	2	3
Age	<60 yrs	60–79 yrs	80 yrs	
Shock: Systolic bp pulse rate	BP >100 mm Hg<100/min	BP >100 mm HgPulse >100/min	BP <100 mm Hg	
Co-morbidity	No major	Cardiac failurelschemic heart disease	Renal failure Liver failure	Metastases
Diagnosis	Mallory–Weiss tear; no lesion; no sign of recent bleeding	All other diagnoses	Upper GI malignancy	
Signs of recent hemorrhage on endoscopy	None, or dark-red spot		Blood in upper GI tract; adherent clot;visible vessel	

Rockall scores help predict risk of rebleeding and death after upper GI bleeding. A score >6 is said to be an indication for surgery, but decisions relating to surgery are rarely taken on the basis of Rockall scores alone.

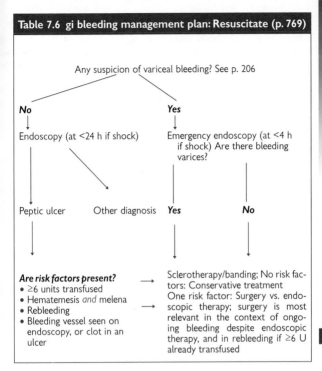

Table 7.6 gi bleeding management plan: Resuscitate (p. 769)

Any suspicion of variceal bleeding? See p. 206

No

Endoscopy (at <24 h if shock)

Peptic ulcer   Other diagnosis

Yes

Emergency endoscopy (at <4 h if shock) Are there bleeding varices?

Yes   **No**

Are risk factors present?
• ≥6 units transfused
• Hematemesis *and* melena
• Rebleeding
• Bleeding vessel seen on endoscopy, or clot in an ulcer

→ Sclerotherapy/banding; No risk factors: Conservative treatment
One risk factor: Surgery vs. endoscopic therapy; surgery is most relevant in the context of ongoing bleeding despite endoscopic therapy, and in rebleeding if ≥6 U already transfused

219

Upper GI bleeding 2 and bleeding varices

Endoscopy should be arranged after resuscitation, within 4 h if variceal hemorrhage is suspected or bleeding is ongoing, and otherwise within 12–24 h of admission. It can identify the site of bleeding, be used to estimate the risk of rebleeding, and to administer endoscopic treatment. Stigmata of high-risk rebleeding lesions for PUD include actively bleeding vessel (60%), adherent clot (40%), visible vessel (20%), flat spot (10%), and clean base (5%). **Rebleeding** Since rebleeders have increased mortality, identify these patients and monitor them closely for signs of rebleeding.

Guidelines for considering surgery

• Severe bleeding or bleeding despite transfusing 6 U if >60 yrs (8 U if <60 yrs)
• Rebleeding
• Active bleeding at endoscopy that cannot be controlled
• Rockall score >6 (p. 218)

Varices Portal hypertension causes dilated collateral veins (varices) at sites of porto-systemic anastomosis. Varices are most prevalently in the distal esophagus, but may also be found in the stomach (gastric varices), around the umbilicus (caput medusa — rare) and in the rectum (rectal varices) and duodenum (duodenal varices). Varices develop in patients with cirrhosis once portal pressure (measured by hepatic venous pressure gradient) is >10 mm Hg; if >12 mm Hg, variceal bleeding may develop; associated with a mortality of 30–50% per episode.

Causes of portal hypertension can be divided into: *Prehepatic:* Portal vein thrombosis; splenic vein thrombosis, arterioportal fistula, splenomegaly. *Intrahepatic:* Cirrhosis; fulminant hepatitis, veno-occlusive disease, Budd–Chiari syndrome, schistosomiasis (common worldwide); sarcoidosis; myeloproliferative diseases; congenital hepatic fibrosis, metastatic malignancy. *Posthepatic:* Budd–Chiari syndrome, right-heart failure, constrictive pericarditis, inferior vena cava web.

Risk factors for variceal hemorrhage: Increased portal pressure; variceal size, endoscopic features of the variceal wall, e.g., fresh clot, red wale sign, etc.; and Child–Pugh score ≥8 (see Table 7.12).

Suspect varices as a cause of gi bleeding if there is alcohol abuse or cirrhosis. Look for signs of chronic liver disease, encephalopathy, splenomegaly ± ascites.

Prophylaxis (primary): Variceal hemorrhage occurs annually in 5–15% of patients with varices and cirrhosis. 2007 American Association for the study of Liver Disease (AASLD) guidelines[3] recommend primary prophylaxis for patients with large varices or small varices at risk for bleeding with: (1) Nonselective β-blockers (propranolol or nadolol) titrated to maximum tolerated dose. (2) Endoscopic ligation (banding) is indicated for large and at risk varices. Banding reduces risk of first bleeding when compared with β-blockers. Endoscopic sclerotherapy is no longer recommended as complications outweigh benefits. *Secondary:* After an initial variceal bleed, risk of further bleeding is high. Options are (1) and (2) as above, + transjugular intrahepatic portosystemic shunting (TIPS) or surgical shunts. TIPS is also used in uncontrolled variceal hemorrhage. Consider surgical shunts if TIPS is impossible for technical reasons.

220

Acute variceal bleeding: Get expert help at the bedside.

- Resuscitate until hemodynamically stable or Hg goal of 8 g/dL. Beyond this, increased rebleeding and mortality rise. Avoid excess saline infusion. Correct clotting abnormalities with vitamin K and FFP.
- Start IVI of octreotide (for 5 d).
- Endoscopic therapy: Band ligation is recommended when possible. Banding may be impossible when visualization is poor due to rapid bleeding.
- If bleeding uncontrolled, a Minnesota tube or Sengstaken–Blakemore tube should be placed by someone with experience—or TIPS as above (see Table 7.7).

In cirrhotic patients with active GI bleed, initiate antibiotic treatment to reduce mortality; recommended agents include ceftriaxone and norfloxacin.

3 Garcia-Tsao G, et al. AASLD Practice Guidelines: Prevention and management of gastroesophageal varices and variceal hemorrhage in cirrhosis. *Hepatology.* 2007;46(3):922–938.

Table 7.7 Balloon tamponade with a Sengstaken–Blakemore tube

In life-threatening variceal bleeding, this can buy time to arrange transfer to a specialty liver center.

It uses balloons to compress gastric and esophageal varices.

Before insertion, inflate balloons with a measured volume (120–300 mL) of air giving pressures of 60 mm Hg (check with a sphygmomanometer).

- Deflate, and clamp exits.
- Pass the lubricated tube and inflate the gastric balloon with the predetermined volume of air in stomach. Tug gently back into position against the upper stomach. Inflation of the gastric balloon within the esophagus will lead to perforation. If there is any question as to location, confirm with x-ray.
- Inflate the esophageal balloon. Check pressures (should be 20–30 mm Hg higher on the trial run). This phase of the procedure is dangerous: Do not overinflate the balloon (risk of esophageal necrosis or rupture). Often, hemodynamic stability can be achieved with inflation of the gastric balloon alone. Again, may confirm position with imaging.
- Many balloons come with a helmet to properly attach and apply tension to the balloon to maintain tamponade. Tie or tape to patient's helmet or forehead to ensure the gastric balloon impacts gently on the gastroesophageal junction.
- Place the esophageal aspiration channel on continuous low suction and arrange for the gastric channel to drain freely.

Leave in situ for just enough time to stabilize, transfer, or determine definitive treatment course. These tubes should be removed within 24 h; long duration risks necrosis and perforation. Various other techniques of insertion may be used, and tubes vary in structure. *Do not try to pass one yourself if you have no or little experience:* Ask an expert; if unavailable locally, call a specialist liver center and transfer urgently.

Endoscopy and biopsy

Upper GI endoscopy *Diagnostic indications*

- Dyspepsia, especially if >50 yrs old
- Gastric biopsy (suspected malignancy)
- Duodenal biopsy (e.g., celiac disease)
- Hematemesis
- Persistent vomiting
- Iron-deficiency anemia.

Therapeutic: Primarily injection/coagulating of bleeding lesions. Also:

- Banding of esophageal varices
- Dilatation of strictures (esophageal, pyloric)
- Palliation of esophageal cancer (stent insertion, laser therapy, mucosal resection therapy)
- Palliation of malignant obstruction (stent insertion)
- Removal of foreign bodies
- Radiofrequency ablation of Barrett esophagus
- Placement of feeding tubes

Preprocedure: NPO after midnight except for medications. Obtain informed written consent. Advise the patient not to drive for 24 h if sedation is being given. Arrange follow-up.

Procedure: Conscious sedation may be given (e.g., midazolam 2 mg IV; monitor O_2 saturation with a pulse oximeter). Anesthesia-directed sedation may be given (e.g., propofol) for selected cases. The pharynx may be sprayed with local anesthetic, and a flexible endoscope is swallowed. Continuous suction must be available to prevent aspiration. *Complications:* Transient sore throat, amnesia following sedation, perforation (<0.1%), cardiorespiratory arrest (<0.1%).

Duodenal biopsy is the gold standard for diagnosing celiac disease. Endoscopy with biopsy is also useful in investigating unusual causes of malabsorption (e.g., giardiasis, lymphoma, Whipple's disease, amyloid, eosinophilic gastroenteritis, or microscopic colitis).

Colonoscopy *Diagnostic indications:* Lower GI bleeding, iron deficiency, persistent diarrhea, biopsy of a known lesion or polyp, to assess for Crohn's or UC, colorectal cancer surveillance, *Strep. bovis* endocarditis.

Therapeutic indications: Polypectomy, lower GI bleeding treatment, treating IBD strictures with dilation, treating malignant obstruction (stenting), pseudo-obstruction or volvulus (decompression).

Preparation: Various prep solutions exist. Most commonly used is polyethylene glycol solution (1 gallon).

Procedure: Sedation and analgesia are given before a flexible colonoscope is passed per rectum around the colon.

Complications: Abdominal discomfort, incomplete examination, perforation (0.2%), hemorrhage after biopsy or polypectomy.

Transjugular or ultrasound-guided percutaneous liver biopsy *Indications:* Abnormal LFT, chronic viral hepatitis, alcoholic hepatitis, AIH, suspected cirrhosis, suspected carcinoma, biopsy of hepatic lesions, investigation of FUO.

Preprocedure: NPO after midnight. Check clotting (International Normalized Ratio [INR] <1.3) and platelet count (>100 × 10^9/L). Obtain written consent. Prescribe analgesia.

Procedure: Sedation (e.g., diazepam 5 mg IV) may be given, but usually not required. If percutaneous, ultrasound guidance is recommended, the liver borders are percussed and local anesthetic (2% lidocaine) is injected to the region of maximal dullness in the midaxillary line during expiration that correlates with target area on ultrasound. Breathing is rehearsed, and a needle biopsy is taken with the breath held in expiration. Afterward the patient lies on the right side for 2 h, then in bed for 6 h while regular pulse and BP observations are taken. Transjugular biopsies are recommended for patients with ascites, low platelets, morbid obesity, etc., in whom the percutaneous approach may be difficult to perform safely. Some academic centers perform transluminal endoscopic peritoneoscopy and liver biopsy; added advantages include direct visualization and immediate treatment of any bleeding lesion. Still in early research trials.

Complications: Local pain, pneumothorax/hemothorax, bleeding (<0.5%), death (<0.1%), biopsy of adjacent organ (e.g., gallbladder, kidney).

Radiological and other GI procedures

Abdominal ultrasound is used for the investigation of abdominal pain, abnormal LFT, jaundice, hepatomegaly, or abdominal masses. Patients should be NPO by mouth for 4 h before the scan to allow visualization of the gallbladder. Pelvic ultrasound requires the bladder to be full. Ultrasound may also be used to guide diagnostic biopsy or therapeutic aspiration.

Endoscopic retrograde cholangiopancreatography *Diagnostic indications:* With the advent of MRCP (below), diagnostic ERCP is uncommonly performed. Indications to perform ERCP prior to MRCP are for therapeutic intervention or when clinical suspicion is high for therapeutic intervention. Indications for ERCP include cholangitis, jaundice with dilated intrahepatic ducts, recurrent pancreatitis, symptomatic choledocholithiasis, biliary obstruction, biliary strictures. *Preprocedure:* Check clotting and platelet count. NPO after midnight. Obtain informed consent. Sedation is accomplished similarly to other endoscopic procedures. *Procedure:* A catheter is advanced from a side-viewing duodenoscope via the ampulla into the common bile duct and/or pancreatic duct. Contrast medium is injected and x-rays taken to show lesions in the biliary tree and pancreatic ducts. *Complications:* Pancreatitis, bleeding, cholangitis, perforation. *Mortality:* <0.2% overall; 0.4% if stone removal.

Small bowel follow-through After bowel preparation, barium is ingested and serial x-ray films are taken every 30 min until barium reaches the cecum. Enhanced films are taken of areas of interest (e.g., terminal ileum).

Small bowel enema After bowel preparation, barium is introduced via duodenal intubation. Although technically more demanding than a barium follow-through, this method results in better mucosal definition.

Barium enema Always do a rectal exam first ± rigid sigmoidoscopy and biopsy. Preparation is per colonoscopy (p. 222). For double-contrast barium enema, barium and air are introduced per rectum. Special views may be needed to visualize the areas of interest. Gastrografin may be used instead of barium in suspected colonic obstruction. It may show diverticular disease or cancers (e.g., an irregular "apple-core" narrowing of the lumen). In Crohn's disease, look for "cobblestoning," "rose thorn" ulcers, colonic strictures with rectal sparing. *Disadvantages:* Significant radiation dose; no biopsy possible.

Computed tomography is indicated if ultrasound is technically difficult or nondiagnostic. It allows better visualization of retroperitoneal structures but requires skilled interpretation. Oral or IV contrast may be given to enhance definition. The main disadvantage is the high radiation dose.

Magnetic resonance imaging provides superior soft tissue imaging and enables the distinction of benign and malignant lesions. The other advantage over CT is the lack of radiation. Disadvantages are that patients with pacemakers and certain metal implants cannot be scanned and that the scanner itself can induce claustrophobia.

Magnetic resonance cholangiopancreatography

MRCP enables in vivo anatomic exploration of the main pancreatic duct. Horizontal sections provide helpful radioanatomic information. The technique nevertheless remains limited by poor spatial resolution. MRCP had a sensitivity of 83% and a specificity of 99% for diagnosing common bile duct stones, and according to some authorities, is the investigation of choice—partly, no doubt, due to lack of side effects.

Endoscopic ultrasound An ultrasound transducer is placed at the tip of an endoscope, allowing for unprecedented visualization of the GI tract and its adjacent structures. The layers of the GI tract can be discerned (allows for unprecedented evaluation of submucosal lesions) and adjacent organs (pancreas, mediastinal structures). A fine-needle aspiration (FNA) or core biopsy can be accomplished through the endoscope, allowing for tissue acquisition. EUS has revolutionized cancer diagnosis and staging of esophageal, pancreaticobiliary, gastric, and colorectal cancers.

Imaging via a wireless enteroscopy capsule This capsule is swallowed and sends images to a recorder worn by the patient. It allows for visualization of the small bowel mucosa and is indicated for obscure GI bleeding, detection of inflammatory bowel disease (IBD), etc. Recently, it is approved for evaluation of the esophagus as well. Robotic biopsy and therapeutic procedures are not yet possible.

Deep bowel enteroscopy with double balloon, single balloon, or spiral enteroscopy. An enteroscope (a long endoscope) and an added balloon-like device can be used in tandem to allow the scope to be inserted deep into the small bowel. The entire length of small bowel can be reached in most cases. The sequential advancement of balloon and scope allows for plication and folding of the bowel to shorten the length and advance the scope further. This technique is useful to reach the small bowel and provide diagnosis of small bowel diseases such as lymphoma or Crohn's with ERCP in patients with Roux-en-Y gastric bypass or therapy for bleeding. It can also be used in retrograde fashion to advance a scope through the colon and into the distal ileum.

Liver failure

Definitions Acute liver failure may occur suddenly in the previously healthy liver, precipitating elevated INR (≥1.5), rapid deterioration of liver function, onset of encephalopathy, or change in mental status] *Acute hepatic failure* is liver failure of <26 wks duration.

Liver failure more commonly may occur as a result of decompensation of chronic liver disease; i.e., *acute-on-chronic hepatic failure*. Many terms are used, including *fulminant* hepatic failure, which refers to severe acute liver injury with synthetic dysfunction and encephalopathy occurring within 8 wks of the onset of symptoms. *Subfulminant* hepatic failure refers to impaired synthetic function and encephalopathy occurring within 9–26 wks (<6 months).

Immediately upon development of acute liver failure (<26 wks duration): Elevated INR (≥1.5) and encephalopathy in a patient: Must initiate contact with a transplant center as early transfer essential.

Causes *Infections:* Viral hepatitis, yellow fever, leptospirosis.

Drugs: Acetaminophen overdose, halothane, isoniazid.

Toxins: Amanita phalloides mushrooms, carbon tetrachloride.

Vascular: Budd–Chiari syndrome, veno-occlusive disease.

Others: Primary biliary cirrhosis, hemochromatosis, autoimmune hepatitis, α_1-antitrypsin deficiency, Wilson's disease, fatty liver of pregnancy, malignancy, drug-induced liver disease.

Clinical features *Hepatic encephalopathy* is graded as follows:

Grade I	Altered mood or behavioral changes, day-night reversal, hyperreflexia
Grade II	Increased drowsiness or hypersomnia, confusion, slurred speech, asterixis
Grade III	Stupor, incoherence, restlessness or severe agitation, clonus, arousable to vocal stimuli
Grade IV	Coma, decerebrate posturing.

Patients determined to have encephalopathy should be transferred to the icu. Intubate when reaches grade III to IV encephalopathy.

Other features: Jaundice, fetor hepaticus (sweat has pungent smell), constructional apraxia (ask the patient to draw a five-pointed star). Signs of chronic liver disease suggest acute-on-chronic hepatic failure.

Investigations

Blood tests: inr/prothrombin time (pt), blood type and screen, CBC (infection, GI bleed); chemistry (renal failure); LFT (bilirubin, AST/ALT, and alk phos); pregnancy test, hepatic synthetic function (albumin, bilirubin) amylase, lipase; glucose (hypoglycemia), acetaminophen level, ethyl alcohol (ETOH) level, consider aspirin level if suspected overdose, hepatitis serologies (anti-HAV IgM, HBsAg, anti-Hbc IgM, anti-HEV, anti-HCV, HCV RNA, HSV1 IgM, VZV, ferritin and iron studies, α_1-antitrypsin level, serum ceruloplasmin level, amylase, lipase, antinuclear antibody (ANA), anti-smooth muscle antibodies (ASMA), immunoglobulin level, toxicology screen, ABG, arterial lactate, ammonia.

Microbiology: Blood culture; urine culture; HIV-1, HIV-2; if ascites, then cell count/culture of ascites; ascitic neutrophils >250/mm³ indicates spontaneous bacterial peritonitis (SBP). Total ascitic white blood cells (WBCs) >500/mm³ also indicates SBP.

Radiology: CXR, abdominal ultrasound; Doppler flow studies of the portal vein and hepatic artery (and hepatic vein, in suspected Budd–Chiari). CT brain to exclude other causes of altered mental status

Neurophysiological studies: Electroencephalogram (EEG) may show diffuse high-voltage slow waveforms.

Management Beware of sepsis, hypoglycemia, and encephalopathy[4]:

* Nursing care with a 20–30-degree head elevation in fulminant hepatic failure to reduce intracranial pressure (ICP) and avoid aspiration. May also protect the airway by inserting an nasogastric (NG) tube and removing any blood or other contents from stomach.
* Monitor temperature, pulse, respiratory rate (RR), BP, pupils (uncal herniation due to ↑ ICP in fulminant hepatic failure), urine output hourly.
* Check CBC, chemistry, LFTs, and INR daily.
* Give 10% dextrose IV, 1 L/12 h to avoid hypoglycemia. Give 50 mL 50% dextrose IV if blood glucose <60 mg/dL (perform every 1–4 h in acute liver failure).
* Treat the cause, if known (e.g., acetaminophen poisoning [p. 790]).
* If malnourished, obtain nutrition help (e.g., diet rich in carbohydrate- and protein-derived calories, preferably orally; give thiamine and folate supplements as needed.
* Hemofiltration or hemodialysis, if renal failure develops (see Table 7.8).
* Avoid sedatives or other drugs with hepatic metabolism.
* Communicate early with your nearest liver transplant center regarding the appropriateness of transfer (see Table 7.9).

Prognosis Poor prognostic factors: Grade III or IV encephalopathy, age >40 yrs, albumin <3.0 g/dL, drug-induced liver failure (see Table 7.10), subfulminant hepatic failure worse than fulminant failure—only 65% survival post-transplantation.

4 Lee W, Larson A, Stravitz, RT. AASLD Position Paper: The management of acute liver failure: update 2011. *Hepatology.* 2005; 41:1179–1197.

Table 7.8 Treating the complications of acute hepatic failure

Bleeding: Vitamin K 10 mg/d IV at least 1 dose; platelets and/or FFP for active bleeding or procedures; PRBCs as needed; recombinant activated Factor VII for invasive procedures

Infection: Until sensitivities are known, give ceftriaxone 1–2 g/24 h IV. Avoid gentamicin or other nephrotoxic meds (increases risk of renal failure).

Ascites: Fluid restriction, low-sodium diet, diuretics, daily weights

Hypoglycemia: Check blood glucose regularly and give 50 mL of 50% glucose IV if levels fall below 60 mg/dL. Monitor plasma K^+.

Encephalopathy: Avoid sedatives; 20–30-degree head elevation in acute hepatic failure; lactulose to alter the gut flora and thus reduce nitrogen (ammonia) production. Aim for three soft stools a day; be careful with oral neomycin—may worsen renal failure; consider oral rifaximin instead.

Cerebral edema: Give mannitol IV bolus at 0.5–1.0 g/kg. Hyperventilation in times of impending herniation. Consider hypertonic saline, barbiturates, corticosteroids, or physician-induced hypothermia.

Hepatorenal syndrome (HRS): On presentation, check volume status, most patients need fluid resuscitation to maintain adequate intravascular volume. If BP fails to respond, then initiate norepinephrine in volume-refractory hypotension. Vasopressin can be used as adjunct to norepinephrine refractory hypotension. Goal mean arterial pressure (MAP) >75, CPP 60–80. Protect renal function with adequate BP, avoid nephrotoxins. If dialysis is needed, recommend continuous filtration.

Table 7.9 King's College Hospital (UK) criteria for liver transplantation

Acetaminophen related fulminant hepatic failure (FHF)	Arterial pH <7.3 following fluid resuscitation, regardless of the stage of encephalopathy
	Or all of the following:
	INR >6.5
	Creatinine >3.4 mg/dL
	Grade III or IV encephalopathy
Non-acetaminophen-related FHF	INR >6.5
	Or three out of five of the following:
1 Drug/toxin-induced liver failure, *or* indeterminate cause	**3** >1 wk duration of jaundice prior to onset of encephalopathy
2 Age <10 or >40	**4** INR >3.5
	5 Bilirubin >17 mg/dL

In some centers, transplantation is either *cadaveric* or from *live donors* (e.g., right lobe).

Table 7.10 Prescribing in liver failure

Avoid opiates and benzodiazepines if possible. Be careful with diuretics (increases risk of encephalopathy) and avoid oral hypoglycemic agents. Warfarin effects are enhanced, therefore monitor the INR closely. Avoid IV saline solutions which are hypotonic. Hepatotoxic drugs include acetaminophen, methotrexate, phenothiazines, isoniazid, azathioprine, estrogen, 6-mercaptopurine, salicylates, tetracycline, mitomycin, and several other antibiotics, antivirals, antifungals, antidepressants, etc. When in doubt, refer to the specific medication's package insert concerning potential adverse effects when prescribing a new medicine.

Cirrhosis

Cirrhosis implies irreversible liver damage. Histologically, there is loss of normal hepatic architecture with fibrosis and nodular regeneration.

Causes Chronic alcohol abuse, chronic viral hepatitis infections, primary biliary cirrhosis, hereditary hemochromatosis, and others: See Table 7.11.

Presentation varies from asymptomatic with abnormal LFTs, to decompensated end-stage liver disease with all its associated complications. *Chronic liver disease:* Leukonychia—white nails without clear demarcation of the lunulae; Terry nails—white proximally, but distal 30% reddened with telangiectasias; hypoalbuminemia with ascites; palmar erythema (hyperdynamic circulation); spider nevi or angiomas; Dupuytren contracture (in alcoholic cirrhosis); gynecomastia; testicular atrophy; parotid gland enlargement; clubbing; hepatomegaly or shrunken/fibrotic liver in late disease.

Complications *Hepatic failure:* Coagulopathy (low levels of factors II, VII, IX, and X cause elevated INR); encephalopathy—asterixis and confusion, coma; hypoalbuminemia (edema, leukopenia, ascites); sepsis (spontaneous bacterial peritonitis); hypoglycemia; GI bleeding; renal failure.

Portal hypertension: Ascites; splenomegaly; portosystemic shunts including esophageal varices (frequently present as a life-threatening upper GI bleed) and "caput medusa" (enlarged superficial periumbilical veins). Increased risk of hepatocellular carcinoma.

Tests *Blood:* LFT: ↔ or ↑bilirubin, ↑AST, ↑ALT, ↑alk phos, and ↑ γ-glutamyl transpeptidase (GGT). Later, with loss of synthetic function, look for ↓albumin ± ↑PT/INR. Low WBC and platelets indicate hypersplenism. *Find the cause:* Ferritin, iron/total iron-binding capacity (p. 231); hepatitis serologies; quantitative immunoglobulins (p. 232); autoantibodies (ANA, AMA, SMA); AFP (p. 219) level; ceruloplasmin (p. 233); α_1-antitrypsin (p. 233).

Liver ultrasound may show hepatomegaly, splenomegaly, focal liver lesion(s), hepatic vein thrombi, reversal of flow in the portal vein, or ascites. *MRI:* Caudate lobe size↑, smaller islands of regenerating nodules, and the presence of the right posterior hepatic notch are more frequent in alcoholic cirrhosis than in virus-induced cirrhosis. MRI scoring systems based on spleen volume, liver volume, and the presence of ascites or varices/collaterals can quantify the severity of cirrhosis in a manner that correlates well with Child–Pugh grades (see Table 7.12).

Ascitic tap should always be performed if ascites is present and fluid should be sent for urgent cell count, C&S: An ascitic neutrophil count of >250/mm³ indicates spontaneous bacterial peritonitis. Also, a total WBC >500/mm³ indicates SBP. *Liver biopsy* confirms the clinical diagnosis. This may be done ultrasound-guided and percutaneously (if the INR ≤1.5 and the platelet count ≥50 K) or via the transjugular route with FFP or activated recombinant Factor VII.

Management *General:* Maintain good nutrition; low-sodium diet (especially if ascites); alcohol abstinence; avoid NSAIDs, sedatives, and opiates; vaccinate against HAV and HBV; cholestyramine may help pruritus (4 g PO bid, 1 h after other drugs). Perform ultrasound every 6 months to screen for hepatocellular cancer (HCC). Consider adding AFP; however, recent data indicate that AFP levels lack sensitivity and specificity for diagnosis or surveillance (p. 236).

Specific treatments: For *hcv-related cirrhosis*, treatment with pegylated interferon-α plus ribavirin and new protease inhibitors improves liver biochemistries and may prevent the development decompensated liver disease and/or HCC. Meta-analyses show some benefit of low-dose ursodeoxycholic acid (URSO) in PBC. There is increased mortality in primary sclerosing cholangitis (PSC) with use of high-dose URSO, and the AASLD recommends against initiation of URSO in PSC. Penicillamine or Trientine for Wilson's disease (p. 233), aggressive phlebotomy for hereditary hemochromatosis.

Ascites: Fluid restriction (<1.5 L/d), low-sodium diet (40–100 mmol/d). Spironolactone (Aldactone), start 50–100 mg/24 h PO (usually given in two divided doses as bid); increase dose q48h to 400 mg/24 h if necessary to control ascites and edema; carefully monitor serum K⁺ levels; chart daily weights, aim for weight loss of ~0.5 kg/d. If response to Aldactone is poor, add furosemide 40–120 mg/24 h PO (usually given in a ratio of 4:10 with Aldactone—e.g., furosemide 40 mg and Aldactone 100 mg, or furosemide 80 mg and Aldactone 200 mg); check BUN/creatinine and serum Na⁺ often. Therapeutic paracentesis with concomitant albumin infusion (6–8 g/L fluid removed) may be tried; albumin infusion during large volume paracentesis may prevent HRS.

Spontaneous bacterial peritonitis: Treatment: E.g., ceftriaxone 1–2 g/24 h or Zosyn 3.375 g q6h (pay special attention to dosing; it depends on degree of liver failure and renal failure; fine-tune antibiotic coverage after the sensitivities are known. *Prophylaxis:* Bactrim DS tab PO 3–5 × a week; norfloxacin 400 mg PO qd; ciprofloxacin 750 mg PO every week.

Prognosis Overall, 5-yr survival is ~50%. Poor prognostic indicators: Encephalopathy, serum Na⁺ <110 mEq/L, serum albumin <2.5 g/dL, ↑INR.

Liver transplantation is the only definitive treatment for cirrhosis. This increases 5-yr survival from ~20% in end-stage disease to ~70%.

Model for End-Stage Liver Disease (MELD) Score: (1–40). Predicts 90-day mortality for cirrhotic patients under consideration for transplant. Calculated via complex formula calculator from basic components: INR, total bilirubin, creatinine (Cr).

Table 7.11 Causes of cirrhosis

- Chronic alcohol abuse
- Chronic HBV or HCV infection
- Autoimmune disease: PBC (p. 220), PSC (p. 221), autoimmune hepatitis
- Genetic disorders: α1-Antitrypsin deficiency (p. 219), Wilson's disease (p. 218), hereditary hemochromatosis (p. 216)
- Others: Budd–Chiari syndrome (hepatic vein thrombosis)
- Drugs: E.g., amiodarone, methyldopa, methotrexate

Table 7.12 Child–Pugh grading and risk of variceal bleeding

Risk ↑↑ if score ≥8

	1 point	2 points	3 points
Bilirubin (mg/dL)	<2	2–3	>3
Albumin (g/dL)	>3.5	2.8–3.5	<2.8
INR	<1.7	1.7–2.3	>2.3
Ascites	None	Slight	Moderate
Encephalopathy	None	1–2	3–4

Alcoholism

An alcoholic is one whose repeated drinking leads to harm in his or her work or social life. Denial is a leading feature of alcoholism, so it may be helpful to query relatives. Screening tests: Mean cell volume (MCV)↑; GGT↑. See Table 7.13.

CAGE questions Screening for alcohol abuse **Have you ever**: Felt you ought to CUT DOWN on your drinking? Had people ANNOY you by criticizing your drinking? Felt bad or GUILTY about your drinking? Had a drink in the AM (eye-opener) to steady your nerves? CAGE is quite good at detecting alcohol abuse and dependence (1 point for each +, more than 2 points is significant; sensitivity, 43–94%; specificity, 70–97%).

Organs affected by alcohol

The liver: (Normal in 50% of alcoholics)

Fatty liver: Acute and reversible, but may progress to cirrhosis if drinking continues (also seen in obesity, DM, and with certain medications). *Cirrhosis:* 5-yr survival is 48% if drinking continues (if not, 77%). *Hepatitis:* TPR↑, anorexia, tender hepatomegaly ± jaundice, bleeding, ascites, WBC↑, INR↓, AST↑, MCV↑, urea↑ (HRS). 80% progress to cirrhosis (hepatic failure in 10%). *Biopsy:* Mallory bodies ± neutrophil infiltrate. *Treatment:* See Table 7.14.

- *CNS:* Poor memory/cognition: Multiple high-potency vitamins IM may reverse it; cortical atrophy; retrobulbar neuropathy; fits; falls; wide-based gait neuropathy; Korsakoff ± Wernicke encephalopathy
- *Gut:* Obesity, diarrhea; gastric erosions; peptic ulcers; varices; pancreatitis (acute and chronic)
- *Blood:* MCV↑; anemia from marrow depression, GI bleeds, alcoholism-associated folate deficiency, hemolysis; sideroblastic anemia
- *Heart:* Arrhythmia; BP↑ cardiomyopathy; sudden death in binge drinkers

Withdrawal signs Pulse↑, BP↓, tremor, fits, hallucinations (*delirium tremens*) may be visual or tactile (e.g., of animals crawling under one's skin).

Alcohol contraindications Driving, hepatitis, cirrhosis, peptic ulcer, drugs (e.g., antihistamines), carcinoid, pregnancy (fetal alcohol syndrome: IQ ↓, short palpebral fissure, absent filtrum, and small eyes).

Management *Alcohol withdrawal:* Admit; do BP + TPR/4 h. Beware BP↓. For the first three days give generous chlordiazepoxide (e.g., 10–50 mg/6 h PO), weaning over 7–14 d. Watch for persistent withdrawal and add benzodiazepine to keep BP stable; if deteriorating consider ICU management with intubation, benzodiazepine or propofol sedation in severe cases as needed. Vitamins required (thiamine, folate, etc.).

Treating established alcoholics may be rewarding, particularly if they really want to change. If so, *group therapy* or self-help (e.g., Alcoholics Anonymous) may be useful.

Relapse: 50% will relapse in the months following initiation of treatment: *Anxiety, insomnia, and craving* may be intense, and is mitigated by *acamprosate.* *CI:* Pregnancy, severe liver failure, creatinine >120 mmol/L. *SE:* Diarrhea and vomiting (D&V), libido ↑ or ↓. Dose example: 666 mg/8 h PO if >60 kg and <65yrs old.

Reducing pleasure that alcohol brings (and decreasing craving): *Naltrexone* 50 mg/24 h PO can halve relapse rates. *SE:* Vomiting, drowsiness, dizziness, cramps, arthralgia. *CI:* Liver failure. It is costly. Confer with experts if drugs are to be used.

Table 7.13 Patterns of lab tests in alcoholic and other liver disease

	AST *Aspartate aminotransferase*	ALT *Alanine aminotransferase*	MCV *Mean cell volume*
Alcoholic liver disease	↑↑ *(twice as high as alt)*	↑	↑↑
Hepatitis C (HCV)	↑ or ↔*	↑↑ *(higher than ast)*	↔
Nonalcoholic fatty liver disease	↑	↑↑	↑ or ↔

*In HCV, AST:ALT ratio is typically <1; ratio may reverse if cirrhosis develops. GGT may be ↑↑ in alcoholic liver disease, but is rather nonspecific.

Table 7.14 Managing alcoholic hepatitis

- Stop alcohol consumption (for withdrawal symptoms, if chlordiazepoxide by the oral route is impossible, try lorazepam IM).
- High-dose B vitamins IV
- Optimize nutrition (35–40 kcal/kg/d nonprotein energy) + 1.5 g/kg/d of protein (use ideal body weight for calculations; e.g., if malnourished). This prevents encephalopathy, sepsis, and some deaths.
- Daily weight; LFT; basic metabolic panel (BMP); INR. If creatinine↑, get help with this hepatorenal syndrome (i.e., renal failure where the underlying pathology is hepatic). Na⁺↓ is common, but water restriction may make matters worse.
- Culture ascites fluid; give appropriate antibiotics in the light of sensitivities.
- If no active infection or GI bleeding consider adjunct medical therapy with Maddrey score >32: Prednisolone 40 mg/d for 5 d tapered off over 3 wks *MAY* help. Pentoxifylline may be helpful for acute alcoholic hepatitis. Liver transplantation is not an option for patients with acute alcoholic hepatitis or without history of documented abstinence, but some centers may consider them after 6 months of rehab/abstinence.

Maddrey Score = 4.6 (patient's PT − control PT) + total bilirubin (mg/dL) (poor prognosis if score ≥32).

Hereditary hemochromatosis

Hereditary hemochromatosis (HH) is an inherited disorder of iron metabolism in which increased intestinal iron absorption leads to its deposition in multiple organs (joints, liver, heart, pancreas, and pituitary). Middle-aged males are more frequently and severely affected than women, in whom the disease tends to present ~10 yrs later (menstrual blood loss is protective). Disease onset is usually at 40–50 yrs in men and 50–60 yrs in women.

Genetics HH is one of the most common inherited diseases in those of Northern European ancestry (carrier rate of ~1 in 10 and a frequency of homozygosity of ~1:200–1:400). The gene responsible for most HH is the HFE gene located on chromosome 6. Two major mutations are termed C282Y and H63D. C282Y accounts for 60–100% of HH, and H63D accounts for 3–7%, with compound heterozygotes accounting for 1–4%. Penetrance is unknown but is clearly <100%.

Clinical features Asymptomatic early on, then fatigue, weakness, lethargy and arthralgias (MCP and large joints) usually develop. Later, look for slate-gray skin pigmentation, DM ("bronze diabetes"), and stigmata of chronic liver disease. Hepatomegaly early on; small and shrunken cirrhotic liver later; heart failure (dilated cardiomyopathy) and conduction disturbances; hypogonadism (pituitary dysfunction, or via cirrhosis) and associated osteoporosis. Other endocrinopathies include hyporeninemic hypoaldosteronism.

Tests *Blood:* Abnormal LFT, ↑serum ferritin; ↑serum iron-to-TIBC ratio; transferrin saturation >60%, often >80%. HFE genotyping. Blood glucose to look for DM. *Joint x-rays* may show chondrocalcinosis. *Liver biopsy:* Perl stain quantifies iron loading (hepatic iron index [HII] >1.9 mcmol/kg/yr) and assesses disease severity. *MRI* also helps estimate hepatic iron loading. Do *ekg* and *echo* if you suspect cardiomyopathy.

Management *Phlebotomize* ~1 U/wk until mildly iron-deficient. Iron will continue to accumulate, so maintenance phlebotomy (1 U q2–3 months) is needed for life. Maintain hemoglobin at about 10–12 g/dL, serum ferritin 50–100 ng/mL, and transferrin saturation <50%. *Other monitoring:* Diabetes; Hb_{A1c} levels may be falsely low as phlebotomy reduces the time available for Hb glycosylation. *Over-the-counter self-medication:* Make sure that vitamin preparations etc. contain no iron. *Screening:* Test serum ferritin, transferrin saturation, and genotype in first-degree relatives. Prevalence of iron overload in asymptomatic C282Y homozygotes is 4.5 per 1,000 persons screened. Fewer than 10% of C282Y homo will develop severe iron overload and organ damage.

Prognosis Phlebotomy returns life expectancy to normal if noncirrhotic and nondiabetic. Arthropathy may not improve or even worsen. Gonadal failure is irreversible. In noncirrhotic patients, phlebotomy may improve liver histology. Cirrhotic patients have >10% chance of developing HCC. Sources vary on the exact risk: Some authorities quote 30%, others 22%. One cause of variability is varying cofactors: Age >50 yrs increases risk by 13-fold; being HBsAg positive by fivefold, and alcohol abuse by twofold.

Secondary hemochromatosis may occur in any hematological condition where many transfusions (~80 U) have been given. To reduce the need for transfusions, find out if the hematological condition responds to erythropoietin or marrow transplantation before the irreversible effects of iron overload become too great.

Autoimmune hepatitis

AIH is an inflammatory liver disease of unknown cause characterized by suppressor T-cell defects with autoantibodies directed against hepatocyte surface antigens. This disease is a steroid-responsive hepatitis. Two types are distinguished by the presence of circulating autoantibodies:

Type I	Affects both adults or children
	Antinuclear antibodies (ANA) and/or
	Anti-smooth muscle antibodies (ASMA) positive in 80%. Other autoantibodies associated with type I include: Anti-soluble liver Ab (ASLA), anti-dsDNA Ab, and p-ANCA.
Type II	Affects children; generally girls and some young women
	Anti-liver/kidney microsomal type 1 (ALKM-1) antibodies. Other autoantibodies associated with type II include: Antiliver cytosol antigen (ALC-1)

Clinical features Predominantly affects young and middle-aged women. 25% of patients present with acute hepatitis and features of an autoimmune disease (e.g., fever, malaise, urticarial rash, polyarthritis, pleurisy, or glomerulonephritis). The remainder present insidiously or are asymptomatic and diagnosed incidentally with signs of chronic liver disease. Amenorrhea is

Associations

Pernicious anemia	Autoimmune hemolysis	Ulcerative colitis (UC)
Diabetes	Glomerulonephritis	Human leukocyte antigen (HLA) A1, B8, & DR3 haplotype
Autoimmune thyroiditis	PSC	PBC

common.

Tests Abnormal LFT (AST/ALT↑), hypergammaglobulinemia (especially IgG), positive autoantibodies: ANA, ASMA, ALKM-1, etc. (see above). Anemia, leukopenia, and thrombocytopenia indicate hypersplenism. Liver biopsy shows a mononuclear infiltrate (usually plasma cells) within the portal, then periportal areas. This may be followed by piecemeal necrosis, bridging fibrosis, or cirrhosis. ERCP helps exclude PSC if the alk phos is disproportionately elevated.

Diagnosis depends on excluding other diseases as there is no pathognomonic sign or lab test. There is genuine overlap with PBC. Diagnostic criteria exist but are not fully validated.

Management Prednisone 30–40 mg/d PO for 1 month; decrease by 5 mg a month to a maintenance dose of 5–10 mg/d PO. Corticosteroids can sometimes be stopped after a few years, but relapse occurs in 50–86%. *Azathioprine* (50–100 mg/d PO) may be used alone as a steroid-sparing agent or in combination with lower doses of prednisone. Remission is achievable in 80% of patients within 3 yrs. *10- and 20-yr survival rates:* >80%. The goal is to achieve a sustained remission without the need for further drug therapy; achievable in 10–40% of patients overall.

Second-line therapies: Mycophenolate mofetil, budesonide, cyclosporin, tacrolimus, ursodeoxycholic acid, methotrexate, cyclophosphamide, 6-mercaptopurine, and free radical scavengers.

Liver transplantation is indicated for decompensated cirrhosis, but recurrence may occur. Post-transplant 10-yr survival rate is 75%.

Wilson's disease/hepatolenticular degeneration

A rare inherited disorder with toxic accumulation of copper (Cu) in liver and CNS (especially basal ganglia; e.g., globus pallidus hypodensity ± putamen cavitation). It is treatable, so screen all young patients with evidence of liver disease. *Genetics:* Autosomal recessive (gene on chromosome 13; codes for a copper transporting ATPase, ATP7B). Twenty-seven mutations are known; HIS1069GLU is the most common.

Signs Children usually present with *liver disease* (hepatitis, cirrhosis, fulminant hepatic failure); young adults often start with *CNS signs:* Tremor, dysarthria, dysphagia, dyskinesias, dystonias, purposeless stereotyped movements (e.g., hand clapping), dementia, parkinsonism, micrographia, ataxia/clumsiness. *Affective features:* Depression/mania, labile emotions, ↑ libido, personality changes. *Cognitive/behavioral:* Memory deficits, quick to anger, slow to solve problems, decline in IQ. *Psychosis:* Delusions, mutism. *Kayser-Fleischer rings:* Cu deposits in the cornea around the iris (Descemet membrane), pathognomonic but not always present; may need slit lamp to detect. *Also:* Hemolysis, blue lunulae (nails), polyarthritis, hypermobile joints, gray skin, hypoparathyroidism.

Tests Serum copper and ceruloplasmin usually low. 24 h urinary copper excretion is elevated (>100 mcg/24 h, normal <40 mcg). Liver biopsy: Elevated hepatic copper content. Molecular genetic testing can confirm the diagnosis. MRI: Basal ganglia degeneration (± frontotemporal, cerebellar, and brainstem atrophy).

Management *Diet* Low-copper diet (avoid shellfish, nuts, chocolate, mushrooms, organ meat). *Chelation:* Lifelong penicillamine (1,000–1,500 mg/24 h in 2–4 divided doses for the first 4–6 months; then maintenance dosing at 750–1,000 mg/24 h in 2 divided doses). *se:* Nausea, rash, leukopenia, anemia, thrombocytopenia, hematuria, nephrotic range proteinuria, lupus. Watch closely for those patients with a known penicillin (PCN) allergy—they will likely have a reaction to penicillamine as well. Monitor CBC and urinary Cu (and protein) excretion. Stop if WBC is <2.5 × 10⁹/L or platelets falling to <100 k. *Alternative:* Trientine dihydrochloride 750–1,500 mg/24 h in 2–3 divided doses (*se:* Rash; sideroblastic anemia). *Adjunct* Zinc. *Liver transplant* if *severe* liver disease. *Screen siblings* as asymptomatic homozygotes need treatment.

ALF If presentation with acute liver failure, refer to transplant center immediately. Development of refractory coagulopathy, hemolytic anemia, and renal insufficiency due to copper build up may only respond to plasma exchange transfusion or transplant. Transplant is curative.

Prognosis Precirrhotic liver disease is reversible. Neurological damage less so. Death occurs from liver failure, variceal hemorrhage, or infection (the typical complications associated with end-stage liver disease).

α₁-Antitrypsin deficiency

α₁-Antitrypsin is one of a family of serine protease inhibitors controlling inflammatory cascades. It is synthesized in the liver, making up 90% of serum α-globulin on electrophoresis. α₁-antitrypsin deficiency is the chief genetic cause of liver disease in children. In adults, its deficiency causes emphysema, chronic liver disease, and HCC. *Other associations:* Asthma, pancreatitis, gallstones. Decreased risk of stroke. *Prevalence:* 1:2,000–1:7,000.

Genetics *Carrier frequency:* 1:10. Genetic variants are typed by their electrophoretic mobility as *medium* (M), *slow* (S), or *very slow* (Z). S and Z types are due to single amino acid substitutions at positions 264 and 342, respectively. These result in diminished production of α_1-antitrypsin (S = 60%, Z = 15%). The normal genotype is PIMM, the homozygote is PIZZ; heterozygotes are PIMZ and PISZ.

Symptomatic patients (e.g., *cholestatic jaundice/cirrhosis; dyspnea* from emphysema) usually have PIZZ genotype. **nb:** Cholestasis often remits in adolescence. In adults, cirrhosis ± HCC affects 25% of all α_1-antitrypsin-deficient individuals >50 yrs.

Tests *Serum α_1-antitrypsin* levels are low. *Liver biopsy:* Periodic acid Schiff (PAS) positive; diastase-resistant globules. *Phenotyping* by isoelectric focusing requires expertise to distinguish SZ and ZZ phenotypes. *Prenatal diagnosis* is possible by DNA analysis of chorionic villus samples obtained at 11–13 wks gestation. DNA tests are likely to find greater use in the future.

Management *Supportive* for emphysema and hepatic complications. Smoking cessation; consider *augmentation therapy* with human α_1-antitrypsin if FEV1 <80% of predicted (expensive!) ± *liver transplant* in decompensated cirrhosis.

Primary biliary cirrhosis

In PBC, the interlobular, intrahepatic bile ducts are damaged by chronic granulomatous inflammation causing progressive cholestasis, cirrhosis, and portal hypertension. *Cause:* Possibly autoimmune. *F:M ratio approaches* 9:1. *Prevalence:* 19–51 cases per million population. *Peak presentation:* ~50 yrs.

Clinical features 50–60% of patients are asymptomatic and diagnosed only after finding ↑alk phos on routine LFTs. Lethargy and pruritus are the most common symptoms in symptomatic patients, and they may precede jaundice by months to years. *Signs:* Jaundice, skin pigmentation (due to melanosis), xanthelasma, xanthomata, hepatomegaly, and splenomegaly.

Complications: Osteoporosis is common. Malabsorption of fat-soluble vitamins (A, D, K, E) is uncommon but in cirrhotic patients may result in osteomalacia and coagulopathy. Other complications: Portal hypertension, ascites, variceal hemorrhage, hepatic encephalopathy, HCC (p. 305).

Tests *Blood tests:* ↑Alk phos, ↑GGT and 5′-nucleotidase levels, and mildly ↑AST and ALT; late disease: ↑Bilirubin, low albumin, ↑PT/INR. 98% are AMA M2 subtype positive (highly specific). Other autoantibodies, such as ANA, may occur in low titers. Immunoglobulins are elevated (especially IgM). TSH and cholesterol may be elevated.

Radiology: Ultrasound, and ERCP or MRCP to exclude extrahepatic cholestasis.

Liver biopsy: Granulomas around the intrahepatic bile ducts, progressing to cirrhosis. Classically, nonsuppurative destructive cholangitis and destruction of interlobular bile ducts.

Treatment *Symptomatic:* Pruritus: Try cholestyramine 4 g PO bid–tid. Diarrhea (usually from steatorrhea): PRN Imodium or loperamide; can also use pancreatic enzymes as there is often an associated pancreatic insufficiency as well. Osteoporosis prevention (p. 305).[5]

Specific: Fat-soluble vitamin prophylaxis: Vitamins A, D, and K. Consider *ursodeoxycholic acid* (UDCA), 13–15 mg/kg/d to all patients, which may obviate the need for *liver transplantation*, which is the last recourse for patients with end-stage disease and/or intractable pruritus. Recurrence in the graft

---

5. Lindor et al. AASLD Practice Guidelines: Primary biliary cirrhosis. *Hepatology.* 2009;50(1):291–308.

may occur but appears not to influence graft success. Other therapies that have been tried besides UCDA include colchicine and methotrexate.

Prognosis Once jaundice develops, survival is <2yrs. In one study, at 2 yrs post-transplant, predicted survival without retransplant was 55% and actual survival was 79%. At 7 yrs, these figures were 22% and 68%, respectively.

Primary sclerosing cholangitis

PSC is a disorder of unknown cause characterized by inflammation, fibrosis, and strictures of both the intra- and extrahepatic bile ducts. Immunological mechanisms are implicated. *Associations:* 80% of PSC patients also have UC, but only 5% of UC patients have PSC; also associated with human leukocyte antigen (HLA)-A1, B8, and DR3.

Clinical features Chronic biliary obstruction and secondary biliary cirrhosis lead to liver failure and death (or transplantation) over ~10–12 yrs.

Symptoms: Patients may be asymptomatic and diagnosed incidentally after finding an elevated alk phos on routine LFTs, or patients may experience fluctuating symptoms such as jaundice, pruritus, right upper quadrant (RUQ) abdominal pain, and fatigue. *Signs:* Jaundice, hepatomegaly, portal hypertension.

Complications: Bacterial cholangitis, cholangiocarcinoma (10–15% lifetime risk), ↑risk of colorectal cancer in those patients with concomitant UC, 30% of patients in some series have an overlap syndrome with type 1 AIH (p. 232). See Table 7.15.

Tests *Blood:* ↑Alk phos initially followed by ↑bilirubin; hypergammaglobulinemia (often first manifested as an elevated serum total protein level); AMA negative, but ANA, ASMA, and p-ANCA may be +ve. *ercp or mrcp* show multiple strictures of the biliary tree (characteristic "beaded" appearance). *Liver biopsy* shows a fibrous obliteration of the bile ducts with concentric replacement by connective tissue in an "onion skin" fashion. AASLD recommends against routine liver biopsy in PSC with typical radiographic/cholangiographic findings, only biopsy if elevated LFTs out of proportion to typical.

235

Management *Drugs:* Corticosteroids and other immunosuppressives have shown little benefit in stopping the progression of disease and delaying the need for liver transplantation; UCDA is no longer recommended at any dose for treatment of PSC. Cholestyramine 4 g PO bid/tid for pruritus; Antibiotics (ciprofloxacin) for bacterial cholangitis and for prophylaxis before invasive GI procedures (like ERCP).

Table 7.15 Disease associations

Primary biliary cirrhosis (PBC)	Primary sclerosing cholangitis (PSC)
• Thyroid disease	• Ulcerative colitis (5% of those with UC have PSC; 80% of those with PSC have UC)
• Rheumatoid arthritis	
• Sjögren's syndrome (70%)	
• Keratoconjunctivitis, sicca syndrome	• Crohn's disease (much rarer); HIV infection
• Progressive systemic sclerosis	
• Renal tubular acidosis	
• Membranous glomerulonephritis	

Endoscopic or radiologic stenting helps symptomatic dominant strictures. *Liver transplantation* is indicated in end-stage disease. Recurrence occurs in 20%; 5-yr graft survival is >60%.

Liver tumors

The most common liver tumors are secondary (metastatic) tumors. They frequently arise from primary malignancies in the breast, lung, or gastro-intestinal tract. Primary hepatic tumors are much less common and may be benign or malignant (see Tables 7.16 and 7.17).

Symptoms Fever, malaise, anorexia, weight loss, RUQ pain (due to liver capsule stretch). Jaundice is late (except with cholangiocarcinoma). Benign tumors are often asymptomatic; if they are large enough, they may cause symptoms due to sheer mass effect. Tumors may rupture, causing life-threatening intraperitoneal hemorrhage.

Signs Hepatomegaly (smooth or hard and irregular; e.g., metastases, cir-rhosis, HCC). Look for signs of chronic liver disease and evidence of dec-ompensation (jaundice, ascites). Feel for an abdominal mass or primary lesion. Listen for an arterial bruit over the liver (HCC).

Tests *Blood:* CBC, PT/INR, LFTs, hepatitis serologies, AFP level (↑ in 80% of HCC), carcino-embryonic antigen (CEA) level.

Imaging: Ultrasound or CT to identify lesions and guide diagnostic biopsies. MRI is better for distinguishing benign from malignant lesions. ERCP and biopsy/brushings should be performed for suspected cholangiocarcinoma.

Biopsy under ultrasound or CT guidance may achieve a histological diagno-sis; exercise extreme care and caution, as seeding along biopsy tract may occur.

Other investigations for metastases (e.g., CXR, mammography, endoscopy, colonoscopy, CT, marrow biopsy) are tailored according to the suspected primary.

Liver metastases signify advanced disease for any primary malignancy. Treatment and prognosis vary with the type and extent of primary tumor. Chemotherapy may be effective (e.g., for lymphomas, germ cell tumors). Small, solitary metastases may be amenable to resection. In most, treatment is palliative. Prognosis: <6–9 months.

Hepatocellular carcinoma HCC is a malignant tumor of hepatocytes accounting for 90% of primary liver cancers. Rare in the West (2–3% of all cancers), but more common in China and sub-Saharan Africa (40% of cancers).

Causes: Cirrhosis, due to any underlying cause (e.g., alcohol, chronic viral hepatitis, PBC, hereditary hemochromatosis, etc.); in the United States, HCV-associated liver disease is a more common cause than HBV; yet in Asia and Africa, chronic HBV-associated liver disease is the more common underlying etiology; other causes include aflatoxin, parasites (*Clonorchis sin-ensis*), drugs (anabolic and contraceptive steroids).

Management of HCC: Liver transplantation as treatment for HCC with newer selection criteria (e.g., ≤3 tumor nodules that are no more than 3 cm in diameter, or a single nodule less <5 cm and without vascular inva-sion) show better outcomes are being achieved than previously reported. Local radiofrequency ablative therapy and intra-arterial chemoembolization are reasonable options with decent 5-yr survival rates for those patients who are not surgical candidates. Sorafenib is a multikinase inhibitor that is effective in multifocal HCC. It increases time to progression and survival, but is expensive. It is first-line treatment for those who cannot get resection, ablation, or transplant; those with local invasion into vessels; or more than the allotted number of lesions for transplant.

Prognosis: Often <6 months without any intervention—95% 5-yr mortality. A subtype of HCC known as fibrolamellar HCC, which occurs in children/young adults, has a better prognosis (60% 5-yr survival).

Prevention is key. Ensure HBV vaccination (see Table 7.18). Do not reuse needles. Reduce exposure to aflatoxins (antihumidity measures such as sun-drying to reduce spread of this common fungal contaminant in stored maize); this is especially important for those who harbor chronic HBV (risk is highly synergistic).

Cholangiocarcinoma Biliary tree malignancy; ~10% of liver primaries. One-third are intrahepatic cholangiocellular cancers, and two-thirds are extrahepatic ductal cholangiocarcinomas.

Causes: PSC: Occurs in 8–13% of these patients; congenital biliary cysts; biliary-enteric drainage surgery.

The patient: Fever, abdominal pain (±ascites), malaise, bilirubin↑; alk phos↑↑, jaundice.

Pathology: Usually slow-growing. Most are distal extrahepatic or perihilar. A Klatskin tumor is a nodular cholangiocarcinoma arising at the bifurcation of the common hepatic duct; it is frequently associated with a collapsed gallbladder.

Management: 70% are not surgically resectable. Of those that are resectable, 76% recur. *Surgery:* E.g., major hepatectomy + extrahepatic bile duct excision + caudate lobe resection. *Postop problems:* Liver failure (15%), bile leak (17%), GI bleeding (6%), wound infection (6.5%). *Palliative stenting* and decompression of an obstructed extrahepatic biliary tree—percutaneously or via ERCP—improves quality of life. *Prognosis:* ~5 months.

Benign tumors *Hemangiomas* are the most common benign liver tumors. They are often an incidental finding on ultrasound or CT scan and do not require treatment. Biopsy should be avoided! *Hepatocellular adenomas* are common.

Table 7.16 Primary liver tumors

Malignant	Benign
HCC	Cysts
Cholangiocarcinoma	Hemangioma
Angiosarcoma	Adenoma
Hepatoblastoma (children)	Focal nodular hyperplasia
Fibrosarcoma	Fibroma
Leiomyosarcoma	Leiomyoma

Table 7.17 Origin of secondary liver tumors

Common in males	Common in females
Stomach	Breast
Lung	Colon
Colon	Stomach
	Uterus

Causes: Anabolic steroids, oral contraceptives, pregnancy. Only treat if symptomatic. Other common benign tumors of the liver include focal nodular hyperplasia; like hepatocellular adenomas, they commonly occur in women, but oral contraceptives do not seem to be implicated as an underlying cause.

Ulcerative colitis

UC is a relapsing and remitting inflammatory disorder of the colonic mucosa. It may affect just the rectum (proctitis) or extend proximally to involve part or the entire colon (pancolitis) without small bowel involvement. However, in 10–15% of patients it may involve the terminal ileum/ileocecal valve due to "backwash ileitis." *Pathology:* Hyperemic/hemorrhagic granular colonic mucosa ± "pseudopolyps" formed by inflammation. Punctate ulcers may extend deep into the lamina propria. *Histology:* See *biopsy*, below. *Cause:* Likely multifactorial etiology involving interplay of environmental factors, genetic susceptibility, and immune system dysregulation. *Incidence:* 19.2/100,000 person years in North America. Bimodal age of onset, most patients diagnosed between 15–30, and 10–15% after age 50. More UC patients tend to be former smokers than Crohn's.

Symptoms Gradual onset of diarrhea ± blood and mucus. Crampy abdominal discomfort is common; bowel frequency is related to severity of disease (see below). Systemic symptoms are common during attacks, e.g., fever, malaise, anorexia, weight loss. Urgency and tenesmus occur with rectal disease. Proctitis may occasionally present as obstipation or constipation associated with urgency/tenesmus.

Signs May be none: In acute, severe UC: Fever, tachycardia, and a tender, distended abdomen. *Extraintestinal signs* Clubbing, aphthous oral ulcers, erythema nodosum (PLATE 18), pyoderma gangrenosum, conjunctivitis, episcleritis, iritis, large joint arthritis, sacroiliitis, ankylosing spondylitis, fatty liver, PSC, cholangiocarcinoma and, very rarely, renal stones, osteomalacia, nutritional deficiencies, and systemic amyloidosis.

Tests *Blood:* CBC, erythrocyte sedimentation rate (ESR), c-reactive protein (CRP), BMP, LFT, and blood cultures. Consider iron studies. *Stool:* Fecal leukocytes, fecal lactoferrin and calprotectin (correlate with disease activity), ova and parasites, routine culture, *C. difficile* toxin. To exclude infectious diarrhea (*C. difficile*, *Salmonella*, *Shigella*, *Campylobacter*, *E. coli*, amebae). *Abdominal x-ray:* No fecal shadows, mucosal thickening (islands), colonic dilatation (toxic dilatation >6 cm), perforation. *Sigmoidoscopy:* Inflamed, friable mucosa. *Rectal biopsy:* Inflammatory infiltrate, goblet cell depletion, glandular distortion, mucosal ulcers, crypt abscesses. *Barium enema:* Loss of haustra, granular mucosa, shortened colon. Never do a barium enema during an acute colour attack. *Colonoscopy* shows disease extent and allows biopsies to be taken.

Complications Perforation and bleeding are two serious complications. Increased risk of arterial and venous thromboembolism. Others include:

- "Toxic megacolon," which is dilatation of colon (mucosal islands, colonic diameter >6 cm).
- Colonic cancer: Risk approaches 15% with pancolitis for 20 yrs; increased risk after 8+ years of having UC. Yearly colonoscopy surveillance with biopsy for dysplasia and early cancer is recommended after 8 yrs of colitis. Annual surveillance if patient has both UC and PSC from time of diagnosis. Some centers perform chromoendoscopy (spraying of colon mucosa with dye to increase yield and better target biopsies to areas with lesions).

Management: Goals of treatment are induction and maintenance of remission, reduced use of steroids, mitigated cancer risk, improved overall quality of life, and, when possible, mucosal healing.

To decide on treatment, classify severity (mild, moderate, severe, fulminant) and location (distal or total):

Mild UC: <4 stools/day, with or without blood, no signs toxicity, normal ESR

Moderate UC: >4 stools per day, may have bloody stools, minimal signs toxicity

Severe UC: >6 bloody stools/d, signs of toxicity

Fulminant UC: >10 bloody stools per day, toxicity, abdominal tenderness and distension, requires transfusion, colon dilated on x-ray films. (Toxicity is fever, tachycardia, anemia, or ↑ESR.)

Treatment is based on many factors and should be coordinated in consult with gastroenterology.

Treat mild distal UC:

Induce remission: Topical mesalamine, topical steroids, oral aminosalicy-lates—likely use combination of oral and topical (mesalamine topical > topical steroids or oral aminosalicylates (5-ASA) (i.e., Asacol MR® in 400- or 800-mg tabs, many others Lialda, Apriso, etc.). If all these measures fail, consider oral prednisone (40–60 mg/day) or infliximab.

Maintain remission: Mesalamine suppositories for proctitis, enemas for distal colitis. *Alternatives:* Sulfasalazine, mesalamine, balsalazide, Note combo of oral and topical is better than either alone. Topical steroids do *not* maintain remission. Can also consider thiopurine (6-MP) or azathioprine (AZA) (2–2.5 mg/kg/d PO) or infliximab.

Treat mild-moderate extensive (total colon) uc:

Induce remission: oral sulfasalazine 4–6 g/d or 5-ASA to 4.8 g/d. Oral steroids if refractory to 5-ASA (prednisone 40–60 mg/d; if response, then taper). Biologic agents, infliximab (Remicade® monoclonal antibody given IV), use if steroid refractory, steroid-dependent despite AZA or reaction to 6 MP/AZA or adalimumab (Humira). *Before using biologics, exclude latent TB, histoplasmosis, HBV, demyelinating disease, active infection, congestive heart failure (CHF), recent malignancy.*

Reference: Sandborn et. al. One-year Maintenance Outcomes Among Patients with Moderately-to Severely Active Ulcerative Colitis who

Responded to Induction Therapy with adalimumab:subgroup analyses from ULTRA 2. Alimentary Pharmacology and Therapeutics Volume 37, Issue 2, pages 204–213, January 2013.

Maintain remission: Acute attack controlled, sulfasalazine, olsalazine, mesalamine, balsalazide maintenance therapy. Slowly taper steroids if they were used. AZA/6MP may help taper steroids. Infliximab maintenance every 8 wks.

Moderate UC: If no improvement after 2 wks, treat as a severe UC.

Severe UC: If relatively well, but severe symptoms and refractory to oral steroids, 5-ASA or topicals, then consider infliximab. If systemically unwell and passing >6 motions daily, hospitalize. Act rapidly:
- Initiate nutritional assessment, enteral feeding is better than parenteral if tolerated.
- Initiate IV hydration (e.g., 1 L of 0.9% saline + 2 L dextrose-saline/24 h, + 20 mmol K$^+$/L; less if elderly).
- Consider steroids like hydrocortisone or Solu-Medrol.
- Avoid narcotics or anticholinergics where possible
- Start rectal steroids (e.g., hydrocortisone 100 mg in 100 mL 0.9% saline/12 h PR).
- Monitor T°, pulse, and BP; record stool frequency/character.
- Twice-daily exam: Document distension, bowel sounds, and tenderness.
- Obtain daily CBC, ESR, CRP, BMP, LFTs, ± abdominal x-ray.
- Assess stool culture and *C. diff* toxin assay, consider CMV testing if has been on immunosuppression prior to admission.
- Consider the need for blood transfusion (if Hb <10 g/dL) and parenteral nutrition (if severely malnourished). Give IV vitamins.
- Consult with gastroenterology and surgery is important during admission.
- If improving in 5 d, transfer to oral prednisolone (40 mg/24 h) with an adjunct, such as thiopurine or biologic.
- *If not improving within 3–5 days of hospitalization and initiation of steroid IV therapy consider additional options: Colectomy, cyclosporine, infliximab. Also, must have patient evaluated by a surgeon with high volume of colon surgeries.*
- *Indications for surgery*: Suspected dysplasia or carcinoma, severe colitis unresponsive to medical therapy or medically intolerable side effects, perforation, massive hemorrhage, toxic megacolon
- *Procedures:* With acute disease and a toxic patient, subtotal colectomy is recommended by most guidelines. Other surgeries for nontoxic refractory UC include: Total proctocolectomy with end-ileostomy, total proctocolectomy with ileal pouch, and anal anastomosis surgery.

Drug side effects to know:
- *Sulfasalazine:* Sulfapyridine intolerance—headache, nausea, anorexia, and malaise. Other allergic/toxic SE: Fever, rash, hemolysis, hepatitis, pancreatitis, paradoxical worsening of colitis, and reversible oligospermia. Follow CBC.
- *5-ASA:* Dyspepsia, nausea ± headache can occur. Rare hypersensitivity reactions: Worsening colitis, pancreatitis, pericarditis, nephritis
- *Steroids:* Cushingoid, emotional-psychiatric, infections, glaucoma, cataracts, GI mucosal injury, impaired wound healing, osteopenia, osteonecrosis, hyperglycemia, atherogenesis, infections
- *Cyclosporine:* Nephrotoxicity; K$^+$↑; BP↑ (do BMP, LFT, cholesterol, and BP often; stop if raised and get expert help). Low cholesterol levels (<120 mg/dL) is a relative contraindication to cyclosporine use.
- *Biologics:* Infections: histoplasmosis, coccidiomycosis and *Listeria*, reactivation of TB, drug-induced lupus or psoriasis, hepatotoxicity, worsening of CHF, infusion site reactions
- *AZA/6MP:* Must follow LFT CBC in these patients. Bone marrow toxicity, allergic reactions, pancreatitis, and serious infections. Onset of drug takes 3–6 months for full effect. Enzyme responsible for inactivation of the 6-MP

is thiopurine S-methyltransferase (TPMT). Levels of TPMT can be commercially obtained and can vary among ethnic groups (10% of the population is heterozygous for the gene), and TPMT levels correlates inversely with 6-TGN levels (the active form of azathioprine). Measurement of thiopurine metabolites, 6-TGN, and 6 MMP can help determine adequate dosing and avoid hepatotoxicity. Also must follow annual skin exams; higher rate of skin cancers in patients taking AZA/6MP.

Crohn's disease

Crohn's disease is a chronic inflammatory GI disease characterized by transmural granulomatous inflammation. It may affect any part of the gut, but favors the terminal ileum and proximal colon. Unlike UC, there may be unaffected bowel between areas of active disease (skip lesions).

Cause: Likely multifactorial etiology involving interplay of environmental factors, genetic susceptibility, and immune system dysregulation. Mutations of the NOD2/CARD15 gene increases risk autosomal recessive. *Prevalence:* 319/100,000. Active smoking is associated with worse outcomes Smoking increases risk 3–4-fold. **Symptoms and signs** Diarrhea, abdominal pain, and weight loss are common. Fever, malaise, anorexia occur with active disease. Look for aphthous ulceration, abdominal tenderness, right iliac fossa mass, perianal abscesses/fistulae/skin tags, anal/rectal strictures.

Extraintestinal signs: Clubbing, erythema nodosum (PLATE 18), pyoderma gangrenosum, conjunctivitis, episcleritis, iritis, large joint arthritis, sacroiliitis, ankylosing spondylitis, fatty liver, primary sclerosing cholangitis, cholangiocarcinoma (rare), renal stones, osteomalacia, malnutrition, amyloidosis.

Complications Small intestinal obstruction; toxic dilatation (colonic diameter >6 cm); abscess formation (abdominal, pelvic, or ischiorectal); fistulae, e.g., colovesical (bladder), colovaginal, perianal, enterocutaneous; perforation; rectal hemorrhage; colonic carcinoma.

Tests *Blood:* CBC, ESR, CRP, BMP, LFT, blood culture. Serum iron, B$_{12}$, and red cell folate if anemia. *Markers of activity:* Hb↓; ↑ESR; ↑CRP; ↑WBC; ↓albumin, fecal calprotectin, fecal lactoferrin.

Stool microscopy/culture and Clostridium difficile toxin (cdt) to exclude infectious diarrhea (*C. difficile, Salmonella, Shigella, Campylobacter, E. coli*).

Colonoscopy and biopsy should be performed even when the mucosa is macroscopically normal (20% have microscopic granulomas).

Small bowel imaging: To detect proximal and distal small bowel disease (strictures, small bowel dilatation, inflammatory mass, abscess or fistula). Studies include small bowel follow-through, CT enterography, MR enterography. *Barium enema:* may show "cobblestoning', "rose thorn" ulcers, and colonic strictures with rectal sparing.

Management Table 7.19 presents a reasonable treatment algorithm, however, medications and doses need to be individualized for each patient. Severity is harder to assess than in UC. Severe symptoms (fever; pulse↑; ↑ESR; ↑CRP; ↑WCC; ↓albumin) merit admission. Endoscopic findings do not reflect overall severity of a Crohn's flare. Recommend consult with gastroenterology to guide therapy.

Mild attacks: Patients are symptomatic but systemically well. Consider induction with ileal release budesonide (9 mg/day), conventional steroids, AZA/6MP. Reassess in clinic for response. (See TPMT data from UC chapter.) If symptoms resolve on oral steroids, taper. Budesonide and steroid can induce induction, but not maintenance. Long term steroid-sparing regimens favored. *Moderate to severe attacks:* Prednisone 40 mg/d until resolution of symptoms and return of weight gain. AZA/6MP can maintain steroid-induced remission; can consider parenteral methotrexate for steroid dependent or steroid-refractory disease. Anti-tumor necrosis factor

(TNF) monoclonal antibodies (infliximab, adalimumab, certolizumab) are effective in those who have not responded to initial therapy. (AZA/6MP, anti-TNF can be used for maintenance of remission).

Severe/fulminant attacks or disease: Admit for IV steroids, NPO, and IV hydration (e.g., 1 L 0.9% saline + 2 L dextrose-saline/24 h, + 20 mmol K⁺/L, less if elderly). Consult gastroenterology. Then consider:

- IV steroids: Hydrocortisone or Solu-Medrol

Table 7.19 Therapies in Crohn's disease

Azathioprine (2–2.5 mg/kg/d PO) or 6MP (1–1.5 mg/kg/d PO) are steroid-sparing agents. Need monitoring of LFT, CBC. Should check TPMT enzyme level prior to initiating therapy.

Aminosalicylates: Little use in Crohn's

Elemental diets: Are as good as steroids in active disease in children, but are unpalatable and relapse is more common.

Methotrexate: 25 mg IM weekly for induction of remission and complete withdrawal from steroids in patients with refractory Crohn's disease. NNT ≈ 5. There is no evidence on lower doses. Monitor LFTS for methotrexate-induced hepatotoxicity.

Biologics: Infliximab, adalimumab, and certolizumab; used for moderate to severe Crohn's. Can be for induction and maintenance.

Surgery: 50–80% of patients need 1 operation in their life.

Indications for surgery:
- Failure to respond to medical therapy
- Intestinal obstruction from strictures
- Intestinal perforation
- Local complications (fistulae, abscesses)

Surgery is never curative: The aim is limited resection of the worst areas. Bypass and pouch surgery is *not* done in Crohn's (increases risk of recurrence).

- Treat rectal disease, if present, with rectal steroids twice daily.
- Antibiotics can be useful if abscess, fistulae, or perforation are identified.
- Monitor T°, pulse, BP, and record stool frequency/character.
- Perform physical examination twice daily.
- Obtain daily CBC, ESR, CRP, BMP, and plain abdominal x-ray.
- Consider need for transfusion (if Hb <10 g/dL) and parenteral nutrition.
- If improving after 5 d, transition to oral steroid for taper.
- If no response (or deterioration) during IV therapy, seek surgical advice.

Irritable bowel syndrome

IBS is used to describe a heterogeneous group of abdominal symptoms for which no organic cause can be found. IBS patients show an exaggerated response to stimuli like meals, distension, stress, etc.

Clinical features Patients are usually 20–40 yrs old, and females are more frequently affected than males. *Symptoms:* Classic patient symptoms: A (abdominal pain), B (bloating or abdominal discomfort), C (change in bowel habit) present and stable for at least 6 months. Diagnostic criteria (modified from Rome criteria) IBS is likely if:

- Pain or discomfort is either
  - Relieved by defecation or
  - Associated with alternating stool form (loose and hard)
- and (need to have at least two of the following):
  - Altered stool passage (straining, urgency, incomplete evacuation),
  - Abdominal bloating, distension, tension or hardness,
  - Symptoms worse with eating,
  - Passage of mucus
- Nausea, dyspareunia; pain in the back, thigh, or chest; urinary frequency; depression can also support the diagnosis.
- Symptoms are chronic (>3 months over 12-month period), and may be exacerbated by stress, menstruation, or gastroenteritis.

Table 7.20 Management of IBS[6,7]

Confirm diagnosis:
1) Take a **good history and physical** with a thorough examination. Exclude symptoms of other illnesses.
2) Elicit history to exclude any **red-flag** symptoms.
3) May perform **testing**
   For all: Celiac panel (anti-TTG Ab, antiendomysial Ab)
   For IBS with no red flags: No other testing
   For IBS with red flags: CBC, ESR, CRP, Thyroid studies, ova and parasites. Refer to gastroenterology. Colonoscopy and imaging.
   (British guidelines also recommend CBC, ESR, and CRP if symptoms of diarrhea are predominant without red flags; American guidelines recommend against further testing without red flags and also recommend against celiac testing for those with IBS–constipation.)

Management:
For typical IBS (no red flags) **dietary and lifestyle changes** (adjust diet to avoid trigger foods, reduce or increase fiber as appropriate, increase exercise as tolerated, provide reassurance and follow-up care) and initiate **medications** (antispasmodics, antimotility, laxatives, TCA or SSRI.)

For those with IBS and red flags, may also consider further investigation:
- If diarrhea is prominent, check: LFT; stool culture and testing, fecal fat; B12/folate; antiendomysial ab; TSH; colonoscopy should include random biopsies.
- If constipation is prominent, consider rectal exam, anorectal motility testing, gut transit testing.
- Further investigation should be guided by severity of symptoms and can also include:
- Upper GI endoscopy (dyspepsia, reflux)
- Duodenal biopsy (celiac disease); e.g., if anti-endomysial antibodies +ve.
- Giardia tests (p. 544) (it often triggers IBS)
- Small bowel radiology (Crohn's disease)
- MRCP or EUS (chronic pancreatitis)
- Transit studies and anorectal physiological studies are rarely used.

6 Drossman, D, Camilleri M, Mayer EA, Whitehead WE. AGA Technical Review on Irritable Bowel Syndrome. *Gastroenterology.* 2002;123 (6): 2108–2131.
7 Khan S, Chang, L. Diagnosis and management of IBS. *Nat Rev Gastroenterol Hepatol.* 2010;7: 565–581.

Table 7.20 (Continued)

When to Refer:
Just because one meets criteria for IBS, it doesn't mean the patient will never have another disease or disorder. If symptoms change or intensify, if depression becomes severe, if red-flag symptoms are evoked, if pain is found to be cyclical and coincide with menstrual cycle, continue investigation as appropriate.

Treatment Be honest with patients. They have a disorder, it will not cause malignancy, but it may cause symptoms. Careful explanation and reassurance are vital. *Create a good relationship with your patient.*

Food intolerance: Can experiment with limited exclusion diets (difficult to maintain). Encourage patient to keep a food diary.

Constipation (p. 200): Increase fiber intake gradually; can lead to bloating

Diarrhea: Bulking agent ± loperamide 2 mg after each loose stool; max 16 mg/d; *se:* Colic, nausea, dizziness, constipation, bloating, ileus

Dyspeptic symptoms: May respond to metoclopramide or antacids

Psychological: Emphasize positive aspects and prognosis: In 50%, symptoms go away or improve after 1 yr; <5% worsen. Symptoms are still troublesome in the rest at 5 yrs. *Tricyclic antidepressants* (low dose) are often helpful; as are *psychotherapy, cognitive-behavioral therapy.* Explain that all forms of stress (sexual, physical, or verbal abuse) perpetuate IBS.

Signs: Examination is often unremarkable although generalized abdominal tenderness is common. Insufflation of air during endoscopy may reproduce the pain.

Markers of organic disease: Referral and further workup for anyone >50 with new onset symptoms; anyone with red-flag symptoms (rectal bleeding, nocturnal diarrhea, weight loss, family history of cancer, anemia, masses, fistulae, markers, or history suggestive of IBD) (i.e., it may well not be IBS). Age >40 yrs; history <6 months; anorexia; weight↓; waking at night with pain/diarrhea; mouth ulcers; rectal bleeding; abnormal investigations. *Management:* See Table 7.20.

Carcinoma of the pancreas

Epidemiology: Fourth most common cause of cancer-related death in the United States; highly lethal; 36,800 deaths in United States in 2010. *Typical patient:* >60 yrs old. *Risk factors:* Smoking, alcohol, DM, family history. *Pathology:* Most are ductal adenocarcinoma (metastasize early; late presentation). 60% arise in the pancreas head, 15% the tail, and 25% in the body. A minority arise from the ampulla of Vater (ampullary tumor) or pancreatic islet cells (insulinoma, gastrinoma, glucagonomas, somatostatinomas, VIPomas); these have a better prognosis.

Symptoms and signs Tumors in the head of the pancreas classically present with painless obstructive jaundice. Tumors in the body and tail present with epigastric pain, which typically radiates to the back and may be relieved by sitting forward. Either may cause anorexia, weight loss, DM, or acute pancreatitis. Rare features include thrombophlebitis migrans, marantic endocarditis, hypercalcemia, Cushing's syndrome, ascites (peritoneal metastases), portal hypertension (splenic vein thrombosis), nephrotic syndrome (renal vein metastases). *Signs:* Jaundice + palpable gallbladder (Courvoisier's "law": Painless jaundice + palpable GB implies a diagnosis other than gallstones), epigastric mass, hepatomegaly, splenomegaly, lymphadenopathy, ascites.

Tests *Blood:* Cholestatic jaundice. CA 19-9 is elevated in pancreatic cancer but is nonspecific and not indicated as a screening test. *Imaging:* Ultrasound or CT scan show a pancreatic mass ± dilated biliary tree ± hepatic metastases. Staging CT or endoscopic ultrasound. ERCP can delineate the biliary tree anatomy and localize the site of obstruction if necessary. MRI is helpful

Histology: Obtainable by endoscopic ultrasound with fine-needle aspiration (FNA), ultrasound- or CT-guided percutaneous biopsy.

Treatment Most ductal carcinomas present with metastatic disease; <10% are suitable for radical surgery. *Surgery:* Consider pancreatoduodenectomy if patient is able to tolerate surgery and the tumor is <3 cm and without metastases. Postop morbidity is high (mortality <5% in experienced hands). *Postop chemotherapy* delays disease progression. *Palliation of jaundice:* Endoscopic (ERCP) or percutaneous stent insertion if symptoms of cholangitis, severe symptoms of hyperbilirubinemia, or if unresectable disease. Plan for chemo or palliation; otherwise discuss options with surgeons. Rarely, palliative bypass surgery is indicated for duodenal obstruction or unsuccessful ERCP. *Pain relief:* Disabling pain may be relieved by opiates or radiotherapy. Celiac plexus infiltration with alcohol may be done at the time of palliative surgery, percutaneously or via endoscopic ultrasound.

Prognosis Mean survival <6 months. 5-yr survival rate: <2%. Overall 5-yr survival after Whipple procedure 5–14% (see Figure 7.3). Patients with the rarer ampullary or islet cell tumors have a better prognosis.

Nutritional disorders

Scurvy is due to lack of vitamin C in the diet. *Is the patient poor, pregnant, or on an odd diet?* Signs: (1) Listlessness, anorexia, cachexia. (2) Gingivitis, loose teeth, and foul-smelling breath (halitosis). (3) Bleeding from gums, nose, hair follicles, or into joints, bladder, gut.

Diagnosis: No test is completely satisfactory.

Treatment: Dietary education; ascorbic acid 250 mg/d PO.

Beriberi presents with heart failure with generalized edema (wet beriberi) or neuropathies (dry beriberi) due to lack of vitamin B_1 (thiamine).

Pellagra (lack of niacin). *Classical triad:* Diarrhea, dementia, dermatitis (± neuropathy, depression, insomnia, tremor, rigidity, ataxia, fits). It may occur in carcinoid syndrome and anti-tuberculosis (TB) treatment. It is endemic in China and Africa. *Treatment:* Education, electrolyte replacement, nicotinamide. Look for other vitamin deficiencies.

Xerophthalmia This vitamin A deficiency is a major cause of blindness in the tropics. Conjunctivae become dry and develop oval or triangular spots (Bitot's spots). Corneas become cloudy and soft. Give vitamin A 200,000 IU stat PO, repeat in 24 h and a week later (halve dose if <1 yr old; quarter if <6 months old); get special help if pregnant; vitamin A embryopathy must be avoided. Re-educate and monitor diet.

Carcinoid tumors

A diverse group of tumors of argentaffin cell origin (neuroendocrine tumors), by definition capable of producing 5HT. *Common site:* Appendix (25%) or rectum. They also occur elsewhere in the GI tract, ovary, testis, and bronchi. Tumors may be benign but 80% >2 cm will metastasize. *Symptoms and signs:* Initially few. GI tumors can cause appendicitis, intussusception, or obstruction. Hepatic metastases may cause RUQ pain. Carcinoid tumors may secrete adrenocorticotropic hormone (ACTH; Cushing's syndrome); 10% are part of multiple endocrine neoplasia (MEN)-1 syndrome and 10% occur with other neuroendocrine tumors. Carcinoid *syndrome* occurs in 10%.

Carcinoid syndrome usually implies hepatic involvement. *Signs:* Paroxysmal flushing (± migrating wheals—bright red color on the face, chest, trunk, and extremities lasting 10–30 min), abdominal pain, diarrhea, tricuspid incompetence, and pulmonary stenosis. *CNS effects:* Numerous (e.g., *enhanced* ability to learn new stimulus–response associations). *Carcinoid crisis* occurs when a tumor outgrows its blood supply and mediators flood into vasculature; this is life-threatening.

Diagnosis *Useful tests:* 24 h urine 5-hydroxyindoleacetic acid↑ (5HIAA, a 5HT metabolite; levels change with drugs and diet: Discuss with lab). If liver metastases are not found, try to find the primary (CXR; chest/pelvis MRI/CT) as curative resection may be possible. Plasma chromogranin A, which is present in chromaffin granules of neuroendocrine cells, is suggested as primary biomarker for diagnosis of neuroendocrine tumors (reflects tumor

Figure 7.3 Whipple procedure

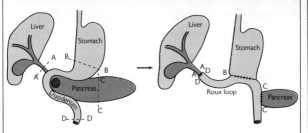

(a) Areas of reflection of different parts (b) Postoperation Whipple procedure may be used for removing masses in the head of the pancreas—typically from pancreatic carcinoma, or, less commonly, a carcinoid tumor.

mass, can follow treatment response); CT and MRI scans, ^{111}Indium octreotide scintigraphy (OctreoScan); positron emission tomography (PET) or PET-CT.

Treatment *Carcinoid syndrome:* Octreotide and lanreotide (somatostatin analogues) block release of tumor mediators and counters peripheral effects. Effects lessen over time. *Other options* Loperamide or cyproheptadine for diarrhea; ketanserin (experimental $5HT_2$ antagonist) for flushing; interferon-α. *Tumor therapy:* Surgical debulking (e.g., enucleation) or embolization of hepatic metastases can decrease symptoms. These must be done with octreotide on-board to avoid precipitating a massive carcinoid crisis. Crisis is treated with high-dose octreotide and careful management of fluid balance. *Median survival:* 5–8 yrs; 38 months if metastases are present, but may be *much* longer (~20 yrs); two-thirds of patients with neuroendocrine tumors have stable disease for up to 5 years.

Gastrointestinal malabsorption

Symptoms Diarrhea, ↓weight, steatorrhea (fatty stools, difficult to flush). *Deficiency signs:* Anemia (↓Fe, B_{12}, folate), bleeding (↓vitamin K), edema (↓protein).

Common causes: Celiac disease, Crohn's, chronic pancreatitis. *Others causes include:* ↓Bile (primary biliary cirrhosis); ileal resection; biliary obstruction. *Treatment* E.g., cholestyramine.

Pancreatic insufficiency: Chronic pancreatitis, pancreas cancer, cystic fibrosis.

Small bowel mucosa: Celiac and Whipple diseases, tropical sprue, radiation enteritis, small bowel resection, brush border enzyme deficiencies (e.g., lactase insufficiency), drugs (metformin, neomycin, alcohol), amyloid.

Bacterial overgrowth: Spontaneous (especially in elderly), in jejunal diverticula, postop blind loops. Try fluoroquinolones, Bactrim.

Infection: Giardiasis, diphyllobothriasis (B_{12} malabsorption), strongyloidiasis.

Intestinal hurry: Postgastrectomy dumping, post-vagotomy, gastrojejunostomy.

Tests CBC (MCV↓, macrocytosis), ↓Ca^{2+}(↓vitamin D due to fat malabsorption), ↓Fe, ↓folate, ↑PT (↓vitamin K), celiac serology (below). *Stool:* Sudan stain for fat globules, stool microscopy for infestation. *Ba follow-through:* Diverticula, Crohn's, radiation enteritis. *Breath hydrogen analysis:* Bacterial overgrowth; take samples of end-expired air; give glucose; take more samples at half-hour intervals. If there is overgrowth, there is increased exhaled hydrogen. *Small bowel biopsy:* Use endoscopy; *MRCP* biliary obstruction, chronic pancreatitis.

Tropical malabsorption *Typical causes:* Giardia intestinalis, Cryptosporidium parvum, Isospora belli, Cyclospora cayetanensis, and the microsporidia. *Tropical sprue:* Villous atrophy and malabsorption occurring in the Far and Middle East and Caribbean (rare in Africa); the etiology is unknown. Tetracycline and folic acid may be helpful.

Celiac disease is a T-cell mediated autoimmune disease of the small bowel in which gluten (alcohol-soluble proteins in wheat, barley, rye, ± oats) intolerance causes villous atrophy and malabsorption. *Associations:* HLA DQ2 in 95%; the rest are DQ8; autoimmune disease; dermatitis herpetiformis.

Presentation: Steatorrhea/offensive stools, other abdominal pain, bloating, nausea/vomiting, aphthous ulcers, angular stomatitis, weight↓, fatigue, weakness, iron-deficiency anemia, osteomalacia, poor growth (children). One-third are asymptomatic, so have a low threshold for evaluating patients for celiac disease. Occurs at any age (peaks in infancy and 50–60 yrs).

Diagnosis: Antibodies: (anti-gliaden, transglutaminase, antiendomysial—an IgA antibody; 95% specific, unless the patient is IgA-deficient). Duodenal biopsies done at endoscopy (as good as jejunal biopsy if >4 samples taken). Villous atrophy, reversing on gluten-free diet (along with ↓symptoms and antibodies).

Treatment: Lifelong gluten-free diet. Rice, maize, soya, potatoes, +/− oats, and sugar are OK. Gluten-free biscuits, flour, bread, and pasta are available. Verify diet by endomysial antibody tests. Refer to a nutritionist.

Complications: Anemia, secondary lactose-intolerance, GI T-cell lymphoma (rare, suspect if worsening despite diet), malignancy (gastric, esophageal, bladder, breast, brain), myopathies, neuropathies, hyposplenism, osteoporosis.

Chronic pancreatitis

Epigastric pain "bores" through to back; bloating, steatorrhea, ↓weight, DM.

Causes: in general: TIGAR-O: Toxic metabolic, Idiopathic, Genetic, Autoimmune, Recurrent and severe acute pancreatitis, Obstruction.

More specific: ANNAHEIM criteria: Alcohol consumption (excessive, increased, or moderate); Nicotine (pack-years of smoking); Nutritional factors (hyperlipidemia or high-fat diet); Hereditary factors (hereditary pancreatitis, familial pancreatitis, early–onset idiopathic, late-onset idiopathic, tropical pancreatitis, possible gene mutations PRSS1, CFTR, or SPINK 1); Efferent duct factors (pancreatic divisum, annular pancreas, pancreatic duct obstruction [tumor], post-traumatic pancreatic duct scars, sphincter of Oddi dysfunction); Immunologic factors (autoimmune pancreatitis, Sjögren-associated, IBD-associated, chronic pancreatitis with PSC or PBC, and miscellaneous factors (hypercalcemia, hyperparathyroidism, chronic renal failure, drugs, toxins).

Tests: Ultrasound (dilated biliary tree; stones); if normal consider CT/MRCP or EUS [>6 criteria of chronic pancreatitis on EUS had a positive predictive value of 85%]. *Plain film:* Speckled pancreatic calcification; glucose↑; breath tests (above).

Drugs: Recommend stopping smoking and alcohol. Can give analgesia (± celiac-plexus block). Pancrelipase; e.g., Creon®; fat-soluble vitamins (e.g., Multivite®), and vitamin D (1,000 units daily). *Diet:* Low fat (+ no alcohol) may help. *Surgery:* For unremitting pain; narcotic abuse (beware of this); weight↓; pancreatectomy or pancreaticojejunostomy, some research centers investigating total pancreatectomy with autoislet cell transplant.

Renal medicine

Matthew Foy, M.D. and Sumeska Thavarajah, M. D.

Contents

Introduction to nephrology

Web links for estimating glomerular filtration rate (GFR)

The four-variable Modification of Diet in Renal Disease **(MDRD)** equation estimates GFR based on age, sex, race, and serum creatinine (**www.nephron.com**). Another estimate of creatinine clearance uses serum creatinine (SCr), sex, and ideal body weight (IBW; muscle bulk is important). See **www.globalrph.com/crcl.htm**. It is based on the Cockcroft-Gault equation:

$CrCl \approx (140 - age) \times IBW/(SCr \times 72)$ ($\times 0.85$ for females).

IBW in (kg) is 50 kg + 2.3 kg for each inch of height over 5 ft for men. IBW is 45.5 kg + 2.3 kg for each inch over 5 ft for women. *Units:* SCr (mcmol/L)/8.4 = SCr (mg/dL). *Example:* A 70-yr-old white woman with a serum creatinine of 1.3 mg/dL has an estimated GFR of 43 mL/min/1.73 m^2 by the four-variable MDRD equation. For Cockcroft-Gault, the same woman standing at 5 feet, 4 inches would have an estimated GFR of 41 mL/min.

Renal disease typically presents with one or more of a short list of clinical syndromes, listed below. One underlying pathology may have a variety of clinical presentations.

1 *Proteinuria and nephrotic syndrome:* Normal protein excretion is <150 mg/d. Nonpathologic increases to ~300 mg/d can be seen in orthostatic proteinuria (related to posture); during fever, during pregnancy, or after exercise. *Proteinuria* (excessive urine protein excretion) is a sign of glomerular or tubular disease. *Nephrotic syndrome* is the triad of proteinuria (>3 g/d [p.248]), hypoalbuminemia (albumin <3.5 g/dL), and edema. Hyperlipidemia is often seen.

2 *Hematuria and nephritic syndrome: Hematuria* (blood in the urine) may arise from anywhere in the renal tract. It may be *macroscopic, microscopic,* or detected as *hemoglobinuria. Nephritic syndrome* comprises hematuria and proteinuria, although often in subnephrotic range. It may be associated with hypertension (HTN), peripheral edema, oliguria, and acute kidney injury (AKI) (ARF). The question of who to refer hematuria patients to (urologist or nephrologist) is discussed on p. 236.

3 *Oliguria and polyuria: Oliguria* is a urine output of <400 ml/d. It is a normal response to severe fluid restriction. *Pathologic causes:* Reduced renal perfusion, renal parenchymal disease, urinary tract obstruction. *Polyuria* is the excretion of larger than normal volumes of urine (generally >3 L/d), usually from high fluid or solute intake. Pathological causes include diabetes mellitus (DM), diabetes insipidus (p. 306), disorders of the renal medulla (urinary concentrating defect), and supraventricular tachycardia.

4 *Flank pain and dysuria:* Flank pain is usually due to postrenal obstruction, acute pyelonephritis, polycystic kidneys, or renal infarction. Severe flank pain (aka renal colic) may be associated with fever and vomiting and may radiate to the abdomen, groin, or upper thigh. It is usually caused by a renal calculus, clot, or sloughed papilla. Urinary *frequency* and *dysuria* (pain on passing urine) are symptoms of cystitis.

5 *Acute renal failure (ARF)/AKI* is significant decline in renal function occurring over hours to days, detected by a rising serum creatinine and urea nitrogen, with or without oliguria. AKI usually occurs secondary to reduced blood flow to the kidneys (hypotension, hypovolemia, sepsis, abdominal compartment syndrome), urinary obstruction, or intrinsic renal disease.

6 *Chronic kidney disease (CKD):* Kidney damage >3 months as defined by structural or functional abnormalities of the kidney, with or without ↓ GFR or a GFR <60 mL/min/1.73 m^2 body surface area. It is classified according to GFR into five categories: Stage 1 (kidney damage with normal GFR >90 mL/min), stage 2 (60–89 mL/min), stage 3 (30–59 mL/min), stage 4 (15–29 mL/min), and stage 5 (<15 mL/min). There is poor correlation between symptoms and signs of CKD. Progression may be so insidious that patients attribute symptoms to age or other illnesses. Severe CKD may not present with any symptoms. End-stage renal failure is a degree of renal failure that, without renal replacement therapy, would result in death.

7 *Microalbuminuria* is a silent harbinger of serious renal (and cardiovascular) risk. In one study, 30% of those with type 2 DM died within ~5 yrs of developing microalbuminuria.

251

Urine

Examine fresh urine (<1 h old) whenever you suspect renal disease.

Dipsticks

- *Hematuria:* Causes: Infections (cystitis, either bacterial or BK and JC virus; pyelonephritis, prostatitis; tuberculosis (TB); schistosomiasis; urethritis), calculi, neoplasia (kidney, bladder, prostate, urethra), trauma (commonly from Foley placement in a hospitalized patient), glomerulonephritis, interstitial nephritis, polycystic kidney disease, papillary necrosis (sickle-cell disease, NSAIDs), medullary sponge kidney, vasculitis, vascular malformation, cyclophosphamide, hemophilia. Anticoagulation should not cause hematuria at usual therapeutic goal levels. *Tests:* Urine dipstick and microscopic exam, culture, 24 h urine collection (protein, creatinine clearance); CBC, erythrocyte sedimentation rate (ESR), c-reactive protein (CRP), blood urea nitrogen (BUN), creatinine. *Others:* Clotting factors, hemoglobin (Hb) electrophoresis; computed tomography (CT) pyelogram with and without IV contrast or renal ultrasound ± renal biopsy. *Management plan:* Usually refer to urologist for urothelial malignancy evaluation if >40 yrs or other high risk (smoker, cyclophosphamide, dye worker). Refer to nephrologist if risk of urothelial malignancy is low and risk of glomerulonephritis is not negligible (e.g., <40 yrs old, ↑ serum creatinine, ↑BP, proteinuria, systemic symptoms, family history of renal disease). *False +ve dipstick hematuria:* Free Hb, myoglobin, bacterial peroxidase *False negative:* Ascorbic acid, old dipsticks. NB: Urine concentration can affect detection rates. *Red urine:* Beets, porphyria, rifampin, phenazopyridine, phenolphthalein (found in some laxatives).
- *Proteinuria:* Normal protein excretion is <150 mg/d (may rise >300 mg/d in fever, or with exercise). *Causes:* Urinary tract infection (UTI), orthostatic proteinuria, primary and secondary glomerular disease (systemic lupus erythematosus [SLE], amyloidosis, DM, pregnancy), interstitial disease, hemolytic-uremic syndrome, multiple myeloma. *Tests:* Blood pressure (BP), urine dipstick (only detects *albumin*, not other proteins, such as light chains; in this instance, use the sulfosalicylic acid test) and microscopic exam; 24 h urine collection (protein excretion, creatinine clearance). Spot urine protein-to-creatinine ratio (ratio of 1 ≈ urine protein excretion of 1 g/24 h if patient has ~1 g urine creatinine excretion), renal ultrasound, serum complement, or others (antinuclear antibodies [ANA]; rapid plasma reagin [RPR]; hepatitis C, hepatitis B, HIV, protein electrophoresis [SPEP, UPEP]). If abnormal, consider renal biopsy.
- *Microalbuminuria:* Albumin excretion 30–300 mg/24 h or spot urine sample value of 30–300 mg/ mg creatinine. *Causes:* DM, ↑BP.
- *Other substances Glucose:* DM (serum glucose levels >200 mg/dL), pregnancy, Fanconi's syndrome, proximal tubule damage. *Ketones:* Starvation, ketoacidosis. *Leukocytes:* UTI, vaginal discharge, interstitial nephritis. *Nitrites:* Enterobacteriaceae infection, high-protein meal. *Bilirubin:* Obstructive jaundice. *Urobilinogen:* Prehepatic jaundice. *Specific gravity:* Normal range: 1.000–1.030 (dilution and concentration). Fixed range of ~1.010 is *isosthenuria* and indicative of interstitial renal disease process, such as sickle cell anemia, severe CKD. *PH:* Normal range: 4.5–8 (acid–base balance: Urease producing bacteria and distal RTA may cause alkaline urine).

Microscopy Collect a fresh urine specimen via clean catch or from Foley catheter. Centrifuge 10 mL for 5 min at 2,000–3,000 rpm. Invert tube, emptying most of urine, then resuspend pellet in few drops of urine. Put a drop of centrifuged urine sediment on a microscope slide, cover with a coverslip, and examine under low (100×) and high (400×) power for leukocytes, rbcs, bacteria, crystals, and casts.

Leukocytes: >10/mm^3 in an unspun urine specimen is abnormal. *Causes:* Cystitis, urethritis, prostatitis, pyelonephritis, interstitial nephritis, TB, renal calculi, glomerulonephritis.

Red cells: >3–5 red blood cells (RBCS)/high-powered field in two-thirds of morning specimens. *Causes:* See hematuria.

Casts are cylindrical bodies formed in the lumen of distal tubules as cells or other elements and are embedded in Tamm–Horsfall protein.

Finely granular and hyaline casts (clear, colorless) are found in concentrated urine, fever, after exercise, or with loop diuretics and pathologic conditions.

Densely granular casts: Acute tubular necrosis (ATN), GN, or interstitial nephritis.

Fatty casts: Heavy proteinuria. Under polarized light, show Maltese-cross appearance.

Red cell casts are a hallmark of glomerulonephritis (GN). May be seen with interstitial nephritis or vasculitis.

White cell casts occur in pyelonephritis, interstitial nephritis, atheroembolic disease, and rarely proliferative glomerulonephritis.

Epithelial cell casts occur in ATN.

Crystals are common in old or refrigerated urine and may not signify pathology. Cystine crystals are diagnostic of cystinuria. Oxalate crystals in fresh urine may indicate ethylene glycol poisoning in patients with severe metabolic acidosis (see Figure 8.1). Medications (sulfonamides, indinavir, acyclovir).

24 h urine for creatinine ± protein excretion. Take blood creatinine simultaneously to calculate creatinine clearance. Can check 24 h urine for Na$^+$, K$^+$, for electrolyte disorders, or stone risk profile for recurrent stones.

Figure 8.1 Urine microscopy

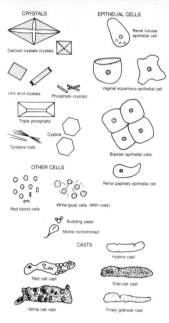

CRYSTALS

Calcium oxalate crystals

Uric acid crystals   Phosphate crystals

Triple phosphate

Cystine

Tyrosine rods

OTHER CELLS

Red blood cells

White (pus) cells (with rods)

Budding yeast

Motile trichomonad

EPITHELIAL CELLS

Renal tubular epithelial cell

Vaginal squamous epithelial cell

Bladder epithelial cells

Renal papillary epithelial cell

CASTS

Hyaline cast

Red cell cast

Granular cast

White cell cast

Finely granular cast

Principle source: M. Longmore An Atlas of Microscopy rcgp.

When you find red cells, consider their morphology to understand where in the GU tract they come from. If >80% of RBCs are dysmorphic G1 cells, suspect glomerular bleeding and look hard for red cell casts. Acanthocytes are RBCs with donut shapes, target configurations, and membrane protrusions or blebs. Acanthocyturia of >5% is considered indicative of glomerular hematuria. www.uninet.edu/cin2003/conf/nguyen/nguyen.html

Urinary tract imaging

Kidney, ureters, bladder (KUB) x-ray Look at kidneys, path of the ureters, and bladder. Abnormal calcification may be related to calculi (only 80% of stones are visible on plain films: See CT below), dystrophic calcification; e.g., in carcinomas or TB (uncommon) and nephrocalcinosis. Note: Plain abdominal film focuses more on bowel, not urinary system, and may miss stones.

Ultrasound is the usual initial image in renal medicine. May be performed with Doppler. Abnormal parenchyma if echogenicity is greater than that of the liver. It shows:

• *Renal size. Small* (<9 cm) implies CKD; *large* in renal masses, benign cysts[1]; hypertrophy if other kidney missing, polycystic kidney disease, amyloidosis, diabetes, and lymphomatous infiltration

1 Cysts may be inherited, developmental, or acquired; e.g., polycystic kidney disease, medullary sponge kidney, multicystic dysplastic kidney, medullary cystic disease, tuberous sclerosis, renal sinus cysts, von Hippel-Lindau's disease.

- *Hydronephrosis*, which indicate renal obstruction or reflux
- *Perinephric collections* (trauma, postrenal biopsy)
- *Transplanted kidneys* (collections, obstruction; color Doppler indicates perfusion)
- *Bladder residual volume*
- *Power Doppler ultrasound* evaluates for renal artery stenosis.

Advantages: Fast, cheap, independent of renal function, no IV contrast or radiation risk. *Disadvantages:* Intraluminal masses, such as transitional cell carcinomas (TCC) in the upper tracts, may not be seen; not a functional study; only suggests obstruction when there is dilatation of the collecting system (~1–2% of obstructed kidneys have nondilated systems).

Disadvantages: May miss obstruction and hydroureter early on in the disease.

Helical noncontrast/CT is gold standard for diagnosis of renal colic. Noncontrast scans are 97% sensitive for calculi and show other pathologies. CT allows detailed characterization of masses (solid or cystic, contrast enhancement, calcification, local/distant extension, renal vein involvement); renal trauma (hemorrhage, devascularization, laceration, urine leak); retroperitoneal lesions. CT urogram for hematuria uses IV contrast to visualize collecting system if noncontrast CT is negative.

Intravenous urogram/pyelogram (IVU/IVP) A study for defining anatomy (especially pelvi-calyceal) and for detecting pathology distorting the collecting system. It yields limited functional information. Abdominal films are taken before and after IV contrast, which is filtered by the kidney, reaching the renal tubules at ~1 min (nephrogram phase). Later images show contrast in the system (pyelogram), ureters, and bladder. Detects papillary necrosis, medullary sponge kidney. *Side effects (SE):* Flushing, nausea, rash, contrast nephropathy (Caution: Risks include preexisting CKD, DM).

Retrograde pyelography is good at showing anatomy of the pelvi-calyceal systems and ureters and for detecting pathology, such as transitional cell carcinoma (TCC). Contrast is injected via a ureteric catheter.

255

Percutaneous nephrostomy The renal pelvis is punctured with imaging guidance. Diagnostic images are obtained following contrast injection. A nephrostomy tube may then be placed to allow drainage of an obstruction above the bladder.

Renal arteriography Still the gold standard for renal artery stenosis. Can perform pressure monitoring across stenosis for significant pressure change for borderline lesions. Therapeutic indications include angioplasty, stenting, and selective embolization (bleeding tumor, trauma, or arteriovenous [AV] malformations).

Magnetic resonance imaging (MRI) offers improved soft tissue resolution; it may be used to clarify equivocal noncontrast CT findings. Magnetic resonance angiography (**MRA**) is useful in imaging renal artery stenosis. Avoid gadolinium in severe CKD.

Radionuclide imaging scans quantify each kidney's contribution to renal function and can detect renal scarring ($^{99}TC^mDTPA$, diethylenetriamine penta-acetic acid). Radiolabeled metal chelators such as ^{51}Cr-EDTA (ethylenediaminetetraacetic acid), ^{125}I iothalamate, or $^{99}Tc^mDTPA$, can also measure GFR.

Renal biopsy

See Table 8.1.

Table 8.1 Renal biopsy

Most acute kidney injury is due to prerenal causes or ATN, and recovery of renal function typically occurs over the course of a few weeks. Renal biopsy should be performed if knowing histology will influence management. Once CKD is long-standing with small kidneys, risks of bleeding from biopsy may be increased and therapy may be limited.

Indications for renal biopsy:

- What is the cause of this acute kidney injury (p. 268)?
- Investigating isolated hematuria with normal renal function and minimal proteinuria to rule out glomerulonephritis is nephrologist-dependent. Is persistent hematuria in this scenario from IgA nephropathy, thin basement membrane disease, or hereditary nephropathy?
- What is the cause of this heavy proteinuria (e.g., >2–3 g/d) when diabetic nephropathy is unlikely?
- Renal dysfunction post-transplantation: Is the cause rejection, drug toxicity, or recurrence of renal disease?

Preprocedure: Check cbc, coagulation profile. Obtain written informed consent. Hold aspirin, NSAIDs, and anticoagulation at least 7 d prior to procedure if possible.

Relative contraindications (CI):

1 One kidney or horseshoe kidney
2 Morbidly obese
3 Uncontrolled HTN (systolic >160 mm Hg)

In these instances, consider open procedure or CT-guided biopsy.

Procedure: Biopsy may be performed with real-time ultrasound using needle guides, with the patient lying in the prone position and the breath held. May also be performed by radiology via transjugular approach or surgically via laparoscopic or open techniques for those who are obese or who are at increased risk for bleeding. Samples should be sent to pathology for routine stains, immunofluorescence, and electron microscopy. A clear indication on the request form of why the test has been done (e.g., exclude amyloidosis) will help in the selection of special stains, immunofluorescence, and use of electron microscopy.

Postprocedure: Bed rest for 6–24 h. Monitor pulse, BP, symptoms, and urine color. Bleeding is the main complication with nephrectomy and death (~1/1,000 cases).

Urinary tract infection

Definitions *Bacteriuria:* Bacteria in the urine may be asymptomatic or symptomatic. *UTI:* The presence of a pure growth of 10^3 colony forming units (CFU)/mL or $>10^3$ of uropathogen with pyuria and symptoms. *UTI sites:* Bladder (*cystitis*), prostate (*prostatitis*), or kidney (*pyelonephritis*). Up to one-third of women with symptoms do not have bacteriuria; a condition known as *urethral syndrome*. *Classification:* UTIs may be classified as *uncomplicated* (normal renal tract and function) or *complicated* (most male patients, abnormal renal tract, impaired renal function, impaired host defenses, virulent organism). A *recurrent UTI* is a further infection with a new organism. A *relapse* is a further infection with the same organism.

Risk factors Female sex, sexual intercourse, diaphragm or spermicide contraceptive, DM, immunosuppression, pregnancy, menopause, urinary tract obstruction (p. 260), nephrolithiasis, instrumentation, or malformation.

Organisms *E. coli* is the most common (~80% in the community but <41% in hospital). Others include *Staphylococcus saprophyticus, Enterococcus faecalis, Proteus mirabilis, Klebsiella* spp., *Enterobacter* spp., *Acinetobacter* spp., *Pseudomonas aeruginosa,* and *Serratia marcescens.* In men <35, should consider sexually transmitted infections (STIs; e.g., *N. gonorrhoea* or *C. trachomatis*) as cause of prostatitis. See Table 8.2.

Symptoms *Cystitis:* Frequency, dysuria, urgency, hematuria, suprapubic pain. *Acute pyelonephritis:* Fever, rigors, vomiting, loin pain and tenderness. *Prostatitis:* Flu-like symptoms, low backache, few urinary symptoms, swollen, boggy, tender prostate.

Signs Fever, abdominal or flank tenderness, renal mass, distended bladder, enlarged prostate.

Tests Microscopic exam for leukocytes or dipstick test for leukocyte esterase or nitrites. May treat uncomplicated empirically if symptoms consistent with acute uncomplicated UTI. If complicated, UTI, pyelonephritis, uncertainty of diagnosis, child, pregnancy, ill-appearing, or if recent recurrence after therapy, send a fresh clean-catch specimen to the lab for culture and sensitivity. Should avoid first morning void for sample. A pure growth of $>10^5$ cfu/ml is diagnostic for complicated UTIs or if bacteria is not always pathogenic. Two consecutive cultures with same bacteria are required for asymptomatic patients in complicated UTIs. If $<10^3$ cfu/ml and pyuria, the result is significant. Cultured organisms are tested for sensitivity to a range of antibiotics.

Blood tests: CBC, BUN, creatinine, blood cultures, if systemically ill-appearing.

Ultrasound, IVP, CT pyelogram/cystoscopy: Consider for UTI in infants, children, or men; recurrent UTI; pyelonephritis; unusual organism; persistent fever; persistent or gross hematuria. *Ultrasound or IVP?* Ultrasound may miss stones, papillary necrosis, and clubbed calyces. Can do ultrasound first because it avoids contrast agents and radiation.

Treatment *Advice:* Drink plenty of fluids, urinate often, double void (going again after 5 min), postintercourse voiding, wipe front to back after micturition. *Antibiotics:* Know your local pattern of resistance: Increasingly, options are narrowing. *Cystitis:* Trimethoprim/sulfamethoxazole (tmp/smx) 160/800 mg bid po ×3 d). Alternative: Quinolone antibiotics (norfloxacin 400 g po bid or ciprofloxacin 250 mg po bid). Longer courses (10–14 d) may be needed in complicated UTI (see above) if fever present. Sensitivity profile determines treatment, although quinolones may be used empirically for severe symptoms.

Acute pyelonephritis: Tmp/smx or quinolones orally unless severe gi symptoms, hemodynamic instability, significant systemic symptoms, noncompliance.

Prostatitis: Acute: ≥35, Ciprofloxacin 500 mg/d PO for 10–14 d. If <35 (or suspected STI), Ceftriaxone 250 mg IM × 1, then doxycycline 100 mg bid × 10 d. *Chronic:* Ciprofloxacin 500 mg PO/12 h × 4 weeks.

Pregnancy: Ask OB.

Prevention: Antibiotic prophylaxis, either continuous or postcoital. Self-treatment with 1–3 d course as symptoms start is an option. Cranberry juice may inhibit adherence of *E. coli* to bladder cells, but needs further assessment.

For patients with renal transplant, end-stage renal disease (ESRD), and indwelling urologic devices, medication choices may need to be adjusted based on clinical scenario and culture data.

Table 8.2 Causes of sterile pyuria

Renal TB (do three early morning urines).	
Inadequately treated UTI	Papillary necrosis from DM, analgesic excess, sickle cell
Appendicitis	UTI with fastidious culture requirement
Calculi, prostatitis	Interstitial nephritis, polycystic kidney
Bladder tumor	Chemical cystitis

Renal calculi (nephrolithiasis)

Renal stones (calculi) consist mainly of crystal aggregates. Stones form in the collecting ducts and may be deposited anywhere from renal pelvis to urethra. See Table 8.3.

Epidemiology *Prevalence:* 0.2%. Lifetime incidence: Up to 12%. *Peak age:* 20–50 yrs. ♂:♀ >4:1. *Risk factors:* Dehydration, UTI with urease producing organisms, hypercalcemia, hypercalciuria, hyperoxaluria, hypocitraturia, hyperuricosuria, small intestinal disease or resection, chronic diarrhea, cystinuria, distal renal tubular acidosis, gout, drugs (triamterene, indinavir), family history, anatomic abnormality (medullary sponge kidney).

Types of stone Calcium (usually oxalate ~75% with pure calcium phosphate rare [5%]), struvite (ammonium magnesium phosphate ± calcium phosphate ~15–20%), uric acid (~10%), cystine (~1%), drug (acyclovir, indinavir, sulfadiazine).

Clinical features Vary widely from asymptomatic to multiple symptoms. *Pain:* Stones in the kidney cause flank pain. Stones in the ureter cause ureteric colic. This classically radiates from the flank to the groin and is associated with nausea and vomiting. Bladder or urethral stones may cause pain on micturition or interruption of urine flow. *Infection* may be acute, chronic, or recurrent. It may present with cystitis (frequency, dysuria), pyelonephritis (fever, rigors, flank pain, nausea, vomiting), or pyonephrosis (infected hydronephrosis). *Other:* Hematuria, sterile pyuria, anuria from obstructing bladder calculi or ureteral calculi with solitary functioning kidney.

Tests *Blood*: BUN, creatinine, electrolytes, Ca^{2+}, PO_4^{3-}, intact parathyroid hormone (PTH) if hypercalcemic, uric acid. *Urinalysis:* Urine ph (normal range 4.5–8). Acidic urine ↑uric acid stone formation and alkaline urine ↑ phosphate stone formation). *24 h urine: Best done in the outpatient setting with patient consuming usual diet;* Ca^{2+}, sodium, sulfate/urea nitrogen reflects animal protein/protein intake, phosphate, uric acid, citrate, pH, oxalate, volume, creatinine for accuracy of collection.

Imaging: Noncontrast helical CT is the imaging modality of choice for stones. Renal ultrasound excludes hydronephrosis or hydroureter. Abdominal KUB film (kidneys + ureters + bladder).

Management Stones not causing obstruction between attacks of renal colic may be managed conservatively. Advise patient to increase fluid intake and strain urine to retrieve stone for biochemical analysis. Note that stones often take ≥30 d to pass. *Ureteric stones* <5 mm in diameter usually pass spontaneously. They may need to be fragmented or removed endoscopically from below. If >5 mm, <50% pass spontaneously. *Pelvicaliceal stones* <5 mm do not need treatment unless causing obstruction or infection. Stones <2 cm in diameter are suitable for lithotripsy. Stones >2 cm are usually removed by percutaneous or cystoscopic methods. *Renal colic:* Give IV fluids if unable to tolerate oral fluids; analgesia and antibiotics if evidence of infection. *Seek urological help urgently if evidence of obstruction.* Procedures include retrograde stent insertion, nephrostomy, and antegrade pyelography (p. 255). These may be combined with lithotripsy. Open surgery is rarely needed.

Prevention Drink plenty of fluid to keep urine output >2–3 L/24 h. It may be necessary to drink at night to cause voiding at night.

Calcium oxalate stones:

Hypercalciuria: Low-salt diet(2 g/d); watch animal protein intake; thiazide diuretic.

Hyperoxaluria: Calcium intake (dairy products) with meals; ↓oxalate intake (less tea, chocolate, nuts, strawberries, rhubarb, spinach, nuts); calcium supplements with meals if enteric hyperoxaluria due to small bowel disease with increased absorption of oxalate.

Hyperuricosuria: Restrict dietary purine intake, allopurinol.

Hypocitraturia: Potassium citrate, orange juice or lemonade.

Uric acid: Alkalinize urine if acidic urine PH with goal urine pH >6. Hyperuricosuria; dietary purine restriction or allopurinol.

Struvite: Antibiotics; urologic removal of stones.

Uric acid stones: Urinary alkalinization (to maintain PH >6); allopurinol (100–300 mg/d).

Cystine stones: Vigorous hydration to keep cystine concentration <250–300 mg/L of urine, D-penicillamine, tiopronin, captopril; urinary alkalinization to achieve urine pH >7–7.5.

Table 8.3 Questions for patients with stones

What is its composition? In order of frequency, the likely answer is:

— Calcium oxalate stones: These are spiculated	(radiopaque)
— Calcium phosphate stones are smooth and may be large	(radiopaque)
— Struvite staghorn stone: Large; spiculated	(radiopaque)
— Uric acid: (smooth, brown, and soft)	(radiolucent)
— Cystine stones: Yellow and crystalline	(semiopaque)

Risk factors?

— Diet: Excess salt and animal protein intake for hypercalciuria, calcium restriction with meals; increased oxalate intake (chocolate, tea, nuts, spinach) for hyperoxaluria; increased purine intake for calcium and uric acid stones

— Hypercalciuria/hypercalcemia (e.g., hyperparathyroidism, sarcoidosis, neoplasia, hyperthyroidism, Li^+, vitamin D excess)

— Dehydration: All stones. Acidic urine can lead to uric acid stones

— Medullary sponge kidney

— Primary or secondary hyperoxaluria (excess oxalate gut reabsorption because of small bowel malabsorption)

— Gout and ↑ urine uric acid: Increases both calcium oxalate and uric acid stone risk

— UTI (predisposes to struvite stones with urease splitting organisms and from staghorn calculi)

— Distal renal tubular acidosis: Acidosis leads to low urine citrate, and alkaline urine leads to increased precipitation of calcium phosphate stones. (Sjögren's is secondary distal RTA)

— Cystinuria

— Family history? X-linked nephrolithiasis or Dent's disease: Low-molecular-weight proteinuria, hypercalciuria, nephrocalcinosis?

Is there infection above the stone? Fever? Flank tender? Pyuria?

Urinary tract obstruction

Urinary tract obstruction is common, often reversible, and should be considered in any patient with impaired renal function due to bilateral or unilateral in solitary functioning kidney. It may occur from the renal calyces to the urethral meatus. It may be *partial* or *complete*, *unilateral*, or *bilateral*. Obstructing lesions are *luminal* (stones, blood clot, sloughed papilla, tumor), *mural* (e.g., congenital or acquired stricture, neuromuscular dysfunction, schistosomiasis), or *extramural* (abdominal or pelvic mass/tumor, retroperitoneal fibrosis). Unilateral, partial, or slowly developing obstruction may be asymptomatic (i.e., normal urine output). Bilateral obstruction or obstruction + infection requires urgent treatment. Note that a patient still producing urine does not rule out obstruction.

Clinical features *Acute upper tract obstruction*: Flank pain ± radiation to groin. There may be superimposed infection.

Chronic upper tract obstruction: Flank pain, renal failure, superimposed infection. Polyuria may occur due to impaired urinary concentration.

Acute lower tract obstruction: May be urinary retention; usually presents with severe suprapubic pain, often preceded by symptoms of bladder outflow obstruction. *Exam*: Distended, palpable bladder.

Chronic lower tract obstruction: Symptoms: Urinary frequency, hesitancy, decreased stream, dribbling, overflow incontinence, nocturia, suprapubic fullness. *Signs:* Distended, palpable bladder; enlarged prostate. *Complications:* UTI, urinary retention.

Tests *Blood:* Electrolytes, BUN, creatinine.

Urine: Dipstick and microscopic exam. Urine pH (may be elevated from acidification defect, distal nephron damage). *Ultrasound* (p. 255) is the imaging test of choice. If obstruction is above the bladder, *antegrade or retrograde pyelography/nephrostomy:* Offers therapeutic option of drainage. *Radionuclide imaging* enables functional assessment of collecting system dilation which may be from vesicoureteral reflux, chronic pyelonephritis, pregnancy (R > L), increased urine flow states, instead of true obstruction. *CT and MRI* may help identify location and etiology of obstruction.

Treatment *Drainage is urgent if there is infection above an obstruction.* *Upper tract obstruction:* Acute, nephrostomy. Chronic, ureteral stent or pyeloplasty. *Lower tract obstruction:* Urethral or suprapubic catheter. Treat the underlying cause if possible. Beware of large diuresis after relief of obstruction; a temporary salt-losing nephropathy may occur with the loss of several liters of fluid a day. Monitor vital signs for hypotension, weight, fluid balance, and electrolytes in case IV fluids (e.g., 0.45% ns) required.

Retroperitoneal fibrosis

A disorder that is part of chronic periaortitis, which includes inflammatory abdominal aortic aneurysms and perianeurysmal retroperitoneal fibrosis. In this rare autoimmune condition, there is vasculitis of adventitial aortic vasa vasorum and periaortic small vessels with fibrous tissue embedding the ureters, resulting in progressive obstruction. Primary and secondary causes.

Associations: Drugs (e.g., β-blockers, bromocriptine, methysergide, ergotamines), malignancy (carcinoid, lymphoma, sarcomas, carcinoma of colon, prostate, breast, stomach), infections (TB, histoplasmosis), radiation therapy, surgery (colectomy, hysterectomy), others (trauma, thyroiditis).

Typical patient: Middle-aged men with dull, noncolicky backache with constitutional symptoms of weight loss, fatigue, anorexia, ↑BP, ± edema.

Tests: Blood: Anemia, uremia, ↑ESR, ↑CRP, ANA and few antineutrophil cytoplasmic antibody (anca) +ve.

Imaging: *Ultrasound/IVP:* Dilated ureters (hydronephrosis) + medial deviation of ureters with extrinsic compression, peri-aortic mass. Rarely, ultrasound may be negative. *CT/MRI:* Periaortic mass that entraps ureters (this allows biopsy, which confirms the diagnosis).

Treatment: Retrograde stent placement to relieve obstruction + steroids or other immunosuppressive medications (mycophenolate mofetil, methotrexate) or tamoxifen ± surgery (open/laparoscopic ureterolysis).

Glomerulonephritis

Abbreviations: ANA, antinuclear antibody; ASO, antistreptolysin O titer; BM, basement membrane (glomerular); EM, electron microscopy; *ESRD,* end-stage renal disease; HCV, hepatitis C virus; IF, immunofluorescence.

Introduction The presentation of GN varies widely, from asymptomatic to microscopic or macroscopic hematuria, proteinuria, the nephrotic syndrome, renal failure, or HTN. Diagnosis is usually made on renal histology, interpreted in the light of clinical, biochemical, and immunologic features.

Pathophysiology The nephritic syndromes can perhaps be easiest remembered on the basis of the mechanisms by which injury occurs.

These include: Antibodies directed against the glomerular basement membrane; immune complex–mediated disease; pauci-immune mediated endothelial injury (ANCA-associated and non-ANCA associated); and inherited disorders. (See Figure 8.1)

Tests In general, testing should be directed towards the suspected clinical syndrome. However, the clinical history can often be ambiguous, and serologic testing can help differentiate the diagnoses.

Blood: Complement (C3, C4); CBC; electrolytes, BUN, creatinine; liver-function tests (LFT); ESR. *Autoantibodies:* ANA, ANCA, anti-dsDNA (*double stranded DNA*), anti-GBM (*glomerular basement membrane*); blood culture; ASO; HBsAg; anti-HCV, cryoglobulins, serum electrophoresis (see Figure 8.2). *Urinalysis:* To diagnose glomerular bleeding, look for RBC casts, dysmorphic RBCs, and acanthocyturia (5% of RBCs [p. 252]). Urinalysis dipstick and microscopic exam. *24 h urine* for protein and creatinine excretion/creatinine clearance. Spot urine protein to creatinine ratio for approximation. *Chest x-ray (CXR); renal ultrasound; renal biopsy.*

Management Prompt consultation or referral to a nephrologist is vital to assist with diagnosis and treatment.

Antiglomerular basement membrane

Rare disorder, seen more frequently in Caucasians and with a bimodal age distribution (second and third decades, and sixth and seventh decades). Autoantibodies generated against type IV collagen lead to injury.

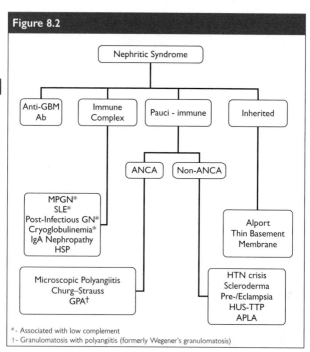

Figure 8.2

Nephritic Syndrome

Anti-GBM Ab — Immune Complex — Pauci-immune — Inherited

Pauci-immune: ANCA / Non-ANCA

MPGN*
SLE*
Post-Infectious GN*
Cryoglobulinemia*
IgA Nephropathy
HSP

Microscopic Polyangiitis
Churg–Strauss
GPA†

Alport
Thin Basement Membrane

HTN crisis
Scleroderma
Pre-/Eclampsia
HUS-TTP
APLA

* - Associated with low complement
† - Granulomatosis with polyangiitis (formerly Wegener's granulomatosis)

Clinical features Over half of patients have rapidly progressive GN with pulmonary involvement (Goodpasture's syndrome) and approximately one-third have isolated GN. Serologic testing for anti-GBM antibodies. Can also find ANCA positivity in 30–40% of patients.

Diagnosis: Renal biopsy: Crescent formation; IF reveals intense linear staining for IgG.

Treatment: Plasmapheresis for pulmonary hemorrhage and consider for renal involvement (if not extensive fibrosis on biopsy and not dialysis dependent in <72 h from presentation), high-dose glucocorticoids, and cyclophosphamide.

Prognosis: Without treatment, progresses quickly to ESRD. Milder forms that do not require dialysis tend to respond to treatment.

Immune complex diseases

IgA nephropathy (Berger's disease) Most common cause of GN

Clinical features Children, young adults, males (2:1).

Presentations Episodic macroscopic gross hematuria 1–2 d after precipitating URI (40–50%). This is sometimes known as *synpharyngitic hematuria*.

Diagnosis Renal biopsy: Mesangial proliferation with +ve immunofluorescence (IF) for IgA and C3. *Prognosis* 4–38% of adults develop ESRD over ~10 yrs. Risk factors for progression include ↑ creatinine, ↑ BP, and >1 g/d proteinuria. *Treatment*: Angiotensin-converting enzyme (ACE)-inhibitors and/or angiotensin receptor blocker (ARB) for HTN or proteinuria. Consider fish oil supplementation. Immunosuppression if active crescents seen on biopsy or proteinuria >2–3 g/d despite ACE inhibitors.

Henoch–Schönlein purpura (HSP) can be regarded as a systemic variant of IgA nephropathy.

Clinical features: Polyarthritis of the large joints, purpuric rash on the extensor surfaces, abdominal symptoms, GN.

Diagnosis: Usually clinical. May be confirmed by finding positive IF for IgA and C3 in skin lesions or renal biopsy (identical to IgA nephropathy). *Prognosis*: 50% remission; 15–20% impaired renal function; 3–5% renal failure.

Treatment: For severe proteinuria and renal failure, consider immunosuppression with steroids.

Lupus nephritis (LN) ~50% of patients with SLE will have renal involvement. There are six classifications of lupus nephritis (Table 8.1). The clinical presentation is widely varied, from microscopic hematuria or mild proteinuria to macroscopic hematuria, nephrotic syndrome, and rapidly progressive renal failure.

Diagnosis: Suggestive lab findings include low C3 and C4 and positive ANA/anti-DNA Ab. Specific diagnosis is confirmed by biopsy. See Table 8.4 for classes of lupus nephritis. In general, it is a proliferative GN, with mesangial and endocapillary involvement, except for membranous type, which should not have endocapillary involvement. A finding of a mixed picture, such as class III/V or class IV/V is not uncommon. Immunofluorescence shows positivity for the five antibodies commonly used (against IgG, IgM, IgA, C3, and C1q) to give a "*full house*" staining pattern. See Table 8.4. Additional biopsy findings can include thrombotic microangiopathy, IC vasculopathy, vasculitis, and interstitial nephritis.

Table 8.4 Classification of lupus nephritis

Class I	Minimal mesangial LN
Class II	Mesangial proliferative LN
Class III	Focal proliferative LN (<50% glomeruli involved)
Class IV	Diffuse proliferative LN (>50% glomeruli involved)
Class V	Membranous LN
Class VI	Advanced sclerosing LN (>90% glomeruli globally sclerosed)

Treatment: Target is to quickly decrease immune activity followed by a more prolonged course of immunosuppression (induction and maintenance therapy). Depending on severity, induction utilizes high-dose glucocorticoids + cyclophosphamide or mycophenolate mofetil. This is followed with maintenance dose glucocorticoids plus additional immunomodulating therapies such as mycophenolate mofetil, azathioprine, calcineurin inhibitors (cyclosporine or tacrolimus). Coordination of care between patient's primary care, nephrologist, and rheumatologist is key.

Prognosis: Worse prognosis is associated with ↑serum creatinine, HTN, nephrotic-range proteinuria; chronic tubulointerstitial disease, extensive crescents on biopsy; delayed initiation of immunosuppression, incomplete remission, or relapse. Despite treatment, 10–30% of patients with proliferative GN will progress to ESRD.

> **Monitoring for renal disease in the patient with sle**
>
> Given that early detection is important in delaying progression of lupus nephritis, close monitoring of SLE patients without active urine sediment is important. Screening of UA for proteinuria or hematuria and monitoring serum creatinine should be performed every 3–6 months for the first several years and then every 6 months to 1 yr thereafter.

Membranoproliferative GN Accounts 8% of children and 14% of adults with nephrotic syndrome. Variable presentation: Hematuria, non-nephrotic proteinuria, slowly progressive glomerular disease, nephrotic syndrome.

Diagnosis: Biopsy shows glomeruli with mesangial proliferation and "double contoured" BM. Three histological types: Type I (subendothelial and mesangial deposits). Type II (intramembranous and mesangial deposits). Type III (subendothelial, mesangial, subepithelial deposits). Reduced serum C3 and C3 nephritic factors are found in most patients (type II more than type I). *Associations:* Hep C, SLE, chronic bacterial infections (endocarditis, visceral abscess, shunt nephritis, syphilis), HBV, schistosomiasis, mixed cryoglobulinemia, monoclonal gammopathy, α_1-antitrypsin deficiency, chronic leukoblastic leukemia (CLL), partial lipodystrophy, complement dysregulation resulting in complement activation. New classification scheme proposed is based on renal biopsy immunofluorescence findings predominantly positive for IgGs (infection, neoplastic or autoimmune etiologies), complement (genetic complement dysregulation), or neither (chronic thrombotic microangiopathy). *Treatment:* In adults, long-term benefit of ASA + Pyridamole, steroids, or other immunosuppressive meds is unclear. Hep C-related treatment (p. 565).

Prognosis: Risk factors for worse prognosis include nephrotic proteinuria, ↑ SCR at presentation, HTN, interstitial fibrosis on biopsy. 50% develop ESRD if untreated.

Acute postinfectious GN Classically occurs 1–3 wks following pharyngitis, or 3–6 wks following skin infection. Although the chief cause is Streptococcus, it can be seen in a variety of bacterial, fungal, parasitic, and viral infections. *Clinical features:* Hematuria, proteinuria, nephritic syndrome, nephrotic syndrome, renal failure (rare). *Renal biopsy:* Hypercellularity, mesangial and endocapillary proliferation, inflammatory cell infiltrate, and cellular crescents in severe cases; IF positive for granular IgG and C3; and subepithelial deposits on EM. *Serology:* ↑ASO; ↓C3. *Treatment:* Antibiotics, diuretics, and antihypertensives as necessary. Dialysis is rarely required. *Prognosis:* Generally good, especially in children. Poorer prognosis in patients >65 and DM with diabetic glomerulosclerosis.

Pauci-immune GN, ANCA-associated granulomatosis with polyangiitis (GPA)/microscopic polyangiitis (MPA) Occurs more in older adults, more commonly in Caucasians. Many have prodrome of a flu-like illness: Fevers, malaise, arthralgias. Renal disease presents with ARF, hematuria, and proteinuria. Upper respiratory involvement more common in GPA, both can have pulmonary involvement. Other organ involvement can include skin (purpura), nervous system (mononeuritis multiplex), heart (pericarditis and conduction abnormalities), and GI tract.

Diagnosis: Serologic testing for ANCA. Although overlap between the syndromes exists, GPA is generally PR3 ANCA +, and mpa is generally mpo ANCA +. Histology shows focal and segmental fibrinoid necrosis and cellular crescents. MPA lacks granulomas. If shows a paucity of immune deposits.

Treatment: High-dose corticosteroids and cyclophosphamide. Consider plasma exchange for pulmonary involvement and severe renal dysfunction (those requiring dialysis). Rituximab without cyclophosphamide can also be considered.

Prognosis: Untreated mortality high (~90% at 2 yrs) versus a 12% mortality at 7–8 yrs in patients treated with cyclophosphamide. Worse renal outcome associated with ↑Cr at presentation, age >65, lack of response to treatment, renal relapse, and ↑ fibrosis on biopsy.

Non-ANCA associated Essentially due to endothelial damage from mechanical injury via thrombotic microangiopathy. See p. 279 for discussion on specific conditions.

Inherited disorders

Thin basement membrane nephropathy (autosomal dominant). There is persistent microscopic hematuria ± minor proteinuria, with normal BP and renal function. *Diagnosis:* Positive family history. *Renal biopsy:* Decreased width of glomerular BM. *Prognosis:* Benign.

Alport syndrome Predominantly X-linked, although autosomal dominant and recessive forms do exist. Caused by a defect in type IV collagen, resulting in progressive glomerulosclerosis of GBM. Patients have persistent microscopic hematuria ± proteinuria, bilateral sensorineural hearing loss, and ocular manifestations involving the lens (lenticonus), retina, or cornea. *Diagnosis:* Positive family history. Can pursue renal biopsy, skin biopsy, or genetic testing. *Renal biopsy:* Findings vary depending on timing of biopsy; early disease may look normal on LM, with progressive disease showing glomerulosclerosis. If utilizes Ab directed against α subunits of type IV collagen and may be useful in diagnosis. On EM, GBM shows thickening and a "basket-weave" appearance. *Prognosis:* ESRD typically occurs between ages 15 and 35 in patients with X-linked or autosomal recessive forms, later for autosomal dominant forms. *Treatment:* Control BP, supportive management of renal failure, dialysis, transplantation.

Rapidly progressive GN (RPGN) ESRD develops over weeks or months if untreated.

Causes: Anti-GBM disease (Goodpasture's), SLE, cryoglobulinemia, Henoch-Schönlein purpura/IgA nephropathy, postinfectious glomerulonephritis, Pauci-immune GN.

See above discussions regarding clinical features, biopsy findings, and treatment. Urgent consultation with a nephrologist is warranted if these entities are suspected.

The nephrotic syndrome

When there is edema, check a urinalysis for protein to avoid missing this diagnosis.

Definition Nephrotic syndrome is the combination of edema, proteinuria (>3 g/24 h), hypoalbuminemia (albumin <3.5 g/dl), and hyperlipidemia. In some cases, this is due to ↑urine protein loss resulting in ↓albumin, hence ↓plasma oncotic pressure (minimal change disease). However, most patients may have a normal or ↑plasma volume, suggesting primary salt retention.

Causes Minimal change disease (common in children and young adults), focal segmental glomerulosclerosis (common in African Americans), membranous nephropathy (common in middle-aged/elderly), DM (the most common cause), amyloidosis, SLE, membranoproliferative GN.

Minimal change glomerulonephritis (MCGN) Commonest cause of nephrotic syndrome in children (76%; 25% of nephrotic adults). *Associations:* Hodgkin's lymphoma; various drugs (NSAIDs). *Clinical features:* Nephrotic syndrome; BP↑; usually little renal impairment; however, acute kidney injury in elderly from ATN or secondary to NSAIDs with interstitial nephritis. *Diagnosis:* Selective proteinuria (especially in children). Renal biopsy shows loss of podocyte foot processes on EM. *Treatment:* Corticosteroids induce remission in >90% of children and 80% of adults (slower response). *Indications for other immunosuppression:* Cyclophosphamide, cyclosporine; frequent relapses; steroid resistance or dependence. *Prognosis:* 1% progress to ESRD.

Focal segmental glomerulosclerosis can be similar to MCGN as only some glomeruli have segmental sclerosis. It may be primary (idiopathic) or secondary (reflux, sickle-cell disease, obesity, HIV, heroin use, renal scarring after glomerulonephritis). *Clinical features:* Nephrotic syndrome, proteinuria, microscopic hematuria, ↓renal function, BP↑. *Renal biopsy:* Segmental areas of glomerular sclerosis, hyalinization of glomerular capillaries, and positive IF for IgM and C3. *Treatment:* 35–60% complete and partial remission to steroids, but prolonged course of high doses (1 mg/kg/d) for >3–4 months may be required. Cyclophosphamide or cyclosporine may be used in steroid-resistant cases. *Prognosis:* 10–40% if subnephrotic, 45–70% if nephrotic progress to ESRD in 10 yrs.

Membranous nephropathy Accounts for 20–30% of nephrotic syndrome in adults, 2–5% in children. *Associations:* Malignancy (adenocarcinoma of colon, lung, breast), drugs (gold, penicillamine), autoimmune (SLE, rheumatoid arthritis [RA]), infections (HBV, syphilis, leprosy). *Signs:* Nephrotic syndrome, proteinuria, hematuria, BP↑, renal impairment. Hypercoagulable state; see below.

Diagnosis: Renal biopsy shows thickened BM, IF +ve for IgG and C3 and subepithelial deposits on EM.

Prognosis: About one-third experience spontaneous remission, one-third have persistent proteinuria but not ESRD, one-third have ESRD over 5–10 yrs.

Treatment: Controversial because of variable natural history. If renal function deteriorates, persistent heavy proteinuria (e.g., >8 g/d for 6 months) consider corticosteroids + chlorambucil (Ponticelli regimen)/cyclophosphamide; cyclosporine, rituximab, others.

Clinical features of nephrotic syndrome

Symptoms Ask about acute or chronic infections, drugs, allergies, systemic symptoms (SLE, malignancy).

Signs: Periorbital/peripheral edema (anasarca); HTN. Rarely, pleural effusions; ascites. Examine for signs associated with secondary causes/hypercoagulable state.

Complications

- Thromboembolism, especially membranous or MPGN (10–40%) with loss of anticoagulant proteins, ↑ of procoagulant proteins, ↑ platelet (PLT) aggregation (deep vein thrombosis [DVT], pulmonary embolism [PE], renal vein thrombosis; central nervous system [CNS] vessels)
- Hyperlipidemia
- AKI, overdiuresis, elderly with minimal change disease, renal vein thrombosis
- ↑Susceptibility to infection, possibly from ↓Ig (peritonitis, pneumococcus)
- Accelerated atherosclerosis

Tests *Urine:* Dipstick (hematuria, proteinuria), microscopy (oval fat bodies, RBCs, casts), culture/sensitivity, 24 h collection (protein excretion, creatinine clearance) or spot urine protein-to-creatinine ratio for approximation, urine protein electrophoresis. *Blood:* Electrolytes, BUN, creatinine, LFT, ESR, CRP, cholesterol, serum electrophoresis, complement (C3, C4), autoantibodies (ANA, anti-dsDNA), HEP B/C serology, VDRL/RPR. *Imaging:* CXR, renal ultrasound. *Renal biopsy:* Usually do in all adults unless suspect diabetic nephropathy (and steroid-unresponsive children or if unusual features).

Treatment

- Monitor BUN, creatinine, electrolytes, BP, fluid balance, weight.
- Fluid restriction (1–1.5 L/d), sodium-restriction (<88 mEq/d or 2 g/d)
- Diet: Target moderate protein intake and avoid excess, with lower end aim of <0.8 kg/d protein.
- Diuretics, e.g., furosemide 40–400 mg/d in bid doses ± metolazone. *Aim for loss of 1 kg/d.* Occasionally, to promote diuresis, you may need very high doses of furosemide (e.g., up to 200 mg iv)± Diuril (up to 500 mg iv) or metolazone.
- Treat HTN with ACE-inhibitors or ARBs; other proteinuric attenuating agents: β-blockers, nondihydropyridine calcium-channel blockers, aldosterone antagonists.
- Persistent nephrotic syndrome: Immunosuppressive medications as above; ACE-inhibitors or ARBs to reduce proteinuria.
- Hypercoagulable state: Prophylactic warfarin is advocated by some at high risk (membranous nephropathy with massive proteinuria >10 g/d); warfarin for thrombosis.
- Hyperlipidemia improves with resolution of nephrotic syndrome. If unresponsive, treatment with an HMG-CoA reductase inhibitors + ACE-inhibitor/ARB may reduce proteinuria further than ACE-inhibitor/ARB alone.

Renal vein thrombosis Clinical prevalence: 6–8% with membranous GN; 1–3% of those with other forms of GN. Radiologic prevalence: 10–40% of patients with membranous GN; 10% other causes. *Clinical features:* Flank pain, hematuria, proteinuria, renal enlargement, and deteriorating renal function. Usually asymptomatic and diagnosed incidentally. 35% have coincident PE. IVC/bilateral renal vein thrombosis with AKI is reported.

Diagnosis: Doppler ultrasound, renal angiography (venous phase), spiral ct, or MRI. *Treatment:* Anticoagulate with warfarin until non-nephrotic proteinuria achieved. Thrombolytic treatment/mechanical thrombolysis for acute severe thrombosis.

Acute kidney injury: Diagnosis

Definition There are numerous definitions of AKI that include a change in urine output and change in creatinine. All the definitions reflect a significant deterioration in renal function occurring over hours or days. AKI may lead to hyperkalemia, acidosis, pulmonary edema, and uremia. Clinically, there may be nausea, vomiting, fatigue, shortness of breath (crackles), chest pain (pericarditis), change in mental status (asterixis), seizures, ↓ urine volume (oliguria <400 cc/d), or no symptoms or signs. Biochemically, AKI is detected by rising creatinine. AKI may arise as an isolated problem; more commonly, it occurs in the setting of circulatory disturbance (e.g., severe illness, sepsis, trauma, or surgery) or in the context of nephrotoxic drugs.

Causes See various sections for details. AKI can be divided into three types

Prerenal (renal hypoperfusion) is usually reversible. Causes are volume depletion, renal vasoconstriction due to medications (NSAIDs, ACE-inhibitor/ARB, calcineurin inhibitors, amphotericin, iodinated contrast dye); hypercalcemia; sepsis; hepatorenal syndrome; decreased effective circulating volume due to hypoalbuminemia; decreased cardiac output due to cardiomyopathy, arrhythmia, or decreased ejection fraction; or decreased perfusion due to intra-abdominal HTN or abdominal compartment syndrome.

Intrinsic (intrarenal)

Tubular: Ischemic ATN is associated with prolonged hypoperfusion (shock), nephrotoxic ATN is associated with aminoglycosides, amphotericin B, iodinated contrast dye, prolonged NSAIDs, ACE-inhibitors, or rhabdomyolysis. Complete recovery of renal function usually occurs within days or weeks.

Vascular: Renal artery/vein occlusion, renal infarction, malignant HTN, atheroemboli.

Glomerular: Acute glomerulonephritis, small vessel vasculitis, hemolytic uremic syndrome—TTP.

Interstitial: Interstitial nephritis, tumor infiltration. Intratubular obstruction (uric acid from tumor lysis syndrome, acyclovir, sulfonamides, indinavir).

Postrenal: AKI is due to urinary obstruction from nephrolithiasis, ↑prostate, pelvic masses; dysfunctional bladder is a potentially treatable cause.

Assessment

1. *Is the kidney injury acute or chronic?* Suspect chronic kidney disease if:
   - History of chronic ill-health or signs of chronic kidney disease
   - Previously abnormal blood tests (prior records, laboratory results)
   - Small kidneys (<9 cm) on ultrasound

The *presence* of anemia, Ca^{2+} ↓, or PO_4^{3-} ↑ may not help to distinguish AKI from CKD, as these can occur subacutely, but their *absence* suggests AKI. Secondary hyperparathyroidism is suggestive of CKD

2. *Is there urinary tract obstruction?*

Obstruction should always be considered as a cause of AKI because it is reversible, and prompt treatment is required to prevent permanent renal damage. Obstruction should be suspected in patients with a single functioning kidney or in those with history of renal stones, anuria, prostatism, or previous pelvic/retroperitoneal surgery. Examine for a palpable bladder, pelvic or abdominal masses, or an enlarged prostate. Remember having good urine output doesn't exclude some component of obstruction. Assess with post-void residual or imaging studies.

Focused history and physical

- History: Urinary changes in output, color. History of urinary tract infections, nephrolithiasis, prior obstruction, hematuria, proteinuria, previous episodes of AKI, medication exposure: NSAIDs, contrast, aminoglycosides, ACE-inhibitors/arbs, or chemotherapy. Recent GI losses, fluid losses, blood loss. Other medical conditions including connective tissue disorders, autoimmune disorders, HTN.
- *Physical examination:* Vital signs, orthostatics, assess jugular venous pressure (JVP), check for bruits, evidence of volume overload, arrhythmias, skin lesions or rashes, joint abnormalities, stigmata of other chronic disease (e.g., liver disease, jaundice, etc.), enlarged bladder, tense/distended abdomen.

Tests *Urine:* Dipstick for leukocytes, nitrite, blood, protein, glucose, specific gravity. *Microscopy* for RBC, WBC, crystals, cellular or granular casts. *Culture and sensitivity. Chemistry:* Sodium, urea nitrogen, creatinine, osmolality; protein (spot/24 h with urine creatinine measurement). *UPEP:* Beware $K^+\uparrow$; LFT. *Blood tests:* Electrolytes, BUN, CR, CBC; clotting; CPK; ESR; ABG; blood cultures. When glomerular disease is suspected, consider complement levels (C3/C4), autoantibodies (ANA, ANCA, anti-dsDNA, anti-GBM, and aso. Suspect myeloma—serum electrophoresis. *CXR:* Pulmonary edema/hemorrhage? *ECG:* Signs of hyperkalemia? *Renal ultrasound:* Renal size or obstruction? Bladder pressure over 12 mm Hg defines increased intra-abdominal pressure and may cause abdominal compartment syndrome.

Distinguishing prerenal failure and ATN

	Prerenal	ATN
Urine Na (mmol/L)	<20	>40
Urine osmolality (mosm/L)	>500	<350
Urine/plasma urea	>8	<3
Urine/plasma creatinine	>40	<20
Fractional Na excretion (%)	<1	>2
BUN/Cr	>20	<20

These indices are of limited clinical use as intermediate values are common, they may be influenced by diuretics and preexisting tubular disease, and "typical" values do not predict renal prognosis. Fractional excretion of urea nitrogen FeUN (<35% prerenal vs. >50%) used for patients on diuretics. *Both FeNa and FeUN are most accurate when patients are oliguric.*

Acute kidney injury: Management

Enlist nephrologist's help. While awaiting this, make sure that urine microscopy results are available.

If shock is the cause, treatment may include volume resuscitation with crystalloids or blood products, pressors for blood pressure support, or inotropic support in setting of poor cardiac output.

Ultrasound: Check for a palpable bladder, but absence of this sign does not rule out obstruction. If it *is* palpable, insert a catheter.

Stop nephrotoxic drugs (e.g., gentamicin, amphotericin B); *any* drug may be nephrotoxic. Peripheral eosinophilia is suggestive of allergic interstitial nephritis (unreliable).

Monitoring

- Check pulse, BP, JVP, CVP (if available), and urine output frequently. Daily fluid balance + weight chart. If euvolemic, match input to losses (urine, vomit, diarrhea, drains) + 500 mL for insensible losses (more if T°↑).
- Correct volume depletion with IV fluid (colloid, saline, or blood [watch plasma ↑K⁺]) as appropriate.
- If the patient is septic, take appropriate cultures and treat empirically with antibiotics. Remove or change any potential sources of sepsis (e.g., central lines).
- Recheck for any nephrotoxic medications; adjust doses of renally excreted medications. NB: When the creatinine is continuing to rise, the effective GFR is 0 mL/min. Dose medications for GFR <10 mL/min.
- *Nutrition*: Aim for calorie intake of 35 kcal/kg/d and protein intake ≈1–1.2 g/kg/d, although some recommend 0.8 g/dk/d if uremic but not on renal replacement therapy. If oral intake is poor, consider nasogastric nutrition early (parenteral if NGT impossible). Restrict dietary sodium intake if volume overloaded to <2 g/d, and if volume depleted, to 2 g/d. Oral potassium intake if hyperkalemic to <50 mEq/d. Phosphate restriction to 600–800 mg/d if hyperphosphatemic.

Treat complications

Hyperkalemia may cause arrhythmias or cardiac arrest. *Electrocardiogram (ECG) changes:* Peaked T waves; small or absent P wave; ↑ P–R interval; widened QRS complex; "sine wave" pattern; asystole (ECG, p. 672).

- Stabilize myocardium if severe hyperkalemia >7 or severe ECG changes (loss of P waves, QRS widening).
  - IV calcium (e.g., 10 mL 10% calcium gluconate IV over 1 min), repeat as necessary until ECG improves.
- Shift potassium into cells
  - IV insulin + glucose (e.g., 10 U regular insulin + 50 mL of 50% glucose IV over 10 min). If not diabetic, consider continuous infusion of D5 to prevent hypoglycemia. Insulin stimulates the intracellular uptake of K⁺, lowering serum K⁺ by 1–2 mmol/L over 30–60 min.
  - ·β-agonists. 10–20 mg by albuterol nebulizer lowers potassium within 30 min; 8 times usual dose and may not work if used alone.
  - Sodium bicarbonate in patient with severe metabolic acidosis to shift potassium in cells, otherwise unlikely benefit.
- Remove potassium. Usually requires one of measures below:
  - Sodium polystyrene sulfonate (Kayexalate) (e.g., 15–60 g PO or PR) to bind K⁺ in the gut. SE: Colonic necrosis of ileus (e.g., recent surgery).
  - Diuretics if responsive
  - Hemodialysis (HD)/continuous renal replacement therapy (crrt); see opposite; latter much slower potassium removal rate is usually required if anuric. CRRT will not remove potassium as quickly as HD.

Pulmonary edema (p. 754):

- High-flow oxygen by face mask
- IV furosemide 200 mg IV as bolus, followed by continuous drip if some response with bolus ± IV chlorothiazide
- Consider inotropes in congestive heart failure due to systolic dysfunction
- If no response, HD/CRRT is necessary.
- Other measures:
- Consider continuous positive airway pressure ventilation (CPAP) therapy.
- Venous vasodilator (e.g., morphine 2.5 mg IV)
- IV nitrates

Bleeding: Impaired hemostasis due to uremic platelets may be compounded by the precipitating cause. In patients with AKI who are actively bleeding, give:

- Fresh frozen plasma, cryoprecipitate, and platelets as needed, if there are clotting problems
- Blood transfusion to maintain Hb >10 g/dL and hematocrit >30%
- Desmopressin to increase release of von Willebrand factor and increase factor VIII activity, normalizing bleeding time

Prognosis for AKI Mortality depends on cause: Burns (80%), trauma/surgery (60%), medical illness (30%), obstetric/poisoning (10%), ICU setting requiring renal replacement therapy (50–80%).

Indications for dialysis

- Severe hyperkalemia (K$^+$ >6.5–7 mmol/L)
- Refractory pulmonary edema
- Severe or worsening metabolic acidosis (pH <7.2 or base excess <–10)
- Uremic encephalopathy or other symptoms (nausea/vomiting)
- Uremic pericarditis
- Toxic ingestions (SALT: Salicylates, Alcohols, Lithium, Theophylline)

Indications for CRRT

CRRT may be preferable in an ICU setting when sudden shifts in volume removal or osmolarity are undesirable.

Indications: Large obligate intake of fluids, ongoing electrolyte abnormalities (rhabdomyolysis, tumor lysis syndrome), drug toxicities/poisoning (lithium, aspirin), elevated intracranial pressure, hemodynamic instability with pressor requirements.

Advantages: Less hemodynamic instability. *Disadvantage:* More expensive than HD and requires ICU setting and elevated clotting.

Chronic kidney disease

Definitions Either GFR of <60 mL/min/1.73 m^2 body surface area or structural or urinary abnormalities (such as proteinuria) that have been present for the last 3 months.

It is classified according to GFR into five categories: Stage 1 (kidney damage with normal GFR >90 mL/min), stage 2 (60–89 mL/min), stage 3 (30–59 mL/min), stage 4 (15–29 mL/min), and stage 5 (<15 mL/min). ESRD is renal failure that would require treatment with either dialysis therapy or renal transplantation.

Causes Almost all causes of renal disease can progress to ESRD *Common:* Diabetes, HTN, chronic glomerulonephritis, polycystic kidney disease, tubulointerstitial disease, vasculitis, renal vascular disease, or amyloidosis.

History Ask about urinary symptoms: Change in output, change in color, hematuria, foamy urine, nocturia, recurrent UTIs, voiding difficulties, previous episodes of AKI especially requiring dialysis. *Other:* HTN (duration, urgencies/emergencies), diabetes, connective tissue disorders (vasculitis, rheumatoid arthritis, scleroderma), vascular disease, infections (HIV, hepatitis, recurrent infections). *General:* Anorexia, weight loss, pruritus.

Physical exam Elevated BP. *Cardiovascular:* cardiomegaly, pericarditis, edema. *Lungs:* Pleural effusion/pulmonary edema. *Skin:* Pallor; jaundice, livedo reticularis, malar rash, purpura, easy bruising; epistaxis; calcifications of skin, eye, calciphylaxis. *Neuro:* Proximal myopathy, peripheral neuropathy, myoclonus, asterixis, encephalopathy, seizures, coma.

Workup *Common tests:* Complete metabolic panel (renal and hepatic panel), intact PTH (assess for metabolic bone disease) urinalysis, urine microscopy, spot urine protein/creatinine ratio. *Further serologic testing* (not

271

needed for everyone): ANA, complement levels, anti-GBM, ANCAs dependent on clinical presentation. *Renal imaging*: Renal ultrasound with Doppler to assess for kidney size (small-scarring/progressive disease; normal or large-amyloidosis, HIV, DM, asymmetry) scarring-renovascular disease, or obstruction. Doppler or MRA for renovascular. *CXR*: Pulmonary infiltrates, pulmonary vascular congestion. *Renal biopsy*: Definitive diagnosis, to help guide management and prognosis. Not necessary in every patient.

Treatment *Refer early to a nephrologist, especially in cases of proteinuria or to assess for reversible conditions*. Regardless of etiology, begin basic management to delay progression of CKD.

HTN: Target blood pressure of <130/80 mm Hg; with proteinuria. ACE-inhibitor/ARB can slow the rate of loss of function even if BP is normal if there is micro-albuminuria. Watch serum creatinine and potassium after start/increase of the ACE-inhibitor/ARB.

Hyperlipidemia: This may contribute to renal damage and increases the risk of cardiovascular disease. Target low-density lipoprotein (LDL) cholesterol of <100 mg/dL.

Proteinuria: The degree of proteinuria and the inability to reduce the levels are significant factors in accelerated loss of renal function. Goal proteinuria is <500 mg/d.

Edema: Appropriate diuretic use (loop diuretics if GFR <35 mL/min and dosing several times daily). As renal function declines, diuretic doses may need to be increased for same effect. Sodium restriction to 2 g/d is important as well.

Anemia: Caused by erythropoietin deficiency. If other causes are excluded and iron stores replete, consider erythropoietin to maintain Hb between 10 and 11 g/dL.

Metabolic bone disease (osteodystrophy): Manifested by hypocalcemia (due to vitamin D deficiency), hyperphosphatemia (decreased excretion), hyperparathyroidism (driven by hypocalcemia, hyperphosphatemia, and PTH resistance), vitamin D deficiency (decreased conversion to 1,25 OH vitamin D). *Hyperphosphatemia*: Management with phosphate restriction (1 g/d), phosphate binders with meals (calcium carbonate and calcium acetate used in stages 3– 5, sevelamer carbonate and lanthanum carbonate used for stage 5) to prevent phosphate absorption. Either 1,25 OH vitamin D or analogue for management of secondary hyperparathyroidism. Target intact PTH stage V 150–300 pg/mL. Other guidelines allow for 150–600 pg/mL in patients on dialysis. In setting of hypercalcemia, calcimimetic can be used for treatment of secondary hyperparathyroidism.

Dietary advice: Individualized based on labs. May need potassium restriction of 40–60 meq/d. Protein restriction of 0.8 g/kg/d for elevated urea levels, acidosis and proteinuria. Sodium restriction to 2 g/d and fluid restriction to 1–1.5 L/d for volume overload. *Acidosis*: Treat with HCO_3, supplements.

Renal replacement therapy planning: Should start at stage IV CKD. Vascular access referral for arteriovenous fistula (AVF) creation if HD planned. If no suitable veins, AVG placement delayed until 6 wks prior to HD. Insert a Tenckhoff catheter 4–6 wks before anticipating need to start peritoneal dialysis (PD). Refer for transplantation unless there is a contraindication.

Figure 8.3

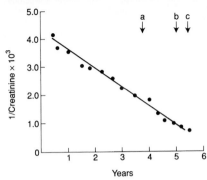

Plot of reciprocal plasma creatinine (mcmol/L) against time in a patient with adult polycystic disease. The letters represent life events: (a) work promotion, (b) arteriovenous fistula, and (c) hemodialysis.

Some patients with CKD lose renal function at a constant rate. Creatinine is produced at a fairly constant rate and rises on an exponential curve as renal function declines, so the reciprocal creatinine plot is a straight line, parallel to the fall in GFR. This is used to monitor renal function and to predict need for dialysis, but there is much individual variation in progression so the plot has limited application. Rapid decline in renal function greater than that expected may be due to infection, dehydration, uncontrolled ↑BP, metabolic disturbance (e.g., Ca^{2+} ↑), obstruction, nephrotoxins (e.g., drugs). Investigation and treatment at this point may delay ESRD.

273

Table 8.5 Prescribing in renal failure

Never prescribe in renal failure before checking through Micromedex or the Physician's Desk Reference for how a drug's dosing should be altered. In AKI, when the creatinine is rising, the effective GFR is 0 mL/min/1.73 m².

Renal replacement therapy

The criterion for initiating dialysis in CKD patients is when GFR falls below 10 mL/min/1.73 m² BSA by using the four-variable MDRD formula, the creatinine clearance estimated by the Cockroft–Gault formula (p. 250), or when patients develop refractory volume overload, hyperkalemia, or uremic symptoms. *Early* preparation is vital, including education about different dialysis modalities and transplantation options. Medical preparation involves hepatitis B vaccination and creating an AVF if HD is the planned option. Choice of HD versus PD depends on medical, social, and psychological factors. **NB:** Kidney function is only partially replaced by dialysis.

Hemodialysis Solute transfer occurs by diffusion and is based on concentration gradients. Blood flows on one side of a semipermeable membrane countercurrent to the dialysate flow to maximize the concentration gradient. Ultrafiltration describes fluid removed during any type of renal replacement therapy. Dialysis prescriptions can be written for a combination of ultrafiltration with dialysis or for either procedure alone. In HD/CRRT, negative pressure across the dialysis membrane removes fluid from filtered blood. *Complications:* Dialysis dysequilibrium syndrome (rapid shift in osmolality), hypotension, arrhythmias, hemolysis, dialysis access complications (poor flow, infection, thrombosis, prolonged bleeding, steal syndrome), infection, vascular access (poor flow, infection)

Peritoneal dialysis PD fluid is introduced into the peritoneal cavity via a Tenckhoff catheter, and uremic solutes diffuse into it across the peritoneal membrane. The peritoneal membrane functions as the dialyzer. Ultrafiltration may be achieved by using osmotic agents (e.g., glucose) in the dialysis fluid of variable strengths. Convection and diffusion both clear uremic toxins. PD clearance is significantly enhanced by residual renal function. Important to ask PD patients about reduced urine output if uremic symptoms arise. This is a good option in patients with low ejection fractions or hypotension as it allows for slow fluid removal.

Continuous ambulatory PD (CAPD): Patient performs manual exchanges of dialysate in which fluid is continuously dwelling in the patient except for filling and draining of dialysate. 2–3 L bags are exchanged usually four times a day to produce, with ultrafiltration, a total dialysate of >10 L/d.

Automated PD: Patient uses a cycler machine that automatically performs exchanges at night. Techniques include continuous cyclic peritoneal dialysis (CCPD), in which there is fluid left in the abdomen during the day, and night intermittent peritoneal dialysis (NIPD), in which the patient has no fluid in abdomen in the daytime. A manual exchange may have to be added to CCPD or NIPD patients if there is poor dialysis clearance.

Problems:

Peritonitis (60% staphylococci, 20% gram-negative organisms, <5% fungi), exit-site infection, catheter malfunction, loss of ultrafiltration, obesity, hyperglycemia; rare, peritoneal-pleural leaks, hernias, back pain, hyperlipidemia.

It may be difficult to achieve adequate clearance in larger patients who have lost residual renal function.

Complications in ESRD patients *Cardiovascular disease* (e.g., coronary heart disease, congestive heart failure, sudden cardiac death, cerebrovascular disease is ↑↑ in dialysis patients and a major cause of mortality). *HTN* persists in 25–30% of patients on HD. Some is related to large fluid gains. Timing of antihypertensive doses in HD patients may need to be altered to allow for fluid removal during the dialysis sessions. *Anemia* is commonly treated with erythropoiesis-stimulating agents and oral or IV iron supplements if deficient. *Bleeding tendency* is due to platelet dysfunction. Acute bleeding is treated with desmopressin and transfusion, as necessary.

CKD: Mineral *bone disorders are* treated with phosphate binders (calcium acetate, calcium carbonate, sevelamer, or lanthanum) for hyperphosphatemia. Secondary hyperparathyroidism with goal IPTH 150 to 300–600 pg/mL is treated with 1,25 dihydroxy vitamin D (calcitriol) PO or IV, paricalcitol (Zemplar) IV or PO (Hectorol) IV or PO, or cinacalcet (Sensipar) PO. Calcitriol and, to a lesser extent, analogs paricalcitol and doxercalciferol may ↑ serum calcium and phosphate. Cinacalcet reduces serum calcium and phosphate. *Infections* are caused by nonsterility with exchanges during PD or vascular access procedures with HD. β_2-microglobulin amyloidosis may cause carpal tunnel syndrome, arthralgia, and fractures. *Acquired renal cystic disease* is seen in patients with long-standing CKD (>90% incidence if on dialysis >5 yrs), and there may be renal malignancy in 4–10%. *Malignancy* is more common in dialysis patients; some tumors are related to the cause of renal failure (e.g., urothelial tumors in analgesic nephropathy). *Aluminum toxicity* due to the use of aluminum-based phosphate binders is now rare (bone disease, dementia, anemia).

Renal transplantation

Table 8.6 Renal transplantation

This is the treatment of choice for ESRD. Each patient requires careful medical assessment and consideration of the advantages and disadvantages of dialysis vs transplantation.

Assessment *Note the following*: Preexisting cardiovascular disease; Screening for diseases that would cause severe disease while patient is immunocompromised and would require treatment or prophylaxis: CMV, VZV, EBV, HBV, Hep C, or TB. ABO blood group and human leukocyte antigen (HLA) tissue typing is required.

• Urological assessment is made, where indicated.

Contraindications Active infection; recently treated cancer (<2 yrs); severe vascular disease, pulmonary disease with FEV_1 <1, severe heart disease; HIV patients are being enrolled for transplantation.

Types of graft *Living related donor* (LRD) grafts offer the advantages of an optimally timed surgical procedure, HLA haplotype matching, and improved graft survival. *Living unrelated donation* is an option that is becoming commonplace. *Deceased donor allografts* are obtained from a brainstem-dead donor and should ideally be transplanted within 24–36 h. Grafts are inserted into an iliac fossa.

Immunosuppressants *Prednisone* + *tacrolimus/cyclosporine* (calcineurin inhibitors) + *mycophenolate mofetil/azathioprine (antiproliferative agents)*. Doses are slowly reduced over the first year. Common side effects with immunosuppressants (prednisone-hyperglycemia, osteoporosis; calcineurin inhibitors, HTN, hyperkalemia, nephrotoxicity; and antiproliferative agents, leukopenia, viral proliferation). *Others*: Sirolimus is an option for calcineurin inhibitor nephrotoxicity (CIN)(risk of pneumonitis, proteinuria, poor wound healing); anti-T-cell antibodies and antithymocyte globulin (polyclonal Ab)/OKT3 (monoclonal ABO, and anti-IL-2 Ab)are used for induction therapy or treatment of rejection.

Complications immediate postsurgery Bleeding thrombosis of renal vasculature, infection, urinary leaks, oliguria.

Later complications: Infections, rejection, malignancy, medication complications.

(Continued)

Table 8.6 (Continued)

Acute rejection (<3–6 months postop): This is characterized by rising serum creatinine ± fever and graft pain. Graft biopsy in acute cellular rejection shows an immune cell infiltrate and tubular damage. *Treatment:* IV high-dose corticosteroids for 3–5 d followed by PO. Cases with vascular component or resistant cases require antithymocyte globulin (ATG) (*SE:* Fevers, chills, anaphylaxis) or monoclonal OKT3 (*SE:* First-dose reaction, pulmonary edema, thrombotic microangiopathy, lymphoproliferative disease) antibody. *Antibody-mediated rejection:* Plasma cell infiltrate with + CD4 staining, plasmapheresis ± IVIG.

Chronic allograft nephropathy (>3 months): Presents with a gradual rise in serum creatinine and proteinuria. Graft biopsy shows vascular changes, glomerular changes, fibrosis, and tubular atrophy. It is not responsive to increased immunosuppression.

Calcineurin inhibitor nephrotoxicity: Afferent arteriole vasoconstriction causes reduced renal blood flow and GFR. There is also chronic tubular atrophy and fibrosis.

Infection: Typically common community infections or those related to ↓t-cell immunity (∵ immunosuppression); e.g., skin infections (fungi, warts, hsv, zoster) and opportunistic (TB, fungi, *P. jiroveci* pneumonia, CMV), others (BK virus).

Malignancy: Immunosuppression causes increased risk of neoplasia ± infection with viruses of malignant potential (EBV, HBV, HHV-8). Typical tumors are squamous cancers, lymphoma (EBV-related), and anogenital cancers.

Atheromatous vascular disease: This is more common in transplant patients than in the general population and is a leading cause of death.

HTN: This occurs in >50% of transplant patients and may be due to diseased native kidneys, immunosuppressive drugs, or dysfunction in the graft. Management is along standard lines (p. 132). Use of ACE-inhibitor/ARB is not contraindicated unless known renal artery stenosis of transplant kidney.

Diabetes: Estimated incidence 24% at 3 yrs post transplant. Corticosteroids and calcineurin inhibitors are factors.

Prognosis 1-yr graft survival: HLA identical 95%; 1 mismatch 90–95%; complete mismatch 75–80%. Average half-life of cadaveric grafts is 8 yrs; 20 yrs for HLA-identical living related donor grafts. Risk of neoplasia is elevated 5× from immunosuppression (e.g., skin cancers, lymphomas).

Interstitial nephritis and nephrotoxins

Interstitial nephritis is an important cause of both acute and chronic renal failure. *Acute interstitial nephritis (AIN):* Typical cause: Allergic reaction to antibiotics: Penicillins/cephalosporins, furosemide (sulfonamides), NSAIDs, allopurinol, rifampin; infection (staphylococci, streptococci, *Brucella*, *Leptospira*); systemic disease (sarcoidosis, Sjögren's syndrome); or no obvious cause. *Clinical features:* Fever, arthralgias, rash (especially if drug-related), eosinophilia, eosinophiluria, AKI or CKD, rarely an associated uveitis (tubulointerstitial nephritis uveitis syndrome or TINU). Except for AKI or CKD, other features may be absent. *Diagnosis:* Biopsy shows mononuclear cell infiltration of the renal interstitium and tubules with eosinophils in drug-induced causes.

Systemic features of fever, rash, and eosinophilia or eosinophiluria are rarely present with NSAIDs, + in ~33–50% of non–penicillin drug induced causes.

Treatment: AKI (p. 269); corticosteroids may be used with systemic disease, but use in drug-induced causes is controversial. Nevertheless, many nephrologists will attempt its use. CKD: None. *Prognosis:* Favorable in AIN if due to drug or systematic disease. *Chronic interstitial nephritis* may be a slowly evolving form of the acute disease or caused by analgesic nephropathy (below), sickle-cell disease, or chronic pyelonephritis/reflux nephropathy with secondary FSGS. NB: Urine may have few WBC/HPF since this has been chronic.

Analgesic nephropathy is associated with the prolonged, heavy ingestion of compound antipyretic analgesics. The incidence of analgesic nephropathy has fallen since the withdrawal of phenacetin. Use of acetaminophen has been associated, but controversial. *Signs:* Urinary abnormalities (proteinuria, hematuria, sterile pyuria); renal colic/obstruction from sloughed papilla; secondary UTI or pyelonephritis from obstruction; chronic kidney disease; HTN. *Diagnosis* is based on a history of excess analgesic use and demonstrating the characteristic renal lesion. *Tests:* CT scan reveals papillary calcifications, ↑ renal size, "bumpy" contours. IVP shows cortical scarring/clubbed calyces; demonstrates papillary necrosis. Biopsy shows chronic interstitial nephritis or capillary sclerosis. *Treatment:* Stop analgesics, antibiotics for infection, drainage for obstruction, dialysis or transplantation for ESRD.

Urate nephropathy *Acute crystal nephropathy* may occur when insoluble purines deposit within the tubules causing blockage or inflammation of the tubules. It is caused by gross uric acid overproduction (e.g., treatment of myeloid tumors) or by inherited diseases (e.g., Lesch–Nyhan syndrome). Diagnosis is by elevated serum uric acid levels of ~15–20 and urine uric acid/urine creatinine >1.

Treatment: Allopurinol, uricase (rasburicase) to ↓uric acid, good fluid intake, alkalinize urine, HD or CRRT if ↑uric acid levels and poor renal function (especially in cases of ongoing uric acid production; e.g., tumor lysis syndrome). *Chronic urate nephropathy* typically affects middle-aged men with gout. May be secondary to lead exposure. *Diagnosis:* X-ray fluorescence or ↑ urine lead levels after EDTA. Histologically, there is interstitial fibrosis with associated vascular changes; crystals are rarely found. *Treatment:* Allopurinol (↓dose in renal impairment); if lead nephropathy, can attempt EDTA to chelate lead with moderate CKD.

Hypercalcemic nephropathy is caused by malignancy (most common), hyperparathyroidism, multiple myeloma, sarcoidosis, vitamin D intoxication. *Clinical features:* Nephrogenic diabetes insipidus (polyuria, polydipsia, dehydration, uremia), symptoms of hypercalcemia (nausea, vomiting, constipation, lethargy, weakness, confusion, coma), pancreatitis. *Investigations:* Creatinine↑, Ca^{2+}↑ (1,25 OH vitamin D, intact PTH, PTH-related peptide, SPEP if clinical suspicion), proteinuria, hematuria, pyuria, hypercalciuria. AXR may show renal calculi/nephrocalcinosis. *Treatment:* IV fluids (3–6 L 0.9% saline/24 h); loop diuretics; IV bisphosphonates (p. 307). Steroids may be useful in sarcoidosis.

Radiation nephritis *Acute radiation nephritis* (within 1 yr of radiotherapy) *Signs:* Hematuria, proteinuria, BP↑, anemia. *Chronic radiation nephritis* may occur after acute radiation nephritis or present with HTN, proteinuria, anemia, or end-stage renal failure (ESRD 2–5 yrs after exposure to radiation). *Treatment:* Control BP, renal replacement therapy for ESRD. *Prevention:* Exclusion or shielding of renal areas during radiotherapy.

Nephrotoxins

Many agents may be toxic to the kidneys and cause ARF (see Table 8.7).

Table 8.7 Nephrotoxins

Exogenous nephrotoxins include:

- Analgesics: NSAIDs/cox-2 inhibitors
- Antimicrobials: *ATN*: Aminoglycosides, amphotericin, pentamidine. *AIN* (potentially all): Penicillins, cephalosporins, sulfonamides. *Tubular obstruction*: Acyclovir, indinavir. *RTA*: Proximal—tenofovir; distal—amphotericin; both—ifosfamide.
- Chemotherapeutic agents: Cisplatin. *ATN*: Mitomycin C-TTP. *Tubular obstruction*: Methotrexate.
- ACE-inhibitors and angiotensin II receptor antagonists (ARBs) may cause glomerular hemodynamic changes.
- Iodinated contrast agents: Especially in diabetic nephropathy, older patients: CKD, AKI (myeloma)
- Organic solvents: Ethylene glycol, hippurate (glue sniffing: Acidosis)
- Insecticides, herbicides, *Amanita* mushrooms, snake venom; all rare
- Immunosuppressants: Cyclosporine, tacrolimus

Endogenous nephrotoxins include:

- Pigments (myoglobin, hemoglobin)
- Crystal deposition/precipitation (urate, phosphate)
- Tumors (immunoglobulin light chains)

Aminoglycosides (e.g., gentamicin, amikacin) are well-recognized nephrotoxins. The typical clinical picture is of nonoliguric renal failure 1–2 wks into therapy. The risk of nephrotoxicity is increased in old age, lowered renal perfusion, preexisting CKD, high dosage or prolonged treatment, and coadministration of other nephrotoxic drugs. These circumstances are common in severely ill patients. Recovery may be full, delayed, or incomplete.

Myoglobin from muscle injury or necrosis (rhabdomyolysis). *Causes:* Trauma, ischemia, immobility, excessive exercise, seizures, myositis, metabolic ($K^+\downarrow$, $\uparrow$ phosphate), medications (fibrates, statins), toxins (alcohol, ecstasy, snake bite, carbon monoxide), malignant hyperpyrexia, neuroleptic malignant syndrome, inherited muscle disorders. *Clinical features:* These may be absent or nonspecific (muscle pain, swelling, or tenderness). *Tests:* Dark brown urine is +ve for blood on dipstick but without RBCs on microscopy. *Blood tests:* $\uparrow$BUN; $\uparrow$creatinine; $\uparrow K^+$; $\downarrow Ca^{2+}$; $\downarrow PO_4^{3-}$; $\uparrow$ck; $\uparrow$ldh; $\uparrow$urate. *Treatment:* Large volumes of IV fluids, urinary alkalinization with IV bicarbonate has been used. Hemodialysis/CRRT may be required.

Renal vascular diseases/secondary hypertension

HTN may be a cause or consequence of renal disease. *Essential HTN:* Investigations (p. 132). *Treatment* (p. 134). *Accelerated (malignant) HTN* may cause ARF. *Treatment* (p. 134). *Pregnancy-induced HTN with proteinuria (preeclampsia):* Edema + proteinuria ± glomerular endotheliosis/obliteration + deposition of fibrin and platelets. *May see:* Hemolysis, elevated liver enzymes, low platelet counts (HELLP). See Table 8.8.

Renal diseases causing HTN Diabetic nephropathy, acute glomerulonephritis, chronic interstitial nephritis, polycystic kidneys, CKD, renovascular disease, acute vasculitis, scleroderma renal crisis, hemolytic uremic syndrome (TTP; see below). As individuals progress to ESRD, even if no preexisting HTN, they will develop HTN. Also, as renal function declines, BP is more difficult to control, requiring increased number of agents.

Renovascular disease *Causes:* Atherosclerosis (65–75%, age >50 yrs, vascular disease); fibromuscular dysplasia (suspect in younger women), trauma, aortic dissection, or medium size vessel vasculitides (Takayasu's or polyarteritis nodosa [PAN]). *History: Atherosclerotic:* Coexistent cardiovascular, cerebrovascular, or peripheral vascular disease; deterioration in renal function after ACE-inhibitor/ARB, sudden ↑ in BP after stable baseline, HTN with asymmetric kidney sizes (>2 cm), severe HTN, recurrent unexplained flash pulmonary edema, proven onset later age (>50). *FMD:* Young onset, sudden-onset HTN in absence of other risk factors. *Examination:* Abdominal, carotid, or femoral bruits; absent leg pulses; grade III–IV hypertensive retinopathy. *Tests:* Renal angiography is gold standard. *Other tests:* Can be center dependent: MRA (avoid gadolinium if EGFR <30 mL/min), CT angiography, Doppler ultrasound are currently used for screening tests for atherosclerotic renal artery disease. These test are poor for detecting fibromuscular dysplasia. CT angiography requires a large amount of potentially nephrotoxic contrast dye. *Treatment:* Percutaneous transluminal renal angioplasty ± stent or renal bypass surgery. Risk of rupture or atheroembolic disease. Recommended for those with refractory disease. Results variable.

Thrombotic microangiopathy Previously thought of as spectrum between hemolytic uremic syndrome (HUS) and thrombotic thrombocytopenic purpura (TTP). *This is a hematologic emergency: Get expert help.*

Thrombotic thrombocytopenic purpura is a pentad of: (1) Fever, (2) fluctuating neurologic signs (microthrombi, e.g., causing seizures, ↓consciousness, ↓vision), (3) microangiopathic hemolytic anemia, (4) thrombocytopenia, (5) AKI. In TTP, there is decreased ADAMTS13 activity (inherited/Ab), leading to unusually large ↑ in von Willebrand factor (vWF) with ↑platelet clumping.

Hemolytic uremic syndrome is characterized by a microangiopathic hemolytic anemia, thrombocytopenia, and AKI. Platelet aggregates stimulated by endothelial damage, causing release of ultra-large multimers of vWF.

279

Thrombotic angiopathy other features: Purpura, GI or intracerebral bleeds, hematuria, proteinuria, BUN/CR ↑.

Causes of thrombotic microangiopathy: Idiopathic, medications (cyclosporine, tacrolimus, OKT3, mitomycin C, 5-fluorouracil, ticlopidine, clopidogrel, quinine, gemcitabine), malignancy (adenocarcinomas), SLE, HIV, pregnancy, bone marrow transplant. *Shigatoxin-associated HUS:* E. coli 0157; *Shigella dysenteriae; Streptococcus pneumoniae).* *Atypical HUS:* Complement factor mutations). *Tests:* Key test: Look at the peripheral smear (fragmented RBC-schistocytes) ↓Hb, ↓platelets, ↑reticulocytes), ↑creatinine, ↑bilirubin, ↑LDH, ↓haptoglobin, hematuria, proteinuria.

Treatment: Plasma exchange may be life-saving with fresh frozen plasma (FFP) for idiopathic TTP, pregnancy, autoimmune disorders, acute drug-induced (quinine, clopidogrel). Cancer-associated and post bone marrow transplant thrombotic microangiopathy is less likely to respond. Immunosuppressive treatment may be used in some cases (idiopathic, autoimmune-associated, adults with severe Shigatoxin-induced cases).

Prognosis: TTP may relapse (depends on underlying cause). Mortality is high, therefore immediate workup is key.

Cholesterol emboli *Suspect in any patient with diffuse atherosclerosis, recent arterial procedures or anticoagulation. Can be spontaneous if high atherosclerotic burden. Prevalence:* 0.3% in unselected autopsies. *Signs:* Livedo reticularis, distal gangrenous lesions, abdominal pain, Hollenhorst plaques in retinal vessels, *progressive* renal failure, eosinophilia, eosinophiluria, hypocomplementemia. Urinalysis may be bland. Cholesterol clefts seen in renal biopsies; they induce inflammation, ischemia, and then fibrosis. *Treatment:* No proven medical therapy; avoid anticoagulants and instrumentation, HMG-CoA reductase inhibitors. *Prognosis:* Often progressive and fatal. A few have regained renal function after dialysis.

Renal tubular disease (see Table 8.9)

Nephrogenic diabetes insipidus is characterized by renal insensitivity to vasopressin, decreased urinary concentration, polyuria, hypernatremia (if water access limited), and, potentially, CKD. It may be *primary* (familial X-linked) or *secondary* to a number of causes:

- Drugs (lithium, ifosfamide, cidofovir, foscarnet, Amphotericin, demeclocycline)
- Metabolic (hypercalcemia, hypokalemia)
- Tubulointerstitial disease (partial obstruction, renal amyloid, Sjögren's, sickle-cell disease)

Fanconi syndrome is a disturbance of proximal renal tubular function resulting in:

- Generalized aminoaciduria
- Phosphaturia
- Glycosuria
- Rickets (children) or osteomalacia (adults)
- Renal tubular acidosis type 2 (proximal); proximal tubular defect leads to inability to reclaim filtered bicarbonate

Inherited causes: Cystinosis, galactosemia, glycogen storage disease type 1, fructose intolerance, Lowe's syndrome, tyrosinemia type 1, Wilson's disease. Idiopathic.

Acquired causes: Myeloma, medications (ifosfamide, tenofovir).

Hereditary hypokalemic tubulopathies *Bartter's syndrome:* Sodium reabsorption defect in ascending limb with mutations in the Na–K–2Cl co-transporter (NKCC2) ROMK channel. (Behaves like a loop diuretic.) May have growth/mental retardation. *Gitelman syndrome:* Sodium reabsorption defect in distal convoluted tubule. *Cause:* Mutations in the distal tubular Na–Cl co-transporter gene (like a thiazide diuretic). Autosomal recessive. Diagnosed later in life, may be asymptomatic.

Table 8.9

Type	Type I Distal	Type II Proximal	Type IV
Characterization	Inability to generate acidic urine in distal nephron	Alone or with Fanconi's syndrome. Defect in H+ secretion, defective HCO_3 reabsorption in proximal tubule and loss of bicarb in urine	Hypoaldosteronism or failure of aldosterone metabolism; Mineralocorticoid deficiency→ increased H secretion in distal nephron resulting in NH_4 excretion
Cause	Sjogren's, amphotericin, SLE, RA, lithium, renal txplt, obstruction, sickle cell disease	Idiopathic, sporadic, multiple myeloma, carbonic anhydrase inhibitors, ifosfamide, tenofovir, heavy metals, renal transplant	Addison's; inborn error of metabolism; DM, chronic interstitial disease; drugs (NSAIDs, K sparing diuretics, ACEi); mineralocorticoid deficiency
Sign	Hyperventilation, low K, nephrocalcinosis	Polyuria, polydipsia, proximal myopathy, osteomalacia, rickets, rare stones and nephrocalcinosis	Hyperkalemia
Diagnosis	Urinary ph>5.3, hyperchloremic metabolic acidosis; hypercalciuria	Hypokalemic Hyperchloremic metabolic acidosis Acidic urine	Urinary ph <5, hyperkalemia hyperchloremic metabolic acidosis
Treatment	Correct hypokalemia; Oral bicarb (1–2 meq/kg/d)	High doses of bicarbonate replacement 3 meq/kg/day	Florinef if acidotic or hyperkalemia

Both are associated with hypokalemia and metabolic alkalosis, hypercalciuria with Bartter's and hypocalciuria with Gitelman's.

Inherited kidney diseases

Autosomal dominant polycystic kidney disease (APKD) *Prevalence:* 1:1,000. *Inheritance:* Autosomal dominant. Genes on chromosomes 16 (PKD1) (accounts for 85%) and 4 (PKD2). *Signs:* Renal enlargement with cysts, abdominal pain, hematuria, UTI, renal calculi, BP↑, CKD. *Extrarenal:* Liver cysts, intracranial aneurysms, subarachnoid hemorrhage, mitral valve prolapse, abdominal hernias. *Diagnosis:* Ultrasound criteria: Between age 15–30, two unilateral or bilateral cysts; age 30–59, two cysts per kidney; >60, four cysts per kidney. *Treatment:* Monitor U&E and BP; treating ↑BP is most important. Treat infections; dialysis or transplantation for ESRD; genetic counseling. *Screening* for intracranial aneurysms: *mra without gadolinium,* if positive family history of aneurysms.

Infantile polycystic kidney disease Prevalence 1:40,000. Autosomal recessive (chromosome 6). *Signs:* Renal cysts; congenital hepatic fibrosis.

Nephronophthisis An inherited medullary cystic disease. The juvenile form (autosomal recessive) accounts for 10–20% of ESRD in children. *Signs:* Polyuria, polydipsia, enuresis, renal impairment, metabolic acidosis, anemia, growth retardation, ESRD. *Extrarenal signs:* Retinal degeneration, retinitis pigmentosa, skeletal changes, cerebellar ataxia, liver fibrosis. The adult form (autosomal dominant; restricted to the kidney) is rare.

Renal phakomatoses *Tuberous sclerosis:* Complex disorder with hamartoma formation in skin, brain, eye, kidney, and heart caused by autosomal dominant genes on chromosomes 9 (TSC1) and 16 (TSC2). *Signs:* Skin: Adenoma sebaceum, angiofibromas, "ash leaf" hypomelanic macules, sacral plaques of shark-like skin (shagreen patch), periungual fibromas; IQ↓; seizures. *von Hippel-Lindau syndrome* is the chief cause of inherited renal cancers. *Cause:* Germline mutations of the VHL tumor-suppressor gene (also inactivated in most sporadic renal cell cancers).

282

Anderson–Fabry disease is X-linked recessive; intralysosomal deposits of trihexoside causing burning pain/paresthesia in the extremities and angiokeratoma corporis diffusum (blue-black telangiectasia in bathing trunk distribution).

Hyperoxaluria *Primary hyperoxaluria* is due to an autosomal recessive inherited enzyme defect (types I and II). Measure 24 h urinary oxalate excretion and creatinine clearance (excretion ↓ in renal failure) for unexplained recurrent calcium oxalate stones. *Secondary hyperoxaluria* is due to small intestine disease/resection, ↓calcium intake, ↑↑oxalate intake (diet, ethylene glycol poisoning), pyridoxine deficiency. *Signs:* Oxalate stones, nephrocalcinosis, renal failure, cardiac conduction defects, cardiomyopathy, subcutaneous calcinosis, peripheral neuropathy, mononeuritis multiplex, retinal changes, synovitis, osteodystrophy. *Treatment:* High fluid intake, restrict dietary oxalate (tea, chocolate, strawberries, rhubarb, beans, celery, nuts), pyridoxine (↓urinary oxalate excretion), hepatic ± renal transplantation.

Cystinuria is the commonest aminoaciduria. *Clinical features:* Cystine stones, abdominal pain, hematuria, renal obstruction, UTI. *Treatment:* ↑Fluid intake, $NaHCO_3^-$ supplements (alkalinizes urine), penicillamine tiopronin (↓cystine excretion).

Renal manifestations of systemic disease

Amyloidosis AL (primary) or AA (secondary) Proteinuria, nephrotic syndrome, progressive renal failure, renal tubular dysfunction. *Diagnosis* (p. 635): For secondary amyloidosis, treat underlying cause (e.g., rheumatoid arthritis).

Diabetes 30–40% of patients on dialysis have diabetic nephropathy. *Pathology:* Nodular capillary glomerulosclerosis (Kimmelstiel–Wilson lesion). Early on, there is renal hyperperfusion associated with ↑GFR and ↑renal size. *Microalbuminuria* (albumin excretion 30–300 mg/d or 30–300 mg/g Cr) occurs 5–15 yrs postdiagnosis and is associated with a normal GFR and a normal but rising BP.

Type 1 DM nephropathy occurs 10–15 yrs postdiagnosis and is characterized by macroalbuminuria (albumin excretion >300 mg/d or 30–300 mg/g Cr), ↓GFR, and ↑BP. *Renal failure* occurs 15–30 yrs postdiagnosis (rare after 30 yrs); there may be nephrotic-range proteinuria (>3 g/d).

Type 2 DM ("maturity onset") nephropathy (see p. 280): >10–30% have nephropathy at diagnosis, and its prevalence rises linearly with time.

Treatment: Good glycemic control delays onset and progression of microalbuminuria but has little effect on established proteinuria. Reducing BP reduces microalbuminuria and attenuates loss of GFR. ACE-inhibitors ± ARBs reduce microalbuminuria and slow progression to CKD, even if normotensive.

Infection-associated nephropathies are common causes of renal disease. Infection-related GNs are characterized by proteinuria/hematuria are associated with endocarditis, bacteremia, shunt nephritis. *Other associated glomerular diseases:* Hepatitis C-membranoproliferative GN; hepatitis B/–syphilis-membranous; HIV/parvovirus-collapsing FSGS.

Vasculitis (p. 416) occurs with HBV, post-streptococcal, staphylococcal, or streptococcal septicemia.

Interstitial nephritis is seen with *E. coli, Staphylococcus aureus, Proteus*, leptospirosis, hantavirus, and schistosomal infections.

Malignancy *Direct effects:* Renal infiltration (leukemia, lymphoma), obstruction (pelvic tumors), metastases. *Indirect:* Hypercalcemia, nephrotic syndrome(membranous nephropathy- solid tumors, minimal change disease-hematologic malignancies), AKI, amyloidosis, glomerulonephritis. *Treatment-associated:* Nephrotoxic drugs, tumor lysis syndrome, radiation nephritis.

Multiple myeloma is characterized by excess production of monoclonal antibody and/or light chains. Bence Jones proteinuria is common. Myeloma kidney is characterized by accumulation of distal nephron casts. Light-chain nephropathy is caused by direct toxic effects of light chains on nephrons. *Clinical features:* AKI, CKD, amyloidosis, nephrotic syndrome, tubular dysfunction, hypercalcemic nephropathy. *Treatment:* Treat AKI (p. 269) and hypercalcemia (p. 675); chemotherapy, dialysis.

Rheumatological diseases *Rheumatoid arthritis (RA) tends to have renal complications as result of medications or long-standing inflammation.* NSAIDs may cause ↓GFR or interstitial nephritis. Penicillamine and gold may induce membranous nephropathy. Tumor necrosis factor (TNF)-α agents may induce crescentic GN. Methotrexate- interstitial disease. Secondary amyloidosis occurs in 15% of RA patients. *SLE* involves the kidney in 40–60% of adults. *Clinical features:* Proteinuria, hematuria, ↑BP, renal impairment, ARF. Lupus nephritis shows a wide variety of histological patterns (p. 264). *Treatment:* Corticosteroids; immunosuppressive meds (cyclophosphamide/ mycophenolate mofetil). *Systemic sclerosis* (p. 412) involves the kidney in 30% of patients. *Clinical features:* Proteinuria, hematuria, ↑BP, renal impairment, "scleroderma crisis" (AKI + malignant HTN) *Treatment:* Control BP (ACE inhibitors); dialysis; transplantation.

Hyperparathyroidism *Nephrocalcinosis:* Deposition of calcium in the renal medulla (seen on plain x-ray). *Renal stones* from associated hypercalciuria.

Sarcoidosis may involve the kidney in a number of ways. *Abnormal Ca2+ metabolism* may cause hypercalciuria, nephrocalcinosis, or nephrolithiasis. *Interstitial nephritis* may present with CKD or AKI. *Glomerular involvement* usually presents with the nephrotic syndrome and is due to membranous glomerulonephritis, other glomerulopathies, or amyloidosis.

Endocrinology

Kendall F. Moseley, M.D.

Contents

The essence of endocrinology

See Table 9.1.

Table 9.1 The essence of endocrinology

- Involves the study of hormones, the many glands that secrete them, and the multiple functions of these hormones on target tissues.
- Endocrine glands include the pancreas, thyroid, parathyroids, adrenals, pituitary and gonads; kidney, bone, and adipose tissue also have endocrine functions.
- Clinical syndromes and endocrine diseases result from deficiencies of hormones (*hypo-* syndromes) and corresponding clinical syndromes associated excessive amounts of hormones (*hyper-* syndromes).
- Primary endocrine disease involves dysfunction of the endocrine gland itself (i.e., primary hypothyroidism = overactive/underactive thyroid gland); central (or secondary) endocrine disease involves dysfunction of the hypothalamus/pituitary with resultant inappropriate signaling to the target endocrine gland (i.e., Cushing's disease).
- Endocrine diseases are identified and diagnosed by measuring levels of hormones or metabolites of hormones in blood or urine samples at the appropriate time of day.
- Measurement of stimulating hormones secreted by the pituitary may be used to distinguish primary from central (secondary) disease (i.e., thyroid-stimulating hormone (TSH) to diagnose primary hypothyroidism and hyperthyroidism; adrenocorticotropic hormone (ACTH) to distinguish between primary and central (secondary) adrenal insufficiency).
- To confirm suspected deficiency of a hormone, administer an agent that stimulates secretion of that hormone before drawing samples for measurement.
- To confirm suspected secretion of excessive amounts of a hormone, administer an agent that suppresses secretion of that hormone before drawing samples for measurement.
- Use radiographic studies to evaluate the anatomic structure and physiologic function of specific endocrine glands only after gland dysfunction has been confirmed by biochemical testing.
- Treat conditions associated with deficiencies of hormones by administering (a) pharmacologic preparations of hormone and hormone analogs, or (b) agents that stimulate secretion of hormones from functional tissue.
- Treat conditions associated with secretion of excessive amounts of hormones by (a) surgically resecting hyperfunctioning tissue, (b) administering agents that target and destroy hyperfunctioning tissue, or (c) administering agents that suppress secretion of hormones from hyperfunctioning tissue.

Type 1 diabetes mellitus

Definition Clinical disease caused by autoimmune destruction of pancreatic islet cells required for secretion of endogenous insulin. Type 1 diabetes mellitus (T1DM) is a disease of insulin deficiency. T1DM usually presents during childhood or adolescence, but may occur at any age (see latent autoimmune diabetes in adulthood [LADA], below). Patients require lifelong treatment with insulin and are prone to developing extreme fluctuations in blood glucose levels (hypoglycemia and hyperglycemia with ketoacidosis). May be associated with specific HLA types (DR3 and DR4) and other autoimmune disorders. Anti-glutamic acid decarboxylase antibodies (anti-GAD) and anti-islet cell antibodies may be detectable at the time of diagnosis and confirm T1DM, if present. Antibody levels may be too low to detect in later-stage T1DM; their absence does not rule out disease. Concordance is >30% in identical twins.

Presentation Usually acute, with ketoacidosis characterized by progressive polyuria, polydipsia, weight loss, fatigue, lethargy, hyperventilation, and a distinctive odor of acetone on the breath. Subacute cases may present with more protracted courses of variable polyuria, polydipsia, and weight loss with associated lethargy and frequent infection(vaginal candidiasis, furunculosis). In adults who present with these symptoms and hyperglycemia, LADA should be suspected. Adults with LADA have T1DM and should be treated, as below. Early in the course of treatment, patients may experience a transient "honeymoon phase" characterized by improved control with reduced daily insulin requirements. Destruction of islet cells will resume and will be permanent.

Diagnosis A suspected diagnosis may be confirmed on the basis of (1) hemoglobin A1c (HbA1c) >6.5% in a certified laboratory, (2) a random plasma glucose >200 mg/dL with associated symptoms (polyuria, polydipsia, weight loss), (3) a fasting plasma glucose >126 mg/dL, or (4) a 75 g oral glucose tolerance test with a 2 h plasma glucose >200 mg/dL.[1] Positive results from tests 2–4 should be verified with repeat testing.

Treatment Insulin, administered as multiple daily injections or through a pump delivering a continuous subcutaneous infusion. Oral medications are not effective in T1DM. Insulin doses should be timed to reproduce normal patterns of basal and postprandial insulin secretion. Monitoring requires frequent self-measurement of blood glucose levels throughout the day (fasting and mealtimes). Intensive control targeting normoglycemic preprandial and postprandial blood glucose levels reduces the risk of developing microvascular complications (described below), but may be associated with more frequent episodes of hypoglycemia. Continuous glucose monitoring (CGM) devices may be helpful in patients with extreme fluctuations in blood glucose ("brittle diabetes"), frequent or dangerous hypoglycemia, or to optimize insulin regimen. See Table 9.2.

Clinical guidelines recommend intensifying treatment to target HbA1c levels <7% to minimize diabetic complications. Aggressive glucose control (HbA1c <6%) is not recommended and may be associated with increased mortality. Note that HbA1c levels reflect average blood glucose control over the course of the previous 8–12 wks. See Table 9.3.

1 American Diabetic Association. American Diabetic Association Clinical Practice Recommendations. *Diabetes Care.* January 2011; 34 (suppl 1).

Table 9.2 Insulin

Available in 100 U/mL preparations. May be drawn up and injected using special syringes (marked in units) or directly injected from preloaded adjustable pen injectors. Five major types available for use.

Rapid-acting insulin analogs *Insulin lispro* (Humalog®), *insulin aspart* (NovoLog®), modified to promote rapid absorption, must be injected immediately before or after eating to cover prandial spike in glucose levels. Dosing schedule: With meals.

Short-acting insulin *Regular insulin*, must be injected 15–30 min before eating. Less commonly prescribed given challenges with timing of insulin and onset of insulin action.

Intermediate-acting insulin (*NPH insulin*), peak effect at 4–10 h, effective duration is 10–16 h. Dosing schedule: Twice daily.

Long-acting insulin analogs *Insulin glargine* (Lantus®), *insulin detemir* (Levemir), modified to promote steady absorption and continuous coverage of glucose levels without peaks. May not be mixed with other types of insulin or insulin analogs. Dosing schedule: Once daily (morning or night), although consider twice-daily dosing for total insulin >40 units to ensure absorption of full dose.

High concentration insulin analogs should only be used in cases of extreme insulin resistance. Humulin R U-500 is only available as a regular form of insulin. Peak effect 2–4 h after administration, duration of action 5–7 h. Should only be prescribed by a diabetologist.

Premixed preparations combine intermediate-acting insulin with short-acting insulin or rapid-acting insulin analogs in specified fractions (i.e., 70/30 NPH insulin/regular insulin, 75/25 NPH/insulin lispro). May be used to minimize daily injections.

Table 9.3 Insulin regimens used to treat type 1 diabetes

General Ideal insulin administration consists of "basal" coverage for 24 h management of blood glucose and "bolus" or "prandial" coverage to manage blood glucose spikes during meals. Persons with T1DM require exogenous insulin at all times given insulin deficiency and risk of diabetic ketoacidosis (DKA).

Continuous insulin administration Available through insulin pumps dosed for time of day, meal intake, and correction of elevated blood glucose levels. Insulin cartridges filled with rapid-acting insulin analogs.

Two daily injections Comprised of (1) intermediate-acting insulin mixed with a rapid-acting insulin analog (or short-acting insulin) before breakfast; and (2) intermediate-acting insulin mixed with a rapid-acting insulin analog (or short-acting insulin) before dinner. Often started by administering two-thirds of the estimated daily dose before breakfast and one-third before dinner.

Three daily injections Comprised of (1) intermediate-acting insulin mixed with a rapid-acting insulin analog (or short-acting insulin) before breakfast; (2) a rapid-acting insulin analog (or short-acting insulin) before dinner; and (3) intermediate-acting insulin at bedtime. May reduce the frequency and severity of overnight hypoglycemia.

Four daily injections Comprised of (1–3) a rapid-acting insulin analog (or short-acting insulin) before breakfast, lunch, and dinner; and (4) a long-acting insulin analog at bedtime.

Prandial doses of rapid-acting insulin analogs may be administered as fixed doses or may be adjusted to account for (a) estimated grams of carbohydrate to be eaten or (b) sliding scale correction formulas based on preprandial blood glucose levels.

(Continued)

Table 9.3 *(Continued)*

Intercurrent illnesses may increase daily insulin requirements despite diminished appetite and reduced caloric intake. During the course of any moderate to severe illness, patients should be instructed to (a) maintain caloric intake, (b) drink large volumes of fluids, (c) check blood glucose levels at least four times daily, and (d) check for urine ketones with home dipstick tests if blood glucose levels are noted to be persistently elevated. Insulin doses may need to be transiently increased to prevent the onset of hyperglycemia, volume depletion, and ketoacidosis.

Type 2 diabetes mellitus

Definition Clinical syndrome characterized by insulin resistance leading to endogenous hyperinsulinemia with eventual β-cell failure and relative insulin deficiency. Over time, the combined effects of insulin resistance and inadequate insulin secretion lead to persistent hyperglycemia. Strongly associated with obesity, physical inactivity, and positive family history. Higher prevalence among certain ethnic groups including African Americans, Latinos, Native Americans, Asian Americans, and Pacific Islanders. Although once considered a disease of adults, incidence of confirmed diagnoses of type 2 diabetes mellitus (T2DM) in children and adolescents is increasing with the obesity epidemic. Concordance is >80% in identical twins.

Presentation Highly variable. At one end of the spectrum, patients may present with mild asymptomatic hyperglycemia identified on routine laboratory testing. At the other extreme, patients with unsuspected and untreated disease may present in advanced, decompensated, hyperosmolar states. Known as the hyperosmolar hyperglycemic state (HHS), it is characterized by severe hyperglycemia, volume depletion, and mental status changes.

Metabolic syndrome is defined by high-density lipoprotein (HDL) cholesterol <40 mg/dL (men) or <50 mg/dL (women), waist circumference >102 cm (men) or >88 cm (women), blood pressure (BP) >130/85 mmHg or active treatment for hypertension, and fasting plasma glucose >100 mg/dL or active drug treatment for elevated blood glucose. Persons with any three of the five criteria have metabolic syndrome. There is a strong link between the metabolic syndrome and subsequent risk of developing T2DM.

Diagnosis Suspected diagnosis.[2] may be confirmed on the basis of (1) HbA1c >6.5% in a certified laboratory, (2) a random plasma glucose >200 mg/dL with associated symptoms (polyuria, polydipsia, weight loss), (3) a fasting plasma glucose >126 mg/dL, or (4) a 75 g oral glucose tolerance test with a 2 h plasma glucose >200 mg/dL. Positive results should be verified with repeat testing. "Pre-diabetes" may be diagnosed when testing reveals (a) HbA1c 5.7–6.4%, (b) a fasting plasma of 100–125 mg/dL glucose (impaired fasting glucose, IFG), or (c) a 2 h plasma glucose of 140–199 mg/dL (impaired glucose tolerance, IGT). There is growing evidence that treatment of prediabetes with lifestyle modification and/or pharmacologic therapy may delay or prevent the progression of disease and end-organ damage.

Testing in asymptomatic patients Should be considered in all overweight adults (body mass index [BMI] >25 kg/m^2) and who have one or more additional risk factors for diabetes (metabolic syndrome, above). Without risk factors, screen adults >45 yrs.

Treatment Must be tailored to the state of disease and severity of hyperglycemia at the time of presentation. See Table 9.4.

Lifestyle modification All patients, regardless of stage of T2DM should be extensively counseled modify both diet and lifestyle. Weight loss (7% body weight) and exercise (150 min/wk moderate exercise) can restore insulin tolerance. Asymptomatic patients with mild or intermittent hyperglycemia may be managed with comprehensive exercise and nutrition therapy targeted to limit glycemic excursions. All patients should receive smoking cessation counseling, if appropriate.

Prediabetes (HbA1c 5.7–6.4%, IFG, IGT) Target weight loss of 7% of body weight, physical activity at least 150 min/wk moderate activity. Consider metformin therapy (see below) in those at high risk for developing diabetes (i.e., HbA1c >6%). Patients with persistent hyperglycemia may need to be started on treatment with oral agents or insulin. Oral agents are preferred as first-line therapy for those with earlier stage T2DM (HbA1c <9%). Oral medications may be used in different combinations to optimize glycemic control. Certain oral agents may be contraindicated in patients with impaired renal or hepatic function. In some cases, patients presenting with severe hyperglycemia ("glucotoxic") initially requiring insulin may be successfully transitioned to oral agents as glucose toxicity subsides and β-cell function is restored.

Pharmacotherapy, insulin In time, most patients who are initially maintained on regimens of oral agents alone eventually require the addition of insulin. Patients presenting with later stage T2DM (HbA1c >9%) often require insulin from the outset. With the exception of metformin (see below), most other oral agents should be discontinued with insulin initiation. Monitoring of blood glucose requires frequent self-measurement. Recommended frequency may vary depending on intensity of treatment and frequency of changes to the regimen. Clinical guidelines recommend intensifying treatment to target HbA1c levels <7%. This may be difficult to achieve in practice. See Table 9.5.

Bariatric surgery May be considered for adults with BMI >35 kg/m^2 and T2DM, particularly with disease that is hard to control with lifestyle interventions and medications or in those with diabetic complications.

Lipid management Measure annual fasting lipid profile. Diet and lifestyle modifications should be implemented for all patients with diabetes. Add statin therapy regardless of lipid panel for (a) diabetic patients with known cardiovascular disease (CVD), (b) patients >40 without CVD but with CVD risk factors (men >50, women >60 and family history, hypertension, dyslipidemia, smoking, or albuminuria). Goal low-density lipoprotein (LDL) is <70 mg/dL if known CVD. In individuals of any age and at low risk for CVD with diabetes, if LDL >100 mg/dL, add statin therapy. Combination therapy with other lipid-lowering agents may be necessary if high-dose statins do not achieve goals.

Antiplatelet agents Consider aspirin therapy (75–162 mg/d) in patients with T1DM or T2DM at increased CVD risk (men >50, women >60 + one additional CVD risk factor = family history, hypertension, dyslipidemia, smoking, albuminuria).

Table 9.4 Noninsulin agents

Eight major classes. Should not be used in T1DM therapy.

Sulfonylureas Stimulate insulin secretion. Effective in patients with early T2DM given medication's dependence on functional β cells. Commonly prescribed preparations include *glipizide* (Glucotrol® 2.5–20 mg/d–bid, Glucotrol XL® 5–10 mg/d), *glyburide* (DiaBeta®, Micronase® 1.25–20 mg/d, Glynase® 0.75–12 mg/d), and *glimepiride* (Amaryl® 1–4 mg/d). Often used in combination with biguanides and thiazolidinediones. Glimepiride may be associated with a lower incidence of hypoglycemia. Preparations are available that combine metformin with glyburide (Glucovance®) and glipizide (Metaglip®). *side effects (SE):* Hypoglycemia, weight gain, increased risk of CV morality. *Contraindications (CI):* DKA, NPO status.

Biguanides Suppress hepatic gluconeogenesis. May help to increase insulin sensitivity in peripheral tissues. *Metformin* is the only biguanide available for use in the United States. Available in regular and long-acting preparations (Glucophage® 500–1,000 mg bid, Glucophage XR® 1,000–2,000 mg qpm). Usually started at a low dose with meals and titrated upward every 2 weeks to maximum dose (2,000 mg/d) to prevent side effects. *Self-limited side effects:* May include nausea, abdominal cramping, and diarrhea. May help to promote weight loss. *CI:* Creatinine >1.5 mg/dL (men), >1.4 mg/dL (women), metabolic acidosis including DKA. Must be held for 4–8 h prior to and following exposure to IV contrast.

Thiazolidinediones PPAR γ-gamma receptor agonists. Increase insulin sensitivity. Available preparations include *rosiglitazone* (Avandia® 4–8 mg/d) and *pioglitazone* (Actos® 15–45 mg/d). May take 3–6 wks to see full effect. *SE:* Transaminase levels should be monitored regularly. May cause weight gain and lower extremity swelling. Rosiglitazone is associated with increased risk of cardiovascular and ischemic events. All thiazolidinediones are associated with bone loss and should be used with caution in patients with osteoporosis. *CI:* Patients with congestive heart failure (New York Heart Association [NYHA] Class III or IV) or impaired hepatic function.

Incretin mimetics GLP-1 agonists available only in SQ injectable form. *Exenatide* (Byetta® 5–10 mcg SQ bid) or *liraglutide* (Victoza® 0.6–1.8 mg/d SQ) should be considered as add-on drugs in T2DM not controlled on 1–2 oral agents. Should not be used as monotherapy. May promote weight loss. Side effects include diarrhea, indigestion, nausea. Reports of pancreatitis. *CI:* Pancreatitis, DKA.

DPP-IV inhibitors Can be used alone or in combination with other oral agents. Can be used in chronic kidney disease, but must be dose-adjusted. *Sitagliptin* (Januvia® 100 mg/d PO) or *saxagliptin* (Onglyza® 2.5–5 mg/d PO). Caution with hepatic disease and history of pancreatitis. *SE:* Headache, nasopharyngitis, URI. *CI:* DKA.

Meglitinides Rapid-acting insulin secretagogues. Must be taken right before meals. May help to control postprandial hyperglycemia. Available preparations include *repaglinide* (Prandin® 0.5–4 mg qac) and *nateglinide* (Starlix® 60–120 mg qac). *SE:* Hypoglycemia, diarrhea, nausea. *CI:* DKA.

α-Glucosidase inhibitors Limit glycemic excursions by inhibiting enzymatic breakdown of carbohydrates. Must be taken with meals. Available preparations include *acarbose* (Precose® 25–100 mg qac) and *miglitol* (Glyset® 25–100 mg qac). *SE:* Bloating and diarrhea. *CI:* Should not be used in patients with inflammatory bowel disease, cirrhosis, DKA, or bowel obstruction.

Amylin analog Available only as SQ injection. *Pramlintide* (Symlin® 60–120 mcg SQ immediately after meals). Side effects include abdominal pain, nausea, vomiting. *CI:* Gastroparesis, hypoglycemia.

Table 9.5 Insulin regimens used to treat type 2 diabetes

General In long-standing T2DM, ideal insulin administration consists of "basal" coverage for 24 h management of blood glucose and "bolus" or "prandial" coverage to manage blood glucose spikes during meals. Additional, sliding-scale insulin may be administered with scheduled prandial doses if premeal blood glucose levels are elevated. Less aggressive management with fewer injections may be possible in early disease when pancreas has some endogenous function. Unlike T1DM, persons with T2DM do not necessarily require exogenous insulin at all times.

Continuous insulin administration Available through insulin pumps dosed for time of day, meal intake, and correction of elevated blood glucose levels. Insulin cartridges filled with rapid-acting insulin analogs.

One daily injection May be added to supplement standing regimens of oral agents. Usually started as a fixed dose of (a) intermediate-acting insulin at bedtime and (b) a long-acting insulin analog at bedtime or before breakfast.

Two daily injections May allow for greater flexibility in making adjustments to accommodate variations in blood glucose levels. Doses administered before breakfast and before dinner may be comprised of (a) intermediate-acting insulin, (b) intermediate-acting insulin mixed with a rapid-acting insulin analog (or short-acting insulin), or (c) premixed preparations combining intermediate-acting insulin with short-acting insulin or rapid-acting insulin analogs.

Multiple daily injection regimens similar to those used to treat patients with T1DM may also be employed to target more intensive control. Total daily insulin requirements tend to be much higher in patients with T2DM. Some patients may require >100 U/d to achieve and maintain adequate glycemic control. Patients with extreme insulin resistance requiring extremely high doses of insulin may benefit from U-500 insulin. This should be prescribed by a diabetologist.

Diabetic retinopathy

Microvascular complication of T1DM and T2DM secondary to changes in retinal blood vessels caused by prolonged exposure to elevated blood glucose levels. Affects most patients with T1DM, although manifestations are usually not detectable until 5 yrs after initial diagnosis. May be detectable in up to 25% of patients with T2DM diabetes at time of presentation. Diabetes is the leading preventable cause of blindness in adults 20–74 yrs of age. See Table 9.6.

Evaluation Individuals with diabetes require yearly retinal exams. They should be performed by an experienced provider. Comprehensive evaluation requires pupillary dilation, slit-lamp examination, and indirect ophthalmoscopy. Examinations limited to direct ophthalmoscopy often miss key findings. Individuals with T1DM should be referred for evaluation within 3–5 yrs of initial diagnosis and yearly thereafter. Individuals with T2DM should be referred at the time of presentation and yearly thereafter. Pregnancy may increase the risk of development or progression of diabetic retinopathy. Comprehensive evaluation should be performed prior to conception and during the first trimester.

Prevention and treatment Intensive control of blood glucose levels may delay the onset or progression of diabetic retinopathy. Adjunctive treatment should target aggressive control of hypertension and hyperlipidemia.

Table 9.6 Stages of diabetic retinopathy

Preretinopathy Subtle dilation of the retinal veins.

Nonproliferative retinopathy Also known as background retinopathy. Weakened areas of retinal capillary walls form outpouchings that may be visible as microaneurysms. Bleeding from these weakened areas in the superficial layer of the retina may produce flame-shaped hemorrhages. Bleeding in deeper layers may produce dot-blot hemorrhages. Leakage of plasma from retinal capillary may lead to formation of yellowish hard exudates. If leakage occurs near the macula, it may lead to swelling identifiable as macular edema.

Preproliferative retinopathy Closure of retinal capillaries leads to focal hypoxia visible as poorly defined soft exudates or cotton wool spots. Retinal veins develop irregular contours.

Proliferative retinopathy Neovascularization with growth of vessels into the vitreous humor. New vessels are weak and prone to rupture. Vitreous hemorrhages may obscure vision. Reabsorption of blood may lead to scarring and traction that may cause retinal detachment. Growth of vessels into the anterior chamber may cause a painful increase in intraocular pressure.

Laser photocoagulation treatment may help arrest identified proliferative retinopathy and macular edema. Symptoms or signs concerning for vitreous hemorrhage, retinal detachment, or changes in intraocular pressure should prompt urgent referral.

Other complications Elevated glucose levels in the aqueous humor may draw fluid out of the lens causing increased stiffness and myopia. Changes are reversible with improved blood glucose control. Patients with diabetes are more prone to develop cataracts.

Diabetic nephropathy

Microvascular complication that develops as a result of changes in glomerular function secondary to prolonged exposure to elevated blood glucose levels. Nephropathy risk is similar in patients with T1DM and T2DM. Diabetes is the cause of almost 50% of cases of end-stage renal disease requiring renal replacement with dialysis or transplantation. Progression may be exacerbated by concomitant hypertension or preexisting renal disease. See Table 9.7.

Table 9.7 Stages of diabetic nephropathy

Stage I Marked by onset of diabetes. Characterized by 30–40% increase in glomerular filtration rate (GFR) with bilateral enlargement of kidneys.

Stage II Normal urinary excretion of albumin (<30 mg/24 h).

Stage III Incipient diabetic nephropathy. Microalbuminuria with urinary excretion of 30–300 mg albumin/24 h.~20% of patients with T1DM who reach this stage will progress to end-stage renal disease within 10 yrs.

Stage IV Overt diabetic nephropathy. Proteinuria with urinary excretion of >0.5 g protein/24 h. Corresponds to urinary excretion of >300 mg albumin/24 h. Protein usually detectable on urine dipstick testing. Marks beginning of progressive decline in GFR.

Stage V End-stage renal disease.

Detection Initial evaluation with quantification of urinary excretion of albumin. This can be assessed by measuring the albumin/creatinine ratio in a random urine specimen ("spot urine microalbumin"). An albumin/creatinine ratio >30 mcg/mg has been proven to be a sensitive and specific predictor of microalbuminuria. Results that are consistent with microalbuminuria or proteinuria should be confirmed on repeat testing within 3 months. Measure serum creatinine at least annually in all adults with diabetes to estimate GFR.

Treatment of hypertensive patients In patients with concomitant hypertension, aggressive control of BP may help to forestall the progressive decline in renal function. Clinical guidelines recommend targeting systolic BPs <130 mm Hg and diastolic BPs <80 mm Hg. Whenever possible, an angiotensin-converting enzyme (ACE)-inhibitor or angiotensin receptor blocker (ARB) should be selected as a first-line antihypertensive agent. ACE-inhibitors and ARBs have been proven to effectively reduce urinary protein excretion in patients with T1DM and T2DM. Persistent cough may be a limiting side effect of ACE-inhibitors. Both agents may precipitate (a) hyperkalemia, which may be particularly severe in patients with hyporeninemic hypoaldosteronism and (b) acute kidney injury in patients with renal artery stenosis. Serum potassium and creatinine levels should be checked 2–3 wks after starting treatment. Additional antihypertensive agents may need to be added in a stepwise fashion to achieve target levels of BP control. Thiazide diuretics may provide an additive effect in patients with preserved renal function (GFR >50 mL/min). A range of different preparations combining ACE-inhibitors and ARBs with thiazide diuretics in varying doses are available. Other classes of agents may be used as well, although attention should be paid to potential complicating side effects (β-blockers may impair recognition of hypoglycemia; α-blockers and centrally acting agents may exacerbate orthostatic hypotension).

Treatment of normotensive patients In patients with T1DM, confirmed microalbuminuria, and normal BP, treatment with an ACE-inhibitor or ARB may delay the onset of proteinuria marking a progression to overt diabetic nephropathy. Similar benefits may accrue in patients with T2DM.

Diabetic neuropathy

Complication that develops as a result of irreversible damage to nerve fibers secondary to prolonged exposure to elevated blood glucose levels. Classification schemes differentiate between peripheral neuropathy and autonomic neuropathy.

Peripheral neuropathy Most common type is distal symmetric polyneuropathy. Manifestation of progressive damage to sensory and motor nerve fibers that may be detected in up to 30% of patients with diabetes. Usually begins in distal lower extremities, extending proximally in a stocking-and-glove distribution. Asymptomatic involvement may be suspected when physical examination of the feet reveals (1) diminished or absent ankle jerk reflexes (usually the first manifestation), (2) diminished proprioception, and/or (3) diminished sensation to light touch with 10 g monofilament testing. Symptomatic involvement may present with pain characterized as paresthesias, hyperesthesias, or burning sensations. May spontaneously resolve or progress to a state of numbness. Other variants include focal mononeuropathy (commonly involving oculomotor nerves), radiculopathy (involving thoracic or lumbar nerve roots), and mononeuropathy multiplex (presenting with asymmetric involvement of multiple peripheral nerves). Intensive control of blood glucose levels may delay progression of peripheral neuropathy, although reversal may not be possible. Pain may respond to staged treatment with tricyclic antidepressants (*desipramine* or *amitriptyline* 25–200 mg qhs), *topical capsaicin cream* (Zostrix® 0.075% cream qid), *gabapentin* (Neurontin® 300–600 mg tid), *pregabalin* (Lyrica® 25–300 mg in 2–3 divided doses), *carbamazepine* (Tegretol® 200–600 mg bid), or *tramadol* (Ultram® 50–100 mg q6h).

Autonomic neuropathy Variable manifestations, depending on distribution and extent of disruption in function of sympathetic and parasympathetic nerve fibers. Cardiovascular involvement may present with evidence of resting tachycardia, exercise intolerance, or orthostatic hypotension (defined as a 20 mm Hg drop in systolic BP or a 10 mm Hg drop in diastolic BP after standing for 2 min). Patients with orthostatic hypotension may report dizziness, weakness, and nausea when standing. Treatment with *fludrocortisone* (Florinef® 0.05–0.1 mg/d) or *midodrine* (ProAmatine® 10 mg tid) may help to relieve symptoms by augmenting intravascular volume with the former and increasing vascular tone with the latter. GI involvement may present with variable symptoms of gastropathy, diarrhea, or constipation. Diabetic gastroparesis is an extreme form of gastropathy that presents with marked dilation and hypotonia of the stomach, with delayed transit of food into the small intestine that may lead to early satiety, regurgitation of undigested food, and problems with coordination of preprandial insulin injections. Delayed transit may be confirmed on gastric emptying studies.Gastric emptying studies should be performed only when blood glucose is under control, as hyperglycemia may lead to false-positive tests. Prokinetic agents used to treat persistent diabetic gastroparesis include *metoclopramide* (Reglan® 5–20 mg 15–60 min qac) and *erythromycin* (50 mg suspension qac). Gastric pacemakers have shown some efficacy in cases of extreme gastroparesis. Severe diabetic diarrhea may respond to treatment with *clonidine* or *octreotide*. Genitourinary involvement may lead to development of a neurogenic bladder. Urinary retention may respond to treatment with *bethanechol* (Urecholine® 10–50 mg tid). Self-catheterization may be necessary in extreme cases. Erectile dysfunction is a common complication of diabetes that may be exacerbated by a range of contributing factors (atherosclerotic disease, hypogonadism, treatment with antihypertensive agents). Affected patients may respond to treatment with phosphodiesterase inhibitors *sildenafil* (Viagra® 25–50 mg × 1), *vardenafil* (Levitra® 2.5–20 mg × 1), and *tadalafil* (Cialis® 5–20 mg × 1). These agents may be contraindicated in patients with known or suspected orthostatic hypotension or coronary artery disease. Individuals with T1DM with significant autonomic neuropathy may have blunted or absent counterregulatory responses to treatment-induced hypoglycemia, a dangerous complication identified as *hypoglycemic unawareness*.

The diabetic foot

The combined effects of (1) distal symmetric polyneuropathy and (2) peripheral vascular disease restricting blood flow to the lower extremities may predispose patients to developing significant complications related to foot injuries. Damage to motor nerve fibers may lead to atrophy and weakness of muscles in the distal lower extremities. Progressive changes may lead to deformities that increase the pressure at prominent points on the soles of the feet. This may lead to development of thick calluses that may ulcerate. To complicate matters, damage to sensory nerve fibers with progressive diabetes may make it difficult for patients to detect foot ulcers or other traumatic injuries to the joints and soft tissues in the foot and ankle. If left untreated, foot ulcers may develop polymicrobial cellulitis, which can progress to osteomyelitis.In many cases, chronic infection is difficult to eradicate in devitalized tissue sites exposed to persistently elevated blood glucose levels. Serious, life-threatening infections in limbs compromised by restricted blood flow may require treatment with surgical amputation. >60% of lower extremity amputations are performed to treat complications of diabetic foot infections.

Prevention Close inspection of the feet should be performed on at least an annual basis to check for evidence of diminished sensation, altered peripheral pulses, joint deformities, signs of tissue damage, or calluses that may be forming at points of direct pressure. All patients should be counseled to perform regular self-inspection of the feet to check for signs of unsuspected trauma or injury. Consider podiatry referral for trimming of toenails to recommended lengths and provision of fitted shoes with adequate support without binding or constricting the feet.

Treatment Should be undertaken with the assistance of a podiatric specialist. Superficial diabetic foot ulcers that do not appear to be infected should be treated with aggressive debridement. Air casting may help to promote healing by relieving direct pressure. Deep ulcers may be probed to check for signs of osteomyelitis. Radiographic evaluation with plain films, magnetic resonance imaging (MRI) scanning, and tagged white blood cell (WBC) studies may help to confirm a suspected diagnosis. Cellulitis and osteomyelitis require treatment with bed rest, surgical debridement, and prolonged courses of IV antibiotics. Bone biopsy is the gold standard to determine the appropriate antibiotic. In cases of chronic wounds complicated by peripheral vascular disease, revascularization may help to promote resolution and healing. Amputation may be necessary if deep infections fail to resolve or if a spreading anaerobic infection or gangrene supervenes.

Hypoglycemia

Strict definition[3] ("Whipple's triad") based on confirmation of (1) a plasma glucose level <50 mg/dL, (2) hyperadrenergic or neuroglycopenic symptoms that occur at the time the low plasma glucose level is detected, and (3) relief of those symptoms corresponding to an increase in the plasma glucose level after administration of oral or IV glucose. Hyperadrenergic symptoms include palpitations, tremulousness, nausea, diaphoresis, and anxiety. Neuroglycopenic symptoms include dizziness, drowsiness, confusion, and dysarthria. Severe neuroglycopenia may result in loss of consciousness and seizures. Symptoms may develop in variable combinations and/or sequences.

295

Causes Most common cause of hypoglycemia is iatrogenic (e.g., treatment with insulin or with insulin secretagogues). Correct treatment-induced hypoglycemia with 15–20 g glucose in conscious patient or glucagon injection in the unconscious patient.Individuals should be given a prescription for and instructions on how to use glucagon pen in case of emergencies. In patients who are not being treated with agents for diabetes, hypoglycemia may be classified as fasting (occurring at any time of day) or postprandial (occurring reproducibly after meals).

Fasting hypoglycemia Distinction must be made between insulin-mediated and non-insulin-mediated mechanisms. Disorders associated with insulin-mediated hypoglycemia include insulinoma, insulin autoantibody production, and factitious administration of insulin or insulin secretagogues. Disorders associated with non-insulin-mediated hypoglycemia include chronic kidney disease, hepatic failure, sepsis, primary adrenal insufficiency, hypopituitarism, neoplasms that produce insulin-like growth factor 2 (IGF-2), and a range of inherited metabolic defects. Mechanisms underlying hypoglycemia associated with exposure to specific pharmacologic agents

---

3 Evaluation and management of adult hypoglycemic disorders: An Endocrine Society Clinical Practice Guideline. *J Clin Endocrinol Metabol.* 2009.

(quinolones, quinine, IV pentamidine, aminoglutethimide) are less clear. Investigation of hypoglycemia usually focuses on sequentially (1) ruling out disorders associated with non-insulin-mediated hypoglycemia, (2) conducting a monitored fast to confirm insulin-mediated hypoglycemia, and (3) determining whether detectable insulin is endogenously secreted or factitiously administered. See Table 9.8.

Insulinoma Very rare. May develop in the setting of multiple endocrine neoplasia type 1 (MEN-1) syndrome (pituitary tumor, parathyroid hyperplasia, pancreatic mass). The majority of confirmed insulinomas represent isolated benign neoplasms. <10% prove to be malignant following pathologic evaluation. Principal treatment is surgical enucleation. Preoperative localization may be difficult. Imaging modalities include computed tomography (CT) scanning, MRI scanning, transabdominal ultrasound, endoscopic ultrasound, and octreotide scanning. Measurement of insulin levels drawn from hepatic veins after arterial administration of calcium gluconate may help to localize regions of excessive secretion. In cases where imaging fails to identify a suspicious mass, intraoperative localization may be attempted through exploration, palpation, and direct ultrasonography. Distal or partial pancreatectomy may be considered as an empiric measure when a suspicious mass cannot be localized, although this will likely commit the patient to lifelong insulin therapy following surgery. Persistent or malignant disease may require treatment with diazoxide to suppress insulin secretion.

Postprandial hypoglycemia Recurrent episodes of hypoglycemia may occur in patients who have undergone upper GI surgical procedures (gastric banding, Roux-en-Y). This can occur immediately following surgery or years after. Transient episodes related to excessive physiologic

Table 9.8 Monitored fast

May be conducted in any inpatient or outpatient setting that allows for monitoring of intake and activity. The patient may drink sugar-free and noncaffeinated beverages. Physical activity should be encouraged.

Protocol
Draw blood samples q6h to measure plasma glucose, insulin, C-peptide, proinsulin, and β-hydroxybutyrate. Once plasma glucose drops to <60 mg/dL, increase frequency of blood draws to every 1–2 h. Terminate the fast once (a) plasma glucose drops to <45 mg/dL *and* the patient has signs/symptoms of hypoglycemia, (b) plasma glucose >45 mg/dL if symptoms present, or (c) 72 h have elapsed without symptoms. At the end of the fast, draw blood samples to measure plasma glucose, insulin, C-peptide, proinsulin, β-hydroxybutyrate, and oral hypoglycemic agents. Then inject 1.0 mg of glucagon IV and measure plasma glucose 10, 20, and 30 min later.

Interpretation
In a blood sample collected when plasma glucose is <55 mg/dL, an insulin level >3 μU/mL may be considered to be inappropriately elevated. An insulinoma may be suspected when a concomitant C-peptide level is >0.6 ng/mL with a proinsulin level >5 pmol/L. Plasma glucose levels that increase by >25 mg/dL or less following administration of glucagon and β-hydroxybutyrate levels of 2.7 mmol suggest mediation of hypoglycemia by insulin (or IGF-1). Factitious administration of insulin may be suspected when C-peptide and proinsulin levels are lower than these thresholds. In situations where factitious administration of insulin secretagogues may be suspected, blood samples can be checked to screen for sulfonylurea exposure.

insulin secretion may occur during the initial onset of T2DM. Self-identified "reactive" hypoglycemia in otherwise healthy individuals is considered a controversial diagnosis. Experimental attempts to provoke and correlate symptoms have reported conflicting results. Oral glucose tolerance testing or mixed meal testing has not proven to reliably reproduce hypoglycemia. Anecdotally, some patients report improvement in symptoms after altering diets to increase intake of protein and complex carbohydrates in smaller portions distributed throughout the course of the day.

Thyroid function tests

Physiology Thyrotropin releasing hormone (TRH) secreted by the hypothalamus stimulates secretion of TSH from thyrotroph cells in the anterior pituitary. TSH binds to receptors on thyrocytes in the thyroid gland, stimulating (a) uptake of iodine, (b) organification of iodine with thyroid peroxidase and thyroglobulin (TG) to, (c) produce thyroxine (T4) and triiodothyronine (T3), followed by (d) secretion of T4 and T3 from the thyroid gland. See Figure 9.1. Most of the T4 and T3 secreted by the thyroid gland bind to transport proteins in the circulation. Free (unbound) T4 is converted to T3 by deiodinase enzymes in peripheral tissues. Free T3 is the active form of thyroid hormone that binds to nuclear receptors to exert different regulatory effects in the target organ. Free T4 and T3 exert negative regulatory feedback on the secretion of TRH from the hypothalamus and the secretion of TSH from the anterior pituitary. There is a log-linear relationship between thyroid hormone levels and TSH levels. The majority of abnormalities of thyroid function in the clinical setting stem from disorders that primarily involve the thyroid gland itself. As such, TSH is an intrinsic assay that provides the most sensitive index of thyroid gland function. See Table 9.9.

Table 9.9 Evaluation of suspected hypothyroidism

1 Check a TSH level
- Normal = euthyroid
- Elevated = likely primary hypothyroidism
- Low = possible central (secondary) hypothyroidism, although rare

1 If the TSH level is elevated, check an unbound (free T4) thyroxine level
- Elevated TSH + low free T4 = primary hypothyroidism
- Elevated TSH + normal free T4 = subclinical hypothyroidism

3 If the TSH level is low, check an unbound (free T4) thyroxine level
- Low TSH + low free T4 = possible central (secondary) hypothyroidism (defect in hypothalamus or pituitary)

4 To confirm diagnosis of autoimmune-mediated hypothyroidism (most common, Hashimoto's thyroiditis), check antithyroid peroxidase and antithyroglobulin antibody titers
- Elevated antithyroid peroxidase and/or antithyroglobulin antibody titers = autoimmune thyroiditis. Negative antibody titers do not rule out autoimmune disease.

> ## Table 9.10 Evaluation of suspected hyperthyroidism
>
> 1 Check a TSH level
>   - Normal = euthyroid
>   - Low = thyrotoxicosis
>   - Elevated = possible central (secondary) hyperthyroidism
> 2 If the TSH level is low, check an unbound (free T4) thyroxine level and a total triiodothyronine (T3) level
>   - Low TSH + elevated free T4, or T3 = thyrotoxicosis
>   - Low TSH + normal free T4, and T3 = subclinical thyrotoxicosis
>   - Elevated TSH + elevated free T4, or T3 = central (secondary) hyperthyroidism (defect in hypothalamus or pituitary)
> 3 Check for findings consistent with manifestations of Graves' disease (goiter, dermopathy, symptoms and signs of thyroid eye disease)
> 4 If no findings consistent with manifestations of Graves' disease are evident, check a radionuclide thyroid uptake and scan study and a thyroglobulin level
>   - Increased, diffuse bilateral uptake (+/− visible pyramidal lobe) = Graves' hyperthyroidism
>   - Normal to increased uptake, focal, "hot" areas of distribution = toxic nodule or toxic multinodular goiter
>   - Low uptake + elevated or normal thyroglobulin = thyroiditis
>   - Low uptake + low thyroglobulin = ingestion of thyroid hormone (factitious hyperthyroidism)

Hyperthyroidism

Definitions Thyrotoxicosis is a systemic syndrome resulting from the manifestations of exposure to excessive levels of thyroid hormone. Hyperthyroidism is defined as thyrotoxicosis caused by increased production and secretion of thyroid hormone from functional thyroid tissue. See Table 9.10.

Symptoms of thyrotoxicosis May include weight loss, heat intolerance, diaphoresis, palpitations, increased appetite, increased frequency of bowel movements, amenorrhea or oligomenorrhea, tremulousness, anxiety, insomnia, and irritability.

Signs of thyrotoxicosis May include resting tachycardia, atrial arrhythmias, warm moist skin, thinning of the hair, onycholysis, low bone mineral density (BMD), proximal muscle weakness, hyperreflexia, a resting tremor, lid lag (defined as a delay in the descent of the upper eyelids on downward gaze; see Table 9.11), and (rarely) hypercalcemia.

Causes of hyperthyroidism Common causes include Graves' disease, toxic multinodular goiter, toxic adenoma, and exposure to large amounts of iodine (IV contrast loads, amiodarone). Rare causes of hyperthyroidism include struma ovarii, metastatic thyroid cancer, and TSH-secreting pituitary adenoma (central hyperthyroidism).

Graves' disease Autoimmune disorder characterized by endogenous production of antibodies that bind to and stimulate TSH receptors (also knows as thyroid-stimulating immunoglobulins). Marked female predominance. Stimulation of TSH receptors may cause significant enlargement of the thyroid gland evident as a goiter with a palpable pyramidal lobe. Increased vascularity of the thyroid gland may be detected as an audible bruit or palpable thrill. Complications believed to be caused by inflammation and

Figure 9.1 Hypothalamic-pituitary-thyroid axis

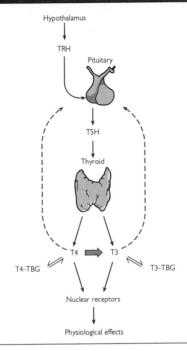

Hypothalamus

TRH

Pituitary

TSH

Thyroid

T4 → T3

T4–TBG

T3–TBG

Nuclear receptors

Physiological effects

antibody-mediated stimulation of fibroblast growth include dermopathy (pretibial myxedema), acropachy, and thyroid eye disease (Graves' ophthalmopathy). Hyperthyroidism may be effectively treated with antithyroid drugs, radioactive iodine ablation, or thyroidectomy. Radioactive iodine treatment may exacerbate active thyroid eye disease. Pretreatment with systemic glucocorticoids may reduce risk. Graves' disease may be associated with other autoimmune conditions in the same patient (T1DM, vitiligo, premature graying of the hair, etc.).

Toxic multinodular goiter Results from the growth of multiple autonomously functioning hyperplastic thyroid nodules. Hyperthyroidism due to multinodular goiter is more common among older individuals and may develop in the setting of a previously euthyroid multinodular goiter. Growth of the thyroid gland substernally may cause compressive thoracic outlet symptoms. Hyperthyroidism in a previously euthyroid patient may be precipitated by exposure to large amounts of iodine. Hyperthyroidism secondary to a multinodular goiter may be treated with radioactive iodine ablation, surgical resection, or antithyroid drugs.

Toxic adenoma A "hot nodule" and resultant hyperthyroidism is due to progressive growth of a single autonomously functioning thyroid nodule. Usually quite large, the nodule may be treated with antithyroid drugs, although radioactive iodine ablation or surgical resection are preferred and definitive. See also Table 9.12.

Table 9.11 Thyroid eye disease

Complication of Graves' disease believed to be caused by antibody-mediated stimulation of fibroblast growth and inflammation in soft tissues of the orbits and eyelids. Inflammation may cause swelling of the eyelids, conjunctival injection, and chemosis. Affected patients may report excessive tearing, ocular irritation, and persistent foreign body or "gritty" sensation of the eye. Swelling of the soft tissues in the orbits may cause protrusion of the eyeballs (proptosis), entrapment of the extraocular muscles with impaired motion, and compression of the optic nerve. Affected patients may report problems with excessive dryness of the eyes, diplopia, and disruptive changes in visual acuity. Risk of developing thyroid eye disease may be increased in patients who smoke.

Evaluation Formal neuro-ophthalmologic evaluation required. Imaging with orbital CT scanning may help to define degree of proptosis and extent of extraocular muscle involvement.

Treatment Management of mild symptoms involves protecting the corneas from exposure and abrasion with artificial tears and ointments to provide adequate lubrication. High-dose systemic glucocorticoids may help to attenuate active inflammation. Progressive diplopia and disruptive changes in visual acuity may require surgical decompression of the orbits. Staged strabismus surgery and eyelid surgery may be considered. Treatments based on the use of orbital irradiation, immunosuppressive agents, and plasmapheresis have been tried with some success. Patients with persistent diplopia may need to wear glasses with corrective prismatic lenses. Thyroidectomy to improve thyroid eye disease is controversial.

Causes of non-hyperthyroid thyrotoxicosis Include ingestion of pharmacologic and nonpharmacologic preparations of thyroid hormone, subacute thyroiditis, and autoimmune thyroiditis.

Subacute thyroiditis Granulomatous inflammation of thyroid tissue. Onset often preceded by a nonspecific viral illness. Patients present with pain localized to thyroid gland that may radiate upward to neck and jaw. The thyroid gland may be slightly enlarged and exquisitely tender to palpation. Inflammation may spread from one lobe to the other. Lab tests may reveal an elevated erythrocyte sedimentation rate (ESR). Thyroid function test profiles typically reveal a hyperthyroid phase (suppressed TSH, elevated free T4 and T3) lasting 1–4 wks caused by release of thyroid hormone, followed by a resolving hypothyroid phase (normal to elevated TSH, low free T4 and T3)lasting 1–3 months, caused by impaired production of thyroid hormone. Hypothyroid phase may be permanent. May require treatment with (a) β-blockers to attenuate thyrotoxicosis and (b) systemic glucocorticoids to alleviate discomfort associated with inflammation.

Subclinical hyperthyroidism Profile of thyroid function test results characterized by a decreased TSH level with normal T4 and T3 levels. Indications for treatment are controversial. Arrhythmias and bone loss associated with TSH <0.1 μIU/mL in elderly individuals, a threshold warranting treatment. Consider mild β-blockade or low-dose antithyroid medications in those with hyperthyroid symptoms to test for amelioration with normalization of thyroid function tests.

Table 9.12 Treatment of hyperthyroidism

β-Blockers May help to attenuate symptoms of thyrotoxicosis while other treatment modalities are being planned or taking effect. Commonly used preparations include *propranolol* (Inderal® 10–40 mg tid, Inderal LA® 60–120 mg/d) and *atenolol* (Tenormin® 25–100 mg/d). β-blocker dose should be titrated to relief of symptoms (palpitations, tremulousness) instead of resting heart rate.

Antithyroid drugs Thioamides that inhibit thyroid hormone production and release from the thyroid gland. Available preparations include *methimazole* (Tapazole 10–60 mg/d) and *propylthiouracil* (PTU 50–200 mg bid-tid). Methimazole offers advantage of once-daily dosing. PTU may be safer during pregnancy and may reduce peripheral conversion of T4 to T3. Doses should initially be titrated to reduce T4 and T3 levels to within normal ranges. Return of suppressed TSH levels to normal range may be delayed. Limiting side effects of both methimazole and PTU may include pruritic rash and hepatotoxicity with elevated transaminase levels or jaundice. Reversible agranulocytosis may develop as a rare complication of methimazole use. Patients should be instructed to stop treatment pending further evaluation if they develop a fever or severe pharyngitis (symptoms of agranulocytosis).

Radioactive iodine ablation Administration of a single oral dose of iodine-131 may be definitive therapy for hyperthyroidism, although multiple doses are sometimes required. Isotope is taken up and organified by hyperfunctioning thyroid tissue. Over time, locally acting β radiation gradually destroys thyrocytes. Calculated doses used to treat Graves' disease based on thyroid gland volume and uptake. High incidence of postablative hypothyroidism requiring lifelong thyroid hormone replacement. Calculated doses may be used to treat toxic adenomas. Higher-range empiric doses are usually used to treat toxic multinodular goiters.

Thyroid surgery Procedures vary depending on indication. Toxic adenomas may be resected, leaving the remainder of the thyroid intact. Toxic multinodular goiters usually require total thyroidectomy, especially when substernal extension may be contributing to compressive symptoms. Subtotal thyroidectomy may be considered in cases of Graves' disease when antithyroid drugs and radioactive iodine are contraindicated or hyperthyroidism is life-threatening (thyroid storm, below).

Thyroid storm Classified based on symptoms or signs (tachycardia/arrhythmias, fever, transaminitis, altered mental status, GI symptoms, and heart failure); requires aggressive therapy with steroids, lithium, super-saturated potassium iodine (SSKI) in addition to β-blockade/antithyroid drugs.

301

Hypothyroidism

A systemic syndrome caused by a deficiency of thyroid hormone. Primary hypothyroidism represents a deficiency of thyroid hormone caused by intrinsic dysfunction of the thyroid gland itself. Central (secondary) hypothyroidism represents a deficiency of thyroid hormone caused by dysfunction of the hypothalamus or pituitary gland.

Symptoms May include weight gain, cold intolerance, dyspnea, constipation, myalgias, arthralgias, fatigue, lethargy, and amenorrhea.

Signs May include bradycardia, pericardial effusion, cool dry skin, hair loss, brittle nails, delayed terminal relaxation of peripheral reflexes, nonpitting edema caused by deposition of glycosaminoglycans(myxedema), anemia, and hyponatremia.

Causes of primary hypothyroidism Common causes include auto-immune thyroiditis, previous radioactive iodine or external beam radiation-induced ablation of thyroid tissue, surgical removal of thyroid tissue, and drug-mediated inhibition of thyroid hormone production and release. Rare causes include congenital absence of thyroid tissue and resistance to thyroid hormone. Most common cause worldwide is iodine deficiency (rare in the United States due to abundant dietary supplementation).

Autoimmune thyroiditis Also known as Hashimoto's thyroiditis. Chronic lymphocytic inflammation often associated with progressive destruction of functioning thyroid tissue. Marked female predominance. Increased preva-lence with age. Autoimmune hypothyroidism is the cause of 95% of cases of primary hypothyroidism. Elevated titers of antithyroid peroxidase and antithyroglobulin antibodies may confirm a suspected diagnosis. May be associated with other autoimmune disorders including T1DM, autoimmune adrenalitis, and vitiligo.

Treatment Thyroid hormone replacement based on administration of pharmacologic preparations of *levothyroxine, or T4* (brand name ver-sions include Levothroid® Levoxyl® Synthroid® Unithroid®; taken daily; available in 25, 50, 75, 88, 100, 112, 125, 137, 150, 175, 200, and 300 mcg color-coded preparations). Usual daily replacement dose is approximately 1.6 mcg/kg body weight. Elderly patients may only require 1 mcg/kg body weight. Preparations of thyroid hormone replacement including T4 and T3 also available (Armour®), although content is variable and TSH harder to monitor. T4 preparations are preferred. Levothyroxine may be started at full replacement doses in patients <50 without evidence of heart disease. In patients with known or suspected heart disease, treatment should be started at a dose of 12.5–25 mcg/d, and should be increased gradually by 12.5–25 mcg increments at 4-wk intervals based on changes in TSH levels. A TSH level should be checked 6 wks after starting a dose or 4 wks after adjusting a dose to assess the adequacy of replacement. Treatment should target maintenance of TSH levels within reference ranges. Coadministration of large doses of calcium supplements, iron supplements, and bile acid res-ins may inhibit absorption of levothyroxine.

Subclinical hypothyroidism Profile of thyroid function test results char-acterized by an elevated TSH level with normal T4 and T3 levels. Indications for treatment are controversial. Concomitant evidence of hypercholester-olemia or underlying autoimmune thyroiditis may provide a rationale for starting treatment with thyroid hormone replacement.

Nonthyroidal illness

When thyroid function tests are checked in the setting of severe nonthyroi-dal illness (i.e., during prolonged hospitalization), secondary changes in TSH and thyroid hormone levels may return profiles that appear to be consis-tent with primary thyroid dysfunction. T3 levels usually decline during the early stages of severe non-thyroidal illness. As illness progresses, T4 levels may also decline. TSH levels are usually normal or suppressed during the early stages of severe non-thyroidal illness. They may rise above the upper limit of the normal range during recovery, producing a profile that may be mistaken for primary hypothyroidism. If thyroid function tests are checked in severely ill patients, clinical correlation is important. The presence of a goiter, history of radioactive iodine treatment, history of pituitary disease, or findings consistent with prior thyroid surgery may help to establish a correct diagnosis. For patients without findings consistent with underlying thyroid dysfunction, retesting 6–8 wks after recovery may be recommended before starting therapy.

Hyperparathyroidism

Physiology Parathyroid hormone (PTH) secreted by the parathyroid glands in response to circulating blood calcium levels. PTH stimulates (a) increased breakdown of bone through activation of osteoclasts, (b) increased reabsorption of calcium (Ca^{2+}) and decreased reabsorption of phosphate (PO_4^-) in the distal tubule of the kidney, and (c) increased production of 1,25-dihydroxyvitamin D. The overall effect is to increase Ca^{2+} levels while decreasing PO_4^- levels. Negative feedback exerted by increased Ca^{2+} levels regulates secretion of PTH. See Table 9.13.

Primary hyperparathyroidism Inappropriate autonomous secretion of PTH due to hyperplastic growth of one or more parathyroid glands. Approximately 80% of cases associated with growth of a solitary adenoma, 15% with hyperplasia of all four glands, 4% with growth of multiple adenomas, and <1% with malignant growth of parathyroid carcinoma. Patients often present with asymptomatic hypercalcemia. Confirmation based on finding an elevated blood Ca^{2+} level in conjunction with an elevated or inappropriately normal PTH level. Complications associated with progressive disease may include (a) osteoporosis and fracture, (b) nephrolithiasis, (c) precipitation or exacerbation of psychiatric symptoms, and (d) GI symptoms. Variants presenting with hyperplasia of all four glands associated with specific MEN syndromes (MEN-1 and -2a). Treatment involves surgical resection of autonomously functioning parathyroid tissue. Surgery is indicated in patients presenting with (a) severe or life-threatening hypercalcemia, (b) osteoporosis or fractures, (c) impaired renal function, or (d) recurrent nephrolithiasis. In asymptomatic cases, evaluation of measured or estimated GFR and dual energy x-ray absorptiometry (DXA) scanning with inclusion of spine, hip, and distal forearm BMD may to help to determine which patients should be referred for surgery.[4] See Table 9.14.

Planned operations may involve exploration and comparison of all four glands to identify hypertrophic tissue or targeted resection of specific glands based on attempted preoperative localization. Studies commonly utilized for preoperative localization include sestamibi scans, MRI scans, CT scans, and neck ultrasonography. Intraoperatively, PTH levels may be measured to track changes following resection of suspect tissue. Solitary adenomas are usually resected in isolation. Confirmed hyperplasia of all four glands

---

Table 9.13 Indications for surgical treatment of asymptomatic primary hyperparathyroidism

- Calcium level >1 mg/dL above lab reference range upper limit of normal
- Bone density T-score at the hip, lumbar spine, or distal radius <-2.5 and/or previous fragility fracture
- Measured or estimated GFR of <60 mL/min
- Age <50 years

---

4 Bilezikian JP et al. Guidelines for the management of asymptomatic primary hyperparathyroidism: Summary statement from the Third International Workshop. *J Clin Endocrinol Metabol.* 2009. 94(2):335–339.

may require resection of up to three and a half glands with reimplantation of residual tissue in an accessible location (forearm, sternocleidomastoid muscle).

Familial hypocalciuric hypercalcemia (FHH) Lab profile may resemble that of primary hyperparathyroidism (elevated vs. inappropriately normal PTH, elevated calcium).Caused by autosomal dominant mutations in the calcium-sensing receptor found in both the parathyroid glands and renal tubules.May be confirmed with positive family history, hypercalcemia at young age, and low 24 h urine calcium level measurement in patient. Ca/Cr clearance ratio <0.01 in 80% of patients. FHH is asymptomatic and without manifestation of end-organ damage (bone loss, kidney disease, etc.).Does not need treatment.

Secondary hyperparathyroidism Presents with a profile of an elevated PTH level in conjunction with a low or normal Ca^{2+} level. Commonly due to vitamin D deficiency (decreased conversion of 25-hydroxyvitamin D to 1,25-dihydroxyvitamin D leads to decreased suppression of PTH secretion and decreased intestinal absorption of Ca^{2+}). Relative hypocalcemia also stimulates increased secretion of PTH to restore and maintain normal Ca^{2+} levels. Secondary hyperparathyroidism also common in patients with chronic kidney disease once estimated GFR declines to <40 mL/min. May respond to treatment with calcium supplementation, phosphate restriction,administration of potent 1,25-dihydroxyvitamin D analogs or calcimimetic drugs like *cinacalcet* (Sensipar® 60–180 mg/d).

Tertiary hyperparathyroidism In patients with chronic kidney disease, prolonged severe secondary hyperparathyroidism may lead to hyperplasia of autonomously functioning parathyroid tissue. Inappropriate secretion of PTH in this setting may lead to hypercalcemia with extracellular Ca^{2+} deposition evident as cutaneous calcification. In extreme cases, this may lead to extremity gangrene as part of a life-threatening syndrome known as *calciphylaxis*. Urgent parathyroidectomy may be required.

Table 9.14 Multiple endocrine neoplasia syndromes

Multiple endocrine neoplasia type 1 (MEN-1) Clinical manifestations include primary hyperparathyroidism, pancreatic tumors, and pituitary adenomas. Autosomal dominant loss-of-function mutation of the MEN-1 tumor suppressor gene. Penetrance of primary hyperparathyroidism characterized by four-gland hyperplasia is 95%. Most common pancreatic tumors are gastrinomas (associated with the Zollinger-Ellison syndrome) and insulinomas. Pituitary adenomas may secrete prolactin or growth hormone or may be nonfunctional.

Multiple endocrine neoplasia type 2a (MEN-2a) Clinical manifestations include medullary thyroid carcinoma (MTC), pheochromocytoma, and primary hyperparathyroidism. Autosomal dominant mutation of the RET proto-oncogene. Different mutations identified in different kindreds. MTC may be diagnosed in 80–100% of affected individuals. Tends to be multicentric. Preceded by hyperplasia of parafollicular C-cells. Pheochromocytomas may develop in 50% of affected individuals. Often bilateral. Rarely malignant. RET proto-oncogene screening is available as a commercial test.

Multiple endocrine neoplasia type 2b (MEN-2b) Clinical manifestations include MTC, pheochromocytoma, and mucosal neuromas (lesions that may be discernible as submucosal masses on the lips, cheeks, tongue, glottis, eyelids, and visible corneal nerves). Affected individuals may present with a characteristic marfanoid habitus. MTC tends to be more aggressive than in MEN-2a, mandating earlier diagnosis and treatment.

Hypoparathyroidism

Characterized by decreased secretion of PTH. Patients may present with symptoms and signs of hypocalcemia including perioral numbness, digital paresthesias, carpopedal spasm, and tetany. Confirmation is based on finding a decreased Ca^{2+} level in conjunction with a low or inappropriately normal PTH level. Commonly due to a complication of surgical procedures that inadvertently lead to removal or destruction of a critical mass of parathyroid tissue. Postoperative hypoparathyroidism may be transient or permanent. Idiopathic hypoparathyroidism caused by autoimmune destruction of parathyroid tissue may develop in conjunction with autoimmune adrenalitis and mucocutaneous candidiasis as part of the type I polyglandular autoimmune syndrome.

Treatment Acute hypocalcemia may require treatment with IV infusions of *calcium chloride* (272 mg of elemental calcium per 10 mL) or *calcium gluconate* (90 mg of elemental calcium per 10 mL). Doses of 200 mg of elemental calcium may be administered over several minutes. Prolonged infusions of 400–1,000 mg of elemental calcium may be administered over 24 h. Chronic hypocalcemia may require treatment with calcium supplementation and vitamin D analog therapy. Patients may require 1,500–3,000 mg of elemental calcium daily in divided doses. Vitamin D analogs that may be used to promote absorption of elemental calcium include *calcitriol* (Rocaltrol® 0.25–1.0 mcg daily–bid) and *ergocalciferol* (50,000 IU daily to weekly). Treatment should target maintenance of calcium levels in low normal ranges. Serum calcium should be closely monitored in cases of possible of transient hypoparathyroidism, as parathyroid gland recovery can lead to dangerous hypercalcemia.

Osteoporosis

Characterized by a loss of bone mass and/or microarchitecture associated with an increased risk of fracture. Proximate cause of >1.5 million fractures annually in the United States. Individuals with osteoporosis and number of fractures will continue to rise as population ages.Up to 40% mortality in the first year following hip fracture. Most common sites of fragility fracture are the vertebral bodies, wrist, and hip.

Risk factors Principal risk factor associated with development of osteoporosis is advancing age. More common in Caucasians and Asians than other ethnic groups. Other risk factors include female sex, low BMI, early menopause, amenorrhea, smoking, alcohol abuse, family history, and a history of minimally traumatic fractures. Iatrogenic risk factors include immobilization, treatment with anticonvulsants, thiazolidinedione use, and prolonged treatment with supraphysiologic doses of glucocorticoids. Disorders associated with development of osteoporosis include primary hyperparathyroidism, T1DM, T2DM, thyrotoxicosis, Cushing's syndrome, rheumatoid arthritis and other chronic inflammatory diseases, malabsorption syndromes (celiac disease, gastric bypass, etc.), hypogonadism, anorexia nervosa, and connective tissue disorders that disrupt synthesis of bone matrix (osteogenesis imperfecta, Ehlers–Danlos syndrome, Marfan's syndrome).

Diagnosis Reliable diagnosis and quantification of bone loss relies on direct measurement of bone density with *Dual-emission X-ray absorptiometry* (DXA) scanning (Table 9.15). Screening evaluation with DXA may show low BMD at one or more sites of interest (lumbar spine, femoral neck, total hip, distal third forearm). Regardless of BMD, likely diagnosis of osteoporosis if an individual presents with a minimally traumatic hip, wrist, or vertebral compression fracture. Asymptomatic presentation may be associated with progressive height loss attributed to vertebral compression fractures. Plain

Table 9.15 DXA scanning

Provides an estimate of areal density of bone measured in g/cm². Most commonly scanned sites are the lumbar vertebrae, hip, and distal forearm. Scoliotic changes, osteoarthritis, hardware, and vertebral compression fractures may distort lumbar vertebral readings and should prompt forearm DXA, which is less distorted by these factors. Generates actual measurements along with T-scores that represent number of standard deviations above or below the mean for healthy young adults. Z-scores represent number of standard deviations above or below mean for representative age group and are used in premenopausal individuals. T-scores have been correlated with associated fracture risk to assign classifications.

WHO definitions
T-score 0 to –1.0 = normal
T-score –1.0 to –2.5 = low BMD(osteopenia)
T-score ≤–2.5 or fragility fracture = osteoporosis

films may reveal low bone mineral density and anterior wedging of vertebral bodies.

Screening The National Osteoporosis Foundation[5] recommends screening with DXA scanning be considered for (a) all women ≥65 or (b) younger postmenopausal women with more than one predisposing risk factor (see above). Screening in men should begin at ≥70 years or in those with more than one predisposing risk factor.

Preventive measures Include regular weight-bearing exercise, maintenance of good nutritional status, adequate calcium intake (>1,000–1,200 mg elemental calcium daily, divided doses), adequate vitamin D intake (600–800 IU daily), smoking cessation, and moderation of alcohol intake. Postmenopausal estrogen replacement therapy is no longer recommended as a preventive measure. See also Table 9.16.

Paget's disease of the bone

Disorder characterized by focally accelerated remodeling of bone resulting in bone overgrowth anddisruption of normal architecture. Affected bone has impaired strength. May be at one (monostotic) or more (polyostotic) sites. Commonly involves the sacrum, spine, femur, skull, and pelvis. May present with bone pain, fractures, deformities, or manifestations of associated neurologic, cardiac, malignant, or metabolic complications. Examination may reveal cutaneous erythema, warmth, and tenderness localized to the soft tissue overlying affected regions. Characteristic findings may include enlargement of the skull, frontal bossing, and bowing of the lower extremities. Associated with an increased risk of fractures, sensorineural deafness, facial palsies, osteoarthritis, and spinal stenosis. Rarely, patients may develop high-output heart failure, hypercalcemia (usually if underlying primary hyperparathyroidism), orosteosarcoma.

Diagnosis Asymptomatic disease detected when routine chemistry panels reveal elevated alkaline phosphatase. Localized symptoms may prompt evaluation with plain films that reveal characteristic ragged lytic lesions and coarsened trabeculae. Radio nucleotide bone scanning may reveal other sites of involvement that may be confirmed with dedicated plain films.

5 National Osteoporosis Foundation, www.nof.org

Table 9.16 Treatment of osteoporosis

Available agents include bisphosphonates, raloxifene, teriparatide, denosumab, and calcitonin.

Bisphosphonates Agents that bind to hydroxyapatite crystals in mineralized bone. Act to inhibit bone resorption by quieting osteoclast activity. Oral bisphosphonates include *alendronate* (Fosamax® 70 mg once a week), *risedronate* (Actonel® 35 mg once a week or 150 mg once a month), and *ibandronate* (Boniva® 150 mg once a month). Monthly dosing may improve compliance and limit risk of side effects. May cause severe esophageal or GI irritation, as well as bone pain or, less commonly, osteonecrosis of the jaw (see below). Should be swallowed with 8 oz of water with directions to remain in an upright position for 30 min afterward. Patients who cannot tolerate oral bisphosphonates (reflux disease, abdominal symptoms, etc.) may be treated with doses of IV *zoledronic acid* (Reclast® 5 mg in 250 mL normal saline [NS] infused over 30 min) administered every 12 months. Side effects of zoledronic acid include first-dose reaction (10–20% patients, self-limited flu-like illness for 2–3 days)and osteonecrosis of the jaw (1 case per 200,000 persons per year) in those receiving high-dose, frequent IV bisphosphonates (multiple myeloma, breast cancer) or those with recent dental procedures (implants, extractions). *CI*: GFR <30 mL/min, hypocalcemia.

Raloxifene (Evista® 60 mg/d). Antiresorptive selective estrogen receptor modulator (SERM) targeting estrogen receptors on the bone, not breast or uterus. May be used to prevent and treat osteoporosis. Often precipitates hot flashes. Associated with an increased risk of deep venous thrombosis. *CI*: History of venous thromboembolic disorders, pregnancy.

Teriparatide (Forteo® 20 mcg SQ daily). Recombinant form of the N-terminal segment of PTH that must be administered as a daily subcutaneous injection. The only anabolic agent that promotes new bone formation. Often consideredwhen patients have continued to lose bone density or sustain fractures during treatment with bisphosphonates. Treatment course limited to 2 yrs and must be followed with an antiresorptive medication (bisphosphonate, denosumab) or rapid bone loss will ensue. Side effects include transient hypercalcemia/hypercalciuria and bone pain. *CI*: Hyperparathyroidism, hypercalcemia, history of skeletal metastases.

Denosumab (Prolia® 60 mg SQ every 6 months). Monoclonal antibody against RANK-L to inhibit osteoclast-mediated bone resorption.Can be used in patients with severe chronic kidney disease.Side effects include dermatitis, bone pain, and weakness; higher rate of infectious complications reported. *CI*: Preexisting hypocalcemia.

Calcitonin (Miacalcin® 200 units intranasally daily). Pharmacologic preparation of salmon calcitonin. Can be administered at home as an intranasal spray. May help to relieve bone pain after an acute osteoporotic vertebral fracture. Tachyphylaxis limits long-term utility in prevention and treatment of osteoporosis.

DXA scanning may be repeated after 1–2 yrs to assess responses to treatment. Comparisons should be based on measurements taken with similar types of equipment loaded with valid databases. BMD changes that are considered significant depend on the calibration of the machine.

Calcium and phosphorus levels are usually normal. Urinary bone turnover markers (N-telopeptides, pyridinoline) are usually elevated.

Treatment Treat biochemically active disease located at sites of high skeletal fragility (spine, weight bearing bones, joints) or in the skull. Also reasonable to treat if alkaline phosphatase >2–4 times upper limit of normal. For symptomatic disease, bone pain may respond to treatment with NSAIDs. Limited courses of treatment with bisphosphonates may help to alleviate symptoms and stabilize deformities. *Alendronate* (Fosamax® 40 mg/d for 6 months) and *risedronate* (Actonel® 30 mg/d PO for 2 months) may be equally effective. IV bisphosphonates include *pamidronate* (Aredia® 30 mg/d × 3d) and or *zoledronic acid* (Reclast® 5 mg IV once).An advantage of IV bisphosphonate administration may be more sustained biochemical remissions (1–2 yrs) compared to oral bisphosphonates. Changes in alkaline phosphatase levels may be tracked over time to assess responses to treatment. Patients who continue to manifest symptoms after an initial course of treatment with a bisphosphonate may respond to subsequent courses of treatment with the same agent. Patients requiring surgery on a pagetic site should be treated prior to surgery with a bisphosphonate to reduce hypervascularity to site and resultant blood loss.

Osteomalacia

Condition characterized by decreased mineralization of bone matrix. May be precipitated by disorders that limit effective reserves of circulating calcium and phosphorus. Impairment of mineralization that occurs during growth may lead to development of rickets associated with short stature (if occurring in childhood), proximal muscle weakness, and bony deformities. Demineralization that occurs after the epiphyses have fused may give rise to bone pain and tenderness. Fractures of the collarbone, ribs, and other "stress fractures" may be associated with osteomalacia, particularly when DXA testing reveals otherwise-normal to fair BMD.

Vitamin D deficiency Most common cause of osteomalacia in adults. Vitamin D stores measured with serum 25-hydroxy vitamin D. Pure nutritional deficiency is becoming more common due to decreased intake of dairy products and rise of vegan diets. Sun is a limited source of vitamin D for most. Malabsorption of vitamin D may occur in the setting of disorders associated with pancreatic insufficiency, impaired biliary secretion, or intestinal malabsorption. Treatment with anticonvulsants may enhance metabolism of vitamin D in the liver, diminishing effective stores of 25-hydroxyvitamin D. In rare instances, severe liver disease may diminish stores of 25-hydroxyvitamin D. In cases where no obvious underlying cause is evident, a confirmed diagnosis of vitamin D deficiency may prompt serologic (positive antiendomysial or anti-tissue transglutaminase antibodies) with confirmatory endoscopic evaluation to check for evidence of unsuspected celiac disease.

Evaluation Should initially focus on measurement of Ca^{2+}, fasting PO_4^-, PTH, alkaline phosphatase, and 25-hydroxyvitamin D levels. Moderate-to-severe cases of vitamin D deficiency may present with secondary hyperparathyroidism characterized by low Ca^{2+} and PO_4, levels in conjunction with elevated PTH and alkaline phosphatase levels. Mild cases may present with normal Ca^{2+}, PO_4^-, and alkaline phosphatase levels in conjunction with normal or slightly elevated PTH levels. Confirmation of a suspected diagnosis based on documentation of a low 25-hydroxyvitamin D level. Although the traditional goal level for 25-hydroxy vitamin D is >30 ng/mL, recent guidelines published by the Institute of Medicine[6] state 25-hydroxy vitamin D level

6 Consensus Report, Institute of Medicine, dietary reference intakes for calcium and vitamin D. November 2010.

>20 ng/mL is sufficient for most adults. Elevated parathyroid hormone or known metabolic bone disease in a patient may prompt supplementation to a 25-hydroxy vitamin D level of >30 ng/mL.

Treatment Vitamin D deficiency repletion requirements may vary depending on the underlying cause and severity of the disorder. Mild cases may respond to repletion with *ergocalciferol* 50,000 IU PO weekly for 6–8 wks, followed by daily administration of a supplement containing 400–800 IU of cholecalciferol. Severe cases associated with persistent malabsorption (gastric bypass, short gut) may require long-term treatment with a combination of calcium supplements and ergocalciferol administered in much higher, supervised doses. Patients with underlying liver disease may require treatment with *calcifediol*, a metabolite of cholecalciferol. Patients with chronic kidney disease often require a combination of ergocalciferol and calcitriol supplementation. Ca^{2+} levels should be monitored during treatment, as vitamin D toxicity may precipitate hypercalcemia.

Hypophosphatemic disorders Persistent renal phosphate wasting may lead to hypophosphatemia with associated osteomalacia. X-linked hypophosphatemic rickets (XLH) is the most common inherited disorder associated with renal phosphate wasting and is caused by a mutation in the PHEX gene. Autosomal dominant hypophosphatemic rickets has a similar presentation and is related to an activating mutation of fibroblast growth factor-23 (FGF-23) gene. Both conditions result in elevated serum FGF-23 levels that promote phosphaturia and inhibit conversion of 25-hydroxy vitamin D to 1, 25-dihydroxy vitamin D. Affected individuals present in early childhood with poor growth complicated by severe rickets, hypophosphatemia, phosphaturia, and low 1,25-vitamin D levels. Defects in dentin may cause tooth decay and dental abscesses. Treatment involves administration of large amounts of supplemental phosphate along with calcitriol taken to prevent secondary hyperparathyroidism. Treatment may not be necessary in asymptomatic adults. Oncogenic osteomalacia represents an acquired form of renal phosphate wasting that may develop in patients diagnosed with benign and malignant mesenchymal tumors producing excess FGF-23. In most cases, resection of neoplastic tissue has proven to be curative, although tumors can be hard to localize.

Cushing's syndrome

Physiology Corticotropin-releasing hormone (CRH) secreted by the hypothalamus stimulates secretion of ACTH from corticotroph cells in the anterior pituitary. ACTH binds to receptors on cells in the zona fasciculata and zona reticularis of the adrenal cortex, stimulating the production and secretion of cortisol and androgens. Basal secretion of cortisol follows a circadian pattern. Cortisol levels fall to nearly undetectable levels in the late evening, then gradually increase to peak after 6–8 h of sleep. Physiologic stress may stimulate increased secretion of cortisol. Most of the cortisol secreted by the adrenal cortex binds to transport proteins in the circulation. Free (unbound) cortisol binds to cytosolic receptors to exert different regulatory effects. Free cortisol exerts negative regulatory effects on the secretion of CRH from the hypothalamus and the secretion of ACTH from the anterior pituitary.

Cushing's syndrome Represents the sequelae of prolonged exposure to chronically elevated glucocorticoid levels. Endogenous Cushing's syndrome is caused by the increased production and secretion of cortisol (hypercortisolemia). Underlying causes may be mechanistically classified as ACTH-dependent (hypercortisolemia driven by increased secretion of ACTH from a pituitary or nonpituitary source) or ACTH-independent (hypercortisolemia that develops as a result of the growth of autonomously functioning adrenal cortex tissue). Iatrogenic Cushing's syndrome may be caused by prolonged exposure to supratherapeutic doses of pharmacologic glucocorticoid preparations. See Table 9.17.

ACTH-dependent Cushing's syndrome Most common cause is growth of an ACTH-secreting pituitary adenoma (Cushing's disease). May also be caused by ectopic secretion of ACTH from other occult neoplasms including small cell lung carcinoma, carcinoid tumors, pancreatic islet cell tumors, medullary thyroid carcinoma, and pheochromocytomas. Rare cases caused by ectopic secretion of CRH.

ACTH-independent Cushing's syndrome Most common cause is growth of an isolated cortisol-secreting adrenal adenoma. May also be caused by secretion of cortisol from functional adrenal carcinomas. Rare cases caused by growth of pigmented micronodules (Carney complex) or macronodular adrenal hyperplasia.

Symptoms May include weight gain, weakness, fatigue, oligomenorrhea, impotence, easy bruising, anxiety, irritability, depression, and impaired concentration. Larger pituitary adenomas may cause blurred or double vision secondary to compression of the optic chiasm.

Signs Most common manifestation is fat deposition in a central distribution with relative sparing of the limbs. Central fat deposition may lead to expansion of the cheeks (producing characteristic "moon" facies), protrusion of supraclavicular fat pads, protrusion of the dorsocervical fat, and truncal obesity. Atrophy of connective tissue in the dermis may lead to facial plethora and development of expanding darkened or violaceous striae (>0.5 cm wide) in the axillae and lower abdominal quadrants. Other manifestations may include hypertension, development or worsening of diabetes, osteoporosis and fracture, proximal muscle weakness, nephrolithiasis, hypertriglyceridemia, and evidence of hirsutism or virilization.

Treatment of ACTH-dependent Cushing's syndrome Confirmation of endogenous hypercortisolism with biochemical testing (see below) should always precede imaging evaluation due to high risk of "incidentaloma" discovery. Treatment then depends on underlying cause and rate of progression. Whenever feasible, confirmed ACTH-secreting pituitary adenomas should be surgically resected. Microadenomas (<1 cm in diameter) can usually be removed via transsphenoidal approaches. Removal of larger macroadenomas may require craniotomy. Success rates following initial surgery vary and are highly dependent on surgical expertise. Persistent disease may require repeat surgery, treatment with external beam radiation, and/ or medical therapies. Successful treatment of ectopic secretion of ACTH depends on accurate localization and surgical resection of functional tissue. In either setting, severe refractory hypercortisolemia may lead to consideration of bilateral surgical adrenalectomy or temporizing use of adrenolytic agents (*mitotane, ketoconazole, metyrapone, etomidate*) to inhibit excessive cortisol production. Surgical or medical eradication of adrenal glands will require monitored steroid replacement.

Treatment of ACTH-independent Cushing's syndrome Principal treatment is surgical resection of cortisol-secreting neoplastic adrenal tissue.

Table 9.17 Evaluation of suspected Cushing's syndrome

1 For the initial evaluation of Cushing's,[7] one of the following tests should be performed to confirm the presence of hypercortisolemia:

- a. Urine free cortisol level, measured in a 24 h urine collection—concomitant measurement of creatinine may confirm adequate collection volume (>1 g/24 h); upper limit of normal range may vary depending on assay used. Perform two collections for verification.
- b. Salivary cortisol level, measured by having the patient chew a cotton pledget to collect 2.5 mL sample of saliva at 11:00 pm. Upper limit of normal range may vary depending on assay used. Two samples should be checked for verification.
- c. Overnight low-dose dexamethasone suppression test. In the normal patient, dexamethasone should suppress ACTH secretion, suppressing cortisol secretion, in turn. Test performed by having the patient take 1 mg of *dexamethasone* (Decadron®) at 11:00 pm, then measuring a cortisol level at 8:00 am the next morning.
  - Cortisol <1.8 mcg/dL = normal response
  - Cortisol >1.8 mcg/dL = hypercortisolemia

2 If the initial test for Cushing's is abnormal, patient should be referred to endocrinology for additional evaluation. In endocrinology, the following steps may be taken:

3 a. If hypercortisolemia has been confirmed, check a plasma ACTH level to distinguish between ACTH-dependent and ACTH-independent Cushing's syndrome.

- Plasma ACTH elevated or inappropriately normal = ACTH-dependent Cushing's syndrome
- Plasma ACTH suppressed = ACTH-independent Cushing's syndrome

b. If ACTH-dependent Cushing's syndrome is suspected, check an overnight high-dose (8 mg) dexamethasone suppression test to distinguish between an ACTH-secreting pituitary adenoma and nonsuppressible ectopic secretion of ACTH. If overnight high-dose dexamethasone suppression test reveals suppression of cortisol by >50% = ACTH-secreting pituitary adenoma.

c. If an ACTH-secreting pituitary adenoma is suspected, consider pituitary MRI scanning. Cases that localize to the pituitary in which there is no lesion on MRI may require inferior petrosal sinus sampling. If ectopic secretion of ACTH is suspected, consider targeted imaging with high-resolution thoracic CT scanning, thoracic MRI scanning, or octreotide scanning to attempt to localize an ACTH-secreting neoplasm

d. If ACTH-independent Cushing's syndrome is suspected, consider targeted imaging with abdominal CT scanning, abdominal MRI scanning, or iodo-cholesterol scintigraphy scanning to identify and characterize adrenal abnormalities.

7 The diagnosis of Cushing's syndrome: An Endocrine Society clinical practice guideline. *J Clin Endocrinol Metabol.* 2008.

Adrenal insufficiency

A systemic syndrome caused by deficiency of hormones secreted by the adrenal cortex. Primary adrenal insufficiency represents a deficiency of cortisol and aldosterone caused by intrinsic dysfunction and/or destruction of the adrenal cortex. Central (secondary) adrenal insufficiency represents a deficiency of cortisol only caused by dysfunction of the hypothalamus or pituitary gland.

Symptoms May vary depending on specific deficiencies and duration of condition. Symptoms associated with deficiency of cortisol may include weight loss, fatigue, weakness, anorexia, nausea, and vomiting. Deficiency of aldosterone may precipitate orthostatic dizziness and lightheadedness with positional changes and salt craving.

Signs Deficiency of cortisol may present with orthostatic hypotension, hypoglycemia, and hyponatremia. Deficiency of aldosterone may present with hyperkalemia, metabolic acidosis, and exacerbation of orthostatic hypotension and hyponatremia. Prolonged primary adrenal insufficiency may eventually cause diffuse hyperpigmentation of the skin and mucous membranes. Auricular-cartilage calcification, splenomegaly, eosinophilia, and tonsillar lymphoid hyperplasia are also observed in long-standing disease.

Causes of primary adrenal insufficiency Common causes include autoimmune adrenalitis, bilateral adrenal hemorrhage, disseminated tuberculosis, and HIV infection. Rare causes include disseminated histoplasmosis, bilateral adrenal metastases, lymphoma, and adrenoleukodystrophy. Most clinically significant cases of primary disease are associated with destruction of >90% of functioning adrenal cortical tissue. In undiagnosed cases, physiologic stress associated with acute illness, infection, trauma, or surgery may precipitate an adrenal crisis.Adrenal crisis (described below) is a medical emergency characterized by fever, refractory hypotension, volume depletion, severe weakness, nausea, vomiting, abdominal pain, and delirium leading to obtundation and coma.

Autoimmune adrenalitis Known as Addison's disease, lymphocytic infiltration of bilateral adrenal glands associated with progressive destruction of functioning adrenal cortical tissue. May be associated with other autoimmune disorders including autoimmune thyroiditis, T1DM, vitiligo, primary ovarian insufficiency, and idiopathic hypoparathyroidism.

Causes of central (secondary) adrenal insufficiency Most common cause is long-term treatment with exogenous steroids leading to suppression of intrinsic hypothalamus-pituitary-adrenal axis.Resection of pituitary tumors for Cushing's can cause permanent ACTH deficiency, although any pituitary process (infiltration, infection, tumor, hemorrhage, ischemia) can cause central adrenal insufficiency. Long-term, high-dose opiate therapy may be associated with central adrenal insufficiency. See Table 9.18.

Adrenal crisis Treatment of a suspected adrenal crisis should not be delayed for any reason. Confirmatory testing may be performed once a patient has been stabilized. Effective therapy incorporates (a) aggressive IV volume repletion with large volumes of isotonic fluid (D5 NS administered as rapidly as possible through a central line or large-bore IVs), (b) concomitant administration of *dexamethasone* (Decadron®) 4 mg IV q12h (other glucocorticoid preparations may interfere with plasma cortisol assays used later to confirm diagnosis), and (c) identification and treatment of precipitating causes.

Treatment Primary and central (secondary) adrenal insufficiency require treatment with glucocorticoid replacement therapy.[8] One commonly

8 Arlt W. The approach to the adult with newly diagnosed adrenal insufficiency. *J Clin Endocrinol Metabol.* 2009. 94(4):1059–1067.

Table 9.18 Evaluation of suspected adrenal insufficiency

1 Perform a cosyntropin (ACTH) stimulation test to evaluate the intrinsic function of the adrenal cortex.
- Cosyntropin stimulation test is performed by measuring a baseline cortisol level, administering 250 mcg of *cosyntropin* (Cortrosyn®) IV, and measuring cortisol levels at 30 and 60 min.
- Peak cortisol (at any time point) >18 mcg/dL = normal response
- Peak cortisol (at any time point) <18 mcg/dL = adrenal insufficiency

2 If adrenal insufficiency has been confirmed, check a plasma ACTH level to distinguish between primary and central (secondary) adrenal insufficiency.
- Plasma ACTH >50 pg/mL = primary adrenal insufficiency
- Plasma ACTH <30 pg/mL = central (secondary) adrenal insufficiency

3 Consider referral to an endocrinologist for complicated cases.

employed regimen is based on twice-daily administration of *hydrocortisone* (Cortef® 7.5–30 mg/d split into two doses, with two-thirds of the daily dose taken before breakfast and one-third taken in the late afternoon). Other regimens are based on once-daily administration of *prednisone* (2.5–10 mg taken before breakfast or at bedtime), or *dexamethasone* (Decadron® 0.25–0.75 mg taken at bedtime). There are no specific tests or assays that provide an accurate index of the adequacy of glucocorticoid replacement. Clinical assessment is required to identify doses that strike a balance between inadequate replacement with residual symptoms and signs of adrenal insufficiency and overreplacement predisposing to iatrogenic Cushing's syndrome. As such, monitor patient weight, blood glucose levels, and overall sense of well-being to monitor and modify therapy. Intercurrent illness, trauma, or planned surgery may require transient doubling of doses of pharmacologic glucocorticoid preparations to meet the demands of superimposed physiologic stress. Patients should be provided with prefilled syringes containing *dexamethasone* (4 mg Decadron® in 1 mL NS) that can be administered intramuscularly or subcutaneously in emergency situations (i.e., illness that prevents PO dosing of home medications). Primary adrenal insufficiency may also require treatment with mineralocorticoid replacement therapy. *Fludrocortisone* (Florinef® 0.1–0.2 mg/d) is the agent of choice. Orthostatic vital signs, serum potassium levels, and plasma renin activity levels may be measured to assess the adequacy of mineralocorticoid replacement.

313

Hyperaldosteronism

Primary aldosteronism Secretion of aldosterone from the zona glomerulosa of the adrenal cortex is mediated by the renin-angiotensin axis. Excessive secretion of aldosterone leads to increased uptake of sodium (Na^+) and increased excretion of potassium (K^+) in the collecting tubules of the kidney. Over time, this may lead to development of hypertension and hypokalemia. See Table 9.19.

Symptoms Tend to be nonspecific. May include fatigue, weakness, headaches, polydipsia, and polyuria.

Signs Hypertension in young adults without personal or family risk factors, hypertension refractory to multiple medications, and concomitant hypokalemia. Note that hypokalemia is not necessary to make a diagnosis of primary hyperaldosteronism and may only be present in later-stage disease.

Causes of primary aldosteronism Approximately 75% of all cases caused by growth of an autonomously functioning, aldosterone-producing adrenal adenoma (also known as Conn's syndrome). The remainder are caused by idiopathic hyperaldosteronism, a condition characterized by bilateral micronodular or macronodular hyperplasia of the adrenal cortex. Rare causes include adrenal carcinoma and glucocorticoid-remediable hypertension.

Treatment of aldosterone-producing adrenal adenomas Mild cases of primary aldosteronism may be treated medically (see medical treatments, below). Localized lesions in the appropriate candidate should be surgically resected by unilateral laparoscopic adrenalectomy. Pre-treatment with *spironolactone* (Aldactone® 12.5–200 mg bid) or *eplerenone* (Inspra® 25–50 mg bid) titrated to control BP for 2–4 wks prior to surgery may reduce risk of perioperative complications associated with changes in BP.

Medical treatment of bilateral disease or idiopathic hyperaldosteronism Long-term medical therapy based on treatment with aldosterone receptor blockers titrated to control BP and normalize serum K+ levels should be employed in these cases. Available agents include *spironolactone* (Aldactone® 12.5–200 mg bid) and *eplerenone* (Inspra® 25–50 mg bid). Patients who cannot tolerate aldosterone receptor blockers may be treated with *amiloride* (Midamor® 5–15 mg bid) in combination with other antihypertensive agents.

Glucocorticoid-remediable aldosteronism (GRA) should be suspected in patients <20 yrs with confirmed primary aldosteronism and in those with a family history of (1) hyperaldosteronism or (2) strokes at a young age (<40). Genetic testing is available. GRA should be managed medically with a low dose of glucocorticoid to normalize BP and serum potassium rather than a mineralocorticoid antagonist.

Table 9.19 Evaluation of suspected primary aldosteronism[9]

1 Screen for inappropriate aldosterone secretion by checking a plasma aldosterone level and a plasma renin activity level[*]
   - Plasma aldosterone >15 ng/dL and/or plasma aldosterone/plasma renin activity ratio >30 = inappropriate aldosterone secretion consistent with possible primary aldosteronism
   - If the results of above testing are not diagnostic and suspicion remains high, refer to endocrinology for possible discontinuation of other confounding medications[**] and retesting.
2 If primary aldosteronism is suspected, refer to endocrinology for one of four confirmatory tests: (1) Oral sodium loading test, (2) saline infusion test, (3) fludrocortisone suppression testing, or (4) captopril challenge test.
3 If primary aldosteronism is confirmed, consider targeted adrenal imaging with abdominal CT scanning, abdominal MRI scanning, or iodo-cholesterol scintigraphy scanning to identify and characterize adrenal abnormalities.
4 If targeted imaging is unrevealing or equivocal, consider bilateral adrenal vein sampling at an experienced center to determine whether lateralization of aldosterone secretion consistent with an aldosterone-producing adrenal adenoma is present.

[*] If the patient is being treated with an aldosterone receptor blocker (spironolactone, eplerenone, amiloride, triamterene)or potassium-wasting diuretic, or is using products derived from licorice root (confections or chewing tobacco), discontinue treatment and wait at least 4 wks before testing.

[**] Withdraw for additional 2 wks: β-blockers, central α2-agonists, NSAIDs, ACE-inhibitors, ARBS, rennin inhibitors, dihydropyridine calcium channel antagonists.

Pheochromocytoma

Represents a rare catecholamine-secreting neoplasm (Table 9.20). ~85% develop within the adrenal medulla, with 5–10% presenting in bilateral distributions and 10% eventually proving to be malignant. Catecholamine-secreting neoplasms that are identified in extra-adrenal locations (abdomen, thorax, head, neck) are called *paragangliomas*. ~15–20% of pheochromocytomas are associated with familial (genetic) disorders: MEN-2 syndromes, von Hippel–Lindau (VHL) syndrome, and neurofibromatosis type 1. Overall, pheochromocytomas account for <0.2% of all cases of newly diagnosed hypertension.

Symptoms Episodic paroxysms that may present with varying constellations of symptoms including episodic headaches, sweating, and palpitations. Other symptoms may include diaphoresis, anxiety, tremulousness, fatigue, nausea, vomiting, abdominal pain, chest pain, polyuria, polydipsia, and visual disturbances.

Signs Sustained or paroxysmal hypertension is characteristic, although 5–15% of patients present with normal BP. Peripheral vasoconstriction during paroxysms may produce transient pallor. Resultant increase in core body temperature may lead to subsequent flushing. Increased ESR, hyperglycemia, and stress-induced cardiomyopathy have been reported.

Table 9.20 Evaluation of suspected pheochromocytoma

1 Screen for increased catecholamine secretion by checking a plasma free metanephrine levels or 24 h urine metanephrine and catecholamine levels.
   - Plasma free metanephrine levels; screening test of choice when available; sensitivity is >99%, specificity is 89%.
   - Urine metanephrine and catecholamine levels (24 h collection). Labetalol, tricyclic antidepressants, levodopa, decongestants, amphetamines, reserpine, ethanol, prochlorperazine, acetaminophen, and buspirone may artifactually increase levels.
   - Normal plasma free metanephrine or urine metanephrine/catecholamine levels = excluded
   - Markedly elevated plasma free metanephrine or urine metanephrine/catecholamine levels (2–4× >normal) = pheochromocytoma
   - Marginally elevated plasma free metanephrine or urine metanephrine/catecholamine levels = increased catecholamine secretion consistent with a possible pheochromocytoma versus other stressor (hypertension, myocardial infarction, sepsis, etc.)
2 If a possible pheochromocytoma is suspected, check repeat plasma free metanephrine levels or urine metanephrine/catecholamine levels.
3 Normal repeat plasma free metanephrine or urine metanephrine/catecholamine levels = excluded
4 Marginally elevated repeat plasma free metanephrine or urine metanephrine/catecholamine levels = increased catecholamine secretion consistent with a possible pheochromocytoma. Consider referral to an endocrinologist who may perform confirmatory tests.
5 If a pheochromocytoma is confirmed, consider targeted adrenal imaging with abdominal CT scanning or abdominal MRI scanning to identify and characterize adrenal abnormalities; pheochromocytomas may show a characteristic bright intensity on T2-weighted MRI images.
6 If targeted imaging is unrevealing or equivocal, consider whole-body imaging with metaiodobenzylguanidine (MIBG), 111-IN-pentetreotide scintigraphy, total body MRI or positron emission tomography (PET) scanning to attempt to localize a suspicious focus of increased catecholamine secretion.

Treatment Surgical resection of benign pheochromocytomas and paragangliomas may be curative. Patients require preoperative treatment with α-blockers started at least 2 wks (and preferably 1 month) prior to planned procedures. Agents used for this purpose include *phenoxybenzamine* (Dibenzyline® 10–100 mg/d) and *doxazosin* (Cardura® 2–8 mg/d). Doses should be titrated every few days to target normotensive BPs. Patient should feel orthostatic if dosing is correct. Intraoperative hypertensive crises may require treatment with *phentolamine* or *nitroprusside*. Postoperatively, patients may require aggressive volume repletion and monitoring for symptoms and signs of incipient hypoglycemia.

MEN-2a and -2b See section on Hyperparathyroidism.

Von Hippel Lindau syndrome Includes pheochromocytoma (frequently bilateral), rarely paraganglioma, with retinal angiomas, cerebellar hemangioblastoma, epididymal cystadenoma, renal and pancreatic cysts, renal cell carcinoma, and pancreatic neuroendocrine tumors. Mutations in the VHL tumor suppressor gene leading to loss of function of VHL protein.

Neurofibromatosis type 1 (NF1) Includes bilateral or unilateral pheochromocytoma, rarely paraganglioma, with neurofibromas, axillary and inguinal freckling, iris hamartomas (Lisch nodules), and café au lait spots. Genetic testing for autosomal dominant mutations in NF1, although not always necessary if clinical phenotype is clear.

Genetic screening Referral to an endocrinologist for genetic testing for familial types of pheochromocytoma and paraganglioma should be made in the following cases:

- Paraganglioma at any site
- Bilateral adrenal pheochromocytoma
- Unilateral pheochromocytoma with family history of pheochromocytoma/ paraganglioma
- Unilateral pheochromocytoma at a young age (<30 years)
- Other clinical findings suggesting genetic syndromes (MEN-2a or -2b, VHL, NF1)

Hirsutism

Defined as new or increased abnormal growth of thick, coarse, pigmented terminal hair in females. May be distributed in regions commonly associated with male secondary sexual characteristics including the face, chest, back, lower abdomen, and inner thighs. May be caused by (a) increased secretion of androgens from the ovaries, (b) increased secretion of androgens from the adrenal cortex, or (c) increased 5α-reductase activity leading to increased conversion of testosterone to dihydrotestosterone at target tissues. Hirsutism may be idiopathic in nature or based on ethnic heritage. Hyperprolactinemia is a rare cause of hirsutism.

Increased secretion of androgens from the ovaries Most common cause is polycystic ovary syndrome (see below). May also be associated with ovarian hyperthecosis or, rarely, the growth of androgen-secreting ovarian neoplasms.

Increased secretion of androgens from the adrenal cortex Most common cause is nonclassic (late-onset) congenital adrenal hyperplasia (CAH) associated with 21-hydroxylase deficiency. May also be caused by Cushing's syndrome, growth of androgen-secreting adrenal adenomas, or growth of adrenal carcinomas.

Evaluation Should initially focus on identification and quantification of abnormal terminal hair growth using a Ferriman- Gallwey score. Patients may need to limit cosmetic treatment for a period to allow for accurate assessment. Reproductive history should focus on identification of significant menstrual irregularities and problems with infertility. Biochemical evaluation of hirsutism should be performed in women (1) with moderate or severe hirsutism, (2) when hirsutism is of rapid and progressive onset to exclude tumor, or (3) if the hirsutism is associated with obesity, irregular menses, or frank virilization (see Table 9.21).

Polycystic ovary syndrome Clinical diagnosis based on identification of a history of significant menstrual irregularities in conjunction with findings consistent with hyperandrogenism (hirsutism, comedonal acne, male pattern balding, etc.). National Institute of Health consensus criteria for the diagnosis of PCOS include: (1) menstrual irregularities due to oligo- or anovulation, (2) clinical (hirsutism, acne, etc.) or biochemical (high serum androgens) evidence of hyperandrogenism, and (3) exclusion of other causes of hyperandrogenism. Only the Rotterdam criteria[12] indicate that polycystic ovaries by ultrasound are necessary for a PCOS diagnosis.

Pathophysiology A complex syndrome in which both genetics and environmental factors contribute to the onset and severity of the condition.In part, may be caused by relative increase in secretion of luteinizing hormone (LH) leading to increased production and secretion of androgens from the ovaries. May lead to enlargement and polycystic thickening of the ovarian capsule. Subsequent conversion of androgens to estrogen may lead to endometrial hyperplasia. Insulin resistance with resultant hyperinsulinemia is frequently found in PCOS, which may also promote androgen secretion by theca cells. Women with PCOS my have genetic predisposition to hyperandrogenism. Groups at risk for PCOS include women with (a) T1DM, T2DM, or gestational diabetes; (b) obesity or insulin resistance; (c) history of premature adrenarche; (d)first-degree relatives with PCOS; or (e)

Table 9.21 Evaluation of hirsutism[10]

1 Check early morning total and free testosterone levels* and dehydroepiandrosterone-sulfate (DHEA-S) levels. If menses are irregular, also check a serum prolactin level.
- Elevated serum prolactin level = consider prolactin-producing pituitary tumor; pituitary MRI may be warranted for further evaluation.
- Total testosterone > upper limit of reference range for females but <150 ng/dL = likely polycystic ovarian syndrome
- Total testosterone >150 ng/dL + DHEA-S <700 mcg/dL = possible androgen-secreting ovarian neoplasm; consider targeted imaging with transvaginal pelvic ultrasonography.

2 Total testosterone >150 ng/dL + DHEA-S >700 mcg/dL = possible Cushing's syndrome, androgen-secreting adrenal adenoma, or adrenal carcinoma; consider formal evaluation for hypercortisolemia (see Cushing's syndrome) or targeted imaging of adrenal glands with abdominal CT or MRI scanning. If nonclassic (late-onset) CAH is suspected, check a base-line 17-hydroxyprogesterone level, administer 250 mcg of *cosyntropin* (Cortrosyn®) IV, then checkrepeat 17-hydroxyprogesterone levels at 30 and 60 min.
- Baseline 17-hydroxyprogesterone >200 ng/dL + stimulated 17-hydroxy-progesterone >1,500 ng/dL = nonclassic CAH

*Free testosterone should be checked in a specialty lab where assays are more accurate.

10 Evaluation and treatment of hirsutism in premenopausal women: An Endocrine Society clinical practice guideline. *J Clin Endolcrinol Metabol.* 2008.

oligo-ovulatory fertility. Women with suspected PCOS should be screened for insulin resistance and other components of the metabolic syndrome.

PCOS and infertility Oligo- or anovulation associated with hyperandrogenism and PCOS often complicates conception.In overweight women, weight loss should be encouraged to lower androgen levels and, often, restore normal ovulation. Pharmacotherapeutic interventions include *clomiphene citrate* (Clomid® 50–100 mg/d × 5 d starting on the fifth day of the menstrual cycle) or *metformin* (Glucophage® 500–1,000 mg bid, Glucophage XR® 1,000–2,000 mg qpm). Some studies show that these agents may be used in combination to help to induce ovulation. Exogenous gonadotropin (LH and follicle-stimulating hormone [FSH]) therapy may also induce ovulation. Patients who do not desire fertility may be treated with oral contraceptives that combine 30–35 mcg of ethinyl estradiol with progestins known to demonstrate minimal androgenic activity (desogestrel, norethindrone). Metformin may also help to manage oligomenorrhea, promote weight loss, and prevent T2DM.

Nonclassic (late-onset) CAH

Condition associated with decreased production and secretion of glucocorticoids due to 21-hydroxylase deficiency that leads to increased secretion of ACTH.[13] Increased ACTH levels stimulate secretion of androgens from the adrenal cortex. Findings consistent with exposure to increased levels of circulating androgens may first become evident at the onset of puberty with premature pubarche, acne, hirsutism, and menstrual irregularities.More common in women of Hispanic, Eastern European Jewish, or Yugoslav descent. Confirmation of CAH based on measurement of baseline and stimulated 17-hydroxyprogesterone levels (see Table 9.21). Treatment for nonclassic CAH aimed at management of hirsutism and oligo- or anovulation.

Antiandrogen therapy *Spironolactone* (Aldactone 50–200 mg/d) acts to inhibit binding of dihydrotestosterone to target receptors. It may be used as a first-line agent or in conjunction with other therapies. Continuous treatment for up to 6 months may be necessary before efficacy can be determined. Cosmetic treatments involving shaving, plucking, waxing, bleaching, electrolysis, or use of depilatories may still be required to achieve desired appearances.

Oral contraceptives In women who do not desire fertility, oral contraceptives may be used alone (or in combination with antiandrogens) for menstrual cycle management and suppression of ACTH and ovarian/adrenal androgens.

Glucocorticoid therapy Given the potential risks and side effects of long-term glucocorticoid therapy, this treatment is usually reserved for women with anovulatory infertility. Treatment usually involves use of *dexamethasone* (Decadron® 0.25–0.75 mg qhs) at doses targeted to suppress ACTH levels.If glucocorticoids are ineffective, other assisted reproduction techniques may be needed to induce ovulation. Glucocorticoid treatment should be discontinued when fertility is no longer desired.

Virilization Constellation of findings that reflect exposure to markedly elevated levels of circulating androgens. Patients may present with frontal (male pattern) balding, deepening of the voice, clitoral enlargement, and increased muscle mass. Presence or rapid onset of signs should raise suspicion of an underlying androgen-secreting ovarian or adrenal neoplasm.

Gynecomastia

Defined as enlargement of breast tissue in males. Transient, self-limited gynecomastia may be evident in up to 70% of males during puberty. Enlargement that persists or presents as a new development in adult males may be considered abnormal. May develop as a result of a range of different underlying disorders that promote relative imbalances between circulating levels of estrogens and androgens (see Table 9.22). Continued exposure to relatively increased circulating levels of estrogens may promote growth of ductal and stromal elements in breast tissue. Usually bilateral. Discernible as a firm concentric ridge of tissue that extends beyond the perimeter of the areola. May be painful, with associated tenderness to palpation.

Evaluation Should focus on (a) quantification of extent of breast tissue, (b) documentation of any history of exposure to possible offending agents, and (c) measurement of total and free testosterone, estradiol, LH, HCG, liver function tests, and TSH levels. If findings consistent with undetected Klinefelter's are evident on exam (tall stature, widened arm span, small testicular size), a karyotype may be performed to confirm a suspected diagnosis. If a suspiciously firm or enlarged breast mass is detected on exam, a mammogram may be considered to check for possible male breast cancer. Elevated serum HCG should prompt testicular ultrasound and urologic referral.

Treatment Should be centered on identification and treatment of underlying disorders. Gynecomastia may persist long after relative balance between circulating levels of estrogens and androgens has been restored. In cases presenting with significant pain, tenderness, or cosmetic deformity, surgical bilateral reduction mammoplasty may be indicated.

Table 9.22 Mechanisms of disorders associated with gynecomastia

- Increased production of sex hormone-binding globulin leads to increased binding of testosterone that decreases circulating free testosterone levels; this may occur in the setting of thyrotoxicosis or chronic liver disease.
- Excessive stimulation of Leydig cells due to exposure to elevated LH levels; leads to increased secretion of estrogens; this condition may develop as a complication of primary hypogonadism associated with Klinefelter's syndrome or adult Leydig cell failure. This may also occur as part of the refeeding syndrome.
- Excessive stimulation of Leydig cells due to exposure to elevated human chorionic gonadotropin (HCG) levels; leads to increased secretion of estrogens; this may be associated with the growth of germ cell testicular neoplasms that secrete excessive amounts of HCG. Also seen in body-builders abusing HCG as a part of an anabolic steroid regimen.
- Inhibition of binding of dihydrotestosterone to target receptors; may be associated with treatment with spironolactone or cimetidine.
- Direct binding of estrogen receptors; may be associated with treatment with digoxin; it may also occur as a result of exposure to phytoestrogens present in marijuana.

Pituitary adenomas

The incidence of detection of sellar masses has increased with more wide-spread use of neuroradiographic imaging to evaluate neurologic symptoms. Dedicated pituitary MRI scanning with gadolinium provides the most accurate assessment of the size and location of a suspected pituitary adenoma. The maximum diameter may be used to classify a suspected pituitary adenoma as a microadenoma (<10 mm) or a macroadenoma (<10 mm). Evaluation requires determining whether a suspected pituitary adenoma is (1) functional (secreting stimulating hormones that may lead to development of characteristic clinical syndromes) or (2) nonfunctional but impairing the normal secretion of hormones by adjacent pituitary tissue.[14] Some functional pituitary adenomas may be treated medically, whereas others require surgery. See Table 9.23.

Evaluation Comprehensive functional evaluation of a suspected pituitary adenoma may incorporate (a) static testing based on measurement of TSH, free T4, prolactin, and IGF-1 levels, and (b) dynamic testing based on performance of an overnight low-dose dexamethasone stimulation test and a GH suppression test. 24 h urine free cortisol levels or salivary cortisol levels may be measured as well.

Nonfunctional pituitary adenomas If a suspected pituitary adenoma proves to be nonfunctional, further evaluation should focus on determining whether its growth may be associated with (a) hypopituitarism, (b) hyperprolactinemia, (c) visual field deficits caused by upward growth with compression of the optic chiasm, (d) cranial nerve palsies caused by lateral extension into the cavernous sinuses, or (e) severe headaches caused by pressure and traction on meningeal structures. Symptomatic nonfunctional pituitary adenomas may require surgery to preserve eyesight or alleviate headaches. Asymptomatic nonfunctional pituitary adenomas may often be followed with serial imaging and visual field testing.

Pituitary apoplexy Hemorrhage into an undetected or previously identified pituitary adenoma may cause sudden pituitary expansion leading to a severe headache. Upward expansion may precipitate compression of the optic chiasm with loss of visual acuity. Lateral expansion may lead to compression of cranial blood vessels and herniation. Expansion within the constrained space of the sella may lead to rapid development

---

Table 9.23 Clinical syndromes associated with functional pituitary adenomas

- Prolactin-secreting pituitary adenoma (prolactinoma) = hyperprolactinemia (high serum prolactin)
- ACTH-secreting pituitary adenoma (Cushing's disease) = ACTH-dependent Cushing's syndrome (high serum ACTH and cortisol)
- Growth hormone (GH)-secreting pituitary adenoma = acromegaly (high serum IGF-1)
- TSH-secreting pituitary adenoma = hyperthyroidism (high serum TSH and free T4)

FSH and LH-secreting pituitary adenomas do not appear to correlate with specific clinical syndromes

---

14 Freda PU, et al. Pituitary incidentaloma: An Endocrine Society clinical practice guideline. *J Clin Endocrinol Metabol.* 2011. 96(4):894–904.

of central (secondary) adrenal insufficiency that may provoke an adrenal crisis. Suspected cases of apoplexy require (a) treatment with stress-dose glucocorticoids, (b) urgent assessment of visual acuity, and (c) urgent neurosurgical decompression versus high-dose steroid administration.

Hypopituitarism

Condition characterized by deficiency of one or more of the stimulating or trophic hormones secreted by the anterior pituitary. May be caused by (1) disorders that disrupt the function of the anterior pituitary itself or (2) disorders that disrupt hypothalamic regulation of the anterior pituitary. The principal stimulating and trophic hormones secreted by clusters of cells in the anterior pituitary include ACTH, TSH, GH, FSH, and LH.

Causes of hypopituitarism Common acquired causes include pituitary surgery, cranial irradiation, head trauma, compression due to growth of pituitary adenomas, or other cranial tumors that impinge upon the sella. Rare causes include hypovolemic pituitary infarction (Sheehan's syndrome), hemochromatosis, disseminated tuberculosis, pituitary abscess, pituitary metastases, lymphocytic hypophysitis, and trauma. There are also inherited, genetic disorders that cause hypopituitarism (POU1F1 defects, PROP1 mutations, etc.).

Evaluation Comprehensive evaluation of suspected hypopituitarism may incorporate (a) targeted imaging with dedicated pituitary MRI scanning; (b) static early morning testing based on measurement of ACTH, TSH, free T4, FSH, LH, testosterone, cortisol, and insulin-like growth factor 1 (IGF-1) levels; and (c) dynamic testing based on performance of a cosyntropin stimulation test and a GH stimulation test.

Central pituitary disorders Deficiencies of pituitary hormones (TSH, LH, FSH, GH, AND ACTH) present clinically in different ways. Clinical presentation will depend on how deficiency of the stimulating and trophic hormones affect target tissues and glands. These disorders are referred to as central or "secondary" forms of clinical syndromes and result from either pituitary or, rarely, hypothalamic dysfunction.

Central adrenal insufficiency Presentation may vary, depending on the acuity of the underlying cause. With rapid deficiency of ACTH (apoplexy, ischemia, trauma), patients may present in adrenal crisis (see above). With more prolonged deficiency of ACTH (tumor, infection, infiltration), the presentation may be insidious and include nonspecific weight loss, fatigue, and weakness. Diagnosis based on confirmation of a cosyntropin-stimulated plasma cortisol <18 mcg/dL in conjunction with a plasma ACTH <30 pg/mL. Condition is treated with glucocorticoid replacement therapy. Mineralocorticoid replacement therapy is usually not necessary, given that aldosterone secretion by adrenals (not controlled centrally) remains intact.

Central hypothyroidism Patients may present with characteristic symptoms and signs reflecting deficiency of thyroid hormone (fatigue, weight gain, dry skin, etc.). Diagnosis based on confirmation of a low or inappropriately normal TSH level in conjunction with a low free T4 level. In some cases, it may be prudent to check a free T4 level measured by equilibrium dialysis to provide verification. Treatment with thyroid hormone replacement required. TSH levels do not provide an accurate index of replacement in this setting. Doses of levothyroxine should be adjusted to target normal free T4 levels

Central hypogonadism Often classified as hypogonadotropic hypogonadism. Manifestations may vary depending on age of onset. Sex steroid deficiency that develops during childhood may lead to delayed or absent onset of puberty. Premenopausal adult females may present with oligomenorrhea or amenorrhea. Diagnosis in females is based on confirmation of low or inappropriately normal FSH and LH levels in conjunction with a previously normal menstrual and reproductive history. Treatment usually involves estrogen and progesterone replacement with oral contraceptives. Conception may require successive courses of ovulation induction and in vitro fertilization. Adult males with hypogonadotrophic hypogonadism may present with variable symptoms that may include a diminished libido, erectile dysfunction, impotence, and an appreciable decline in muscle strength. Examination may reveal diminished growth of facial hair and body hair, decreased muscle mass, low BMD, and fine wrinkles at the corners of the eyes and mouth. Diagnosis in males is based on confirmation of a low or inappropriately normal LH level in conjunction with a low testosterone level. Treatment involves androgen replacement therapy with *testosterone* administered as a 1% topical gel (AndroGel® 5–10 g qam, Testim® 5–10 g qam), a transdermal patch (Androderm® 2.5–10 mg qhs), or an intramuscular depot injection (testosterone cypionate 50–400 mg IM every 2–4 wks). Doses may be adjusted to target testosterone levels in the normal range. Blood counts should be monitored for polycythemia, and prostate-specific antigen (PSA) should be followed.

Central growth hormone deficiency Manifestations may vary depending on age of onset. Growth hormone deficiency that develops during childhood may lead to short stature. Adults may present with low BMD and changes in body composition discernible as an increase in fat mass and decrease in lean body mass. Diagnosis is based on confirmation of a low serum IGF-1 level by itself or in conjunction with an abnormal growth hormone stimulation test. Serum GH should not be measured to screen for GH deficiency and should only be assessed during formal GH stimulation testing. Growth hormone stimulation tests are performed by measuring GH levels before and after administration of glucagon, a provocative agent thought to stimulate GH indirectly via insulin release. A peak GH level <3 ng/mL may be consistent with growth hormone deficiency. Insulin tolerance tests (ITT) also stimulate GH secretion. Both glucagon and ITT testing require careful monitoring of blood glucose levels, as hypoglycemia can occur. Treatment of GH deficiency involves daily administration of subcutaneous injections of *recombinant human growth hormone*. Doses may be adjusted to target normal IGF-1 levels.[15]

Hyperprolactinemia

Physiology Prolactin is constitutively secreted by lactotroph cells in the anterior pituitary. Dopamine secreted by the hypothalamus travels along the pituitary stalk through the hypophyseal portal circulation to bind to dopamine receptors on lactotroph cells. This binding of dopamine inhibits the secretion of prolactin. Several different underlying mechanisms may lead to increased secretion of prolactin with resultant hyperprolactinemia (Table 9.24).

Symptoms Hyperprolactinemia may suppress secretion of gonadotropin releasing hormone (GnRH), effectively inhibiting secretion of FSH and LH. This may lead to development of hypogonadotropic hypogonadism. Premenopausal adult females may present with oligomenorrhea, amenorrhea, or infertility. Elevated prolactin levels in premenopausal females may also stimulate abnormal secretion of milk from one or both breasts, a condition known as *galactorrhea*. Adult males may present with a diminished libido, erectile dysfunction, or impotence.

15 Moltich ME, et al. Evaluation and management of adult growth hormone deficiency: An Endocrine Society clinical practice guideline. *J Clin Endocrinol Metabol*. 2011.96(6):1587–1609.

Table 9.24 Mechanisms of disorders associated with hyperprolactinemia

- Proliferation of lactotroph cells in the form of a prolactin-secreting pituitary adenoma (prolactinoma) leads to increased constitutive secretion of prolactin
- Exposure to agents that inhibit binding of dopamine to dopamine receptors; most commonly implicated agents are those used to treat psychosis (haloperidol, risperidone, chlorpromazine, olanzapine), GI drugs (metoclopramide, cimetidine), opiates (codeine, morphine), and antihypertensive agents (methyldopa, verapamil, reserpine).
- Compression of the pituitary stalk may interrupt passage of dopamine through the hypophyseal portal system; stalk compression may be associated with growth of nonfunctional pituitary adenomas or other sellar and suprasellar masses.
- Increased secretion of prolactin caused by increased secretion of TRH; precise mechanism is unclear; hyperprolactinemia may develop in cases of untreated primary hypothyroidism.
- Macroprolactin is a benign cause of elevated serum prolactin levels. "Big prolactin" forms when 23-kD molecules become glycosylated. Diagnose with serum macroprolactin measurements in patients without symptoms of hyperprolactinemia.
- Rare causes of hyperprolactinemia: Nipple stimulation/chest wall injury, chronic kidney disease, excessive estrogen intake.

Evaluation Initial evaluation should focus on (a) documenting a recent medication history to check for exposure to specific agents and (b) measuring a TSH level to check for primary hypothyroidism. Prolactin >200 ng/mL should raise suspicion for prolactinoma. Further evaluation may require dedicated pituitary MRI scanning with gadolinium to check for the presence of a sellar mass that may represent a prolactin-secreting pituitary adenoma or a nonfunctional pituitary adenoma with stalk compression.

Treatment of prolactin-secreting pituitary adenomas Many prolactin-secreting pituitary adenomas are very responsive to treatment with dopamine agonists alone.[16] Reduction in size with diminished secretion of prolactin may be confirmed in up to 90% of successfully treated patients. *Cabergoline* (Dostinex® 0.5 mg) is preferred as a first-line agent. Usual starting dose is 0.25 mg twice a week. May be advanced as tolerated to 1 mg twice a week. Dose-limiting side effects may include nausea, orthostasis, and cognitive impairment. *Bromocriptine* (Parlodel® 2.5 mg bid-tid) may also be considered as an alternative agent when cost, availability, or intolerance of cabergoline side effects present difficulties. Prolactin levels may be checked 2–3 wks after starting treatment or after adjusting a dose of a dopamine agonist to gauge efficacy. Changes in prolactinoma size may be detected on pituitary MRI scans checked 6–8 wks after starting treatment. In cases where patients require treatment but (1) cannot tolerate therapeutic doses of dopamine agonists or (2) tumor is unresponsive to medical therapy, surgery may be considered. Microadenomas can usually be removed via transsphenoidal approaches. Removal of larger macroadenomas may require craniotomy. Success rates following initial surgery vary. Persistent disease may require repeat surgery and/or treatment with external beam radiation.

16 Melmed S, et al. Diagnosis and treatment of hyperprolactinemia: An Endocrine Society clinical practice guideline. *J Clin Endocrinol Metabol*. 2011. 96(2):273–288.

Treatment of prolactin-secreting pituitary adenomas during pregnancy Increased production and secretion of estrogen during pregnancy may promote growth and expansion of prolactin-secreting pituitary adenomas. Macroadenomas may expand and cause visual field deficits or severe headaches. Women who require treatment of hyperprolactinemia to become pregnant should be placed on bromocriptine due to the greater certainty that it does not cause birth defects. If possible, dopamine agonists should be discontinued in pregnancy. Clinical monitoring every 3 months during pregnancy should include questioning about headaches and visual changes. If the location or size of the prolactinoma requires continued medical management during pregnancy, treatment with *bromocriptine* can be continued or reinitiated. In cases of known macroadenomas, particularly those that abut the optic chiasm, expectant management may focus on considering surgery prior to conception to prevent potential complications. Should visual acuity decline or neurologic symptoms progress during pregnancy, dedicated pituitary MRI scanning and visual field testing may be required to assess tumor growth. If necessary, surgery may be considered during the second trimester.

Acromegaly

A rare systemic syndrome resulting from exposure to excessive levels of GH. The most common cause is proliferation of somatotroph cells in the form of a GH-secreting pituitary adenoma. GH stimulates increased production and secretion of IGF-1 in the liver. Over time, excessive circulating levels of IGF-1 may lead to growth and enlargement of somatic tissues.

Signs Changes in appearance may be insidious, developing gradually over the course of several years (Table 9.25). Review of older photographs may help to establish timing and extent of changes. Overgrowth of soft tissues may lead to coarsening of facial features. Patients and observers may note bossing of the frontal bones, expansion of the nose, enlargement of the tongue (macroglossia), deepening of the voice, and increased prominence of the jaw with resultant spacing of the teeth. Spade-like enlargement of the hands and feet may prompt successive changes in ring and shoe sizes. Carpal tunnel syndrome, skin tag formation, excessive sweating (hyperhidrosis), and hirsutism are also associated with acromegaly. Bone density may be increased in men and premenopausal women. Findings consistent with left ventricular hypertrophy may be evident.

Complications Untreated acromegaly may be associated with the development of hypertension, cardiomyopathy, heart failure, T2DM, hypertrophic cardiomyopathy, colonic neoplasia, and obstructive sleep apnea.

Table 9.25 Evaluation of suspected acromegaly

1 Screen for elevated GH secretion by checking a serum IGF-1 level.
2 If the IGF-1 level is elevated, check a GH suppression test.
   • GH suppression test is performed by measuring a baseline GH level, administering a 75 g oral glucose tolerance test load, then measuring GH levels at 30, 60, 90, and 120 min marks.
      • Peak GH <1 ng/mL = normal response
      • Peak GH >2 ng/mL = acromegaly
3 Consider dedicated pituitary MRI scanning with gadolinium to check for the presence of a sellar mass that may represent a GH-secreting pituitary adenoma. Note that, at the time of diagnosis, many tumors are macroadenomas (>10 mm in size).

Treatment Principal treatment is surgical resection. Smaller macroadenomas can usually be removed via transsphenoidal approaches. Removal of larger macroadenomas may require craniotomy. Success rates following initial surgery vary. Documentation of cure may depend on demonstrating (a) normal postsurgical IGF-1 levels, (b) postsurgical serum GH concentration <2.5 ng/mL, and (c) a postsurgical GH suppression test with a peak GH <1 ng/mL. Persistent disease may require repeat surgery, treatment with external beam radiation, and/or initiation of medical therapy targeted to inhibit secretion of GH from residual pituitary tissue or antagonize growth hormone receptors to inhibit production and secretion of IGF-1.

Medical therapy targeted to inhibit secretion of GH Somatostatin analogs act by binding to somatostatin receptors on target tissues and inhibiting GH secretion. *Octreotide* and *lanreotide* are commercially available somatostatin analogs. Octreotide is available in a short-acting subcutaneous preparation (Sandostatin®) and a long-acting IM preparation (Sandostatin LAR®). Lanreotide is only available as a long-acting analog (Somatuline ®Depot). Limiting side effects of both agents may include nausea, abdominal discomfort, hyperglycemia, and cholelithiasis. Patients who tolerate test doses may be continued on escalating doses of the short-acting preparation or may be switched to the long-acting preparations. Doses may be adjusted every 6–8 wks to target normalization of IGF-1 levels. In some cases, dopamine agonists may also inhibit secretion of GH from residual tissue and may be used alone or in concert with somatostatin analogs. *Cabergoline* (Dostinex® 0.5 mg, usual starting dose 0.25 mg twice a week) has proven to be more effective than other agents when used for this purpose. May be advanced as tolerated to 1 mg twice a week. Dose-limiting side effects may include nausea, orthostasis, and cognitive impairment.

Medical therapy targeted to inhibit production and secretion of IGF-1 *Pegvisomant* (Somavert®) is a modified form of GH that acts by competitively binding to GH receptors, inhibiting the production and secretion of IGF-1 in the liver. Clinical trials have shown that it may effectively normalize IGF-1 levels in patients who have failed to respond to treatment with somatostatin analogs. Can also be used in combination with somatostatin analogs. Side effects of this GH receptor antagonist include nausea, diarrhea, chest pain, and transaminitis that may require discontinuation of the drug.

Diabetes insipidus

Physiology of water balance Increased serum osmolality and decreased effective circulating volume stimulate release of antidiuretic hormone (ADH) from the supraoptic and paraventricular nuclei in the hypothalamus. Circulating ADH binds to receptors in the collecting tubules of the kidney, activating aquaporin channels that mediate increased reabsorption of free water (see figure). Diabetes insipidus is a disorder characterized by decreased reabsorption of free water in the collecting tubules. It may be precipitated by disorders that (1) interrupt the release of ADH from the hypothalamus (central diabetes insipidus) or (2) inhibit the action of ADH in the collecting tubules (nephrogenic diabetes insipidus). See Figure 9.2. Patients present with severe polyuria (urine output >3,000 mL/day) and compensatory polydipsia associated with the excretion of large volumes of dilute urine.

Primary polydipsia Also known as psychogenic polydipsia, is caused by excessive intake of water. Commonly seen in patients with psychiatric illness, although may be induced by hypothalamic injury or infiltration affecting thirst center.

Table 9.26 Water deprivation test

1 Starting after breakfast, hold all intake of fluids. Check the patient's baseline weight, pulse, and BP, and measure a baseline serum osmolality and serum sodium level.
  - Every hour, check the patient's weight, pulse, and BP.
  - Every 2 h, measure a serum osmolality and serum sodium level.
  - With each urine void, measure the urine volume and urine osmolality.

2 Consider terminating the test when one of the following endpoints has been reached*
  - Urine osmolality >600 mosm/kg
  - Serum osmolality >295–300 mosm/kg*
  - Serum sodium >145 meq/dL*

3 Interpretation:
  - Determine the maximum urine osmolality and calculate the percentage increase in urine osmolality following administration of vasopressin, if administered.
  - Maximum urine osmolality >500 mosm/kg = primary polydipsia
  - Maximum urine osmolality <500 mosm/kg = central or nephrogenic diabetes insipidus
  - Maximum urine osmolality <300 mosm/kg + 100–800% ↑ in urine osmolality = complete central diabetes insipidus
  - Maximum urine osmolality <300 mosm/kg + 15–50% ↑ in urine osmolality = partial central diabetes insipidus
  - Maximum urine osmolality >300 mosm/kg + 15–50% ↑ in urine osmolality = partial nephrogenic diabetes insipidus
  - Maximum urine osmolality >300 mosm/kg + <15% ↑ in urine osmolality = complete nephrogenic diabetes insipidus

* Administer desmopressin (10 mcg by nasal insufflation or 4 mcg SQ/IV), then measure the urine volume and urine osmolality with the next urine void before allowing resumption of fluid intake.

Causes of central diabetes insipidus Include neurosurgery, head trauma, growth of suprasellar masses, histiocytosis, neurosarcoidosis, hypothalamic metastases, hypoxic or ischemic events, and idiopathic etiologies.

Causes of nephrogenic diabetes insipidus Include exposure to lithium, hypercalcemia, hypokalemia, and hereditary forms of nephrogenic diabetes insipidus.

Evaluation of polyuria Principal goal is to determine whether elevated urine output is primarily driven by increased intake of free water (primary polydipsia) or by decreased reabsorption of free water (central or nephrogenic diabetes insipidus). Performance of a water deprivation test (Table 9.26) may clarify this distinction while providing clues to the root cause of diabetes insipidus.

Treatment of central diabetes insipidus Identify and treat any reversible conditions that may be interrupting the release of ADH from the hypothalamus. Persistent central diabetes insipidus may require long-term treatment with *desmopressin* (DDAVP®), an ADH analog that has minimal vasopressor activity. Desmopressin is available as a 10 mcg metered nasal spray and in 0.1 mg tablet form. The usual starting dose is one spray (10 mcg) intranasally or 0.05 mg PO taken at bedtime. Doses may be increased incrementally with expansion to twice daily administration to attenuate nocturia and daytime polyuria. Patients should be encouraged to pay attention to and honor their thirst.

Figure 9.2 Nephrogenic action of ADH

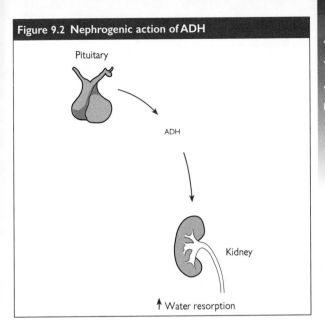

Pituitary

ADH

Kidney

↑ Water resorption

Treatment of nephrogenic diabetes insipidus Identify and treat any reversible conditions that may be inhibiting the action of ADH in the collecting tubules. Persistent nephrogenic diabetes insipidus may respond to treatment with *hydrochlorothiazide* (12.5–25 mg bid), *amiloride* (Midamor® 5–20 mg/d), or NSAIDs. Amiloride may be particularly effective in attenuating polyuria in patients who develop nephrogenic diabetes insipidus associated with exposure to lithium used to treat affective disorders.

Neurology

Jason Rosenberg, M.D.

Contents

Common chief complaints

Specific diseases and conditions

Approach to the neurology patient

Localization

For many neurological conditions, diagnosis begins with localization. In other words, to determine *what* type of pathology a patient is suffering, it is often helpful to start with determining *where* within the nervous system the lesion lies. For example, a patient complaining of weakness might have psychogenic, cortical, cerebellar, myelopathic (spinal cord), neuropathic, neuromuscular junction, or myopathic pathology. Identifying the level of dysfunction within the central or peripheral nervous system is critical for developing an appropriate differential. Diseases that affect the brain and spinal cord (the central nervous system) are distinct from peripheral nervous system pathologies.

Ironically, the proliferation of high-quality imaging techniques has made the traditional approach to the neurological history and examination more important than ever, both in terms of avoiding unnecessary expense and in preventing futile pursuits down blind alleys, chasing after coincidental or spurious findings. Thus, not only is localization critical in implicating a specific disease process or pathology, but localization prior to definitive diagnosis will guide appropriate testing; i.e., whether to order a magnetic resonance imaging (MRI) of the brain, of the cervical spine, of the thoracic spine, of the lumbar spine, or whether to order an electromyographic nerve conduction study (EMG-NCS).

Thus, this chapter opens with the classical neurological approach to the chief concern—*localization*—because it truly matters in the assessment of the individual patient. The anatomy, while admittedly dense and dry, is very much relevant. Clinically relevant examples will be peppered throughout to maintain your interest.

Where is the lesion? Localizing the site of the lesion depends on recognizing the *pattern* of cognitive, cranial nerve, motor, and sensory deficits that occur following lesions at different sites within the nervous system, as revealed by history and examination. The traditional "complete" neurological exam consists of a thorough assessment of mental status and higher cortical function, the cranial nerves, the motor system (bulk, tone, and power), sensation (touch, vibration, proprioception, pain, and temperature), deep tendon reflexes, coordination/cerebellar function, and gait. Techniques of even a neurological screening examination are beyond the scope of this chapter, but for reference, a reasonably thorough documentation of a normal exam is provided in Table 10.1, as are examples of abnormal findings. Weakness associated with aphasia or agnosia localizes the motor lesion to the cortex. Weakness associated with double vision or an asymmetric gag reflex signifies a brainstem lesion. Sensory loss below a segmental dermatome implicates spinal cord pathology. Weakness or sensory loss in the distribution of individual nerves localizes the dysfunction to the peripheral nervous system.

Patterns of motor deficits: Localizing the lesion responsible for weakness is initially dependent on identifying whether the pattern of motor weakness is more consistent with lower or upper motor neuron dysfunction (LMN or UMN; see Tables 10.2 and 10.3). The upper motor neuron is part of the central nervous system (CNS), extending all the way from the homunculus within the cortical motor strip, down through the brainstem, where they decussate (cross the midline) in the lower brainstem medulla, travel down through the spinal cord in white matter tracts, and eventually synapse in the anterior horn of the spinal cord with the lower motor neurons, which in turn extend their axons ipsilaterally through nerve roots and peripheral nerves to specific muscles.

Table 10.1 Neurological exam findings

Example of a normal neurological exam, in detail

Mental status: The patient is alert, attentive, fully oriented, and appropriate in terms of behavior, mood, and affect. Historical ability is good. Language function is normal, with fluent speech, normal comprehension, intact repetition, and no spontaneous or confrontational word finding difficulty. There is no dysarthria. There is no agnosia, apraxia, or neglect. Fund of knowledge is good, and recall is 3/3. There is no right/left confusion, and simple coin calculations are normal. There are no frontal release signs (glabellar, palmar-mental, grasp, snout, root, paratonia).

Cranial Nerves: Olfaction is normal in each nostril (coffee). Pupils are equal, round, and reactive to light and accommodation, without afferent papillary defects. Visual acuity and red color saturation are normal in each eye. Visual fields are full to confrontation. Optic discs are sharp with normal central venous pulsations. Extraocular movements are intact, with normal saccades and smooth pursuits, without nystagmus or any reported diplopia. Facial sensation is normal to pinprick in V1, V2, and V3 distributions bilaterally. Face is symmetric at rest, with equal movement/normal grimace. Hearing is intact to finger rubs bilaterally, with normal vestibular responses to head impulse testing bilaterally. Gag is intact, uvula is midline, and palate elevates symmetrically. Head turn and shoulder shrug are 5/5 bilaterally. Tongue is midline with normal movement and no atrophy or fasciculations at rest.

Motor exam is normal for bulk and tone throughout, and power is 5/5 in the major proximal and distal muscle groups of the bilateral upper and lower extremities. The patient can easily rise from a chair without the use of the arms and is able to walk on toes and on heels. There is no pronator drift and no obit sign. There are no adventitious movements. Deep tendon reflexes are 2+ throughout. There are no Hoffman signs, there is no ankle clonus, and toes are downgoing (negative Babinski).

Coordination is normal for fine finger movements, rapid alternating movements, finger-nose-finger, foot tapping, and heel-to-shin bilaterally. There is no ataxia or dysmetria.

Sensation is normal in the fingers to pinprick and texture, and in the toes to pinprick, vibration, and joint position sense. Romberg is negative.

Station and gait are narrow-based and normal, without limp, ataxia, imbalance, festination, magnetic quality, or reduced arm swing. Tandem gait is normal.

(Such an exam is rarely done or documented this exhaustively; typically a neurologist will actively "tailor" a screening exam to the individual patient and a non-neurologist will document the grossly abnormal findings on brief screening exam.)

Example of a report of pertinent exam findings in a patient with acute onset of new deficits:

The patient is fully awake and appears frustrated but denies pain, saying a few appropriate simple words but with stammering, nonfluent, slurred speech. He is able to follow simple commands and comply with exam testing. The patient blinks to visual threat from both visual fields and appears to feel pinpricks equally on both sides. Eyes move conjugately but appear to be deviated to the left, and there is obvious right facial weakness. There is a marked right-sided flaccid paresis of the arm with reduced reflexes, with weak flexor movement of the elbow only. There is at least 4/5 strength of the right leg throughout, hip flexion and plantar flexion appearing to be the weakest, with slowed foot tapping. Reflexes may be slightly reduced compared to the left, but the right toe is upgoing. The left side is intact in terms of power, coordination, and reflexes. The patient winces to pinprick in the arms and the legs bilaterally. Gait was not tested due to concerns for safety.

(Continued)

Table 10.1 (Continued)

Or, more succinctly:

The fully awake patient has a nonfluent aphasia with decent comprehension, left eye deviation without field cut, and left-sided flaccid hemiparesis face and arm>leg with an upgoing toe and intact sensation.

Given such a report, a neurologist or other experienced provider would immediately suspect an acute left middle cerebral artery (MCA) territory stroke.

Although, classically, UMN weakness is described as having increased muscle tone (specifically, spasticity) and elevated deep tendon reflexes, early in the course of CNS injuries these features may be absent (e.g., immediately after a stroke or spinal cord injury). Due to the variability in UMN findings in acute CNS pathologies, it is necessary for clinicians to additionally recognize colocalizing associated neurological exam findings, as well as specific muscle patterns of weakness seen with lesions affecting the brain or spinal cord.

Lesions of the UMN tracts within the cortex, subcortex, internal capsule, basal ganglia, and brainstem will cause *contralateral* weakness, affecting the side of the body *opposite* the lesion. Cortical lesions affecting neighboring structures may cause additional deficits, such as aphasia (typically left hemisphere) or neglect (typically right parietal lobe). Brainstem lesions typically cause ipsilateral cranial nerve findings. Lesions within the spinal cord—below the medullary decussation—will cause *ipsilateral* UMN type weakness (although, due to its small diameter, lesions commonly will affect both sides of the cord and thus cause bilateral weakness). Cord lesions typically affect all motor levels *below* the pathology. Findings of normal arms and weak, spastic legs would imply thoracic cord pathology; affected arms and legs with normal cranial nerves and cortical function would implicate the cervical cord.

Lesions of the lower motor neurons within the anterior horn of the spinal cord or the axons within the periphery will cause weakness with reduced muscle tone, decreased reflexes, fasciculations, and eventual atrophy. Neuromuscular junction pathologies may cause variable weakness that fluctuates in severity, often worse with activity ("fatigueability"), the classic example being myasthenia gravis. Botulinum toxin affecting the NMJ may cause profound flaccidity.

Ratings of muscle strength are given on a 5-point scale (see Table 10.4) as determined by the examiner on direct confrontational testing. The patient is encouraged to give maximal effort of a given muscle group, attempting to overcome resistance provided by the examiner. Exam technique is important; the examiner must supply an appropriate degree of counterforce for each muscle group being tested (e.g., fingers against fingers; arm against arm; arm and body weight against leg, with appropriate leverage) and must ensure that the tested group is being isolated by selecting an appropriate movement and supporting the patient (see Table 10.5 for more on motor testing).

Behavioral (voluntary malingering or psychogenic) patterns of weakness are notable for a ratcheting or collapsing "give-way" quality rather than a steady level of power. A suggestible patient who responds to encouragement may demonstrate 5/5 muscle strength for a split second before seeming to give out—and such is enough to determine that motor pathways are in fact intact. Another hallmark is distractibility, with involuntary or casually

Table 10.2 UMN lesions

These are caused by damage to motor pathways anywhere from the motor nerve cells in the precentral gyrus of the frontal cortex (the motor strip) through the internal capsule, brainstem, and spinal cord. Typical characteristics are the so-called "pyramidal" distribution of preferential weakness involving physiological extensors of the upper limb (shoulder abduction; elbow, wrist, and finger extension, and the small muscles of the hand) and the flexors of the lower limb (hip flexion, knee flexion, and ankle dorsiflexion and everters). There is little muscle wasting and *loss of skilled fine finger movements* may be greater than expected from the overall grade of weakness. Increased *tone* (spasticity) develops in stronger muscles (arm flexors and leg extensors). It is manifest as resistance to passive movement that can suddenly be overcome (clasp-knife feel). There is *hyperreflexia*: Reflexes are brisk; *plantars are upgoing* (+ve Babinski sign) ± *clonus* (elicited by the examiner rapidly dorsiflexing the foot) is more suggestive of an UMN lesion (1 or 2 rhythmic, downward beats of the foot may be normal); a positive *Hoffmann's reflex*—passive flicking of a finger (examiner rapidly flexes a DIP joint) causes neighboring digits, particularly the thumb, to briefly flex. UMN weakness affects *muscle groups* rather than individual muscles.

Table 10.3 LMN lesions

These are caused by damage anywhere from anterior horn cells in the cord, nerve roots, plexus, or peripheral nerves. The distribution of weakness corresponds to those individual muscles supplied by the involved cord segment, nerve root, part of plexus, or peripheral nerve. A combination of anatomical knowledge, good muscle testing technique, and experience is needed to distinguish them (e.g. a radial nerve palsy from a C7 root lesion, or a common peroneal nerve palsy from an L5 root lesion). The relevant muscles will generally exhibit loss of resistance to rapid passive movements (*hypotonia/flaccidity*) and may show spontaneous involuntary twitching (*fasciculation*). Over time, they will also exhibit loss of bulk, with atrophic wasting. *Reflexes are reduced* or absent, the *plantar responses remain flexor (negative Babinski)*.

Table 10.4 Muscle weakness grading (MRC classification)

Grade 0	No muscle contraction	Grade 3	Active movement against gravity
Grade 1	Flicker of contraction	Grade 4	Active movement against resistance
Grade 2	Some active movement	Grade 5	Normal power (allowing for age)

Because Grade 4 covers such a large range of strength, from marked paresis with substantial disability to nearly normal power, it is often subdivided, with 4-, 4, and 4+ denoting movement against slight, moderate, and stronger resistance respectively. Some examiners also document 5- power as barely below normal.

observed strength demonstrably greater than strength on directed confrontational testing; for example, a patient being able to lift a supposedly plegic leg during testing of balance.

Sensory deficits: Information about the site of a lesion is conferred by the distribution of the sensory loss. Additionally, because specific sensory modalities travel in anatomically discrete pathways, the pattern/type of sensory loss may convey additional information. For example, pain and temperature sensations travel along small fibers in peripheral nerves and spinothalamic tracts in the cord and brainstem and are distinct from joint position and vibration sense (travelling in fast myelinated fibers in the dorsal columns of the cord). Distal, symmetric, length-dependent sensory loss (feet affected more than ankles) suggests a polyneuropathy and may involve all sensory modalities or be more selective, depending on the nerve fiber size involved. Individual nerve lesions are identified by the anatomic territories they innervate, which are more distinctly defined than those of root lesions (dermatomes), which often show considerable overlap (refer to section on peripheral nervous system below). The hallmark of a spinal cord lesion is a sensory level; that is, an area of decreased or absent sensation at and *below* the lesion (e.g., numbness from the mid-trunk down to the toes), but with normal sensation above. Lateralized cord lesions give rise to a Brown-Séquard syndrome, with dorsal column damage on the side of the lesion causing ipsilateral loss of joint position sense, and spinothalamic damage causing reduction of pain and temperature sense on the contralateral side (the other cardinal feature is ipsilateral motor involvement). In thalamic and cortical lesions, sensory loss is contralateral to the lesion and can be confined to more subtle and discriminating sensory functions (pattern/texture detection, graphesthesia, stereognosis).

Nervous system anatomy

The elegance of clinical neurology is a product of nervous system anatomy. Understanding the functions associated with various locations within the central and peripheral nervous system is critical for localization. Although some person-to-person variability exists, most of the so-called higher cortical functions can be mapped to relatively specific locations within the cortex. (Little annoys a neurologist more than hearing from a colleague that a neurological examination is "nonfocal," typically meaning without weakness or sensory loss, when visual system, mental status, or coordination testing may implicate specific areas of brain dysfunction). Gray matter holds neuronal cell bodies (the processors), organized in nuclei or layered structures, and white matter consists of myelinated axons (the wiring). Within the white matter, brainstem, spinal cord, and peripheral nervous system there is limited variability among patients, making localization extremely reliable.

Higher functions of the cortex

Frontal lobe

Hemispheric dominance is defined by the location of Broca's area, which is responsible for the motor production of speech. The vast majority of right-handed individuals have their speech production area within the left hemisphere, whereas left-handed individuals are split ~50:50 between right- and left-hemisphere dominance. The frontal lobes anteriorly are composed of orbitofrontal and dorsolateral regions. These areas are involved in olfaction, visual interpretation, executive planning, and memory. Also within the frontal lobes are the frontal eye fields (FEF) responsible for initiating saccadic eye movements, the FEF on the left responsible for initiating eye movements to the right, and vice versa. Thus, an easily observable sign of a frontal stroke (also visible on imaging studies) is gaze deviation toward the damaged hemisphere (inability to look away) due to damage of the FEF. On the dominant side, Broca's area is responsible for the motor production of speech, whereas the nondominant side the frontal lobe controls prosody (voice inflections with questions and statements). Specific damage to Broca's area will cause stammering, hesitant speech, often with a great degree of frustration as the patient will "know" what he wants to say but be unable to express himself. Posteriorly in the frontal lobe are the premotor and motor strips. These structures are the control center for voluntary face, head, neck, body, and limb movements of the opposite side of the body.

Parietal lobe

The parietal lobes are primarily sensory structures, acting as the primary input for various somatosensory systems and providing significant networks for the interpretation of the incoming information. A significant portion of parietal lobe function is dedicated to visuospatial representations—maps—both of our own bodies and of our surroundings. Hence, a nondominant hemisphere parietal lobe lesion will often cause a hemineglect syndrome, in which patients do not attend to (ignore) the contralateral side (i.e., dressing one half of their body, only speaking to people on one side of the room, etc.). The dominant parietal lobe, particularly Wernicke's area, is also responsible for much of the "meaning" of language. Specific damage to Wernicke's area can cause a "word salad" fluent aphasia, with the patient producing strings of nonsense speech devoid of content, unaware that they neither produce nor comprehend even simple utterances.

Temporal lobe

The temporal lobes have a variety of functions including language, memory, behavior, interpretation of visual inputs, and hearing. Within the temporal lobes are the hippocampi, responsible for consolidation of new memories; damage to them (e.g., from dementia or anoxia) causes amnesia with short-term memory loss. An epileptic focus located within the temporal lobe will often present as complex partial seizures with patients appearing confused and acting strangely.

Occipital lobe

The occipital lobes are dedicated to visual pathways. Information from the retina is carried via the optic nerves and optic tracts to the lateral geniculate nuclei of the thalami. From there, the optic radiations transmit visual field information to the contralateral occipital lobes. Primary visual information is translated into more highly processed forms within the occipital lobes, with parallel streams of abstracted information (color, form, motion, contrast, etc.) being passed along from the initial topographical map of the primary visual cortex. The temporal and parietal lobes assign significance to the structures perceived by the occipital lobes.

Occipital lobe lesions cause contralateral visual field loss (i.e., a right occipital lesion causes impaired perception of visual space to the left of fixation, through *either* eye; the problem is with the TV screen, not the cameras). Bilateral occipital strokes can cause complete cortical blindness (Anton's syndrome), typically with the patient being unaware of her deficit. It may present with disorientation and visual confabulation that may be mistaken for delirium.

Isolated occipital lobe strokes are commonly "missed" by patients as well as well as by providers. The patient may complain of something vaguely wrong with his vision, perhaps in the setting of a slight orbital headache ipsilateral to the stroke. If visual fields are not examined—the simplest way being a quick screen of finger movements in each quadrant distally and finger counting in each quadrant more centrally—the patient may go undiagnosed. As occipital lobe infarctions can be an early sign of a threatened basilar artery occlusion, a missed diagnosis can be disastrous.

Deep nuclei: Basal ganglia, thalamus, hypothalamus

These extracortical collections of gray matter lie deep within the brain. The basal ganglia predominately control motor function, with lesions causing extrapyramidal motor disorders such as parkinsonism (bradykinesia, resting tremor, masked facies), chorea (dancing/jerky movements), and athetosis (writhing). Lesions of the nearby subthalamic nucleus may cause the wildly flinging motions of hemiballismus.

The anatomy of the thalamus is extremely complex, with many subnuclei, but is best known clinically as a relay between ascending sensory pathways and the cortex. Lesions typically affect contralateral sensory modalities from the face and/or body, with loss of sensation or occasionally a central pain syndrome (Dejerine-Roussy syndrome). Damage to the left thalamus sometimes produces aphasia, and to the right may produce neglect.

The hypothalamus is a deep midline structure at the base of the brain, regulating a number of vital "primitive" homeostatic functions including the biological clock, appetite mechanisms, temperature, and release of pituitary hormones. Various distinct cell populations and functions are again clustered into numerous nuclei.

Brainstem

The brainstem is expensive real estate—a number of vital structures and crucial pathways confined to a small, densely packed and complex region of anatomy. Divided into three portions—the midbrain (uppermost), the pons (middle), and the medulla (lowermost)—the brainstem consists of long fiber tracts descending from the brain (motor and modulatory) or ascending from the body (sensory), and relay circuitry to and from the cerebellum. It also houses the various nuclei for the individual cranial nerves, as well as structures dealing with pain and its modulation, consciousness, autonomic function, nausea, balance, and other important somatic functions.

Localization in the brainstem is facilitated by identification of damaged cranial nerve function. For example, a process affecting cranial nerves III or IV would occur in the midbrain, VI or VII the pons, and XI the medulla. Because of the small size and high density of structures, nearby pathways or nuclei are nearly always affected by brainstem lesions, and thus isolated "pure" cranial neuropathies are more usually due to a more distal/peripheral process. The trigeminal nerve (V) has longitudinally extensive nucleus and fiber tracts, meaning that injury anywhere from the midbrain to the upper spinal cord could result in facial sensory symptoms.

Cerebellum

The cerebellum serves as a feedback integrator of complex movements across multiple joints, assists in coordination of speech output, and is involved in eye movements and balance. Its role in cognition is somewhat obscure. Relatively esoteric or subtle signs of specific cerebellar lesions are beyond the scope of this chapter. In general, due to double-decussation of its prominent pathways, cerebellar lesions will cause *ipsilateral* incoordination (dysmetria, ataxia, impaired fine movements, or intentional tremor that worsens as the hand approaches the target). Peripheral/hemispheric lesions tend to affect limbs, and midline lesions the trunk and balance. In cerebellar injury speech may be slowed, monotonous, jerky/arrhythmic, and/or slurred.

Spinal cord anatomy

As opposed to the brain, the spinal cord is organized with white matter tracts coursing along the *outer* portions. The inner, butterfly-shaped gray matter of the spinal cord forms the anterior horn, which houses the motor neuron cell bodies that will project into the periphery. Important to understanding anatomic-clinical correlations is keeping track of where specific white matter tracts decussate (cross the midline). Ultimately, all motor and sensory information will be generated or interpreted within the contralateral brain, but whereas the corticospinal tracts (motor pathways) and ascending dorsal columns (vibration and proprioceptive information) decussate within the medulla, the spinothalamic tracts (pain and temperature information) cross over within the spinal cord itself shortly after entering.

The corticospinal tracts run along the posterolateral portions of the spinal cord. The cell bodies are located within the precentral gyrus and project their axons down to the appropriate level of the spinal cord, crossing over to the contralateral side within the medulla. Within the spinal cord, the fibers travelling down to the legs are located along the outer portions of the corticospinal tract. Thus, extramedullary spinal processes pushing inward (abscess, metastatic tumor) within the cervical or thoracic spine may present with ipsilateral leg weakness.

The dorsal columns that carry vibratory and proprioceptive information are located along the posteromedial aspects of the spinal cord. Lesions of these afferent pathways cause ipsilateral symptoms. These pathways decussate within the medulla, such that lesions above the medulla cause contralateral symptoms. The dorsal columns have two distinct pathways, the fasciculus cuneatus and gracilis. Fibers entering the spinal cord below T6—including from the legs—travel in the fasciculus gracilis, whereas fibers at T6 and above—including from the arms—utilize the more medial fasciculus cuneatus. These are particularly vulnerable to posterior compression and for uncertain reasons, vitamin B_{12} deficiency.

The spinothalamic tracts occupy the anterior-lateral portions of the spinal cord and convey pain and temperature information from the contralateral portion of the body to the postcentral gyrus (the primary sensory cortex). Within the spinothalamic tracts, information from the legs is carried along the outer portions of the tracts. The decussation of the white matter tracts occurs along the most medial anterior portion of the spinal cord, anterior to the central canal. Thus, central spinal cord pathologies (e.g., syringomyelia) can cause a band-like pattern of loss of pain and temperature sensation due to disruption of the crossing spinothalamic fibers at that level. When a significant cervical syrinx (a dilated central canal) affects multiple levels of the central cord, the coalesced bands form a cape-like area of numbness over the shoulders and arms, often resulting in initially unnoticed burn injuries due to inability to distinguish temperature in the hands.

Blood is supplied to the spinal cord via a singular anterior spinal artery and paired posterior spinal arteries. Clinically, patients with anterior spinal artery syndromes will have paraplegia, with loss of temperature and pain below the level of the lesion, but with sparing of vibratory sensation and proprioception.

Cerebral artery territories

A basic knowledge of the anatomy of the blood supply of the brain is helpful in the diagnosis and management of cerebrovascular disease. Knowledge of anatomical-vascular-functional correlation will allow a clinician to implicate a particular artery (or arteries) without imaging. Large arterial territory ischemic strokes will cause dysfunction of a contiguous, wedge-shaped area of brain supplied by the occluded artery (Figure 10.1). For example, a patient with symptoms that localize to both the anterior cerebral and middle cerebral arteries will quickly be assessed as having likely carotid pathology, prompting a search for occlusion or dissection. A patient with significant weakness or sensory loss in the absence of any associated cortical findings will likely be the victim of a small, deep lacunar infarction rather than a large artery or embolic process.

Figure 10.1 Arteries and CNS territories

Carotid artery Internal carotid artery occlusion may cause total infarction of the anterior two-thirds of the ipsilateral hemisphere and basal ganglia (lenticulostriate arteries). With right carotid occlusion, patients will typically have dysprosody, neglect, a right-field cut, rightward eye deviation, flaccid left-sided paralysis, and profound sensory loss. More often, the picture is similar to an MCA occlusion (below).

The cerebral arteries Three pairs of arteries leave the circle of Willis to supply the cerebral hemispheres; the anterior, middle, and posterior cerebral arteries. The anterior and middle cerebrals are branches of the carotid arteries; the basilar artery divides into the two posterior cerebral arteries. These large arteries are essentially end arteries (lacking significant anastomoses), although ischemia due to occlusion of any one of them may be reduced, if not prevented, by retrograde supply from meningeal vessels.

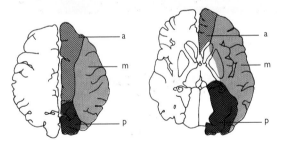

Anterior cerebral artery (a, above): Supplies the frontal and medial part of the cerebral hemispheres (including the "leg" area of the homunculus). Occlusion may cause a weak, numb contralateral leg ± similar, if milder, arm symptom. The face is generally spared. Bilateral infarction may lead to an akinetic mute state due to damage to the cingulate gyri and is also a rare cause of paraplegia. Sometimes both arteries originate from a single carotid.

Middle cerebral artery (m): Supplies the lateral (external) part of each hemisphere, including the face and arm areas of the homunculus. Occlusion may cause contralateral hemiplegia, hemisensory loss mainly of face and arm, contralateral homonymous hemianopia due to involvement of the optic radiation, cognitive change including aphasia if the dominant hemisphere is affected, and visuospatial disturbance (e.g., cannot dress, neglect, gets lost) with nondominant lesions.

337

(Continued)

Figure 10.1 (Continued)

Posterior cerebral artery (p): Supplies the occipital lobe. Occlusion causes contralateral homonymous hemianopia.

Vertebrobasilar circulation: Supplies the cerebellum, brainstem (with the cranial nerve nuclei), and occipital lobes. Depending on specific involvement, occlusion may cause hemianopia, cortical blindness (bilaterally occipital), diplopia, vertigo, nystagmus, hemi- or quadriplegia, unilateral or bilateral sensory symptoms, cerebellar symptoms, hiccups, dysarthria, dysphagia, and coma. Infarctions of the brainstem can produce various eponymous syndromes, a common one being Wallenberg's or lateral medullary syndrome (occlusion of a posterior inferior cerebellar artery, sometimes due to vertebral artery occlusion). Infarction of the lateral medulla and inferior surface of the cerebellum causes vertigo with vomiting, dysphagia, nystagmus, ipsilateral ataxia, paralysis of the soft palate, ipsilateral Horner's syndrome, a crossed pattern of sensory loss (analgesia to pinprick on ipsilateral face and contralateral trunk and limbs), and, interestingly, hiccups.

Subclavian steal syndrome: Subclavian artery stenosis proximal to the vertebral artery may cause blood to be "stolen" by retrograde flow down the vertebral artery, down into the arm, causing brainstem ischemia after exertion. Suspect if the blood pressure (BP) in the arms differs by >20 mm Hg.

Figure 10.2 Cerebral arterial anatomy

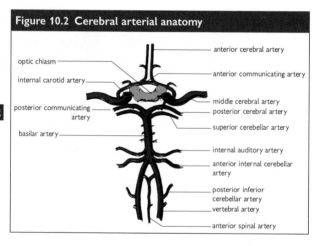

optic chiasm — anterior cerebral artery
internal carotid artery — anterior communicating artery
posterior communicating artery — middle cerebral artery
— posterior cerebral artery
— superior cerebellar artery
basilar artery — internal auditory artery
— anterior internal cerebellar artery
— posterior inferior cerebellar artery
— vertebral artery
— anterior spinal artery

Cerebral blood supply

The brain is supplied by the two internal carotid arteries and the basilar artery (formed by the joining of the two vertebral arteries). These three vessels feed into an anastomotic ring at the base of the brain called the Circle of Willis (Figure 10.2). This arrangement may lessen the effects of occlusion of any single feeder vessel by allowing collateral supply from unaffected vessels. The anatomy of the Circle of Willis is, however, highly variable and is "incomplete" in many people (e.g., missing one or more of the communicating arteries) and thus may in some cases be unable to provide much in the way of redundancy. In other variations, the typically posterior arteries may derive from the anterior supply (e.g., the posterior cerebral arteries originating from the carotid rather than the basilar). Collateral supply from other vessels in the neck may also mitigate occlusions of feeder vessels (e.g., occlusion of the internal carotid in the neck may not cause a large infarction if flow from the external carotid artery enters the Circle of Willis via the facial artery and its anastomosis with the ophthalmic artery).

Peripheral nerves, myotomes, and dermatomes

The peripheral nervous system is made up of sensory and motor nerves that form from the roots emerging from the dorsal and anterior horns of the spinal cord respectively. Some nerves are pure motor (e.g., suboccipital), some pure sensory (e.g., sural), but most are mixed. Pathologies can affect the nerve root, plexus, or peripheral nerve itself. Thus, identifying the root and the nerve that is responsible for each area of sensation and each muscle is vital for localizing peripheral nervous system pathologies. Table 10.5 summarizes motor nerve root innervation (myotomes) and individual peripheral nerve innervation patterns of selected muscles. When trying to discern a C7 lesion from a radial nerve lesion, an examiner could test muscles innervated by the radial nerve, but not C7, such as the brachioradialis. Also, an examiner could test C7 innervated muscles that are not innervated by the radial nerve, such as the flexor carpi radialis, which is innervated by the median nerve.

Table 10.5 Motor testing: Roots, nerves, muscles, actions

Nerve root	Muscle	Test by asking the patient to:
C3, 4	Trapezius	Shrug shoulder (via accessory nerve)
C5, 6	Serratus anterior	Push arm forward against resistance; look for winging of the scapula, if weak
C**5**, 6	Pectoralis major (p. major) clavicular head	Adduct arm from above horizontal and push it forward
C6, **7**, 8	P. major sterno-costal head	Adduct arm below horizontal
C**5**, 6	Supraspinatus	Abduct arm the first 15 degrees
C**5**, 6	Infraspinatus	Externally rotate arm, elbow at side
C6, **7**, 8	Latissimus dorsi	Adduct arm from horizontal position
C5, 6	Biceps	Flex supinated forearm
C**5**, 6	Deltoid	Abduct arm between 15 and 90 degrees
Radial nerve		
C6, **7**, 8	Triceps	Extend elbow against resistance
C5, **6**	Brachioradialis	Flex elbow with forearm half way between pronation and supination
C5, **6**	Extensor carpi radialis longus	Extend wrist to radial side with fingers extended
C6, 7	Supinator	Arm by side, resist hand pronation

(Continued)

Table 10.5 (*Continued*)

Nerve root	Muscle	Test by asking the patient to:
C**7**, 8	Extensor digitorum	Keep fingers extended at metacarpophalangeal (MCP) joint
C**7**, 8	Extensor carpi ulnaris	Extend wrist to ulnar side
C**7**, 8	Abductor pollicis longus	Abduct thumb at 90 degrees to palm
C**7**, 8	Extensor pollicis brevis	Extend thumb at MCP joint
C**7**, 8	Extensor pollicis longus	Resist thumb flexion at interphalangeal (IP) joint
Median nerve		
C6, 7	Pronator teres	Maintain arm pronation against resistance
C6, 7	Flexor carpi radialis	Flex wrist toward radial side
C7, **8**, T1	Flexor digitorum superficialis	Resist extension at proximal interphalangeal (PIP) joint (with proximal phalanx fixed by the examiner)
C7, **8**	Flexor digitorum profundus I & II	Resist extension at index distal interphalangeal (DIP) joint of index finger
C7, **8**, T1	Flexor pollicis longus	Resist thumb extension at interphalangeal joint (fix proximal phalanx)
C8, **T1**	Abductor pollicis brevis	Abduct thumb (nail at 90 degrees to palm)
C8, **T1**	Opponens pollicis	Thumb touches base of fifth fingertip (nail parallel to palm)
C8, **T1**	Lumbrical/interosseus (median & ulnar nerves)	Extend PIP joint against resistance with MCP joint held hyperextended
Ulnar nerve		
C7, **8**, T1	Flexor carpi ulnaris	Flex wrist to ulnar side; observe tendon
C7, C**8**	Flexor digitorum profundus III and IV	Resist extension of distal phalanx of fifth finger while you fix its middle phalanx
C8, **T1**	Dorsal interossei	Finger abduction: Cannot cross the middle over the index finger (tests index finger adduction too)
C8, **T1**	Palmar interossei	Finger adduction: Pull apart a sheet of paper held between middle and ring finger DIP joints of both hands; the paper moves on the weaker side
C8, **T1**	Adductor pollicis	Adduct thumb (nail at 90 degrees to palm)
C8, **T1**	Abductor digiti minimi	Abduct little finger
C8, **T1**	Flexor digiti minimi	Flex the little finger at MCP joint

(Continued)

Table 10.5 (*Continued*)

Lower limb

Nerve root	Muscle	Activity to test:
L**4**, **5**, S1	Gluteus medius & minimus (superior gluteal nerve)	Internal rotation at hip, hip abduction
L5, S1, 2	Gluteus maximus (inferior gluteal nerve)	Extension at hip (lie prone)
L2, **3**, 4	Adductors (obturator nerve)	Adduct leg against resistance

Femoral nerve

L**1**, **2**, 3	Iliopsoas (also supplied via upper lumbar spinal nerves)	Flex hip against resistance with knee flexed and lower leg supported: Patient lies on back
L2, **3**, 4	Quadriceps femoris	Extend at the knee against resistance; start with the knee flexed

Obturator nerve

L2, **3**, 4	Hip adductors	Adduct the leg against resistance

Inferior gluteal nerve

L5, S**1**, S2	Gluteus maximus	Hip extension ("bury heel into the bed") with knee in extension

Superficial gluteal nerve

L4, **5**, S1	Gluteus medius & minimus	Abduction and internal hip rotation with leg flexed at hip and knee

Sciatic: common peroneal* and tibial** nerves

*L**4**, 5	Tibialis anterior	Dorsiflex ankle
*L**5**, S1	Extensor digitorum longus	Dorsiflex toes against resistance
*L**5**, S1	Extensor hallucis longus	Dorsiflex hallux against resistance
*L**5**, S1	Peroneus longus & brevis	Evert foot against resistance
*L**5**, S1	Extensor digitorum brevis	Dorsiflex proximal phalanges of toes
L5, **S1, 2	Hamstrings	Flex the knee against resistance
**L4, 5	Tibialis posterior	Invert the plantarflexed foot
**S1, 2	Gastrocnemius	Plantarflex ankle or stand on tiptoe
L5, S1**, **2**	Flexor digitorum longus	Flex terminal joints of the toes
**S1, 2	Small muscles of foot	Make the sole of the foot into a cup

Quick screening test for muscle power

Shoulder	Abduction	C5		*Hip*	Flexion	L1–L2
	Adduction	C5–C7			Adduction	L2–3
Elbow	Flexion	C5–C6			Extension	L5–S1
	Extension	C7		*Knee*	Flexion	L5–S1

(*Continued*)

Table 10.5 (Continued)

Quick screening test for muscle power

Wrist	Flexion	C7–8		Extension	L3–L4
	Extension	C7	*Ankle*	Dorsiflexion	L4
Fingers	Flexion	C8		Eversion	L5–S1
	Extension	C7		Plantarflexion	S1–S2
	Abduction	T1	*Toe*	Big toe extension	L5

The segment of skin innervated by a particular nerve root is known as a *dermatome*; cutaneous nerves derive from portions of multiple roots. Although nerve root/dermatome distributions tend to be somewhat ill-defined and may overlap, cutaneous nerve distributions tend to be distinctly marginated, crossing multiple dermatomes. Figures 10.3 and 10.4 illustrate the cutaneous innervation of the anterior and posterior skin surface, respectively.

Figure 10.3 Dermatomes and cutaneous nerves

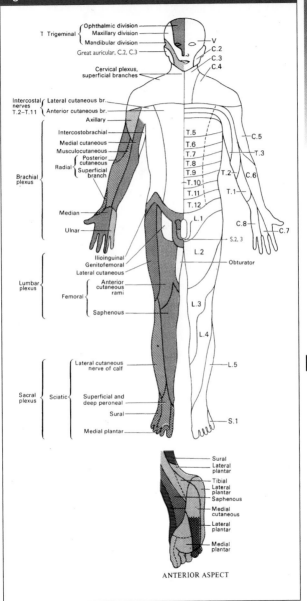

T Trigeminal {
  Ophthalmic division
  Maxillary division
  Mandibular division
}

Great auricular, C.2, C.3

Cervical plexus, superficial branches

Intercostal nerves T.2–T.11 {
  Lateral cutaneous br.
  Anterior cutaneous br.
}

Axillary

Intercostobrachial

Medial cutaneous

Musculocutaneous

Radial {
  Posterior cutaneous
  Superficial branch
}

Brachial plexus

Median

Ulnar

Lumbar plexus {
  Ilioinguinal
  Genitofemoral
  Lateral cutaneous
  Femoral {
    Anterior cutaneous rami
    Saphenous
  }
}

Sacral plexus {
  Sciatic {
    Lateral cutaneous nerve of calf
    Superficial and deep peroneal
    Sural
    Medial plantar
  }
}

V
C.2
C.3
C.4
C.5
T.3
C.6
T.2
T.1
C.8
C.7
T.5
T.6
T.7
T.8
T.9
T.10
T.11
T.12
L.1
S.2, 3
L.2
Obturator
L.3
L.4
L.5
S.1

Sural
Lateral plantar
Tibial
Lateral plantar
Saphenous
Medial cutaneous
Lateral plantar
Medial plantar

ANTERIOR ASPECT

Figure 10.4

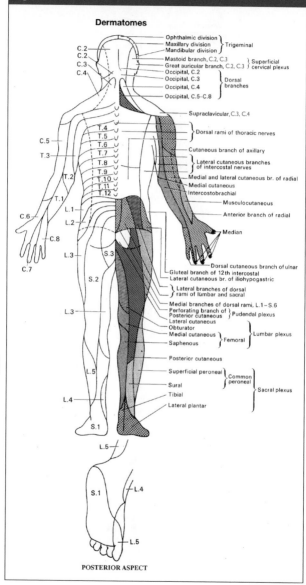

Dermatomes

Ophthalmic division ⎫
Maxillary division ⎬ Trigeminal
Mandibular division ⎭

Mastoid branch, C.2, C.3 ⎫ Superficial
Great auricular branch, C.2, C.3 ⎬ cervical plexus

Occipital, C.2 ⎫
Occipital, C.3 ⎬ Dorsal
Occipital, C.4 ⎬ branches
Occipital, C.5–C.8 ⎭

Supraclavicular, C.3, C.4

Dorsal rami of thoracic nerves

Cutaneous branch of axillary

Lateral cutaneous branches of intercostal nerves

Medial and lateral cutaneous br. of radial

Medial cutaneous

Intercostobrachial

Musculocutaneous

Anterior branch of radial

Median

Dorsal cutaneous branch of ulnar

Gluteal branch of 12th intercostal

Lateral cutaneous br. of iliohypogastric

Lateral branches of dorsal ⎫
rami of lumbar and sacral ⎭

Medial branches of dorsal rami, L.1–S.6

Perforating branch of ⎫ Pudendal plexus
Posterior cutaneous ⎭

Lateral cutaneous

Obturator

Medial cutaneous ⎫ Femoral ⎫ Lumbar plexus
Saphenous ⎭

Posterior cutaneous

Superficial peroneal ⎫ Common
Sural ⎬ peroneal ⎫ Sacral plexus
Tibial ⎭

Lateral plantar

C.2
C.2
C.3
C.4

C.5
T.3

C.6

C.8
C.7

T.4
T.5
T.6
T.7
T.8
T.9
T.10
T.11
T.12

T.2
T.1

L.1
L.2
L.3
S.3
S.2
L.3
L.5
L.4
S.1

L.5

S.1   L.4

L.5

POSTERIOR ASPECT

344

Headache

Every day, thousands of patients visit doctors complaining of headache. It is the top neurological chief complaint in primary care settings, a top-five emergency room chief complaint, and the most common reason for neurological referral. A variety of pathologies can cause *cephalalgia* (head pain), most of which are benign or primary headache syndromes (e.g., migraine, tension-type), but that occasionally may be the harbinger of impending catastrophe (e.g., subarachnoid hemorrhage, meningitis). Recognizing common syndromes as well as indications for evaluating patients for potentially more serious conditions is extremely important for every physician.

At first cut, the goal of assessing a patient with a headache complaint should focus on distinguishing a *secondary* headache—nociceptive pain as a *symptom* of an underlying identifiable pathology—from a *primary* headache, one of the more benign, idiopathic headache *syndromes*.

There are a variety of ways to approach the differential diagnosis for headache. "Red flags" serve to triage patients for further or expedited workup, increasing the likelihood that the patient is suffering from a dangerous or treatable secondary headache. A useful red flag mnemonic—HPAIN (see Table 10.6)—is given. The temporal *pattern* ("P"of HPAIN) of the headache is particularly salient. Sudden onset with rapid time to peak intensity ("thunderclap"—see discussion and differential under subarachnoid hemorrhage), first, worst, or unusual headaches require more urgent triage; a stable pattern of recurring headaches with complete return to baseline each time is seldom a cause for alarm. A brief list of selected headache syndromes based on temporal pattern of presentation is given in Table 10.7. The individual headaches will be discussed below. Migraine, the most clinically prevalent and important, will be discussed separately.

Acute single episode

Meningitis, encephalitis, subarachnoid hemorrhage: If the headache is acute, severe, felt over most of the head and accompanied by meningeal irritation (neck stiffness) ± drowsiness, you must think of meningitis, encephalitis, or a subarachnoid hemorrhage. Emergent head imagining with a computed tomography (CT) scan and possible LP is indicated, possibly with follow up MRI/A/V if unrevealing.

After head injury: Headache is common after trauma. It may be at the site of trauma or be more generalized. It typically lasts approximately 2 wks and is often resistant to analgesia. Bear in mind subdural or epidural hematoma. Worrisome are any drowsiness or any focal neurological signs or symptoms. Chronic post-traumatic headaches may respond to treatment for chronic migraine, and presentation may be complicated by litigation, worker's comp, etc. Paradoxically, they are *more* likely to occur after *minor*

Table 10.6 HPAIN: Identifying headache "red flags"

Host: Particular patient vulnerabilities. Older, immunocompromised or suppressed, cancer, autoimmune disease

Pattern: Sudden and severe ("thunderclap"), first, worst, new onset, steady progression, change in previously stable pattern

Associated systemic symptoms: Fever, stiff neck, weight loss, rash, etc.

Increased by, provoked by, or worsened by: Valsalva, upright posture, exertion, sleeping

Neurological symptoms or signs: Seizure, numbness, weakness, unsteadiness, impaired or double vision

Table 10.7 Differential diagnosis for selected headache syndromes based on presentation

Acute single episode

Meningitis	Fever, photophobia, stiff neck, rash, coma
Encephalitis	Fever, odd behavior, seizures or change in consciousness
Subarachnoid	*Sudden* headache ± stiff neck ± loss of consciousness
Sinusitis	Pressure, tender face + coryza + anosmia + postnasal drip/cough; nearly all cases of isolated recurring "sinus" headaches are misdiagnosed migraines.
Head injury	Cuts/bruises, transient or ongoing ↓consciousness, lucid interval, amnesia
Spontaneous intracranial hypotension (SIH)	Sudden onset, improves with lying flat, worsens when upright.

Acute recurrent attacks

Migraine	Any pre-attack visual or sensory aura (25% of migraineurs). Sensitivity to light, noise, or movement; nausea; throbbing or pounding quality; unilateral or bilateral; typically last hours to a few days
Cluster headache	Typically repeated episodes (1–5+/d) of excruciating pain in one periorbital region, with ipsilateral eye and nose symptoms, lasting for ~30 mins to 2 h, active for ~8 wks followed by weeks of remission
Glaucoma	Rarely. Red eye; sees haloes, fixed big oval pupil; ↓acuity

Acute recurrent attacks
Subacute onset

Giant cell arteritis	Tender scalp; >50 yrs; vision changes, systemic complaints, very elevated erythrocyte sedimentation rate (ESR) or c-reactive protein (CRP)

Chronic headache (pain for >15 d/month for >3 months)

Chronic tension-type headache	"A tight band round my head," otherwise fairly featureless
Chronically elevated intracranial pressure (ICP)	Pseudotumor cerebri/idiopathic intracranial hypertension (IIH), or symptomatic ICP elevation due to hydrocephalus, mass lesion, venous thrombosis. Worse overnight or upon waking; blurred vision, papilledema, and eventual transient visual obscurations; may have pulsatile tinnitus (heartbeat in ears); focal signs if due to a lesion
Rebound headache	Analgesic overuse (>2 d/wk on average, particularly with barbiturates or narcotics) in a known migraineur; develops over months
Chronic migraine aka transformed migraine	Continuous or near continuous underlying smoldering headache, spiking at times to full-blown migraine, in a known migraineur; typically develops over many months to years. Exacerbations respond at times to migraine-specific treatments

rather than severe injury. Rarely are they the result of spinal fluid leaks, accompanying upper neck trauma, or nerve injury.

Sinusitis: Presents with dull, constant, aching pressure over the affected frontal or maxillary sinus, with tender overlying skin ± postnasal drip. Pain is typically a *minor* feature of sinus infection. Ethmoid or sphenoid sinus pain is felt deep in the midline at the root of the nose. Pain worsened by bending over. Often accompanied by coryza; symptoms may last 1–2 wks. Endoscopy or sinus CT scan may verify diagnosis. Role of antibiotics is controversial as most cases are viral.

Acute glaucoma: Mostly observed in elderly, far-sighted people. Constant, aching pain develops rapidly around one eye and radiates to the forehead. Symptoms: Markedly reduced vision in affected eye, nausea, and vomiting. Signs: Red, congested eye; cloudy cornea; dilated, non-responsive pupil. Attacks may be precipitated by sitting in the dark, such as at the movies; by dilating eye-drops; or emotional upset. Seek expert help immediately. If delay in treatment of >1 h is likely, start IV acetazolamide (500 mg over several minutes).

Recurrent acute attacks of headache

Cluster headache: Pain occurs up to seven times every 24 h, each episode lasting 15–160 min. Active cluster periods typically last 4–12 wks and are followed by pain-free periods of months or even 1–2 yrs before another cluster begins. Sometimes there are no remissions. Men outnumber women 3 to 1. Classically, patients are agitated, rocking, or writhing in pain, unlike migraineurs who usually remain quite still and quiet during a headache. May become irrational and injure self or others. *Suicide risk.* Image all cluster-like headache patients with MRI, refer to neurologist or headache subspecialist. Symptoms: Rapid onset severe pain around one eye, which may become watery and bloodshot with lid swelling, lacrimation, facial flushing, and rhinorrhea. Miosis ± ptosis (20% attacks), remaining permanent in 5%. Pain is strictly unilateral and almost always side-locked. Treatment: *Acute attack:* 100% O_2 (10–15 L/min for 20 min) often helps, or *sumatriptan* SC 6 mg at attack's onset. IV or nasal DHE, nasal triptans may be helpful, but oral drugs are typically too slow to act. Indomethacin and intranasal lidocaine are also effective abortive agents. Preventives (NB: Scant quality evidence in literature): Verapamil up to 960 mg/day (checking ECGs at 480 mg and above); lithium; topiramate; divalproex. 2–4-wk steroid taper and ipsilateral greater occipital nerve block with steroids and local anesthetic for bridge therapy.

Trigeminal neuralgia

(TN): Paroxysms of intense, unilateral stabbing facial pain, lasting seconds, typically in V2 (maxillary) and/or V3 (mandibular) distribution. The face may twist with pain (hence the moniker, *tic douloureux*). Pain may recur many times a day and night and can often be triggered by touching the skin of the affected area, by washing, shaving, eating, or talking. TN often presents in older men, with most cases resulting from microvascular compression of the trigeminal nerve roots as they exit the brainstem but can occur due to other mass lesions and multiple sclerosis (MS) as well (consider this especially in a younger, female patient). All patients should be imaged with a high-resolution contrast-enhanced brain MRI, with heavily T2-weighted thin cuts through the brainstem and trigeminal nerves to assess for causative lesions. Treatment: Carbamazepine (start at 100 mg/12 h PO; max 400 mg/6 h; oxcarbazepine working up to as high as 900 mg bid; lamotrigine (slow to titrate but well-tolerated); phenytoin 200–400 mg/24 h; or gabapentin up to 1,800 mg tid. Baclofen may work rapidly for rescue, and, in extreme cases, IV anticonvulsants may be required. The condition is often surgically curable; after imaging, we recommend referring all cases to neurosurgery *early* to discuss options if medications fail or cause intolerable side effects. Interventions may be directed at the peripheral nerve, the trigeminal ganglion (rhizotomy with radiation, radiofrequency, or glycerol lesioning), or the nerve root with surgical microvascular decompression to separate anomalous vessels from the nerve.

Headaches of subacute onset

Giant cell arteritis: Exclude in all patients >50 presenting with a headache that has lasted a few weeks. Look for tender, thickened, pulseless temporal arteries with an extremely elevated ESR. *Ask about* jaw claudication during eating (specific, not sensitive), systemic symptoms (malaise, sweats, muscle aches, weakness of limb girdles/polymyalgia rheumatica), and episodes of vision loss (amaurosis fugax). Prompt diagnosis and immediate treatment with steroids (starting at 60–80 mg of PO prednisone) are essential for avoiding blindness or potential strokes. The temporal arteries should be biopsied to confirm the diagnosis; start steroids *first* to prevent complications, then ensure that adequate 4 cm+ biopsies, ideally bilaterally, are performed within 10 d.

Chronic headaches

Raised ICP: Headache is a complaint of ~50% patients with ↑ICP, whether idiopathic intracranial hypertension (IIH, aka pseudotumor cerebri or "benign" intracranial hypertension) or due to hydrocephalus or other mass lesion. Although variable in nature, headaches are characteristically present on waking or may awaken the patient overnight. They are generally not severe and are worse lying down. If accompanied by other signs of ↑ ICP, such as vomiting, papilledema, seizures, focal deficits, or mental status change, admit the patient urgently for diagnostic imaging. Any space-occupying lesion (neoplasm, abscess, subdural hematoma) may present in this way, as may IIH, or cerebral venous thrombosis. Lumbar puncture is the diagnostic test of choice in patients *with unremarkable imaging*; cerebellar herniation may be risked if there is obstructive hydrocephalus or mass lesion.

Classically, patients with IIH are overweight women of child-bearing age (20-fold elevated risk over general population, but still 100-fold less common than chronic migraine in this group) who have constant dull head pain and vision changes. Think of this diagnosis in those presenting as if with a mass (headache, ↑ ICP, and papilledema) *when no mass is found* and when there is no venous occlusion. Consciousness and cognition are preserved. Opening pressure during LP is elevated. *Cause:* Unknown. Rule out elevated ICP secondary to venous sinus thrombosis (contrast-enhanced MRV, CTV, or angiography are the best studies) or drugs (e.g., tetracycline, minocycline, nitrofurantoin, vitamin A, isotretinoin, danazol, and somatropin).

Treatment: Treatment should be geared toward preserving vision rather than headache. Refer all suspected cases of ICP elevation early and often to ophthalmology; urgent optic nerve sheath fenestration or neurosurgical treatment may prevent permanent blindness. Ophthalmological workup should include funduscopy (ideally with photo documentation), perimetry, and color vision testing. Urgent and even serial lumbar punctures (LPs) (with measurement of the opening pressure) with drainage of 20+ cc of cerebrospinal fluid (CSF) may be indicated in patients with worsening symptoms. Acetazolamide is the mainstay of medical treatment; consider loop diuretics and advise weight loss in all patients. High-dose topiramate may be useful in causing both weight loss and CSF pressure-lowering effects. Surgical shunting or even venous stenting may be indicated in specific cases. *Prognosis:* Often self-limiting. Permanent significant visual loss in 10% (i.e., not so benign), higher if not treated.

Intracranial hypotension: An internal leak of CSF, whether iatrogenic (LP, surgery, overshunting), due to trauma, or spontaneous (SIH), tends to present with a postural headache, worsening when upright and improving when recumbent, particularly with prolonged sleep. Some SIH patients experience thunderclap headache at onset. When mild, the disorder presents as a daily recurring headache absent in the morning that comes on gradually and then worsens toward the end of the day. Valsalva or straining, such as during bouts of cough may exacerbate symptoms, and meningeal irritation may cause increased pain during jarring motions. Rarely, there are associated cranial neuropathies, ataxia, a frontotemporal dementia-like picture, or even a reduced level of consciousness. Patients with certain connective tissue or genetic disorders that cause weakening or outpouchings of the spinal meninges may be particularly susceptible (Ehlers-Danlos, Marfan's, neurofibromatosis). Characteristic imaging findings on contrast brain MRI include signs of downward displacement of brain structures ("sag"), including the cerebellar tonsils (resembling Chiari I malformation), engorgement of vascular structures such as the pituitary and venous sinuses, and avid enhancement of the pachymeninges (dura), which in coronal cross-section through the posterior fossa may resemble a Mercedes-Benz symbol drawn in white. Opening pressure on recumbent LP is often <7 cm H_2O, but may be normal. Leaks can be localized by a variety of techniques. In skull base leaks, CT may reveal fluid in the sinuses, and collection of nasal discharge will test positive for β_2-transferrin, found only in CSF and endolymph but not in mucous. Spinal leaks, often at the cervical-thoracic junction, at dilated nerve root sheaths/Tarlov cysts, or due to osteophytes, can be localized by CT myelography, CSF radiocisternography (include nasal pledgets if skull base leak is suspected) or noninvasively by high-resolution heavily T2-weighted MRI. SIH is well worth knowing about—it may be as common as subarachnoid hemorrhage, is commonly missed, can be extremely disabling, and is entirely curable through interventional procedures such as empiric or radiographically directed epidural blood patch or fibrin gluing.

Chronic daily headache from medication overuse (aka rebound headache): The main culprits are mixed analgesics containing narcotics, the barbiturate butalbital, ergotamine, triptans, and most over-the-counter combination "headache medications" containing caffeine (or even with caffeine-containing beverages). Consider this diagnosis in a migraineur who develops daily headache in the setting of increasing medication usage, *even when the medication is being used to treat another condition.* Typically, patients are using medications >10 times per month over a period of several months, but cases can occur with barbiturates use as infrequent as 5 d per month, and in narcotics in as few as 8 d per month. Acetaminophen and NSAIDs are only rarely implicated. It is a common reason for episodic migraines "transforming" into a daily headache. Aggressive treatment is directed at the underlying migraine condition with initiation of a preventive medication, potentially with a short course of an adjunctive "bridge" therapy of another class (steroid, round-the-clock NSAID), and complete withdrawal of the offending medication(s). *In general, it is best to entirely avoid narcotic and barbiturate-containing analgesics in migraineurs; the syndrome is often easier to avoid than to treat.*

349

Migraine

Because migraine headaches are both severe, causing limitation of routine activities, and prevalent, affecting ~12% of the adult population, they are overwhelmingly the most common headache type coming to attention in any medical setting, including in the ER. It is essential for healthcare providers to recognize the disorder and understand the fundamentals of treatment.

Few other conditions will strike down an otherwise healthy adult, rendering them unable to attend work, school, chores, or social activities. *The overwhelming majority of patients presenting with a chief complaint of episodic, disabling headaches will have migraine, particularly if attacks are accompanied by any nausea or sensitivity to light.*

Symptoms and diagnosis Migraine is a syndrome of episodically recurring, self-limiting headaches accompanied by oversensitivity to other stimuli. See Table 10.8 for formal diagnostic criteria. Only 25% of migraineurs ever experience an aura (see below). The individual headache typically progresses gradually to become at least moderately severe, is often unilateral and described as throbbing or pounding with the heartbeat. The hallmark of migraine is intolerance to other stimuli—photophobia, phonophobia, osmophobia (odor aversion), and exacerbation with routine activities (running up a flight of stairs, bending, jumping). Allodynia (nonpainful stimuli producing pain) is an underrecognized but very common symptom; patients may not be able to brush hair, wear earrings or glasses, or shave due to pain. If patients with recurring headaches say they would prefer to curl up in a ball in a dark, quiet place during attacks, they almost certainly have migraine.

Aura Transient stereotyped episodes of neurological dysfunction caused by the complex underlying phenomenon known as cortical spreading depression, auras are characterized by the *gradual* or *progressive* march of focal neurological symptoms over ~20 mins–1 h, immediately preceding the headache phase of the attack (or sometimes in isolation), usually involving both positive and negative symptomatology. Most typical is the classical visual/occipital lobe aura, consisting of flashing lights or zig-zag lines (+) followed by scotoma (−). Sensory/parietal auras are next most common, with a march of tingling (+) and numbness (−), typically from hand to face. Left hemisphere involvement may lead to language disturbances (aphasia). Bizarre, higher order perceptual distortions (aka Alice-in-Wonderland/Todd syndrome) are of great curiosity but fairly rare.

Brainstem or bilateral symptoms can occur in the relatively uncommon basilar-type migraines. The true neurological weakness of the genetic hemiplegic migraine syndromes is extremely rare. Weakness, brainstem symptoms, or any other unusual or sudden-onset neurological symptoms should prompt workup, unless absolutely characteristic of multiple previous attacks with a firm diagnosis of migraine.

Table 10.8 Migraine diagnostic criteria

The patient must have experienced five headaches lasting 4–72 h meeting the criteria below.

The mnemonic SULTANS (from neurologist Morris Maizel, *AAN Headache Toolkit*) encapsulates the International Classification of Headache Disorders criteria for migraine:

2/4 of:

       Severity is at least moderate

       Uni**L**ateral

       Throbbing or pounding (with heartbeat)

       Activity intolerance

1/2 of:

       Nausea

       Sensitivity to light/sound (phonophobia, photophobia)

In some cases, alterations in mood, energy, or appetite change may occur hours before the aura or headache; these nonfocal symptoms are properly referred to as prodromal.

"Triggers" Individual migraines may be provoked by exposure to certain internal or external stimuli, which may in combination exceed some sort of internal "headache threshold." The fall of estrogen prior to menses, change in sleep schedule, skipping a meal, dehydration, altitude, alcohol, overexertion, irregular or overconsumption of caffeine, stress, and let-down after a stressful period are all potential contributors. Airplane travel across time zones involves a particularly potent combination of triggers.

There is a substantial body of widely propagated but ultimately apocryphal beliefs about so-called dietary migraine triggers, but there is very little evidence for food items provoking individual headaches, including chocolate (thankfully, there is actually randomized controlled trial evidence to the contrary), nuts, cheese, and items containing nitrates, nitrites, or vasoactive amines. Prodromal symptoms may lead a patient to feel unwell or develop cravings. She reaches for a chocolate bar and shortly thereafter develops a headache. The patient falsely attributes the headaches to the snack, when the reverse was true—the impending headache caused her to consume the chocolate! Alcohol is certainly a trigger in many patients, as is possibly monosodium glutamate (MSG) and the artificial sweetener aspartame. Hunger from skipping a meal is probably much more likely to provoke a migraine than any individual food item. While advocating a strict so-called migraine elimination diet may seem harmless, it has close to zero scientific evidence and can lead to social isolation or even the unhealthily obsessive food avoidance of so-called *orthorexia*. It is often more productive to focus efforts on overall lifestyle factors (obesity, sleep hygiene, lack of exercise) and preventive medications.

Differential There are few conditions that are confused with episodic migraines. As mentioned earlier, nearly all cases of recurring "sinus" headaches are in fact migraines that have been misdiagnosed. Cluster headaches are briefer, more excruciating and agitating, often occurring more than once per day. Occipital lobe seizures may present with dramatic visual disturbances followed by postictal headache. It is worth noting that in migraineurs, any *change in headache pattern* may represent the emergence of another underlying pathology that is "setting off" migraine symptoms.

351

Treatment Migraines often strike when the patient is vulnerable due to the buildup of triggers (see above). Lifestyle modification should be recommended or at least considered in all migraineurs. Trigger avoidance, and a generally even-keeled lifestyle devoid of "rocking the boat," may reduce attacks. Obesity, disrupted sleep (whether apnea, insomnia, insufficient sleep, erratic schedule, or otherwise poor sleep hygiene), excess or irregular caffeine consumption, under-treated psychiatric disorders, and use of analgesics more than twice per week are all potentially modifiable risk factors for worsening/more frequent migraines.

Pharmacological prophylaxis If headache frequency is >2 per month, or if individual headaches are severe, have dramatic neurological symptoms, or do not respond well to available acute treatment, the patient should be offered a daily maintenance medication. The analogy to asthma is obvious: Patients who wheeze on rare occasions may be treated with an inhaled β-agonist prn alone; those with more frequent or severe attacks additionally are placed on maintenance medication.

Tip: As a starting point for the patient, ask "Would you consider taking a medication every day to potentially cut your headaches in half?"

Most medications used to prevent migraines are drawn from the "three anti" classes: antihypertensives, antidepressants, and anticonvulsants. Many are used off-label, and *none* was specifically designed as a migraine preventive. *Learn the ins-and-outs (dosing, side effects) of one drug from each class and you will be able to manage most patients without neurological referral.*

If possible, try to choose a drug that will potentially benefit the patient in some other way (e.g., a tricyclic may help insomnia, topiramate may cause weight loss, a β-blocker may treat hypertension) to add secondary benefit and improve compliance. Conversely, avoid medications that might worsen preexisting conditions (e.g., β-blockers in athletes, erectile dysfunction, asthma, or a strong family history of diabetes; divalproex in those with obesity). Try to use once-daily formulations.

In general, do not switch medications until a trial of 2–3 months at maximum recommended or maximal tolerated dose is tried.

- *Antihypertensives:* Propranolol or nadolol 40–160 mg/24 h (gastroesophageal reflux disease [GERD], reduced exercise tolerance, erectile dysfunction, syncope, asthma exacerbation, small risk of weight gain and diabetes mellitus [DM]), verapamil up to 360 mg/24 h (constipation common, peripheral edema), lisinopril up to 40 mg/24 h (cough), candesartan up to 32 mg/24 h
- *Antidepressants:* Nortriptyline or amitriptyline 20–75 mg per night (weight gain, sedation/improved sleep, dry mouth, tachycardia, constipation, avoid in patients with abnormal electrocardiograms [ECGs]), venlafaxine up to 225 mg/24 h (useful to treat comorbid depression; typical antidepressant adverse effects but also sweating and significant withdrawal adverse effects if stopped suddenly or with variable compliance)
- *Anticonvulsants:* Divalproex 500–1,000 mg/24 h (weight gain, hair loss, tremor, GI effects; rare hematologic, hepatic effects; *avoid in potential pregnancy*). Topiramate, working up to as high as 400 mg/24 h if tolerated (paresthesias and weight loss very common; cognitive adverse effects, particularly on language (dysgeusia); may interfere with hormonal contraception at doses >200 mg, increases cleft-lip/palate in pregnancy). Gabapentin up to 3,600 mg/24 h (dose-limiting sedation, peripheral edema)

Acute attack treatment Success in aborting migraine attacks is related to three factors: Speed of administration of the agent (how long from first symptom it takes for medication to be administered), absorption/bioavailability of the agent, and the efficacy of the medication. In general, abortive medications are less effective the longer the patient waits to take them, particularly if the patient progresses to allodynia, when normally nonpainful stimuli such as brushing the hair becomes uncomfortable. "*Waiting to see how bad it gets*" before taking medication is generally counterproductive. Also, there is evidence indicating that many migraineurs have delayed gastric emptying times (related to their nausea), and thus pills or dissolving tablets may not achieve the same rapid bioavailability as injections or nasal sprays. Finally, medications can differ in pharmacology, their relative efficacy, time to onset of analgesia, and half-life.

The triptans are serotonergic *agonists* at $5HT_{1B/D/F}$ receptors. Although they were designed to and do result in constriction of the cranial arteries (and, unfortunately, the coronary arteries to some extent), this effect may not be necessary for their beneficial effects, as they also bind nerve terminals in the trigeminal system (reducing neurogenic inflammation) and potentially in the brainstem itself. There are a variety of formulations including pills, dissolving wafers, injections, and nasal sprays. Nonoral routes may be preferred in patients who awaken with migraines or in those who have severe nausea at onset. Paresthesias or vague feelings of discomfort or even initial exacerbation of headache symptoms are not uncommon, but serious side effects are extremely rare. They are contraindicated in uncontrolled hypertension and known or strongly suspected vascular disease. Although they are labeled as interacting with antidepressants to cause the potentially dangerous serotonin syndrome, there are nearly no rigorously documented cases related to a high incidence of coadministration (see information sheets and publications from the American Headache Society for more information).

All NSAIDs can benefit migraine at sufficient doses (a formulation of ibuprofen and a powdered form of diclofenac are FDA approved), as can acetaminophen, and they can be safely combined with triptans for added efficacy (a sumatriptan-naproxen combination pill is available).

Dopaminergic antiemetics/neuroleptics from metoclopramide to haloperidol have been shown to benefit migraine headache as well as accompanying nausea. IV/IM preparations are often part of so-called "migraine cocktails" in ERs or neurology offices. Acute extrapyramidal side effects including akathisia (an intolerable inner restlessness) and dystonic reactions may be limited by coadministration of diphenhydramine or benztropine, but there is concern about potential for inducing tardive dyskinesia over longer periods of ongoing or repeated use.

Dihydroergotamine (currently available as a nasal spray and in an injectable and IV formulation; soon likely to be available as an inhaled formulation) is often useful in triptan nonresponders and in "rescue" treatment of a patient in status migrainosus (severe migraine for >72 h).

Single doses of dexamethasone up to 20 mg PO or IV have been shown to reduce rate of recurrence within 24–48 h in ER settings.

Altered mental status

Delirium (acute confusional state) Common in hospitalized patients (5–15% patients in general medical or surgical wards), so consider any unexplained behavior change in a hospitalized patient as possible delirium and investigate for possible underlying organic cause(s). There are seven major signs:

1 *Consciousness* is impaired (onset over hours or days). This has been described as an impairment of thinking, attention, and concentration—or more simply as a mild global impairment of cognitive processes associated with a reduced awareness. Level of consciousness *fluctuates* throughout the day, with confusion typically worsening in the late afternoon and at night ("sundowning").

2 *Disorientation* in time (does not know time, day, or year) and place (often more marked)

3 *Behavior*: Inactivity, quietness, reduced speech, and perseveration (repetition of words) or else hyperactivity, noisiness, and irritability

4 *Thinking*: Slow and confused, commonly with ideas of reference or delusions (e.g., accuse staff of plotting against them)

5 *Perception*: Disturbed, often with illusions and visual or tactile hallucinations (unlike in schizophrenia, where auditory modality dominates)

6 *Mood*: Lability, anxiety, perplexity, fear, agitation, or depression

7 *Memory*: Impaired. Later, patients may be amnesic for this episode.

Causes Pain and other psychological states are important cofactors.

- *Infections*: Pneumonia, urinary tract infection (UTI), wounds; IV lines
- *Drugs*: Opiates, anticonvulsants, L-dopa, sedatives, recreational, postanesthesia, cephalosporil antibiotics
- *Alcohol withdrawal* 2–5 d postadmission; may or may not be associated with elevated liver function tests (LFTs) and raised mean cell volume (MCV); history of alcohol abuse); also drug withdrawal.
- *Metabolic*: Hypoglycemia, uremia, liver failure, anemia
- *Hypoxia*: Respiratory or cardiac failure

- *Vascular:* Stroke (particularly bilateral occipital/parietal), myocardial infarction (MI)
- *Intracranial infection:* Encephalitis, meningitis
- *Raised ICP/space-occupying lesions*
- *Epilepsy:* Nonconvulsive status epilepticus (see Table 10.9), postictal states
- *Trauma, head injury* (especially subdural hematoma)
- *Nutritional:* Thiamine, nicotinic acid, or B_{12} deficiency

Rarely, specific focal CNS lesions can present as delirium: Right parietal processes, bilateral "watershed" (hypoperfusion from hypotension) infarcts, bilateral occipital infarcts; visual field examination is critical in detecting these. Nonconvulsive status epilepticus (NCSE) is a potentially underrecognized cause of delirium states (Table 10.9).

Evaluation and workup Once the diagnosis of delirium is established, a thorough attempt to identify the underlying causes should be undertaken. Obtaining vital signs, including oxygen saturation and blood glucose; performing a thorough general physical and neurological exam; and obtaining appropriate lab tests (i.e., electrolytes, arterial blood gas [ABG]) and possibly an electrocardiogram are warranted first steps. Reviewing medication administration records can be extremely helpful in identifying causes of altered mental status.

Management After identifying and treating the underlying cause, aim to:

1 Reduce distress and take measures to prevent accidents/falls. Close monitoring is prudent. Repeated reassurance and orientation to time and place may help.
2 Minimize medication (especially sedatives). If agitated and disruptive, however, some sedation may be necessary. Use haloperidol 0.5–2 mg IM/PO, judiciously. Wait 20 min to judge effect; further doses can be given if needed. Benzodiazepines may be used for nighttime sedation, but can worsen delirium.

Table 10.9 Nonconvulsive status epilepticus as a cause of confusion

NCSE is underdiagnosed and may manifest itself as confusion, oddly hesitant speech, impaired cognition/memory, odd behavior, dreamy state, aggression, or rarely psychosis ± abnormalities of eye movement, after psychosis eyelid myoclonus, or odd postures including the "waxy rigidity" associated with catalepsy. It may or may not occur in the context of classic seizures or ischemic brain injury. Other causes and associations: Drugs (e.g., antidepressants), infections (e.g., arboviruses; HIV; syphilis), neoplasia, dementias, sepsis, sudden changes in calcium levels, renal failure. It may be most common in ICU settings. *Diagnosis:* Electroencephalogram (EEG). *Treatment:* May respond acutely (and diagnostically) to cautiously administered low doses of IV benzodiazepines, as well as anticonvulsants. In general, nonconvulsive status epilepticus is not considered to be as dangerous as generalized convulsive status epilepticus (typically lacks the accompanying metabolic changes). Thus, the treatment algorithm is quite different, with a goal of avoiding iatrogenic overmedication and subsequent need for intubation.

Dizziness

Dizziness and vertigo

Concerns of "dizzy spells" are very common and are used by patients to describe many different sensations. The key to making a diagnosis is to find out exactly what the patient means by "dizzy" and then decide whether or not this represents vertigo.

Does the patient have true vertigo? *Definition:* An illusion of movement, often rotatory, of the patient or their surroundings. In practice, straightforward "spinning" is rare—the floor may tilt, sink, rise, or rock. Vertigo is nearly always worsened by movement, including by standing upright. *Associated symptoms:* Difficulty walking or standing, relief on lying or sitting still, nausea, vomiting, pallor, sweating. Attacks may even cause patients to fall suddenly to the ground. Associated hearing loss, otalgia, or tinnitus implies labyrinth or eighth-nerve involvement. *What is not vertigo:* Faintness or presyncope due to hypotension may be described as dizziness, often with an orthostatic quality and a graying out of vision. Anxiety with associated palpitations, tremor, and sweating may also be described as feeling dizzy, which is complicated by the fact that vertigo is nearly always anxiety provoking. Loss of consciousness during attacks should prompt thoughts of epilepsy or syncope rather than vertigo.

Causes Disorders of the labyrinth, vestibular nerve, vestibular nuclei, or their central connections are responsible for practically all vertigo. Only rarely are other structures implicated (see Table 10.10).

Labyrinthine vertigo *Benign paroxysmal positional vertigo (BPPV):* Displacement of the otoconia (otoliths) from the maculae (the receptor for sensing gravity and other acceleration) into the semicircular canals, the organs that sense head motion. This results in dramatic but transient head-position-related attacks of vertigo. The posterior canal is most often affected. Otoconia settle due to gravitational forces on the lowest part of the labyrinth (which changes with head position), leading to an illusory perception of motion. Classically, patients describe vertigo with rolling over in bed or looking up. The diagnostic Dix-Hallpike (Nylen-Barany) maneuver results in reproduction of symptoms with dramatic upward and outward rotatory nystagmus when the head is tipped backward with the symptomatic ear downward and lowered below the body in supine position. Posterior canal BPPV is easily curable by the modified Epley maneuver, which repositions the particles.

The Dix-Hallpike test is a recommended part of the examination of all patients presenting with dizziness or vertigo, as posterior canal BPPV can be almost miraculously cured noninvasively by what appears to the uninitiated to be a mere parlor trick. There are few other diseases in all of medicine that rely so dramatically on the physical examination for diagnosis, and the laying-on-of-hands for nearly instantaneous cure; such patients are eternally grateful.

Ménière's disease: Recurrent, spontaneous attacks of vertigo, tinnitus, and a sense of aural fullness caused by endolymphatic hydrops, typically resulting in some degree of permanent low frequency sensorineural hearing loss within the first year of onset. Vertigo is severe and rotational, lasts 20 min to hours, and is often accompanied by nausea and vomiting. Drop attacks may rarely be experienced (no loss of consciousness or vertigo, but sudden falling or even flinging to one side). Treatment includes low-salt diet and diuretics, and may progress to surgical or interventional procedures that may be as extreme as deliberate destruction of the dysfunctional vestibular apparatus, allowing for re-equilibration/compensation. Absent hearing loss should cause rethinking of the diagnosis.

Vestibular nerve Damage in the petrous temporal bone or cerebellopontine angle often involves the auditory nerve, causing deafness or tinnitus.

Causes: Trauma, vestibular schwannomas (acoustic neuromas), neuromas, or bony compression such as found in fibrous dysplasia.

Acoustic neuromas: Usually present with slowly progressive hearing loss, with vertigo as a later possible manifestation. With progressive tumor growth, ipsilateral cranial nerves V, VI, IX, and X may be affected (also ipsilateral cerebellum). Paradoxically, there is only rarely VII nerve involvement preoperatively. Signs of ↑ ICP occur late and indicate a large tumor.

Vestibular neuronitis: Abrupt onset of severe vertigo, nausea, and vomiting, with prostration and immobility, perhaps after an upper respiratory infection. No deafness or tinnitus. May be from a virus in the young or a vascular lesion in the elderly (essentially an end-artery stroke of a branch of the anterior inferior cerebellar artery [AICA]). Severe vertigo subsides in days, complete recovery takes 3–4 wks. Some studies indicate that early treatment with steroids can improve chance for and degree of eventual return of function.

Herpes zoster oticus (Ramsay Hunt syndrome): Herpetic eruption of the external auditory meatus from latent varicella zoster virus, with symptoms due to dysfunction of the seventh and adjacent eighth cranial nerves; ear pain with associated facial palsy ± deafness, tinnitus, and vertigo.

Brainstem Infarction of the brainstem (vertebrobasilar circulation) may produce marked vertigo, but other lesions may also be responsible (see Table 10.10). Vertigo is protracted, as are the associated nausea, vomiting, nystagmus, and potential skew deviation (uneven vertical alignment of the eyes). It is exceptional for vertigo to be the only symptom of brainstem disease; multiple cranial nerve palsies and sensory and motor tract defects are commonly also seen. Hearing is typically spared. The aura of basilar-type migraine may cause vertigo along with other transient brainstem symptoms.

Migrainous (also called vestibular migraine, migraine associated vertigo). Migraineurs not uncommonly experience dizziness/vertigo even in headache-free intervals, typically in a patient with susceptibility to motion-sickness, often with intolerance to intricate or moving visual stimuli (visual-evoked vertigo). Only consider the diagnosis in a patient with definite migraine, when routine vestibular testing and brain imaging are normal.

Table 10.10 Causes of vertigo

Vestibular end organs and vestibular nerve
    Ménière's disease
    Vestibular neuronitis (acute labyrinthitis)
    Benign positional vertigo
    Motion sickness
    Trauma
    Ototoxicity (aminoglycosides)
    Herpes zoster oticus (Ramsay-Hunt syndrome)
Brainstem, cerebellum, and cerebellopontine angle
    MS
    Infarction/transient ischemic attack (TIA)
    Hemorrhage
    Migraine aura (basilar-type, uncommon)
    Vestibular schwannoma (acoustic neuroma)
Cerebral cortex
    Vertiginous epilepsy
Alcohol or other intoxication
Migrainous vertigo
Cervical vertigo (controversial; neck symptoms are more commonly a result of a patient keeping the neck stiff to avoid exacerbating vertigo)

Deafness

Simple hearing tests To establish a clinical finding of hearing loss, the examiner should whisper a number increasingly loudly in one ear while blocking the other ear with a finger. The patient is asked to repeat the number. Make sure that failure is not due to misunderstanding.

Rinne's test Place the base of a vibrating 256 (or 512) Hz tuning fork on the mastoid process. When the patient no longer perceives sound, move the fork so that the prongs are 4 cm from the external acoustic meatus. The energy in the fork will be lessening, but the sound will be heard again if air conduction (AC) is better than bone conduction (BC), as in the normal situation. If on the other hand, BC > AC, there is either conductive hearing loss or a false-negative result due to sensorineural deafness with "hearing" of sound in the other ear. Distinguish these possibilities with Weber's test (below). If there is hearing loss and AC is better than BC, this suggests sensorineural deafness.

Weber's test Place a vibrating tuning fork in the middle of the forehead. Ask which side the patient localizes the sound to—or is it heard in the middle? In unilateral sensorineural deafness, the patient will localize the sound to the good side. In conduction deafness, the sound is located to the bad side (as if the sensitivity of the nerve has been turned up to allow for poor AC). Neither of these tests is completely reliable.

Conductive deafness Mechanical in nature, usually due to wax, otosclerosis, or otitis media.

Causes of sensorineural deafness Due to dysfunction of the cochlea or the auditory nerve. Presbycusis (senile deafness, typically higher frequencies); previous noise exposure; Ménière's disease (lower frequency); meningitis; acute labyrinthitis; head injury; acoustic neuroma; MS (rarely); Paget's disease; ototoxic drugs, such as aminoglycosides; autoimmune disorders or vasculitides; maternal infections during pregnancy; several rare congenital syndromes.

Brain MRI can assess for AICA strokes, masses or lesions of the eighth nerve, and the MS-like lesions seen in Susac's syndrome, a vasculitis that presents with sensorineural hearing loss, branch retinal artery occlusions (BRAO, best identified on fluorescein angiography), and focal CNS symptoms.

Tinnitus

This symptom is the perception of ringing, buzzing, or other noises generally without external sound. It is a common phenomenon. In most cases, the sound is an illusory subjective perception of a high-pitched whine, but there are conditions where there is objectively measurable sound.

Causes Unknown, hearing loss (20%), wax, viral, presbyacusis, noise (e.g., gunfire), head injury, suppurative otitis media, post-stapedectomy, Ménière's (often lower pitched/hissing/roaring/staticky), head injury, anemia, hypertension (found in up to 16%, but it may not be causative). *Drugs:* Aspirin or other salicylates, loop diuretics, aminoglycosides (e.g., gentamicin).

Causes of pulsatile tinnitus: i.e., with heartbeat; potentially audible with stethoscope; do MRI. Carotid artery stenosis/dissection, arteriovenous (AV) fistula, glomus jugulare tumors, radiating cardiac murmur, elevated intracranial pressure, dehiscence of temporal bone near a branch of the carotid.

Treatment Identify and treat the underlying pathology if possible. Specific treatments for tinnitus itself are often unsatisfactory and may involve the use of masking hearing devices or white-noise and behavioral conditioning.

Abnormal movements

Dyskinesia (abnormal involuntary movements) Tremor

Rest tremor is rhythmic, present at rest during waking, and abolished on voluntary movement. It occurs in parkinsonism (with rigidity/bradykinesia) and may respond to dopaminergic medications.

Intention tremor is an irregular, large-amplitude shaking worse on reaching out for something, typically more dramatic the closer the movement is to the target. It is typical of cerebellar disease (e.g., MS). Medical treatment is difficult; use of wrist weights or extra-heavy utensils may improve functioning by dampening the oscillations. Some patients may benefit from thalamic deep brain stimulation.

Postural tremor is absent at rest, present on maintained posture (e.g., arms outstretched), and may persist (but is not exaggerated) on movement.

Causes: Familial essential tremor (autosomal dominant; improved with alcohol, β-blockers, primidone, or, in severe cases, with deep brain stimulation), thyrotoxicosis, anxiety, caffeine or other stimulants, withdrawal from alcohol or benzodiazepines.

Chorea, athetosis, and hemiballismus

Chorea: Nonrhythmic, jerky, purposeless movements that flit from one part of the body to another. Causes include Huntington's and Sydenham's chorea (choreoathetoid movements)—a rare complication of streptococcal infection. Chorea gravidarum is a poorly understood condition typically self-limited to pregnancy. The anatomical basis of chorea is uncertain but it is thought of as the pharmacological mirror image of Parkinson's disease (PD) (levodopa worsens chorea). *Hemiballismus:* Large-amplitude, flinging hemichorea (affects proximal muscles) contralateral to a lesion of the subthalamic nucleus (often a lacunar infarction in an elderly diabetic). Recovers spontaneously over months. *Athetosis:* Slow, sinuous, confluent, purposeless writhing movements (especially of the digits, hands, face, tongue), often difficult to distinguish from chorea (some consider chorea-athetosis a continuum). Most common cause is cerebral palsy. Treatment of these adventitious movement disorders is difficult, but recently tetrabenazine has been shown to improve function in Huntington's, although with a significant risk for depression.

Tics

Brief, repeated, stereotyped movements that patients are able to voluntarily suppress for a time, at least until an overwhelming urge "builds up" that is released by the acting out of the movement. Simple tics are common in children, but usually resolve. In *Gilles de la Tourette's syndrome*, multiple motor and vocal tics occur. Consider psychological support; the central α_2 agonists clonidine or guanfacine are first-line treatments, and various antipsychotic agents may be required if tics are severe.

Myoclonus

Sudden involuntary focal or general jerks arising from cord, brainstem, or cerebral cortex, seen in neurodegenerative disease (e.g., lysosomal storage enzyme defects), Creutzfeldt-Jacobs disease (CJD), myoclonic epilepsies (including infantile spasms), and sometimes post spinal cord injuries. Most commonly, multifocal or generalized myoclonus is seen in severe toxic or metabolic disturbances, such as hepatic, renal, or ventilatory insufficiency, or due to medications such as cephalosporins. *Benign essential myoclonus:* General myoclonus begins in childhood as muscle twitches (autosomal dominant and has no other consequences). *Asterixis:* Can be considered a negative myoclonus, the loss of muscle tone. Seen as downward "flap" of outstretched hands from loss of extensor tone. Myoclonus may respond to valproate, levetiracetam, or clonazepam. *Post-anoxic* If seen in a comatose patient after circulatory arrest, prognosis is usually fatal. In post-respiratory arrest (e.g., asthma), survivors may exhibit a stimulus- or action-induced myoclonus, known as the Lance-Adams syndrome. Cause is thought to be selective vulnerability and loss of Purkinje cells.

Dystonia Prolonged muscle contraction causing abnormal posture or repetitive movements due to any number of causes. Dystonia may worsen in conditions of mental or emotional stress. In patients <40 with widespread dystonia, consider a trial of levodopa to rule out *dopa-responsive dystonia* (rare), a genetic disorder. Many patients with dystonia suffer from mutation of the DYT-1 gene. Some dystonia patients respond to high-dose trihexyphenidyl or deep brain stimulation. Cervical dystonia, or spasmodic torticollis, is relatively common, a focal dystonia of the neck musculature resulting in a head tilt or "wry neck." *Blepharospasm*, involuntary contraction of orbicularis oculi, and *writer's cramp* are other focal dystonias. Disabling focal dystonias *may* respond to botulinum toxin injected into the overactive muscles. *Acute dystonia* may occur in young men starting neuroleptics (head jerked back, eyes drawn upward, trismus). Use anticholinergics (benztropine 1–2 mg IV).

Tardive dyskinesia Involuntary chewing and grimacing movements, a dreaded complication due to long-term use of neuroleptic agents (e.g., antipsychotics such as haloperidol or antiemetics such as metoclopramide or prochlorperazine). *Treatment:* Withdraw neuroleptic and wait 3–6 months. The dyskinesia may fail to resolve or may even worsen. If so, consider tetrabenazine 25–50 mg/8 h.

Ischemic stroke

Stroke: Clinical features and investigations

Strokes result from ischemic infarction or bleeding into part of the brain, manifest by rapid onset (instantly, or over minutes) of focal CNS signs and symptoms. It is the major cause of permanent neurological disability and death.

Incidence: There are 700,000 strokes each year in the United States. It is the third leading cause of death behind heart disease and cancer.

Causes:
- Thrombosis-in-situ
- Heart emboli (atrial fibrillation, infective endocarditis, MI). See Table 10.11.
- Atherothromboembolism (often from carotids)
- Ischemia due to hypoperfusion distal to an intracranial stenosis
- CNS hemorrhage (hypertension, trauma, cocaine use)

359

Rare causes: Sudden hypotension ("watershed infarctions" in distal perfusion territories), vasculitis, venous sinus thrombosis. *In young patients suspect:* Thrombophilia, vasculitis, venous-sinus thrombosis, carotid artery dissection (spontaneous or from neck trauma or fibromuscular dysplasia), cardiac defects.

Risk factors Hypertension, smoking, diabetes mellitus, heart disease (valvular, ischemic, atrial fibrillation), peripheral vascular disease, prior TIA or stroke, carotid bruit, hyperlipidemia, excess alcohol, hypercoagulable states.

Signs Sudden onset or a step-wise progression over minutes to hours is typical. In theory, focal signs relate to distribution of the affected artery, but collateral supplies can cloud the issue. *Cerebral hemisphere infarcts* (50%) may cause contralateral hemiplegia that is initially flaccid (floppy limb, falls like a dead weight when lifted), then over days to weeks becomes spastic (UMN); contralateral sensory loss; homonymous hemianopia; dysphasia.

Brainstem infarction (25%) produces a wide range of effects that include quadriplegia, disturbances of gaze and vision, locked-in syndrome (aware, but unable to respond), ataxia, vertigo, and possibly dysphagia. *Lacunar infarcts* (25%) are small infarcts around basal ganglia, internal capsule, thalamus, and pons. Classically, they may cause pure motor, pure sensory, mixed motor and sensory signs; ataxia with hemiparesis; or dysarthria with a clumsy hand. Cognition and cortical functions remain intact.

Evaluation of acute strokes The approach to emergent stroke management has changed dramatically with the advent of thrombolytic therapy. In most cases, the following steps are undertaken, potentially in parallel:

- Stabilize patient
- Establish diagnosis
- Establish time of onset
- Grade severity
- Begin acute thrombolytic therapy:
  - Establish eligibility
  - Establish contraindications
  - Administer if appropriate
- Begin peristroke assessment and management
- Prevent and treat acute post-stroke complications
- Modify secondary risk factor
- Rehabilitate

Establishing the diagnosis of ischemic stroke and the time of onset has become critical for identifying patients who could benefit from the IV or intra-arterial administration of thrombolytics. Thus, the evaluation of a patient presenting with new-onset stroke symptoms includes the following: stabilization (the ABC's of airway, breathing, circulation), evaluation of vital signs, assessment of blood glucose (as hypo- and hyperglycemia can cause focal neurologic deficits), a thorough history and physical, and a noncontrast CT scan of the brain to rule out intracranial hemorrhage. Patients presenting early enough (such that a workup can be completed and therapy initiated within 3 h or, in certain cases, 4.5 h of onset of symptoms) and meeting inclusion criteria without exclusion criteria are candidates for modestly effective IV thrombolytic therapy. If the patient presents in such a way that therapy cannot be administered within 3–4.5 h of symptom onset, then consideration may be given for intra-arterial thrombolysis or clot retrieval (if administration will occur within 6 h of symptoms, or longer in posterior circulation cases).

Diffusion-weighted MRI imaging (DWI) has dramatically improved the detection of early and small strokes and the ability to distinguish stroke from mimics, with high sensitivity and specificity (Figure 10.5). Additional MRI techniques (comparing perfusion deficits to areas of infarction on DWI, for example) may eventually allow for a longer time window in patients with a small central area of infarction but a much larger territory at risk of ischemic death.

After the acute management stage—which also involves ensuring adequate swallowing, nutrition, and treatment of complications such as pneumonia and prophylaxis against deep vein thrombosis (DVT)—physicians need to pursue appropriate evaluations to identify modifiable patient risk factors for future strokes. These tests are meant to improve secondary prevention. They include evaluations for:

- *Hypertension:* Look for retinopathy and enlarged heart on chest x-ray (CXR). Acutely raised BP is common in early stroke. In general, do not treat the elevated pressure acutely. This elevation of BP may be responsible for collateral flow to "at risk" but not yet infarcted brain tissue (the so-called ischemic penumbra). Once the patient is out of the acute post-stroke period, tight BP control, typically with a thiazide diuretic or an angiotensin-converting enzyme (ACE)-inhibitor is a mainstay of secondary prevention).

- *Cardiac source of emboli: Atrial fibrillation (AF):* Emboli from the left atrium may have caused the stroke. Look for an enlarged left atrium (ECG, CXR, echo). *Post-MI:* Mural thrombus is best seen by echocardiography. In stroke from AF or mural thrombus, do CT to exclude a hemorrhagic stroke, then start aspirin; wait before commencing full anticoagulation to avoid bleeds into infracted brain tissue. *SBE/IE:* 20% of patients with bacterial endocarditis present with CNS signs due to septic emboli from valves. Anticoagulation in such cases can potentially lead to disastrous complications from bleeding mycotic aneurysms and must be balanced against risk of clotting from a mechanical valve (if present). Treat as endocarditis; seek input from both neurology and cardiology.
- *Carotid artery stenosis:* In carotid territory stroke/TIA, randomized trials show clear benefit of carotid endarterectomy or stenting, so expert bodies affirm that 80% stenosis (on Doppler ultrasound) merits angiography ± interventions in appropriate patients.

Table 10.11 Cardiac causes of stroke

Cardioembolic causes are the source of stroke in >30% of patients in population studies. If identified, cardioembolic sources can dramatically change secondary prevention strategies.

- Atrial fibrillation (AF) ↑ risk of stroke fivefold (5–12% per year, depending on comorbidities). This risk rises with age, duration of AF, hypertension, and heart failure—and if the AF follows rheumatic fever. Left ventricular dilatation, left atrial enlargement with stasis, and mitral valve disease particularly increases risk for stroke; this risk can be largely reduced by anticoagulation. Aspirin may be preferable for those at low risk of stroke (<65, no concurrent vascular risk factors, no history of cerebral events), or for those with high risk of hemorrhage. Aim for an International Normalized Ratio (INR) of 2.0–3.0 (stroke risk is twice as much for those with an INR of 1.7 as opposed to 2).
- Newer non-warfarin anticoagulants (e.g., dabigatran, rivarobaxan, apixaban) have been developed. They generally do not require therapeutic monitoring, but lack of reversibility, which may be a serious issue in the event of acute intracranial hemorrhage or other bleeding complication. Although they do have their own issues in terms of specific drug interactions and use in hepatic or renal failure, it is possible that one or more may eventually prove superior to warfarin.
- Studies of extended-wear cardiac telemetric or event monitors have shown a significant proportion of otherwise cryptogenic strokes may be caused by otherwise asymptomatic paroxysmal atrial fibrillation and should be considered in such cases.
- External cardioversion is complicated in 1–3% by peripheral emboli: Pharmacological cardioversion may carry similar risks.
- Prosthetic valves risk major emboli; anticoagulate (INR 2.5–3.5).
- Acute myocardial infarct with large left ventricular wall motion abnormalities on echocardiography predispose to left ventricular thrombus. Emboli arise in 10% of these patients in the next 6–12 months; risk is reduced by two-thirds by anticoagulation.
- Paradoxical systemic emboli via the venous circulation in those with patent foramen ovale and atrial and ventricular septal defects can occur.

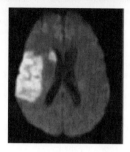

Figure 10.5 Diffusion-weighted MRI of brain revealing right sided, MCA territory infarct

The treatment of stroke will vary somewhat depending on the etiology, but in almost all cases patients will be started on an antiplatelet agent (aspirin), a statin, and possibly a thiazide diuretic, ACE-inhibitor or angiotensin receptor blocking agent. DVT prophylaxis is indicated during hospitalization and rehabilitation. Dysphagia screens for anyone with facial weakness or cognitive impairments should be done on admission to identify patients at increased risk for aspiration. Based on numerous large studies, there is no indication for empiric anticoagulation or "heparinization" in stroke patients. The addition of heparin in all stroke patients seems to help as many individuals as it harms, making its "standard" use impractical and unwarranted.

- *Diabetes mellitus:* Stroke in the setting of elevated blood glucose may have worsened outcome. Tight control of blood sugar from immediately after stroke is recommended for initial outcome as well as secondary prevention.
- *Hyperlipidemia:* Acute, high-dose statin (HMG-CoA reductase inhibitor) therapy has been shown to reduce risk in myocardial infarction; many neurologists take the same approach presumptively in stroke. Statins reduce risk of second stroke, probably even in the absence of significant hypercholesterolemia.
- *Giant cell arteritis:* If ESR is extremely elevated or there is a history of subacute headache, tender scalp (not necessarily temporal), or symptoms consistent with polymyalgia rheumatica, give steroids promptly, then biopsy within 10 d.
- *Syphilis:* Look for active, untreated disease.

Central retinal artery occlusion (CRAO) is an ophthalmological emergency that should be considered as a stroke of the retina. It presents with sudden, painless monocular visual loss and an often initially bland funduscopic exam with an afferent pupillary defect (positive swinging flashlight test). Promptly administered systemic or catheter-directed thrombolytic therapy may prevent permanent blindness (the time window for administration may extend to 24 hours, the but earlier the better). Giant cell (temporal) arteritis must be on the differential diagnosis of causes, along with carotid and embolic disease.

Transient ischemic attack

The sudden onset of focal CNS signs or symptoms due to temporary occlusion, usually by emboli, of part of the cerebral circulation, is termed a TIA if symptoms fully resolve within 24 h (TIAs are typically much shorter, resolving in far less than an hour) *and* there is no subsequent evidence of infarct on MRI. As vascular events, they are the harbingers of impending stroke or even MI. If they are recognized for what they are and preventive measures are prompt, a disastrous infarction may be averted. Simple scoring systems such as ABCD² (see Table 10.12) have been developed that may predict risk of subsequent stroke and facilitate triage in terms of the need for expedited workup (older patients, those with hypertension or diabetes, or those with long duration symptoms). It cannot be strongly enough emphasized *that it is much better to prevent a stroke than to treat one after it has occurred.* Whereas TIA is a warning shot across the bow, a stroke is a sinking ship.

Symptoms Attacks may be single or many. Symptoms may be the same or different on each occasion and depend on the specific arterial territory involved. Symptoms are sudden onset and typically last <30 minutes. Anything that lasts >2 hours or so will often be revealed by subsequent MRI imaging to involve infarction of tissue, even in cases of near complete improvement. In carotid disease, in addition to the expected contralateral weakness/numbness and higher cortical function deficits (dominant: Language; nondominant: Neglect or visuospatial problems) be alert for amaurosis fugax (one eye's vision is blotted out "like a curtain descending over my field of view"), representing a transient occlusion of the ophthalmic artery (the first branch of the internal carotid).

Signs *No CNS signs 24 h after an attack.* Listen for carotid bruits, although their absence does not rule out a carotid source of emboli. Tight stenoses often have *no* bruit. Listen for cardiac murmurs suggesting valve disease and identify AF.

Causes The same as for ischemic stroke.

Differential diagnosis of brief, focal CNS symptoms: *Migraine* aura (symptoms spread and intensify over minutes, typically involving both *positive* and negative phenomena, as opposed to TIA in which symptoms are negative only); *focal seizure* (symptoms typically spread over *seconds* and often include twitching and jerking). Any episodic cause of dizziness

363

Table 10.12 ABCD² score for risk of stroke after tia

Points	Age of Pt	BP	Clinical Features	Duration	Diabetes
0	<60	Normal	Other than below	<10 mins	No DM
1	≥60	≥140/90	speech disturbance w/o weakness	10–59 mins	DM present
2			unilateral weakness	≥60 mins	
			ABCD² score:		
		1–3 (low)	4–5 (mod)	6–7 (high)	
2 day risk		1.0%	4.1%	8.1%	
7 day risk		1.2%	5.9%	11.7%	

(see above) may to some extent mimic vertebrobasilar insufficiency. Sometimes the problem lies in the peripheral nerves. Rare mimics of TIAs: *Malignant hypertension, hypoglycemia, MS, intracranial lesions, somatization.*

Tests TIAs should be urgently evaluated in a manner similar to acute strokes. An inpatient admission should be considered if the TIA was recent, given the 12% rate of stroke within 30 d following a TIA, perhaps utilizing additional information based on ABCD[2] or similar scoring.

Treatment Treat exactly as if the patient has had a true ischemic stroke but made a full recovery, with appropriate secondary stroke prevention measures.

Intracerebral hemorrhage

10–20% of all strokes are hemorrhagic. The pathophysiology and management of hemorrhagic strokes are completely different from ischemic strokes, yet initial clinical presentations can be identical. Thus, it is imperative that all patients presenting with symptoms of an acute stroke rapidly undergo brain imaging—typically a noncontrast head CT—to quickly diagnose intracerebral hemorrhages (ICH). Hypertension, drug use, head trauma, and vascular malformations are risk factors for ICH, with hypertension being the most common cause of spontaneous intracerebral hemorrhage. Common locations of hypertensive ICH include the basal ganglia, thalamus, and cerebellum. Lobar or cortical hemorrhages should prompt a search for another underlying lesion or amyloid disease.

The treatment of patients with ICH begins with evaluation of the airway, breathing, and cardiovascular status. If the patient is stable, then directed therapy for the hemorrhage is initially focused on preventing expansion of the hematoma. Two factors, if left uncontrolled, can lead to dramatic worsening of the patient—hypertension and coagulopathies. Patients who present with an ICH and elevated BP should have a careful but rapid reduction in their BP following the guidelines used to treat hypertensive emergencies. If the patient is known to be on anticoagulation, has a known bleeding disorder, or has coagulation profiles that are noted to be abnormal, then transfusion with fresh frozen plasma should be instituted (specific coagulopathies or drugs can be treated differently).

There are various scales prognosticating functional outcome after ICH. In general, patients with larger intracerebral hemorrhages, unstable vitals at presentation, diminished level of consciousness (as measured by the Glasgow Coma Scale), and the presence of intraventricular extension do much worse. If patients survive the initial hemorrhage and do not suffer further bleeding, then the outcome will dictated by the amount of ↑ ICP and tissue damaged. Newer studies suggest that catheter-directed thrombolytic therapy into the ventricles or even into the clot itself may improve outcomes.

Subarachnoid hemorrhage

Spontaneous arterial bleeding into the subarachnoid space is often a catastrophic event and always a neurological emergency.

Incidence 8/100,000/yr; typical age: 35–65. **Causes** Rupture of saccular aneurysm is the most common cause (80%), with arteriovenous malformations accounting for ~15%. An underrecognized condition known as reversible cerebral vasoconstriction syndrome (RCVS) may be responsible for focal, cortical subarachnoid hemorrhage (SAH), particularly when presenting as thunderclap headache. Benign venous events may be the cause of small perimesencephalic SAH. *Associations:* Smoking, hypertension, alcohol abuse, bleeding disorders, mycotic aneurysm, postinfective endocarditis. Lack of estrogen (postmenopausal) has also been implicated. *Genetics:* Close relatives of those with SAH have a 3–5-fold increase in risk for SAH.

Berry aneurysms *Common sites:* Junction of the posterior communicating with the internal carotid (or of the anterior communicating with the anterior cerebral) or bifurcation of the middle cerebral artery. 15% are multiple. Some are hereditary. Skin biopsy may reveal type 3 collagen deficiency and identify relatives at risk. *Associations:* Polycystic kidneys, coarctation of the aorta, Ehlers–Danlos syndrome (hypermobile joints + ↑ skin elasticity), fibromuscular dysplasia.

Clinical features *Symptoms:* Sudden (peaking within seconds) devastating "thunderclap" headache "The worst headache of my life," often occipital. Vomiting, collapse (± seizures), and coma frequently follow. Coma/drowsiness may last for days. Up to 15% of patients die by the time they reach the hospital; overall mortality at 6 months is near 50%, and one-third or so of survivors will have residual neurological deficits (mortality risks at presentation are given in Table 10.13). *Signs:* Neck stiffness; retinal and subhyaloid hemorrhage; or focal neurologic findings, particularly a pupil, involving complete third-nerve palsy.

Differential In primary care, only 25% of those with severe, thunderclap headache have SAH. A number of other potentially devastating or treatable conditions can present with thunderclap: intracerebral bleeds, cerebral venous thrombosis, ischemic stroke, large artery dissection, colloid cyst of the third ventricle, SIH, RCVS. Although most cases will ultimately prove to be migraine or idiopathic, *thunderclap headache should always be considered a neurological emergency.* All patients deserve brain imaging, vascular imaging, and LP before ascribing the presentation to something innocuous.

Sentinel headache SAH patients may earlier have experienced a sentinel headache, perhaps due to a small warning leak from the offending aneurysm (~6%), but the picture is clouded by recall bias. As corrective surgery is more successful in the least symptomatic patients, be suspicious of any *sudden* headache, particularly if associated with neck or back pain.

Tests CT (early) shows subarachnoid or ventricular blood (Figure 10.6) but misses approximately 2% of small bleeds. Delay >1 wk progressively drops the sensitivity of CT to 50%. If a CT scan is negative, then a LP should *always* be performed in suspected cases of SAH to analyze the CSF for blood or blood breakdown products. Always send two tubes (the first and last) for cell counts to help differentiate traumatic taps from SAH. The CSF in SAH is uniformly bloody in the early stages of SAH, and the supernatant is stained xanthochromic (yellow) after a few hours due to hemoglobin breakdown to bilirubin. The diagnosis is easy (and outcome unfortunate) in a neurologically devastated patient; it is the patient presenting with headache alone who may be misdiagnosed and who stands the most to lose. Vascular imaging is needed to establish the presence, number, location, size, and type of aneurysm (including anatomic suitability for clipping vs. coiling). Noninvasive MR and CT angiographic techniques have improved to the point where they are nearly as useful as the gold standard invasive four-vessel angiogram.

Management Obtain a neurosurgical opinion (immediately if ↓level of consciousness, progressive focal deficit, or cerebellar hematoma suspected). Bed rest, BP control (maintain within normal range). Repeat CT if deteriorating. Re-examine CNS often. Prevent the need for straining with stool softeners. Maintain euvolemia. *Vasospasm* due to the presence of irritating blood around the large vessels of the brain can lead to stroke. Treatment includes nimodipine, induced hypertension, hypervolemia, and hemodilution ("triple H therapy"). In extreme cases, intra-arterial therapy may be required. Nimodipine (60 mg/4 h PO for 3 wks, or 1 mg/h IVI) is a Ca^{2+} antagonist that improves outcome (give to all if BP allows). The definitive management of a cerebral aneurysm involves either surgical clipping of the aneurysm or intravascular coiling of the aneurysm lumen. The sooner the better, as *rebleeding* is a common mode of death in those who have had a subarachnoid hemorrhage. Rebleeding occurs in 30%, often in the first few days. Ultimate outcome is strongly correlated with the patient's neurological status on initial presentation.

Many unruptured aneurysms are diagnosed incidentally on imaging studies; management is discussed in Table 10.14.

Table 10.13 Mortality in subarachnoid hemorrhage based on Hunt and Hess grading

Grade	Signs	Mortality (%)
I	None	0
II	Neck stiffness and cranial nerve palsies	11
III	Drowsiness	37
IV	Drowsy with hemiplegia	71
V	Prolonged coma	100

Almost all the mortality occurs in the first month. Of those who survive the first month, 90% survive a year or more.

Table 10.14 Unruptured aneurysms

The management of unruptured cerebral aneurysms is controversial, based on conflicting data series. In general, the risk of rupture is felt to be between 0.5 and 1.5% per year (thus, odds favor intervention in younger patients and expectant management in those with an otherwise short life expectancy). There is some data to suggest that irregularly shaped, larger, and posterior circulation aneurysms have higher rupture rates. Careful consultation with a neurosurgeon and interventional neuroradiologist is warranted whenever unruptured aneurysms are discovered, even incidentally.

Figure 10.6

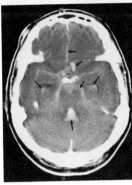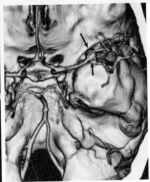

Blood from a ruptured aneurysm occupies the interhemispheric fissure (top arrow), a crescentic intracerebral area presumably near the aneurysm (next arrow down), the basal cisterns (third arrow down, right of midline), the lateral ventricles (temporal horns, the two lateralmost arrows), and the fourth ventricle (bottom arrow).

CT images can be manipulated to show only high-density structures such as bones and arteries containing contrast. Here is a middle cerebral artery aneurysm.

We thank Professor Peter Scally for these CT images and the commentaries on them.

Intracranial venous thrombosis

Isolated sagittal sinus thrombosis (47% of patients) *Presentation:* Headache, vomiting, seizures, papilledema (one cause of intracranial hypertension and is in the differential diagnosis of pseudotumor cerebri/IIH). If venous infarction or bleeding supervenes, focal neurologic deficit will be seen (e.g., hemiplegia). Sagittal sinus thrombosis is usually accompanied by thrombosis of other sinuses; e.g., *lateral (transverse) sinus thrombosis* (35%, with VI and VII cranial nerve palsies, field defect, ear pain), *cavernous sinus thrombosis* (see below), *sigmoid sinus thrombosis* (cerebellar signs, lower cranial nerve palsies), *inferior petrosal sinus* (V and VI cranial nerve palsies—Gradenigo's syndrome).

Cortical vein thrombosis This may cause venous infarcts (± focal signs), encephalopathy, seizures, and headache (including thunderclap). It usually occurs with concurrent sinus thrombosis, but may be an isolated event. Venous angiomas—otherwise benign, dilated vascular structures—may be predisposed to thrombosis.

Predisposing factors In 30%, no cause is found. Hypercoagulable states, genetic and acquired, such as pregnancy and the postpartum period, are risks factors for cerebral vein thrombosis (Table 10.15).

Differential diagnosis (See subarachnoid differential diagnosis list) Pseudotumor cerebri/IIH, RCVS.

Evaluation

Cerebral venous thrombosis is commonly missed at initial presentation, as the initial "dry" noncontrast head CT often appears normal, and the signs can be subtle on a routine noncontrast MRI (without MRV) as well. Check that there are no signs of meningitis. Do an emergency MRI or CT scan. If CT is normal, proceed to LP, measuring the opening CSF pressure. If high, and the headache is persisting, but no subarachnoid bleed, suspect cerebral vein thrombosis especially if presentation is acute or there are predisposing factors. Get further imaging. A contrast CT may show the "empty delta" sign, in which a transversely cut sinus shows a contrast filling defect (dark) in its triangular cross section. Although angiography is the gold standard, MRV (best with contrast) and CTV (reconstruction of a carefully timed contrast CT) are being utilized as noninvasive screening tools with considerable success.

Management Although there is a paucity of randomized trial data on the treatment of intracerebral venous thrombosis, the standard of care is to anticoagulate with heparin, *even in the setting of intracerebral hemorrhage*. Manage ↑ ICP and seizures as indicated. Catheter-based interventional radiographic procedures may be successful in individual cases, but are not widely available or well studied.

Cavernous sinus thrombosis is a potentially grave condition typically resulting from the extension of nearby bacterial infection (e.g., meningitis, sinusitis, dental, orbital cellulitis). It may present with cranial neuropathies (facial sensory disturbance and diplopia are common; III, IV, V1, V2, VI, and sympathetics may be affected), chemosis (swollen conjunctiva), exophthalmos, and often obtundation. Dedicated imaging studies are diagnostic and, even with immediate antibiotic treatment, this septic thrombophlebitis is often fatal.

Jugular vein thrombosis may occur as the result of central line placement, especially in critically ill patients or in the setting of other hypercoagulable issues. It may result in elevated ICP and may propagate intracranially.

Septic jugular vein thrombosis (Lemierre's) may occur as the result of oral or pharyngeal infections, including peritonsillar pathology.

Branch or central retinal vein occlusion presents with visual loss and dramatically abnormal retinal exam, often with hemorrhage. Macular edema, ischemia, and complications due to neovascularization may result.

Subdural hematoma

Consider this very treatable condition in all whose conscious level fluctuates and also in those having an "evolving stroke"—especially if on anticoagulants. Bleeding is from bridging veins between cortex and venous sinuses (vulnerable to deceleration injury), resulting in accumulating hematoma between dura and arachnoid. This gradually raises ICP, shifting midline structures away from the side of the clot and, if untreated, eventual tentorial herniation and coning.

Most subdurals are secondary to trauma but they can occur without. The trauma may have been so minor or have happened so long ago that it is not recalled. The elderly are particularly susceptible, as brain atrophy makes bridging veins more vulnerable. Others at risk are those prone to falls (epileptics, alcoholics), those on long-term anticoagulation, and those with spinal fluid leaks.

Symptoms Development of a subdural hemorrhage may be insidious so be alerted by a fluctuating level of consciousness (present in 35%). Typical complaints are of physical and intellectual slowing, sleepiness, headache, personality change, and unsteadiness.

Signs ↑ ICP. Localizing neurological symptoms (e.g., unequal pupils, hemiparesis) occur late and often long after the injury (63 d average).

CT Shows clot ± midline shift (but beware bilateral isodense clots). Look for crescent-shaped collection of blood over one hemisphere. The sickle-shape differentiates subdural blood from epidural hemorrhage.

Differential Evolving stroke, cerebral tumor, dementia.

Treatment Evacuation of symptomatic acute SDH via burr holes usually leads to full recovery. Minor cases can be managed with close observation.

Epidural hematoma

Suspect this if, after head injury, conscious level falls or is slow to improve. Extradural bleeds are commonly due to a fractured temporal or parietal bone causing laceration of the middle meningeal artery and vein, typically after trauma to a temple just lateral to the eye. Any tear in a dural venous sinus will also result in an extradural bleed. Blood accumulates between bone and dura.

Symptoms and signs Look for a rapid deterioration of consciousness after any head injury that initially produced no loss of consciousness or after initial drowsiness post-injury seems to have resolved. This "lucid interval" pattern is typical of epidural bleeds. It may last a few hours to a few days before a bleed declares itself by a deteriorating level of consciousness caused by a rising ICP. Increasingly severe headache, vomiting, confusion, and seizures can follow, accompanied by a hemiparesis with brisk reflexes and an upgoing plantar response. If bleeding continues, the ipsilateral pupil dilates and coma deepens, a bilateral spastic paraparesis develops, and breathing becomes deep and irregular. Death follows a period of coma and is due to respiratory arrest. Bradycardia and raised BP are late signs.

Tests CT reveals hematoma that is often lens-shaped (biconvex; the blood forms a more rounded shape because the tough dural attachments to the skull tend to keep it more localized). Skull x-ray may be normal or show fracture lines crossing the course of the middle meningeal vessels. Skull fracture after trauma greatly increases the risk of an extradural hemorrhage and should lead to prompt CT.

Management Stabilize and transfer promptly (with skilled medical and nursing escorts) to a neurosurgical unit for clot evacuation. Care of the airway in an unconscious patient and measures to reduce ICP often mandate intubation, hyperventilation and administration of IV mannitol or hypertonic saline.

Meningitis

Meningitis, an inflammation of the lining surrounding the brain, can be caused by a variety of pathologies. Bacteria, viruses, fungi, mycobacteria, medications, and tumors can all cause acute meningitis. Depending on the etiology, the presentation will vary dramatically. Bacterial meningitis classically causes fulminant illnesses with severe headaches, photophobia, and meningeal symptoms; viral and drug-related etiologies tend to have milder symptoms; fungal and mycobacterial infections can be indolent; whereas meningeal carcinomatosis is often accompanied by radicular or cranial nerve findings. Other cases of aseptic meningitis are due to autoimmune or vasculitic diseases, such as systemic lupus erythematosus, sarcoidosis, rheumatoid arthritis, Wegener's/antineutrophil cytoplasmic antibody (ANCA)+, Behçet's, or Vogt-Koyanagi-Harada.

The evaluation of suspected infectious meningitis (fever, headache, stiff neck, nausea, photophobia) hinges on CSF sampling via LP. A significant body of research has investigated the necessity for obtaining CT prior to LP in order to mitigate risk for iatrogenic herniation due to CSF withdrawal from the thecal sac. There are conflicting priorities. An abundance of data indicate that antibiotic administration should be given as early as possible to improve outcome, but treatment prior to LP may sterilize the CSF, thus rendering a specific microbiological diagnosis impossible. Treatment delay, such as for obtaining CT scan, may worsen outcomes. Thus, the Infectious Disease Society of America has formulated a consensus statement regarding management of patients with suspected bacterial meningitis. If a patient is immunocompromised, has a CNS disease, develops a seizure during presentation, or has papilledema, alteration of consciousness, or a focal neurologic deficit, then they should have blood cultures drawn, therapy initiated, and a head CT performed *before* the LP is performed. If all of those features are absent, then the patient should have urgent blood cultures drawn, an urgent LP performed, and empiric therapy initiated.

Empiric therapy for bacterial meningitis includes IV dexamethasone and an antibiotic regimen based on the patient's age and risk factors (Table 10.16).

In the United States in 2012, an outbreak of severe and sometimes lethal fungal meningitis occurred as the result of injection of contaminated steroid solution from a compounding pharmacy for various spinal procedures; delay from the procedure to symptom onset was many weeks.

Once the CSF is obtained, it can be analyzed to determine whether it is consistent with a bacterial, viral, fungal, mycobacterial, neoplastic, or drug-related etiology. This interpretation *must* include an assessment of the clinical situation as the patterns of CSF findings may not be classic.

In general, bacterial meningitis is associated with higher CSF white blood cell (WBC) counts with a predominance of polymorphonuclear cells, whereas viral and other meningitides have predominantly lymphocytes but can present early with neutrophils. The typical features of CSF in a variety of pathologies are summarized in Table 10.17.

Table 10.16 Bacterial meningitis organisms and empiric treatment

Predisposing factor	Common organisms	Empiric antibiotics
Age <1 month	*Streptococcus agalactiae, Escherichia coli, Listeria mono-cytogenes, Klebsiella* sp.	Ampicillin plus cefotaxime or ampicillin plus an aminoglycoside
Age 1–23 months	*Streptococcus pneumoniae, Neisseria meningitides, S. agalactiae, Haemophilus influenzae, E. coli*	Vancomycin plus a third-generation cephalosporin
Age 2–50 yrs	*N. meningitides, S. pneumoniae*	Vancomycin plus a third-generation cephalosporin
Age >50 yrs	*S. pneumoniae, N. meningitides, L. monocytogenes,* aerobic gram-negative bacilli	Vancomycin plus ampicillin plus a third-generation cephalosporin
Basilar skull fracture	*S. pneumoniae, H. influenzae,* group A β-hemolytic streptococci	Vancomycin plus a third-generation cephalosporin
Penetrating head trauma	*Staphylococcus aureus,* coagulase-negative staphylococci, aerobic gram-negative bacilli (including *Pseudomonas aeruginosa*)	Vancomycin plus cefepime, vancomycin plus ceftazidime, or vancomycin plus meropenem
Post neurosurgery	Aerobic gram-negative bacilli (including *P. aeruginosa*), *S. aureus,* coagulase-negative staphylococci	Vancomycin plus cefepime, vancomycin plus ceftazidime, or vancomycin plus meropenem
CSF shunt	Coagulase-negative staphylococci, *S. aureus,* aerobic gram-negative bacilli, *Propionibacterium acnes*	Vancomycin plus cefepime, vancomycin plus ceftazidime or vancomycin plus meropenem

Table 10.17 CSF in meningitis

	Cell count	Differential	Protein	Glucose
Bacterial	++++	Polys	++	Low
Viral	+++	Lymphocytes	+	Low to normal
Fungal	+++	Monocytes	+++	Low
Mycobacterial	++	Variable	+++	Low
Neoplastic	+	Variable	++	Very low
Drug related	++	Variable	+	Normal

Encephalitis

Whereas meningitis is caused by inflammation within the lining *around* the brain (the meninges), encephalitis is caused by inflammation *within* the brain parenchyma. Encephalitis can be caused by both infectious and noninfectious etiologies, but classically the term "encephalitis" refers to infectious causes while the term "cerebritis" is used to identify noninfectious inflammatory processes within the brain.

Infectious causes of encephalitis include viral, bacterial, fungal, and mycobacterial pathogens, but viruses are by far the most common cause of acquired encephalitis worldwide. The differential of viruses varies depending on geography, with arboviral pathogens (mosquito-borne viruses) changing dramatically from country to country. Within the United States, the most common identifiable cause of nonepidemic encephalitis is herpes (HSV1), a devastating illness that can lead to amnesia, seizures, and death.

Typically, encephalitis presents with fever, photophobia, altered sensorium or behavior, and variable degrees of meningeal symptoms. In this setting, a patient should be initiated on IV acyclovir therapy for possible HSV encephalitis while a LP is performed. Besides testing for cell count, protein, glucose, Gram stain, and bacterial culture, an HSV polymerase chain reaction (PCR) should be sent. This highly sensitive and specific test is the gold standard for identifying patients with HSV encephalitis. Caution should be taken, however, due to the false-negative rate that occurs within the first 3–4 d of symptoms. In the appropriate clinical setting, when a high pretest probability occurs, a negative HSV PCR should not be an indication to stop acyclovir therapy, but rather a second LP should be performed and a second HSV PCR obtained.

West Nile arbovirus has emerged and spread in recent years throughout much of the world, with seasonal epidemics in the United States, and it may present with (meningo-) encephalitis and/or a poliomyelitis-like picture of flaccid weakness. Fortunately, the vast majority of exposures result in mild or subclinical disease.

Autoimmune encephalitis is increasingly being recognized as a cause of subacute, non-infectious, progressive encephalitis. Limbic encephalitis presenting with personality changes, bizarre behavior, amnesia, and/or difficult seizures is typical; cerebellar or other degenerative syndromes can be seen as well. Paraneoplastic as well as non-paraneoplastic associated antibodies have been identified. Voltage gated potassium channel (VGKC) and anti-NMDA receptor antibodies are frequently implicated; anti-GAD, anti-AMPA receptor, and anti GABA receptor antibodies have also been reported. Antibodies against other intracellular neuronal antigens may be markers rather than pathogenic. Search for and treatment of underlying malignancies (especially testicular, breast, small cell lung, and ovarian) should be undertaken, and aggressive immunological treatments are often warranted. Commercial test panels are available for both serum and CSF analysis.

Multiple sclerosis

This typically relapsing/remitting disorder consists of plaques of demyelination (and, as is increasingly apparent with pathological studies and newer imaging techniques, axon loss and even destruction of gray matter) at sites throughout the CNS (but not peripheral nerves). Pathogenesis involves focal disruption of the blood–brain barrier and associated autoimmune response, and myelin damage as well as neurodegenerative and regenerative processes.

Epidemiology MS affects ~350,000 people in the United States, with a ♀:♂ ratio of 2:1. The peak age of onset is in the 20s and 30s, making MS one of the most common causes of disability in young adults. MS is more common in temperate climates, with some data suggesting an increased prevalence as you move farther away from the Equator, and with newer studies suggesting that early-life vitamin D deficiency may account for this link. There is also a strong genetic influence within MS, with monozygotic twins having a 30% concordance rate and dizygotic twins having a 5% concordance rate. Children of patients with MS have a 3–5% rate of MS, compared to the background rate of 0.2% in Caucasian populations.

Presentation is initially usually monosymptomatic due to a *clinically isolated syndrome (cis)*: Unilateral optic neuritis (pain on eye movement and rapid deterioration in central vision); numbness or tingling in the limbs; leg weakness or brainstem or cerebellar symptoms, such as diplopia or ataxia. Less often, there may be more than one symptom. *Uhthoff's phenomenon*, symptoms worsening with heat (e.g., a hot bath) or exercise, may be present.

Progression/prognosis: Early on, relapses may be followed by remission/full recovery. With time, remissions are incomplete, so disability accumulates. This form of *relapsing remitting multiple sclerosis* (RRMS) occurs in 80% of patients. Primary progressive MS is more relentless and seems to respond poorly to therapy. *Poor prognostic signs:* Older males; motor signs at onset; many relapses early on; many MRI lesions.

Examination Look carefully for CNS deficits other than the presenting problem. Lhermitte's symptom (paresthesia/pain in the back or limbs on flexing of the neck due to demyelination the cord) may be positive (also in cervical spondylosis or B_{12} deficiency). Reduced perception of the color red in one eye or an afferent papillary defect may indicate prior optic neuritis. Internuclear ophthalmoplegia (disconjugate movements due to reduced amplitude or velocity of adduction of one or both eyes, best noted on rapid side-to-side saccades to the extremes of gaze; additionally there is typically abducting nystagmus) is characteristic of brainstem involvement in the disease. When mild, patients may not report.

Diagnosis This is clinical, requiring demonstration of lesions disseminated in time and space, unattributable to other causes (Table 10.18). Isolated CNS deficits are never diagnostic but may become so if a careful history reveals previous episodes (e.g., unexplained blindness for a week). Before the advent of MRI, making the diagnosis of clinically definite MS required more than one clinical episode. Utilizing MRI techniques, the diagnosis of clinically definite MS can be made after only one clinically apparent demyelinating event, based on subsequent appearance of other radiographic lesions. This ability is important due to data that suggest early immunomodulatory treatment can alter the course of the disease. Additionally, patients with optic neuritis or other CIS with additional characteristic imaging lesions at the time of presentation may benefit from disease-modifying therapy without meeting formal criteria for definite disease.

Differential diagnosis includes neuromyelitis optica (see below), CNS Sjögren's syndrome, acute disseminated encephalomyelitis (a monophasic but sometimes fulminate demyelinating condition), Susac's and other vasculitis or autoimmune disorders affecting the CNS.

Tests None is pathognomonic; the quest for reliable serological and CSF biomarkers is ongoing. *CSF:* Typically, the CSF of patients with MS will show normal cell counts or a mild pleocytosis (up to 50 lymphocytes/mm³), but, rarely there can be more profound elevations. A white blood cell count >50 cells/mm³ should prompt consideration for alternate diagnoses. The protein level is usually normal or mildly elevated, rarely >100 mg/L. Evidence of inflammation restricted to the CNS can be demonstrated by comparing CSF to serum, with IgG index and especially oligoclonal bands on electrophoresis showing utility. Although not specific for MS, the presence of two or more oligoclonal bands in the CSF that are not present in the serum can increase confidence in the diagnosis in the right clinical setting. Delayed visual, auditory, and somatosensory evoked potentials can provide information regarding previous demyelinating events that are not identified on clinical exam. *MRI* is sensitive but not specific for plaque detection and may exclude other causes (e.g., cord compression). Correlation of MRI with clinical condition is poor. Some studies have identified *antibodies to myelin oligodendrocyte glycoprotein* (MOG) and *myelin basic protein* (MBP) in patients with a single MS-like clinical lesion as being predictive of conversion to clinically definite MS. It is likely that other disease markers will be identified. Visual evoked potentials may show delayed peaks in prior optic neuritis. Optical coherence tomography (OCT), a noninvasive retinal imaging modality, as well as specific MRI techniques, may serve as useful surrogate markers for disease activity, potentially guiding therapy before clinical evidence of relapse or progression.

Treatment *Methylprednisolone:* 1 g/d for 3–5 d given IV shortens relapses, but does not alter the overall prognosis, except in the case of initial optic neuritis. Repeated treatments with IV steroids can lead to risk of avascular necrosis (osteonecrosis).

Disease-modifying agents: After a slow start, development of new agents and new treatment regimens aimed at halting disease progression or otherwise protecting against damage are showing promise, with the welcome availability of newer disease-modifying oral agents attracting great attention; there are few areas of neurological therapeutics making faster advances. Treatment of the disease has *de facto* become a subspecialty in its own right. *Interferonβ (infβ-1b; infβ-1a):* Trials show that these can reduce relapses by 30% in active RRMS. They also reduce lesion accumulation on MRI. Their power to diminish disability remains controversial, as does benefit in secondary and primary progressive MS. Side effects include flu-like symptoms (low-grade fevers, myalgias, fatigue), depression, and site reactions. Monitoring of liver functions tests is indicated. Development of antibodies against these agents has the potential to reduce efficacy. *Glatiramer acetate:* A copolymer comprising a random mix of four amino acids—glutamate, lysine, alanine, and tyrosine. Some data suggest that glatiramer acetate exerts its therapeutic effect by shifting a patient's immune system from predominately a Th1 response to a more protective Th2 response. Side effects include site reactions and an idiosyncratic episode of flushing, palpitations, and chest pain that can last for 20 min after injection. This response is not an allergy, and it is safe to continue treatment. No blood tests need to be followed on this therapy. *Oral agents* have recently been developed to great fanfare, but they, too, have serious risks beyond that of infection. Fingolimod, a sphingosine 1-phosphate receptor modulator, has won FDA approval, but carries major risks for dangerous bradycardia (potentially fatal), macular edema, reduced lung function, and other serious adverse effects mandating a specific risk evaluation and mitigation strategy in the United States. Teriflunomide, a drug similar to one long used in rheumatological disease, has recently been approved as well and carries lower risks of major complications. An oral psoriasis treatment, dimethyl fumarate, has shown significant activity against the disease. Cladribine has been withdrawn from the U.S. and European markets due to safety concerns (cancer) but is available in other countries. Where these newer agents fit in the armamentarium is as yet uncertain (timing, mono- or polytherapy, etc.). *IV immunological agents* can have rapid and dramatic benefit, but with significant risks—*natalizumab* can lead to potentially devastating or even fatal progressive multifocal leukoencephalopathy from reactivation of latent JC virus in the brain; *mitoxantrone* has dose-limiting cardiotoxicity. Other, more aggressive immunosuppressant strategies may be employed in aggressive cases, sometimes combining multiple agents. Many newer monoclonal antibodies currently utilized for other immunological and hematological diseases are being tested for activity against MS. *Symptomatic management*

Table 10.18 2010 Revised McDonald criteria for diagnosing MS

Presentation	Additional data needed
≥2 attacks; objective clinical evidence of ≥2 lesions or objective clinical evidence of 1 lesion with reasonable historical evidence of a prior attack	None; clinical evidence will do (imaging evidence desirable; must be consistent with MS)
≥2 attacks; objective clinical evidence of 1 lesion	Dissemination in *space (DIS)*, shown by: + MRI criteria; or await a further clinical attack implicating a different CNS site
1 attack; objective clinical evidence of ≥2 lesions	Dissemination in *time (DIT)*, shown by: Simultaneous presence of asymptomatic gadolinium-enhancing and nonenhancing lesions at any time; or a new T2 and/or gadolinium-enhancing lesion(s) on follow-up MRI, irrespective of its timing with reference to a baseline scan; or await a second clinical attack
1 attack; objective clinical evidence of 1 lesion (clinically isolated syndrome)	Dissemination in *space* and *time*, demonstrated by: For DIS: + MRI; or await a second clinical attack implicating a different CNS site and For DIT: Simultaneous presence of asymptomatic gadolinium-enhancing and nonenhancing lesions at any time; or a new T2 and/or gadolinium-enhancing lesion(s) on follow-up MRI, irrespective of its timing with reference to a baseline scan; or await a second clinical attack
Insidious neurological progression suggestive of MS (PPMS)	1 year of disease progression (retrospectively or prospectively determined) plus 2 of 3 of the following criteria: • 1. Evidence for DIS in the brain based on ≥1 T2 lesions in the MS-characteristic (periventricular, juxtacortical, or infratentorial) regions • 2. Evidence for DIS in the spinal cord based on ≥2 T2 lesions in the cord • 3. Positive CSF (OCBs and/or elevated IgG index

If the criteria are fulfilled and there is no better explanation for the clinical presentation, the diagnosis is MS; if suspicious, but the criteria are not completely met, the diagnosis is "possible MS"; if another diagnosis arises during the evaluation that better explains the clinical presentation, then the diagnosis is "not MS.'"

Attacks: These must last >24 h, be focal, patient-reported, or objectively observed events typical of an acute inflammatory demyelinating event, without fever or infection.

MRI abnormality:
≥1 T2 lesion in at least 2 of 4 MS-typical regions of the CNS (periventricular, juxtacortical, infratentorial, or spinal cord)

involves lifestyle and pharmacological therapies to treat fatigue, neurogenic/spastic bladder, and tremor, as well as gait problems and other physical impairments. Fampridine (4-aminopyridine) has been shown to improve impaired walking in patients with MS, but with risk for seizure.

Transverse myelitis

Transverse myelitis is an inflammatory demyelinating disease restricted to the spinal cord. Patients present with acute to subacute onset of myelopathic symptoms. There are usually prominent motor, sensory, and bowel/bladder symptoms. This disease is usually monophasic, but some patients experience recurrences. Risk factors for recurrence include underlying autoimmune conditions such as Sjögren's or serology suggestive of an underlying condition (e.g., positive SSA/anti-Ro or SSB/anti-La antibodies). In the appropriate clinical setting of a acute/subacute myelopathy, imaging (MRI with gadolinium) must be obtained to rule out compressive lesions, intrinsic masses, or vascular lesions, and a LP should be obtained to confirm evidence of inflammation (i.e., mild pleocytosis or elevated IgG index). Absence of an enhancing lesion on MRI or pleocytosis within the CSF should prompt a search for an alternative diagnosis.

Differential diagnosis Longitudinally extensive transverse myelitis across multiple spinal levels can occur in Sjögren's, lupus, sarcoidosis, or neuromyelitis optica, whereas shorter segments are more typical for MS. An MRI of the brain should be obtained to evaluate the patient for possible MS. White matter lesions within the brain in association with a spinal cord demyelinating event could indicate that the myelopathy is in fact the first symptom of MS. Other pathologies that should be considered include neuromyelitis optica (see below), dural AV fistula, sarcoidosis, spinal cord tumor, spinal cord infarct (venous and arterial), and compressive myelopathies.

Treatment of transverse myelitis has two components, specific treatments to reduce the degree of inflammation and supportive care given to all patients with spinal cord pathology. Specifically for the transverse myelitis, high-dose IV steroids (1 g/d methylprednisolone for 5 d) is the standard of care. For patients not improving on this therapy, plasmapheresis and/or pulse-dose cyclophosphamide is indicated.

Neuromyelitis optica (Devic's)

Neuromyelitis optica (Devic's syndrome) is a demyelinating condition that is primarily restricted to the optic nerves and the spinal cord. Clinically, it presents as either an optic neuritis (diminished vision in one eye accompanied by pain with movement of that eye) or as an episode of transverse myelitis. Some patients diagnosed as having transverse myelitis will actually go on to have the initial diagnosis of Devic's syndrome after they have an episode of optic neuritis. MRI of the entire CNS with gadolinium is warranted to evaluate for evidence of MS. Patients with neuromyelitis optica (NMO) tend to progress more rapidly than MS patients and do not respond to interferons or glatiramer acetate. A circulating IgG antibody to aquaporin 4 (anti-NMO) has been identified in a large number of NMO patients, suggesting a humoral etiology. Thus, these patients may respond best to plasmapheresis, IV immunoglobulin (IVIG), or immunosuppressants with humoral activity. Immunomodulatory monoclonal antibody therapies are being tested for potential disease-modifying effects, but none is yet part of a standard or approved treatment regimen.

Dementia

The hallmark of dementia is *impaired cognition with intact consciousness* (unlike delirium). Most causes are progressive and irreversible. The key is a good history: Ask spouse, relatives, or friends about *progressively* impaired cognition/memory. Get *objective* evidence. Histories usually go back months or years. There is worsening forgetfulness, and normal tasks of daily living are done with increasing incompetence, such as going to the store several times in a day and then being baffled as to why there is a great quantity of food in the kitchen. Sometimes the patient will exhibit personality change such as apathy, uncharacteristic rudeness, or literalness. For objective evidence, do tests of cognitive functioning.

Epidemiology Rare <55 yrs. 5–10% prevalence >65 yrs. 20% prevalence >80 yrs, and 70% in those >100 yrs.

Common causes *Alzheimer's disease (AD)*; see below. *Vascular dementia:* ~25% of all dementias. It represents the cumulative effects of many small strokes. Look for evidence of vascular pathology (hypertension, past strokes, focal CNS signs). Onset is sometimes sudden, and deterioration is often stepwise (vs. slowly progressive).

Lewy body dementia: Characterized by Lewy bodies in brainstem *and* neocortex, *fluctuating* cognitive loss, alertness, and attention; parkinsonism; detailed visual hallucinations; falls; loss of consciousness/syncope. It is the third most common dementia (15–25%) after AD and vascular causes. Neuroleptics in these patients *often* cause neuropsychiatric symptoms. Parkinsonism is poorly responsive to levodopa.

Frontotemporal dementia: Frontal and temporal atrophy without Alzheimer histology. *Signs:* Behavioral/personality change; early preservation of episodic memory and spatial orientation; disinhibition; hyperorality, stereotyped behavior, and emotional unconcern.

Rarer causes: Alcohol/drug abuse, Huntington's, CJD, Parkinson's, corticobasal ganglionic degeneration, HIV, cryptococcosis, subacute sclerosing panencephalitis (SSPE), progressive leukoencephalopathy.

Ameliorable causes Hypothyroidism, vitamin B_{12} deficiency, thiamine deficiency (alcoholics), pellagra (B_3/niacin deficiency) syphilis, some cerebral tumors (e.g., parasagittal meningioma), chronic subdural hematoma, normal-pressure hydrocephalus (dilatation of ventricles without signs of ↑ ICP, possibly due to obstructed CSF flow from subarachnoid space; CSF shunts help if patients respond positively to high-volume LP; it is suggested by incontinence early-on and gait apraxia), intracranial hypotension (rarely).

377

Tests Before consigning a patient to the diagnosis of an irreversible dementia, make absolutely certain that no treatable cause of progressive mental status decline is missed, however unlikely. Assess for underlying or superimposed delirium. Complete blood count, ESR, electrolytes, LFTs, ammonia level, TSH, B_{12}, RPR/FTA, HIV, CT/MRI, and consider EEG. Treat depression if present. Nuclear imaging studies (single proton emission CT [SPECT], positron emission tomography [PET] with amyloid labeling) and spinal fluid sampling ($A\beta_{42}$, tau, others) may be useful in specific instances to confirm a specific neurodegenerative etiology.

Alzheimer's disease

This leading cause of dementia is currently having a huge impact on our health care system, nursing home system, and society. As our population continues to live longer, a greater portion will suffer from this disease, requiring increasing attention from their children and families. *Mean survival* 7–10 yrs from onset. Suspect Alzheimer's in adults with enduring, acquired deficits of visual-spatial skill ("he gets lost easily"), memory, and cognition; e.g., tested by mental test scores + other neuropsychometric tests.

Cause The pathological hallmarks of AD is accumulation of β-amyloid peptide (a degradation product of amyloid precursor protein), progressive neuronal damage, intraneuronal neurofibrillary tangles, increasing numbers of senile plaques, and loss of the neurotransmitter acetylcholine from damage to an ascending forebrain projection (nucleus basalis of Meynert; connects with cortex).

Risk factors *Defective genes* on chromosomes 1, 14, 19, 21; the apoE4 variant is linked to earlier age of onset. Family history confers risk. Incidence is also linked to diabetes, cardiovascular risk factors (smoking, hypertension), depression, obesity; exercise (physical and mental, including educational level) may be protective.

Presentation Gradual and relentless decline in memory capabilities and cognition, behavioral change (e.g., aggression, wandering, disinhibition), delusions, apathy, depression, irritability. There is no standard natural history. Toward end stage, often, but by no means invariably, patients become sedentary, taking little interest in anything. Wasting, mutism, incontinence ± seizures may occur.

Diagnosis The absolute diagnosis of Alzheimer's is based on pathology on biopsy or autopsy. Clinically, neurocognitive testing can identify patients with dementia that is consistent with an Alzheimer's type. Various disease biomarkers (spect, specific labels used with pet scans; increased csf ratios of tau or phospho-tau to $A\beta_{42}$, mri morphometry, particular panels of mental status tests) are being developed, but so far none has proven reliable or widely applicable for definite disease, let alone presymptomatically.

Treatment The standard of care for AD is cholinergic therapy with cholinesterase inhibitors. These medications do not cure or reverse the effects of this dementing illness, but rather slow the progression and delay nursing home placement. A new class of drug, the NMDA receptor antagonist (memantine), has also shown efficacy for delaying the cognitive decline seen in ad. Effective disease-modifying treatments have been frustratingly slow in coming, with many promising compounds and approaches falling by the wayside. Otherwise, care is supportive.

Epilepsy

Epilepsy is a recurrent tendency to spontaneous, intermittent, abnormal electrical activity in part of the brain, manifest as episodic *seizures*. These may take many forms, but for a given patient they tend to be stereotyped. *Convulsions* are the motor signs of electrical discharges. Many of us would have seizures in abnormal metabolic circumstances (e.g., severe hyponatremia, hypoxia [reflex brief anoxic convulsions after syncope]), but some patients have a low threshold for having seizures and do not require metabolic stresses to have a convulsion.

Presentation There may (rarely) be a *prodrome* lasting hours or days preceding the seizure. It is not part of the seizure itself: The patient or others notice a change in mood or behavior. An *aura*, which *is* part of the seizure, may precede its other manifestations. The aura may be a strange feeling in the gut, or a sensation or an experience such as *déjà vu* (disturbing sense of familiarity), or strange smells, or flashing lights. This implies a partial seizure (a focal event), often, but not necessarily, caused by temporal lobe epilepsy. After a partial seizure involving the motor cortex (Jacksonian convulsion) there may be temporary weakness of the affected limb(s) (Todd's palsy). After a generalized seizure, patients experience a headache, myalgias, confusion, and lethargy, the so-called postictal state.

Diagnosis First, since most seizures are not witnessed by medical personnel, confirming that a reported event was in fact a seizure is not a trivial matter. A detailed description from a witness of the event is crucial. Better still, *with* the proliferation of digital cameras and mobile phones with video capabilities, it is still possible to educate family members about the importance of capturing a spell for later inspection. Although a diagnosis based on history is never 100% accurate, certain historical features can increase the odds that an event was epileptic versus syncopal. The presence of prolonged tonic–clonic activity, automatisms, or tongue biting is suggestive of an ictal event. Syncopal events are often preceded by feelings of light-headedness, vision changes, and/or diaphoresis. One or two clonic movements after syncope are not abnormal and can be mistaken for an epileptic event. A more complete differential of recurrent movements includes nonepileptic (psychogenic) seizures, tetanus, posturing, rigors, neuroleptic malignant syndrome, myoclonic jerks, tremors, hemiballismus, dyskinesias, dystonias, migraine auras, and metabolic derangements. The attack's onset is the key for determining what type of seizure is occurring—partial or generalized. If the seizure begins with focal features, it is a partial seizure, however rapidly it generalizes.

Types *Partial onset seizures:* Simple partial seizures, complex partial seizures, and secondary generalized seizures. These are often lesional in etiology. *Generalized onset seizures:* Absence seizures, myoclonic seizures, clonic seizures, tonic seizures, tonic–clonic seizures, and atonic seizures. These are often genetic or developmental disorders, with widespread abnormal neuronal dysfunction.

Causes Often none is found. *Physical:* Trauma, space-occupying lesions, stroke, hypertension, tuberous sclerosis, systemic lupus erythematosus (SLE), polyarteritis nodosa (PAN), sarcoid, vascular malformations, Alzheimer's. *Metabolic:* Alcohol or benzodiazepine withdrawal; hyperglycemia or hypoglycemia, hypoxia, uremia, hypernatremia, hyponatremia, hypercalcemia, liver disease, drugs (e.g., phenothiazines, tricyclics, cocaine). *Infections:* Encephalitis, syphilis, cysticercosis, HIV.

Workup Careful history, toxic-metabolic assessment, imaging, and EEG are indicated for a first seizure (Table 10.19).

Table 10.19 Evaluation of adult with first-ever suspected seizure

Overriding goals: (1) Determine whether the event was in fact a seizure or some other paroxysmal event. (2) Assess for urgent, dangerous, treatable pathology or toxic/metabolic derangement. (3) Determine risk for subsequent seizures (epilepsy, requiring ongoing anticonvulsant therapy) versus likelihood of a one-time event.

Obtain as much history as possible from patient and witnesses. Try to form an opinion as to whether the witness is reliable. *Video* of the spell, if available, is invaluable.

You must attempt to establish a cause. Adult-onset seizures, particularly with focal features, are often "symptomatic"; i.e., secondary to another structural pathology (or cardiac-, metabolic-, or drug-related problem).

Clues from the history may point to an obvious illness or other toxic/metabolic cause for the seizure. If not, then these tests may help: Urine, electrolytes, LFTs, glucose, calcium, phosphorous, coagulation profiles, and serum and urine toxicology screens. Measure serum levels of medications. If the patient is not alert on presentation, consider screening for common antiepileptics in case the patient is a known seizure patient on medication and subtherapeutic.

Consider LP if CT shows no signs of ↑ ICP and there are signs or symptoms of a CNS infection.

(Continued)

Table 10.19 (Continued)

Imaging: Don't assume that if one CT scan is normal, there is no structural lesion. MRI/MRA should be obtained in all patients to assess for small areas of cortical dysgenesis, tumors, vascular malformations, or cavernomas. Significant cortical or juxtacortical abnormalities increase risk for subsequent seizures.

Routine EEG can help establish risk for subsequent seizure—if positive for focal or generalized spikes, a subsequent seizure much more likely. Emergent EEG only in cases of suspected status epilepticus, including nonconvulsive.

You must give advice against driving (laws vary by state as to physician responsibility for reporting), occupational hazards, bathing, swimming, and reproductive issues if the patient is a woman of childbearing age. Document your discussion.

The decision to initiate antiepileptic therapy after a first, unprovoked seizure should be individualized to the patient. Neurologic consultation is indicated.

Epilepsy: Management

Involve patients in all decisions. Compliance depends on communication and doctor–patient concordance issues. Living with epilepsy creates many problems (inability to drive, swim, or bathe alone, or operate machinery) and fears (loss of control, risk of sudden death) and medication issues.

Therapy Treat initially with one drug (with one doctor in charge) only. Increase doses until seizures are controlled, toxic effects are manifest, or maximum drug dosage reached. Beware of drug interactions, including with hormonal contraceptive therapies. Most specialists would not recommend treatment after one generalized seizure with normal EEG and imaging (in all comers, approximately 50% would have a second seizure in the next few years), but would start treatment after two, at which point epilepsy is likely. Discuss options with the patient. If your patient has only one seizure every 2 yrs, he or she may accept the risk (particularly if there is no need to drive or operate machinery) rather than have to take drugs every day.

Commonly used drugs

Carbamazepine: Has indications for partial epilepsy. Starting dose is 400 mg/d (divided into bid dosing) with a maximum dose of 2,400 mg/d (in divided doses). Side effects include rash, nausea, diplopia, dizziness, fluid retention, hyponatremia, blood dyscrasias. Levels tend to fall over time as the drug induces its own metabolism. Many drug interactions.

Gabapentin: Not a particularly potent agent, especially in monotherapy. Has indications for partial epilepsy as an adjunctive agent. Typical doses begin at 300 mg/d and can be titrated to a maximum dose of 3,600 mg/d (divided into tid dosing). Side effects include weight gain, edema, somnolence, and rarely heart failure. *Pregabalin* is a more effective drug with a similar side-effect profile.

Lamotrigine: Has indications for generalized and partial epilepsy. Usual starting dose for adults is 25 mg bid, titrating as recommended to a maximum of 400 mg/d (total dose). *Slow titration limits use in patients experiencing frequent seizures who need to be brought under rapid control.* Side effects include rash, Stephens–Johnson syndrome, dizziness, headaches, aplastic anemia, and toxic epidermal necrosis, but, in general, it is well tolerated and has relatively few cognitive effects. Caution when used in conjunction with valproate, as this will reduce the clearance of lamotrigine (slower/lower titration required). More aggressive/rapid titration is required when given with carbamazepine.

Levetiracetam: Has indications for partial epilepsy and myoclonic epilepsy, but is also useful for seizure disorders with secondary generalization. Usual dosing begins at 250 mg or 500 mg bid and can be titrated to a maximum dose of 1,500 mg bid. Side effects can include irritability and rarely psychosis.

Oxcarbazepine: Has indications for partial epilepsy. Starting doses are between 300 and 600 mg/d with a maximum dose of 2,400 mg/d (divided into bid dosing). Side effects include headaches, dizziness, hyponatremia, and ataxia.

Phenytoin: Has indications for generalized or partial epilepsy. Initial maintenance doses are around 300 mg/d with dosing being altered based on presence or absence of side effects, efficacy, and serum levels of the drug. Side effects include coarsening of facial features, gum hypertrophy, blood dyscrasias, nystagmus, and ataxia. Significant drug interactions.

Topiramate: Has indications for generalized and partial seizures. Starting doses are between 25 and 50 mg/d with a maximum dose of 400 mg/d (divided into bid dosing). Side effects include cognitive slowing, weight loss, renal stones, glaucoma, metabolic acidosis, and paresthesias (related to the drugs partial carbonic anhydrase inhibition activity). *Teratogenic, with increased risk for cleft lip/palate. Zonisamide is a similar drug.*

Valproate: Has indications for generalized and partial epilepsy. Starting dose is approximately 250 mg tid with a maximum daily dose of 3,000 mg/d (in divided doses). Side effects: Sedation, tremor, weight gain, hair thinning, ankle swelling, hyperammonemia (causing encephalopathy), and hepatic failure. *Do not use in pregnancy or in patient planning pregnancy.*

Lacosamide: A newer, very potent drug, available in PO and IV form. Dizziness is common, and cardiac conduction delay can occur.

Newer generation agents are coming online with regularity, some with more specific indications (e.g., rufinamide for Lennox-Gastaut syndrome).

Therapeutic monitoring Epilepsy patients are mostly monitored clinically, with a seizure diary and surveillance for side effects. Routine drug levels are seldom helpful in the well-controlled patient without side effects, and turnaround time for test results of newer antiepileptic agents is unacceptably long for rapid decision making. In patients with ongoing seizures, a high therapeutic level could occur with refractory epilepsy but might also raise suspicion nonepileptic seizures. Moderate levels might indicate safety to increase dosing. Extremely low levels might indicate lack of compliance. In patients with obvious side effects, drug levels may not be necessary to decrease dosing.

Changing drugs *Indications:* On inappropriate drug; side-effects unacceptable; treatment failure. *Method:* Begin new drug at its starting dose, overlapping with the first (being mindful of drug interactions) unless the patient is experiencing toxicity, in which case rapid discontinuation may be indicated. Titrate the second drug to a mid-therapeutic level, then begin a slow wean off the first if desired.

Devices and procedures Vagus nerve stimulators are effective for certain types of epilepsy. Newer implantable seizure detection and prevention devices are being developed. In appropriate cases, epileptic foci can be surgically resected after careful brain mapping. Many studies have shown that partial temporal lobectomy can greatly improve quality of life for selected patients with temporal lobe epilepsy. Corpus callosotomies are seldom performed except in extreme cases. Newer implantable devices are being developed that may be able to detect and even potentially prevent impending seizures.

Status epilepticus

Management

Status epilepticus (SE) has traditionally been defined as continuous seizure activity for 20–30 min or two seizures occurring without interval return to neurological baseline. Although >90% of all seizures will stop within 2 min, some are prolonged. No emergent therapy is needed for a normal, self-limited seizure. Prolonged convulsive seizures, however, are medical emergencies given the risk of death with status epilepticus. In addition to airway issues and potential brain injury, serious metabolic derangements can rapidly result. Once identified, the management of a patient with SE begins with assessment of the airway, acquisition of a rapid blood glucose determination (to rule out hypo- and hyperglycemia as easily treatable causes of SE), and establishment of IV access. Labs should be sent for a complete blood count, electrolytes including calcium, ABG, LFTs, toxicology, renal function, and antiepileptic drug concentrations.

While labs are being analyzed, treatment of SE is initiated with the administration of 0.1 mg/kg of lorazepam intravenously at a rate of 2 mg/min. If seizures continue, the patient should be "loaded" with an anticonvulsant, typically with phenytoin or fosphenytoin (lower hemodynamic and extravasation risks) at a dose of 20 mg/kg or 20 PE/kg,[1] respectively. If seizures continue despite this load, an additional 10 mg/kg of phenytoin or 10 PE/kg of fosphenytoin should be administered. At this stage, the use of anesthesia should be considered in conjunction with continuous EEG monitoring. Remember that once a patient is paralyzed for intubation the clinical signs of seizures are lost and frequent or continuous EEG monitoring is needed to guide therapy.

Various other agents may be used. Divalproex, various barbiturates, levetiracetam, and lacosamide are all available in IV formulations. Propofol as an agent frequently used during intubation can also be helpful at "breaking" a seizure.

382

Parkinson's disease and parkinsonism

Parkinsonism is a syndrome of *tremor, rigidity, bradykinesia (slowness)*, and loss of postural reflexes. **Prevalence** 1:200 in people >65.

Tremor 3–6 Hz (cycles per sec). It is most marked *at rest* during wakefulness and coarser than cerebellar tremor. It is typically a "pill rolling" of thumb over fingers.

Rigidity Increased resistance to passive stretch of muscles throughout range of movement (*lead-pipe*); tone may be broken-up by tremor (*cogwheel rigidity*). Unlike in spasticity, rigidity is present equally in flexors and extensors and is not velocity-dependent.

Bradykinesia Slowness of movement initiation with progressive reduction in speed and amplitude of repetitive actions; also monotonous speech. Expressionless face. Short shuffling steps with flexed trunk as if forever a step behind one's center of gravity (*festinating gait*). Feet as if frozen to the ground. Decreased blink rate. Micrographia (small writing).

---

1 PE = phenytoin equivalents

PD is one cause of parkinsonism; due to degeneration of substantia nigra dopaminergic neurons. Symptoms usually start between 50 and 70 yrs and progress steadily. A large proportion of patients will end up with some degree of dementia within 10 yrs. A number of single-gene mutations have been implicated, as have environmental chemical exposures, particularly pesticides and certain solvents.

Due to motor involvement, reduced reaction times, and associated visuospatial impairments, and side effects from medications (including sleep attacks on dopaminergic agonists), patients with PD suffer from significantly impaired driving ability even early in the course of the disease. *Surrender of driving license may be medically appropriate.*

Other causes of parkinsonism include medication exposures such as neuroleptics (e.g., metoclopramide, prochlorperazine, haloperidol) Lewy body dementia (hallmarks including fluctuating levels of cognition and alertness, visual hallucinations, dementia due to executive dysfunction early in course); rarely postencephalitis; supranuclear palsy (Steele–Richardson–Olszewski syndrome, with absent vertical gaze, both upward and downward, and dementia); multisystem atrophy (MSA) (formerly Shy–Drager syndrome), with prominent orthostatic hypotension; carbon monoxide poisoning; Wilson's disease; communicating hydrocephalus; welding (manganese); and microvascular ischemic disease.

Management of PD The goal of therapy is to treat symptoms, restoring function while minimizing side effects. The mainstay of this approach utilizes dopamine precursors and dopamine agonists. Start drugs when PD is seriously interfering with life (not too soon, as levodopa's effects wear off with time; explain this to patients and let them choose). Use the lowest dose giving symptom relief without troublesome SEs.

In general, L-dopa is the most effective agent for motor symptoms (indeed, it can be nearly miraculous when first started). The active L-dopa is given with a peripheral dopa decarboxylase inhibitor (in the form of a single tablet of carbidopa/levodopa) to increase efficacy and reduce GI and other side effects. With progression of the disease and prolonged use, however, more frequent dosing is required, and there tends to be a simultaneous narrowing of the therapeutic window between the patient being in an unacceptable "off" state (with severe bradykinesia and tremor) and frankly dyskinetic due to side effects from the drug. As PD progresses, strategies that augment delivery of levodopa into the nervous system can be utilized to improve therapeutic effects. Catechol-o-methyl transferase (COMT) inhibitors (tolcapone and entacapone) can be used to reduce the peripheral and central degradation of L-dopa. Other side effects of levodopa include orthostasis, and absorption is reduced with food.

A therapeutic trial of carbidopa/levodopa is generally warranted even in cases of seemingly atypical parkinsonism, titrating from 25/100 mg half-tablet tid with food, up to a maximum of 2 tablets tid without food over a couple of weeks. Lack of responsiveness is the hallmark of non-PD parkinsonism.

Many neurologists take the approach of utilizing dopamine agonists in younger patients to spare levodopa for later. The dopamine agonists currently used are either ergotamine derivatives (pergolide and bromocriptine) or nonergotamines (pramipexole, ropinirole, rotigotine). Although these have a lower rate of dyskinesias than L-dopa, they tend to be less effective for severe symptoms. Side effects can include bizarre, compulsive behavioral disorders (hypersexuality, gambling, shopping), as well as troublesome sleep attacks. Rotigotine is available in a transdermal patch that may avoid fluctuations that plague oral agents.

MAO-B inhibitors (selegiline, rasagiline) are often useful, particularly adjunctively. Anticholinergic agents can be added to PD therapy regimens in an attempt to improve tremor control. Drugs utilized for this include trihexyphenidyl, benztropine, and biperiden. Amantadine has been shown to be useful in PD by helping early mild symptoms and later by controlling some dyskinesias.

In patients with symptoms that progress to become refractory to medical management, surgical interventions are available. These include implantable deep brain stimulators (DBS) of the globus pallidus pars interna or subthalamic nucleus, and lesional surgery (thalamotomy, pallidotomy, subthalamotomy).

Nonmotor symptoms of PD may be sufficiently severe to warrant specific treatment, including associated depression, constipation, and drooling (due to reduced swallowing). Postural instability tends not to respond well to medication.

Apomorphine injections can serve to "rescue" patients who are "frozen" in an "off" state.

As yet, neuroprotective or disease-modifying strategies have not been definitively proven effective.

Tremor

Tremors are involuntary movements involving rapid oscillations. They can be classified based on when they appear—i.e., at rest, during assumption of a posture, or with activity. Classically, rest tremors are seen in PD and other parkinsonian states. Postural and action tremors include essential tremor, metabolic disorders (e.g., hyperthyroidism, hypoglycemia, pheochromocytoma) and medication-related tremors (e.g., lithium). One of the most common neurologic causes of tremor is essential tremor.

Essential tremor (ET) is a kinetic/postural tremor usually seen in the upper extremities, sometimes involving the head, neck, and voice as well. Generally, it is characterized by low-amplitude, high-frequency movement that can be disabling in its most severe forms. Often, patients identify other family members with similar tremors. More than half of patients will report improvement in the tremor after consumption of alcoholic beverages. Primidone and propranolol are the mainstays of therapy for patients with ET. Responses are seen in 50–75% of patients. Other anticonvulsants are sometimes used (gabapentin, topiramate), and thalamic DBS can be very helpful in severe cases.

Non-ET tremor can be difficult to treat. Sometimes weighted silverware or wrist weights can be used to reduce oscillations. Severe intentional tremor from MS may respond to thalamic DBS.

Neuromuscular disease

Neuromuscular diseases involve pathologies of the nerve roots, plexuses, nerve axons, myelin sheaths, neuromuscular junctions, and muscles. Patients will complain of weakness, numbness, or both. Cramping may be present. The pattern of dysfunction is the clinical key to identifying neuromuscular conditions. Electrophysiology studies (nerve conduction and electromyography) serve as an extension of the clinical exam—*they do not replace it!*

For example, once a peripheral neuropathy is identified, there is no clinical means to determine whether the pathology is demyelinating or axonal. A variety of different diseases—often autoimmune—cause demyelinating conditions and would be treated quite differently than axonal pathologies. A nerve conduction study would identify if there were reduced conduction velocities (indicative of demyelination) versus low amplitudes (signifying axonal loss).

The *pattern* of nerve weakness and numbness is crucial for determining where within the peripheral nervous system pathology exists. A mononeuropathy will give symptoms confined to one nerve distribution. A systemic condition causing a polyneuropathy classically affects the longest nerves first, giving predominantly distal symptoms (toes prior to ankles).

The following section reviews neuromuscular disease from a clinical standpoint.

Mononeuropathies

These are lesions of individual peripheral and cranial nerves. There are a variety of causes, including trauma, diabetes, heavy metal exposure, infections such as leprosy, and vasculitides. If more than one peripheral nerve is affected, the term *mononeuritis multiplex* is used. Causes include diabetes, vasculitis, infections, amyloidosis, rheumatoid arthritis, paraneoplastic syndromes, and a variety of hereditary diseases.

Median nerve C6–T1 *At the wrist* (e.g., lacerations; carpal tunnel syndrome—see Table 10.20): Weakness of abductor pollicis brevis and sensory loss over the radial 3½ fingers and palm. Lesions confined to the anterior interosseous nerve: Weakness of flexion of the distal phalanx of the thumb and index finger. *Proximal lesions* (e.g., at the elbow) may show combined defects.

Ulnar nerve C7–T1 Vulnerable to elbow trauma and at the wrist. *Signs:* Weakness/wasting of medial (ulnar side) wrist flexors; weakness/wasting of the interossei (cannot cross the fingers) and medial two lumbricals (claw hand); wasting of the hypothenar eminence, which abolishes finger abduction and sensory loss over the medial 1½ fingers and the ulnar side of the hand. Flexion of fourth and fifth DIP joints is weak. *Treatment:* See Table 10.21. With lesions at the wrist (digitorum profundus intact), claw hand is more marked.

Radial nerve C5–T1 This nerve opens the fist. Damaged by compression against the humerus (commonly seen with humeral fractures). Test for wrist and finger drop with elbow flexed and arm pronated. *Sensory loss:* Variable; test dorsal aspect of root of thumb.

Sciatic nerve L4–S2 Damaged by pelvic tumors or fractures to pelvis or femur. Lesions affect the hamstrings (knee flexors) and all muscles below the knee (foot drop), with loss of sensation below the knee laterally.

Common peroneal nerve L4–S2 Frequently damaged as it winds round the fibular head by trauma or tight-fitting casts. Lesions lead to inability to dorsiflex the foot (foot drop), evert the foot, extend the toes—and sensory loss over dorsum of foot.

Tibial nerve S1–3 Lesions lead to an inability to stand on tiptoe (plantar flexion), invert the foot, or flex the toes. Sensory loss over the sole.

Table 10.20 Carpal tunnel syndrome: The most common mononeuropathy

Nine tendons and the median nerve compete for space within the wrist. Compression is common, especially in women who have narrower wrists but similar-sized tendons to men.

The patient: Aching pain in the hand and arm (especially at night) and paresthesias in the thumb, index, and middle fingers, all relieved by dangling the hand over the edge of the bed and shaking it. Some patients experience referred pain into the forearm and shoulder. There may be sensory loss and weakness of abductor pollicis brevis with or without wasting of the thenar eminence. Light touch, two-point discrimination, and sweating may be impaired.

Associations: Pregnancy, rheumatoid arthritis, DM, hypothyroidism, dialysis, trauma.

Tests: Neurophysiology helps by confirming the lesion's site and severity (and likelihood of improvement after surgery). Maximal wrist flexion for 1 min (Phalen's test) may elicit symptoms but is unreliable. Tapping over the nerve at the wrist induces tingling (Tinel's test; also rather nonspecific).

Treatment: Splinting of the wrist for 3–6 months may help. If not, local steroid injection may be temporizing. Surgical decompression (traditional or minimally invasive) is quite effective in the long run, but at the expense of slight reduction in grip strength and initial immobility during recovery.

Table 10.21 Managing ulnar mononeuropathies from entrapments

The ulnar nerve is in an anatomically precarious position and is subject to compression at multiple sites around the elbow. Most commonly, compression occurs at the epicondylar groove or at the point where the nerve passes between the two heads of the flexor carpi ulnaris muscle (true *cubital tunnel syndrome*). Trauma can easily damage the nerve against its bony confines (the medial condyle of the humerus—the "funny bone"). Normally, the ulnar nerve suffers stretch and compression forces at the elbow that are moderated by its ability to glide in its groove. When normal excursion is restricted, irritation ensues. This may cause a vicious cycle of perineural scarring, consequent loss of excursion, and progressive symptoms—without there being any antecedent trauma.

Rest and avoiding pressure on the nerve helps but if symptoms continue, nighttime soft elbow splinting (to prevent flexion to >60 degrees) is warranted for a few months. For chronic neuropathy associated with weakness, or if splinting fails, a variety of surgical procedures have been tried. For moderately severe neuropathies, decompressions *in situ* may help initially but subsequently fail. Medial epicondylectomies are effective in 50% (there is a high rate of recurrence). SC nerve reroutings (transpositions) may be tried. IM and submuscular transpositions are more complicated, but the latter may be preferable.

Compressive ulnar neuropathies at the wrist (*Guyon's canal*—between the pisiform and hamate bones) are less common, but they can also result in disability. *Thoracic outlet compression* is another cause of a weak, numb hand. Electromyography (EMG) helps define the anatomic site of lesions.

Polyneuropathies

Polyneuropathies are generalized disorders of peripheral nerves (including cranial nerves) whose distribution is usually bilaterally symmetrical and widespread—typically a distal pattern of muscle weakness and sensory loss (known as "stocking-glove anesthesia"). They may be classified by time course (acute or chronic), by the functions disturbed (motor, sensory, autonomic, mixed), or by the underlying pathology (demyelination, axonal degeneration, or both). Guillain–Barré syndrome (GBS), for example, is a subacute, predominantly motor, demyelinating neuropathy, whereas chronic alcohol abuse leads to a chronic, initially sensory then mixed, axonal neuropathy. Differential based on motor vs. sensory predominance is given in Table 10.22 and a more thorough list in Table 10.23.

Symptoms *Sensory neuropathy:* Numbness; "feels funny"; tingling or burning sensations often affecting the extremities first ("stocking-glove" distribution). There may be difficulty handling small objects such as a needle.

Motor neuropathy: Often progressive (may be rapid) weakness or clumsiness of the hands; difficulty walking (falls; stumbling); respiratory difficulty. Signs are those of an LMN lesion: Wasting and weakness most marked in the distal muscles of hands and feet (foot or wrist drop). Reflexes are reduced or absent. Involvement of the respiratory muscles may be shown by a diminished vital capacity.

Cranial nerves: Difficulties swallowing; speaking; double vision; changes in facial sensation, facial weakness.

Diagnosis The history is vital; make sure you are clear about the illness's time course, the precise nature of the symptoms, any antecedent or associated events (e.g., gastrointestinal or respiratory symptoms preceding GBS, weight loss in cancer, arthralgia from a connective tissue disease), travel, sexual history (infections), alcohol use, medications, and family history. Pain is typical of neuropathies due to DM or alcohol. *Examination:* Do a careful neurological examination looking particularly for lower motor signs (weakness, wasting, reduced or absent reflexes); any sensory loss should be carefully mapped out for each modality. Make use of a peripheral nerve/myotome/dermatome chart, such as those presented earlier in this chapter, to assist in localization (Table 10.5; Figures 10.3 and 10.4). Do not forget to assess the autonomic system and cranial nerves. Look also for signs of trauma (e.g., finger burns) indicating reduced sensation. Scuff marks on shoes may suggest foot drop. If there is palpable nerve thickening, think of leprosy or Charcot–Marie–Tooth. Examine other systems for clues to the cause, such as for signs of alcoholic liver disease.

387

Tests Complete blood count, glucose, hemoglobin A1C, LFT, thyroid function tests, B_{12}, protein electrophoresis, ANCA (p- & c-), antinuclear antibodies (ANA), CXR, urinalysis, and consider a LP in the appropriate clinical setting (concern for GBS or chronic inflammatory demyelinating polyradiculoneuropathy [CIDP]). In a patient with a distal sensory neuropathy and no clear cause, obtain a glucose tolerance test to identify patients in a "prediabetic" state (which is a significant cause of peripheral

Table 10.22 Motor vs. sensory polyneuropathy

Mostly motor	Mostly sensory
GBS	Diabetes mellitus
Lead poisoning	Uremia
Charcot–Marie–Tooth syndrome	Leprosy

Table 10.23 Causes of polyneuropathies

Inflammatory
GBS, CIDP, sarcoidosis

Metabolic
Diabetes mellitus, renal failure, hypothyroidism, hypoglycemia, mitochondrial disorders

Vasculitides
Polyarteritis nodosa, rheumatoid arthritis, Wegener's granulomatosis

Malignancy
Paraneoplastic syndromes (especially small cell lung cancer), polycythemia vera

Infections
Leprosy, syphilis, Lyme disease, HIV

Vitamin deficiencies and excesses
Lack of vitamins B_1, B_6, B_{12} (alcoholics), folate; also excess of B_6 (>100 mg/d)

Inherited
Refsum's syndrome, Charcot–Marie–Tooth syndrome, porphyria, leukodystrophy (and many more)

Toxins
Lead, arsenic

Drugs
Alcohol, cisplatin, isoniazid, vincristine, nitrofurantoin. Less frequently: Metronidazole, phenytoin

Others
Paraproteinemias including multiple myeloma, amyloidosis, prediabetic states (impaired glucose tolerance)

neuropathy). Consider specific genetic tests for inherited neuropathies (e.g., Charcot–Marie–Tooth syndrome), lead levels, and antiganglioside antibodies. Nerve conduction studies are necessary for distinguishing demyelinating from axonal neuropathies.

Treatment Treat the underlying cause if possible (e.g., withdraw precipitating drug; tight glucose control in diabetes). Involve physical therapists and occupational therapists. Care of the feet and shoe choice is important in sensory neuropathies to minimize trauma and subsequent disability. In GBS and CIDP, IV immunoglobulin helps. Steroids and other immunosuppressants may help vasculitic neuropathy.

Although there are no treatments available to improve the *negative* symptoms of numbness/sensory loss, there are a variety of strategies for managing the *positive*, painful symptoms of neuropathy such as paresthesia (burning, tingling), hyperesthesia (increased pain sensitivity), or allodynia (nonpainful stimuli being perceived as painful). Tricyclic antidepressants (particularly nortriptyline, which is inexpensive and has a low number-needed-to-treat), serotonin-norepinephrine reuptake inhibitor (SNRI) drugs, and many of the anticonvulsants (gabapentin; pregabalin may be preferred due to relatively benign risk profiles) are useful for this purpose. NSAIDs tend not to help much, but the combination mu-opioid agonist/norepinephrine reuptake inhibitors, such as tramadol and tapentadol, may be useful. Chronic opioid therapy can be beneficial for neuropathic pain, but with attendant risks of tolerance, dependency, etc. Where pain is peripherally mediated, topical treatments (lidocaine patches or creams) should be tried. A high-potency capsaicin patch preparation can result in prolonged pain relief through destruction of unmyelinated C-fibers.

Bell's palsy

An *idiopathic* palsy of the facial nerve (VII) resulting in a unilateral facial weakness or paralysis. Other causes of a facial palsy must be excluded before a diagnosis of Bell's palsy is made. Possible etiologies for Bell's palsy include a viral neuropathy (HSV1 has been implicated) and idiopathic inflammation.

Incidence ~20/100,000/yr; risk increases in pregnancy (three-fold) and diabetes (~five-fold).

Symptoms Onset of facial weakness is rapid and may occur with or be preceded by pain below the ear. Weakness worsens for 1–2 d before stabilizing, and pain resolves within a few days. Accompanying *subtle* trigeminal sensory loss may be noted. *Any more dramatic trigeminal loss or any other accompanying cranial neuropathies must prompt a search for underlying etiology.* Symptoms and signs are unilateral. If bilateral, consider other diagnoses (e.g., sarcoidosis, infiltrative meningeal disease, Lyme disease; see Table 10.24). Patients will experience weakness of the face, including the periocular muscles (difficulty closing the eye), drooling, impaired taste on the anterior tongue, and hyperacusis (the perception of loud sounds due to a paralysis of the stapedius muscle that normally dampens sounds).

Natural history Those patients with incomplete paralysis and no axonal degeneration typically recover completely within a few weeks (approximately 85% of patients with Bell's palsy). Those with complete paralysis nearly all fully recover too but ~15% have axonal degeneration. Recovery frequently begins only after 3 months, may be incomplete, fail to happen at all, or else will be complicated by the formation of aberrant reconnections producing synkinesis (e.g., eye blinking is accompanied by unintentional synchronous upturning of the mouth, or smiling accompanied by involuntary eye closure). Misconnection of parasympathetic fibers can produce so-called crocodile tears, when eating stimulates unilateral lacrimation. Cutting the tympanic branch of IX solves this problem (rarely needed).

The House-Brackmann scale is commonly used to score patients with Bell's palsy and can prognosticate recovery. The scale has six grades (1–6), with grade 1 being normal and grade 6 describing a patient with no movement whatsoever.

389

Tests *Electroneurography* at 1–3 wks can predict delayed recovery by identifying axonal degeneration but does not influence management.

MRI and *LP* help rule out other diagnoses (only needed in atypical presentations, such as bilateral Bell's palsy or a facial nerve palsy in the presence of concomitant cranial neuropathies). In the appropriate setting, consider testing for other disorders, such as Lyme.

Management If presentation is within 6 d of onset, prednisone (1 mg/kg/d for 5–10 d) is relatively safe and probably effective in improving facial function outcomes in patients. Acyclovir, however, is considered by the American Academy of Neurology Practice Guidelines to be safe (in combination with prednisone) and *possibly* effective in treating Bell's palsy. Protect the cornea with artificial tears, lubrication, or overnight taping or moisture chambers if there is any evidence of drying. If ectropion is severe, lateral tarsorrhaphy (partial lid-to-lid suturing) can help.

Table 10.24 Other causes of a VII nerve palsy

Infection
　Ramsay Hunt syndrome (cephalic herpes zoster). This is a peripheral
　　facial nerve palsy accompanied by a painful erythematous vesicular
　　rash in the ear (zoster oticus) or in the mouth, often with vertigo.
　　(Famciclovir 500 mg/8 h PO + prednisolone may be indicated.)
　Lyme disease
　HIV
　Meningitis
　Polio
　TB
　Chronic meningitis (e.g., fungal)

Brainstem lesions
　Brainstem tumor
　Stroke
　MS

Cerebellopontine angle lesions
　Acoustic neuroma, meningioma

Systemic disease
　Diabetes mellitus
　Sarcoidosis (facial palsy is the most common CNS sign of sarcoidosis)
　GBS

ENT and other rare causes
　Orofacial granulomatosis—recurrent VII palsies
　Parotid tumors
　Cholesteatoma
　Otitis media
　Trauma to skull base
　Pregnancy/delivery, via intracranial hypotension

Neuromuscular junction disorders

Myasthenia gravis (MG) is an antibody-mediated, autoimmune disease
with too few functioning acetylcholine receptors on muscle, leading to
muscle weakness. Antiacetylcholine receptor antibodies are detectable in
80–90% of patients and cause depletion of functioning postsynaptic receptor sites. A fraction of the remainder will have antibodies to muscle specific
kinase, MuSK.

Presentation: Can present at any age as worsening muscular fatigability. If
<50 yrs, myasthenia is more common in women, associated with other
autoimmune diseases and thymic hyperplasia. >50 yrs, it is more common in
men and associated with thymic atrophy or, rarely, a thymic tumor. Muscle
groups commonly affected (most likely first): Extraocular, bulbar, face, neck,
limb girdle, trunk. Look especially for ptosis, diplopia,"myasthenic snarl"
on smiling. On counting aloud to 50, the voice weakens. Reflexes are normal. Weakness may be exacerbated by pregnancy, infection, overtreatment,
change of climate, emotion, exercise, gentamicin, opiates, tetracycline, quinine, quinidine, procainamide, and many other medications.

Associations: Thymic tumor, hyperthyroidism, rheumatoid arthritis, SLE.

Diagnosis: In the clinically appropriate situations, obtain an antiacetylcholine
receptor antibody titer and anti-MuSK if normal. Although the titer itself
does not correlate with disease severity, a positive test is highly suggestive,
and the rise or fall in titer can be used to track the success of treatment.

Additional tests include a repetitive stimulation EMG to look for decremental responses, a single-fiber EMG to look for "jitter," and, more rarely, the Tensilon test. This pharmacologic test uses the administration of edrophonium (an anticholinesterase) to determine whether a patient's symptoms would improve with more acetylcholine at a neuromuscular junction. The test is difficult to assess, somewhat nonspecific, and has significant associated risks (bradycardia, e.g.) and hence is rarely used. Once the diagnosis of MG is established, a CT scan of the chest is obtained to rule out thymic tumors. In patients with MG even without thymic tumors, thymectomy can cause remission or significant improvement and are worth considering in patients who are suitable surgical candidates.

Treatment options: Symptomatic control with an anticholinesterase (e.g., *pyridostigmine* 60–450 mg/24 h PO) taken through the day. Side effects include diarrhea, salivation, lacrimation, vomiting, miosis, and even weakness. Immunosuppression with prednisone, azathioprine, cyclosporin, and mycophenolate have all been utilized with success. Also, both plasmapheresis and IVIg have been used on 2–4 wk schedules for patients with difficult to control symptoms or in patients suffering from myasthenic crises.

Myasthenic crisis is characterized by weakness significant enough to cause respiratory compromise. This occurs in 10–20% of patients at some time in the course of their disease and can be triggered by preceding infections. Plasmapheresis is commonly used to treat patients in crisis.

Lambert–Eaton myasthenic syndrome

This typically occurs in association with small cell lung cancer (Lambert–Eaton syndrome) or, less commonly, with other autoimmune disease. Unlike MG, it affects especially proximal limbs and trunk (rarely the eyes), there is *hyporeflexia*, only a slight response to edrophonium, repeated muscle contraction may lead to increased muscle strength and reflexes, and it is the presynaptic membrane that is affected (the carcinoma provokes production of antibodies to Ca^{2+} channels).

Other causes of muscle fatigability Polymyositis, SLE, botulism, Takayasu's disease (fatigability of the extremities due to ischemia from vasculitis).

391

Myopathies

Signs and symptoms *Muscle weakness* Rapid onset suggests a toxic, drug, or metabolic cause. *Excess fatigability* (weakness increases with exercise) may suggest MG versus storage disease myopathy. *Myotonia* (delayed muscular relaxation after contraction, e.g., unable to release grip or rapidly let go of a handshake) is characteristic of myotonic disorders. *Spontaneous pain* at rest occurs in inflammatory disease, as does local tenderness. Pain on exercise suggests ischemia or metabolic myopathy (e.g., McArdle's disease). *Fasciculation* (spontaneous, irregular, and brief contractions of part of a muscle) suggests anterior horn cell or root disease. Look carefully for evidence of systemic disease. *Tests:* Consider EMG with or without muscle biopsy and investigations relevant to systemic causes (e.g., TSH). Many genetic disorders of muscle can be detected by DNA analysis, and muscle biopsy is now reserved for when genetic tests are nondiagnostic (e.g., Duchenne's or myotonic dystrophy).

There are five main categories of myopathy

1 *Muscular dystrophies* are a group of genetic diseases with progressive degeneration and weakness of specific muscle groups. The primary abnormality may be in the muscle membrane. Secondary effects are marked

variation in size of individual fibers and deposition of fat and connective tissue. The most common is *Duchenne's muscular dystrophy* (sex-linked recessive—30% from spontaneous mutation) and is (almost always) confined to boys. The Duchenne gene is on the short arm of the X chromosome, and its product, dystrophin, is absent (or present in only very low levels). Serum creatine kinase is raised >40-fold. It presents usually around 4 yrs of age with increasingly clumsy walking, progressing to difficulty in standing and respiratory failure. Some survive beyond 20 yrs. There is no specific treatment. Genetic counselling is vital. *Fascioscapulohumeral muscular dystrophy* (Landouzy–Dejerine) is almost as common. *Inheritance:* Autosomal dominant (4q35). *Typical age of onset:* 12–14 yrs. *Early symptoms:* Inability to puff out the cheeks, difficulty raising the arms above the head (e.g., changing light-bulbs). *Signs:* Weakness of face, shoulders, and upper arms (often asymmetric with deltoids spared), with or without foot-drop and/or winging of the scapula. 20% of patients will need a wheelchair by 40 yrs.

2 *Myotonic disorders* are characterized by myotonia (tonic spasm of muscle). Muscle histology shows long chains of central nuclei within the fibers. The chief disorder is *myotonic dystrophy* (autosomal dominant). *Typical onset:* 25 yrs with weakness (hands, legs, sternocleidomastoids) and myotonia. Muscle wasting and weakness in the face results in a long, haggard appearance. *Other features*: Cataracts, frontal baldness (men), atrophy of testes or ovaries, cardiomyopathy, mild endocrine abnormalities (e.g., DM), and mental impairment). Most patients die in middle age of intercurrent illness. Genetic counseling is important.

3 *Acquired myopathies of late onset* are often a manifestation of systemic disease. Look carefully for evidence of carcinoma, thyroid disease (especially hyperthyroidism), Cushing's disease, hypo- and hypercalcemia.

4 *Inflammatory disorders:* Inclusion-body myositis, polymyositis, dermatomyositis, other auto-immune myopathies.

5 *Toxic myopathies:* Alcohol, statins (etiology may be partially auto-immune), steroids, chloroquine, colchicine, procainamide, zidovudine, vincristine, cyclosporin, hypervitaminosis E, cocaine.

Myelopathies

The time course of symptom onset is critical for evaluating patients with myelopathic spinal cord symptoms (UMN weakness, a sensory level, and/ or bowel/bladder dysfunction). In the acute setting, compressive lesions must be ruled out because of the urgent indication for surgical intervention. Traumatic spinal cord injuries are currently treated with massive doses of steroids, while nontraumatic, noncompressive myelopathies are evaluated and treated very differently. Certain facts about the patient's history are critical for determining the etiology of the myelopathy. For example, a patient with a T10 sensory level and spinal cord dysfunction after an angiogram most probably has suffered an anterior spinal artery occlusion and spinal infarct due to disruption of blood supply in the artery of Adamkiewicz.

Differential of noncompressive myelopathy Acute and subacute pathologies include arterial infarct, venous hypertension (with or without infarct), transverse myelitis, MS, neuromyelitis optica, spinal cord ischemia related to spinal AV malformations, fistulas, and various spinal tumors (primary and metastatic). A gadolinium-enhanced MRI of the spine and brain and LP can be used to identify to causative process. Evidence of inflammation (enhancing lesion on MRI, pleocytosis, elevated protein, oligoclonal bands or IgG Index) supports the diagnosis of TM, MS, or NMO. In cases where an acute myelopathy has no clear cause, a spinal angiogram must be considered if a vascular malformation is suspected

Space-occupying lesions in the brain

Signs Features of ↑ ICP, evolving focal neurologic symptom (Table 10.25), seizures, false localizing signs, cognitive or behavioral change and local effects (e.g., proptosis). *Raised ICP:* Headache, vomiting, papilledema (only in 50% of tumors), altered consciousness (the most common finding in patients with ↑ ICP). *Seizures:* Seen in about 50% of tumors. Suspect in all adult-onset seizures, especially if focal or with a localizing aura or postictal weakness (Todd's palsy). *False localizing signs:* These are caused by ↑ ICP. Cranial nerve VI palsy is most common due to its long intracranial course. *Subtle personality change:* Irritability, lack of application to tasks, lack of initiative, socially inappropriate behavior may be seen early in the process, but are nonspecific.

Causes

Tumor (primary or secondary), aneurysm, abscess (25% multiple), chronic subdural hematoma, granuloma (e.g., tuberculoma), cyst (e.g., cysticercosis, arachnoid). *Tumor histology:* 30% secondary (breast, lung, melanoma; 50% multiple). Primaries include astrocytoma, glioblastoma multiforme, oligo-dendroglioma, ependymoma (all <50% 5-yr survival), cerebellar hemangio-blastoma (40% 20-yr survival), meningioma (generally benign).

Differential diagnosis Stroke, head injury, vasculitis (SLE, syphilis, PAN, giant cell arteritis, etc.), MS, encephalitis, postictal (Todd's palsy), metabolic, or electrolyte disturbances. Also, obstructive hydrocephalus (e.g., from colloid cyst of the third ventricle), venous sinus occlusion, and idiopathic intracranial hypertension.

Tests CT; MRI (good for posterior fossa masses). Consider biopsy. Extreme caution with LPs (performed only if absolutely necessary) due to risks of cerebellar herniation through the foramen magnum)—see discussion above.

Tumor management *Benign:* Complete removal if possible but some may be inaccessible. *Malignant:* Complete removal of gliomas is difficult as resection margins are rarely clear, but surgery does give a tissue diagnosis and allows debulking pre-radiotherapy. If a tumor is inaccessible but causing hydrocephalus, a ventriculo-peritoneal shunt may be used to reduce ICP. Radiotherapy is used postop for gliomas or metastases and as sole therapy for some tumors if surgery is impossible. Chemotherapy is used in gliomas with limited benefit. Intracranial, chemotherapy-impregnated wafers have improved outcome somewhat. Dexamethasone 4 mg/8 h PO for vasogenic cerebral edema. Prophylactic administration of antiepileptics in patients with newly diagnosed brain tumors is not recommended due to a lack of efficacy and the presence of side effects. *Enzyme-inducing antiepileptics may reduce effectiveness of certain chemotherapeutic agents.*

Prognosis Complete removal of a benign tumor achieves cure but the prognosis of those with malignant tumors is poor.

Table 10.25 Localizing signs

Temporal lobe Seizures (complex partial ± automatisms), hallucinations (smell, taste, sound, *déjà vu*), complex partial with automatisms, dysphasia, field defect (contralateral upper quadrantanopia), forgetfulness, psychosis, fear/rage, hypersexuality.

Frontal lobe Hemiparesis, seizures (focal motor seizures, i.e., aversive seizures involving head and eyes), personality changes (indecent, indolent, indiscreet), positive grasp reflex (fingers drawn across palm are grasped) significant only if unilateral, aphasia (Broca's area), loss of smell unilaterally. *Orbitofrontal syndrome:* Lack of empathy, disinhibition, diminished social skills, overeating, rash actions (mania), unconscious imitation of postures observed in others.

Parietal lobe Hemisensory loss, diminished two-point discrimination, astereognosis (inability to recognize object in hand by touch alone), sensory inattention, aphasia, Gerstmann's syndrome (i.e., left–right disorientation), finger agnosia, acalculia, and agraphia).

Occipital lobe Contralateral visual field defects (homonymous hemianopia); hallucinations such as palinopsia (persisting or recurring images, once the stimulus has left the field of view).

Cerebellum ('DASHING') **D**ysdiadochokinesis, **a**taxia (truncal), **s**lurred speech, **h**ypotonia, **i**ntention tremor, **n**ystagmus, **g**ait abnormality.

Dysdiadochokinesis is impaired *rapidly alternating* movements (e.g., pronation–supination).

Cerebellopontine angle Usually vestibular schwannoma. Ipsilateral deafness; nystagmus; reduced corneal reflex, facial weakness; ipsilateral cerebellar signs, papilledema, and cranial nerve VI palsies.

Midbrain (e.g., pineal gland tumors or midbrain infarction) Failure of up or down gaze; dissociated pupil responses, with constriction on near gaze but not to light; convergence retraction nystagmus on attempted upgaze.

Neuroradiology

Fast-moving technological advances in neurological imaging have revolutionized neurological diagnosis and treatment, shedding light where there once was darkness—but sometimes generating more heat than light.

CT works by identifying x-ray attenuation of materials, measured in Hounsfield units (HU) (e.g., bone +1,000, water 0, and air –1,000 HU). The x-ray attenuation of a pixel is revealed as a shade of gray. At the extremes, high attenuation is white and low attenuation is black. The attenuation of biological soft tissues is in a narrow range from about +80 for blood and muscle, to 0 for CSF, and down to –100 for fat. IV contrast may be given, demonstrating initially an angiographic effect, the high attenuation contrast in the vessels making them appear white. Later, if there is a defect in the blood–brain barrier, as with neoplasms or infection, contrast will extravasate, giving an enhancing white area in the cerebrum or cerebellum. Some intracranial components do not have a blood–brain barrier and thus will enhance (e.g., the pituitary gland and choroid plexus).

Compared to MRI, CT is good at showing acute hemorrhage and fractures and is much easier to perform in ill or anesthetized patients—so it is invaluable in emergencies. Modern scanners can obtain a whole head view in seconds, and there are basically no contraindications to a noncontrast scan. Fresh blood is of higher attenuation (whiter) than brain tissue. Attenuation of hematomas declines as hemoglobin breaks down so that a subacute subdural hematoma at 2 wks may appear isodense to adjacent brain, making it difficult to detect. A chronic subdural hematoma will be of relatively low attenuation.

CT is commonly performed in acute stroke to exclude hemorrhage (before giving thrombolytics). An area of ischemia will not show up distinctly for several hours or so, and will appear as low-attenuation cytotoxic edema (intracellular edema mainly confined to the gray matter).

Tumors and abscesses may share radiographic features—ring-enhancing mass, surrounding vasogenic edema, and mass effect. Vasogenic edema is extracellular and spreads through the white matter. Mass effect can cause compression of the sulci and ipsilateral ventricle. It may also cause subfalcine, transtentorial, or tonsillar herniation.

One indication for CT scan is acute, severe headache. If there is concern about subarachnoid hemorrhage, a noncontrast CT may show acute blood. Even if it does not, it will show if the basal cisterns are normal and therefore LP is probably safe.

In MRI, an image is made by disturbing an atomic nucleus in a strong magnetic field by using a radiofrequency pulse at the resonant frequency and detecting the signal as the nucleus (usually hydrogen) returns to equilibrium. The resulting noninvasively obtained anatomic and pathological information is unrivaled, but the technique has drawbacks as well (Table 10.26). The chief clinically useful image sequences are:

- *T1-weighted images:* Give good anatomical detail to which the T2 image can be compared/related. Fat is brightest (↑ signal intensity) other tissues are darker to varying degrees. Flowing blood appears black ("flow voids"). Bone is dark. Gadolinium contrast agent can be given to "enhance" vascular lesions or areas of blood-brain barrier breakdown.
- *T2-weighted images:* These provide the best detection of pathology, with most pathology having some edema fluid and therefore appearing white. Fat and fluid appear brightest. Again, fat is bright and bone is dark.
- *FLAIR or TIRM:* These sequences are similar to T2-weighted images and highlight pathology far better but remove the bright signal of CSF, which might otherwise obscure small lesions adjacent to sulci or ventricles.
- *HEME, gradient echo, or susceptibility weighted imaging:* All these sequences highlight blood products (or calcium deposits) as black. They are very sensitive to the point of picking up previously asymptomatic "microbleeds" in amyloidosis or mild head trauma but tend to "overcall" the size of small lesions.
- *DWI and apparent diffusion coefficient (ADC):* Most useful for revealing and dating acute strokes. DWI imaging will reveal acute cytotoxic injury (ischemic infarction) as bright signal within minutes of onset, out to ~14 d. ADC will reveal ischemic injury as dark signal out to ~7 d.
- *Perfusion weighted imaging:* Serial slices timed around injection of gadolinium contrast medium reveal areas of the brain that are oligemic. In the setting of a stroke, an area of reduced blood flow *without* corresponding DWI brightness is "at risk" but not yet infarcted and thus potentially salvageable. Often an "ischemic penumbra" surrounds an area of acute stroke.
- *MRA, MRV:* MR scanners can reveal vasculature through various techniques, each with its own advantages and limitations. In general, images obtained from noncontrast studies are related to *flow*, rather than anatomic lumen size. MRV and neck MRA studies are best performed with contrast enhancement, but MRA of the Circle of Willis is adequately obtained without contrast.

395

- *Other:* A host of other specialized MR techniques have been developed that can highlight specific anatomy and pathology. *MR neurography* can reveal peripheral nerves and plexus, *diffusion tensor imaging* can highlight the integrity of white matter tracts, and *morphometry* and other volumetric imaging can reveal specific areas of atrophy or hypertrophy (often referenced to a standardized"brain map"). Novel sequences can reveal the otherwise undetectable early gray matter involvement of MS, as well as clinically asymptomatic white matter lesions. *MR spectroscopy* can show us constituent molecular components of the brain in specific regions of interest (distinguishing, e.g., areas of demyelination from areas of tumor or of cell death or of abscess). *Functional MRI* techniques can reveal regional brain activation in real time, by way of detecting changes in regional blood flow or blood oxygenation status.

In **PET** and **SPECT** nuclear medicine techniques, images are created by detection of the decay of radioactive atoms attached to an injected molecular label. PET has superior spatial and far superior temporal resolution, but generally requires an on-site accelerator for generating isotopes. Areas of hypo- or hypermetabolism can reveal seizure foci, distinguish abscess from tumors, or reveal patterns suggestive of specific types of dementia. Specific labels have been developed that bind amyloid- or dopamine-producing neurons, of potential use in Alzheimer's and Parkinson's diseases, respectively.

Table 10.26 Advantages and disadvantages of MRI imaging

Advantages of MRI	Disadvantages of MRI
Nonionizing radiation	High cost
Shows vasculature without contrast	Claustrophobia (in magnet tunnel for 15–60 min—sedation may be needed)
Images can easily be produced in any plane, e.g., sagittal or coronal	Motion artifact and longer time for image acquisition
Visualization of posterior fossa and other areas prone to bony artifact on CT, e.g., at the craniocervical junction. MRI images the posterior fossa extremely well.	Unhelpful in imaging calcium
	Unsuitable for those with ferromagnetic foreign bodies (pacemakers, CNS vascular clips, cochlear implants, valves, shrapnel, etc.)
High inherent soft-tissue contrast	Difficult in anesthetized patients
Precise staging of malignancy, e.g., involvement of bone marrow	Gadolinium may be harmful in patients with renal failure
	Imaging artifacts may be misinterpreted as abnormal findings

Rheumatology and musculoskeletal conditions

Lanaya W. Smith M.D. and John A. Flynn, M.D., M.Ed., M.B.A.

Contents

Important points in assessing for rheumatic disease

Is there a history to suggest inflammation?

• Morning stiffness (>30 min)
• Joint swelling, warmth, or redness
• Loss of function.

How many joints are involved?

• One = monoarthritis
• Several (2–4) = oligoarthritis
• Many (>4) = polyarthritis

Are there any extra-articular manifestations?

Also consider age, gender, occupation, family history, ancestry (e.g., systemic lupus erythematosus [SLE] is more common in women and African Americans).

• *Presenting symptoms*		• *Rheumatological and related diseases:* E.g., Crohn's/ulcerative colitis (UC) in ankylosing spondylitis; psoriasis, gonorrhea, or reactive arthritis
Joints	Morning stiffness	
	Clinical synovitis (rheumatoid arthritis [RA])	
	Pattern of distribution; mono vs. polyarticular	
	Swelling; loss of function	

Extra-articular	Rashes, photosensitivity (SLE)	• *Current and past drugs:* Disease modifying drugs, e.g., methotrexate etc.
	Raynaud (SLE; scleroderma poly- and dermatomyositis)	• *Family history:* Arthritis; psoriasis (psoriatic arthritis, ankylosing spondylitis)
	Dry eyes or mouth (Sjögren's)	• *Social history:* Functioning, e.g., dressing, writing, walking, activities of daily living (ADLs), social support, home adaptations
	Diarrhea/urethritis (Reactive arthritis)	
	Red eyes, e.g., ankylosing spondylitis,	
	Nodules or nodes (RA, sarcoid, SLE, tuberculosis [TB], and gouty tophi)	
	Mouth/genital ulcers (Behçet's)mouth ulcers also with SLE Weight loss (e.g., TB arthritis)	

Features of inflammatory arthritis Pain, stiffness (especially morning), synovitis, destruction of the joint on x-ray, loss of function.

Causes—*Monoarthritis*	*Polyarthritis (e.g., >4 swollen painful joints)*
Septic arthritis (e.g., staph, strep, Gram-negative bacilli, gonococci, TB)	Viruses, e.g., mumps, rubella, parvovirus B19, Chikungunya, EBV, hepatitis B, enteroviruses, HIV, α-viral arthropathy
Psoriatic and reactive arthritis	
Trauma (hemarthrosis)	Rheumatoid (RA) or osteoarthritis (OA)
Calcium pyrophosphate dihydrate (CPPD) crystals; gout	Spondyloarthritis
	Connective tissue diseases (e.g., scleroderma, SLE)
Osteoarthritis	Crystal arthropathies (gout, CPPD)
Monoarthritic presentation of a polyarticular disease (e.g., RA)	Poststreptococcal reactive arthritis Sarcoidosis

399

Assessment

Assess extent of joint involvement (include spine), symmetry, disruption of joint involvement, limitation of movement, effusions and periarticular involvement. *Associated features* : Dysuria or genital ulcers, skin or eye involvement, lungs, kidneys, heart, GI (e.g., mouth ulcers, bloody diarrhea), and central nervous system (CNS).

Urine: Urine protein/creatinine (or 24 h urine protein) representing at least 500 mg of protein/24 h or red blood cell casts.

Adjunct therapy for proteinuria (angiotensin-converting enzyme [ACE]-inhibitors or angiotensin receptor blocker [ARB])

Radiology: Look for erosions, calcification, loss of joint space, changes in underlying bone (e.g., periarticular osteoporosis, sclerotic areas, osteophytes) of affected joints. Image sacroiliac joints if considering a spondyloarthritis (irregularity of lower third); chest x-ray (CXR) in RA, SLE, vasculitis, and TB. In septic arthritis, x-rays may be normal, as may be erythrocyte sedimentation rate (ESR) and c-reactive protein (CRP; if CRP ↑, expect it to fall with treatment).

Septic arthritis Consider septic arthritis in any acute monoarthritis. Features may be less overt if immunosuppressed or if underlying joint disease. Aspirate the joint. Look for blood, crystals, and pus (polarized light microscopy, culture, Gram stain). Sepsis may damage a joint within 24 h. If in doubt, treat initially for sepsis, as described below.

Joint aspiration: Microscopy (+culture): Any blood, crystals, or pus? Do polarized light microscopy for urate or CPPD crystals (p. 409).

Blood: Culture if sepsis is possible. CBC, ESR, uric acid, urea, and creatinine if systemic disease. Rheumatoid factor, antinuclear antibody, and other autoantibodies (p. 414). Consider HIV serology.

Treatment is determined by the cause. If *septic arthritis* is suspected, provide analgesia, immediate antibiotics, imaging, and surgical intervention (washing) if necessary. Oxacillin or cefazolin for meth-sensitive staph; vancomycin if meth resistance is suspected, third-generation cephalosporin if gram-negative organisms are suspected, until sensitivities are known. Look for atypical mycobacteria and fungi if HIV +ve. Request infectious disease consultant for how long to continue treatment (e.g., 2 wks IV, then 3 wks PO).

Repeat aspiration (arthrocentesis) if no improvement (falling joint white blood cells [WBCs] and culture becoming sterile), then consider lavage and arthroscopic debridement(e.g., for knee) or open (e.g., for hip or shoulder; this allows biopsy; helpful for TB). Ask for orthopedic consult. If a joint prosthesis is *in situ*, get orthopedic consult before aspiration. Try to determine the source of infection. Is there immunosuppression or a focus of infection (e.g., pneumonia, as in 50% of those with pneumococcal arthritis)?

Synovial fluid analysis

Table 11.1 Synovial fluid analysis

Aspiration of synovial fluid is primarily used to look for infection or crystals (gout and CPPD crystal arthritis.

	Appearance	Viscosity	WBC/mm³	Neutrophils (%)
Normal	Clear, colorless	↑	≤200	None
Noninflammatory[a]	Clear, straw	↑	≤5000	≤25
Hemorrhagic[b]	Bloody, xanthochromic	Varies	≤10,000	≤50
Acutely inflamed[c]	Turbid, yellow	↓		
• Crystal			~14,000	~80
• Rheumatic fever			~18,000	~50
• RA			~16,000	Varies
Septic	Turbid, yellow	↓		
• TB			~20,000	~70
• Gonorrheal			~10,000	~60
• Septic (nongonococcal)[d]			~50,000	~95

[a] E.g., degenerative joint disease
[b] E.g., tumors, hemophilia, trauma
[c] E.g., Reactive arthritis, CPPD crystals, SLE
[d] Includes staphs, streps, and *Pseudomonas* (e.g., postop)

Back pain

This is very common and often self-limiting; *but be alert to "red flags" that may indicate serious underlying causes* (see Table 11.2). Key points in the history: (1) *Onset:* Sudden (related to trauma?) or gradual? (2) Are there motor or sensory symptoms? (3) Is bladder or bowel affected? Pain that is worse with movement and relieved by rest is often mechanical. If it is worse after rest, an inflammatory cause should be considered, such as ankylosing spondylitis. (4) Constitutional symptoms (fever, weight loss, night sweats).

Examination (1) With the patient standing (legs straight), gauge the extent and smoothness of lumbar forward/lateral flexion and extension. (2) *Neurological decits:* Perianal sensation; upper and lower motor neuron (UMN and LMN) signs in legs (p. 392); (3) signs of generalized disease suggest malignancy.

Nerve root impingement causes pain in relevant dermatomes and can be worsened by bending forward. A positive straight leg raising sign occurs when a supine patient experiences pain in buttock/back/other leg when lifting leg to <45 degrees. It suggests lumbar disc herniation impinging on nerve roots. (Its sensitivity is ~0.9 and its specificity is 0.2.)

Neurosurgical emergencies

Acute cauda equina compression: Alternating or bilateral root pain in legs, saddle anesthesia (i.e., bilaterally around anus) and disturbance of bladder or bowel function

Acute cord compression: Bilateral pain, LMN signs at level of compression, UMN and sensory signs below, sphincter disturbance. *Causes* (same for both types of compression): Bony metastasis (look for missing pedicle on x-ray), myeloma, cord or paraspinal tumor, TB (p. 552), abscess. *Urgent treatment needed to prevent irreversible loss:* Laminectomy for disc protrusions; decompression for abscess; radiotherapy for tumors.

Tests *Magnetic resonance imaging (MRI)* is the best way to image cord compression, myelopathy, spinal neoplasms, cysts, hemorrhages, and abscesses. CBC, ESR (↑ in myeloma, infections, tumors), prostate specific antigen (PSA), and bone scan "hot spot" suggest neoplastic diagnoses.

Causes Age determines the most likely causes.
- *15-30 yrs:* Herniated disc, trauma, fractures, ankylosing spondylitis (AS) (p. 402), spondylolisthesis (e.g., L5 shifts forward on S1)
- *30-50 yrs:* Degenerative spinal disease, herniated disc, malignancy (lung, breast, prostate)
- *>50 yrs:* Degenerative, osteoporosis compression fracture, Paget's, malignancy, myeloma (request serum electrophoresis), lumbar spinal stenosis

Rarer causes: Cauda equina tumors, spinal infection (usually staphylococcal, also TB).

Treatment Specific causes need specific treatment. For most back pain, a specific cause is not found, so treat empirically. Avoid precipitants; arrange physical therapy. Analgesia and normal activities are better than bed rest. In certain patients there are roles for disc, epidural, or nerve root injections and surgical procedures, such as foraminotomy, stabilization, or laminectomy.

Features of serious causes of back pain

- Young (<20 yrs) or old (>55 yrs)
- Trauma
- Alternating sciatica
- Bilateral sciatica
- Weak legs
- Weight loss
- Fever of unknown origin (FUO); ESR↑ (>25 mm/h)
- Systemic steroids or immunosuppressive use

- Progressive, continuous, nonmechanical pain
- Constitutionally ill; drug abuse; HIV +ve
- Spine pain in *all* directions of movement
- Localized bony tenderness
- CNS deficit at more than one root level
- Pain or tenderness of thoracic spine
- Bilateral nerve impingement
- Past history of malignancy

Table 11.2 Inflammatory versus mechanical back pain

Inflammatory back pain is associated with ankylosing spondylitis and other forms of spondyloarthritis (psoriatic, inflammatory bowel disease [IBD], and reactive arthritis).

When determining if the back pain is inflammatory in nature, the following features should be sought:

- Onset of pain is usually <40 years of age and is insidious.
- Pain persists for >3 months (i.e., it is chronic).
- The back pain and stiffness worsen with immobility, especially at night and early morning.
- The back pain can be alternating in nature: "buttock to buttock."
- The back pain and stiffness tend to ease with physical activity and exercise.
- NSAIDs are effective in relieving pain and stiffness in most patients.

Spondyloarthritis

Investigations Diagnosis of spondyloarthritis (SPA) is clinical, supported by radiology findings (may be normal in early disease). Look for irregularities, erosions, or sclerosis affecting both sides of the lower third of the sacroiliac joints. See Table 11.3. *Later:* Squaring of the vertebra, "bamboo spine," erosions of the apophyseal joints, obliteration of the sacroiliac joints (sacroiliitis also occurs in reactive arthritis, Crohn's disease, psoriatic arthritis, *Brucella* arthritis). *Other tests:* CBC (normochromic anemia), ESR↑, ↑CRP. A new classification criterion has been developed for SPA.

Ankylosing spondylitis (AS) *Prevalence:* 0.25–1%. *Men present earlier:* ♂:♀ ≈ 6:1 at 16 yrs and ≈ 2:1 at 30 yrs. >85% are human leukocyte antigen (HLA) B27 +ve.

Symptoms: The typical patient is a young man presenting with low back pain, spinal morning stiffness, and progressive loss of spinal movement (spinal ankylosis) who later develops kyphosis and cervical ankylosis. Other features and associations:

- Chest wall expansion ↓
- Chest pain

- Hip involvement
- Knee involvement

- Enthesitis of calcaneal, tibial or ischial tuberosities, or plantar fascia
- Crohn's/UC
- Amyloid

- Carditis; iritis; recurrent sterile urethritis
- Aortic valve disease
- Psoriaform rashes

- Osteoporosis

Treatment: Exercise, not rest, for backache; physical therapy regimens to maintain posture and mobility. Trial NSAIDs 4–6 wks; if unsuccessful, change to another class before moving to anti-tumor necrosis factor (TNF) therapy. Sulfasalazine and methotrexate help peripheral arthritis and enthesitis but not spinal inflammation. Efficacy is proved with anti-TNF therapies. Rarely, spinal osteotomy is useful. Difficult-to-fix osteoporotic spinal fractures can occur.

Enteropathic spondyloarthritis Inflammatory bowel disease (Crohn's and UC) are associated with spondyloarthritis. Avoid etanercept.

Psoriatic arthritis Often asymmetrical, involves distal interphalangeal (DIP) joints, spine, typically causing dactylitis (sausage digits). X-ray changes can be misinterpreted as OA. Associated with synovitis, acneiform rashes, palmoplantar pustulosis, hyperostoses, and (sterile) osteomyelitis (SAPHO). Responds to NSAIDs, methotrexate, cyclosporin, and anti-TNF-α therapy (p. 406).

Reactive arthritis *Presentation:* Secondary to *Chlamydia trachomatis* urethritis, *Campylobacter jejuni, Salmonella, Shigella,* and *Yersinia* species. Typically, a young man with recent nonspecific urethritis, which may be asymptomatic; it may also follow dysentery. Often large joint, lower limb mono- or oligoarthritis or enthesitis; it may be chronic or relapsing. *Also:* Iritis, keratoderma blenorrhagica (brown, aseptic abscesses on soles and palms), and circinate balanitis—painless serpiginous penile rash; mouth ulcers; enthesitis (plantar fasciitis, Achilles tendonitis) and aortic regurgitation. *Tests:* ESR and CRP ↑ or normal. Culture stool if diarrhea. Obtain sexual history. *X-rays:* Periostitis at ligamentous entheses; enthesopathic erosions. *Management:* Rest; splint affected joints; NSAIDs or steroids. Consider sulfasalazine or methotrexate. Rarely, TNF inhibitor.

Table 11.3 Features common to spondyloarthritis

1 Seronegativity (rheumatoid factor –ve)
2 Pathology in spine (spondylo-) and sacroiliac (SI) joints; i.e., "axial arthritis."
3 Asymmetrical large-joint oligoarthritis (i.e. few joints) or monoarthritis
4 Inflamed tendon ligament union sites (enthesitis); e.g., plantar fasciitis, Achilles tendonitis, costochondritis, or digit (finger and toe) tendon sheaths (dactylitis)
5 Extra-articular manifestations; e.g., uveitis, psoriaform rashes, Crohn's, UC
6 HLA B27 association (84–96% of those with AS)

Different forms of spondyloarthritis show much overlap with one another. They are treated with physical and occupational therapy, advice on posture, NSAIDs, sulfasalazine, methotrexate, and TNF inhibitors.

Rheumatoid arthritis

Typically, RA has a persistent, symmetrical distribution but does not have to be symmetric! Persistent symptoms >6 months. To recognize early disease, look for morning stiffness >30 min, + antibodies, + squeeze test across metacarpophalangeal/metatarsal (MCP/MTP)joints. *Later:* Deforming, polyarthritis often affecting hands and feet. *Peak onset:* Fifth decade. ♀:♂ > 2:1. *Prevalence:* 0.5–1% (higher in smokers). *Genetics:* HLA DR4 linked in Caucasians.

Presentation Typically swollen, painful, and stiff hands and feet, especially in the morning. This can fluctuate and larger joints become involved. Less common presentations are:

- Recurring monoarthritis of various joints
- Persistent monoarthritis (often of one knee)
- Systemic illness (pericarditis, pleurisy, weight↓) with minimal joint problems at first (more common in men)
- Sudden onset of widespread arthritis

Palindromic RA : The onset of RA is episodic, with one to several joints being affected sequentially for hours to days, with symptom-free periods in between

Signs At first, swollen fingers and MCP joint swelling or pain and swelling of the feet "positive squeeze test." The first site for erosive change can be the metatarsals. Later, ulnar deviation at MCPs and dorsal wrist subluxation. Boutonnière and swan-neck deformities of fingers (see Figure 11.1) or Z-deformity of thumbs. Hand extensor tendons may rupture and adjacent muscles waste. Foot changes are similar. Larger joints may be involved. Atlantoaxial joint subluxation may threaten the cervical spinal cord. (See Plate 20.)

Extra-articular Anemia, nodules, lymphadenopathy, vasculitis, carpal tunnel syndrome, multifocal neuropathies, splenomegaly (5%, but only 1% have *Felty syndrome*: Splenomegaly and granulocytopenia). *Eyes*: Episcleritis, scleritis, keratoconjunctivitis sicca. *Other signs*: Pleurisy, pericarditis, pulmonary fibrosis, osteoporosis, amyloidosis. Associated with increased risk of ischemic heart disease and lymphomas.

Diagnosis New international criteria have been developed with the purpose of establishing an earlier diagnosis of RA. A scoring system is based on joint distribution, symptom duration, and the presence of serologies and acute-phase reactants.

See: Http://www.rheumatology.org/practice/clinical/classification/ra/ra_2010.asp

X-rays Increased soft tissue, juxta-articular osteoporosis, widened joint space. *Later:* Bony erosions ± subluxation ± complete carpal destruction.

Blood tests ESR↑; hemoglobin (Hb)↓; mean cellular volume (MCV) ↔; WBC↓; platelets↑. *Rheumatoid factor* often –ve at start, becoming +ve in 80% (also +ve in: Sjögren's syndrome (80%), SLE (30%), systemic sclerosis (30%); antinuclear antibodies (ANA) +ve in 30%.

Anti-CCP (cyclic citrullinated peptide) can be seen in early polyarthritis when RF negative, indicating early RA. This has a high specificity and a high positive predictive value for RA.

Treatment Encourage regular exercise, physio- and occupational therapy.

Treat to target! *The goal is to achieve very low disease activity or remission:*

- Prevent joint damage and deformity
- *Early* disease recognition
- Fewer swollen and tender joints
- Normal acute-phase reactants

- *Early* start of disease-modifying therapy and control of the disease
- Most erosions happen within the first few years of the disease.
- Assistive devices and appropriate orthotics (e.g., wrist splints)
- Intra-articular steroids
- *Oral drugs*: If no contraindication (asthma, active peptic ulcer) start an NSAID. Often, NSAIDs, such as ibuprofen 400 mg/8 h after food, do not control symptoms or are not tolerated (GI bleeds). Patients who need low-dose aspirin ± prednisone may also need regular proton pump inhibitor. One cannot predict which NSAID a patient will respond to: Different ones can be tried. Disease-modifying antirheumatic drugs (DMARDs) should be considered early (see Table 11.4). Regular monitoring is vital.
- Steroids may reduce joint damage and control difficult symptoms (e.g., prednisone 5 mg/d PO), but place in treatment schema is controversial. One problem is reduced bone density over long periods.
- Manage cardiovascular risk factors (p. 89) because atherosclerosis is accelerated.
- Surgery to relieve pain, improve function, and to prevent disease complications (e.g., radial-carpal fusion, joint replacements)

Adult-onset Still's disease (AOSD) is a systemic inflammatory disorder characterized by fever, skin rash, polyarthralgias or polyarthritis, sore throat, hepatosplenomegaly, lymphadenopathy, leukocytosis, liver enzyme elevation, and high serum level of ferritin. No specific diagnostic test is available. The clinical diagnosis is based on pattern recognition and exclusion of other conditions. Treatment requires suppression of inflammation: NSAIDs, IL-1 inhibition (Anakinra). See Table 11.5 for forms of arthritis not associated with rheumatoid factor.

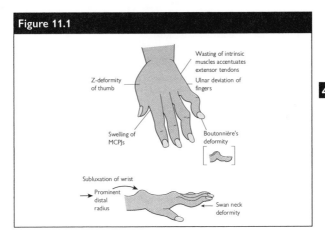

Figure 11.1

Z-deformity of thumb

Wasting of intrinsic muscles accentuates extensor tendons

Ulnar deviation of fingers

Swelling of MCPJs

Boutonnière's deformity

Subluxation of wrist

Prominent distal radius

Swan neck deformity

Table 11.4 Influencing biological events in RA

The chief biological event is inflammation. Monocytes traffic into joints, cytokines are produced, fibroblasts and endothelial cells are activated, and tissue proliferates. Inflammatory fluid is generated (synovial effusion), and cytokines and cellular processes erode cartilage and bone. Cytokines also produce systemic effects: Fatigue, accelerated atherosclerosis, and accelerated bone turnover.

Disease-modifying drugs (DMARDs) Drugs that alter the course of disease and slow joint destruction.

Traditional DMARDs

Methotrexate (MTX), sulfasalazine, leflunomide, and hydroxychloroquine First-line therapy is commonly MTX.

- *Sulfasalazine:* Common side effects (SE): Nausea, headaches, diarrhea, marrow↓, reversible sperm count↓, rash, G6PD deficiency, oral ulcers.
- *Methotrexate:* Avoid in liver disease, pregnancy, and excessive alcohol consumption; caution if preexisting lung disease. SE: Mucositis, nausea, fatigue/lethargy, pneumonitis (rare; can be life-threatening), aspartate aminotransferase/alanine aminotransferase (AST/ALT) ↑. Give concurrent folate supplements (e.g., folic acid 1 mg/d, PO).
- *Cyclosporin:* SE: Nausea, tremor, gingival hypertrophy, hypertension, renal impairment/hypertension
- *Leflunomide:* Reduces autoimmune effects (takes months to work). For first 6 months, do CBC and chemistry monthly. Stop if platelets < 150 × 10⁹/L; WBC < 4 × 10⁹/L, or AST↑ by >3-fold or rashes. SE: liver function tests (LFT) ↑, alopecia, diarrhea, infections
- *Azathioprine:* SE: Marrow↓, nausea, LFT↑, oncogenic (do TPMT[1] test first).
- *Hydroxychloroquine (HCQ):* SE: Rash, diarrhea, While on HCQ, ophthalmic evaluation should occur every year. After 5 years, 1 in 5,000 patients can experience retinopathy.

Anticytokine therapy *Tumor necrosis factor-α (TNF)* is a key cytokine overproduced in RA synovium. Infliximab (chimeric murine/human anti-TNF antibody given IV every 8 wks), etanercept (TNF-α receptor/Ig Fc fusion protein given 25 mg SC twice weekly or 50 mg weekly), and *adalimumab* (fully human anti-TNF monoclonal given as 40 mg SC every 2 wks). SE: Rashes, nausea, diarrhea, and infections (e.g., reactivation of TB). ANA and even SLE-type illness can evolve. Long-term safety issues are unclear (?increased risk of cancer, multiple sclerosis) but responses can be striking compared with other DMARDs.

Immune modulator therapy *Abatacept* (binds to CD86 and CD80 receptors on antigen presenting cells with down-regulation of T cell activation; given IV every 4 wks). SE: Exacerbation of COPD, headaches, nausea. Rituximab (a monoclonal antibody that binds to CD20 antigen on B lymphocytes reducing B cell function). Given in combination with methotrexate and prednisone as two separate IVs 2 wks apart. SE: Fevers, chills, headache, rash, nausea, hepatitis B reactivation, and progressive multifocal leukoencephalopathy (PML) reported.

(Continued)

---

1 Thiopurine methyl transferase—deficiency of this enzyme can lead to bone marrow suppression in the setting of azathioprine use.

Table 11.4 (Continued)

TNF Antagonists	T-cell modulators:
Adalimumab	Abatacept
Etanercept	
Infliximab	
Golimumab	
Certolizumab Pegol	
IL-1 antagonist	**B-cell depletion**
Anakinra	Rituximab
Janus kinase inhibitor	**IL-6 antagonist**
Tofacitinib	Tocilizumab

Table 11.5 Forms of arthritis not associated with rheumatoid factor (sero −ve)

Lyme disease, Behçet's, leukemia, pulmonary osteoarthropathy, endocarditis, acromegaly, Wilson's disease, familial Mediterranean fever, sarcoid, hemophilia, sickle-cell, hemochromatosis, and infections, as from:

Poststreptococcal	Hepatitis B	Rubella
Parvovirus B19	Chl. pneumoniae	Ureaplasma; HIV
Vibrio parahaemolyticus	Borrelia burgdorferi	Clostridium difficile

Chronic arthritis in children (i.e., before 16 yrs) takes several forms and is classified into juvenile idiopathic arthritis (JIA) subforms:

- Systemic arthritis (or Still's disease)
- Oligoarthritis (1–4 joints affected in first 6 months)
- Polyarthritis (RhF −ve, ANA +ve)
- Polyarthritis (RhF +ve)
- Psoriatic arthritis
- Enthesitis-related arthritis at ligament/tendon insertion into bone.

NB: JIA shares only some features with RA:

JIA shares these in common with RA:	JIA and RA differ in these ways:
Both display destructive arthritis	RA is more likely to run in families
Autoimmune with autoantibodies	RA is more homogeneous than JIA
Both have HLA associations	RA has poorer outcomes than JIA

Children with chronic arthritis need regular ophthalmic review to detect occult uveitis, as well as regular monitoring of growth and development.

Osteoarthritis

OA is the commonest joint condition. Women are prone to symptomatic OA ($\female : \male \approx 3:1$). *Mean age at onset:* 50 yrs. OA is usually primary, but may be secondary to any joint disease/injury or some diseases (e.g., hemochromatosis).

Signs and symptoms In single joints, pain on movement, worse at end of day; background pain at rest; minimal stiffness; joint instability. In polyarticular OA with Heberden nodes ("nodal OA"), the most commonly affected joints are DIP, thumb metacarpophalangeal joints, cervical and lumbar spine, and knee. There may be joint tenderness, derangement ± bony swelling (e.g., Heberden nodes; i.e. bony lumps at DIP joints), poor range of movement, and some (usually limited) synovitis.

Imaging/tests *Radiology:* Loss of joint space, subchondral sclerosis and cysts, osteophytes. *CRP* usually normal.

Treatment Acetaminophen for pain. If ineffective, try NSAIDs. Reduce weight; use walking aids, supportive footwear; physical therapy. Do exercises (e.g., regular quadriceps exercises in knee OA) and keep active. Joint replacement for end-stage OA.

Fibromyalgia

Fibromyalgia is a chronic, widespread pain disorder. Fibromyalgia is not due to inflammation but to abnormal nerve conduction that causes pain. Tai Chi twice daily has been shown to be beneficial in reducing pain.[2] Three medications have been FDA-approved for fibromyalgia: pregabalin, duloxetine, and milnacipran. Narcotics are of no benefit in fibromyalgia and can paradoxically increase pain.

Crystal-induced arthritis

Gout In the acute stage, there is severe pain, redness, and swelling of the joint—often the metatarsophalangeal joint of the big toe (podagra). Attacks are due to the deposition of monosodium urate crystals in and around joints and may be precipitated by trauma, surgery, starvation, infection, or diuretics. With long-term hyperuricemia, after repeated attacks, urate deposits (tophi) develop (e.g., finger pads, tendons, joints, pinna). "*Secondary*" *causes:* Polycythemia, psoriasis, leukemia, cytotoxics, renal impairment, long-term alcohol excess.

Diagnosis depends on finding urate crystals in tissues and synovial fluid (serum urate not always ↑). *Synovial fluid microscopy:* Negatively birefringent crystals; neutrophils (+ingested crystals). X-rays may show only soft-tissue swelling in the early stages. Later, well-defined "punched out" lesions are seen in juxta-articular bone. Sclerotic reaction develops later creating an "overhanging edge" or "rat-bite" erosion. Joint spaces are preserved until late. *Prevalence:* ~0.5–1%. $\male : \female \approx 5:1$. (See PLATE 16.)

Treating acute gout Use an NSAID unless contraindicated (e.g., peptic ulcer, renal insufficiency). Steroids are effective (prednisone 30–40 mg PO with rapid taper over 6–10 d). Oral colchicine for acute gout flare treatment; use low-dose colchicine 1.2 mg followed by 0.6 mg in 1 h (1.8 mg total). Low-dose colchicine has both maximum plasma concentration and early gout flare efficacy comparable with that of high-dose colchicine, with a better safety profile.[3]

2 Zhang F, et al. A randomized trial of tai chi for fibromyalgia. *N Engl J Med.* 2010;363:2265–67.

Preventing attacks The goal is to lower uric acid levels: Avoid prolonged fasts, alcohol excess, and high purine food. Lose weight. Allopurinol inhibits xanthine oxidase, metabolized by the kidney. Consider reducing serum urate with long-term allopurinol, but not until 3 wks after an attack. Start with regular NSAID or colchicine cover (0.6 mg/d PO) as introduction of allopurinol may cause gout attack. *Allopurinol dose:* Start at low dose (100 mg/24 h PO), adjust monthly in light of serum urate levels to achieve <6 mg/dL or <5 mg/dL for tophaceous gout. Haste makes waste! Typically 300–400 mg/24 h for mild disease; up to 400–600/d for severe disease. SE: Rash, fever, WBC↓. If simple treatment fails, refer to a rheumatologist. *Febuxostat:* 40 mg/d metabolized by the liver, PO administration. This is a therapeutic alternative when allopurinol is not tolerated (monitor for cytopenias and monitor liver function).

Uricase: A recombinant mammalian uricase, reduces number of tophi. Acutely lowers uric acid levels in patients refractory to conventional therapy. Must check for G6PD deficiency. *Dose:* IV 8 mg/mL (2 mL) infuse over 2 h every 2 wks. SE: Gout flare, infusion reaction, antibody formation (anti-PEG antibodies). Uric acid increase after infusion may indicate antibody formation.

Calcium pyrophosphate dihydrate arthritis

Risk factors:

• Dehydration	• Intercurrent illness	• Hyper-parathyroidism	• Myxedema
• PO_4^{3-}↓; Mg^{2+}↓	• Osteoarthritis	• Hemo-chromatosis	• Acromegaly

Acute CPPD monoarthritis (pseudogout): Similar to gout; affects different joints (mainly wrist, knee, ankles). *Chronic CPPD:* Destructive changes like OA, but more severe; affects knees (also wrists, shoulders, hips). Can present as polyarthritis (pseudorheumatoid). See Figure 11.2.

Tests: Polarized light microscopy of joint fluid; crystals are weakly positively birefringent. Associated with soft-tissue calcium deposition on x-ray; e.g., triangular ligament in wrist or in knee cartilage (chondrocalcinosis). If arthrocentesis is performed, it can be blood tinged. *Treatment:* NSAIDs help but are rarely sufficient and often contraindicated in the elderly; consider steroid joint injection for mono-arthritis, oral or parenteral administration for >2 joints with taper over 1–2 wks. For chronic disease, consider colchicine 0.6 mg/d to prevent flares. See Table 11.6.

Table 11.6 Prescribing NSAIDs: Patient education

Most patients prescribed NSAIDs do not need them all the time, but some patients obediently take them continuously, as prescribed, with potential serious side effects, such as GI bleeding. Explain to your patients that:

- Drugs are for relief of symptoms: *On good days none may be needed.*
- Abdominal pain may be a sign of impending problems: Stop the medication and notify your physician.
- Ulcers may occur with no warning: *Report black stool or light-headedness at once.*
- Don't supplement prescribed NSAIDs with ones bought over the counter (e.g., ibuprofen): Mixing NSAIDs can increase risks greatly.
- Smoking and alcohol increases NSAID risk.

3 Terkeltaub RA. High versus low dosing of oral colchicine for early acute gout flare: Twenty-four hour outcome of the first multicenter, randomized, double-blind, placebo-controlled, parallel-group, dose comparison study. A&R 2010;62:1060–1068.

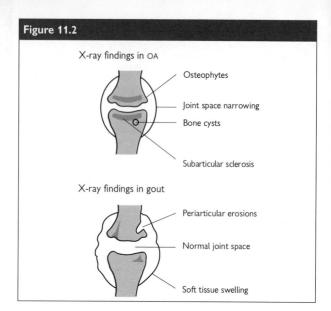

Figure 11.2

X-ray findings in OA

- Osteophytes
- Joint space narrowing
- Bone cysts
- Subarticular sclerosis

X-ray findings in gout

- Periarticular erosions
- Normal joint space
- Soft tissue swelling

Autoimmune connective tissue diseases

Included under this heading are SLE, diffuse/limited cutaneous systemic sclerosis, primary Sjögren's syndrome, idiopathic inflammatory myopathies, undifferentiated connective tissue disease, and relapsing polychondritis. They overlap with each other, may affect many organ systems, and often respond to immunosuppressives.

Systemic lupus erythematosus

SLE is a non-organ-specific autoimmune disease in which autoantibodies are produced against a variety of autoantigens (e.g., ANA). Immunopathology results in polyclonal B-cell secretion of pathogenic autoantibodies and subsequent formation of immune complexes that deposit in sites such as the kidneys. ♀:♂ ≈ 9:1.

Prevalence ~0.2%. *Common in:* Pregnancy; African-Americans; Asians, and if HLA B8, DR2 or DR3 +ve. ~10% of relatives of SLE patients are affected. It is a remitting and relapsing illness, with peak age at diagnosis being 30–40 yrs. Precipitants of lupus flares that should avoided include the sun, echinacea, alfalfa sprouts, melatonin, garlic, and granulocyte colony stimulating factor. *Clinical features:* See Table 11.7. In addition: T°↑ (77%), splenomegaly, lymphadenopathy, alopecia (in 70%) recurrent abortion, retinal exudates, fibrosing alveolitis, myalgia (50%), anorexia (40%), myositis, migraine (40%), ESR↑ (CRP often ↔: Think of SLE whenever someone has a multisystem disorder and ESR↑ but CRP normal).

Serologies >95% are ANA +ve. High titer of antibodies directed against double-stranded DNA is nearly exclusive to SLE. Its absence does not exclude it. 11% have false +ve syphilis serology from IgG anticardiolipin antibodies. Antibodies to Ro (SS-A), La (SS-B), and U1 ribonuclear protein help define overlap syndromes (e.g., with Sjögren's).

Monitoring activity *Important tests:* (1) ESR, (2) complement C3↓, C4↓; C3d↑ denotes degradation products of C3, hence it moves in the opposite direction,(3) double-stranded (anti-DS) DNA antibody titers, (4) urinalysis with spot protein/Cr ratio, and (5) CBC.

Drug-induced lupus This can be caused by isoniazid, hydralazine (in slow acetylators), procainamide, chlorpromazine, minocycline, TNF inhibitors. Lung and skin signs prevail over renal and CNS signs. It remits if the drug is stopped. Sulfonamides and birth control pills may exacerbate idiopathic SLE.

Antiphospholipid syndrome SLE may occur with arterial or venous thrombosis, livedo rash, stroke, adrenal hemorrhage, migraine, miscarriages, myelitis, myocardial infarct, multi-infarct dementia, and cardiolipin antibodies. *Presentation:* Abdominal pain (55%), blood pressure (BP)↓ (54%), fever (40%), nausea (31%), weakness (31%), altered mental status (19%). Venous thrombi occur more often if lupus anticoagulant is +ve; arterial thrombi occur if IgG or IgM antiphospholipid antibody or anti-b₂ glycoprotein 1 +ve.

Treatment Refer to a rheumatologist. NSAIDs, sun-block creams.
- *Hydroxchloroquine:* Reduces flares by 50%, reduces end-organ damage, reduces progression to renal on CNS involvement, reduces lipids, reduces thrombotic risk, and improves survival 200 mg bid. *SE:* Irreversible retinopathy; annual ophthalmic referral is recommended.
- *High-dose prednisone* is kept for severe episodes of SLE (~1 mg/kg/24 h PO with rapid tapering)
- 15 yrs after the diagnosis of lupus, 80% of permanent organ damage in SLE is secondary to prednisone.[4] Any dose of prednisone >6 mg increases later organ damage by 50%.[5]
- The side effects of prednisone include but are not limited to muscle loss and weakness, cataracts, osteonecrosis, osteoporotic fracture, osteoporosis, diabetes, dyslipidemia, weight gain, obesity, hypertension, and memory loss.
- For lupus flare, consider intramuscular triamcinolone(100 mg IM)instead if initiating or increasing oral steroids; no more than quarterly.[6]
- *Mycophenolate mofetil* for lupus nephritis; when used with hydroxchloroquine improves three-fold the complete renal response.[7] Also found to be superior to azathioprine in maintaining a renal response and in preventing relapse.[8]
- *Azathioprine* 1–2.5mg/kg/d PO can be a "steroid-sparer" *SE:* Lymphoma.
- *Belimumab* for active musculoskeletal or cutaneous autoantibody-positive SLE. Inhibits B-lymphocyte stimulator. 10 mg/kg monthly IV. SE: Infusion reaction, nausea, diarrhea.
- *Cyclophosphamide:* Monthly intravenous (IV) cyclophosphamide (750 mg/m² body surface) for 6 months has been the standard induction regimen for lupus nephritis, followed by a maintenance regimen of quarterly infusions for 2 yrs.[9]

411

4 Gladman D, et al. Accrual of organ damage over time in patients with systemic lupus erythematosus. *J Rheumatol.* 2003;30: 1955–1959.
5 Thamer M, et al. Prednisone, lupus activity and permanent organ damage. *J Rheumatol.* 2009;36:560–564.
6 Danowski A, et al. Flares in lupus: Outcome Assessment Trial (FLOAT), a comparison between oral methylprednisolone and intramuscular triamcinolone. *J Rheumatol.* 2006;33:57–60.
7 Ibid.
8 Dooley MA, et al. Mycophenolate versus azathioprine as maintenance therapy for lupus nephritis. *N Engl J Med.* 2011;17(365): 1886–1895.
9 Petri M., et al. High-dose cyclophosphamide versus monthly intravenous cyclophosphamide for systemic lupus erythematosus: A prospective randomized trial. *Arthritis Rheum.* 2010;62(5):1487–1493.

Table 11.7 Revised criteria for diagnosing SLE

Malar rash (butterfly rash): Fixed erythema, flat or raised, over the malar eminences, tending to spare the nasolabial folds.

Discoid rash: Erythematous raised patches with adherent keratotic scaling and follicular plugging ± atrophic scarring. Think of it as a three-stage rash affecting ears, cheeks, scalp, forehead, and chest: Erythema → pigmented hyperkeratotic edematous papules → atrophic depressed lesions.

Photosensitivity on exposed skin representing unusual reaction to light.

Oral ulcers: Oral or nasopharyngeal ulceration.

Arthritis: Nonerosive arthritis involving "2 peripheral joints, characterized by tenderness, swelling, or effusion. Joint involvement is seen in 90% of patients. Deforming arthropathy may occur due to capsular laxity (Jaccoud arthropathy). Aseptic bone necrosis also occurs.

Serositis: (a) Pleuritis (pleuritic pain or rub; 80% of all patients have lung function abnormalities; 40% have dyspnea), (b) pleural effusion, or (c) pericarditis (electrocardiogram [ECG], pericardial rub, or evidence of pericardial effusion).

Renal disorders: (a) Persistent proteinuria >0.5 g/d (or >3+ on dipstick) or (b) *cellular casts;* may be red cell, granular, or mixed.

CNS disorders: (a) Seizures, in the absence of causative drugs or known metabolic imbalance (e.g., uremia, ketoacidosis) or (b) *psychosis* in the absence of causative drugs/metabolic derangements, as above.

Hematological disorders: (a) *Hemolytic anemia* with reticulocytosis or (b) *leukopenia* (i.e., WBC <4 × 10^9/L on ≥2 occasions), or (c) *lymphopenia* (i.e., <1.500 × 10^9/L on ≥2 occasions), or (d) *thrombocytopenia* (i.e., platelets <100 ×10^9/L in the absence of a drug effect).

Immunological disorders: (a) Anti-DNA antibody to native DNA in abnormal titer, or (b) *anti-Sm* antibody to Sm nuclear antigen, or (c) antiphospholipid antibody +ve based on:
    (1) an abnormal serum level of IgG or IgM anticardiolipin antibodies,
    (2) positive result for lupus anticoagulant using a standard method, or
    (3) false-positive serological test for syphilis, +ve for >6 months and confirmed by *Treponema pallidum* immobilization or fluorescent treponemal antibody absorption tests.

Antinuclear antibody: Positive in 95%.

Diagnose SLE in the appropriate clinical setting if ≥4 out of the 11 criteria are present, serially or simultaneously.

Renal transplantation may be needed; nephritis recurs in ~50% on biopsy, but is a rare cause of graft failure (graft survival is 87% at 1 yr and 60% at 5 yrs). *Rituximab can be used for certain types of refractory severe SLE.*

Systemic sclerosis Scleroderma is a connective tissue disease that is characterized by functional and structural abnormalities that involve changes in the skin, blood vessels, muscles, and internal organs. Scleroderma means hard skin. The disease can cause abnormal growth of connective tissue, the proteins that support the skin and organs. Symptoms of scleroderma include but are not limited to *Raynaud phenomenon* (constriction of blood vessels in the hands or feet with cold exposure or stress), esophageal and

GI dysmotility, *sclerodactyly* (thickening of the digital skin), telangiectasia, dyspnea, and calcium deposits in connective tissues.

There are several forms: Localized scleroderma (morphea, linear morphea, linear scleroderma) mainly affecting the skin and subcutaneous tissues. *Limited cutaneous systemic sclerosis* has limited skin involvement typically of only the fingers (sclerodactyly), less frequent fibrosis complications in other organs, but more significant vascular disease overall. Associates primarily with anticentromere antibodies. *Diffuse cutaneous systemic sclerosis:* "Diffuse" defines skin involvement; often associated with lung (anti-Topo I [scl-70] antibodies), cardiac, and renal changes. Higher risk for lung fibrosis and renal disease. *Therapy:* Calcium antagonists, ACE-inhibitors and ARB for Raynaud's. Meticulous BP control (ACE-inhibitors) if any renal crisis. Endothelin-1 receptor blockade (bosentan, ambrisentan, sildenafil, tadalafil) if pulmonary hypertension.

Undifferentiated connective tissue disease (UCTD) The existence of conditions characterized by the presence of clinical and serological manifestations suggestive of systemic autoimmune diseases but not fulfilling the classification criteria for defined connective tissue disease.

Patients who do not meet criteria for lupus and have UCTD may benefit from hydroxychloroquine. There is a 10% risk of progression of undifferentiated connective tissue disease to SLE over 10 yrs.[10] Researched showed that hydroxychloroquine (Plaquenil) may prevent later lupus in patients who do not meet four SLE criteria.

Sjögren's syndrome is a systemic disease in which the defining clinical features are dry mouth (xerostomia) and dry eyes (keratoconjunctivitis sicca) due to chronic lymphocytic infiltration of salivary and lacrimal glands. Lymphocytic infiltrates replace functional epithelium, leading to decreased exocrine secretions (exocrinopathy).It may occur either alone or associated with other autoimmune diseases, like RA or SLE. There can be an associated polyarthritis. Characteristic autoantibodies (anti-Ro/SS-A and anti-La/SS-B) are produced. May affect the nervous system with peripheral neuropathy, a length-dependent or non-length dependent neuropathy. There is an associated increased risk for lymphoma.

Relapsing polychondritis attacks the pinna, nasal septum ± larynx (stridor). *Association:* Aortic valve disease; arthritis; vasculitis. *Treatment:* Steroids.

413

Polymyositis and dermatomyositis

Both conditions cause symmetrical, proximal muscle weakness from muscle inflammation. Can be associated with malignancy (in 9–23%). Dysphagia, dysphonia, facial edema, or respiratory weakness may develop.

Skin signs Macular rash (if over back and shoulder, the *shawl sign* is +ve). A lilac-purple *(heliotrope rash)* on cheeks, eyelids, and light-exposed areas in 25% ± nail-fold erythema *(dilated capillary loops)* and erythematous papules over extensor surfaces of phalanges *(Gottron papules;* pathognomonic if CK↑ + muscle weakness). Also *mechanic's hands* (rough, cracked skin on the lateral and palmar surfaces of the fingers and hands, with irregular "dirty" lines, particularly in the antisynthetase syndrome [anti-Jo1]).

Systemic signs Fevers, Raynaud's; lung involvement (20%); polyarthritis/arthralgia (40%); calcifications; retinitis (like cotton-wool patches); myocardial involvement (myocarditis, arrhythmias); dysphagia; and gut dysmotility.

10 James JA, et al. Hydroxychloroquine sulfate treatment is associated with later onset of systemic lupus erythematosus. *Lupus.* 2007;16:401–409.

Diagnosis Muscle enzymes (ALT, CK, and aldolase) ↑ in plasma; electromyography (EMG) shows fibrillation potentials; muscle biopsy. *Autoantibody (ab) associations:* Myositis-specific: Anti-Mi-2, anti-Jo1 (look for lung fibrosis as well). *Overlap syndromes:* Scleroderma with dermatomyositis (e.g., anti-PM-Scl +ve) or polymyositis/alveolitis (e.g., anti-Jo1 +ve). *Differential diagnosis:* Subacute weakness from inclusion-body myositis, muscular dystrophies, SLE myositis, polymyalgia, systemic sclerosis, endocrine/metabolic myopathies, rhabdomyolysis.

Management Investigate extensively for malignancy; get expert help; rest and prednisone help (start with 1 mg/kg/24 h PO). Immunosuppressives (p. 406) and cytotoxics are also used early (e.g., azathioprine, methotrexate, cyclophosphamide, or cyclosporin). High-dose immune globulin has a role. Dapsone can help skin disease. A more aggressive form with prominent vasculitis occurs in children.

Antisynthetase syndrome Up to 30% of patients with DM or PM have a group of clinical findings called "the antisynthetase syndrome." These findings include Raynaud's phenomenon, mechanic's hands, arthritis, and interstitial lung disease. These patients often have antisynthetase antibodies that are highly specific. *Antisynthetase autoantibodies:* Anti-Jo-1, Anti-PL-7, Anti-PL-12, Anti-EJ, Anti-OJ, Anti-KS, Anti-Zo, Anti-Ha. See Table 11.8.

Inclusion body myositis (IBM) Affects men more than women. The mean age at onset of symptoms is ~60 yrs. Patients with IBM present with the insidious onset of weakness. The average duration of symptoms before diagnosis is about 6 yrs. Proximal lower extremity weakness is usually the first sign, with subsequent involvement of upper extremity and distal muscle groups. Proximal muscle weakness is typically more pronounced. Weakness is accompanied by myalgias in about 40% of cases. Muscle atrophy usually progresses in parallel with the duration and severity of weakness. Some patients, however, have profound atrophy of the upper arms or quadriceps. The muscles look "scooped out."

Statin myopathy In addition to inducing a self-limited myopathy, statin use is associated with an immune-mediated necrotizing myopathy (IMNM), with autoantibodies that recognize 200-kd and 100-kd autoantigens. Statins upregulate the expression of HMG-COA reductase (HMGCR), the major target of autoantibodies in statin-associated IMNM. Regenerating muscle cells express high levels of HMGCR, which may sustain the immune response even after statins are discontinued.

Table 11.8 Plasma autoantibodies: Disease associations

Antinuclear antibody (ANA)	+ve in (%)	Smooth muscle antibody (SMA)	+ve in (%)
SLE	95	Chronic active hepatitis	40–90
RA	32	Primary biliary cirrhosis	30–70
JIA (p. 407)	76	Idiopathic cirrhosis	25–30
Chronic active hepatitis	75	Viral infections	80
Sjögren's syndrome	68	(Low titers)	
Systemic sclerosis	64	"Normal" controls	3–12
"Normal" controls	0–2	(↑ with age: 20% at 70 yrs)	

(Continued)

Table 11.8 (Continued)

Gastric parietal cell antibody		Mitochondrial autoantibodies, AMA	
Pernicious anemia (adults)	>90	Primary biliary cirrhosis	60–94
Atrophic gastritis		Chronic active hepatitis	25–60
Females	60	Idiopathic cirrhosis	25–30
Males	15–20	"Normal" controls	0.8
Autoimmune thyroid disease	33		
"Normal" controls	2–16		

Myositis-associated autoantibodies:

PM-Scl   *PM or DM/SSc overlap*

U1RNP

Anti-SRP: Severe, acute, resistant necrotizing myopathy

Anti-Mi-2 DM with rash > muscle symptoms, treatment responsive

Anti-HMGCR (anti-200/100) HMGCR Necrotizing myopathy related to statin use in majority; most patients are statin-exposed, but myopathy also reported in a minority of statin-naive patients

Anti-MDA5 (anti-CADM 140) CAM (cancer-associated myositis), DM with rapidly progressive lung disease.

Antisynthetase antibodies

Anti Jo-1, Anti PL-7, Anti PL-12, Anti EJ, Anti-OJ, Anti –KS, Anti –Zo, Anti-HA

Thyroid antibodies	Microsomal (%)	Thyroglobulin (%)	
Hashimoto's thyroiditis	70–91	75–95	
Graves' disease	50–80	33–75	
Myxedema	40–65	50–81	
Thyrotoxicosis	37–54	40–75	
Juvenile lymphocytic thyroiditis	91	72	
Pernicious anemia	55		
"Normal" controls (50% in older women)	10–13	6–10	

Rheumatoid factor	+ve in (%)		
RA	70–80	Juvenile arthropathy	
Sjögren's syndrome	≤80	Infective endocarditis	≤50
Felty's syndrome	≤100	SLE	≤40
Systemic sclerosis	30	"Normal" controls	5–10

(Continued)

ANCA-associated vasculitis: Two types:

- *Classical antineutrophil cytoplasmic antibody (c-ANCA): Target:* Serine protease 3: +ve in granulomatosis with polyangiitis (p. 416) in >90% of patients.
- *Perinuclear antineutrophil cytoplasmic antibody (p-ANCA): Target:* Myeloperoxidase; +ve in ~80% pauci-immune crescentic glomerulonephritis (p. 261) and systemic vasculitides (e.g., microscopic polyangiitis, a vasculitis of kidney ± lung, p-ANCA +ve in ~75%).

NB: Churg–Strauss may be associated with p- and c-ANCA.

Vasculitis and polyarteritis nodosa

Vasculitis, defined as any inflammatory disorder of blood vessels (typically noninfectious), can affect vessels of any organ. It may be occlusive (necrotizing, as in SLE) or nonocclusive, as in Henoch–Schönlein purpura (p. 263). It can occur *de novo*, as in polyarteritis (see Table 11.9), Churg–Strauss, Behçet's, giant cell arteritis (GCA), Takayasu's, and granulomatosis with polyangiitis (formerly known as Wegener's), be caused by drugs (cocaine) or infection (syphilis is an endarteritis obliterans), or be mediated by complement activation induced by immune complexes in autoimmunity (e.g., SLE, RA). *Consider vasculitis as a diagnosis for any unidentified multisystem disorder.* Organ involvement can be from acute vasculitis or end-organ damage resulting from recurrent vasculitis.

Features seen in many vasculitides

- *General:* Fever, malaise, weight↓, arthralgia, myalgia, ESR↑
- *Skin:* Purpura, ulcers, livedo reticularis, nail bed infarcts, digital gangrene
- *Eyes:* Episcleritis, ulceration, visual loss
- *ENT:* Epistaxis, nasal crusting, stridor, deafness
- *Pulmonary:* Hemoptysis, dyspnea
- *Cardiac:* Loss of pulses, heart failure, myocardial infarction, angina
- *GI:* Abdominal pain (any viscus may infarct), malabsorption because of chronic mesenteric ischemia
- *Renal:* BP↑ hematuria, proteinuria, casts, acute/chronic renal failure
- *Neurological:* Mononeuritis multiplex, sensorimotor neuropathy, hemiplegia, seizures, psychoses, confusion, cognition↓, fluctuating mood, odd behavior

Diagnosis is based on clinical findings, supported by histological and occasionally angiographic findings. ANCA may be +ve (p. 416).

Treatment Treat hypertension meticulously. Refer to experts. Use high-dose prednisone and cyclophosphamide if major organ involvement.

Granulomatosis with polyangiitis (GPA) has a predisposition for certain organs. The classic organs involved are the upper respiratory tract (sinuses, nose, ears, and trachea), lungs, and kidneys. May develop recurrent ear infections, hearing loss, nasal crusting, epistaxis, and septal perforation. The bridge of the nose can collapse, resulting in a "saddle–nose deformity."

Inflammation can occur in different parts of the eye with episcleritis, scleritis, or uveitis, as well as inflammation behind the eye causing an orbital pseudotumor with proptosis. Infiltrates can be seen on chest x-ray, and there can be bleeding in the lungs. Inflammation can happen in the kidney as well. Glomerulonephritis can lead to hematuria, proteinuria, and renal

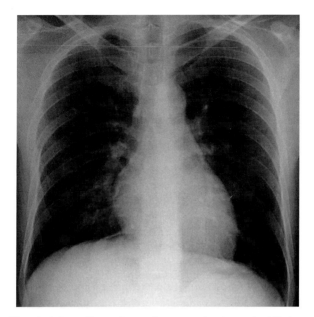

Plate 1. A few millilitres of gas in the peritoneal cavity can be difficult to see. The best way is with a CXR after remaining erect for 10 min. This may be a small pneumoperitoneum at the right cardiophrenic angle. Check with another view or a CT if necessary. If you strongly suspected a perforated ulcer and the CXR and AXR showed no signs of pneumoperitoneum, could you exclude the diagnosis? No. Only 75% of perforations have evidence of pneumoperitoneum.

The authors and publishers would like to thank Peter Scally for permission to use these plates taken from Scally, P. (1999) *Medical imaging: an Oxford core text*. Oxford University Press, Oxford

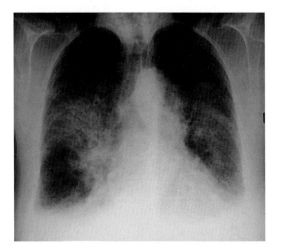

(a)

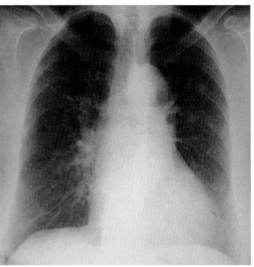

(b)

Plate 2. (a) (b) Two radiographs, 4 days apart. *Lungs*: The major abnormality in the initial film is in the lungs; perihilar opacities that are poorly defined. This is consolidation. But what is the cause? Pulmonary oedema, infection, or blood? The lungs are filled with fluid and unable to expand fully. *Pleura*: The hemidiaphragms are not visible because of pleural effusions, seen curving up the side walls. *Mediastinum*: The heart is enlarged. *Hila, bones, soft tissues*: normal. These are the changes of severe left heart failure. The pulmonary venous pressure has been so high that fluid has flowed from the capillaries, into the interstitium, and then into the alveoli. Look at how the lungs have expanded and the heart borders and hemidiaphragms have sharpened up after treatment.

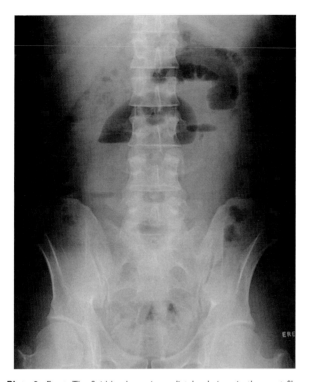

Plate 3. Erect. The fluid levels are immediately obvious in the erect film, but let's approach it in a systematic way. *Gas* can be seen in the colon from the rectum back to the caecum. The stomach bubble is barely visible. That leaves several loops with fluid levels to be explained. They must be small intestine, being centrally placed and with a few valvulae conniventes. The loops are dilated, 3 cm wide, and are probably ileum as the valvulae conniventes are less pronounced here than in the jejunum. By comparison, if the large bowel was obstructed it would show as a few peripheral loops, often over 5 cm in diameter, containing faeces and showing a haustral (scalloped) pattern. Folds in the mucosa of the colon do not extend completely across the lumen. No sign of *calcification in the biliary tree or urinary tract*. The *bones* and *soft tissues* are normal. We would be looking for evidence of a cause of small bowel obstruction: a hernia, surgical clips, or any other signs of surgery.

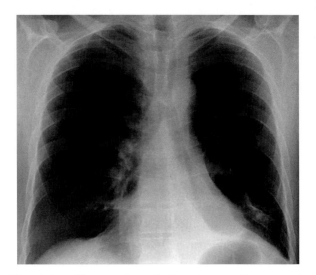

Plate 4. *Lungs*: These are of normal volume. Fewer markings are seen in the left lung except at the base. *Pleura*: Following the pleura reveals loss of the clarity of the left hemidiaphragm. *Mediastinum*: In the mediastinum the left main bronchus is pulled down and there is a triangular opacity behind the heart on the left. This is a collapsed left lower lobe. It also depresses the left *hilum*. *Bones*: Check the bones for metastatic disease because the left lower lobe bronchus may be obstructed by a neoplasm. *Soft tissues*: appear unremarkable.

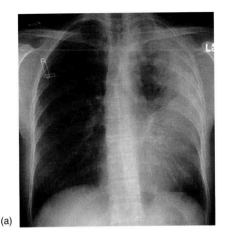

(a)

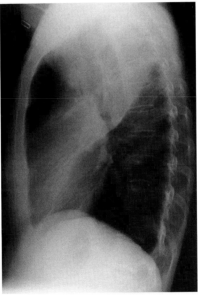

(b)

Plate 5. (a) (b) *Lungs*: Normal lung volumes. A poorly defined opacity in the left lung obliterates the left heart border and therefore is in the upper lobe. The air-bronchogram indicates consolidation. *Pleura*: The pleura in the right hemithorax seem normal. *Mediastinum*: This is central but the oblique fissure on the lateral film is bowed inferiorly because of a slight increase in volume. *Hila*: The left hilum is not visible. *Bones, soft tissues*: normal. Left upper lobe pneumonia (lobar pneumonia). Pneumonia is an infection of the lung, classified as lobar, broncho, and atypical. Usually the pathology progresses through four stages: congestion, red hepatization, grey hepatization, and resolution. This would be one of the stages of hepatization.

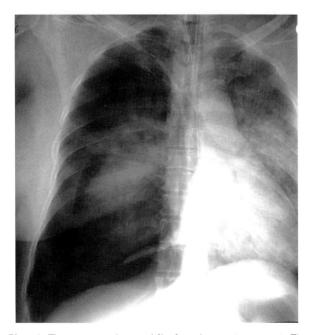

Plate 6. This is a great educational film from the intensive care unit. The inexperienced doctor could be distracted by the poor quality, badly centred film. The technicians do the best they can under difficult conditions. To ask for another in this instance would be a mistake. There is adequate information to make a life-saving decision. After checking the name of the patient, see that the tubes and lines are well positioned—the endotracheal and nasogastric tubes and the right subclavian central venous line. *Lungs*: The left lung shows consolidation. The right hemithorax is too black and hyperexpanded. Right hemidiaphragm is depressed. *Pleura*: The pleural recess is seen at the right base. *Mediastinum*: This is shifted to the left, obstructing venous return and decreasing cardiac output, a threat to life. Is it being pushed or pulled? *Hila, bones, and soft tissues*: Check these structures. Is the endotracheal tube down the right main bronchus, inflating the right lung and collapsing the left? No. Is the right lung collapsed? Yes. Right tension pneumothorax. Beware of the half-toning of the hemidiaphragm in a supine film. In the supine position, a pneumothorax will be anterior and the lung will fall posteriorly. A chest tube is needed immediately. The consolidation in the left lung could be a result of any of the causes of the acute respiratory distress syndrome (ARDS). Consolidation/collapse often occurs in intubated patients at the left base. Suction catheters to clear the lungs pass down the ETT and preferentially into the right main bronchus.

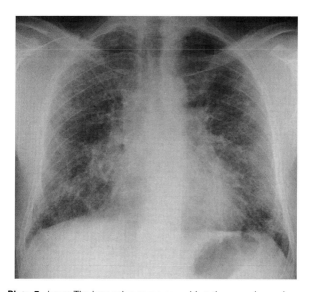

Plate 7. *Lungs*: The lung volumes are normal but the parenchyma shows increased markings that extend out to the chest wall. Normally vessels (arteries and veins) are only seen for 80% of the distance from hilum to pleura. The bronchi should barely be visible. *Pleura*: Following the pleura demonstrates that the heart borders are poorly defined, reflecting interstitial disease in the lung adjacent to the heart. *Mediastinum*: The mediastinal structures themselves are normal. *Hila*: The hila are difficult to interpret. So what? It is not unusual to be missing a piece of information when making a clinical decision. No need for wringing of hands and gnashing of teeth. Either go ahead without it or, if it is essential, find it. In this case, further information is available by comparison with old films or by requesting a CT. *Bone* and *soft tissues*: No abnormality. This is interstitial lung disease. It has a similar appearance to the interstitial oedema of moderate left heart failure but without a big heart. Check the previous film to see if it is acute. It was not. The diagnosis in this example is fibrosing alveolitis.

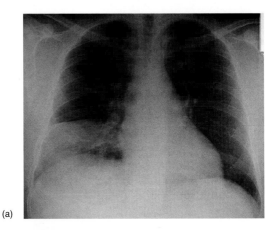

(a)

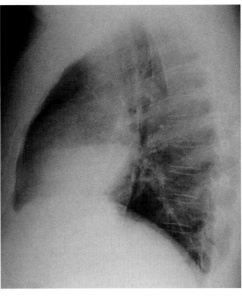

(b)

Plate 8. (a) (b) *Lungs*: An opacity can be seen at the base of the right lung. *Pleura*: The silhouette of the pleura over the right hemidiaphragm is lost because of adjacent lung disease. The right heart border is also unclear. *Mediastinum, hila, bones, soft tissues*: normal. The middle lobe has two segments. The consolidation of lobar pneumonia here involves principally the lateral segment. The medial segment is affected to a lesser extent, shown by the loss of clarity of the right heart border. Also well seen on the lateral projection, but the PA view has adequate information.

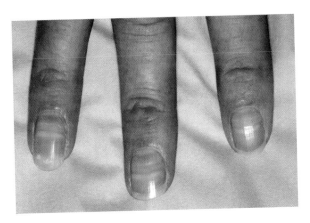

Plate 9. Beau's lines.

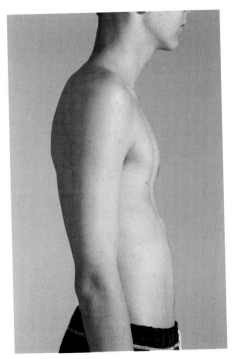

Plate 10. Pectus excavatum. The medical term for funnel or sunken chest. Associations: scoliosis; restrictive spirometry; Marfan's syndrome; Ehlers–Danlos syndrome (plate 24).

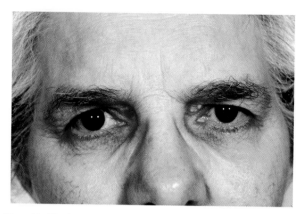

Plate 11. Xanthelasma. *Xanthos* is Greek for yellow, and *elasma* means plate. Xanthelasma are lipid-laden yellow plaques congregating around the lids. They are typically a few mm wide, and signify hyperlipidaemia.

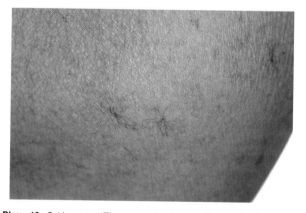

Plate 12. Spider naevi. These consist of a central arteriole, from which numerous vessels radiate (like the legs of a spider). These fill from the centre. They occur most commonly in skin drained by the superior vena cava. Up to 5 are said to be normal (they are common in young females). Causes include liver failure, contraceptive steroids, and pregnancy (ie changes in oestrogen metabolism).

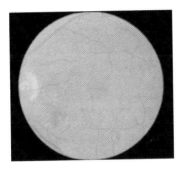

Plate 13. Diabetes, background retinopathy. There are scattered blot haemorrhages and sparse hard exudates but vision is normal.

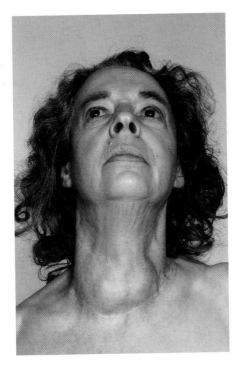

Plate 14. Nodular goitre.

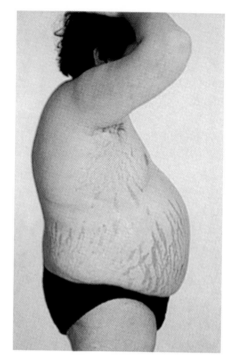

Plate 15. Cushing's disease. Signs of Cushings include purple abdominal striae and wasting, eg in the thighs.

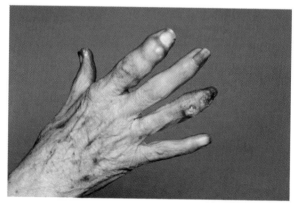

Plate 16. Tophaceous gout.

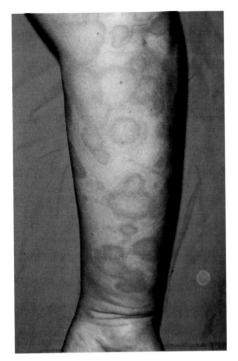

Plate 17. Erythema multiforme. Target lesions eg caused by drugs, herpes or mycoplasma.

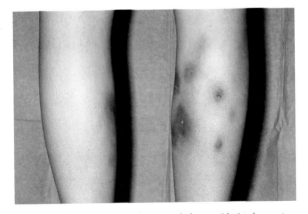

Plate 18. Erythema nodosum. Causes include sarcoidosis, drugs, streps, TB, and UC/Crohn's disease.

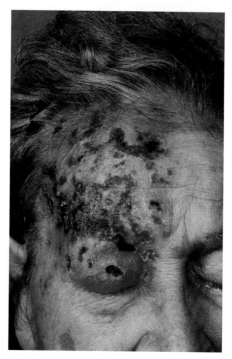

Plate 19. Shingles (herpes zoster) involving the ophthalmic (Vi) division of the trigeminal nerve.

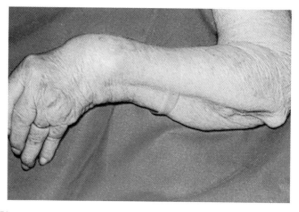

Plate 20. Rheumatoid arthritis. Note ulnar deviation of fingers.

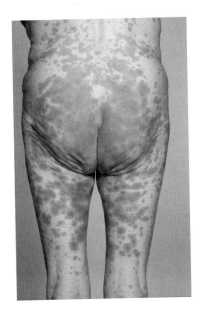

Plate 21. Drug reaction.

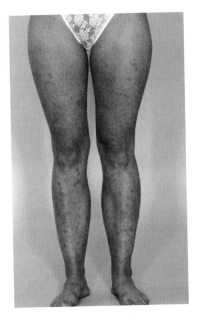

Plate 22. Vascultic skin rash from Behcet's disease.

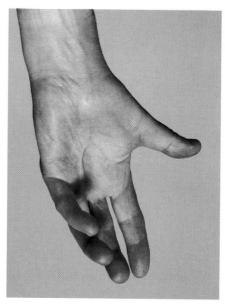

Plate 23. Dupuytren's contracture.

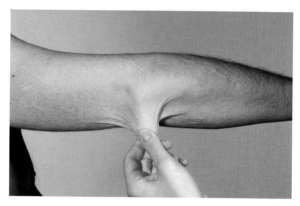

Plate 24. Ehlers–Danlos syndrome. Note the hyperelasticity of the skin. Associations: aneurysms; GI bleeds/perforations; hypermobile joints; flat feet. It is a disorder of collagen.

Table 11.9 Polyarteritis nodosa (PAN)

PAN is a necrotizing vasculitis that causes aneurysms of medium-sized arteries. ♂:♀ ≈ 2:1. Sometimes PAN is associated with HBSAG.

Signs and symptoms

- *General features*: Fevers, abdominal pain, malaise, weight↓, arthralgia
- *Renal*: 75% of cases. Main cause of death. Hypertension, hematuria, proteinuria, renal failure, intrarenal aneurysms, vasculitis
- *Vascular*: BP↑; claudication
- *Cardiac*: 80% of cases. Coronary arteritis and consequent infarction. ↑BP and heart failure. Pericarditis. In Kawasaki's disease (childhood PAN variant), coronary aneurysms occur.
- *Pulmonary*: Pulmonary infiltrates and asthma occur in vasculitis (some say that lung involvement is incompatible with PAN, calling it then Churg—Strauss syndrome).
- *CNS*: 70% of cases. Mononeuritis multiplex, sensorimotor polyneuropathy, seizures, hemiplegia, psychoses
- *GI*: 70% of cases. Abdominal pain (any viscus may infarct), malabsorption because of chronic ischemia
- *Skin*: Urticaria, purpura, infarcts, livedo reticularis, nodules
- *Blood*: WBC↑, eosinophilia (in 30%), anemia, ESR↑, CRP↑

Diagnosis This is most often made from clinical features in combination with renal or mesenteric angiography. ANCA is classically negative.

Treatment Treat hypertension aggressively. Refer to rheumatology. Use high-dose prednisone, then cyclophosphamide.

failure. *Treatment for limited disease*: Patients can be treated with trimethoprim/sulfamethoxazole, which may help to eradicate *S. aureus* colonization of the nasal cavity. *Treatment for systemic ANCA-associated vasculitis:* Remission induction with oral cyclophosphamide 2 mg/kg/d (adjust for the elderly and renal insufficiency) α 6 months and prednisone 1 mg/kg/d α 1 month followed by tapered dose. Initiate maintenance therapy with a steroid-sparing agent like MTX or azathioprine for 1 yr after the 6-month treatment course with cyclophosphamide.

Behçet's disease involves small, medium, and large arteries and veins. HLA–B51 is a risk factor. Uveitis, painful aphthous, scrotal or vaginal ulcers. Arthritis or arthralgias are common. Pustular skin lesions after trauma (pathergy). CNS involvement with headaches, aseptic meningitis, confusion, strokes, and personality changes. (See Plate 22.)

Polymyalgia rheumatica

Polymyalgia rheumatica (PMR) is common in those >70 yrs who have symmetrical aching and morning stiffness in shoulders and proximal limb muscles for >1 month ± mild polyarthritis, tenosynovitis (e.g., carpal tunnel syndrome [p. 386]; occurs in 10%), depression, fatigue, fever, weight↓, and anorexia. It may come on suddenly or over the course of weeks. It overlaps with GCA. ♀:♂ ≈ 2:1 **Tests** ESR usually >40 mm/h; CK usually ↔; alk phos↑; mild anemia **Differential diagnosis** Recent onset RA; hypothyroidism, primary muscle disease, occult malignancy or infection, neck lesions, bilateral subacromial impingement lesions, spinal stenosis. **Treatment** Prednisone 15–20 mg/24 h PO; decrease dose slowly after symptoms have been controlled at least 1 month (in light of symptoms and ESR). Most need steroids for "2 yrs. Preventing osteoporosis is essential (p. 305).

Giant cell (temporal) arteritis

GCA has PMR symptoms in up to 25% of people. Common in the elderly, it is rare under 55 yrs. **Symptoms** Headache, scalp and temporal artery tenderness (e.g., on combing hair), jaw claudication, amaurosis fugax, or sudden blindness in one eye. **Tests** ESR↑, CRP↑, platelets↑, alk phos↑, anemia. If you suspect GCA, do an ESR, start prednisone 1 mg/kg/24 h PO *immediately*. Some advocate higher doses IV (up to 1,000 mg) if visual symptoms (ask an ophthalmologist). Osteoporosis prophylaxis is essential. Get temporal artery biopsy (several cm in length because skip lesions occur) in the next few days. *NB:* The immediate risk is blindness, but longer term, the main cause of death and morbidity in GCA is steroid treatment! Reduce prednisone after 5–7 d in light of symptoms and ESR; increase dose if symptoms recur. *Typical course:* 1–2 yrs, although it can reoccur.

Oncology

Daniel Laheru, M.D.

Contents

Introduction

Since Richard Nixon signed the National Cancer Act on December 23, 1971 to focus and prioritize federal resources to advance cancer clinical and basic science research, there have been a number of notable achievements in cancer treatment, particularly in solid tumors such as germ cell tumors and hematologic malignancies including Hodgkin's lymphoma, acute lymphoblastic leukemia, acute myelogenous leukemia, and chronic myelogenous leukemia.

The sequencing and analysis of the human genome in 2001, followed by the sequencing of a number of cancers including colorectal cancer, breast cancer, brain tumors, pancreas and neuroendocrine cancers, and head and neck cancers provided researchers with the critical tools to begin to identify and differentiate cancer from normal tissue at the genetic level. Although the implications of these landmark projects are still being realized, it is evident that the identification of critical genes and proteins involved in cell division and growth and metastasis are just the beginning. The full comprehension of how these genes control nonlinear cellular signaling matrices has become the new discovery and treatment paradigm in oncology. The potential has raised expectations for unprecedented progress in the near future. However, even as better treatments are being developed, the best treatment remains earlier diagnosis and improved screening methods for those at risk. This review will provide only a general overview of the epidemiology, genetics, screening, and treatment of some select cancers.

Looking after people with cancer

Table 12.1 Looking after people with cancer

No rules guarantee success, but there is no doubt that getting to know your patient, making an agreed management plan, and seeking out the right expert for each stage of treatment (with emphasis now in multi-discipline care) *all* need to be central activities in oncology. These issues focus around communication with patients and families but also with a team of disease-specific experts across disciplines including surgery, medical and radiation oncology, pathology, radiology, interventional disciplines, social work, nutrition, palliative care, and pain services.

Psychological support Examples include:

- Allowing the patient to express anger, fear—or any negative feeling (anger can anesthetize pain).
- Counseling (e.g., with a breast cancer nurse for mastectomy preparation)
- Cognitive and behavioral therapy reduces psychological morbidity associated with cancer treatments.
- Group therapy reduces pain, mood disturbance, and the frequency of maladaptive coping strategies.
- Meta-analyses have suggested that psychological support can have some effect on improving outcome measures such as survival.

Advice on breaking bad news

1 Choose a quiet place where you will not be disturbed.
2 Find out what the patient already knows or surmises (often a great deal).
3 Find out how much the person wants to know. You can be surprisingly direct about this. "Are you the sort of person who, if anything were amiss, would want to know all the details?"
4 Give some warning (e.g., "there is some bad news for us to address").
5 Share information about diagnosis, treatments, and prognosis. Specifically list supporting people (e.g., nurses) and facilities (e.g., hospices). Try asking "Is there anything else you want me to explain?" Don't hesitate to go over the same ground repeatedly. Allow denial: Don't force the conversation.
6 Listen to any concerns raised; encourage the airing of feelings.
7 Summarize and make a plan. Offer availability.
8 Follow through. The most important thing is to leave the patient with the strong impression that you are with him or her.

Don't imagine that a single blueprint will do for everyone. Be prepared to use *whatever* the patient gives you. This requires close observation of verbal and nonverbal cues. Because humans are very complex, we all frequently fail. Don't be put off: Keep trying.

Epidemiology

The incidences of selected most-common cancers for men and women worldwide are identified in Table 12.2. These numbers do not include carcinoma in situ of any site except urinary bladder, nor do they include basal and squamous cell cancers of the skin. The incidence reflects an overall increase when compared to recent years. This is thought to be secondary to the continuing growth and aging of the worldwide population, as well as to external environmental factors such as smoking.

The expected worldwide deaths are identified in Table 12.3. Breast cancer remains the most common cause of cancer (23% of total cancer cases) and cancer death (14% of total cancer deaths) in women worldwide. In developing countries, breast cancer is now also the leading cause of cancer death, surpassing cervical cancer over the past decade. Lung cancer remains the most common cause of cancer (17% of total cancer cases) and cancer death (23% of total cancer deaths worldwide) in men worldwide.

Mortality rates have slightly increased across all four major cancer sites in men and in women, except for female lung cancer, in which rates have been stable. The incidence trends are mixed, reflective of the recent initiatives in public policy or awareness and screening. Many cancers, including pancreas, breast, and prostate cancers, have continued to demonstrate slight increases every year. Lung cancer incidence rates are declining in men and leveled off for the first time in women after increasing for many decades. Colorectal cancer incidence rates are slightly increasing/stable in Western countries. The incremental decrease in incidence rates of prostate cancer and female breast cancer in at least Western countries may be attributable to increased screening through prostate-specific antigen (PSA) testing (for prostate cancer) and mammography (for breast cancer),although currently there is significant controversy regarding the utility of early prostate cancer screening using PSA. Conversely, the slight increase in colorectal cancer incidence may represent the fact that screening tests such as colonoscopy are still completed in the minority of eligible individuals. The increase in female breast cancer incidence may also reflect increased use of hormone replacement therapy and/or increased prevalence of obesity. An additional cancer that has noted a slight increase for unclear reasons is hepatocellular cancer.

Table 12.2 New worldwide cancer incidence of selected cancers for 2011.

Male	Female
1. Lung and bronchus (1,095,200)	1. Breast (1,383,500)
2. Prostate (903,500)	2. Colon and rectum (570,100)
3. Colon and rectum (663,600)	3. Cervix and uteri (529,800)
4. Stomach (640,600)	4. Lung and bronchus (513,600)
5. Liver (522,400)	5. Stomach (349,000)
6. Esophagus (326,600)	6. Corpus uteri (287,100)
7. Bladder (297,300)	7. Liver (225,900)
8. Non-Hodgkin's lymphoma (199,600)	8. Ovary (225,500)
9. Leukemia (195,900)	9. Thyroid (163,000)
10. Oral cavity (170,900)	10. Non-Hodgkin's lymphoma (156,300)

Data modified from Jemal A. Global cancer statistics. *CA Cancer J Clin.* 2011;Mar-Apr: 61(2):69–90.

Table 12.3 Estimated worldwide deaths of selected cancers for 2011.

Male	Female
1. Lung and bronchus (951,000)	1. Breast (458,400)
2. Liver (478,300)	2. Lung and bronchus (427,400)
3. Stomach (464,400)	3. Colon and rectum (288,100)
4. Colon and rectum (320,600)	4. Cervix uteri (275,100)
5. Esophagus (276,100)	5. Stomach (273,600)
6. Prostate (258,400)	6. Liver (217,600)
7. Leukemia (143,700)	7. Ovary (140,200)
8. Pancreas (138,100)	8. Esophagus (130,700)
9. Urinary bladder (112,300)	9. Pancreas (127,900)
10. Non-Hodgkin's lymphoma (109,500)	10. Leukemia (113,800)

Data modified from Jemal A. Global cancer statistics. *CA Cancer J Clin*. 2011;Mar-Apr: 61(2):69–90.

Oncology and genetics

The majority of cancers are believed to be sporadic. However, a number of gene mutations that predispose to cancer have been identified. Much progress has been made at understanding a number of cancers at the genetic level, although it is beyond the scope of this chapter to provide a comprehensive review of this. However, some of the genetic underpinnings for some of the most common and notable cancers have recently been described (see Table 12.4).

Familial colorectal cancer ~20% of those with colorectal cancer (CRC) have a family history of the disease. There have been a number of hereditary syndromes identified from this group, including familial adenomatous polyposis (FAP) and hereditary nonpolyposis colorectal cancer (HNPCC). The genes responsible for these syndromes have also been identified and characterized. FAP accounts for <1% of hereditary CRC but is the best characterized cancer genetic syndrome. The identified genetic mutation has been mapped to chromosome 5 and is known to be autosomal dominant. FAP is characterized by innumerable colonic adenomas at an early age, with the development of overt cancer in 100% of patients by age 40–50. Patients who have a mutation in the locus for FAP [adenomatous polyposis coli (APC) gene] or who have one or more first-degree relatives with FAP or an identified APC mutation are at considerable risk and require yearly colonoscopies at an early age. As the incidence of developing CRC is essentially 100% in patients with FAP and because of the elevated risk of developing metachronous (i.e., with lesions occurring at different times) CRC, these patients are often recommended one of three prophylactic surgeries: (1) total proctocolectomy with ileostomy, (2) total proctocolectomy with ileal pouch-anal anastomosis (IPAA), or (3) colectomy with ileorectal anastomosis (IRA).

Of the hereditary syndromes, HNPCC (Lynch syndrome I and II) is the most common, accounting for ~2–7% of the total. Patients with HNPCC typically develop CRC later than patients with FAP, with age of onset during the fourth and fifth decades. The genetic alterations are more heterogeneous than for FAP, with the majority of individuals linked to chromosomes 2, 3, and 7. The molecular fingerprint of HNPCC is the microsatellite instability (MSI) phenotype, which is a germline mutation caused by a number of genes, particularly MLH1 and MSH2. MSH2/MLH1 gene testing is the gold standard, but, for a variety of reasons including cost, this testing is performed in only selected cases. The diagnosis of HNPCC is complex as it is based initially on both clinical evaluation and a careful assessment of family history, followed by MSI and MSH2/MLH1 testing only if strict clinical criteria have been met. Despite a complex diagnosis algorithm, such screening is thought to underestimate the true incidence of HNPCC.

Familial breast cancer In breast cancer, numerous studies have shown that the risk of developing breast cancer increases if a first-degree relative is diagnosed with breast cancer. For example, if a mother or sister has been diagnosed with bilateral breast cancer and the age at diagnosis was premenopause, the absolute risk to other first-degree relatives approaches 50%. If the diagnosis in the affected relative was postmenopause, the risk is reduced to ~10%. ~5% of women with breast cancer report a family history. BRCA1 (mapped to chromosome 17) and BRCA2 (mapped to chromosome 13) mutations account for most cases of breast cancer. Of note, BRCA2 mutations predispose carriers to a number of cancers including pancreas and colorectal, prostate, gastric, oral cavity, hepatobiliary, and ovarian cancers, as well as melanoma. The risk of developing male breast cancer is higher in individuals with BRCA2 mutations, whereas the risk of developing ovarian cancer is higher in individuals with BRAC1 mutations. Most of the identified mutations within each of these genes are associated with loss of function, suggesting that BRCA1 and BRCA2 are tumor suppressor genes.

Familial prostate cancer ~5% of those with prostate cancer have a family history: The genetic basis is multifactorial. There is a modestly elevated lifetime risk of prostate cancer for male carriers of BRCA1 and BRCA2 mutations, although the molecular basis of this remains to be elucidated. Mutations in BRCA1/BRCA2 or in the genes on chromosomes 1 and X do not account for all family clusters of prostate cancer, so it is clear that other genes must be involved. In one twin study, 42% of the risk was found to be genetic.

Genetic tests can also tell if chemotherapy is likely to work: Chemotherapy fails in 17% of colon cancer patients (i.e., those with certain mutations).[1]

---

1 Shown by the microsatellite instability status being "high-frequency." Microsatellites are stretches of DNA in which a short section is repeated several times. 5-FU chemotherapy only improves survival in microsatellite-stable or low-frequency microsatellite unstable tumors. Gallinger S. *N Engl J Med.* 2003; 249: 209.

Table 12.4 Examples of cancers with a familial predisposition

Cancer/syndrome	Gene	Chromosome	
Breast and ovarian cancers	BRCA1	17q	(p. 423)
	BRCA2	13q	
HNPCC	MSH2	2p	(p. 423)
	MLH1	3p	
	PMS2	7p	
Familial polyposis (colorectum)	APC	5q	
von Hippel–Lindau (kidney, CNS)	VHL	3p	
Carney complex	PRKAR1A	17q	
Multiple endocrine neoplasia type I (pituitary, pancreas, thyroid)	MEN1	11q	(p. 304)
Multiple endocrine neoplasia type 2	RET	10q	(p. 304)
Basal cell nevus syndrome (CNS, skin)	PTCH	9q	
Retinoblastoma (eye, bone)	Rb	13q	
Li–Fraumeni syndrome (multiple)	TP53	17p	
Neurofibromatosis type I (CNS; rare)	NF1	17q	
Neurofibromatosis type 2 (common) (meningiomas, auditory neuromas)	NF2	22	
Familial melanoma	INK4A	9p	

Screening: Colorectal and breast cancer

It is intuitive that the earlier any cancer is identified, the higher the likelihood of a curative treatment. The development of a screening test for cervical cancer (the Pap smear) has been the paradigm for an effective screening test. This has proven to be true in a number of cancers but has also proven to be surprisingly elusive or controversial in others. It is again beyond the scope of this general review to comprehensively identify screening guidelines for all cancers. Rather, a few of the most common or deadliest cancers will be highlighted. The results are summarized in Table 12.5.

Table 12.5 Screening tests and recommendations for screening

Cancer	Screening test	Recommendations
CRC	Colonoscopy	Starting at age 50 if no risk factors, repeat every 10 yrs
Breast cancer	Mammography	Starting at age 40, repeat yearly
Lung cancer	CT scan	No recommendations
Pancreas cancer	EUS	No recommendations, EUS investigational for high risk families
Prostate cancer	PSA	No recommendations

Screening for colorectal cancer

Data from a number of randomized and non-randomized studies would currently support options including fecal occult blood testing (FOBT) in combination with sigmoidoscopy or colonoscopy alone. The test of choice remains controversial.

A recently published study from the Veteran's Administration medical system performed colonoscopy on 2,885 patients at 13 different Veterans Affairs Medical Centers to determine whether or not the patients had invasive cancer, large colon polyps, or colon polyps that had visible or microscopic signs suggesting they were precancerous. These findings were called "advanced neoplasia" if they were found on the colonoscopic examination. The participants also underwent FOBT before the colonoscopy. The researchers then performed colonoscopy and made careful observations of their findings in the sigmoid colon and rectum (the regions of the colon that would usually be seen through the sigmoidoscope; examination of the rectum and sigmoid colon during the colonoscopy was defined as a surrogate for a sigmoidoscopy), and their findings throughout the remainder of the colon (which would usually be seen only with the colonoscope). The researchers then determined what percentage of cases detected by colonoscopy were also detected by the FOBT tests and were seen in the area usually examined with the sigmoidoscope, the two less extensive screening techniques.

Among patients who had advanced neoplasias detected by their colonoscopy, an FOBT detected only 24% of the patients with advanced neoplasias; sigmoidoscopy would have detected 70%; and combined testing would have detected 76%, meaning that about 25% of all the patients with advanced neoplasias detected by colonoscopy would have been missed if a colonoscopy was not performed.

Why, then, do most clinical-practice guidelines provide a number of options and not recommend colonoscopy exclusively? The first reason is that the standard of care evidence required to support screening with colonoscopy without reservation is not all derived from randomized trial data. Evidence-based guidelines frequently restrict their highest recommendations to technology that has been proved in large-scale, randomized trials to reduce the burden of illness. Fecal occult-blood testing has been studied in this way; colonoscopy has not. The second reason relates to adherence to recommendations and patients' preferences. Colonoscopy may be uncomfortable and requires a preparative bowel cleansing schedule. However, if the colonoscopy is negative, it need be performed only once every 10 yrs, whereas other tests, such as sigmoidoscopy, must be performed more frequently. The third reason is risk. An earlier study in this same patient population reported the risk of serious complications, including bleeding and perforation, was ~0.3%.

The fourth reason is economic. A mathematical model of the costs and consequences (measured in terms of life expectancy) of 22 screening strategies for colorectal cancer has been published incorporating not only the cost of the screening test (e.g., colonoscopy was assumed to cost $1,012) but that of all subsequent events (e.g., the treatment of metastatic cancer). They suggest that if the cost of colonoscopy could be reduced by 23%, the expenditure required to achieve one more year of life with screening colonoscopy would be substantially reduced, and such screening would be made more economically attractive.

The fifth reason why colonoscopy is not recommended or covered is availability. The current supply of clinicians trained in colonoscopy may not be adequate to screen everyone who turns 50, let alone the large population between 50 and 75 yrs of age who have not been screened.

The American Cancer Society (ACS) recommends that people without risk factors, such as a family history of the disease or inflammatory bowel disease, begin screening at age 50. The ACS has three preferred options for screening of people at average risk:

- A colonoscopy every 10 yrs
- A yearly FOBT combined with flexible sigmoidoscopy every 5 yrs
- A double contrast barium enema every 5 yrs

Screening for breast cancer

The current screening guidelines for breast cancer recommend screening mammography for women aged 50–69. Within the United States, the recommendations include women ≥40. However, there is some recent debate regarding these guidelines with respect to the recommendation of screening at age 40. A number of randomized clinical trials have demonstrated that screening mammography reduces the risk of developing breast cancer by about 20–35% in women aged 50–69 yrs, with slightly less benefit in women aged 40–49. Women in their 40s have a lower incidence of developing breast cancer, as well as having denser breast tissue that could lower the sensitivity of the screening mammography. As such, it has been suggested, based on statistical modeling, that to prevent one breast cancer death after 14–20 yrs, between 500 and 1,800 women who are 40 yrs of age would need to undergo regular screening mammography.

Screening: Lung, pancreatic, and prostate cancer

Screening for lung cancer

The earliest screening methods for lung cancer included sputum for cytology and/or chest radiography and were, on the whole, disappointing since these interventions failed to detect a significant reduction in lung cancer mortality. However, improved imaging modalities, such as high resolution CT have provided new opportunities. Like all screening tests for cancer, the possible benefits must be weighed against the potential risk of the test; the harm of false-positive tests, given the subsequent additional tests that may be required to follow-up suspicious screening evaluations; and the additional costs. For example, lung cancers classically appear on CT scans as noncalcified nodules. However, over 80–90% of noncalcified nodules identified by CT are benign. A strategy proposed by the Early Lung Cancer Action Project was to determine the rate of growth of nodules.

For noncalcified nodules that were <1 cm in diameter, high-resolution CT scanning was repeated at 3 months. Among individuals who were referred for needle biopsy on the basis of lung growth, the positive predictive value was 90%. In addition, the use of PET scanning integrated with traditional CT imaging has been proposed as a useful complement. A number of comprehensive studies have since been completed. The National Lung Screening Trial (NLST) randomized 53,454 persons at high risk for developing lung cancer (age 55–74, had a cigarette smoking history of at least 30 pack-years, and, if previous smokers, had quit within the past 15 yrs) to either three low-dose CT scans at 1-yr intervals or CXR at same intervals. The rate of positive screening was 24% in the CT group versus 6.9% in the CXR group. 96% of the positive CT findings and 94% of the positive findings on CXR were false positive. There were 247 deaths from lung cancer per 100,000 person-years in the CT group versus 309 deaths from lung cancer per 100,000 person-years in the CXR group, representing a 20% relative risk reduction in death.[2] In contrast, the Prostate, Lung, Colorectal Cancer and Ovarian (PLCO) screening trial randomized 154,00 patients considered high risk to either annual CXR × 4 yrs or observation. No improvement in lung cancer mortality was identified.[3]

Currently, neither the ACS nor the U.S. Preventive Services Task Force recommend that CT scanning be performed in asymptomatic but at-risk individuals.

Screening for pancreas cancer

As has been the story for other cancers, CT scanning has not proven to be sensitive enough in diagnosing early pancreas cancer. Endoscopic ultrasonography is currently used in investigational studies for screening and early detection of familial pancreatic cancer and its precursors. Endoscopic ultrasonography (EUS) is a standard, diagnostic, predominantly outpatient technique that involves endoscopy plus high-frequency ultrasound imaging of the pancreas (parenchyma and ducts; unlike ERCP, which images the ducts) and adjacent areas from the upper gastrointestinal tract. Tissue sampling can also be readily performed from multiple sites under EUS guidance without accompanying pain or need for local anesthesia (unlike percutaneous fine-needle aspiration) with a high diagnostic yield for pancreatic lesions and lymph node metastases. When used for screening high-risk individuals, EUS imaging can be followed by biopsy of pancreatic masses, cystic lesions, or evidence of intraductal papillary mucinous neoplasm (IPMN) and collection of pancreatic secretions from the duodenum for molecular marker analysis following secretin stimulation. A recent study for individuals considered at high risk for developing pancreas cancer (defined as a study patient having ≥3 first-degree family members with pancreas cancer) using EUS as a screening modality identified one early invasive pancreas cancer and one preinvasive cancer.

Screening for prostate cancer

Screening for prostate cancer remains controversial. Although there has been a decline in prostate cancer mortality, this is thought to be a function of improved treatment as opposed to improved early screening. The PLCO screening trial randomized 76,693 men to either annual screening with PSA for 6 yrs and digital rectal exam for 4 yrs versus no testing. At the most recent follow-up at 7–10 yrs there was no reported difference in

2 Aberle DR, et al. Reduced lung cancer mortality with low-dose computed tomography screening. N Engl J Med. 2011;365(5):395–409.

3 Oken M, et al. Screening by chest radiography and lung cancer mortality: The Prostate, Lung, Colorectal, and Ovarian (PLCO) randomized trial. JAMA. 2011;306(17):1865–1873.

mortality.[4] In addition, the European Randomized Study of Screening for Prostate Cancer (ERSPC) randomized 182,000 patients to either PSA at an average of once every 4 yrs versus a control group. Although there was a reduction in prostate cancer mortality, the study determined that for every one death from prostate cancer prevented, 1,410 patients would need to be screened and 48 patients would need to be treated. The U.S. Preventive Services Task Force does not recommend routine screening for prostate cancer with digital rectal examination (DRE), serum PSA, or transrectal ultrasound of the prostate. The ACS, the American College of Physicians, and the American Urological Association recommend that clinicians advise patients of the risks and benefits of screening to assist them in deciding whether or not to have these tests performed. In general, men ≥50 yrs with a reasonable certainty of a 10-yr life expectancy should be screened annually or biennially. Patients with an elevated risk of disease (e.g., African Americans and those with a family history) should be screened beginning at an earlier age (45 yrs).

Oncological emergencies

A patient who becomes acutely ill can often be made more comfortable with simple measures, but some problems require specific treatment.

Spinal cord compression Requires urgent and efficient treatment to preserve neurological function. A high index of suspicion is essential.

Causes: Typically extradural metastases. *Others:* Extension of tumor from a vertebral body, direct extension of the tumor, or fracture. *Signs and symptoms:* Back pain with a root distribution, weakness and sensory loss (a level may be found), bowel and bladder dysfunction. *Tests:* Urgent MRI. *Management:* Dexamethasone 8–16 mg IV then 4 mg/6 h PO. Discuss with neurosurgeon and clinical oncologist immediately.

Superior vena cava (SVC) obstruction with airway compromise SVC obstruction is not an emergency unless there is tracheal compression with airway compromise: Usually there is time to plan optimal treatment, and this is to be preferred, rather than rushing into therapy that may not be beneficial. *Causes:* Typically lung cancer; rarely from causes of mediastinal enlargement (e.g., germ cell tumor), lymphadenopathy (lymphoma), thymus malignancy, thrombotic disorders (e.g., Behçet's or nephrotic syndromes), thrombus around an IV central line, hamartoma, ovarian hyperstimulation, fibrotic bands (lung fibrosis after chemotherapy). *Signs and symptoms:* Dyspnea, orthopnea, swollen face and arm, cough, plethora/cyanosis, headache, engorged veins. *Pemberton's test:* On lifting the arms over the head for >1 min, there is increased facial plethora/cyanosis, JVP↑ (nonpulsatile), and inspiratory stridor. *Tests:* Sputum cytology, CXR, CT, venography. *Management:* Get a tissue diagnosis if possible, but bronchoscopy may be hazardous. Give dexamethasone 4 mg/6 h PO. Consider balloon venoplasty and SVC stenting; e.g., prior to radical or palliative chemo- or radiotherapy (depending on tumor type).

Hypercalcemia

Affects 10–20% of patients with cancer and 40% of those with myeloma. *Causes:* Lytic bone metastases, production of osteoclast activating factor, 1-α-hydroxylase activity of 25 hydroxy vitamin D in lymphomas, or PTH-like hormones by the tumor. *Symptoms:* Lethargy, anorexia, nausea,

4 Andriole G et al. Mortality results from a randomized prostate-cancer screening trial. *N Engl J Med.* 2009;360:310–319.

polydipsia, polyuria, constipation, dehydration, confusion, weakness. Most obvious with serum Ca^{2+} >12 mg/dL. *Management:* Rehydrate with 3–4 L of 0.9% saline IV over 24 h. Avoid diuretics. Give bisphosphonate IV (consider maintenance therapy, IV or PO). Best treatment is control of underlying malignancy. In resistant hypercalcemia, consider calcitonin. See Table 12.6.

Raised intracranial pressure Due to either a primary CNS tumor or metastatic disease. *Signs and symptoms:* Headache (often worse in the morning), nausea, vomiting, papilledema, seizures, focal neurological signs. *Tests:* Urgent CT is important to diagnose an expanding mass, cystic degeneration, hemorrhage within a tumor, cerebral edema, or hydrocephalus due to tumor or blocked shunt, since the management of these scenarios can be very different. *Management:* Dexamethasone 4 mg/6 h PO/IV, radiotherapy, and surgery as appropriate depending on cause.

Tumor lysis syndrome Rapid cell death on starting chemotherapy for rapidly proliferating leukemia, lymphoma, myeloma, and some germ cell tumors can result in a rise in serum urate, K^+, and phosphate, precipitating renal failure. Prevention is with good hydration and *rasburicase* or *allopurinol* 24 h *before* chemotherapy; dose example if renal function is good: 300 mg/12 h PO. If creatinine >1.2 mg/dL: 100 mg on alternate days.

Inappropriate ADH secretion (p. 669); febrile neutropenic regimen (p. 625)

Table 12.6 Treating hypercalcemia with bisphosphonates

Ensure adequate hydration (e.g., with 0.9% saline IVI). Zoledronic acid and pamidronate are two options.
Disodium pamidronate

Calcium (mg/dL; corrected)	Single-dose pamidronate (mg)
<12	30
12–14	60
>14	90

Infuse slowly, e.g., 30 mg in 300 mL 0.9% saline over 3 h via a large vein. Max dose: 90 mg. Response starts at ~3–5 d, peaking at 1 wk.
SE: Flu-like symptoms, bone pain, $PO_4^{3-}\downarrow$, bone pain, myalgia, nausea, vomiting, headache, lymphocytopenia, $Mg^{2+}\downarrow$, seizures (rare).
Zoledronic acid is significantly more effective in reducing serum Ca^{2+} than previously used bisphosphonates. Usually, a single dose of 4 mg IVI over 2 h will normalize plasma Ca^{2+} within a week. A higher dose should be used if corrected Ca^{2+} is 12 mmol/L. *SE:* Flu-like symptoms, bone pain, $PO_4^{3-}\downarrow$, confusion, thirst, taste disturbance, nausea, pulse↓, WBC↓, creatinine↑.

Symptom control in severe cancer

Pain Do not under treat with analgesia: Aim to *prevent* or *eliminate* pain.

Types of pain Don't assume that the cancer is the cause (abdominal pain, e.g., may be from constipation). Seek the mechanism. Pain caused by nerve infiltration and damage via local pressure may respond to amitriptyline (e.g., 10–50 mg at night) rather than opioids. Bone pain (e.g., presenting with back pain) may respond to NSAIDs, radiotherapy, or a nerve block.

Identify each symptom and type of pain.

Management (1) Pain is affected by mood, morale, and meaning. Explain its origin to both the patient and relatives, and plan rehabilitation goals. (2) Use oral analgesics if possible—aim to prevent pain with regular prophylactic doses (e.g., q4h); do not wait for pain to recur. (3) Modify the pathological process where possible (e.g., radiotherapy, hormones, chemotherapy, surgery).

With analgesia, work up the pain ladder until pain is relieved (see Table 12.7). Monitor response carefully. Laxatives and antiemetics are often needed with analgesics. *Adjuvant analgesics:* NSAIDs, steroids, muscle relaxants, anxiolytic, antidepressants.

Giving oral morphine: Start with aqueous morphine 5–10 mg/4 h PO. A double dose at night can be used to promote 8 h of sleep. Most patients need no more than 30 mg/4 h PO. A few need much more. Aim to change to extended-release morphine (e.g., MS-Contin tablets q12h) when daily morphine needs are known. In morphine-resistant pain (persisting when 60 mg/4 h is given), consider adjuvant analgesics, methadone, or ketamine (specialist use only).

Vomiting: Prevent from before the first dose of chemotherapy, to avoid anticipatory vomiting before the next dose. Give orally if possible, but if severe vomiting prevents this, give rectally or subcutaneously. *Agents to try:* Metoclopramide 10 mg/8 h PO; ondansetron 4–8 mg/8–12 h PO/IV; haloperidol 0.5–2 mg/24 h (max 5 mg).

Shortness of breath: Consider supplementary O_2 or morphine. Use of relaxation techniques and benzodiazepines can be effective. Assess for pleural or pericardial effusion. If there is significant pleural effusion, consider thoracocentesis ± pleurodesis. If there is a malignant pericardial effusion, consider pericardiocentesis (p. 147), pericardiectomy, pleuropericardial windows, external beam radiotherapy, percutaneous balloon pericardiotomy, or pericardial instillation of immunomodulators or sclerosing bleomycin.

Venipuncture problems: Repeated venipuncture with the attendant risk of painful extravasation and phlebitis may be avoided by insertion of skin tunneled catheter (e.g., a Hickman line)—a single or multilumen line—into a major central vein (e.g., subclavian or internal jugular). It is inserted using a strict antiseptic technique. Patients can look after their own lines at home and give their own drugs. Problems include infection, blockage (flush with 0.9% saline or dilute heparin, e.g., every week); axillary, subclavian, or superior vena cava thrombosis/obstruction; and line slippage. Even more convenient portable delivery devices are available, allowing drugs to be given at a preset time without the patient's intervention.

Table 12.7 The analgesic ladder

Rung 1	Nonopioid	Aspirin; acetaminophen; NSAID
Rung 2	Weak opioid	Codeine, dihydrocodeine, dextropropoxyphene, tramadol, oxycodone (some place this on rung 3)
Rung 3	Strong opioid	Morphine, diamorphine, hydromorphone, fentanyl ± adjuvant analgesics.

If 1 drug fails to relieve pain, move up ladder; do not try other drugs at the same level. In new, severe pain, rung 2 may be omitted.

IV delivery of opioids, haloperidol, cyclizine and metoclopramide, and hyoscine, giving 24 h cover. Or suppositories (below) or *fentanyl transdermal patches:* If not previously exposed to morphine, start with one low-strength patch (25 mcg/h). Remove after 72 h, and place a new patch at a different site. 25, 50, 75, and 100 mcg/h patches are made. $t_{\frac{1}{2}} \approx 17$ h.
Suppositories can also be used if unable to tolerate oral route. For pain: Try oxycodone 30 mg suppositories (e.g., 30 mg/8 h ≈ 30 mg morphine).
Agitation: Try diazepam 10 mg/8 h suppositories.

Other agents and procedures to know about (alphabetically listed)

- *Bisacodyl tablets* (5 mg), 1–2 at night, help opioid-induced constipation.
- *Cholestyramine* 4 g/6 h PO (1 h after other drugs) helps itch in jaundice.
- *Enemas*, e.g., arachis oil, may help resistant constipation.
- H_2*-antagonists* (e.g., cimetidine 400 mg/12 h PO) help gastric irritation; e.g., associated with gastric carcinoma.
- *Haloperidol* 0.5–5 mg/24 h PO helps agitation, nightmares, hallucinations, and vomiting.
- *Hydrogen peroxide* 6% cleans an unpleasant-feeling coated tongue.
- *Hyoscine hydrobromide* 0.4–0.6 mg/8 h SC or 0.3 mg sublingual helps with vomiting from upper GI obstruction or bronchial congestion.
- *Low-residue diets* may be needed for postradiotherapy diarrhea.
- *Metronidazole* 400 mg/8 h PO mitigates anaerobic odors from tumors; so do charcoal dressings (Actisorb®).
- *Nerve blocks* may lastingly relieve pleural or other resistant pains.
- *Polyethylene glycol* sachets 2–4/12 h for 48 h to shift resistant constipation with overflow.
- *Naproxen* 250 mg/8 h with food: Fevers caused by malignancy or bone pain from metastases (consider splinting joints if this fails).
- *Spironolactone* 100 mg bd PO + bumetanide 1 mg/24 h PO for ascites.
- *Steroids: Dexamethasone:* Give 8 mg IV stat to relieve symptoms of superior vena cava or bronchial obstruction, or lymphangitis carcinomatosa. Tablets are 2 mg (≈15 mg prednisolone). 4 mg/12–24 h PO may stimulate appetite, reduce ICP headache, or induce (in some patients) a satisfactory sense of euphoria.
- *Supplemental humidified O_2* helps hypoxic dyspnea.
- *Thoracocentesis* (± bleomycin pleurodesis) helps in pleural effusion.

Cancer therapy

It is beyond the scope of this chapter to provide a comprehensive review of treatment options for each malignancy. However, as noted earlier, there have been some remarkable achievements in the management of some solid tumors, such as germ cell tumors. The sensitivity of germ cell tumors to platinum-based chemotherapy, together with radiation and surgical measures, has led to a cure rate of >99% in early stage disease.

Cancer management Management requires a multidisciplinary team, and communication is vital. Most patients wish to have some part in decision making at the various stages of their treatment and to be informed of their options. Patients are becoming better informed through self-help groups and access to the Internet. Most patients undergo a variety of treatments during the treatment of their cancer, and your job may be to orchestrate these.

Surgery In many cases, a tissue diagnosis of cancer is made with either a biopsy or formal operation to remove the primary tumor. Although it is sometimes the only treatment required in early tumors of the GI tract, soft tissue sarcomas, and gynecological tumors, it is often the case that best results follow the combination of surgery and chemotherapy. Surgery also has a role in palliating advanced disease.

Chemotherapy Cytotoxics should be given under expert guidance by people trained in their administration. Drugs are often given in combination with a variety of intents. *Neoadjuvants* to shrink tumors to reduce the need for major surgery (e.g., mastectomy). There is also a rationale that considers early control of micrometastasis. *Primary therapy* as the sole treatment for hematological malignancies. *Adjuvants* to reduce the chance of relapse (e.g., breast and bowel cancers). *Palliative* to provide relief from symptomatic metastatic disease and possibly to prolong survival.

Important classes of drugs include:

• *Alkylating agents* (e.g., cyclophosphamide, chlorambucil, busulfan)
• *Antimetabolites* (e.g., methotrexate, 5-fluorouracil)
• *Vinca alkaloids* (e.g., vincristine, vinblastine)
• *Antitumor antibiotics* (e.g., actinomycin d, doxorubicin)
• *Others* (e.g., etoposide, taxanes, platinum compounds)

Side effects depend on the types of drugs used. Nausea/vomiting are most feared by patients and are preventable or controllable in most. Alopecia can also have a profound impact on quality of life. Neutropenia is most commonly seen 10–14 d after chemotherapy (but can occur within 7 d for taxanes), and sepsis requires immediate attention (p. 625).

Extravasation of a chemotherapeutic agent: Suspect if there is pain, burning, or swelling at infusion site. *Management:* Stop the infusion, attempt to aspirate blood from the cannula, and then remove. Administer steroids and consider antidotes. Elevate the arm and mark site affected. Review regularly and apply steroid cream. Apply cold pack (unless a vinca alkaloid, in which case a heat compress should be applied).

As was also noted earlier, what has impeded systematic progress in achieving similar successes in other cancers has been the realization that the molecular signaling pathways that ultimately lead to cell proliferation and growth were largely unrecognized. The identification of molecular target-specific therapy would provide the potential of maximal therapeutic benefit while minimizing toxicity to normal cells.

Ligand-dependent or -independent growth factor receptors Activate downstream signaling pathways via their ability to phosphorylate and thereby activate downstream proteins to effect unregulated cellular proliferation. As such, inhibitors of receptor kinases with high specificity are currently being tested as anticancer drugs. The discovery of the molecular defect associated with the constitutively active tyrosine kinase fusion protein BCR-ABL, which results from the reciprocal DNA exchange between the long arms of chromosomes 9 and 22 [t(9;22) Philadelphia chromosome], has been identified in >90% of patients with CML. The clinical features of CML and the biology of BCR-ABL have recently been elegantly summarized. The variability in the breakpoint on chromosome 22 is well described and has implications for the disease phenotype. As a result, BCR-ABL inhibition represented an ideal target for drug therapy. This strategy has been validated in clinical trials of CML with imatinib that culminated in its approval in May 2001 by the FDA. In the chronic phase, the hematologic response rate is 95% and cytogenetic response rates range from 50–80%, depending on the stage of disease. Moreover, response rates were also high in blast crisis patients, despite the presence of multiple oncogenic abnormalities in addition to BCR-ABL.

Epidermal growth factor receptor (EGFR) Includes a family of receptor tyrosine kinases comprised of four related receptors: EGFR (ErbB1/EGFR/Her1), ErbB2 (Her2/neu), ErbB3 (Her3), and ErbB4 (Her4). The formation of receptor homo- or hetero-dimerization through either ligand-dependent or -independent activation leads to constitutively activated receptor signaling and has been associated with amplification of downstream signals involving a number of nonlinear cellular pathways. The end product of this signaling cascade leads to increased cellular proliferation, migration, tissue stromal invasion, resistance to apoptotic signals, and angiogenesis. In addition, EGFR is overexpressed in a significant percentage of solid tumors and is believed to be a marker for poor prognosis and decreased survival. These properties provide the rationale for the development and testing of EGFR inhibitors. Inhibitors to EGFR have already been tested in clinical trials with FDA approval in 2003 of the oral EGFR tyrosine kinase inhibitor gefitinib (Iressa®, AstraZeneca) for third-line therapy of advanced non-small cell lung cancer. Many important challenges for the use of EGFR small-molecule inhibitors remain, including identifying appropriate surrogate markers of activity and in best integrating these therapies with other treatment modalities. Cetuximab (Erbitux®, Imclone Systems) is an IgG1 monoclonal antibody against EGFR that has demonstrated activity in patients with Irinotecan-refractory colorectal cancer. Cetuximab has also shown response to treatment and improvement in progression-free progression in patients with locally advanced head and neck cancer refractory to platinum-based chemotherapy. The association of an acne-like rash with activity of drug has been suggested.

The formation of new blood vessels to keep pace with growing tumors is an enormously complicated process that occurs in response to a vast array of molecular signals, including oxygen tension (hypoxia inducing factor) and growth factors such as fibroblast growth factor (FGF), transforming growth factor α and β (TGF-α and TGF-β), tumor necrosis factor-α (TNF-α), insulin growth factor, and platelet-derived growth factor (PDGF). Vascular endothelial growth factor (VEGF) signaling is a critical rate-limiting step in angiogenesis.

Inhibitors to VEGF have already been approved in CRC (bevacizumab) and in breast cancer (trastuzumab) and have been examined in lung, renal, pancreas, head and neck, hepatocellular cancer, and non-Hodgkin's lymphoma in ongoing trials.

Mutations to other driver pathways such as BRAF and translocations between alk and EML-4 are thought to occur at lower frequencies in non-small cell lung cancer. Mutations to other driver pathways such as BRAF and translocations between alk and EML-4 are thought to occur at lower frequencies in non-small cell lung cancer. There are now approved drugs that target inhibitors of alk tyrosine kinase (crizotinib) in non-small cell lung cancer. Mutations in BRAF are thought to occur at higher frequencies in other cancers such as melanoma. As such, inhibitors of BRAF specifically targeting mutations at V600E in melanoma (vemurafenib) have been tested and approved in the United States in 2011.

In addition, there has been a better understanding of the complex relationship that affects the balance between antigen recognition and development of immune tolerance between the immune system and cancer. In the past few years, there has been FDA approval of the CTLA-4 inhibitor Ipilimumab (Yervoy; in 2011) for melanoma and for the autologous immunotherapy treatment consisting of prostatic acid phosphatase (PAP)linked to the immune cell activator GM-CSF known as sipuleucel-T (Provenge; approved in 2010).

Radiotherapy

Radiotherapy uses ionizing radiation to produce free radicals that damage DNA. Normal cells are better at repairing this damage than are cancer cells, so are able to recover before the next dose (or fraction) of treatment.

Radical treatment is given with curative intent. The total doses given range from 40 to 70 Gy (1 Gy = 100 cGy = 100 rads) in 15–35 daily fractions. Some regimens involving giving several smaller fractions a day with a gap of 6–8 h. Combined chemoradiation is used in some sites (e.g., anus and esophagus) to increase response rates.

Palliation aims to relieve symptoms. Doses: 8–30 Gy, given in 1, 2, 5, or 10 fractions. Bone pain, hemoptysis, cough, dyspnea, and bleeding are helped in >50% of patients.

Early reactions occur during or soon after treatment.
- *Tiredness:* Common after radical treatments; can last weeks to months.
- *Skin reactions:* These vary from erythema to dry desquamation to moist desquamation to ulceration; on completing treatment, use moisturizers.
- *Mucositis:* All patients receiving head and neck treatment should have a dental check-up before commencing therapy. Avoid smoking, alcohol, and spicy foods. Antiseptic mouthwashes may help. Soluble analgesics are helpful. Treat oral thrush.
- *Nausea and vomiting:* Occur when stomach, liver, or brain is treated. Try a dopamine antagonist first. If unsuccessful, try 5HT3 antagonist.
- *Diarrhea:* Usually after abdominal or pelvic treatments. Maintain good hydration. Avoid high-fiber bulking agents; try loperamide.
- *Dysphagia:* Thoracic treatments.
- *Cystitis:* Pelvic treatments. Drink plenty of fluids. NSAIDs.
- *Bone marrow suppression:* More likely after chemotherapy or when large areas are being treated. Usually reversible.

Late reactions occur months or years after the treatment.
- *CNS: Somnolence:* 6–12 wks after brain radiotherapy. Treat with steroids. *Spinal cord myelopathy:* Progressive weakness. MRI is needed to exclude cord compression. *Brachial plexopathy:* Numb, weak, and painful arm after axillary radiotherapy. Reduced IQ can occur in children receiving brain irradiation if <6 yrs.
- *Lung:* Pneumonitis may occur 6–12 wks after thoracic treatment (e.g., with dry cough ± dyspnea). *Treatment:* Prednisolone 40 mg reducing over 6 wks.
- *GI: Xerostomia* (reduced saliva). Treat with pilocarpine 5 mg/8 h or artificial saliva. Care must be taken with all future dental care as healing

is reduced. *Benign strictures of esophagus or bowel*: Treat with dilatation. Fistulae need surgical intervention.

- GU: *Urinary frequency* from small fibrosed bladder after pelvic treatments. *Fertility*: Pelvic radiotherapy (and cytotoxics) may affect fertility, so ova or sperm storage should be considered. This is a complex area: Get expert help. In premature female menopause or reduced testosterone, replace hormones. Vaginal stenosis and dyspareunia. Impotence can occur several years after pelvic radiotherapy.
- *Others:* Panhypopituitarism following radical treatment involving pituitary fossa. Children need hormones checked regularly, as growth hormone may be required. Hypothyroidism may follow neck treatments (e.g., for Hodgkin's lymphoma). Cataracts. Secondary cancers (e.g., sarcomas usually ≥10 yrs later).

Surgery

Susan L. Gearhart, M.D.

Contents

Introduction

The goal of the following chapter is to give the reader some insight into commonly managed surgical disorders. This chapter is not intended to be comprehensive. A great emphasis has been placed on the perioperative management of the surgical patient. This is particularly timely given the development of American College of Surgeons National Surgical Quality Improvement Program (ACS NSQIP). This program contains several recommendations, based on peer-reviewed studies, to improve surgical outcomes for patients. Further information regarding this program can be obtained through the ACS NSQIP website: http://site.acsnsqip.org

Surgical terms

Commonly used surgical terms are listed in Figure 13.1.

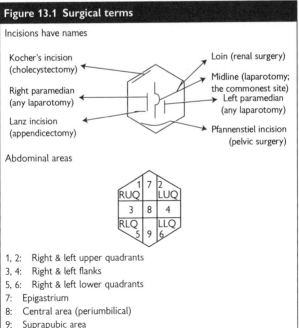

Figure 13.1 Surgical terms

Incisions have names

Kocher's incision (cholecystectomy)

Right paramedian (any laparotomy)

Lanz incision (appendicectomy)

Loin (renal surgery)

Midline (laparotomy; the commonest site)

Left paramedian (any laparotomy)

Pfannenstiel incision (pelvic surgery)

Abdominal areas

1	7	2
RUQ		LUQ
3	8	4
RLQ		LLQ
5	9	6

1, 2: Right & left upper quadrants
3, 4: Right & left flanks
5, 6: Right & left lower quadrants
7: Epigastrium
8: Central area (periumbilical)
9: Suprapubic area

439

(Continued)

Figure 13.1 (Continued)

Abscess	A cavity containing pus
Angio-	To do with tubes or blood vessels
-ectomy	The surgical removal of something, e.g., appendectomy
Chole-	To do with bile
Cyst	A fluid-filled sac
Docho-	To do with ducts

Fistula An abnormal communication between two epithelial surfaces; e.g., enterocutaneous between the bowel and the skin; endothelial in arteriovenous fistulae); gastrocolic fistula (stomach/colon). Fistulae may close spontaneously but will not do so in the presence of chronic inflammation, distal obstruction, epithelialization of the tract, foreign bodies, or malignant tissue.

Ileus Used in this book to mean adynamic bowel (e.g., no bowel sounds).

Lith Stone; e.g., nephrolithotomy (cutting kidney open to get to a stone).

Ostomy An opening usually made to create a new connection between two conduits or between a conduit and the outside world (e.g., colostomy: The colon is made to open onto the skin (p. 462). Stoma or mouth.

Otomy Surgical opening; e.g., laparotomy (opening of abdomen).

Plasty A remolding or reforming of something to make it work; e.g., pyloroplasty relieves pyloric (gastric outlet) obstruction.

Percutaneous Entering through the skin (invasive).

Sinus A blind ending tract typically lined by epithelium from which it opens.

Stent Artificial tube inserted into a biological tube to keep it open.

Trans Going across a structure.

Ulcer An abnormal break in an epithelial surface.

The preoperative evaluation

The purpose of the preoperative evaluation is:

1 To determine the need for surgical intervention
2 To assess the anesthetic risk to the patient
3 To coordinate surgical, anesthetic, and nursing care for the safety of the patient.

The care team may require additional testing to determine if surgery is indicated and safe to perform. For example, a 64-yr-old man with a newly diagnosed rectal cancer and a history of smoking will need local staging with an ultrasound (US) exam of the tumor, a computed tomography (CT) scan of the abdomen and pelvis to evaluate for metastatic disease, a chest X-ray, electrocardiogram (ECG), and the following laboratory work: CBC, comprehensive panel, prothrombin time (PT), partial thromboplastin time (PTT). If the patient has cardiac risk factors, an echocardiogram and/or cardiac stress test may need to be performed. For further assessment of any pulmonary conditions, pulmonary function tests may be necessary as well. More discussion is included with the individual descriptions of the disorders or diseases.

Preoperative tests

Commonly oredered preoperative tests are listed in Table 13.1.

Table 13.1 Preoperative tests

Use the history and examination as well as local protocols as your guide.

Blood tests

Routine blood tests include CBC, comprehensive panel, and coagulation profile (PT, PTT) in most patients. If hemoglobin (Hgb) <10 g/dL, tell anesthesiologist. Investigate/treat as appropriate. A comprehensive panel is particularly important if the patient is starved, diabetic, on diuretics, has significant burns, has hepatic or renal diseases, has an ileus, or is parenterally fed.

In healthy adults <45 yrs of age, no preoperative testing may be necessary. Recommendations are based on the guidelines put forth by most institutions. The only exception is β-human chorionic gonadotropin (HCG) which is mandatory in *all* premenopausal women.

Cross-matching: Type and cross is recommended for most major surgical cases. For major cardiac, vascular and spine cases, up to 6 units should be available for surgery.

Specific blood tests: Liver function tests (LFTs) in jaundice, malignancy, or alcohol abuse.

Urinalysis: Routine prior to prosthetic device insertion as well as routine abdominal surgery.

β-HCG: Mandatory in *all* premenopausal women.

Drug levels: As appropriate (e.g., digoxin, Dilantin, lithium).

Coagulations studies: In liver disease, disseminated intravascular coagulation (DIC), massive blood loss, patients already on valproic acid, warfarin, or heparin.

Sickle test: In those from Africa, West Indies, or Mediterranean—and others whose origins are in malarial areas (including most of India).

Thyroid function tests: In those with thyroid disease who have not had annual testing.

Additional tests

Chest x-ray (CXR): If known smoker, evidence of cardiopulmonary disease, pathology or symptoms, possible lung metastases, or ≥50 yrs old.

ECG: Patients with prior coronary revascularization or admission to a hospital for cardiac reasons. Asymptomatic males >45, females >55 without significant comorbidities (diabetes, obesity, hypertension).

Echocardiogram (ECG)/stress test: Any patient with cardiac symptoms (chest pain, shortness of breath [SOB]), known cardiac disease (particularly heart failure) that has not been evaluated recently or has progressed in symptoms to assess adequacy of medical therapy.

Pulmonary function test (PFT): Chronic smoker, known pulmonary disease, sleep apnea, especially before thoracic surgery

Lower or upper extremity venous duplex: Patients with a history of VTE (venothrombotic events), prolonged hospitalizations, malignancy, inflammatory bowel disease, etc. (see deep vein thrombosis [DVT] prophylaxis). If positive test, may consider vena cava filter prior to operation.

(Continued)

Preoperative medical assessment

Begin with the medical history of the patient and family and a general review of systems. Assess cardiopulmonary system, exercise tolerance, existing illnesses, drugs, and allergies. Assess past history of myocardial infarction, diabetes, asthma, hypertension, rheumatic fever, epilepsy, jaundice. Assess any specific risks: Is the patient pregnant? Has there been previous anesthesia? Were there any complications? Family history may be relevant, as in malignant hyperthermia, myotonic dystrophy, porphyria, cholinesterase problems, sickle-cell disease.

Drugs: Any drug/antiseptic/latex allergies? Inform the anesthesiologist about all drugs, even if over-the-counter.

Antibiotics: Tetracycline, neomycin and others may ↑ neuromuscular blockade.

Anticoagulants: Tell the surgeon. See Cardiac Risk Assessment regarding anticoagulation and cardiac stents. Avoid epidural, spinal, and regional blocks.

Anticonvulsants: Give as usual preop. Postop, give drugs IV (or by NGT) until able to take orally. *Valproate:* Give usual dose IV. *Phenytoin:* Give IV slowly (<50 mg/min; monitor ECG). IM phenytoin absorption is unreliable.

Avastin (BEV): Should be stopped 1 month prior to surgery; may cause coagulopathy.

Antihypertensives: Chronic use should be continued. Consider calcium-channel blockers in patients who have contraindication to β-blockade.

β-blockers: Continue up to and including the day of surgery as this precludes a labile cardiovascular response.

Estrogen replacement or oral contraceptives: Stop 4 wks before major surgery because of the risk of thromboembolic event and ensure alternative contraception is used.

Diabetic medicine: Insulin therapy/oral hypoglycemic. See Glucose Management in the Diabetic Patient.

Digoxin: Continue up to and including morning of surgery. Check for toxicity (ECG; plasma level); do plasma K^+ and Ca^{2+} (succinylcholine ↑K^+ and can lead to ventricular arrhythmias in the fully digitalized).

Diuretics: Beware hypokalemia, dehydration.

Herbal Supplements: Should be stopped 1 month prior to surgery; may cause coagulopathy

Levodopa: Possible arrhythmias when patient under GA.

Lithium: Get expert help; it may potentiate neuromuscular blockade and cause arrhythmias.

MAOI: Get expert help as interaction with opiates and anesthetics may cause hypotensive/hypertensive crises.

Eye-drops: Many be absorbed; anticholinesterases ↑(succinylcholine).

Tricyclics: These enhance epinephrine and arrhythmias.

Difficult Airway Management
Predictors of difficult intubation

I do not know of any area of medicine where proper preparation is more important in preventing complications. The overall incidence of difficult intubation is reportedly 5.8%. The incidence for obese patients is 15.8%. Currently, the best method of determining the potential for a difficult airway includes the patient's history and physical exam. Any patient who has had a difficult intubation in the past is given an alert bracelet indicating this. Furthermore, a history of maxillofacial trauma, reconstructive surgery, or radiation should alert the anesthetist of potential difficulties. Is the neck unstable (e.g., arthritis complicating intubation)? Is the neck/jaw immobile (intubation risk)? Other assessment tools include the following:

Mallampati classication: Estimates the size of the tongue relative to the oral cavity; alone this test is marginally helpful.

Thyromental distance: Distance from thyroid notch to mentum (<4–6 cm) is an indication of mouth opening capability

Sternomental distance: Distance from sternum to mentum (<12.5–13.5 cm) is an indication of mouth opening capability

Mouth opening: Ability to visualize the glottis on mouth opening; inconsistent

Wilson risk score: Simple summation of risk factor; somewhat reliable score is ≤2

Most operating rooms will have an airway management team that includes anesthesiologists, surgeons, nurses, and technicians. A dedicated difficult airway cart should be readily accessible to the team and should contain items that would assist in an airway emergency(ask anesthesia coordinator).

Cardiac risk assessment

The American College of Cardiology and the American Heart Association have published guidelines regarding cardiac risk assessment in noncardiac surgery in 1996; these were updated in 2002. The European Society of Cardiology and the European Society of Anesthesiology have also published similar guidelines in 2010. Some of these guidelines have been summarized here.

Preoperative risk stratication:

1. Low risk (<1% risk of myocardial infarction (MI) or death)

   Type of procedures: Breast, endocrine, eye, genitourinary (GU)—minor, gastrointestinal(GI)—minor, plastic/reconstructive, orthopaedic-minor
2. Intermediate risk (1–5% risk of MI or death

   Types of procedures: GI-major, GU-major, vascular (carotid, endo-vascular, peripheral vascular angioplasty), head and neck, neurologic/orthopedic-major, transplant (lung, renal, liver)
3. High risk (>5% risk or MI or death)

   Types of procedures: Open abdominal aorta, peripheral vascular surgery

Lee Index: Clinical factors predictive of cardiac complication following surgery:

1. Ischemic heart disease
2. Heart failure
3. Stroke/transient ischemic attack
4. Diabetes requiring insulin therapy
5. Renal dysfunction/hemodialysis
6. High-risk surgery

1 point assigned to each clinical factor. For total points assigned, estimated incidence (% per 100 cases) of major cardiac complication is as follows:

0 point 0.4%
1 point 0.9%
2 points 7%
≥3 points 11%

Noninvasive preoperative testing: Active, uncontrolled bleeding or high Aims at providing information on three cardiac risk markers: lv function, myocardial ischemia, and valve abnormalities. Should occur if two of the three following factors are true in any patient:

1 Intermediate clinical predictors are present (Canadian class 1 or 2 angina, prior MI, compensated or prior heart failure, diabetes, renal insufficiency)
2 Poor functional capacity (<4 metabolic equivalent levels on Duke Activity Status Index AJC 1989)
3 High surgical risk procedure (emergency major operation, aortic or peripheral vascular disease (PVD) surgery, prolonged surgery with large fluid shifts)

Several studies have demonstrated that a left ventricular ejection fraction (LVEF) <35% is associated with an increased risk of a coronary event in patients undergoing noncardiac surgery.

Invasive perioperative evaluation: Recommended for the following patients prior to undergoing surgery:

1 Patients with suspected or known coronary artery disease (CAD) who have demonstrated a high risk of adverse outcome based on noninvasive testing
2 Unstable angina or angina not responsive to medical therapy
3 Equivocal noninvasive test results in patients undergoing high-risk surgery
4 Urgent noncardiac surgery while convalescing from an acute mi
5 Perioperative MI
6 Candidate for liver, lung, or renal transplant ≥40 yrs, as part of evaluation for transplantation, unless noninvasive testing reveals high risk for adverse outcome
7 Patients should undergo preoperative coronary bypass grafting before high-risk surgery if their long-term outcome would be improved

Other factors:

1 Prior to surgical intervention, severe hypertension (diastolic >110 mm Hg) should be controlled.
2 Symptomatic stenotic lesions (mitral or aortic) are associated with risk of perioperative severe heart failure and should be treated with intense medical therapy or surgical correction when possible.
3 Arrhythmias and conduction abnormalities: Management is identical to nonoperative setting; however, pacemakers and implantable cardioverter defibrillator (ICDs) will need to be programmed off prior to surgery because of the concern of electrocautery use.

4 Medical therapy, particularly β-blockade, should be started days prior to planned surgery and continued postoperatively with a dose titrated to achieve a resting heart rate around 50–60 bpm. Patients who have a contraindication to β-blockade (chronic obstructive pulmonary disease [COPD]) may be started on α-adrenergic agonists.

5 Some studies indicate that maintenance of normothermia and adequate analgesia prevents cardiac events.

6 Because 95% of coronary events may be silent, postoperative ECG monitoring should be performed in high-risk patients.

All patients who smoke should be encouraged to discontinue smoking prior to surgery.

Prophylactic antibiotics and bowel preparation

The rate of wound infection following surgery ranges from <5% for clean cases without entry into the GI tract to >50% for intra-abdominal perforation. Successful prevention has been demonstrated with the use of IV antibiotics only.

Preoperative mechanical bowel preparation In the era of routine IV antibiotics, mechanical bowel preparation prior to surgery has not shown to be beneficial in the prevention of anastomotic complications or wound infections. However, most surgeons find it more aesthetically pleasing, and it facilitates bowel anastomosis and the identification of intraluminal lesions. The mechanical bowel preparations utilized, either polyethylene glycol 4 L or MiraLax, do not cause significant electrolyte abnormalities and therefore are beneficial in patients with cardiac disease or renal insufficiency, and in the elderly.

Previously, sodium phosphate hypertonic solutions were utilized; however, dehydration and significant electrolyte abnormalities($\uparrow$ Na, $\uparrow$ Phos, K, Ca) have led to the removal of these preparations from the market.

Preoperative oral antibiotics There has been much debate over the use of preoperative oral antibiotics, especially with the use of IV antibiotics. Currently, there are sufficient data to suggest that the use of preoperative oral antibiotics is beneficial in the prevention of surgical site infections, and their use is endorsed by many surgical societies.

Preoperative iv antibiotics The surgical literature supports the routine use of IV antibiotics in the prevention of wound infections. To be effective, the dose should be given 1 h prior to incision. Meta-analysis has demonstrated that a single dose is all that is necessary, although frequently three doses are given.

1 First-generation cephalosporin is given in noncontaminated surgery without entry into the GI tract(e.g., Ancef 1 g q6h while in the operating room).

2 Second-generation cephalosporin is given in cases in which limited contamination is expected, including entry into the GI tract. This antibiotic covers aerobic and anaerobic bacteria (e.g., cefotetan 2 g q6h while in the operating room).

3 For penicillin-allergic patients, cephalosporins should be avoided as well (5% cross-reactivity). Alternatives include clindamycin or vancomycin.

4 For intra-abdominal perforation, coverage with a third-generation cephalosporin and metronidazole, a broad-spectrum penicillin, or fluoroquinolone is acceptable (e.g., cefuroxime 1.5 g and metronidazole 500 mg).

Venothromboembolic risk assessment and prevention

Table 13.2 lists the current method of risk assessment for venous thromboembolic disease.

Table 13.2 Risk factors for venous thromboembolic disease

Serious risk factors

- Age >60
- Cancer undergoing treatment
- Previous DVT and pulmonary embolism (PE)
- Stroke with paresis (>3 months)
- Trauma
- Heart and respiratory failure
- Prolonged procedure (>2 h)
- Inherited or acquired hypercoagulability

Other risk factors

- Immobility
- Central venous catheterization
- Acute medical illness or sepsis
- Myeloproliferative disorder
- Inflammatory bowel disease
- Nephrotic syndrome
- Obesity (body mass index [BMI] >30 kg/m^2)
- Smoking
- Estrogen use
- Varicose veins

Contraindications to prophylaxis for venous thromboembolic disease include

- Active, uncontrolled bleeding or high risk of bleeding
- Systemic anticoagulation
- Bacterial endocarditis or pericarditis
- Severe head trauma
- Malignant hypertension
- Threatened abortion
- Severe thrombocytopenia
- Heparin or enoxaparin: Heparin-induced-thrombocytopenia
- Enoxaparin: Spinal tap, epidural instrumentation
- Sequential compression device (SCD): Open wound or extremity with DVT

Risk categories and management See Table 13.3.

Table 13.3 Risk categories → Prophylaxis

Low risk → **Early mobilization**
- Minor/vascular/laparoscopic/urologic procedures <2 h
- Age <40 yrs
- NO additional risk factors

Moderate risk → **Heparin 5,000 U SC tid (first dose to be given 2 h prior to surgery) ± TEDS and SCDs**
- Minor/laparoscopic/gynecological surgery
- Age <40 yrs
- With additional risk factors

     or

- Minor surgery
- Age 40–60 yrs
- No additional risk factors

     or

- Major surgery
- Age <40 yrs
- NO additional risk factors

High risk → **Heparin 5,000 U SC tid (first dose to be given 2 h prior to surgery) or enoxaparin 40 mg SC qd**
± TEDS and SCDs
- Any surgery
- Any age >60 yrs
- NO additional risk factors

     or

- Minor surgery
- Age 40–60 yrs
- With additional risk factors

Very high risk → **Heparin 5,000 U SQ tid (first dose to be given 2 h prior to surgery) or enoxaparin 40 mg SC** qd *and* **TEDs and SCDs**
- Major surgery
- Serious risk factors (≥2)

     or

- Major surgery
- Age >60 yrs
- With any additional risk factor

447

Informed consent

The purpose of the informed consent is to document that a discussion was undertaken between the surgeon and the patient with regards to the planned procedure. This discussion is paramount with regards to the patient–physician relationship. During this discussion, the physician should feel confident that the patient has a reasonable expectation of what is going to be done at the time of surgery. The patient should be informed of the known foreseeable complications. The patient should also be informed of the alternatives to surgery. All questions should be answered. It is mandatory in many institutions that one-sided surgeries be marked with the surgeon's initials and the agreement of the patient prior to incision (i.e., nephrectomy).

Perioperative IV fluid and electrolyte management

The goal of fluid therapy is the normalization of hemodynamic parameters and the body fluid electrolyte composition.

Intraoperative fluids

With the exception of major hemorrhage, avoid taking a patient to surgery without adequate resuscitation. Anesthesia compounds shock by inhibiting normal baroreceptor function, causing vasodilatation and depressing cardiac contractility.

Most patients can tolerate a 500 mL blood loss; however, loss in excess of this may require transfusion.

For third-space losses as a result of tissue trauma, isotonic solution such as lactated Ringer's should be used for replacement. Colloids are expensive and provide no added benefit.

Postoperative fluids

A normal requirement is 2–3 L/24 h, which allows for urinary, fecal, and insensible loss. This maintenance therapy should be supplemented by replacement of the additional fluids needed to replace ongoing third-space losses.

Monitoring fluid status is best accomplished through close following of vital signs, urinary output, and central venous pressure (CVP) monitoring.

Urine output: Should be maintained at a level >0.5 mL/kg/h.

The first 24 h: Isotonic solutions (0.9% saline) should be given initially because of ongoing third-space losses.

A standard postoperative regimen: (One of many; 2 L 5% dextrose with 0.45% saline/24 h. Add K$^+$ postop (20 mEq/L). More K$^+$ is needed if losses are from the gut (e.g., diarrhea, vomiting or high NG tube output, intestinal fistula, high-output stoma). More saline is appropriate for those at risk of hyponatremia: See Table 13.4.

When to increase the above regimen
- *Dehydration:* This may be by 5 L if severe. Replace this slowly.
- *Shock:* All causes, except for cardiogenic shock
- *Operative losses:* Check operation notes for extent of bleeding.
- *Losses from gut:* Replace nasogastric tube (NGT) aspirate volume with 0.45% saline with 20 mEq/L potassium.
- *Insensible losses:* Feverish patients and burns
- *Pancreatitis;* There are large pools of sequestered fluid that should be allowed for.
- *Losses from surgical drains:* Check fluid charts and replace significant losses.
- *Low urine output* (the night after surgery) is commonly due to inadequate infusion of fluids; however, the possibility of bleeding must always be considered. Check jugular venous pressure (JVP), operative drains, proper Foley function and insert if not present, and review for signs of cardiac failure. The fractional excretion of urine sodium (Fe$_{Na}$) can be used to determine how well the kidneys are processing sodium. If(Fe$_{Na}$) <1%, prerenal; if (Fe$_{Na}$) >1% consider intrinsic renal disease(acute tubular necrosis [ATN]). Treatment for prerenal disorder is to increase IV rate. For patients with cardiac disease or intrinsic renal failure, further workup of organ-specific disorder is warranted (echocardiogram or renal US). If evidence of bleeding, transfuse and check coagulation factors. If in doubt, a fluid challenge may be indicated: 500 mL of 0.9% saline over 30 min or

200 mL of colloid (Hespan® or albumin) over 30–60 min, with monitoring of urine output. Then you may increase IV rate (e.g., to 1 L/h of 0.9% saline for 2–3 h).

- Further monitoring with a CVP line or CVP Swan–Ganz catheter may be necessary.

Guidelines for success (p. 667)

- Be simple. Chart losses and replace them. Know the urine output. Aim for 60 mL/h; 30 mL/h is the minimum in adults (0.5 mL/kg/h).
- Measure plasma electrolytes if the patient is ill. Regular electrolytes are not needed in young people with good kidneys unless patient has ongoing losses (vomiting, diarrhea).
- Start oral fluids as soon as possible; the kidney is smarter than the best doctor.

What fluids to use

Hemorrhagic/hypovolemic shock (p. 745): Insert two large IV cannulas (14 or 16 G) for fast fluid infusion. Start with crystalloid (e.g., 0.9% saline) or colloid until blood is available. The advantage of crystalloids is that they are cheap, but they do not stay as long in the intravascular compartment as colloids because they equilibrate with the total extracellular volume (dextrose is useless for resuscitation as it rapidly equilibrates with the enormous intracellular volume). In practice, the best results are achieved by combining crystalloids and colloids. Aim to keep the hemoglobin >8 mg/dL, and urine flowing at >30 mL/h. Monitor pulse and blood pressure (BP) often.

Septicemic shock: Infuse isotonic (0.9% saline) fluids to replace third-space losses. Consider hypertonic saline (3%).

Heart or liver failure: Avoid sodium loads.

Excessive vomiting, diarrhea: Use 0.9% saline and replace losses, including K^+. (See chart.)

Urine output↓ (oliguria): Aim for output of >30 mL/h in adults (½ mL/kg/h). Anuria means a blocked catheter. Flush or replace catheter. Oliguria is usually due to inadequate replacement of lost fluid. Treat by increasing fluid input. Acute renal failure may follow shock, nephrotoxic drugs, transfusion, or trauma.

- Review fluid chart and examine for signs of volume depletion.
- Urinary retention is also common, so examine for a palpable bladder.
- Establish normovolemia (a CVP line may help here; normal is 0–5 cm H_2O relative to sternal angle); you may need 1 L/h IVI for 2–3 h.
- Catheterize bladder (for accurate monitoring).

If intrinsic renal failure (see Fe_{Na}, above) is suspected, refer to a nephrologist early.

449

Electrolyte concentrations (meq/l)

Location	Na^+	K^+	Cl^-	HCO_3^-	H^+	Rate (ML/d)
Salivary	50	20	40	30	–	Up to 1 L
Gastric	100	10	140	–	100	Up to 4 L
Bile	140	5	100	60	–	Up to 1 L
Pancreatic	140	5	75	100	–	Up to 1 L
Duodenal	140	5	80	–	–	Up to 2 L
Ileum	140	5	70	50	–	Up to 2 L
Colon	100	70	15	30	–	–

Electrolyte management in the surgical patient

Tables 13.4, 13.5, 13.6, and 13.7 detail the management of electrolytes in the surgical patient.

Table 13.4 Hypo- and hypernatremia

Hyponatremia The most common cause is excess free fluid. Symptoms related to hyponatremia include nausea, headaches, weakness, cognition↓, coma, death. Hyponatremia results from infusion of 5% dextrose in H_2O, thiazide diuretics, inappropriate antidiuretic hormone (ADH) secretion.

Treatment (p. 668): 0.9% saline IVI; check electrolytes every 2 h; aim to bring Na^+ up to 130 mmol/L by 1–2 mmol/L per hour. Diuretics may be useful in acute hyponatremia, or if the patient is symptomatic.

Hypernatremia The most common cause is excess free water loss. Less common in surgical patients. Diabetes insipidus (depressed ADH secretion) can result from head trauma. Symptoms occur when Na^+ exceeds 160 mEq/ML; symptoms include irritability, restlessness, fever, seizures.

Treatment: Free water is administered to correct Na^+ at a rate of 0.7 mEq/L/h.

Table 13.5 Hypo- and hyperkalemia

Potassium is the major intracellular cation and is the major determinant of intracellular osmolality.

Hypokalemia A result of total body depletion (diarrhea, hyperaldosteronism) or intracellular redistribution (acute alkalosis, glucose and insulin administration, catecholamine excess). Symptoms include muscle weakness, ileus, arrhythmias; ECG may demonstrate flattened T waves, depressed ST segments, prolonged QT, U waves.

Treatment: Replace K^+ at 10 mEq/h. A drop of 1 mEq/ML in the serum K^+ level represents a total body loss of ~100 mEq. Correct acid–base abnormalities.

Hyperkalemia In the postop patient, usually the result of diminished renal function. Also seen in crush and reperfusion injuries after vascular surgery. Acute elevation in K^+ can result from depolarizing muscle relaxants (e.g., succinylcholine)

Treatment: ECG changes (peaked T waves) paresthesia, and weakness should be treated with a rapid infusion of calcium gluconate, 1 ampule of sodium bicarbonate, and 50 g glucose along with 10 U of regular insulin, which will temporize for 30 min. Need ICU monitoring. Definite treatment includes K^+-wasting diuretics or K^+–Na^+ exchange resin (Kayexalate) 40 g in 100 mL of sorbitol. Alternatively, hemodialysis should be performed.

Table 13.6 Hypo- and hypercalcemia

Hypocalcemia In the postop patient, hypocalcemia is usually secondary to inadvertent or planned total parathyroidectomy. After the resection of a parathyroid adenoma, hypocalcemia may be secondary to temporary nonfunction of existing glands as a result of atrophy. Other causes include acute pancreatitis and pancreatic fistulas, vitamin D deficiency, renal failure. Symptoms occur with serum level <8 mg/dL and include muscle cramps, perioral tingling, paresthesia, laryngeal stridor, tetany, seizures, psychotic behavior. Check for hyperactive deep tendon reflexes: Chvostek sign and Trousseau sign. ECG changes include prolonged QT interval caused by prolongation of the ST segment.
Treatment: Verify if not secondary to a low albumin (check ionized calcium). IV calcium gluconate or calcium chloride (can burn in the IV). Should not be administered at a rate >50 mg/min (2.5 mEq/min). Oral replacement with calcium gluconate, citrate, or carbonate (TUMs), as well as vitamin D supplementation to increase GI absorption.

Hypercalcemia Primary hyperparathyroidism as a result of a parathyroid adenoma is the most common cause of hypercalcemia. Other causes include chief cell hyperplasia, renal failure, paraneoplastic syndrome, familial hyperkalemia. Symptoms include muscle fatigue, weakness, personality disorders, psychoses, coma, hypertension, shortening of QT interval on ECG, nausea, vomiting, abdominal pain, nephrocalcinosis, and lithiasis ("bones, stones, and abdominal groans").
Treatment: Serum Ca^+ >14 mg/dL must be dealt with immediately. Hydration with 0.9% or 0.45% saline with 20 mEq of K^+ intravenously at 200–300 mL/h to promote diuresis. Furosemide will enhance Ca^+ excretion. Long-term treatment requires resection of the parathyroid adenoma or the tumor. Metastatic bone disease resulting in hypercalcemia may respond to mithramycin or calcitonin. Metastatic breast disease or hematogenous disease may respond to steroids. ESRD patients on dialysis may respond to a low-calcium dialysate.

Table 13.7 Hypo- and hypermagnesemia

Hypomagnesemia Prolonged period of IV fluid without Mg^{2+} replacement is the most common cause in the postoperative period. Symptoms are similar to hypocalcemia. Hypokalemia may develop.
Treatment: Large deficits are best managed by IV doses infusion with up to 4 g. For mild deficits, magnesium can be given orally.

Hypermagnesemia Renal failure is the primary reason. Symptoms include depressed neuromuscular function.
Treatment: Calcium antagonizes the effects of magnesium, so a slow IV of 5–10 mEq of calcium is used in acute cases.

The control of pain

The control of postoperative pain is essential and must be individualized (Table 13.8). Numerous studies have indicated that patients recover more quickly and have less complications and a better experience if their pain is well controlled.

Guidelines for success Review and chart each pain carefully and individually.

• Identify and treat the underlying pathology wherever possible.
• Give regular doses rather than on an as-required basis.
• Choose the best route: Oral, PR, IM, epidural, SC, inhalation, or IV.
• Explanation and reassurance contribute greatly to analgesia.
• Allow the patient to be in charge. This promotes well-being and does not lead to overuse. Patient-controlled continuous parenteral morphine delivery systems are useful.

Non-narcotic analgesia Acetaminophen: 650 mg/6 h PO. Caution in liver impairment. Recently, IV acetaminophen (1 g) was approved by the FDA for use in the United States for postoperative pain management. NSAIDs (e.g., ibuprofen 400 mg/8 h PO or Toradol® 15–30 mg IV/6–8 h) are good for musculoskeletal pain and work well as an adjunct to the more potent narcotics. *Contraindications (CI)*: Peptic ulcer, clotting disorder, anticoagulants, renal insufficiency (Toradol). *Cautions:* Asthma, renal or hepatic impairment, pregnancy, and the elderly. Aspirin is contraindicated in children due to the risk of Reye's syndrome.

Opioid drugs for severe pain Morphine (e.g., 2–4 mg/2–4 h IV push) or oxycodone (5–10 mg/4 h PO) or derivatives of these medications are best. Meperidine (Demerol®) is also useful on a short-term basis. Long–term use of meperidine can result in central nervous system (CNS) hyperexcitability. These are controlled drugs.

Side effects of opioids: These include nausea, respiratory depression, constipation, cough suppression, urinary retention, BP↓, and sedation (do not use in hepatic failure or head injury). Dependency is a problem, especially with longer acting drugs such as OxyContin. Naloxone may be needed to reverse the effects of excess opioids (p. 790).

Patient-controlled analgesia Morphine or fentanyl is given through an IV pump, which is controlled by the patient. IV infusion allows the patient to receive the pain medication within 2–5 min. The patient is allowed just so much medication every hour. Side effects are nausea, pruritus, and ileus. Patient-controlled analgesia (PCA) is only effective if the patient is properly educated on its use. Family members must be discouraged from administering the drug for the patient.

Epidural analgesia Opioids and anesthetics are given into the epidural space by infusion or as boluses. Ask the advice of the Pain Service (if available). *Side effects (SE):* Thought to be more localized: Watch for respiratory depression; neuromuscular weakness, difficulty voiding, local anaesthetic-induced autonomic blockade (BP↓).

Adjuvant treatments E.g., radiotherapy for bone cancer pain; anticonvulsants, antidepressants, or steroids for nerve pain; antispasmodics (e.g., hyoscine [Buscopan®] 10–20 mg/8 h) for intestinal, renal, or bladder colic. Transcutaneous electrical nerve stimulation (TENS), local heat, local or regional anesthesia, and neurosurgical procedures (e.g., excision of neuroma) may be tried but can prove disappointing. Treat conditions that exacerbate pain (e.g., constipation, depression, anxiety).

Table 13.8 Why is controlling postoperative pain so important?

- *Psychological reasons*: Pain control is a humanitarian undertaking.
- *Social reasons*: Pain relief makes surgery less feared by society.
- *Biological reasons*: There is evidence for the following sequence: Pain → autonomic activation → ↑ adrenergic activity → arteriolar vasoconstriction → reduced wound perfusion → ↓ tissue oxygenation → delayed wound healing → serious or mortal consequences.

Deep vein thrombosis and swollen legs

DVTs occur in ~20% of surgical patients and many nonsurgical patients. 65% of below-knee DVTs are asymptomatic; these rarely embolize to the lung.

Risks Age, pregnancy, synthetic estrogen, surgery (especially pelvic/orthopedic), past DVT, malignancy, obesity, immobility, thrombophilia (p. 638). See Table 13.9.

Signs Calf warmth/tenderness/swelling, mild fever, pitting edema.

Differential diagnoses Cellulitis (may coexist); ruptured Baker's cyst (both may coexist).

Tests *D-dimer blood tests* are sensitive but not specific for DVT. They are also elevated in infection, pregnancy, malignancy, and postop. A –ve result, combined with a low pre-test clinical probability score is sufficient to exclude (see below). DVT. If D-dimer is elevated or the patient has a high/intermediate pre-test clinical probability score, do compression US. If this is –ve, a repeat US may be performed at 1 wk to catch early but propagating DVTs. Venography is rarely necessary. Do thrombophilia tests if there are no pre-disposing factors, in recurrent DVT, or if there is a family history of DVT.

Prevention Stop oral contraceptive pills (OCPs) 4 wks preop. Mobilize early. See above.

Treatment Meta-analyses have shown LMWH (e.g., enoxaparin 1.5 mg/kg/24 h SC) to be superior to unfractionated heparin (dose guided by aPTT [p. 574]), but extensive ileofemoral thrombi may still require unfractionated heparin because such patients were excluded from the trials. Start warfarin simultaneously, stopping heparin when International Normalized Ratio (INR) is 2–3; treat for 3 months if postop (6 months if no cause is found; lifelong in recurrent DVT or thrombophilia). Inferior vena cava filters may be used in active bleeding, or, when anticoagulants fail, to minimize risk of pulmonary embolus. Preventing postphlebitic change: Thrombolytic therapy (to reduce damage to venous valves) and graduated compression stockings have both been tried, but neither has been conclusively shown to be beneficial.

Swollen legs

Bilateral edema implies systemic disease with ↑ venous pressure (right heart failure) or intravascular oncotic pressure (any cause of albumin decrease, so test the urine for protein). It is dependant (distributed by gravity), which is why legs are affected early, but severe edema extends above the legs. The exception is the local increase in venous pressure occurring in IVC obstruction: The swelling neither extends above the legs nor redistributes. *Causes:* Right-heart failure (p. 128). Low albumin. *Venous insufficiency*: Acute (e.g., prolonged sitting; see Table 13.10) or chronic, with hemosiderin-pigmented, itchy, eczematous skin ± ulcers. Vasodilators (e.g., nifedipine). Pelvic mass. Pregnancy—if BP↑ + proteinuria, diagnose pre-eclampsia: Find an obstetrician urgently. In all the above, both legs need not be affected to the same extent.

Unilateral edema: Pain ± redness implies DVT or inflammation; e.g., cellulitis or insect bites (any blisters?). Bone or muscle may be to blame; e.g., trauma (check sensation and pulses: A compartment syndrome with ischemic necrosis needs prompt fasciotomy), tumors, or necrotizing fasciitis.

Table 13.9 Pre-test clinical probability scoring for DVT

In patients with symptoms in both legs, the more symptomatic leg is used.

Clinical feature	Score
Active cancer (treatment within last 6 months or palliative)	1 point
Paralysis, paresis, or recent cast immobilization of leg	1 point
Major surgery or recently bedridden for >3 d in last 4 wks	1 point
Local tenderness along distribution of deep venous system	1 point
Entire leg swollen	1 point
Calf swelling >3 cm compared to asymptomatic leg (measured 10 cm below tibial tuberosity)	1 point
Pitting edema (greater in the symptomatic leg)	1 point
Collateral superficial veins (nonvaricose)	1 point
Alternative diagnosis as likely or more likely than that of DVT	2 points

3 or more points: High probability; 1–2 points: Intermediate probability; 0 or fewer points: Low pre-test probability of DVT.

Table 13.10 Air travel and DVT

In 1954, Homans first reported an association between air travel and venous thromboembolism. Recently, the supposed risk of DVT and subsequent pulmonary emboli associated with air travel (the so-called "economy-class syndrome") has been the subject of much public scrutiny. Factors such as dehydration, immobilization, reduced oxygen tension, and prolonged pressure on the popliteal veins resulting from long periods in confined aircraft seats have all been suggested to be contributory factors. Although the evidence linking air travel to an increased risk of DVT is still largely circumstantial, the following facts may help answer questions from your patients, family, and friends:

- The risk of developing a DVT from a long-distance flight has been estimated at 0.1–0.4/1,000 for the general population.
- There is an increased risk of pulmonary embolus associated with long-distance air travel.
- Compression stockings may decrease the risk of DVT, although they may also cause superficial thrombophlebitis.
- The role of prophylactic aspirin is still under investigation.
- Measures to minimize risk of DVT include leg exercises, increased water intake, and refraining from alcohol or caffeine during the flight.

Impaired mobility suggests trauma, arthritis, or a Baker's cyst.

Nonpitting edema is edema you cannot indent.

Treatment Treat the cause. Giving diuretics to everyone is not an answer. Ameliorate dependent edema by elevating the legs (ankles higher than hips; do not just use foot stools); raise the foot of the bed. Graduated support stockings may help (*CI*: Ischemia).

Glucose management and the diabetic patient

Hyperglycemia results from surgical trauma. Although insulin levels are appropriately elevated, the tolerance of insulin-sensitive tissues is reduced. The importance of good glucose regulation (<130 mg/dL) in the postoperative period has led to a significant decrease in wound infection rates.

Insulin-dependent diabetes mellitus (e.g., type 1 diabetes mellitus)

- Patients are often well informed about their diabetes; involve them fully when managing their diabetic care.
- Stress or concurrent illness increases basal insulin needs.
- Always try to put the patient first on the list (surgery, endoscopy, bronchoscopy, etc.). Inform the surgeon and anesthetist early.
- Stop all long–acting insulin the night before. Get IV access before you need it urgently. If surgery is in the morning, stop all SC morning insulin. If surgery is in the afternoon, have the usual short-acting insulin in the morning at breakfast. No medium- or long-acting insulin.
- Check blood glucose hourly. Aim for 100 mg/dL during surgery.
- Check electrolytes and glucose preop. Start an IV of 1 L of 5% dextrose with 20 mmol KCL/8 h. Dextrose saline can be given if Na^+ low, but do not give only saline; dextrose may need constant infusion to maintain blood glucose.
- Start an infusion pump with 50 U short-acting insulin in 50 mL 0.9% saline. Give according to sliding scale (below), adjusted in the light of blood glucose.
- Postop, continue IV insulin and dextrose until patient is tolerating food. Finger-stick glucose every 2 h. Switch to usual SC regimen.

Practical hints

- Some prefer to control blood sugar with a glucose-potassium-insulin (GKI) infusion.
- If the patient is having minor surgery and thus will definitely be able to eat postop, IV insulin may not be necessary. Some advocate giving the patient a small glucose drink early on the morning of surgery and delaying his morning insulin dose and breakfast until after the procedure.
- If in doubt, check with the anesthesiologist.

455

Non-insulin-dependent diabetes mellitus (type 2 diabetes)

- These patients are usually controlled on oral hypoglycemics (p. 290). If diabetes is poorly controlled, treat as for type 1 diabetes.
- Do not give long-acting sulfonylureas 24 h prior to surgery, as they can cause prolonged hypoglycemia on fasting.
- Beware of lactic acidosis in patients on biguanides (e.g., metformin). It is recommended to hold dose of metformin 24 h prior to surgery.
- If the patient can eat postoperatively, simply omit tablets on the morning of surgery and give postop with a meal.
- If the patient is having major surgery with restrictions to eating postop, check fasting glucose on the morning of surgery and start IV or SC insulin given according to sliding scale. Postop, consult the diabetic

team as the patient may need a phase of insulin to supplement his oral hypoglycemics.

Diet-controlled diabetes is usually no problem although the patient may temporarily become insulin-dependent postop. Monitor finger-stick glucose before meals and bedtime. Avoid giving 5% dextrose IVI as a fluid replacement as blood glucose will rise.

IV insulin sliding scale (This is only a guide; values are in mg/dL):

Finger stick glucose (mg/dL)	IV soluble insulin	Alternative SC insulin
<60	None (50% glucose IV)	None (50% glucose IV)
60–130	No insulin	No insulin
131–180	1 U/h	2 U SC
181–250	2 U/h	4 U SC
251–350	3 U/h	6 U SC
>351	6 U/h	8 U SC

Blood transfusion and blood products

Blood should only be given if strictly necessary, and a preoperative discussion regarding its use should be always undertaken.

• Know *and use* local procedures to ensure that the right blood gets to the right patient at the right time.
• Take blood for cross-matching from only one patient at a time. Label immediately. This minimizes risk of wrong labeling of samples.
• When giving blood, monitor temperature and BP every ½ h.

Type and screen requests Find your local guidelines for elective surgery. Obtaining cross-matched blood is easier if the patient has already been typed and screened. No units are set up for the patient when only a type and screen is requested. Furthermore, blood typing and screening may identify antibodies in a patient's blood that may require additional testing.

Whole blood (rarely used) *Indications:* Exchange transfusion; grave exsanguination: Use cross-matched blood if possible, but if not, use "universal donor" group O Rh -ve blood, changing to cross-matched blood as soon as possible. Blood >2 days old has no effective platelets.

Red cells (packed to make hematocrit ~70%) Use to correct anemia or blood loss. 1 U ↑ Hb by 1–1.5 g/dL. In anemia, transfuse until Hb ~8 g/dL.

Platelet transfusion (p. 632) not usually needed if not bleeding or count is >20 × 10^9/L. If surgery is planned, get advice if <60 × 10^9/L.

Fresh frozen plasma (ffp) Use to correct clotting defects; e.g., DIC (p. 625), warfarin overdosage, liver disease. It is expensive and carries all the risks of blood transfusion. Do not use as a simple volume expander.

Human albumin solution (plasma protein fraction) is produced as 4.5% or 20% protein solution and is basically albumin to use for protein replacement. Both the solutions have much the same Na$^+$ content, and 20% albumin can be used temporarily in the hypoproteinemic patient (e.g., liver disease; nephrotic) who is fluid overloaded without giving an excessive salt load.

Others Cryoprecipitate (a source of fibrinogen); coagulation concentrates (self-injected in hemophilia); immunoglobulin (anti-D).

Complications of transfusion Management of acute reactions (see Table 13.11):

• *Early (within 24 h):* Acute hemolytic reactions (e.g., ABO or Rhesus incompatibility), anaphylaxis, bacterial contamination, febrile reactions (e.g., from HLA antibodies), allergic reactions (e.g., itch, urticaria, mild fever), fluid overload, transfusion-related acute lung injury (TRALI)—basically ARDS due to anti-leukocyte antibodies in donor plasma.

• *Delayed (after 24 h):* Infections (e.g., viruses [hepatitis B/C, HIV], bacteria, protozoa, prions), iron overload (treatable with desferrioxamine), graft-versus-host disease, and *posttransfusion purpura*, potentially lethal fall in platelet count 5–7 d post-transfusion requiring specialist treatment with IV immuno-globulin and platelet transfusions.

Massive blood transfusion This is defined as replacement of an individual's entire blood volume (>10 U) within 24 h. *Complications:*

Table 13.11 Transfusion reactions

A rapid spike of temperature (>40°C) at the start indicates that the transfusion should be stopped (suggests intravascular hemolysis or bacterial contamination). For a slowly rising temperature (<40°C), slow the IVI—this is most frequently due to antibodies against white cells.

Acute transfusion reactions	Action
Acute hemolytic reaction (e.g., ABO incompatibility) Agitation, T°↑ (rapid onset), ↓BP, flushing, abdominal/chest pain, oozing venopuncture sites, DIC	STOP transfusion. Check identity and name on unit; tell hematologist; send unit + CBC and electrolytes, PT, PTT, cultures and urine (hemoglobinuria) to lab. Keep IV line open with 0.9% saline. Treat DIC.
Anaphylaxis Bronchospasm, cyanosis, BP, soft-tissue swelling	SLOW or STOP the transfusion. Maintain airway and give oxygen. Transfer to ICU and contact code team for intubation.
Bacterial contamination T°↑ (rapid onset), ↓BP, and rigors	STOP the transfusion. Check identity against name on unit; tell hematologist and send unit +CBC, electrolytes, clotting, cultures, and urine to lab. Start broad-spectrum antibiotics.
TRALI (transfer related acute lung injury) Dyspnea, cough; CXR "white out"	STOP the transfusion. Give 100% O₂. Treat as acute respiratory distress syndrome (ARDS, p. 174). Donor should be removed from donor panel.
Nonhemolytic febrile transfusion reaction Shivering and fever usually 30–60 min after starting transfusion	SLOW or STOP the transfusion. Give an antipyretic (e.g., Tylenol® 1 g). Monitor closely. If recurrent, use leukocyte-depleted blood or white blood cell (WBC) filter.
Allergic reactions Urticaria and itch	SLOW or STOP the transfusion; give diphenhydramine 25–50 mg IV/PO q6–8h. Monitor closely.
Fluid overload Dyspnea, hypoxia, tachycardia, ↑JVP, and basal crepitations	SLOW or STOP the transfusion. Give oxygen and a diuretic (e.g., furosemide 40 mg) IV initially. Consider CVP line and exchange transfusion.

457

Platelets↓, Ca^{2+}↓, clotting factors↓, K^+↑, hypothermia. Current guidelines recommend transfusing fresh frozen plasma (FFP) to packed red blood cells (PRBCs) at a 1:1 or 1:2 ratio.

Transfusing patients with heart failure If Hb 5 g/dL with heart failure, transfusion with packed red cells is vital to restore Hb to safe level (e.g., 6–8 g/dL) but must be done with great care. Give each unit over 4 h with (furosemide, e.g., 40 mg slow IV/PO; do not mix with blood) with alternate units. Check for ↑JVP and basal lung crackles; consider CVP line.

There is a role for patients having their own blood stored preop for later use; however, the lifespan of autologous blood will be less than that of fresh blood (autologous transfusion). Erythropoietin (EPO) can be used to increase the yield of autologous blood in normal individuals. See Table 13.12.

Table 13.12 Blood transfusion and Jehovah's witnesses

These patients are likely to refuse even vital transfusions on religious grounds. These views must be respected, but complex issues can arise, especially if the patient is a child. Alternative methods of hemoconcentration should be offered to these patients. These methods include preoperative erythropoietin and iron and intraoperative normovolemic hemodilution. Consultation with hematology and anesthesiology preoperatively is recommended.

Nutritional support

>25% of hospital inpatients may be malnourished. Weight loss of >10% of normal body mass may compromise the host by altering the ability to heal wounds or develop an immune response to infection. Operative mortality is increased in patients with weight loss of >20–25% of total body weight. In contrast, patients with normal body composition who are not hypermetabolic do not require nutritional intervention for up to a period of 5–7 d of inadequate intake.

Why are so many hospital patients malnourished?
1 Increased nutritional requirements (e.g., sepsis, burns, surgery)
2 Increased nutritional losses (e.g., malabsorption, output from stoma)
3 Poor intake (e.g., dysphagia, sedation, coma)
4 Effect of treatment (e.g., nausea, diarrhea)
5 Enforced starvation (e.g., prolonged npo periods)

Identifying the malnourished patient
History: Recent weight change; recent reduced intake; diet change (e.g., recent change in consistency of food); nausea, vomiting, pain, diarrhea that might have led to reduced intake.

Examination: Examine for state of hydration; dehydration can go hand-in-hand with malnutrition, and overhydration can mask the appearance of malnutrition. Evidence of malnutrition: Poor skin turgor (e.g., over biceps); no fat between folds of skin; hair rough and wiry; pressure sores; sores at corner of mouth. Body mass index (BMI) <19 kg/m² suggests malnourishment.

Investigations: Low albumin, prealbumin, and transferring levels are suggestive of poor nutritional status.

Calculations of needs: To estimate caloric needs, the basal metabolic rate is estimated based on height, weight, age, and gender. A stress factor is added to account for the increased demands in hospitalized patients, and 1,000 kcal should be added per day when weight gain is desired.

Protein requirements: ~1–2 g/kg/d will maintain a positive nitrogen (N) balance. The optimal N-to-calorie ratio is 1:150. Divide total kcal necessary by 150 to get grams of N. Then multiply the grams of N by 6.25 to calculate grams of protein needed per day.

The remainder of requirements is based on the kcals needed.

Remember:	Carbohydrates 3.4 kcal/g
	Protein 4 kcal/g
	Fat 9 kcal/g

Most patients are well-nourished with 2,000–2,500 kcal (20–40 kcal/kg) and 7–14 g nitrogen every 24 h. Even catabolic patients rarely need >2,500 kcal. Very high calorie diets (e.g., 4,000 kcal/24 h) can lead to fatty liver. If a patient requires nutritional support, seek help from dietician.

Prevention of malnutrition Assess nutrition state and weight on admission and possibly weekly thereafter. Identify those at risk (see above). Nutritional supplements high in caloric count will assist with improving nutritional status.

Enteral nutrition (i.e., nutrition given into gastrointestinal tract). If at all possible, give nutrition by mouth. An all-fluid diet can meet requirements (but get advice from dietitian). If a patient has a limited capacity to swallow but has passed a swallowing study (e.g., after stroke), consider a pureed diet before abandoning food by mouth.

Tube feeding: This is giving liquid nutrition via a tube (e.g., placed endoscopically, radiologically, or surgically directly into stomach; i.e., gastrostomy or into the jejunum). Use nutritionally complete, commercially prepared feeds. Standard feeds (e.g., Nutrison standard®, Osmolite®) normally contain 1 kcal/ML and 4–6 g protein per 100 mL. Most people's requirements are met in 2 L/24 h. Specialist advice from a dietitian is essential. Nausea and vomiting is less of a problem if feeds are given continuously via pump, but these may have disadvantages compared with intermittent nutrition. For various methods of tube feedin, see Figure 13.2.

Guidelines for success
- Use jejunal tube feeding when possible.
- Keep height of bed at 30 degrees to avoid aspiration risk.
- Build up feeds gradually to avoid diarrhea and distension.
- Weigh weekly, check blood glucose and plasma electrolytes (including phosphate, zinc, and magnesium, if previously malnourished).
- Working closely with a dietitian is essential.

459

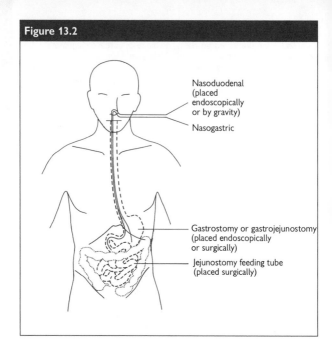

Figure 13.2

Nasoduodenal (placed endoscopically or by gravity)

Nasogastric

Gastrostomy or gastrojejunostomy (placed endoscopically or surgically)

Jejunostomy feeding tube (placed surgically)

Parenteral (IV) nutrition

Do not undertake parenteral feeding lightly: It has risks. Specialist advice is vital. Only consider it if the patient is likely to become malnourished without it. This normally means that the gastrointestinal tract is not functioning or is not available (e.g., bowel obstruction or fistula) and is unlikely to function for at least 7 d. Parenteral feeding may supplement other forms of nutrition (e.g., in active Crohn's disease when insufficient nutrition can be absorbed in the gut) or be used alone (total parenteral nutrition—TPN). Even if there is GI disease (e.g., pancreatitis), studies show that enteral nutrition is safer, cheaper, and at least as efficacious.

Administration Nutrition is normally given through a central venous line as this usually lasts longer than if given into a peripheral vein. A peripherally inserted central catheter (PICC line) is another option. Insert under strictly sterile conditions and check its position on x-ray. This line is then dedicated for the administration of nutrition only.

Requirements There are many different regimens for parenteral feeding. Most provide ~2,000 kcal and 10–14 g nitrogen in 2–3 L; this usually meets a patient's daily requirements of 20–40 kcal/kg and 0.2 g nitrogen/kg. ~50% of calories are provided by fat and 50% by carbohydrate. Regimens comprise vitamins, minerals, trace elements, and electrolytes; these will normally be included by the pharmacist.

Complications

Sepsis: E.g., *Staphylococcus epidermidis* and *Staphylococcus aureus, Candida, Pseudomonas,* infective endocarditis.) Look for spiking pyrexia and examine wound at tube insertion point. If central venous line-related sepsis is suspected, the safest course of action is always to remove the line. Do not attempt to salvage a line when *S. aureus* or *Candida* infection has been identified.

Thrombosis: Central vein thrombosis may occur, resulting in pulmonary embolus or superior vena caval obstruction. Heparin in the nutrient solution may be useful for prophylaxis in high-risk patients.

Metabolic imbalance: Electrolyte abnormalities (including K+, calcium, phosphate, zinc, magnesium), plasma glucose, deficiency syndromes.

Mechanical: Pneumothorax; embolism from CVP tip.

Guidelines for success

- Work closely with nutrition team and pharmacist.
- Practice meticulous sterility. Do not use central venous lines other than for nutrition. Remove the line if you suspect infection. Culture the line on removal.
- Review fluid balance at least twice daily and requirements for energy and electrolytes daily.
- Check weight, fluid balance, and urine glucose daily throughout period of parenteral nutrition. Check plasma glucose, creatinine, and electrolytes (including calcium and phosphate), and take full blood count daily until stable and then three times a week. Check LFT and lipid clearance three times a week until stable and then weekly. Check zinc and magnesium weekly throughout.
- Do not rush. Achieve the maintenance regimen in small steps.

Drains, wounds, and stoma care

Drains

Surgical drains: Abdominal drains placed in surgery are usually closed suction drains (Jackson–Pratt). These drains can also be open drains such as a Penrose. Open drains are more commonly associated with infection. Surgical drains should always be brought out of an incision separately from the primary incision because of the risk of infection to the primary incision. The purpose of an abdominal drain is to collect fluid that may accumulate after surgery. Common sites to drain include the pelvis, the lateral gutters, and any procedure performed around the pancreas. Drains are also placed above the fascia to drain the subcutaneous tissue, especially if skin flaps have been mobilized. Drains are usually removed when the output has dropped. Routine drain care includes drain site care and drain stripping. To strip a drain, the fluid in the drain is squeezed through the tubing using the fingertips to push the fluid into the drain reservoir. Several studies have been performed looking at the benefit of drains in the abdomen and very few have demonstrated a benefit; however, individual surgeons continue to use drains. Another important point about drain management: When cracking or advancing a drain, the drain is removed from the body in increments of 1–2 inches a day. The drain must then be resecured.

External drains: Drainage tubes may also be placed radiographically to drain collection. In general, these drains are not closed suction drains. Care of these drains includes flushing with sterile saline 2–3 times a day.

Tube thoracostomy: Performed to evacuate an ongoing production of air/fluid into the pleural space or fluid that is too viscous to be aspirated by thoracentesis.

If there is a question of a tension pneumothorax, a 14- or 16-g angiocatheter should immediately be placed in the second or third intercostal space in the mid-clavicular line on the affected side.

Posterior thoracostomy: To drain hemothorax, pneumothorax (also anterior thoracostomy), persistent pleural effusion, and empyema. After application of local anesthesia, the incision is placed in the sixth intercostal space along the anterior axillary line. Placement of the tube occurs by entering the pleural in the fifth intercostal space and directing the tip posteriorly.

Anterior thoracostomy: For an anterior approach, the tube is placed over the fourth rib along the mid-clavicular line. Avoid injury to the intercostal artery and vein by entering the pleural space above the rib.

The tube thoracostomy is then connected to a Pleuravac®.

Tube thoracostomy removal: When the drainage is low and there is no longer a pneumothorax or air leak, the chest tube can be removed. The patient is asked to take a deep breath and perform a Valsalva. An airtight dressing is placed over the site once the tube has been removed.

Wounds

All surgical procedures involve the creation of a wound. Factors that prevent wounds from healing include lack of good blood supply (smoking and micro-vascular damage), infection, malnutrition, immunosuppression (diabetes, HIV), radiation, and age.

Clean wounds created at the time of elective surgery can be closed primarily. Sutures used for wound closure should be placed in tissue with good tensile strength, such as the dermis or fascia.

Contaminated wounds: Emergent surgery with free intra-abdominal contamination is best closed by secondary intention. Healing by secondary intention involves closure of a wound by the natural biologic forces of wound contraction. These wounds are dressed with antiseptic gauze moistened with saline. Once the wound has granulated with pink healthy tissue, other forms of dressing can applied to accelerate healing.

Stomas

A stoma is an artificial union made between two conduits (e.g., a choledochojejunostomy) or, more commonly, between a conduit and the outside of the body (e.g., a colostomy, in which feces are made to pass through a hole in the abdominal wall into an adherent plastic pouch). When choosing the site for a colostomy, avoid areas in scars, the area around the waistline, and creases. The patient should be sitting at the time of stoma marking.

The *stoma nurse* is expert in fitting secure, odorless devices. Ensure patients have their nurse's phone number for use before and after surgery. Nurse visits are more useful than any doctor's in explaining what is going to happen and what the colostomy will be like, and in troubleshooting postop problems.

1 *Loop colostomy:* A loop of colon is exteriorized, opened, and sewn to the skin. A rod under the loop prevents retraction and may be removed after 5–7 d. This is often called a *defunctioning colostomy,* but this is not strictly true as feces may pass beyond the loop. A loop colostomy is used to protect a distal anastomosis or to relieve distal obstruction. It is often temporary and is more prone to complications than end colostomies. A colostomy does not need to protrude very far from the skin because the efflux is not as irritating as in more proximal stomas, such as in ileostomy."

2 *End colostomy:* The bowel is divided; the proximal end is brought out as a stoma. The distal end may be resected (e.g., abdominoperineal excision of the rectum), left in the abdomen (Hartman's procedure), or exteriorized, forming a "mucous fistula."

3 *Double-barrelled (Paul-Mikulicz) colostomy:* The colon is brought out as two openings (similar to a mucus fistula).

Ileostomies protrude from the skin and emit fluids that contain active enzymes (so skin needs protecting). These stoma are made to protrude (Brooke) more than a colostomy stoma because of the risk of skin irritation. Furthermore, because the colon is not in continuity, the risk of dehydration is great. Patients must be instructed on careful fluid management. End ileostomy usually follows proctocolectomy, typically for IBD. Loop ileostomy can be used to temporarily protect distal anastomoses. Most stomal complications do not require emergent surgery. Work closely with your stoma therapist. See Table 13.13.

Table 13.13 Complication Management

Early:	*Early:*
• 1. Hemorrhage at stoma site	1. More commonly seen in cirrhotic patients; may require suture ligation of subcutaneous vessel
• 2. Stoma ischemia	
• 3. High output (especially ileostomies—can lead to ↑ K⁺ and dehydration)	2. Monitor bowel below the fascia for ischemia.
Delayed:	3. Replace with normal saline (NS).
• 1. Obstruction (failure at operation to close lateral space around stoma)	*Delayed:*
	1. IV support
	2. Product change
• 2. Dermatitis around stoma site	3. Topical or systemic immunosuppression
• 3. Pyoderma	4. Sugar to stomal prolapse to assist in reduction
• 4. Stoma prolapse	
• 5. Parastomal hernia	5. Stoma belt
• 6. Fistula	6. Monitor output to determine course.
• 7. Stoma retraction/stenosis	7. Stoma dilation and possible revision
• 8. Psychological problems	8. Stoma support group

Thyroid disease, hepatic failure, steroids, anticoagulation, and surgery

Thyroid hormone exerts primary influences on growth and metabolism. It is not a primary mediator of the host response to injury and infection. Frequently, thyroid hormones levels are low in severe illness.

463

Thyroid surgery for hyperthyroidism Life-threatening thyrotoxicosis may be precipitated by any operation but especially after thyroidectomy for hyperthyroidism. It is best to bring hyperthyroid patients into a euthyroid state before surgery. If severe, give propylthiouracil 50–200 mg q4h for 1 wk followed by 200–400 mg/d for an additional 5 wks prior to surgery or until euthyroid. Aqueous iodine oral solution (Lugol's solution), 0.1–0.3 mL/8 h PO, well-diluted with milk or water, can also be started prior to surgery.

Mild hyperthyroidism Start propranolol 80 mg/8 h PO and Lugol's solution as above at the first consultation. Stop Lugol's solution on the day of surgery but continue propranolol for 5 d postop.

Thyroid storm Severe thyrotoxicosis may result from surgical stress or trauma. The patient may be tachycardic, febrile, and have an altered mental status. Supplemental oxygen should be given to the patient, as well as propanolol and hydrocortisone. There is a 10–20% mortality rate associated with thyroid storm.

Hepatic failure and surgery

Patients with hepatic failure are particularly prone to developing oliguria after surgery. The cause of this can be multifactorial and includes prerenal azotemia, acute renal failure, and the hepatorenal syndrome. The cause of the hepatorenal syndrome is unknown but may be related to intrahepatic blood flow redistribution, cortical ischemia, and inappropriate activation of the renin-angiotensin system. Development of this syndrome is suggestive of a grim outcome.

Preoperative preparation

- Consider arterial line and CVP line to ensure an adequate intravascular volume intra- and postoperatively.
- Insert a urinary catheter.
- Check clotting and give prophylactic vitamin K (p. 621).

During surgery

- Measure urine output.
- Alert anesthesiologist to the removal of large quantities of ascites, which may lead to hypovolemia. Consider giving 0.9% saline IV to match the urine output.
- Measure urine output and urine and serum electrolytes and follow closely. Low urine sodium concentration (<10 mEq/L) with normal urine osmolality may suggest prerenal azotemia or the hepatorenal syndrome.
- Give 0.9% saline at rate to match fluid lost through NGT, as well as maintenance fluid.
- Intraoperative ascites drains may be placed to help with anastomotic healing and wound closure. Drain output should be matched ½ cc per CC output with 0.9% normal saline. Spironolactone (50–100 mg q6–8h) may be used to assist in treating ascites.
- Give furosemide if urine output is poor despite adequate intravascular volume.

Surgery in those on steroids or anticoagulants

Steroids: Patients with a history of steroid use in the 6 months prior to surgery may need extra exogenous steroids to cope with the added stress of surgery and the potential for adrenal insufficiency. The amount needed depends on the extent of the surgery and the preop dose of steroids. *Major surgery:* Typically, give hydrocortisone 50–100 mg IV with the pre-med and then q8h IV/IM for 2 d. Then return to previous medication. *Minor surgery:* Prepare as for major surgery except that hydrocortisone is given for 24 h only. Adrenal insufficiency results in hypotension. If this is encountered without an obvious cause, it may be worthwhile giving a dose of 50 mg hydrocortisone IV.

Those on stable long-term anticoagulants (warfarin and aspirin): All long-term anticoagulants should be stopped 5–7 d prior to surgery. Presently, there are enough alternatives that no patient should be on a long-term anticoagulant at the time of surgery. Discuss these issues when arranging consent. Vitamin K or FFP may be needed in emergency surgery. Patients with artificial valves requiring anticoagulation (particularly mitral) and newly placed cardiac stents should be placed on an alternative shorter acting anticoagulant prior to surgery, such as SQ fractionated heparin (Lovenox) or IV unfractionated heparin.

Postoperative care

Postoperative complications and management

Fever: Mild fever in the first 24 h is typically from atelectasis (needs prompt respiratory therapy, not antibiotics); tissue damage, or necrosis but an elevated in temperature >24 h postop should stimulate an infection evaluation. Check the CXR for pneumonia, the wound, the urine, and the abdomen for signs of peritonitis (e.g., anastomotic leakage). Examine sites of IV cannula and central venous access for signs of infection. Check the legs for DVT. Send blood for CBC, electrolytes, and culture. Send the urine for analysis. Consider CXR, abdominal CT, and lower extremity duplex depending on the clinical findings.

Confusion: This may manifest as agitation, disorientation, and attempts to leave hospital, especially at night. Gently reassure the patient in well-lit surroundings (p. 354). The common causes are:

- Hypoxia (pneumonia, atelectasis, CHF, PE)
- Infection (see above)
- Drugs (opiates, sedatives, and many others)
- Alcohol withdrawal
- Urinary retention; MI or stroke
- Liver/renal failure

Occasionally, sedation is necessary to examine the patient; consider midazolam (antidote: Flumazenil) or haloperidol 0.5–2 mg IM. Reassure relatives that postop confusion is common and reversible.

Shortness of breath or hypoxia Any previous lung disease?

Have patient sit up. Give oxygen, monitoring peripheral O_2 saturation by pulse oximetry. Examine for evidence of:

- Pneumonia/pulmonary collapse/aspiration
- Pulmonary edema (MI or fluid overload)
- Pulmonary embolism (p. 188)
- Pneumothorax (p. 189; due to CVP line or intercostal anaesthetic block).

Do CBC, arterial blood gases, CXR, and ECG. Manage according to findings.

BP↓ If severe, tilt bed head down and give O_2. Check pulse rate and measure BP yourself; compare it with that prior to surgery. Postop ↓BP is commonly due to hypovolemia resulting from inadequate fluid input so check fluid chart and replace losses, usually with colloid initially. Monitor urine output; consider catheterization. A CVP line may be useful to monitor fluid resuscitation. Hypovolemia may also be caused by hemorrhage so review wounds and abdomen. If severe, return to operating room for hemostasis. Beware cardiogenic causes and look for evidence of MI and PE. Consider sepsis and anaphylaxis.

Urine output↓ (oliguria) Aim for output of >30 mL/h in adults (½ mL/kg/h). Anuria frequently means a blocked or obstructed catheter. Flush or replace catheter. Oliguria is usually due to inadequate replacement of lost fluid. Treat by increasing fluid input. Acute renal failure may follow shock, nephrotoxic drugs, transfusion, or trauma.

- Review fluid chart and examine for signs of volume depletion.
- Urinary retention is also common, so examine for a palpable bladder.
- Establish normovolemia (a CVP line may help here; normal is 0–5 cm H_2O relative to sternal angle); patient may need 1 L/h IVI for 2–3 h.
- If intrinsic renal failure is suspected, refer to a nephrologist early.

Nausea/vomiting Any mechanical obstruction, paralytic ileus, or emetic drugs (opiates, digoxin, anesthetics)? Consider abdominal x-ray (AXR), NGT, and antiemetic.

Other postop complications Pain (p. 452), DVT (p. 453), PE (p. 188), wound dehiscence, bleeding (see Table 13.14).

Follow-up for surgical patients
1 Prior to discharge, all patient should be given instructions for follow-up. Determine what further care is needed for the patient.
2 If patients have skin staples, these are usually removed 10–14 d after surgery.

465

Table 13.14 Postoperative bleeding

- *Primary hemorrhage*: I.e., continuous bleeding, starting during surgery. Replace blood loss. If severe, return to the operating room for adequate hemostasis. Treat shock vigorously (p. 745).
- *Reactive hemorrhage*: Hemostasis appears secure until BP rises and bleeding starts. Replace blood and reexplore wound.
- *Secondary hemorrhage* occurs 1–2 wks postop and is the result of infection.

Table 13.15 Discharging patients after day-case surgery

After day-case surgery, don't discharge until "LEAP-FROG" is established:

Lucid, not vomiting, and cough reflex established
Easy breathing; easy urination
Ambulating
Pain relief + postop drugs dispensed + given. Do they understand doses?
Follow-up arranged
Rhythm, pulse rate, and BP checked one last time. Is trend satisfactory?
Operation site checked and explained to patient
Give the primary care provider a call

3 If a patient has a stoma, this should be attended to by a stoma therapist by at least 4 wks after surgery because the size of the stoma often changes.

4 If patient is being treated for a cancer and requires further adjuvant therapy, the oncologist appreciates a check from the surgeon prior to initiating therapy.

For day-case surgery, see Table 13.15.

The acute abdomen

An acute abdomen refers to any sudden manifestation of a nontraumatic disorder involving pain in the abdominal area for which urgent surgical exploration may be necessary and repeated examination is essential.

Begin by obtaining a careful history of the pain Ask about the location of the pain, any spreading or shifting, duration, mode of onset, progression, character (dull, sharp, crampy), and any other associated symptoms including nausea, vomiting, diarrhea, obstipation, constipation, hematuria, etc.

Types of pain

Visceral pain is mediated by the afferent C fiber and usually is felt in the midline. It is slow in onset and dull. It can be elicited by distension, inflammation, or ischemia.

Parietal pain is mediated by both C fibers and A delta nerve fibers. Abdominal parietal pain is more focused as a result of direct irritation of the somatically innervated parietal peritoneum by pus, bile, GI secretions, etc. It is conventionally described as occurring in four abdominal quadrants (see Figure 13.4).

Other relevant aspects of history include:

- Medical and surgical history
- Menstrual history
- Drug history
- Family history
- Travel history

Physical exam *Observe patient:* Lying still or writhing, pallor, sweating, feverish? Inspect the abdomen for distension, bruising; look for gray Turner's sign for hemorrhagic pancreatitis. *Auscultate for bowel sound:* Hypoactive indicates intra-abdominal infection; hyperactive sounds are noted in bowel obstruction. Palpate in a sequential pattern with the most tender area being touched last. Specific signs on palpation include:

- *Guarding:* Peritoneal inflammation causing rectus muscle rigidity.
- *Rebound tenderness:* Discomfort is felt upon releasing your hands from gentle pressure; acute appendicitis.
- *Murphy's sign:* Palpation in the right subcostal area while inspiring causes abrupt arrest of inspiration secondary to pain; acute cholecystitis.
- *Iliopsoas sign:* Active flexion or passive extension of the hip illicit pain; psoas abscess in Crohn's disease.
- *Obturators sign:* Internal or external rotation of the flexed thigh may cause discomfort in the groin area; incarcerated obturator hernia.
- *Costovertebral angle tenderness:* Punch tenderness of the costovertebral angle; renal colic.

Tests CBC, electrolytes, amylase, LFT, β-HCG, urinalysis; laparoscopy may avert open surgery. CT can be helpful provided it is readily available and causes no delay.

Preop care Anesthesia compounds shock, so resuscitate properly first, unless blood is being lost faster than it can be replaced in ruptured ectopic pregnancy or a leaking abdominal aneurysm (p. 475). Also do the following:

1 Establish good IV access (two 18-g IVs) and begin resuscitation with 0.9% saline.
2 Insert Foley and NGT.
3 Type and cross-match.
4 ECG, AXR, CXR
5 Begin broad-spectrum antibiotics if infection is suspected.
6 Consent and manage pain.

Clinical syndromes that usually require urgent surgical exploration

- *Rupture of an organ:* Spleen, aorta, ectopic pregnancy. Shock secondary to cardiovascular collapse (e.g., faints or orthostatic BP↓ by " 20 mm Hg on standing) is a leading sign. Abdominal swelling may be seen. Delayed rupture of the spleen may occur weeks after trauma.
- *Peritonitis:* Perforation of peptic ulcer, diverticulum, appendix, bowel, or gall bladder. *Signs:* Prostration, shock, lying still, tenderness (± rebound/percussion pain), board-like abdominal rigidity, guarding, and no bowel sounds. Erect CXR may show gas under the diaphragm on the right side usually or free intraperitoneal air (see Figure 13.3). *NB:* Acute pancreatitis (p. 487) may cause these signs, but does not require a laparotomy, so always check serum amylase.

Syndromes that may not require urgent exploration

- *Local peritonitis:* E.g., diverticulitis, cholecystitis, salpingitis, and appendicitis. If abscess formation is suspected (palpable mass, fever, and WBC↑), arrange a diagnostic US or CT. Drainage can be percutaneous (US- or CT-guided) or by laparotomy. Look for a "sentinel loop" on the plain AXR.

- *Colic* is a regularly waxing and waning pain caused by muscular spasm in a hollow viscus; e.g., gut, ureter, uterus, or gallbladder. (In the latter, pain is often dull and constant.) Colic causes restlessness, unlike peritonitis.

Other causes of abdominal pain that may masquerade as an acute surgical abdomen in which surgery is not indicated

Myocardial infarction	Pneumonia (p. 160)	Sickle-cell crisis (p. 618)
Gastroenteritis or urinary tract infection (UTI)	Tabes (p. 576)	Pheochromocytoma (p. 315)
Diabetes mellitus (p. 268)	Zoster (p. 558)	Malaria (p. 549)
Pneumococcal peritonitis	Tuberculosis (p. 552)	Typhoid fever (p. 590)
Henoch–Schönlein	Porphyria (p. 682)	Cholera (p. 585)
Narcotic addiction	Thyroid storm	*Yersinia enterocolitica* (p. 583)
	PAN (p. 417)	Lead colic

Accuracy in diagnosing acute abdomen is ~45% so always maintain a high index of suspicion. It is better to have a negative surgical exploration than to miss a surgical emergency. With newer minimally invasive techniques in surgery, patients recover quickly. These diagrams go over the causes of an acute abdomen manifested as free intra-abdominal air or peritonitis.

Intestinal ischemia

Acute onset of severe abdominal pain should always suggest the idea of bowel ischemia. Etiology can be classified as the following:
- *Occlusive:* Strangulated bowel, large-vessel embolic or thrombotic event, ligation of the IMA during aortic surgery
- *Vasospastic:* Small-vessel nonocclusive intestinal ischemia, ischemic hepatitis, pancreatitis, acalculous cholecystitis
- *Inflammatory:* Lupus, Behçet's disease, angioedema

Acute intestinal ischemia The most common cause is arterial embolism. Emboli originate from the heart in >75% of cases and lodge preferentially just distal to the origin of the superior mesenteric artery (SMA) (see Figure 13.5). Low-flow states usually reflect poor cardiac output but there may be other factors, such as DIC. Venous thrombosis is uncommon and tends to affect smaller lengths of bowel. The incidence of acute colonic ischemia after aortic surgery is 5–9%. Other risk factors include atrial fibrillation, recent myocardial infarction, valvular heart disease, recent cardiac or vascular catheterization, atherosclerotic disease, hypercoagulable state.

A classical clinical triad of occlusive ischemia: Acute severe abdominal pain, no abdominal signs, and rapid hypovolemia (causing shock). Pain tends to be constant and central or in the right lower quadrant. The degree of pain is often out of proportion to the clinical signs.

Nonocclusive ischemia: Ischemic colitis; usually presents with generalized abdominal pain, anorexia, bloody stools, and abdominal distension.

Tests: There may be Hb↑ (due to plasma loss), WBC↑, modestly elevated plasma amylase, elevated lactate, elevated creatine phosphokinase (CPK), and a persistent metabolic acidosis. Early on, the AXR shows a gasless abdomen. Arteriography helps, but many diagnoses are made at laparotomy. CT/MR angiography may provide a noninvasive alternative to conventional arteriography.

Treatment: Fluid replacement, antibiotics (broad spectrum) secondary to the risk of translocation and, usually, heparin. If arteriography is performed, thrombolytics may be infused locally via the catheter. At surgery, dead bowel must be removed. What needs to be removed can be a difficult surgical decision and often the Woods' lamp can help. Revascularization of potentially viable bowel should be attempted but is difficult. A second-look laparotomy may be required.

Chronic intestinal ischemia Small bowel chronic ischemia is typically due to SMA disease. Less common causes of ischemia include vasculitis, trauma, radiotherapy, and strangulation (e.g., hernias). Chronic ischemia presents quite a different picture from acute ischemia, with severe, colicky postprandial abdominal pain ("gut claudication") with weight loss (food hurts). Auscultation may reveal abdominal bruits. Diagnosis can be made by duplex US scan of the aorta or on angiography. Treatment requires revascularization with either endovascular or open surgical techniques.

Colonic ischemia usually follows low flow in the watershed areas between the inferior mesenteric artery and the superior mesenteric branches . Griffith's (splenic flexure) and Sudeck's (rectosigmoid) points (see Figure 13.5). Patients present with left-sided abdominal pain and bloody diarrhea. There may be fever, tachycardia, blood per rectum, and a leukocytosis. Usually this "ischemic colitis" resolves, but it may progress to gangrenous ischemic colitis. Colonoscopy will demonstrate a spectrum of findings beginning with hyperemia and ending with frankly dead mucosa. Barium enema may show "thumb-printing" indentation of the barium due to submucosal swelling. CT will demonstrate diffuse colonic thickening. Symptoms may be mild and result in stricture formation. Treatment may be supportive, with fluid replacement and antibiotics, or involve surgical removal of the colon with formation of an ileostomy in severe cases.

Gangrenous ischemic colitis This may follow ischemic colitis and is signaled by more severe pain, peritonitis, and hypovolemic shock. After resuscitation, necrotic bowel should be resected and a colostomy or ileostomy formed.

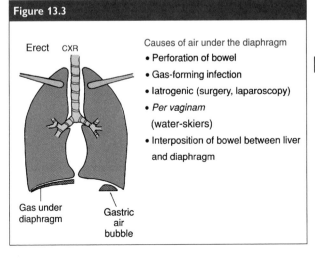

Figure 13.3

Erect CXR

Causes of air under the diaphragm
- Perforation of bowel
- Gas-forming infection
- Iatrogenic (surgery, laparoscopy)
- *Per vaginam*
  (water-skiers)
- Interposition of bowel between liver
  and diaphragm

Gas under diaphragm

Gastric air bubble

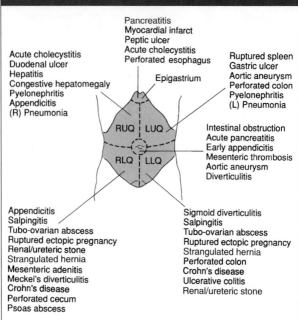

Figure 13.4 The causes of parietal pain in the four quadrants of the abdomen

Pancreatitis
Myocardial infarct
Peptic ulcer
Acute cholecystitis
Perforated esophagus

Acute cholecystitis
Duodenal ulcer
Hepatitis
Congestive hepatomegaly
Pyelonephritis
Appendicitis
(R) Pneumonia

Epigastrium

Ruptured spleen
Gastric ulcer
Aortic aneurysm
Perforated colon
Pyelonephritis
(L) Pneumonia

RUQ LUQ

RLQ LLQ

Intestinal obstruction
Acute pancreatitis
Early appendicitis
Mesenteric thrombosis
Aortic aneurysm
Diverticulitis

Appendicitis
Salpingitis
Tubo-ovarian abscess
Ruptured ectopic pregnancy
Renal/ureteric stone
Strangulated hernia
Mesenteric adenitis
Meckel's diverticulitis
Crohn's disease
Perforated cecum
Psoas abscess

Sigmoid diverticulitis
Salpingitis
Tubo-ovarian abscess
Ruptured ectopic pregnancy
Strangulated hernia
Perforated colon
Crohn's disease
Ulcerative colitis
Renal/ureteric stone

Gastrointestinal bleeding

GI bleeding is manifested as hematemesis, melena, or hematochezia. Melena can be from a gastroduodenal source, as well as from the colon. Small bowel bleeding is rare (<5%). The most common causes of gastrointestinal bleeding are listed below:

Upper gastrointestinal tract:

- Peptic ulcer disease
- Gastritis
- Gastric neoplasia
- Mallory–Weiss syndrome (see Table 13.16)
- Delafore lesion
- Varices

Small intestinal bleeding:

- Angiodysplasia
- Meckel's diverticulum
- Crohn's enteritis
- Neoplasia
- NSAID abuse

Large intestinal bleeding:
- Diverticulosis (30–50%)
- Colitis—inflammatory, infectious, or ischemic (20%)
- Angiodysplasia (10%)
- Arteriovenous (AV) malformations
- Anorectal disease
- Neoplasia

Initial management Directed toward resuscitation and includes the following:

1 Establish IV access with two large-bore IVs (16 g).
2 Draw blood for type and cross-match, CBC, PT, PTT, and electrolytes.
3 NGT aspirate to rule out (R/O) upper GI source, although can be inaccurate.
4 Foley catheterization and O administration is based on the severity of the bleed.
5 Obtain history regarding the use of warfarin, Plavix, aspirin, or NSAIDs.

Diagnostic tests For bleeding <1 cc/min: esophagogastric-duodenoscopy (EGD) and colonoscopy

For bleeding ≥1 cc/min: Angiography for localization and possible treatment, radionucleotide bleeding scan, endoscopic evaluation, surgery.

Therapeutic interventions Most causes of upper gastrointestinal bleeding are managed endoscopically with either electrocautery, heater probe, banding, or injection of epinephrine. Similarly, lower tract bleeding can also be managed endoscopically but more frequently will require surgery.

Arterial embolization or coiling is routinely performed for gastroduodenal bleeding because of the low risk of end-organ ischemia. However, only highly selective embolization can be performed for colonic bleeding secondary to the risk of ischemia following embolization (20%).

Surgical intervention for colonic bleeding from a source that has *not* been identified either colonoscopically or angiographically is a *subtotal colectomy*. If the bleeding source has been identified, a colonic segmentectomy can be performed. The decision of whether to re-anastomose the bowel is based on the overall health of the patient and the amount of bleeding that has occurred. A transfusion requirement of >10 units is associated with a higher anastomotic leak rate.

The collateral arterial blood supply to the intestinal tract

Figure 13.5

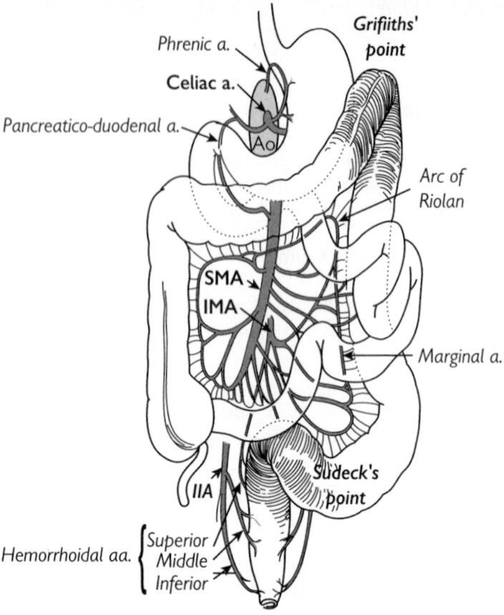

Phrenic a.

Grifiiths' point

Celiac a.

Pancreatico-duodenal a.

Ao

Arc of Riolan

SMA
IMA

Marginal a.

IIA

Sudeck's point

Hemorrhoidal aa. { Superior Middle Inferior

Table 13.16 Mallory–Weiss syndrome

A 1–4 cm submucosal tear occurring at the gastroesophageal junction usually following forceful retching. The lesion is diagnosed on EGD. Brisk bleeding will require surgical repair by the creation of an open high gastrotomy and oversewing the bleeding ends. Alternatively, with less brisk bleeding, the lesion can be controlled with endoscopic electrocautery.

Trauma

Trauma is the leading cause of death in the United States for individuals <45 yrs. Death as a result of trauma can occur immediately as a result of hemorrhage, severe head injury, loss of airway, pneumothorax, and fatal heart injury. Other causes of death can be less immediate and include sepsis and multiple organ system failure. Surgical training under the auspices of Advanced Trauma Life Support (ATLS) has produced an algorithm for maximizing the care of the trauma patient. The basics of this algorithm are the ABCDE of primary survey in trauma care:

A. Airway and cervical spine protection An airway can be maintained with a simple jaw thrust and bagging. A definitive airway can be established either by orotracheal, nasotracheal, or surgical means and is indicated in apnea, inability to maintain airway or oxygenation by other means, and for airway protection in inhalation injuries, head injuries, etc.

i. Spinal cord injuries must be assumed in all patients and therefore inline manual cervical traction should be used during intubation.

ii. A surgical airway should be performed through the cricothyroid membrane when oral or nasotracheal intubation cannot be successfully performed.

B. Breathing and ventilation Expose the chest to assess breathing. Keep an eye out for the following disorders that will inhibit adequate breathing:

i. *Tension pneumothorax:* Hypotension with distended neck veins; treat initially with large-bore IV placed in the second intercostals space in the mid-clavicular line.

ii. *Flail chest:* Multiple rib fractures often associated with pneumothorax and pulmonary contusion.

iii. *Massive hemorrhage and hemothorax:* Requires thoracostomy and possibly thoracotomy if >1,000 cc drain immediately or patient becomes hemodynamically unstable.

iv. *Open pneumothorax:* Initial treatment is the placement of a sterile occlusive dressing taped on three sides with a flutter valve. Definite treatment is a chest tube.

C. Circulation

i. *Shock:* Recognize and resuscitate with 0.9% NS or LR. Assume hemorrhage and be prepared to give O-neg blood. Other causes of shock in trauma include tamponade, tension pneumothorax, air embolus, myocardial contusion, and spinal cord injury resulting in neurogenic shock. *Cardiac tamponade* can be diagnosed on bedside US (focused assessment with sonography for trauma—FAST). Management usually requires pericardial window.

ii. Interventions:

1. Apply direct pressure to external bleeding.
2. Two large-caliber IVS and possibly cordis for large-volume rapid infusion.
3. Infusion of warmed crystalloid using 3:1 rule and give type-specific or O-neg blood for class III or IV shock (see Table 13.17).
4. Send patient's blood for type and cross-match, hemoglobin, chemistries, β-HCG in female patients.

Table 13.17 Classes of shock

Class I. Blood volume loss <15% associated with mild tachycardia
Class II. Blood volume loss 15–30%. Signs include tachycardia, tachypnea, ↓ pulse pressure
Class III. Blood volume loss of 30–40%. Marked tachycardia and tachypnea, hypotension and confusion
Class IV. Blood volume loss of >40%. Severe tachycardia, hypotension, narrow pulse pressure, obtundation

---

Table 13.18 Glasgow Coma Scale

Assessment of eye opening (1–4)
Assessment of verbal response (1–5)
Assessment of motor response (1–6)
If total is >8, high potential for severe CNS injury.

D. Disability Refers to a brief neurologic assessment via a measurement for the level of consciousness, also known as the Glasgow Coma Scale (see Table 13.18). Altered mental status may be the result of hypoxia, shock, drugs, alcohol, but consider injury to the central nervous system until proven otherwise.

E. Exposure Undress the patient to evaluate every area to make sure no injury is missed. Broken bones are commonly missed in the intoxicated trauma patient. Once this is done, the patient should be covered to prevent hypothermia.

Following the primary survey for trauma, a secondary survey is undertaken. This begins with an AMPLE history: Allergies, Medicines, Past medical and surgical history, Last meal, Exposures (tetanus). A complete head-to-toe examination is performed and vital signs are reassessed. Any further interventions are arranged.

F. FAST (Focused Assessment with US in Trauma) Exam Bedside US examination of the chest and abdomen to evaluate for free fluid in the pericardium or abdomen.

Indications: Thoracoabdominal trauma in an unstable patient.

Evaluation: Rapid, sequential exam of the pericardial sac, right upper quadrant (RUQ) interface between the liver and kidney, left upper quadrant (LUQ) splenorenal fossa, pelvic area around bladder.

Aortic aneurysm and dissection

Aortic aneurysm True aneurysms are abnormal dilatations of arteries. They should be distinguished from "false" aneurysms, which are collections of blood around a vessel wall (e.g., following trauma). Aneurysms may be fusiform or sac-like (e.g., berry aneurysms in the Circle of Willis).

Common sites: Aorta, iliac, femoral, and popliteal arteries. Atheroma is the usual cause; also connective tissue disorders (e.g., Marfan's, Ehlers–Danlos) and infections (e.g., endocarditis or tertiary syphilis). *Complications from aneurysms:* Rupture, thrombosis, embolism, pressure on other structures, infection.

Symptomatic and ruptured abdominal aortic aneurysm (AAA)

Signs and symptoms: Intermittent or continuous abdominal pain (radiates to back, lower abdomen, or groins), collapse, an expansile abdominal mass (i.e., the mass expands and contracts: Swellings that are pulsatile merely transmit the pulse; e.g., nodes overlying arteries), and mottling over the lower extremities. Other associated findings in patients with AAA include hypertension ~40%, peripheral aneurysms ~20%. The main differential diagnoses are myocardial infarction and pancreatitis. If in doubt, assume a ruptured aneurysm.

Management:

1 Start two large-bore IVs.
2 Send type and cross-match for 12 units, CBC, electrolytes, ECG, and, if in doubt, cross-table lateral plain film of the abdomen, which will demonstrate aortic calcification.
3 Take the patient to the operating room. Do not order other investigations. You will waste precious time.
4 The patient is prepped and draped while awake and only put to sleep when the surgeon is ready to cut. Surgery involves clamping the aorta above the leak (usually at the diaphragmatic hiatus). Alternatively, a large-bore Foley can be placed in the proximal end of the aorta and inflated to temporarily tamponade the bleeding. A Dacron® graft (e.g., "tube graft" or, if significant iliac aneurysm also, a "trouser graft" with each "leg" attached

to an iliac artery) may be used to replace the ruptured aorta. Presently, the role of endoluminal placement of stent grafts for ruptured AAA is being investigated (see below).

Outcomes: Mortality when treated: 21–70%; untreated: 100%.

Asymptomatic AAA

Prevalence: 3% of those >50 yrs. Trials suggest that aneurysms <5.5 cm across might safely be monitored by regular examination and US/CT. Risk of rupture below this size is <1%/ yr, compared with ~25%/yr for aneurysms >6 cm across. Aneurysms larger than this, rapidly expanding (>1 cm/ yr), or symptomatic should be considered for elective surgery. It should be noted that ~75% of aneurysms monitored in this way will eventually need repair. Elective operative mortality is ~5%. Studies show that age >80 yrs is not a reason to decline surgery.

Open elective and emergent operations can be avoided by the placement of an endoluminal stent, also known as EVAR (endovascular aneurysm repair). 60% of all aneurysm repairs are done via EVAR. Indicated in patients with suitable anatomy and at high risk for conventional repair. 50% will not have suitable anatomy. EVAR is associated with shorter hospital stays and fewer transfusions than conventional surgery. There is also a risk that the stent will leak.

Types of Endoleaks

Type	Description
I	Inadequate seal at proximal or distal attachment site
II	Flow into aortic aneurysmal sac from branch vessel (lumbar)
III	Endograft fabric tear or failure of seal between component grafts
IV	Endograft fabric porosity

Preparation for surgery is similar to the above preparation, with the addition of a preoperative cardiac and pulmonary evaluation. A mechanical bowel prep is preferred. Urinalysis should be performed and antibiotics given prior to incision.

Postoperative care and complications: Patients will usually spend time in the ICU postoperatively. Peripheral pulses are monitored. The most common complications following aortic surgery include:

1 *Renal insufficiency:* Usually hypovolemic, but you must be concerned about injury from aortic cross-clamping leading to embolization.
2 *Ischemic colitis:* Secondary to inferior mesenteric artery (IMA) ligation. Can start as early as 12 h after surgery.
3 *Spinal cord ischemia:* Occurs when the blood supply to the distal spinal cord is compromised and results in paraplegia. The injured artery is the artery of Adamkiewicz and can arise anywhere from T8 to L4.

Aorta dissection

Blood splits aortic media with sudden tearing chest pain (± radiation to back). As dissection unfolds, branches of the aorta occlude, leading sequentially to hemiplegia (carotid), unequal arm pulses and BP, paraplegia (anterior spinal artery), and anuria (renal arteries). Aortic valve incompetence and myocardial ischemia may develop if dissection moves proximally. Aortic dissection is classified according to the Stanford classification (Table 13.19).

Management: Type A dissections: Because of the risk of intrapericardial rupture and left ventricular failure, all patients with type A dissections should be considered for surgery. Cross-match 10 U blood; do ECG and CXR (expanded mediastinum is rare). Perform CT/MRI or transesophageal echocardiography (TEE). Admit to ICU. *If hypertensive:* Keep systolic at

Table 13.19 Stanford classification

Type A. Primary intimal tear located in the ascending aorta
Two-thirds of all dissections
Ehlers–Danlos syndrome, Marfan's
Type B. Dissection limited to the descending thoracic aorta with the intimal tear located near the subclavian artery
One-third of all dissections
Ruptured atherosclerotic plaque

~100–110 mm Hg; labetalol (p. 135) or esmolol (p. 122; t½ is ultra-short) by IVI is helpful here. Perioperative mortality: 12%.

Type B dissections: May extend and cause symptoms as a result of poor flow to peripheral vessels. Symptomatic extension is treated surgically or by endovascular techniques with fenestration, stenting, or bypass. To prevent extension, antihypertensive therapy is started.

Limb ischemia

Chronic ischemia is due to atherosclerosis. Its chief feature is *intermittent claudication* (from the Latin meaning "to limp"). Cramping pain is felt in the calf, thigh, or buttock after walking for a fairly fixed distance (the claudication distance). Ulceration, gangrene, and foot pain at rest (e.g., burning pain at night relieved by hanging legs over side of bed) are cardinal features of critical ischemia. See Figure 13.6.

Signs: Absent pulses; cold, white leg(s); atrophic skin; punched out ulcers (often painful); postural color change.

Tests: Exclude DM, arteritis (erythrocyte sedimentation rate/c-reactive protein [ESR/CRP]). Do CBC (anemia, infection), electrolytes (renal disease), lipids (dyslipidemia), syphilis serology, ECG (cardiac ischemia). Do coagulation profile and type and cross-match if planning arteriography. *Ankle—brachial pressure index (Doppler):* Normal = 1. Claudication = 0.9–0.6. Rest pain = 0.3–0.6. Impending gangrene ≤0.3 or ankle systolic pressure <50 mm Hg. Do *arteriography, digital subtraction arteriography, or color duplex imaging* to assess the extent and location of stenoses and the quality of distal vessels (run off). If only distal obliterative disease is seen, with little proximal atheroma, suspect arteritis, previous embolus, or diabetes mellitus.

Management: Symptoms improve with conservative treatment; i.e., quit smoking, lose weight, get more exercise—ideally a supervised exercise program. Treat diabetes, hypertension (avoid β-blockers), and hyperlipidemia. Aspirin has a role. Vasodilators rarely help.

Percutaneous transluminal angioplasty is good for short stenoses in big arteries (a balloon is inflated in the narrowed segment). Stents maintain artery patency after angioplasty and are beneficial for iliac artery disease. If atheromatous disease is extensive but distal run off is good (i.e., distal arteries filled by collateral vessels), the patient may be a candidate for arterial reconstruction by a bypass graft. Vein grafts are often used but prosthetic grafts are an option. Aspirin helps prosthetic grafts to remain patent; warfarin may be better after vein grafts and in high-risk patients.

Sympathectomy (chemical or surgical) may help relieve rest pain. It may not be appropriate in diabetic patients with peripheral neuropathy.

Amputation may relieve intractable pain and death from sepsis and gangrene. The decision to amputate must be made by the patient, usually against a background of failed alternative strategies. The level of amputation must be high enough to ensure healing of the stump. Rehabilitation should be started early with a view to limb fitting.

Acute ischemia may be due to thrombosis in situ (in ~41%), emboli (38%), graft/angioplasty occlusion (15%), or trauma. There is little difference in presenting signs. *Mortality: 22%. Amputation rate: 16%.*

Figure 13.6

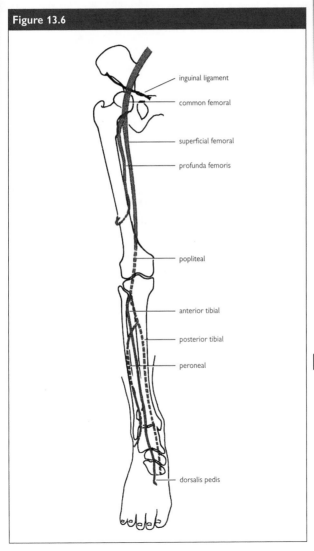

inguinal ligament

common femoral

superficial femoral

profunda femoris

popliteal

anterior tibial

posterior tibial

peroneal

dorsalis pedis

Signs and symptoms: The 5 Ps: The limb is **p**ulseless, **p**ainful, **p**allid, **p**araesthetic, and **p**aralyzed. Onset of fixed mottling implies irreversibility. Emboli commonly arise from the heart (infarcts, atrial fibrillation [AF]) or an aneurysm (aorta, femoral, or popliteal). The limb may be red, but only when dependent, leading to disastrous misdiagnosis of gout or cellulitis.

Management: This is an emergency and may require urgent surgery or angioplasty. Ischemia of <12 h is associated with 93% limb salvage rate, whereas ischemic time of >12 h is associated with only a 78% limb salvage rate and a 30% mortality. If diagnosis is in doubt, do urgent arteriography. If the occlusion is embolic, the options are surgical embolectomy (Fogarty catheter) or local thrombolysis (e.g., t-PA [p. 622]). Anticoagulate with heparin before and after either procedure. Later, look for the embolic source: Echocardiogram; US of aorta and popliteal and femoral arteries. Ischemia following trauma and acute thrombosis may require urgent reconstruction.

Acute appendicitis

Appendicitis is primarily a disease of adolescents and young adults and is uncommon in individuals >55 yrs. The ♀:♂ ratio is 1.2:1.5. Although the incidence of acute appendicitis approaches 20% in some reports, there has been a notable decline in the incidence for all age groups over the past 30 yrs.

Pathogenesis Epidemiologists have demonstrated that genetic, dietary, and infectious factors are associated with development of acute appendicitis. Appendiceal inflammation results from luminal obstruction of the appendiceal orifice lymphoid hyperplasia, fecalith, or filarial worms. This inflammation allows for invasion of GI organisms through the appendix wall. There may also be impaired ability to prevent invasion.

Symptoms Often referred to as the "great masquerader," the diagnosis of acute appendicitis is not always straightforward. A careful review of symptoms is essential. See Table 13.20.

Pain is the most important symptom. In general, as inflammation begins, central abdominal colic occurs as a result of stimulation of the visceral pain fibers. Once the peritoneum becomes inflamed, the pain shifts to the right lower quadrant (RLQ) and becomes more constant. On examination, RLQ point tenderness (↑ pain on palpation) or rebound tenderness (↑ pain on release) may be present. Look for Rovsing's sign (pain more in the RLQ than in the left LQ (LLQ) when the LLQ is pressed). RLQ pain may also be elicited on rectal exam. In women, do a vaginal examination: Does she have cervical motion tenderness or discharge? Reexamine frequently if unsure of diagnosis.

Table 13.20 Other signs and symptoms of appendicitis

- Tachycardia
- Lying still
- Flushing
- Low-grade fever
- Leukocytosis
- Anorexia
- Rare vomiting, diarrhea, or constipation

Essential studies

CBC: To evaluate for a leukocytosis

Urinalysis: Evaluate for WBCs and bacteria indicating bladder infection (can be misleading), and red blood cells (RBCs), which may suggest kidney stone.

β-*HCG*: R/O pregnancy (ectopic)

Additional studies

Abdominal X-rays: Usually demonstrates a paucity of gas in the RLQ. May also see fecalith.

Abdominal CT scan: Highly sensitive (0.94) for appendiceal inflammation (thickening of appendiceal wall) but cannot always separate acute and chronic inflammation.

CT signs of acute appendicitis:

1. Thick wall >2 mm
2. Increased diameter (7 mm) with target sign
3. Appendicolith (seen in 25%)
4. Phlegmon, abscess, or free fluid

Abdominal US: Sensitive for evaluation of ovarian cyst or abscess, hydrosalpinx.

Differential diagnosis	Cholecystitis	Crohn's disease
Ectopic pregnancy	Diverticulitis	Ovarian cyst or abscess
Mesenteric adenitis	Salpingitis	Kidney stone
Cystitis	Menstrual cramps	Meckel's diverticulitis

Complications of acute appendicitis Perforation (does not appear to cause later infertility in girls), appendix mass, appendix abscess.

An appendix mass may result when an inflamed appendix becomes covered with omentum or loops of small bowel. The mass is palpable on exam and easily seen on abdominal CT scan. Some advocate early surgery, but initial management is usually conservative—NPO and antibiotics (e.g., cefuroxime 1.5 g/8 h IV and metronidazole 500 mg/8 h IV). Mark out the size of the mass and proceed to drainage if the mass develops into an abscess (see below). If the mass resolves, some perform an interval (i.e., delayed) appendicectomy. See Table 13.21.

An appendix abscess may result if an appendix mass fails to resolve. Signs of abscess formation include enlargement of the mass or the patient becoming more toxic (pain↑, temperature↑, pulse↑, WBC↑). Treatment usually involves drainage, either surgical or percutaneous (under radiological guidance). Antibiotics alone may bring about resolution (e.g., in >90% of children).

Table 13.21 Appendicitis in pregnancy

Appendicitis occurs in ~1/1,000 pregnancies. Mortality is higher, especially from 20 wks of gestation. Perforation (15–20%), and ↑ fetal mortality from ~1.5% (for simple appendicitis) to ~30%. As pregnancy progresses, the appendix migrates, so pain is often less well localized. Prompt assessment is vital; laparotomy should be performed by an experienced surgeon.

Surgical treatment

Once decision is made to operate, make patient NPO and hydrate with NS. Metronidazole 1 g/8 h + cefuroxime 1.5 g/8 h, 1–3 doses IV starting 1 h preop reduces wound infections. Appendectomy is performed laparoscopically or through a RLQ incision at McBurney's Point (one-third the distance between the anterior superior iliac crest and the umbilicus). Some surgical hints include:

- Laparoscopic appendectomy reduces recovery time and incidence of wound infections, but increases risk of intra-abdominal abscesses.
- If the appendix is perforated, most advocate closing the fascia but leaving the wound open for closure by secondary intention.
- If the appendiceal stump is difficult to locate and close, and the appendix has ruptured, leave a drain because patient is at risk to develop GI leak and fistula.
- If the appendix is associated with an unusual mass, always think of carcinoid or cystadenoma of the appendix. These tumors may cause luminal obstruction and lead to appendicitis. Larger tumors (>2 cm) will require formal right hemicolectomy, which should be performed at the time of surgery or once pathology is confirmed.

Diverticular disease

A *diverticulum* is an out-pouching of the wall of the gut. The term *diverticulosis* means that diverticula are present, whereas *diverticular disease* implies that they are symptomatic. *Diverticulitis* refers to inflammation within a diverticulum. Although diverticula may be congenital or acquired and can occur in any part of the gut, by far the most important type is acquired colonic diverticula, to which this section refers.

Pathogenesis Most occur in the sigmoid colon, with 95% of complications at this site, but right-sided, as well as small bowel diverticula, do occur. Lack of dietary fiber is thought to lead to high intraluminal pressures that force the mucosa to herniate through the muscular bowel wall near where vessels penetrate the wall. Nearly 50% of the population in the Western world >50 has diverticulosis.

Symptoms 15–30% of patients with diverticulosis have symptomatic diverticular disease. The most common symptoms is LLQ pain. Pain usually occurs after eating and persists. Associated symptoms include low-grade fever, diarrhea or obstipation, and anorexia. Rarely do patients experience nausea or vomiting. On exam, LLQ point and rebound tenderness may be present.

Complications of diverticular disease

Free perforation: A free communication exists between the colon and the peritoneal cavity. There is ileus, peritonitis ± shock. Free fluid in air is noted on imaging studies.

Hemorrhage: Is usually sudden and painless. It is a common cause of big rectal bleeds. Bleeding usually stops with bed rest.

Fistula:

- Colovesical: Complaints of pneumaturia (air in urine stream) or fecaluria (feces in urine stream)
- Colovaginal: Complaints of fecal vaginal discharge
- Coloenteric: Complaints of persistent diarrhea

Abscess: E.g., with swinging fever, leukocytosis, and localizing signs (e.g., boggy rectal mass).

Postinfective strictures may form in the sigmoid colon and present with large bowel obstruction.

Studies CBC, urine analysis and culture.

Uncomplicated diverticulitis:

- ABD and pelvic CT scan initially
- Colonoscopy or barium enema once symptoms resolve to R/O cancer.

Complicated diverticular disease:

- AXR to R/O free air
- CT cystogram to R/O colovesical fistula
- Barium enema to R/O colovaginal fistula
- Small bowel series to R/O coloenteric fistula
- Colonoscopy to R/O cancer.

Treatment

Uncomplicated diverticular disease:

- A 7–14 d course of IV or oral antibiotics (ciprofloxacin 500 mg bid and Flagyl® 250–500 mg PO tid)
- Keep NPO till pain resolves.
- Avoid narcotics, which may constipate.
- Encourage a *high-fiber diet* with dietary supplements (Metamucil®)
- *Antispasmodics* such as Bentyl® 10 mg PO 4α a day.
- Repetitive attacks requiring hospitalization of documented diverticular disease should be treated with either laparoscopic or open surgical resection of the diseased colon.
- Recurrence of LLQ pain after surgery is more common in patients who have not had a complete resection of the distal sigmoid and in patients with irritable bowel syndrome (IBS) as well as diverticular disease.

Complicated diverticular disease

Free perforation: Laparotomy, a Hartman's procedure may be used (temporary end colostomy + partial colectomy or "perforectomy"). It is sometimes possible to do on-table colon lavage via the appendix stump, then immediate anastomosis (so avoiding repeat surgery to close the colostomy).

Hemorrhage: Transfusion may be needed. Highly selective embolization or colonic resection may be necessary after locating bleeding points by angiography or colonoscopy (cautery ± local epinephrine injections may obviate the need for surgery). If bleeding site is identified and surgery is necessary, a limited resection can be performed. Otherwise, a total abdominal colectomy with either an ileostomy or ileorectal anastomosis is performed.

Fistula: Treatment is surgical (e.g., laparoscopic or open colonic resection, as well as removal of the fistula). Successful laparoscopic resection is less likely when a fistula is present. The most common site for a colovesical fistula is the dome of the bladder. The trigone may on occasion be involved and, if so, consider urology consult for stents and reconstruction. Consider urology consult for stents and reconstruction.

Abscess: Antibiotics ± CT- or US-guided drainage may be needed. This should be followed by definitive resection in 6 wks or sooner if no clinical improvement (<25%).

Postinfective strictures: Stent colon if necessary and prep if possible to perform a primary anastomosis.

Hernias

Any congenital or acquired defect in a musculoaponeurotic structure through which an epithelialized or peritonealized sac protrudes. Hernias involving bowel are said to be *irreducible* if they cannot be pushed back into the right place. This does not mean that they are either necessarily obstructed or strangulated. Gastrointestinal hernias are *obstructed* if bowel contents cannot pass through them—the classical features of intestinal obstruction soon appear. *Strangulated* hernias are a result of ischemia to the bowel and require urgent surgery. See Figure 13.7.

Sites of hernias

Inguinal hernia: See p. 483.

Pantaloon hernia: Both indirect and direct inguinal hernias occurring in the same patient.

Femoral hernia: Bowel enters the femoral canal, presenting as a mass in the upper medial thigh or above the inguinal ligament, where it points down the leg, unlike an inguinal hernia, which points to the groin. They occur more often in women than men and are likely to be irreducible and to strangulate. *Anatomy:* The neck of the hernia is felt below and lateral to the pubic tubercle (inguinal hernias are above and medial to this point). The boundaries of the femoral canal are anterior and medial to the inguinal ligament; laterally to the femoral vein and posteriorly to the pectineal ligament. The canal contains fat and Cloquet's node. *Treatment:* Surgical repair is recommended.

Paraumbilical hernias: These occur just above or below the umbilicus. Risk factors are obesity and ascites. Omentum or bowel herniates through the defect. Surgery involves repair of the rectus sheath.

Epigastric hernias: These pass through the linea alba above the umbilicus.

Incisional hernias; These follow breakdown of muscle closure after previous surgery (seen in 11–20%). If obese, repair is not easy. A randomized trial of repairs favored mesh over suture techniques.

Spigelian hernias: These occur at the lateral edge of the rectus sheath, below and lateral to the umbilicus.

Lumbar hernias: These occur through one of the lumbar triangles.

Richter's hernia: This involves bowel wall only—not lumen.

Obturator hernias: These occur through the obturator canal. Typically, there is pain along the medial side of the thigh in a thin woman.

Levator hernias: These occur when fat or rectum balloons out the levator muscles of the pelvic floor

Other examples of hernias

- Of the nucleus pulposus into the spinal canal (slipped disc)
- Of the uncus and hippocampal gyrus through the tentorium (tentorial hernia) in space-occupying lesions
- Of the brainstem and cerebellum through the foramen magnum (Arnold–Chiari malformation)
- Of the stomach through the diaphragm (hiatal hernia [p. 209])
- Of the terminal (intravesical) portion of the ureter into the bladder, with cystic ballooning between the mucosa and muscle layers. This is a *ureterocele* and results from stenosis of the ureteral meatus.

Symptoms

- Reducible hernias are associated with a dull ache and bulge that go away with recumbency and worsen with physical activity. A neuralgia can occur from injury to a sensory nerve lying at the site of the hernia (i.e., ilioinguinal nerve and the inguinal hernia or obturator nerve and the obturator canal).
- Incarcerated or strangulated hernias (5%) will be associated with more severe pain, nausea, and vomiting.

Figure 13.7 Some examples of hernias

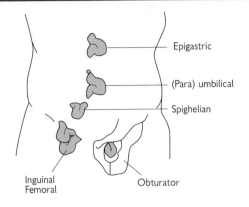

- Epigastric
- (Para) umbilical
- Spighelian
- Inguinal Femoral
- Obturator

Reproduced with permission from PA Grace & N Borley 2002, 'Surgery at a Glance', Blackwell Science

Treatment

- Symptomatic hernias should be considered for operative repair. Patients should be encouraged to lose weight and to stop smoking to improve the outcome of hernia repair. Several trials of laparoscopic repair for large incarcerated hernias using in-lay versus on-lay mesh have demonstrated improved outcomes.
- If incarcerated, a trial of gentle reduction with manual pressure can be attempted.
- Strangulated hernias should be operatively repaired immediately.

Inguinal hernias

Indirect hernias pass through the internal inguinal ring as a result of incomplete closure of the processus vaginalis at birth (see Table 13.22 and Figure 13.8). Direct hernias enter through the posterior wall of the inguinal canal through an acquired defect in the transverses abdominus aponeurosis and transversalis fascia. Overall, indirect hernias are more common than direct hernias. However, direct hernias are more common in adults and indirect are more common in children. The anatomic landmark distinguishing these hernias is the inferior epigastric artery: Indirect is lateral, direct is medial through *Hesselbach's triangle*: Medial edge of rectus abdominis, lateral edge of inferior epigastric artery, and inferior edge of inguinal ligament.

Predisposing conditions include chronic cough, constipation, urinary obstruction, heavy lifting, ascites, previous abdominal surgery, prematurity.

Relations of the inguinal canal

Floor: Inguinal ligament
Roof: Fibers of transversalis and internal oblique
Front: External oblique aponeurosis + internal oblique for the lateral
Back: Laterally, transversalis fascia; medially, conjoined tendon

Table 13.22 Contents of the inguinal canal

- Spermatic cord in men
- Round ligament in women
- Testicular artery
- Deferential vessel
- Pampiniform plexus of veins
- Ilioinguinal nerve
- Genital branch of the genitofemoral nerve
- Cremasteric artery and muscle
- Internal spermatic fascia

Examining the patient Always look for previous scars, feel the other side, and examine the external genitalia. Then ask: Is the lump visible? If so, ask the patient to reduce it; if he cannot, make sure that it is not a scrotal lump. Ask him to cough. Inguinal hernias appear inferomedial to the external ring. If no lump is visible, feel for a cough impulse. If there is no lump, ask the patient to stand and repeat the cough.

Irreducible hernias You may be called because a long-standing hernia is now irreducible and painful. It is always worth trying to reduce these yourself to prevent strangulation and bowel necrosis (a grave event, demanding prompt laparotomy). Use the flat of the hand, direct the hernia from below, up toward the contralateral shoulder. Sometimes, as the hernia obstructs, reduction requires perseverance, which may be rewarded with a gurgle from the retreating bowel. This can spare unnecessary surgery.

Surgical repairs Advise patients to diet and stop smoking preop. Laparoscopic and open mesh techniques (e.g., Lichtenstein repair) have replaced other methods briefly described here:

Shouldice repair: Multilayered suture involving both anterior and posterior walls of the inguinal canal

Bassini repair: Floor of inguinal canal approximates the rectus sheath and to the shelving edge of the inguinal ligament (Poupart ligament)

McVay repair or Cooper's ligament repair approximates the floor of the inguinal canal to Cooper's ligament between the pubic tubercle to the femoral vein.

In mesh repairs, a polypropylene mesh reinforces the posterior wall. Recurrence rate is lower (<2% mesh vs. 10% no mesh). Local anaesthetic techniques have led to day-case ambulatory surgery. Laparoscopic repair is also possible and gives similar recurrence rates. This can be done through the peritoneal cavity or through a pre-peritoneal approach. There is less postoperative pain and an earlier return to work after a laparoscopic repair, and undiagnosed contralateral hernias can be identified. Care must be taken to avoid injury to the iliohypogastric nerve, which may occur by placing a holding tack too far laterally along the abdominal wall. This results in severe chronic pain.

Figure 13.8

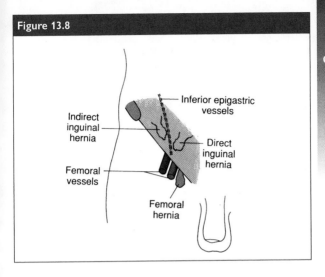

Labels in figure:
- Indirect inguinal hernia
- Inferior epigastric vessels
- Direct inguinal hernia
- Femoral vessels
- Femoral hernia

Benign diseases of the biliary tract

Bile contains cholesterol, bile pigments (from broken-down Hb), and phospholipids. If the concentrations of these vary, different kinds of stones may be formed. Stones cause chronic inflammation ± colic. See Figure 13.9.

- *Pigment stones:* Most common type of stone worldwide; small, friable, and irregular. *Causes:* Hemolysis
- *Cholesterol stones:* Most common type of stone in the United States; large, often solitary. *Causes:* Female sex, age, obesity
- *Mixed stones:* Faceted (calcium salts, pigment, and cholesterol)

Gallstone prevalence 8% of those >40 yrs. 90% remain asymptomatic and for these no treatment is commonly offered.

Biliary colic Follows stone impaction in the neck of the gall bladder (GB), which may cause epigastric or RUQ pain after eating fatty foods.

Acute cholecystitis Pain, fevers, and WBC↑ with +ve US findings is suggestive of cholecystitis. Other symptoms include nausea and vomiting. If the stone moves to the CBD, jaundice may occur.

Murphy's sign: Press over the RUQ. Ask the patient to breathe in. This causes pain and arrest of inspiration as an inflamed GB is impinged. It is only +ve if the same test in the LUQ does not cause pain.

Acalculous cholecystitis Pain, fever, and WBC↑ with biliary stasis and delayed GB emptying on hepatic iminodiacetic acid (HIDA) without evidence of stones. Commonly seen in critically ill, immunosuppressed patients and in patients on TPN.

Chronic cholecystitis Vague abdominal discomfort, distension, nausea, flatulence, and intolerance of fats may also be caused by reflux, ulcers, irritable bowel syndrome, relapsing pancreatitis, or tumor (stomach, pancreas, colon, GB). US is used to image stones, and to assess common

bile duct (CBD) diameter. Magnetic resonance cholangiopancreaticogram (MRCP, p. 222) is increasingly being used to check for stones in the CBD.
Complications of gallstones

Obstructive jaundice with CBD stones: RUQ pain and jaundice; unusual to have a total bilirubin >10 mg/dL.

Cholangitis: Bile duct infection usually resulting from a blocked duct. Charcot's triad RUQ pain, jaundice, and fevers; Reynolds' pentad with the addition of hypotension and mental status changes; worse prognosis.

Gallstone ileus: A stone perforates the GB entering the duodenum; it may then obstruct the terminal ileum. X-ray shows air in CBD, small bowel fluid levels, and a stone. Duodenal obstruction is rarer (Bouveret's syndrome).

Pancreatitis: See p. 487.

Empyema of the gallbladder: The obstructed GB fills with pus.

Mirizzi syndrome: Impaction of the cystic duct with a large stone causing obstruction of the CBD.

Tests WBC, RUQ us (thickened GB wall, pericholecystic fluid, and stones), HIDA cholescintigraphy to check for GB emptying (useful if diagnosis uncertain after US).

MRCP images the bile duct for the presence of stones. Gallstones are only radiopaque on plain abdominal films in ~10% of cases.

Medical management NPO, pain relief (avoid morphine, which may cause sphincter of Oddi dysfunction), IV fluids, and antibiotics if evidence of inflammation/infection; common organisms include *E. coli,* Enterococci, and *Klebsiella* (e.g., cefuroxime 1.5 g/8 h IV and metronidazole 500 mg/8 h IV, or Zosyn 3.375 mg/6 h IV).

Surgical treatment Cholecystectomy (e.g., laparoscopic). If US or MRCP shows a dilated CBD with stones, endoscopic retrograde cholangiopancreatography (ERCP) with sphincterotomy is used to remove stones, usually prior to surgery or at the time of surgery with CBD exploration (if there is no obstruction/cholangitis). A stone-trapping basket on the end of a choledochoscope introduced through the cystic duct at laparoscopy can be done. In suitable candidates, do laparoscopic cholecystectomy within 72 h; early surgery is associated with fewer complications and lower conversion rates to open cholecystectomy. *Mortality:* <1%. If delayed, relapse occurs in 18%. Otherwise, operate after 6–12 wks. In elderly or high-risk patients unsuitable for surgery, percutaneous cholecystostomy may be useful; cholecystectomy can still be performed at a later date.

Complications of laparoscopic cholecystectomy

Injury to the right hepatic duct, accessory duct, or common bile duct: All will require drainage of biloma and possible intrahepatic biliary drain. Depending on the site of injury, reconstruction with a Roux-en-Y choledochojejunostomy may have to be performed.

Figure 13.9

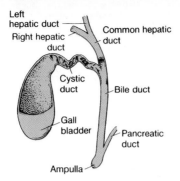

Left hepatic duct
Right hepatic duct
Common hepatic duct
Cystic duct
Bile duct
Gall bladder
Pancreatic duct
Ampulla

Reproduced from Cunningham. *Manual of Practical Anatomy*, 14th ed., Vol. 2. New York: Oxford University Press, 1997; 138, with kind permission.

Pancreatitis

Pancreatic inflammation results in injury to the gland and the surrounding retroperitoneal tissue; most common in adults >30 yrs. Overall mortality is 6–20%. There may be rapid progression from a phase of mild edema of the pancreas associated with fluid sequestration to one of necrotizing pancreatitis. In fulminating cases, the pancreas is replaced by gray-black necrotic material. Death may be from shock, renal failure, sepsis, or respiratory failure, with contributory factors being protease-induced activation of complement, kinin, and the fibrinolytic and coagulation cascades. May be acute or chronic.

Causes "GET SMASHED": *G*allstones, *E*thanol, *T*rauma, *S*teroids, *M*umps, *A*utoimmune (PAN), *S*corpion venom, *H*yperlipidemia ($\uparrow Ca^{2+}$, hypothermia), *E*RCP(also emboli), *D*rugs (e.g., azathioprine, asparaginase, mercaptopurine, pentamidine, didanosine, diuretics); also pregnancy. Often none is found.

Symptoms Gradual or sudden severe epigastric or central abdominal pain (radiates to back); vomiting with signs of gastric outlet obstruction are prominent.

Signs Tachycardia, fever, jaundice, shock, ileus, rigid abdomen ± local/generalized tenderness and periumbilical discoloration *Cullen's sign* or, at the flanks, *Grey Turner's sign*.

Tests No test is pathognomonic. Serum amylase elevation (amylase may be normal even in severe pancreatitis as amylase starts to fall within the 1st 24–48 h; levels may be abnormally elevated secondary to renal failure or alternative source—salivary gland, fallopian tube). Serum lipase is derived from pancreatic acinar cells, and elevation may indicate acinar cell injury. Blood gases. Biochemical analysis. *Abdominal Ims:* No psoas shadow (retroperitoneal fluid↑), "sentinel loop" of proximal jejunum (solitary air-filled dilatation). CT helps assess severity. US (if gallstones). ERCP. *Differential diagnosis:* Any acute abdomen (p. 466), myocardial infarct.

Management

- NPO (may need NGT)
- IV fluid resuscitation with 0.9% saline until vital signs are satisfactory and urine flows at >30 mL/h. If shocked or elderly, consider CVP. Insert a urinary catheter.
- *Analgesia:* Demerol 75–100 mg/4 h IM, or morphine (a better analgesic, but *may* cause Oddi's sphincter to contract more) + prochlorperazine.
- Hourly pulse, BP, and urine flow; daily CBC, *Comprehensive panel:* Glucose, amylase, lipase, blood gas—about one-third of patients will have respiratory compromise. Supplemental O_2 if $P_aO_{2\downarrow}$ is low.
- In suspected abscess formation or pancreatic necrosis (on contrast-enhanced CT), consider parenteral nutrition ± laparotomy and debridement. Antibiotics may help in *severe* disease.
- ERCP + gallstone removal may be needed if there is progressive jaundice.

Prognosis (See Table 13.23.) Several grading systems exist. Presently, the APACHE II score is used to assess the likelihood of mortality. Some patients suffer recurrent pancreatitis so often that near-total pancreatectomy is contemplated. Evidence is accumulating that oxidant stress is important here, but initial clinical trials of free radical scavengers have been disappointing.

Complications *Early:* Shock, ARDS (p. 185), renal failure, DIC, $Ca^{2+}\downarrow$ (10 mL of 10% calcium gluconate IV [slow replacement] is rarely necessary; albumin replacement has also been tried), glucose↑ (transient; 5% need insulin). *Later (>1 wk):* Pancreatic necrosis, pseudocyst (fluid in lesser sac, e.g., at ≥6 wks), with fever, a mass, and persistent ↑amylase/LFTs. It may resolve or need drainage, externally or into the stomach (may be laparoscopically). Abscesses need draining. Bleeding is from elastase eroding a major vessel (e.g., splenic artery); embolization of the artery may be life-saving. Thrombosis may occur in the splenic and gastroduodenal arteries, or in the colic branches of the SMA, causing bowel necrosis.

Table 13.23 Ransom criteria

On admission
- Age >55 yrs
- WBC >16,000/uL
- Glucose >200 mg/dL
- LDH >350 IU/L
- SGOT >250 IU/L

After 48 h
- Hct ↓ 10%
- BUN ↑ 5 mg/dL
- Ca^{2+} <8 mg/dL
- P_aO_2 <60 mm Hg
- Base deficit >4 mEq/L
- Fluid sequestration >6 L
- Mortality is 30% if 3 criteria met, 40% for 5–6 criteria, 100% for 7–8.

Intestinal obstruction

This disorder is the result of inability of normal secretions and waste to pass through the GI tract. It is best to separate intestinal obstruction into two major sites, small intestinal and large intestinal obstruction.

Symptoms Both large and small intestinal obstruction are associated with anorexia and colicky abdominal pain with distension. In small bowel obstruction, vomiting occurs earlier, distension may be less. In large bowel obstruction, the pain is more constant. Obstipation is common but constipation need not be absolute (i.e., no feces or flatus passed). Fever is an ominous sign and when associated with localized peritonitis, always worry about strangulation.

Causes *Small bowel:* Adhesions are the number one cause in the United States; hernias (external/internal) are the most common worldwide. Also, intussusception, Crohn's disease, radiation enteritis, gallstone ileus, tumor, foreign body.
Large bowel: Tumor, sigmoid or cecal volvulus, feces, diverticular or ischemic stricture.

Physical exam Examine for distension and borborygmi, auscultate for bowel sounds—no bowel sounds may indicate ileus without obstruction; high-pitched bowel sounds are the hallmark of obstruction.

Tests

- CBC, electrolytes (K^+ and Mg^{2+})
- Urine analysis and culture—a UTI may cause ileus.
- AXR (plain AXR) look for abnormal gas patterns (gas in the fundus of stomach and throughout the large bowel is normal).
- On erect AXR, look for horizontal fluid levels within the small bowel, as well as central gas shadows and no gas in the large bowel. Small bowel is identified by valvulae conniventes that completely cross the lumen (large bowel haustral folds do *not* cross all the lumen's width). In large bowel obstruction, AXR shows gas proximal to the block (e.g., in cecum) but not in the rectum.
- Abdominal and pelvic CT scan with oral contrast may demonstrate dilated loops of bowel to a transition point followed by compressed loops of bowel. Be careful in immediately administering IV contrast because often these patients are dehydrated and may have renal insufficiency.

Management

General principles: The site, speed of onset, and completeness of obstruction determine therapy. Strangulation and large bowel obstruction require surgery soon. Paralytic ileus and incomplete small bowel obstruction can be managed conservatively, at least initially.

489

- *Conservative options:* Pass NGT and give IV fluids to rehydrate and correct electrolyte imbalance (p. 667). Recurrent small bowel obstruction requiring hospitalization may be better served with exploratory laparotomy.
- *Surgery:* Strangulation requires emergency surgery, as does *closed loop obstruction*—large bowel obstruction with tenderness over a grossly distended cecum (>8 cm), which occurs when the ileocecal valve remains competent despite bowel distension. Usually, large volumes of IV fluid must be given. For less urgent large bowel obstruction, there is time for an enema to determine if a complete or partial obstruction exists and to try to clear the obstruction and correct fluid imbalance.

Sigmoid volvulus occurs when the bowel twists on the mesentery, and it can produce a severe, rapid strangulated obstruction. There is a characteristic AXR with an "inverted U" loop of bowel. It tends to occur in the elderly, constipated patient, and it is often managed by sigmoidoscopy and insertion of a flatus tube, but sigmoid colectomy is sometimes required.

If sigmoid volvulus can be decompressed, it is recommended that the colon be prepped and removed during the same hospitalization.

Cecal volvulus is similar but less common than sigmoid volvulus. It is found in patients with a mobile cecum. Treatment is surgical resection or cecal pexy.

Pseudo-obstruction resembles mechanical GI obstruction but no cause for obstruction is found. *Predisposing factors:* Malignancy, electrolyte disturbances (e.g., ↓K+), recent surgery. *Presentation:* Nausea and postprandial bloating. Acute colonic pseudo-obstruction is called *Ogilvie's syndrome*. This is common in the elderly, institutionalized patient. *Treatment:* Manage conservatively. Neostigmine or colonoscopic decompression is sometimes useful in acute cases. Weight loss is a problem in chronic pseudo-obstruction. There is a case for investigating the cause by colonoscopy or water-soluble contrast enema in most instances of suspected mechanical obstruction.

Rectal prolapse (procidentia)

Full-thickness concentric prolapse of the rectum through the anus; in contrast to mucosal prolapse seen with hemorrhoidal disease. True incidence is unknown but ♀:♂ ratio is 6:1 in patients >60. In children, be concerned about cystic fibrosis.

Symptoms Prolapse of the rectum usually with defecation; patients often have constipation, fecal incontinence, and uterine and bladder prolapse.

Exam Have patient do enema while in the clinic and observe prolapse. Assess strength of sphincter muscles and evaluate for anterior compartment prolapse. Perform colonoscopy to look for possible lead point and for possible solitary rectal ulcer.

Management Stool bulking agents (fiber). Surgery is mainstay. Two approaches, either transperineal or transabdominal. Best result with transabdominal but depends on health of patient. Colonic resection recommended if constipation is present. Incontinence improves in 80% of patients with repair of prolapse alone.

Transperineal procedures
- Delorme: Rectal mucosectomy
- Altemeier: Full-thickness rectal resection transanally
- Tirsch wire: Suture around the anus

Transabdominal approaches
- Ripstein rectopexy: Anterior mesh rectopexy
- Open suture rectopexy or Laparoscopic Wells procedure: Presacral suture rectopexy
- Frykman-Goldberg: Sigmoid resection with presacral suture rectopexy
- Anterior resection

Fecal incontinence

Inability to control the loss of gas or stool per anus. In women, the majority of cases are the result of obstetrical injury (forceps, vacuum, third- and fourth-degree tears). Prevalence is 0.5–11%. Requires frequent pad usage.

Anatomy The internal sphincter is innervated by intestinal myenteric plexus and is under involuntary control; it provides a large portion of anal tone, which is further increased by the external sphincters innervated by the pudendal nerve and under voluntary control.

Exam Patulous anus and anal excoriation.

Tests
• Pudendal nerve terminal motor latency to document functioning nerves
• Transrectal US to demonstrate sphincter defects
• Anorectal manometry to record resting and squeeze tone

Management Imodium will increase internal sphincter tone.

Surgical correction with overlapping sphincteroplasty has a 50% 5-yr success rate. Can be repeated. Newer options include sacral stimulation and the artificial bowel sphincter.

Hemorrhoids

The anus is lined by mainly discontinuous areas of spongy vascular tissue—the anal cushions—which contribute to anal closure. Viewed from the lithotomy position, their positions are at 3, 7, and 11 o'clock or right anterior and posterior and left lateral. Hemorrhoids are attached by smooth muscle and elastic tissue to the supporting structure of the anal canal, but are prone to displacement and disruption, either singly or together. The effects of gravity (our erect posture), increased anal tone, and straining at stool may make them become both bulky and loose and so protrude. They are vulnerable to trauma and bleed readily from the capillaries of the underlying lamina propria, hence their name—*hemorrhoids* (meaning "running blood" in Greek). Because the bleeding is from capillaries, it is bright red. (Hemorrhoids are *not* varicose veins.)

Symptoms The patient notices bright red rectal bleeding, often coating stools or dripping into the pan after defecation. There may be mucous discharge and pruritus ani. Severe anemia may occur. Often patients complain of mass that needs to be pushed back into the anus. If patient complains of pain, either fissure or thrombosed hemorrhoid* is present. As there are no sensory fibers above the dentate line (squamomucosal junction), hemorrhoids are not painful unless they thrombose when protruded. Fissures and hemorrhoids commonly occur together.

Exam
• *Abdominal examination* to R/O other diseases
• *Rectal examination:* Prolapsing hemorrhoids are obvious.
• *Proctoscopy* to see the internal hemorrhoids
• *Sigmoidoscopy* to identify rectal pathology higher up (you can get no higher up than the rectosigmoid junction).

Classification and treatment All patients should be instructed in the use of a high-fiber diet and refraining from straining and long trips to the bathroom (see Table 13.24).

Infrared coagulation: Applied for 1.5–2 sec, 3–8 times to localized areas works by coagulating vessels and tethering mucosa to subcutaneous tissue.

Sclerosants: (2 mL of 5% phenol in oil injected above the dentate line) *SE:* Impotence; prostatitis.

Rubber band ligation: Do fewer than three band-treatments per session; a cheap treatment, but needs skill. Banding produces an ulcer to anchor the mucosa (see: Pain, bleeding, infection).

Conventional hemorrhoidectomy: Excision and ligation of vascular pedicles. Done as day-case surgery, needing ~2 wks off work. *SE:* Hemorrhage or stenosis.

Stapled hemorrhoidectomy: Results in a quicker return to normal activity than conventional surgery because of less pain. Will not remove large protruding anal tags (fourth-degree).

Table 13.24 Hemorrhoidal classification and treatment

Stage	Definition	Treatment
I	Enlarged with bleeding	Fiber
		Suppositories
		Sclerotherapy
II	Protrusion with spontaneous reduction	Fiber
		Suppositories
		Banding
III	Protrusion requiring manual reduction	Fiber
		Banding
		Conventional or stapled hemorrhoidectomy
IV	Irreducible protrusion	Fiber
		Stapled hemorrhoidectomy in selected cases
		Conventional hemorrhoidectomy

*Treatment of prolapsed, thrombosed hemorrhoid is with excision if <72 h, otherwise analgesia, sitz baths, and bed rest. Pain usually resolves in 2 wks.

Anal fissure

Anal fissure is a midline longitudinal split in the squamous lining of the lower anus, often, if chronic, with a mucosal tag at the external aspect—the "sentinel pile." 90% are posterior (anterior ones follow parturition) and are perpetuated by internal sphincter spasm. Defecation is very painful and spasm may constrict the rectal artery, making healing difficult.

Causes

Primary cause: Diarrhea or hard stools, acquired disorder.
Rare causes: Syphilis, herpes, trauma, Crohn's, anal cancer, psoriasis; more common in the lateral location.

Exam

Examine with a bright light. Do a digital rectal exam ± sigmoidoscopy. Groin nodes suggest a complicating factor (e.g., immunosuppression from HIV).

Treatment Try 2% lidocaine ointment, extra dietary roughage + good anal toilet, sitz baths. Glyceryl trinitrate ointment (0.2–0.3%) or 0.2% nifedipine ointment relieves pain and ischemia caused by chronic fissures and spasm and can prevent need for surgery, but may cause headache. If conservative measures fail, consider day-case lateral partial internal *sphincterotomy*. Manual anal dilatation (under general anesthesia) is also used but has fallen out of favor due to increased risk of postop anal incontinence (24.3% vs. 4.8% for lateral sphincterotomy).

Pilonidal sinus/cyst Obstruction of natal cleft hair follicles ~6 cm above the anus, with ingrowing of hair; excites a foreign-body reaction and may cause secondary tracts that open laterally ± abscesses, with foul-smelling discharge.

Treatment is excision of the sinus tract ± primary closure, but is unsatisfactory in 10% of patients. Complex tracts can be laid open and packed individually, or skin flaps can be used to cover the defect.

Anal ulcers are rare. Consider Crohn's disease, anal cancer, TB, syphilis.

Skin tags seldom cause trouble but are easily excised.

Anorectal abscess/fistula is usually caused by enteric organisms (rarely *S. aureus* or tuberculosis [TB]). *Location:* Perianal (~45%), ischiorectal (30%), intersphincteric (>20%), supralevator (~5%). Redness and swelling may spread well into the buttock. Do incision and drainage, usually under GA unless small perianal (+ fistulotomy if needed, e.g., in Crohn's disease). *Associations:* DM, Crohn's, malignancy. Don't rely on antibiotics.

Anal cancer *Increased risk:* Syphilis, anal warts (herpesvirus [HPV] 16, 6, 11, and 18 implicated), anoreceptive homosexuals (often young). *Histology:* Squamous cell (80%); rarely, basaloid, melanoma, or adenocarcinoma. The patient may present with bleeding, pain, bowel habit change, pruritus ani, masses, and stricture. *Differential diagnosis:* Condyloma acuminata, leucoplakia, lichen sclerosus, Bowen's, Paget's, or Crohn's disease. *Treatment:* Radiotherapy + 5-FU + mitomycin/cisplatin is usually preferred to anorectal excision and colostomy, and 75% of patients retain normal anal function.

Gastric and duodenal ulcer disease

Ulcerative disease of the stomach and duodenum has declined in incidence sharply from levels seen in 1960. Risk factors include smoking, NSAID use, *Helicobacter pylori*, and increased acid production or a defect in mucosal defense.

Symptoms Cardinal feature is epigastric pain described as burning, stabbing, or gnawing relieved by eating or antacids. Other associated symptoms include nausea, vomiting, bleeding, weight loss. Differential diagnosis includes cholelithiasis, pancreatitis, pancreatic cancer, MI, and gastric neoplasia.

Evaluation
- Barium swallow and upper GI study
- EGD: Biopsy for neoplasia and *H. pylori*
- Recurrent peptic ulceration in unusual places; think of Zollinger–Ellison syndrome (gastrinoma). Do secretin stimulation test.

Medical management
- Treat *H. pylori*
- Antihistamines
- Proton pump inhibitors
- Prostaglandin analogues
- Sucralfate
- Antacids

493

Surgical management

Operative intervention is reserved for the treatment of complicated ulcer disease (intractability, hemorrhage, perforation, obstruction).

Operations for benign gastric ulceration

Elective operation for gastric fundus ulceration is rarely needed as ulcers respond well to medical treatment, stopping smoking, and avoidance of NSAIDs. Emergency surgery is sometimes needed for hemorrhage or perforation. Hemorrhage is usually treated by underrunning the bleeding ulcer base or excision of the ulcer. If the former is done, then a biopsy should be taken to exclude malignancy. Perforation is usually managed by excision of the hole for histology, then closure. Prepyloric ulceration is considered peptic disease and an anti-acid procedure should be considered, especially if the patient has been on acid suppression therapy.

Gastric carcinoma

Curative surgical options include D_1 resection (removal of tumor and perigastric lymph nodes) and D_2 resection (removal of the D_1 tier of lymph nodes and the next tier out, along the celiac axis). There is considerable controversy as to which should be performed, as some studies have shown worse morbidity and mortality for D_2 resections performed in Western countries. It is likely that the results reflect the lack of dedicated specialists, such as those in Japan, where gastric carcinoma is particularly common. D_2 resections should therefore only be performed in specialist centers.

Partial gastrectomy (the Billroth operations)

Billroth I: Partial gastrectomy with simple re-anastomosis (rejoining).

Billroth II (Polya gastrectomy): Partial gastrectomy. The duodenal stump is oversewn (leaving a blind loop), and anastomosis is achieved between the proximal jejunum and the stomach remnant (Figure 13.10).

Physical complications of gastrectomy and peptic ulcer surgery

See Table 13.25.

Recurrent ulceration: Symptoms are similar to those experienced preoperatively but complications are more common and response to medical treatment is poor. Further surgery with a total gastrectomy may be necessary. Consider Zollinger–Ellison syndrome.

Abdominal fullness: Feeling of early satiety (perhaps with discomfort and distension) improving with time. Advise patient to take small, frequent meals.

Dumping syndrome: Fainting and sweating after eating due to food of high osmotic potential being dumped into the jejunum; causes rapid fluid shifts. "Late dumping" is due to rebound hypoglycemia and occurs 1–3 h after meals. Both tend to improve with time but may be helped by eating less sugar and more guar and pectin (slows glucose absorption). Acarbose may also help to reduce the early hyperglycemic stimulus to insulin secretion.

Bilious vomiting: This is difficult to treat but often improves with time.

Diarrhea: May be disabling after vagotomy. Codeine phosphate may help.

Gastric tumor: A rare complication of any surgery that affects acid production.

Amylase elevation: If associated with abdominal pain, this may indicate afferent loop obstruction after Billroth II surgery (requires emergency surgery).

Metabolic complications

Weight loss: Often due to poor calorie intake.

Bacterial overgrowth ± malabsorption (the blind loop syndrome) may occur.

Anemia: Usually from lack of iron hypochlorhydria and stomach resection. B_{12} levels are frequently low but megaloblastic anemia is rare.

Osteomalacia: There may be pseudofractures that look like metastases.

Table 13.25 Complications of peptic ulcer surgery				
	Recurrence (%)	Dumping (%)	Diarrhea (%)	Metabolic
Partial gastrectomy	2	20	1	++++
Vagotomy and pyloroplasty	7	14	4	++
Highly selective vagotomy	>7	6	<1	0
(These values are approximate based on the literature)				

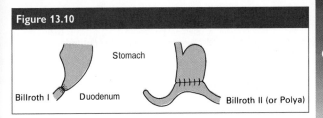

Figure 13.10

Stomach

Billroth I   Duodenum

Billroth II (or Polya)

Surgery for duodenal ulcer

Peptic ulcers usually present as epigastric pain and dyspepsia (p. 208). There is no reliable method of distinguishing clinically between gastric and duodenal ulcers. Although management of both is usually medical in the first instance (with *H. pylori* eradication [p. 208]), surgery still has a role.

Surgery is usually only required for complications such as *hemorrhage, perforation*, and *pyloric stenosis*, although it may be considered for the few patients who are not responsive/tolerant to medical therapy.

Several types of operation have been tried but, as with any operation, one must consider efficacy, side effects, and mortality.

Elective surgery may be undertaken for patients who are intolerant of or fail to respond to medical treatment:

- *Highly selective vagotomy:* May be useful in patients unable to tolerate medical treatment. The vagus supply is denervated only where it supplies the lower esophagus and stomach. The nerve of Latarjet to the pylorus is left intact; thus, gastric emptying is unaffected.
- *Vagotomy and pyloroplasty:* A vagotomy reduces acid production from the stomach body and fundus and reduces gastrin production from the antrum. However, it interferes with emptying of the pyloric sphincter and so a drainage procedure (e.g., pyloroplasty) must be added. This operation is now almost obsolete and is only performed in exceptional circumstances.
- *Gastrectomy* is rarely required in the modern management of peptic ulcer disease.

Emergency surgery may be required for the following complications:

- *Hemorrhage* may be controlled endoscopically by adrenaline injection, cautery, laser coagulation, or heat probe. Operation should be considered for severe hemorrhage or rebleeding, especially in the elderly. At surgery, the bleeding ulcer base is underrun or oversewn. Occasionally, the gastroduodenal artery must be ligated.
- *Perforation:* Most patients undergo surgery, although some advocate an initial conservative approach (NPO, NG tube, IV antibiotics) in patients without generalized peritonitis. This can prevent surgery in up to 50% of such cases. If emergency surgery is required, laparoscopic repair of the hole will usually suffice. *H. pylori* eradication should be commenced postop.
- *Pyloric stenosis:* This is a late complication, presenting with vomiting of large amounts of food some hours after meals. (Adult pyloric stenosis is a complication of duodenal ulcers and has nothing to do with congenital hypertrophic pyloric stenosis.)

Treatment: Endoscopic balloon dilatation, followed by maximal acid suppression, may be tried in the first instance (NB: 5% risk of perforation). If this is unsuccessful, a drainage procedure (e.g., gastroenterostomy or pyloroplasty) ± highly selective vagotomy may be performed, often laparoscopically. The operation should be done after correction of the metabolic defect (hypochloremic, hypokalemic metabolic alkalosis).

Surgery for gastroesophageal reflux disease

Fundoplication for gerd

The goal of surgery for GERD is to reestablish lower esophageal sphincter tone and prevent continued esophageal inflammation.

Indications

- Failure of medical therapy
- Barrett's esophagus without dysplasia
- Recurrent pneumonia secondary to aspiration
- Mechanically defective sphincter

Evaluations

- Videoesophagram
- Upper GI endoscopy
- Esophageal manometry and 24 h pH monitoring.

Multivariant analysis has shown that three factors are significant predictors of an excellent to good outcome for antireflux surgery: (1) an abnormal 24 h pH score, (2) the presence of symptoms of heartburn and regurgitation, (3) a clinical response to acid suppression therapy. Large hiatal hernias and long-term chronic disease maybe associated with a shortened esophagus. Failure of laparoscopic fundoplication is higher in patients with a shortened esophagus.

Procedure Gastric fundoplication involves wrapping the gastric fundus around the lower esophagus, closing the hiatus, and securing the wrap in the abdomen. There are various types of procedure: Nissen (360-degree wrap), Toupet (270-degree posterior wrap), Watson (anterior hemifundoplication). Now usually performed laparoscopically which, when performed in specialist centers, is at least as effective at controlling reflux as open surgery but with lower resulting morbidity. Wound infections and respiratory complications are also more common in open surgery, and the incidence of dysphagia is similar for the two procedures.

Obesity surgery

Patients are eligible for surgical management of morbid obesity if their BMI is >40 without a comorbidity and ≥35 with comorbidity. Surgical treatment can result in one-half to one-third of weight being lost within the first 1–1.5 years following surgery. This requires a great deal of patient education and cooperation. Many comorbidities will reverse.

Comorbidity of obesity

- Cardiovascular dysfunction
- Non-insulin dependent diabetes
- Respiratory insufficiency
- Increased intra-abdominal pressure leading to GERD, urinary incontinence, venous stasis
- Nephrotic syndrome
- Pseudotumor cerebri
- Degenerative osteoarthritis
- Cholelithiasis
- Infectious complications

- Sexual hormone dysfunction
- Colon cancer
- Psychosocial impairment

Indications for bariatric surgery for morbid obesity

- BMI ≥40 kg/m^2
- BMI 35–40 kg/m^2 with significant comorbidities
- Unsuccessful attempt at weight loss by nonoperative means
- Clearance by a dietician and mental health expert
- No medical contraindications to surgery

Surgical procedures include:

- Gastric procedures—restrictive:
  - Gastroplasty: Horizontal stapling, vertical banded gastroplasty (VBGP)
  - Gastric bypass: Formation of a small gastric pouch that is drained via a gastrojejunostomy
  - Laparoscopic vertical sleeve gastrectomy
- Small bowel bypass—malabsorptive:
  - Jejunoileal bypass: Obligatory malabsorption associated with numerous complications (cirrhosis) and now avoided.
  - Partial biliopancreatic bypass: Both restrictive and malabsorptive with small gastric pouch emptying into small bowel without pancreatic and biliary secretions (because contents empty into terminal ileum, thus minimizing absorption).

Complications associated with obesity surgery (<15%)

- Pulmonary emboli
- Anastomotic leak
- Bowel obstruction from internal hernia
- Vitamin B$_{12}$, calcium, iron, vitamin D, protein deficiencies

Breast lumps and breast cancer

Incidence and Mortality (2011) Most common non-skin cancer in women in the United States; estimated new cases 230,480. Second leading cause of cancer death, with estimated death of 40,000. Risk of death is on the decline since 1990 due to screening.

History The presenting complaint is a mass, bloody nipple discharge, pain, change in the skin of the breast, or abnormal mammogram (most common).

Risk factors Age; obesity; consuming more than one acholic beverage per day. Menstrual history: Parity; age of first childbirth; use of hormone replacement therapy, birth control pills, or tamoxifen. Family history of breast or ovarian cancer.

Examination Inspect the breast (arms both up and down) noting contour of the breast, nipple/areolar complex, skin overlying the breast (specifically for redness or dimpling), and symmetry. For abnormalities identified, note symmetry, fixation to the skin or chest wall, and characteristics of the lump. Nodal evaluation of the axillary, supraclavicular, and cervical basins.

Investigations Annual mammography is recommended for all women beginning at age 40 and for high- risk women beginning at age 30, consider MRI. Clinical examination is crucial and all suspicious of abnormalities, whether suspicious by imaging or physical examination, must undergo biopsy, preferably by core needle biopsy

Imaging includes: Mammography, US, MRI; many breast cancers are identified by breast imaging and have no symptoms.

Abnormalities of the breast *Causes of lumps:* Fibroadenoma, cyst, cancer, fibroadenosis, mastitis, galactocele, abscess, fibrocystic change;

non-breast lumps; lipoma, fat necrosis, and sebaceous cyst. *Causes of nipple discharge:* Duct ectasia (green/red, often multiple ducts and bilateral), intraductal papilloma/adenoma/carcinoma (bloody/brown, often single duct and unilateral), lactation. *Abnormal mammogram ndings:* Microcalcification, architectural distortion of density, asymmetric density. Mammograms are classified by birad levels (see Table 13.26). *Causes of abnormal mammogram:* Fibroadenoma, cyst, cancer, ductal carcinoma in-situ, atypical hyperplasia, radial scar, columnar cell hyperplasia.

Management Core needle biopsy is used to diagnose most abnormalities identified on either mammogram or physical examination. If there are discordances between the abnormal finding and the pathology, excisional biopsy is performed. If there is concordance and the pathology is benign, no further investigation is necessary with the following exceptions. For mastitis, continue breast-feeding if lactating and treat with antibiotics. Abscesses must be drained and wound care initiated. If the finding is atypical hyperplasia, excisional biopsy is recommended and consider of the use of tamoxifen for prevention. For nipple discharge, microdochectomy/total duct excision. See Figure 13.11.

Breast cancer

Genetic factors: Brac1, brac2 are responsible for 5–10% of breast cancer; widespread testing is not recommended unless strong family history of breast or ovarian cancer.

TNM *Staging:*

- TIS *in situ;* T1 <2 cm; T2 2–5 cm; T3 >5 cm; T4 fixed to chest wall or skin or/and inflammatory breast cancer.
- N0 negative nodes; N1 1–3 positive nodes; N2 4–10 positive nodes; N3 >10 positive nodes.
- M0 no metastases; M1 metastases present.

Early breast cancer including DCIS: Wide local excision (WLE) with radiation therapy (RT) *or* mastectomy plus or minus reconstruction, with sentinel lymph node biopsy or axillary lymph node dissection. WLE plus RT has equal survival but higher local recurrence rates compared to mastectomy. Consider endocrine therapy.

Staging

Assess liver function test and calcium levels; CT scan of the chest and abdomen and bone scan. A positron emission tomography (PET) scan may be used. Staging reserved for high-risk patients or those with symptoms.

Table 13.26 Mammogram birad levels	
Birads Level	**Finding**
0	Needs additional imaging and/or comparison to prior studies
1	Negative
2	Benign finding
3	Probable benign finding <2% risk of cancer, short-term follow-up recommended
4	Suspicious abnormality for cancer 2–95%. Should be seen right away
5	Highly suspicious abnormality >95% likely for cancer. Appropriate action should be taken
6	Known biopsy-proven adenocarcinoma

Figure 13.11

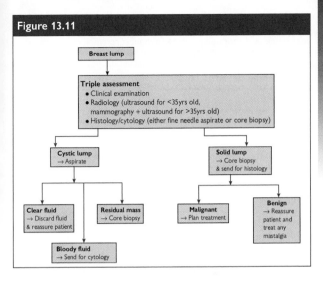

Adjuvant therapy *Radiation therapy* for all patients with WLE; post-mastectomy RT to the chest wall for T3 or T4 and N2 or N3 tumors. RT results in reduced local regional recurrence. *Chemotherapy* improves survival, with the most common combination being doxorubicin-based, with taxanes added for high-risk patients. Herceptin is used for *HER-2 neu*-positive disease. *Endocrine therapy* for those patients who are estrogen or progesterone receptor-positive. Tamoxifen is most commonly used for 5 yrs postoperatively. Aromatase inhibitors may also be used in postmenopausal women with possibly fewer side affects. In premenopausal women with estrogen receptor-positive tumors, ovarian ablation/suppression can be considered.

Treatment of metastatic disease: RT can be used for metastatic lesions at high risk for functional deficit; hormonal therapy is effective in many patients with estrogen receptor-positive disease; after failure of one hormonal therapy, switching to another may be effective.

Preventing breast cancer deaths

Promoting breast awareness: Mammography: The detection rates of mammography are 6.4 cancers per 1,000 healthy women >50. Breast cancer screening with mammography decreases deaths in women >50 by 25%. Prevention with the use of tamoxifen is possible for high-risk women (equal to the risk of a women of 60), resulting in a 50% risk reduction.

Sentinel lymph node biopsy is used in staging breast cancer patients. For those patients who are sentinel lymph node-negative, no addition surgery is completed in the axilla; for those who are positive, a completion axillary dissection is performed. Sentinel lymph node biopsy has a 2% risk of lymphedema with minimal risk of functional deficit of the arm. Axillary lymph node dissection has a risk of lymphedema of 10–20%, with 20% of patients having functional deficit of the arm. The sentinel lymph node procedure is completed as follows: A vital blue dye and/or radiocolloid is injected either peri-tumorally or in the retroareolar area; an incision is made in the axilla and a γ-probe or visual inspection is used to identify and remove the sentinel lymph node for pathologic assessment. Multicenter trials report identification rates >90% and false-negative rates <12%.

Colorectal adenocarcinoma

Incidence and mortality (2011) Third most common cancer diagnosed and second most common cause of cancer deaths in the United States, with 141,000 estimated cases and 49,000 deaths annually.

Predisposing factors Neoplastic polyps, UC, Crohn's, familial adenomatous polyposis, previous cancer, low-fiber diet. NSAIDs may be protective.

Genetics: No close relative affected: Colorectal cancer risk is 1:50. One first-degree relative affected: Risk = 1:17; if two are affected, 1:10 (refer when 10 yrs younger than the youngest affected relative).

Polyps are lumps that appear above the mucosa. There are two types:
- *Non-neoplastic:* Hyperplastic, inflammatory, lymphoid aggregate, hamartoma (juvenile polyps, Peutz–Jeghers' syndrome)
- *Neoplastic:* Tubular or villous adenomas: Malignant potential, especially if >2 cm.

Symptoms of polyps: Asymptomatic, passage of blood/mucus per rectum. They should be biopsied and removed. Most can be reached by the flexible colonoscope to avoid the morbidity of colectomy. Check resection margins are clear of tumor.

Presentation of cancer *Left-sided:* Bleeding per rectum, altered bowel habit, tenesmus, mass (60%). *Right-sided:* Weight loss, anemia, abdominal pain. *Either:* Abdominal mass, obstruction, perforation, hemorrhage, fistula. See Figure 13.12 and Table 13.27.

Tests CBC (microcytic anemia); fecal occult blood (FOB); proctoscopy, sigmoidoscopy, barium enema, or colonoscopy (can be done virtually by CT); LFT, CT/MRI; liver US. Carcino-embryonic antigen (CEA) levels may be used to monitor disease and effectiveness of treatment (p. 680). If polyposis in family or strong family history, consider genetic testing.

Spread Local, lymphatic, hematogenous (liver, lung, bone), or transcoelomic.

Surgical treatment Surgery is considered curative for Stage I and II disease. Attention to technique may reduce local recurrence rates.

Hemicolectomies: Right is for cecal tumors, ascending or proximal transverse colon (extended right including the middle colic artery). Left is for tumors in the distal transverse colon, descending colon, and proximal sigmoid colon. *Anterior resection* is for distal sigmoid or high rectal tumors. *Abdomino-perineal (a-p) resection* is for tumors low in the rectum that are abutting or invading the sphincter muscles: Permanent colostomy and removal of rectum and anus. *Low anterior resection* for tumors of the mid and low rectum. Stapling devices are helpful. *Radiotherapy and chemotherapy (neoadjuvant)* is used preop in stage II or III rectal cancer to reduce local recurrence and increase sphincter preservation rates. *Adjuvant therapy* is reserved generally for stage III and IV colon cancer and in stage II-IV rectal cancer. *Chemotherapy:* Usually 5-FU-based chemotherapy ± folinic acid and newer agents (e.g., irinotecan, oxaliplatin) for 6 months postop; increases survival in patients with stage III or IV colorectal cancer. Adjuvant chemotherapy in stage II (T3N0) colon tumors is beneficial in young patients with more aggressive histology (see Table 13.28).

Patients with resectable hepatic metastases (<4), >1-yr disease-free interval, and no extrahepatic spread will have improved survival following hepatic metastectomy.

Screening guidelines are listed in Table 13.29.

Table 13.27 Signs and symptoms of colorectal cancer

- Persistent change in bowel habit for >6 wks
- Persistent rectal bleeding any age, with no obvious external evidence of benign anal disease
- Iron-deficiency anemia without an obvious cause and Hb <10 g/dL
- An easily palpable abdominal or rectal mass

Figure 13.12 Location of cancers of the large bowel

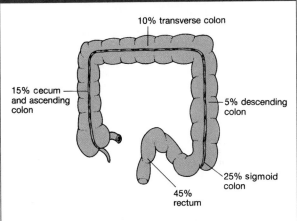

10% transverse colon

15% cecum and ascending colon

5% descending colon

25% sigmoid colon

45% rectum

NB: These are averages: Black females tend to have more proximal neoplasms, whereas white males tend to have more distal neoplasms.

Table 13.28 Survival for colon and rectal cancer (SEER data 1988–2000)

Stage	Colon, 5 yr (%)	Rectal, 5 yr (%)
I (T1-T2, N0,M0)	74	74
IIA (T3, N0,M0)	67	65
IIB (T4a, N0, M0)	59	52
IIC (T4b, N0, M0)	37	32
IIIA (T1–2, N1, M0) (T1, N2a, M0)	73	74
IIIB (T3–4a, N1,M0) (T2-T3, N2a,M0) (T1–2, N2b,M0)	46	45
IIIC (T4a, N2a, M0) (T3–4a, N2b, M0) (T4b, N1–2,M0)	28	33
IV (Tx, Nx, M1)	6	6

Pancreatic cancer

Pancreatic cancer is divided into neoplasms of the exocrine pancreas and endocrine pancreas (Table 13.30). Exocrine pancreatic cancer is more common. Pancreatic ductal adenocarcinoma is the tenth leading new cancer diagnosis and the fourth leading cause of cancer death in the United States. In 2012, it is estimated that there will be 43,920 new cases, and 37,390 will die from pancreatic cancer.

Neoplasms of the exocrine pancreas Pancreatic ductal cancer is more common in men, African Americans, and individuals >70. The only known risk factor is smoking. Other factors that suggest an association are family history, chronic pancreatitis, and previous gastric surgery. 70% of pancreatic ductal cancers occur in the head (periampullary), 15% occur in the body, 10% occur in the tail, and 5% are diffuse. The most common presentation for periampullary tumors is painless jaundice. Other associated symptoms include weight loss, epigastric pain, nausea, and vomiting.

Tests Bilirubin, alk phos, CA 19–9. Contrast enhanced spiral CT, endoscopic US, ERCP, staging laparoscopy.

Treatment Surgical resection, when possible, provides the greatest survival benefit. For tumors of the head, a pancreaticoduodenectomy (*Whipple procedure*) is done. Small resectable tumors (<2 cm) of the head of the pancreas result in a 18–24% 5-yr survival. For tumors of the tail, a distal pancreatectomy ± splenectomy is performed. These tumors tend to be much larger at the time of diagnosis because patients are largely asymptomatic. Palliation for periampullary cancer can be achieved with gastrojejunostomy and hepaticojejunostomy at the time or attempted resection, or with transhepatic stents.

Adjuvant chemotherapy with 5-FU-based regimens and radiation has been shown to improve survival following curative resection for pancreatic cancer. For unresectable cancer, neoadjuvant chemoradiation may convert the tumor to a resectable lesion.

The primary treatment of endocrine tumors of the pancreas is excision. If disease is unresectable, systemically active therapy can be directed at the products of the tumors (e.g., H_2 receptor blockers in Zollinger–Ellison syndrome, diazoxide in insulinomas, somatostatin analogues).

Table 13.30 Neoplasms of the endocrine pancreas

Islet cell type	Hormone	Syndrome	Clinical features	Diagnostic test	% Malignant
α cell	Glucagon	Glucagonoma	Migratory rash, diabetes, diarrhea	↑ Glucagon after tolbutamide	Nearly 100
β cell	Insulin	Insulinoma	Hypoglycemia, mental confusion	↑Insulin	10
δ cell	Somatostatin	Somatostatinoma	Dyspepsia, diabetes, gallstones, steatorrhea	↑ Glucose without ↑Ketones	Nearly 100
δ_2 cell	VIP	VIPoma	Diarrhea?	—	40
G cell	Gastrin	Gastrinoma	(Zollinger–Ellison) Severe peptic ulcer disease (PUD), diarrhea	↑gastrin after secretin 70	

Thyroid nodules and cancer

The single thyroid nodule is a common problem; ~10% will be malignant.

Causes Cyst, adenoma, discrete nodule in multinodular goiter, malignancy.

Examination Watch the neck during swallowing water. Stand behind and feel thyroid for size, shape, tenderness, and mobility. Percuss for retrosternal extension. Any nodes? Bruits? If the thyroid is enlarged, is the thyroid smooth or nodular? Is the patient euthyroid, thyrotoxic (p. 298), or hypothyroid (p. 302)? Check TSH,T3, and T4 levels.
- *Smooth, nontoxic goiter:* Endemic (iodine deficiency); congenital; goitrogens; thyroiditis; physiological; Hashimoto's thyroiditis
- *Smooth, toxic goiter:* Graves' disease
- If >4 cm across, malignancy is more likely.
- *Multinodular goiter:* Usually euthyroid but hyperthyroidism may develop. Hypothyroidism and malignancy are rare.

Tests US, to see if nodule is solid, cystic, calcified, or part of a group of nodules.

Radionucleotide scans may show malignant lesions as hypofunctioning or "cold," whereas a hyperfunctioning "hot" lesion suggests adenoma.

Fine-needle aspirate (FNA) Can be done in the office or by US guidance (most common). 70–90% will be diagnostic. No clinical/lab test is good enough to tell without doubt if follicular neoplasms found on FNA are benign, so such patients are referred for surgery.

Thyroid neoplasia Uncommon malignancy but the most common endocrine cancer. Affects women more than men, ages 25–65. Most common presentation is a cold nodule on US. Risk of cancer in nodule is 12–15%. Increased risk in those <40 yrs and with calcifications of the nodule noted on US.

Known risk factors (1) History of radiation (2) History of goiter. (3) Family history of thyroid disease (multiple endocrine neoplasia [MEN]-2a, -2b). (4) Female. (5) Asian.

Five types:
- *Follicular:* 25%. Middle-aged; spreads early via blood (bone, lungs). Well-differentiated. Treat by total thyroidectomy, T4 suppression, and radioiodine (^{131}I) ablation.
- *Anaplastic:* Rare. $\female:\male \approx$ 3:1. Elderly; poor response to any treatment. In the absence of unresectable disease, excision + radiotherapy may be tried.
- *Medullary:* 5%. Sporadic (75%) or part of MEN syndrome (p. 304). May produce calcitonin. They do not concentrate iodine. Do thyroidectomy + node clearance (do pheochromocytoma screen preop). External beam radiotherapy should be considered to prevent regional recurrence.
- *Papillary:* 60%. Often seen in the young; spread to nodes and lung. Total thyroidectomy (to remove nonobvious tumor) ± node excision + radioiodine to ablate residual cells may all be needed. Give T4 to suppress TSH. Prognosis is better if young and female.
- *Lymphoma:* 5%. $\female:\male \approx$ 3:1. May present with stridor or dysphagia. Do full staging pretreatment (chemoradiotherapy). Assess histology for mucosa-associated lymphoid tissue (MALT) origin (associated with a good prognosis).

Thyroid surgery indications Pressure symptoms, hyperthyroidism, carcinoma, cosmetic reasons. Render euthyroid preop, by antithyroid drugs and/or propranolol. Check vocal cords by indirect laryngoscopy pre- and postop.

Early complications Recurrent laryngeal nerve palsy, hemorrhage (if compresses airway, instantly remove sutures for evacuation of clot), hypoparathyroidism (check plasma Ca^{2+} daily, usually transient), thyroid storm (symptoms of severe hyperthyroidism; treat by propranolol PO or IV, antithyroid drugs, and iodine [p. 782]).

Late complications Hypothyroidism.

Esophageal cancer

Benign tumors make up 1%; most are common leiomyoma or GIST. The incidence of esophageal cancer is on the rise, especially in Western countries. The types of esophageal cancer include squamous cell, adenocarcinoma, and small cell cancer. The most common presenting symptoms are dysphagia and weight loss.

Squamous cell cancer of the esophagus
• More common worldwide
• Associated with cigarette use and alcohol
• More common in the proximal one-third of the esophagus

Adenocarcinoma
• More common in the United States
• Associated with Plummer–Vinson syndrome, obesity, reflux esophagitis ± Barrett's esophagus (there is a 44-fold increased risk of adenocarcinoma if severe reflux for >10 yrs).

Evaluation
• Barium swallow
• EGD with biopsy
• Endoscopic US
• CT scan
• Staging laparoscopy (see Table 13.31)

Treatment

Resection:
• Transthoracic (radical) resection with en-bloc lymphadenectomy; three incisions
• Transhiatal resection; easier to perform

Reconstruction:
• Gastric pull-up with pyloroplasty based on the right gastric artery
• Colonic interposition

Adjuvant therapy:
• Given preoperatively (neoadjuvant) or postoperatively for stage II or III tumors
• Cisplatin, 5-FU
• Radiation
• Palliation with metal stents for stage IV disease

505

Table 13.31 Staging for esophageal cancer and 5-yr survival		
TNM	*Stage*	*5-yr survival*
TisN0M0	0	100
T1N0M0	I	85
T2N0M0, T3N0M0	IIA	45
T1N1M0, T2N1M0	IIB	20
T3-T4N1-2M0	III	10
Any T, Any N M1	IV	<4

Gastric cancer

The incidence of gastric cancer, unlike esophageal, has dropped dramatically in the past 70 yrs (~70%). Risk factors include lower economic status; smoking; consumption of salted, smoked foods; atrophic gastritis; genetic factors (HNPCC), *H. pylori*.

Adenocarcinoma accounts for >90%; others include squamous cell, carcinoid, GIST, lymphoma.

Pathology The adenocarcinoma may be polypoid, ulcerating, or leather bottle-type (linitis plastica). Some are confined to mucosa and submucosa, so-called early gastric carcinoma.

Presentation symptoms Often nonspecific. Dyspepsia (p. 208) lasting >1 month in patients aged 40–50 yrs demands GI investigation. *Others:* Weight loss, vomiting, dysphagia, anemia. *Signs suggesting incurable disease:* Epigastric mass, hepatomegaly, jaundice, ascites (p. 227), large left supraclavicular (Virchow's) node (Troisier's sign), acanthosis nigricans. Spread is local, lymphatic, blood-borne, and transcoelomic; e.g., to ovaries (Krukenberg tumor).

Evaluation

- EGD with multiple biopsies; always biopsy ulcers
- Endoscopic US
- CT scan/MRI to evaluate for metastatic disease (see Table 13.32)

Treatment

- Endoscopic mucosal resection may remove early cancers limited to the mucosa.
- Surgical resection with gross negative margins of 6 cm
- Need at least 15 lymph nodes harvested to determine the nodal status of the disease
- Adjacent organs should be resected en-bloc only if involved with tumor *and* only one organ is involved.
- Stage II and IIIA may benefit from a more extensive nodal dissection D_2 (12 lymph node stations) versus D_1 (6 lymph node stations) with an improved 5-yr survival, 80% versus 55%, respectively.
- Reconstruction is performed with a Roux-en-Y end-to-side esophagojejunostomy.
- Adjuvant therapy includes radiation and 5-FU-based chemotherapy.

Table 13.32 Staging for gastric cancer	
TNM	*Stage*
TisN0M0	0
T1N0M0	IA
T1N1MO, T2N0M0	IB
T1N2M0, T2N1M0, T3N0M0	II
T2N2M0, T3N1M0, T4N0M0	IIIA
T3N2M0	IIIB
T4N1–3M0, T1–3N3M0, or M1	IV

Cutaneous neoplasms

Cutaneous neoplasms are the most commonly diagnosed tumor in the United States, with 600,000 new cases annually. The most common cutaneous neoplasms include:

- Basal cell cancer
- Squamous cell cancer
- Melanoma:
  - Accounts for 5% of all skin cancers but leads to 65% of all skin cancer-related deaths

The evaluation and treatment of cutaneous neoplasms is based on whether the lesion is melanoma or nonmelanoma skin cancer.

Melanoma

Risk factors:

- Fair complexion
- Sun exposure
- Previous history of melanoma
- Dysplastic nevi syndrome
- Large congenital nevi have a 5–20% lifetime risk of developing melanoma
- Xeroderma pigmentosum

Types of melanoma:

- Lentigo maligna (~10–15%), least aggressive
- Superficial spreading (~70%)
- Nodular melanoma (~15–30%), most aggressive
- Acryl lentiginous melanoma (~2–8%), seen in greater percentage of darker-skinned individuals (African Americans, Asians, Hispanics)

Most common sites:

- Women: Legs
- Men: Back of body

Depths of invasion	Staging: JCC	~5-yr survival* (%)
<0.75 mm	Stage IA	99
0.76–1.5 mm	Stage IB	90
1.5–4 mm	Stage IIA	75
>4 mm	Stage IIB	65
Any depth + 1 nodal station	Stage III	40
Any depth + >1 nodal station	Stage IV	0
Or disseminated disease		
*Dependent on site as well		

Treatment

Wide local excision is the primary method of local control of the lesion. The margin of excision is based on the thickness of the lesion (Table 13.33). For advanced stage (III and IV), chemotherapy in the form of immunotherapy is currently offered in addition to surgery, with a modest response.

Sentinel lymph node dissection indications: (1) Primary melanoma ≥1 mm because >10% chance of lymph node spread, (2) clinically negative nodal basin, (3) no evidence of distant disease.

Procedure: Should be performed concurrently with wide local excision because improves accuracy. An intradermal injection with technetium-sulfur-colloid is performed around the lesion.

Table 13.33 Appropriate margins for wide local excision of primary melanoma

Thickness of primary lesion	Margin
Melanoma in situ	5 mm
<1 mm	1 cm
1–4 mm	2 cm
>4 mm	≥2 cm

The sentinel node is located by use of a γ-probe to identify the site of a hot focus (≥10α background counts); the use of isosulfan blue dye will also allow for easier identification of the sentinel node.

Lymphadenectomy: Indications and procedure: (1) Patients with known nodal disease determined clinically or on sentinel node dissection. Intermediate thickness melanoma and sentinel node cannot be performed. (2) Nodal dissections should be complete. (3) The risk of upper or lower extremity lymphedema associated with an axillary or inguinal dissection is ~10%.

Sites of spread or recurrence: Local, distant cutaneous sites (in transit), distant nodal sites, lung, liver, brain, bone, gastrointestinal tract, thyroid.

Adjuvant therapy: Interferon, dacarbazine, temozolomide, immunotherapy, radiation for palliation.

Nonmelanoma skin cancer
Risk factors:
- Chemical carcinogens
- HPV
- Previous skin radiation

Basal cell carcinoma
- Most common
- Little or no aggressive potential

Squamous cell carcinoma (scc)
- Contain keratin pearls
- *Bowen's disease:* In situ cancer that occurs around the anus
- *Queyrat erythroplasia:* In situ cancer that occurs around the penis
- *Marjolin's ulcer:* Aggressive SCC in old scar

Treatment
- *Mohs surgery:* For basal cell and SCC in certain hard-to-reconstruct areas; layered excision of tumor to limit the amount of tissue removed
- SCC requires 1 cm margin
- Adjuvant therapy
  - Chemotherapy: Mitomycin, 5-FU, cisplatin (anal)
  - Radiation

Common urological disorders

Torsion of the testis
The aim is to recognize this condition early on so that prompt surgical intervention can be undertaken to preserve both the fertility and hormonal function of the involved testis.

If in any clinical doubt, and timely color Doppler US is not available, surgical exploration is mandatory. A missed torsion is one of the most common reasons for medical malpractice claims!

Symptoms Sudden onset of pain in one testis, which makes walking uncomfortable. (Pain in the abdomen, nausea, and vomiting are common.)

Signs Inflammation of one testis: It is tender, hot, and swollen. The testis may lie high and transversely. Torsion may occur at any age but is most common at 11–30 yrs.

Tests Doppler US (may demonstrate lack of blood flow to testis). Isotope scanning was used but its use has declined with the widespread availability of color Doppler US.

Treatment Ask consent for possible orchiectomy + *bilateral* fixation (orchiopexy). At surgery, a scrotal incision is made to expose and untwist the spermatic cord. If the color of the testis returns and it pinks up, return it to the scrotum and fix *both* testes to the scrotum. If you are unsure of the status of the testis, incise the tunica albuginea; if you see bright red blood then the blood supply has been reconstituted.

Differential diagnosis Primarily, epididymitis but here the patient tends to be older and there may be symptoms of urinary infection, and more gradual onset of pain. Also consider testis tumor, trauma, and an acute hydrocele. NB: *Torsion of the hydatid of Morgagni:* Remnants of the Müllerian ducts; occurs a little earlier and causes less pain (the patient can often walk with no pain, unlike in testicular torsion) and its tiny blue nodule may be discernible through the scrotal skin. It is thought to be due to the surge in gonadotrophins that signal the onset of puberty. *Idiopathic scrotal edema* is a benign condition and is differentiated from torsion by the absence of pain and tenderness.

Urinary retention and benign prostatic hyperplasia

Retention means not emptying the bladder (*obstruction* or *decreased detrusor power*).

Acute retention The bladder is usually tender, containing ~600 mL of urine. The cause in men is usually prostatic obstruction; e.g., precipitated by anticholinergics, "holding it," constipation, pain, anaesthetics, alcohol, infection (p. 257).

Examine: Abdomen, PR, perineal sensation (cauda equina compression).

Investigations: Midstream urine, analysis and culture, CBC, and prostate-specific antigen (PSA) (p. 681). Renal US and bladder US.

Tricks to aid voiding: Analgesia, privacy on hospital wards, ambulation, standing to void, voiding to the sound of running taps—or in a hot bath.

If the tricks fail: Catheterize (p. 720) and drain bladder. After about 7 d, trial without catheter may work (esp. if <75 yrs old and <1 L drained or retention was triggered by a passing event [e.g., general anaesthesia]).

Prevention: Finasteride reduces prostate size and retention risk.

Chronic retention is more insidious. Bladder capacity may be >1.5 L. *Presentation:* Overflow incontinence, acute on chronic retention, a lower abdominal mass, UTI, or renal failure. Prostatic enlargement is the common cause. *Others:* Pelvic malignancy, rectal surgery; DM; CNS disease [e.g., transverse myelitis/MS]; zoster (S2–S4). Only catheterize the patient if there is pain, urinary infection, or renal impairment (e.g., urea >12 mmol/L). Institute definitive treatment promptly. Intermittent self-catheterization is sometimes required. Both bladder and renal US may be informative.

Catheters and catheterization (p. 720).

Prostate cancer (p. 511).

Benign prostatic hypertrophy (BPH) is common (24% if aged 40–64; if older, 40%). Decreased urine flow (e.g., <15 mL/s) is associated with frequency, urgency, and voiding difficulty.

Managing BPH:

- History: Severity of symptoms and impact on life. Rectal examination.
- Effect on bladder/kidneys: US (residual volume↑, hydronephrosis).
- Electrolytes: Renal function.
- MSU: R/O infection.
- R/O cancer: PSA, transrectal US ± biopsy. Then consider:
  - *Transurethral resection of the prostate* (TURP, a common operation; 14% become impotent). Cross-match 2 U. Consider perioperative antibiotics (e.g., cefuroxime 1.5 g/8 h IV, 3 doses). Beware excessive bleeding postop and clot retention. ~20% of TURPs need redoing within 10 yrs. See Table 13.34.
  - *Transurethral incision of the prostate* (TUIP) involves less destruction than TURP and less risk to sexual function while achieving similar clinical improvement in symptoms. It achieves its effect by relieving pressure on the urethra. It is perhaps the best surgical option for those with small glands (<30 g; i.e., ~50% of those operated on in some areas).
  - *Retropubic prostatectomy* is an open operation.
  - *Transurethral laser-induced prostatectomy* (TULIP).
  - *Drugs* may be useful in mild disease, and while awaiting TURP:
  - α-Blockers: Tamsulosin 400 mcg/24 h PO. Alternatives: Alfuzosin, doxazosin, terazosin. These decrease smooth muscle tone (prostate and bladder). *SE:* Drowsiness, depression, dizziness, BP↓, dry mouth, ejaculatory failure, extrapyramidal signs, nasal congestion, weight↑. They are the drugs of choice.

Table 13.34 Advice for patients concerning transurethral prostatectomy

Preop consent issues may center on risks of the procedure:

- Hematuria/hemorrhage
- Infection; prostatitis
- Hematospermia
- Impotence (~10%)
- Hypothermia
- Incontinence (10%)
- Urethral trauma/stricture
- Clot retention near strictures
- Post TURP syndrome (T°↓; Na⁺↓)
- Retrograde ejaculation (common)

Postoperative advice:

- Avoid driving for 2 wks after the operation.
- Avoid sex for 2 wks after surgery. Then get back to normal. The amount ejaculated may be reduced (as it flows backward into the bladder—harmless, but may cloud the urine). It means you may be infertile. Impotence may be a problem after TURP, but do not expect this: In some men, erections improve. Rarely, orgasmic sensations are reduced.
- Expect to pass blood in the urine for the first 2 wks. A small amount of blood colors the urine bright red. Do not be alarmed.
- At first, you may need to urinate *more* frequently than before. In 6 wks, things should be much better, but the operation cannot be guaranteed to work (8% fail, and lasting incontinence is problem in 6%; 12% may need repeat TURPs within 8 yrs, compared with 1.8% of men undergoing open prostatectomy).
- If feverish, or if urination hurts, take a sample of urine to your doctor.

- 5α-reductase inhibitors: Finasteride (5 mg/d PO ↓testosterone's conversion to dihydrotestosterone). It is excreted in semen, so warn to use condoms. Women should avoid handling crushed pills. *SE*: Impotence; libido↓. Effects on prostate size are limited and slow so, if α-blockers fail, many try surgery next.
- *Wait and see* is an option, but risks incontinence, retention, and renal failure.

Urinary tract malignancies

Renal cell carcinoma (hypernephroma, Grawitz tumor) Arises from the proximal renal tubular epithelium.

Epidemiology: 90% of renal cancers; mean age 55 yrs; ♂:♀ = 2:1.

Clinical features: 50% are incidental findings during abdominal imaging for other symptoms. Hematuria, flank pain, abdominal mass, anorexia, malaise, weight loss, PUO may occur. Rarely, invasion of left renal vein compresses the left testicular vein causing a left varicocele. Spread may be direct (renal vein), via lymph nodes, or hematogenous (bone, liver, lung).

Tests: Blood: CBC (polycythemia from erythropoietin secretion); ESR; electrolytes, alk phos.

Urine: RBCs; cytology.

Imaging: US; CT/MRI; renal angiography (if partial nephrectomy or palliative embolization are being considered; angiography can be done by CT); IVP (filling defect in kidney ± calcification); CXR ("cannon ball" metastases).

Treatment: Nephron sparing versus radical nephrectomy either open or laparoscopic, depending on the size of tumor. Metastatic disease is reason to consider immunotherapy with interferon-α or interleukin-2.

Prognosis: 5-yr survival: 45%.

Transitional cell carcinoma (TCC) may arise in the bladder (50%), ureter, or renal pelvis. *Epidemiology:* Age >40 yrs; ♂:♀ = 4. *Risk factors:* Smoking, drugs (cyclophosphamide, phenacetin), industrial carcinogens (azo-dyes, β-naphthalene). Schistosomiasis is a risk factor for squamous cell carcinoma of the bladder. *Presentation:* Painless hematuria; frequency, urgency, dysuria, or urinary tract obstruction. *Diagnosis:* Urine cytology, IVP, cystoscopy + biopsy, CT/MRI scan. *Treatment:* See *bladder tumors* (p. 514). *Prognosis:* Varies with clinical stage/histological grade: 10–80% 5-yr survival.

Wilms' tumor (nephroblastoma) is a childhood tumor of primitive renal tubules and mesenchymal cells. It presents most commonly with an abdominal mass and hematuria. *Investigations:* US with careful examination of the renal vein; CT/MRI scan. May biopsy only if tumor is massive and preoperative chemotherapy will be given. *Treatment:* Nephrectomy, with adjunctive radiotherapy and chemotherapy depending on pathological stage. *Prognosis:* 90% 5-yr survival.

Prostate cancer is the second most common malignancy of men. *Incidence:* Rises with age: 80% in men >80 yrs (in autopsy studies). *Associations:* ↑testosterone, +ve family history. Most are adenocarcinomas arising in the peripheral pro-state. Spread may be local (seminal vesicles, bladder, rectum) via nodes or hematogenous (sclerotic bony lesions). *Symptoms:* May be asymptomatic or nocturia, hesitancy, poor stream, terminal dribbling, or urinary obstruction. Weight↓ ± bone pain suggests metastases. *Digital rectal exam:* May show a hard, irregular prostate. *Diagnosis:* ↑PSA (p. 681;

511

normal in 30% of small cancers); transrectal US and biopsy; bone scan; CT/MRI. See Tables 13.35 and 13.36.

Treatment *Local disease:* Which is better: *Radical prostatectomy, radiotherapy* or *watchful waiting* with serial PSA monitoring? One trial (N = 695) found radical prostatectomy improved disease-specific mortality, but not overall survival when compared with watchful waiting. Radical surgery does risk erectile dysfunction and incontinence. Some centers recommend brachytherapy for local disease. *Metastatic disease:* Hormonal drugs may give benefit for 1–2 yrs. Gonadotrophin-releasing analogues; e.g., 12-weekly goserelin (10.8 mg SC as Zoladex LA®) first stimulate, then inhibit pituitary gonadotrophin output. *Alternatives:* Cyproterone acetate, flutamide, diethylstilboestrol. *Symptomatic treatment:* Analgesia; treat hypercalcemia; radiotherapy for bone metastases or spinal cord compression.

Prognosis 10% die in 6 months, but 10% live >10 yrs. *Screening:* Rectal examination; PSA; transrectal US. There are problems with all (p. 681).

Table 13.35 Advice to asymptomatic men asking for a PSA test

The prostate lies below the bladder and surrounds the tube taking urine out. Prostate cancer is common in older men. Many men >50 (to whom this advice applies) consider a PSA test on their blood to detect prostatic cancer. *Is this a good idea?*

The test itself has no side effects, provided you don't mind giving blood and time. There is indirect evidence of benefit of screening from the United States, where fewer radical prostatectomies reveal cancer-affected lymph nodes than do those done before widespread PSA-based screening. Intensive screening and treatment for prostate cancer does not, however, appear to be associated with lower prostate-specific mortality in retrospective studies.

Table 13.36 Prognostic factors in prostate cancer

A number of prognostic factors are used to help determine whether watchful waiting or aggressive therapy should be undertaken in prostate cancer. These include age, overall general health and risk factors, pretreatment PSA level, tumor stage (as measured by the TNM system), and tumor grade (as measured by its Gleason score). Gleason grading is from 1–10, with 10 being the highest grade and carrying the poorest prognosis. A pathologist determines the Gleason grade by analyzing histology from two separate areas of tumor specimen, then adds them to get the total Gleason score for the tumor. Scores from 8–10 suggest an aggressive tumor; 5–7 suggest intermediate grade; whereas from 2–4 suggest indolent tumor. Patients with high Gleason scores (6–7) are more likely to be treated aggressively, especially if they are young and/or have higher stage disease.

Urinary incontinence

Think twice before inserting a urinary catheter.

Carry out rectal examination to exclude fecal impaction.

Is the bladder palpable after voiding (retention with overflow)? Do not think of people as either dry or incontinent but as incontinent in certain circumstances (i.e., stress-cough, laughing). Attending to these circumstances is as important as focusing on the physiology.

Incontinence in men Enlargement of the prostate is the major cause of incontinence: Urge incontinence (see below) or dribbling may result from the partial retention of urine. TURP may weaken the bladder sphincter and cause incontinence. Troublesome incontinence needs specialist assessment.

Incontinence in women

- *Functional incontinence* occurs when physiological factors are relatively unimportant. The patient is "caught short" and too slow in finding the toilet because of immobility or unfamiliar surroundings.
- *Stress incontinence:* Leakage of urine due to incompetent sphincter. Leakage typically occurs when intra-abdominal pressure rises (e.g., coughing, laughing). The key to diagnosis is the loss of small (but often frequent) amounts of urine when coughing, etc. Examine for pelvic floor prolapse. Look for cough leak with the patient standing and with full bladder. Stress incontinence is common during pregnancy and following childbirth. It occurs to some degree in about 50% of postmenopausal women. In elderly women, pelvic floor weakness (e.g., with uterine prolapse or urethrocele) is the most common cause.
- *Urge incontinence* is the most common type seen in hospital practice. The urge to pass urine is quickly followed by uncontrollable complete emptying of the bladder as the detrusor muscle contracts. Large amounts of urine flow down the patient's legs. In the elderly, it is usually related to detrusor instability (a urodynamic diagnosis) or organic brain damage. Look for evidence of stroke, Parkinson's, dementia. *Other causes:* Urinary infection, diabetes, diuretics, senile vaginitis, urethritis.

In both sexes, incontinence may result from diminished awareness due to confusion or sedation. Occasionally, incontinence may be purposeful (e.g., preventing admission to an old people's home) or due to anger.

Management Check for: UTI, diabetes mellitus, diuretic use, fecal impaction. Do urine analysis and culture. *Stress incontinence:* Pelvic floor exercises may help. Intravaginal electrical stimulation may also be effective, but is not acceptable to many women. A ring pessary may help uterine prolapse while awaiting surgical repair (this must be preceded by cystometry and urine flow rate measurement to exclude detrusor instability or sphincter dyssynergia). Surgical options for stress incontinence include Burch colposuspension and sling procedures; a variety of minimal-access techniques (e.g., involving tension-free vaginal tape) have also been tried but remain unproven.

If urge incontinence: Examine for spinal cord and CNS signs (including cognitive test) and for vaginitis—treat with estriol 0.1% cream (e.g., Ovestin®, one applicator dose twice weekly for a few months)—consider cyclical progesterone if prolonged use, if no hysterectomy, to avoid risk of uterine cancer. The patient (or caregiver) should complete an incontinence chart for 3 d to obtain the pattern of incontinence. Maximize access to toilet; advise on toileting regimen (e.g., every 4 h). The aim is to keep bladder volume below that which triggers emptying. Drugs may help reduce nighttime incontinence but are generally disappointing. Consider aids (absorbent pad; bedside commode).

Do urodynamic assessment before any surgical intervention.

Bladder tumors

What appear as benign papillomata rarely behave in a purely benign way. They are almost certainly indolent transitional cell (urothelial) malignancies. Adenocarcinomas and squamous cell carcinomas are rare in the West (the latter may follow schistosomiasis). Histology is important for prognosis: Grade 1, differentiated; grade 2, intermediate; grade 3, poorly differentiated. 80% are confined to bladder mucosa and only ~20% penetrate muscle (increases mortality to 50% at 5 yrs).

Presentation Painless hematuria (see Table 13.37), recurrent UTIs, voiding irritability.

Associations Smoking, aromatic amines (rubber industry), chronic cystitis, schistosomiasis (↑risk of squamous cell carcinoma), pelvic irradiation, and history of Cytoxan exposure.

Tests Urine: Microscopy/cytology (cancers may cause sterile pyuria).
• IVP may show filling defects ± ureteric involvement.
• Cystoscopy with biopsy is diagnostic.
• Bimanual examination under anesthesia (EUA) helps assess spread.
• CT/MRI or lymphangiography may show involved pelvic nodes.

Staging Complex and changing (EUA, examination under anaesthesia)

Tis	Carcinoma *in situ*	Not felt at EUA
Ta	Tumor confined to epithelium	Not felt at EUA
T1	Tumor in mucosa or submucosa	Not felt at EUA
T2	Superficial muscle involved	Rubbery thickening at EUA
T3	Deep muscle involved	EUA: Mobile mass
T4	Invasion beyond bladder	EUA: Fixed mass

Treatment of transitional cell carcinoma (tcc)

Tis/Ta/T1: 80% of all patients. Electrocautery via cystoscope. Consider intravesical chemotherapeutic agents (e.g., mitomycin C) for multiple small tumors or high-grade tumors. Immunotherapy with intravesical BCG is useful in high-grade tumors and carcinoma *in situ*.

T2-3: Radical cystectomy is the gold standard. Radiotherapy gives worse 5-yr survival rates than surgery, but preserves the bladder. Salvage cystectomy can be performed if radiotherapy fails, but yields worse results than primary surgery. Postop chemotherapy (e.g., M-VAC: Methotrexate, vinblastine, Adriamycin, and cisplatin) is toxic but effective. Methods to preserve the bladder with transurethral resection/partial cystectomy + systemic chemotherapy have been tried, but long-term results are disappointing. The patient should have all these options explained by a urologist *and* an oncologist.

T4: Usually palliative chemo-/radiotherapy. Chronic catheterization and urinary diversions may help to relieve pain.

Cystectomy complications include sexual and urinary malfunction. To avoid a urostomy, a continent urinary reservoir may be made from the patient's ileum.

Follow-up History, examination, and regular cystoscopy. *High-risk tumors*: Every 3 months for 2 yrs, then every 6 months. *Low-risk tumors*: First follow-up cystoscopy after 9 months, then yearly.

Tumor spread Local, to pelvic structures; lymphatic, to iliac and para-aortic nodes; hematogenous, to liver and lungs.

Survival This depends on age at surgery. For example, the 3-yr survival after cystectomy for T2 and T3 tumors is 60% if 65–75 yrs old, falling to 40% if 75–82 yrs old (in whom the operative mortality is 4%). With unilateral

Table 13.37 Is asymptomatic microscopic hematuria significant?

Dipstick tests are often done routinely as part of a new admission. If microscopic hematuria is found, but the patient has no related symptoms, what does this mean? Before rushing into a barrage of investigations, consider:

- A meta-analysis found incidence of urogenital disease (e.g., bladder cancer) was no higher in those with asymptomatic microhematuria than in those without.[1]
- Asymptomatic microscopic hematuria is the sole presenting feature in only 4% of bladder cancers, and there is no evidence that these are less advanced than malignancies presenting with macroscopic hematuria.
- When monitoring those with treated bladder cancer for recurrence, microscopic hematuria tests have a sensitivity of only 31% in those with superficial bladder malignancy, in whom detection would be most useful.
- Although 80% of those with flank pain due to a renal stone have microscopic hematuria, so will >50% of those with flank pain but no stone.

The conclusion is not that urine dipstick testing is useless, but that results should not be interpreted *in isolation*. Smokers and those with a +ve family history for urothelial malignancy may be investigated differently from those with no risk factors (e.g., US, cystoscopy ± referral to a renal physician in some patients), but in a young fit athlete, the diagnosis is more likely to be exercise-induced hematuria.

---

pelvic node involvement, only 6% of patients survive 5 yrs. The 3-yr survival with bilateral or para-aortic node involvement is nil.

Massive bladder hemorrhage may complicate treatment; consider alum solution bladder irrigation (safer than formalin): It is an in-patient procedure.

Gynecology

Disorders of the vulva The vulva is the area surrounding the vagina that is loosely covered by skin and is affected by pathologic processes that affect squamous epithelium.

Benign disorders: Bartholin's gland cyst or abscess: Obstruction of the mucus-secreting gland surrounding the vagina leads to superinfection; polymicrobial, needs marsupialization and antibiotics. Undrained abscess of either Bartholin's gland or perianal glands may lead to necrotizing fasciitis. More common in diabetics, immuno-compromised, and a history of atherosclerotic disease.

Premalignant and malignant conditions: Vulvar intraepithelial neoplasia (VIN): Presents either asymptomatically or with pruritus. Appearance is white and red papular or macular rash. 5% acetic acid may help visualize. Document lesions and biopsy. Often associated with human papilloma virus (HPV). Look for perianal lesions as well.

Histological grade : VIN I (mild dysplasia), VIN II (moderate), VIN III (severe dysplasia or carcinoma in situ). *Treatment*: Local excision, CO_2 laser

1 *JAMA* 1989, Sep 1;262(9):1214–1219.

Vulvar cancer: 5% of female genital malignancies; look for vaginal and ano-rectal involvement. VIN is usually a precursor lesion. 90% squamous cell, also melanoma. Inguinal and pelvic lymph nodes involved in 20% of cases if lesion is <2 cm, 40% of cases if lesion is >2 cm. *Treatment:* Unilateral lesions <2 cm can be treated with WLE. All others are treated with WLE and bilateral inguinal/femoral lymphadenectomy. If node-negative, 5-yr survival approaches 90%; inguinal node metastases, ~40%; pelvic nodes, ~20%.

Disorders of the vagina

Benign disorders: Pelvic organ prolapse: Secondary to weakness in pel-vic support. Risk factors include pregnancy and childbirth, increased in intra-abdominal pressure (respiratory disease, obesity), postmenopausal atrophy, and connective tissue disorder.

Presentation: Pelvic pressure, coital difficulty, backache, protrusion from the vagina, vaginal spotting, urinary incontinence, fecal incontinence or obstructed defecation.

Evaluation: Clinical exam, urodynamics, radiographic studies include cysto-colpoproctography, dynamic pelvic MRI.

Treatment: Pessary if unfit for surgery. Abdominal suspension procedures including sacrocolpopexy or sacrocolpoperineopexy.

Premalignant or malignant conditions:

Vaginal cancer: Rare, most are extensions from either vulvar or cervical can-cers. Usually squamous cell (90%), adenocarcinoma, sarcoma (DES expo-sure), melanoma in 10%. Surgery has a limited role. Radiation therapy is the mainstay. Poor survival rates.

Disorders of the uterus

Benign disorders: Hyperplasia or uterine polyps:

Presentation is abnormal uterine bleeding. Laser or cauterization of the endometrium is the method of treatment.

Leiomyoma (fibroids): 25% of women in reproductive years have fibroids. Risk of malignant degeneration is <0.5%. GnRH analogs, myomectomy, embolization, hysterectomy are all methods of treatment.

Cervicitis: Common organisms include *Trichomonas vaginalis, Chlamydia trachomatis, N. gonorrhoeae, Herpes simplex virus. Presentation:* Vaginal dis-charge, pruritus. *Clinical findings:* Yellow discharge and erythematous cervix on inspection. Cervical motion tenderness on bimanual exam. Treatment is antibiotics and education.

Pelvic inflammatory disease (PID): Spread of organisms in the endocervix through the endometrium to the fallopian tubes and beyond. Common organisms include *Chlamydia trachomatis, N. gonorrhoeae, Haemophilus influenzae.* Criteria for diagnosis include lower abdominal pain, mucopu-rulent cervical discharge on exam, bilateral adnexal tenderness. Associated findings include fever, leukocytosis. *Treatment:* For questionable diagnosis, laparoscopy is helpful. There are usually erythematous tubes, with a sticky exudate. Antibiotics are the mainstay treatment. Outpatient treatment is ceftriaxone 250 mg intramuscular and doxycycline 100 mg bid for 10–14 d. Reexamine outpatients within 48 h. A tubo-ovarian abscess is the most severe form of PID. Inpatient antibiotics will resolve abscess in 75%; drain-age is necessary either operatively or via interventional radiology in 25%.

Malignant disorders

Cervical cancer

~20% of female genital cancers. Adenocarcinoma (90%) or squamous cell cancer (10%). Spreads primarily through direct extension and into the regional pelvic lymph nodes. Treatment is either radiotherapy or surgery with similar 5-yr survival rates. Localized disease has a 5-yr survival rate of 80–90%; metastatic disease to the lymph nodes, ~40% 5-yr survival.

Endometrial cancer: Most common female genital cancer. Risk factors include nulliparity, obesity, delayed menopause, chronic anovulation, and unopposed postmenopausal estrogens. Presenting symptom is bleeding. Types include adenocarcinoma (90%).

Evaluation includes transvaginal US and endometrial sampling. Treatment of localized disease is surgical and includes extrafascial abdominal hysterectomy and bilateral salpingo-oophorectomy. Poorly differentiated endometrial cancer and extension into the cervix or beyond the superficial myometrium should undergo selective pelvic and periaortic lymph node sampling. Additional radiotherapy is commonly employed in these patients. 5-yr survival for superficial stage I disease is 80%; stage II disease is 60%; 30% for advanced disease.

Disorders of the ovary

Benign disorders:

Benign follicular, corpus luteal, and theca lutein cysts are the most common. Usually disappear with new menstrual cycle or oral contraception. Cysts >10 cm are unlikely to disappear.

Teratoma: Commonly seen in women of reproductive age. Often bilateral. Ovarian cystectomy is recommended treatment.

Serous or mucinous cystadenoma: Benign epithelial tumors. Treated with cystectomy or oophorectomy. Intraoperative frozen section may be important to determine whether these cysts contain malignant cells. If so, and the patient is postmenopausal, bilateral oophorectomy and hysterectomy is recommended.

Ectopic pregnancy: Risk factors include history of PID, use of infertility drugs, intrauterine contraceptive device. Any women of childbearing age with lower abdominal pain should have a β-HCG drawn. Small ectopic pregnancies may be treated with methotrexate. Laparoscopy or laparotomy is otherwise performed.

Malignant disorders:

Ovarian cancer: 25% of all female genital cancers. Risk factors include ↑ age, ↓ fertility, family history, Peutz–Jeghers' syndrome, Turner's syndrome. Presentation is often late and consists of abdominal pain and swelling, GI symptoms, adnexal mass.

Evaluation: CBC, chemistry, CA-125, α-fetoprotein, CT, IVP.

Treatment: Abdominal hysterectomy with bilaterally salpingo-oophorectomy, lymphadenectomy, and tumor cytoreduction. Adjuvant chemotherapy (Taxol) and/or radiation are given for advanced disease. 5-yr survival from epithelial ovarian cancer is 70% for stage I, 30% for stage II, and <15% for stage III and IV.

Infectious diseases (ID)

Shmuel Shoham, M.D.

Contents

U.S. notifiable diseases

Table 14.1 Notifiable infectious diseases in the U.S. (adults)

Arthropod-borne viral infections:

California serogroup virus, Dengue

Eastern equine encephalitis, Powassan virus, St. Louis encephalitis, West Nile virus

Diarrheal/enteric infections:

Cholera, cryptosporidiosis, cyclosporiasis, giardiasis, hemolytic uremic syndrome (post-diarrheal), salmonellosis, Shiga toxin-producing *Escherichia coli* (STEC), shigellosis

Disseminated diseases of food/water/livestock origin:

Brucellosis, listeriosis, trichinellosis (trichinosis), typhoid fever, vibriosis

HIV infection

Infections preventable by routine vaccination:

Diphtheria, measles, mumps, pertussis, rubella, varicella (morbidity and death)

Respiratory tract-predominant infections:

Coccidioidomycosis, *Haemophilus influenzae* (invasive disease), hantavirus pulmonary syndrome, legionellosis, novel influenza A virus infections, psittacosis, Q fever, severe acute respiratory syndrome-associated coronavirus (SARS-COV), *Streptococcus pneumoniae* (invasive disease), tuberculosis

Parasitic infections:
Babesiosis, malaria

Potential agents of bioterrorism/biowarfare:
Anthrax, botulism, plague, smallpox, tetanus, viral hemorrhagic fevers (Ebola, Marburg, Crimean-Congo hemorrhagic fever, Guanarito, Junin, Lassa, Lujo, Machupo, Sabia, and yellow viruses)

Sexually transmitted infections:
Chancroid, *Chlamydia trachomatis* infection, gonorrhea, syphilis

Tick-borne bacterial infections:

Anaplasma phagocytophilum, Ehrlichia chaffeensis, Ehrlichia ewingii, lyme disease, spotted fever, rickettsiosis, tularemia

Viral hepatitis infections:

Hepatitis A, B, C

Other:

Hansen's disease (leprosy), meningococcal disease, rabies, toxic-shock syndrome, vancomycin-intermediate or -resistant *Staphylococcus aureus* (VISA, VRSA)

Note: Classifications in blue are for guidance only. There is extensive overlap between groups

National Notifiable Infectious conditions (United States Department of HHS, CDC)

Pathogens

Table 14.2 Examples of bacterial pathogens from different classes

Gram-positive cocci
Coagulase-positive staphylococci:
S. aureus
Coagulase-negative or intermediate:
S. lugdunensis
Coagulase-negative:
S. epidermidis
Streptococci[a]:
β-Hemolytic streptococci:
S. pneumoniae, S. mitis spp.
Other streptococci:
Nutritionally variant streptococci:
Abiotrophia defectiva, Granulicatella sp.,
Anaerobic streptococci

Gram-positive bacilli
Aerobes:
Bacillus anthracis, B. cereus
Corynebacterium diphtheriae
Listeria monocytogenes
Nocardia species
Other coryneforms (diphtheroids)
Anaerobes:
Clostridium botulinum, C. difficile, C. perfringens, C. tetani
Actinomyces israelii, A. Naeslundii, A. odontolyticus, A. viscosus

Gram-negative cocci
Neisseria meningitidis, N. gonorrhoeae
Moraxella catarrhalis

Gram-negative bacilli
Acinetobacter baumannii complex
Bordetella pertussis
Brucella species
Burkholderia cepacia
Campylobacter species
Citrobacter species
Edwardsiella tarda

Obligate intracellular bacteria
Anaplasma phagocytophilum
Bartonella bacilliformis, B. henselae, B. quintana
Chlamydia trachomatis, C. psittaci, C. pneumoniae
Coxiella burnetii
Ehrlichia chaffeensis, E. ewingii
Legionella pneumophila
Mycoplasma pneumoniae
Rickettsia rickettsii (RMSF), *R. prowazekii*

β-hemolytic streptococci:
S. pyogenes (Group A),
S. dysgalactiae (Group C, G)
β- or γ-hemolytic:
S. agalactiae (Group B)
β- or γ-Hemolytic:
S. bovis spp. (Group D),
S. salivarius spp.
β-, β-, or γ-hemolytic:
S. anginosus spp. (Group A, C, F, G), S. mutans spp.
Enterococci (γ-hemolysis):
E. faecalis, E. faecium

Gram-negative bacilli (cont.)
Enterobacter species,
Escherichia coli (multiple pathotypes)
Francisella tularensis
Haemophilus influenza, H. parainfluenza, H. ducreyi
Hafnia alvei
Helicobacter pylori
Klebsiella species
Morganella morganii
Pantoea agglomerans
Pasteurella multocida
Plesiomonas shigelloides
Proteus species
Providencia species
Pseudomonas aeruginosa
Salmonella enterica (many serotypes)
Serratia marcescens Shigella spp.
Stenotrophomonas maltophilia
Vibrio cholerae, V. parahaemolyticus, V. vulnificus
Yersinia species
Anaerobes:
Bacteroides species,
Fusobacterium species, Prevotella species, Porphyromonas spp.

Mycobacteria
M. tuberculosis
M. leprae
M. bovis
M. abscessus, M. avium complex, M. chelonae, M. fortuitum, M. marinum, M. kansasii

(Continued)

Table 14.2 (Continued)

	Spirochetes
	Treponema pallidum (syphilis)
	Leptospira species (leptospirosis)
	Borrelia burgdorferi (Lyme), *Borrelia* species, other (relapsing fever)

[a] Streptococci are classified according to hemolytic pattern (β, green; β, clear; γ, nonhemolytic), by Lancefield antigen group (A–G), or by species (e.g., *S. pyogenes*).

Table 14.3 Viruses

Herpes viruses (double-stranded DNA)

	Normal host	Immunocompromised
Herpes simplex virus 1 (HSV–1)	Orolabial > genital, meningoencephalitis, keratitis	More severe and recurrent mucocutaneous disease
Herpes simplex virus 2 (HSV–2)	Genital > orolabial more, recurrent aseptic meningitis, keratitis	More severe and recurrent mucocutaneous disease
Varicella zoster virus (VZV)	Varicella, zoster (reactivation)	More severe and recurrent disease, Central nervous system (CNS), retinal disease
Cytomegalovirus (CMV)	Mononucleosis syndrome	Nonspecific viral syndrome, GI, liver, CNS, retina, lung, bone marrow manifestations
Epstein–Barr virus (EBV)	Mononucleosis syndrome, lymphoma, nasopharyngeal carcinoma	Lymphoma, post-transplant lymphoproliferative disease
Human herpes virus 6 and 7 (HHV–6, HHV–7)	Infants: Fever followed by rash, may have CNS involvement with seizures (known as roseola infantum, sixth disease)	Similar to CMV infection
Human herpes virus 8 (HHV–8)	Asymptomatic carriage	Kaposi's sarcoma

Polyoma viruses (double-stranded DNA)

	Normal host	Immunocompromised
BK virus	Asymptomatic carriage	Hemorrhagic cystitis, nephropathy
JC virus	Asymptomatic carriage	Progressive multifocal leukoencephalopathy (PML)

(Continued)

Table 14.3 (*Continued*)

Pox viruses (double-stranded DNA)

Variola	Smallpox (eradicated)
Vaccinia	Used for vaccination to protect against smallpox
Molluscum contagiosum	Pearly skin papules

Hepatitis viruses

Hepatitis A (RNA)	Acute, sometimes fulminant infection
Hepatitis B (DS DNA)	Self-resolving or chronic infection
Hepatitis C (RNA)	Self-resolving, or more commonly chronic infection
Hepatitis D (RNA)	Accelerates hepatitis B
Hepatitis E (RNA)	Acute, sometimes fulminant infection

Single-stranded DNA virus

Parvovirus B19	Fever with slapped-cheek appearance in kids (erythema infectiosum; fifth disease), arthritis in adults, red blood cell aplasia in immunocompromised and patients with RBC disease

Retroviruses

HIV–1	Major cause of HIV disease/AIDS worldwide
HIV–2	Uncommon cause of HIV disease/AIDS, predominantly found in West Africa, immunodeficiency develops more slowly and is milder compared with HIV–1
HTLV–1	Mostly asymptomatic, 5% develop adult T-cell leukemia (ATL) 1% myelopathy/tropical spastic paraparesis (HAM/TSP)
HTLV–2	Associated with intravenous drug use (IVDU), not clearly associated with disease

Orthomyxoviruses (SS RNA)

Influenza virus A, B, C	Major causes of respiratory viral infections

Paramyxovirus (SS RNA)

Parainfluenza	Major causes of respiratory viral infections
RSV	Can cause severe disease in bone marrow transplant recipients

Other viruses frequently associated with respiratory tract infection

Rhinoviruses	Major cause of common cold
Metapneumovirus	Respiratory tract infections
Adenovirus (>50 serotypes)	Respiratory, GI, bladder, conjunctivae or skin manifestations
Enteroviruses	Coxsackie A, B, echovirus (meningitis, gastroenteritis, pericarditis, pleuritis, rash)
Coronaviruses	Respiratory and GI infections

(*Continued*)

Table 14.3 (Continued)

Mosquito-borne viruses	
Dengue	Endemic in urban areas of many developing countries, fever, headache, myalgias, bone pain
Yellow fever	Parts of Africa, South America; vaccine preventable
Encephalitis viruses	Eastern equine, St. Louis, Western equine, West Nile, Japanese encephalitis (vaccine preventable)
Viruses frequently associated with GI illness	
Noroviruses	Major cause of gastroenteritis; cruise ships, cafeterias
Rotavirus	Major cause of diarrhea
Viruses preventable by routine vaccinations	
Measles	Outbreaks in unimmunized populations
Mumps	Causes fevers, myalgias, parotitis
Rubella	Intrauterine disease associated with major congenital abnormalities
Polio	Outbreaks continue in Asia, Africa
Viruses transmitted by animal exposure	
Rabies	Bats, raccoons, foxes, dogs and cats; encephalitis
Herpes B	Monkeys, severe CNS infection
Monkeypox	Exotic pets, fever, rash
Orf	Goat and sheep, skin infection
Hantavirus	Rodents, severe pulmonary disease
Ebola, Marburg	Bats, bushmeat, hemorrhagic virus, high mortality
Rift valley, Congo-Crimean HF, Alkhurma viruses	Livestock slaughter and consumption of raw milk
Lassa virus	Rodents, West Africa, fevers, bleeding
Avian influenza	Domestic poultry, high mortality
Lymphocytic choriomeningitis virus (LCM)	Rodents, CNS infection

Fungal pathogens

Yeasts:

Candida albicans
Other *Candida* spp. (e.g., *C. glabrata, C. parapsilosis, C. krusei, C. tropicalis*)
Cryptococcus neoformans, C. gattii

Filamentous fungi:

Aspergillus fumigatus
Other *Aspergillus* spp. (e.g., *A. flavus, A. niger, A. terreus*)
Fusarium spp.
Zygomycetes (mucormycosis)
Dark molds (e.g., *Bipolaris* spp., *Alternaria* spp., *Ochroconis* spp.)

Endemic mycoses:

Histoplasma capsulatum
Blastomyces dermatitidis
Coccidioides immitis

Dermatophytes:

Trichophyton rubrum, T. tonsurans
Microsporum canis

Travel advice

The majority of travel-related illnesses are not infections but due to other events such as motor vehicle accidents or flare of an underlying illness. Many infections can be avoided with adherence to prevention methods. *Advice to travelers is more important than vaccination.* This is extremely important in foreign-born travelers who are returning to their country of origin after living in the United States for many yrs. An understanding of the traveler's health history, itinerary, and expected activities abroad is essential to providing good advice. Topics to cover include general safety and hygiene, illegal drug use, food and water safety, prevention of arthropod bites, animal avoidance, safer sex practices, and malaria prophylaxis and counterfeit drugs. **Travelers' diarrhea, typhoid, malaria, and dengue are major concerns.**

Traveler's diarrhea (affects 30–70% of travelers): Common causes: Noroviruses, rotavirus, enteroviruses, *E. coli, Campylobacter jejuni, Salmonella, Shigella,* and *Vibrio.*

Prevention: Hand hygiene: Cleanse hands with soap and water or alcohol gel before handling food and after contact with animals, infants, or toilet facilities. **Water/beverages safety**: Avoid ingesting tap water (including during brushing teeth) unless sure it is not contaminated. If in doubt, water should be boiled, disinfected, or filtered. In many developing countries, assume that all nonbottled water is unsafe. With bottled water, ensure the rim is clean and dry. Avoid ice, including popsicles or flavored ice that may have been made with contaminated water. Boiled beverages that are still hot (e.g., tea and coffee), commercially prepared beverages in sealed containers, and pasteurized drinks are generally safe. **Food safety:** Fully cooked food that is still hot is safest. Avoid food and beverages obtained from street vendors, buffets, salads, and raw fruits and vegetables that cannot be peeled. Travelers should peel their own fruit. If you cannot wash your hands, discard the part of the food that you are holding. Meals cooked in homes of friends and relatives are usually safer than restaurant food. **Vaccination:** Typhoid (see travel vaccine table).

Treatment: Consider advising higher risk travelers to have **antimicrobial therapy** on hand (ciprofloxacin, levofloxacin, or azithromycin for 1–3 d). **Antimotility drugs** (e.g., loperamide or diphenoxylate) can be used for symptom relief until the antibiotics take effect. **Fluid and electrolyte replacement** is an important adjunct, especially in children and in those with chronic medical conditions.

Mosquito-, tick-, and other arthropod-borne infections: Malaria, dengue, yellow fever, Japanese encephalitis, chikungunya, tick borne infections

Prevention: Avoid areas in the midst of outbreaks, use protective clothing and shoes, check for ticks, and use bed nets as appropriate, use repellents (DEET, picaridin, oil of lemon, eucalyptus, IR3535).
Vaccinations: Yellow fever, Japanese encephalitis (see travel vaccine table)

Malaria chemoprophylaxis

Medication	Start time before entry to malarious area	Stop time after leaving area	Usage areas
Atovaquone 250 mg/ Proguanil 100 mg/d	1–2 d	7 d	All
Chloroquine 500 mg (salt)/wk	7–14 d	28 d	**Chloroquine sensitive areas only**
Doxycycline 100 mg/d	1–2 d	28 d	All
Hydroxychloroquine 400 mg (salt)/wk	7–14 d	28 d	**Chloroquine sensitive areas only**
Mefloquine 250 mg (salt)/wk	≥14 d	28 d	All except parts of SE Asia

If area has poor medical care and traveler is not pregnant, consider carrying reliable supply regimen of atovaquone/proguanil or artemether/lumefantrine for presumptive self-treatment. Medical care should be sought as soon as possible.

Vaccines for adult travelers

First make sure patients are up-to-date on their routine immunizations. Vaccine needs differ by details of travel and traveler's health status.

Vaccine	Schedule	booster
Yellow fever (**LIVE VIRUS**)	1 dose SQ	10 yrs
Typhoid	Vi capsular: IM α 1	2 yrs
	Ty21a (**LIVE**): PO every other day α 4	5 yrs (repeat series)
Tetanus (previously vaccinated)	1 dose IM	10 yrs
Inactivated Polio (previously vaccinated)	1 dose SQ	10 yrs
Rabies pre-exposure	3 doses IM: d 0,7,21–28	

Meningococcal quadrivalent	MCV4: 1 dose IM	3–5 yrs
	MPSV4: 1 dose SQ	
Japanese encephalitis JE-VC	2 doses IM: d 0 and 28	1 year
Hepatitis A	2 doses IM	
	HAVRIX: D 0 and 6–12 months	
	VAQTA: Day 0 and 6–18 months	
Hepatitis B	3 doses IM: Day 0, 1 month, 4–6 months	

Suggested vaccines: Africa: Meningitis, typhoid, diphtheria, tetanus, polio, hepatitis A ± yellow fever (many countries insist on it for entry). **Asia:** Meningitis (quadrivalent vaccine against meningitis A, C, W135, and Y for Saudi Arabia), typhoid, diphtheria, tetanus, polio, hepatitis A; consider rabies and encephalitis. **S. America:** Typhoid, diphtheria, tetanus, polio, hepatitis A ± yellow fever. **Travel if immunocompromised:** Avoid live vaccines. Hepatitis B vaccine.

CDC 2012 Yellow Book

Overview of antimicrobial susceptibility

Table 14.5 Susceptibility of some bacteria to certain antibiotics

Agents	vre	E. faecalis	MRSA	MSSA	Coagulase Neg. Staph.	B-hemol. Strep.	S. Viridans	S. pneumoniae	L. monocytogenes	H. influenzae	E. coli	Klebsiella spp.	Serratia spp.	Enterobacter spp.	Pseudomonas aeruginosa	Oral anaerobic flora	Gut anaerobic flora	atypicals
PCN -G	0	2	0	0	0	**2**	1	2	1	0	0	0	0	0	0	2	0	0
Ampicillin	0	**2**	0	0	0	**2**	1	2	**2**	1	1	0	0	0	0	1	0	0
Ampicillin/sul	0	2	0	2	0	2	1	2	2	2	1	1	0	0	0	2	2	0
Oxacillin	0	0	0	**2**	1	1	1	1	0	0	0	0	0	0	0	0	0	0
Piperacillin/taz	0	2	0	2	0	2	2	1	0	2	2	2	2	1	2	2	2	0
Cefazolin	0	0	0	2	0	2	1	1	0	2	2	2	0	0	0	1	0	0
Cefotetan	0	0	0	1	0	2	2	1	0	2	2	2	0	0	0	2	1	0
Ceftriaxone	0	0	0	1	0	2	2	**2**	0	**2**	2	2	2	1	0	1	0	0
Cefepime	0	0	0	1	0	2	2	2	0	2	2	2	2	1	2	1	0	0
Aztreonam	0	0	0	0	0	0	0	0	0	2	2	2	2	1	2	0	0	0
Ertapenem	0	0	0	1	0	2	2	2	0	2	2	2	2	2	0	2	2	0
Meropenem	0	1	0	1	0	2	2	1	1	2	2	2	2	2	2	2	2	0
Ciprofloxacin	0	0	0	0	0	1	1	0	1	2	2	2	2	2	2	2	0	2
Moxifloxacin	0	0	0	1	0	2	2	2	0	2	2	2	2	2	1	2	1	2
Gentamicin	0	0	0	0	0	0	0	0	0	2	2	2	2	2	2	0	0	0

(Continued)

Table 14.5 (Continued)

Agents	vre	E. faecalis	MRSA	MSSA	Coagulase Neg. Staph.	B-hemol. Strep.	S. Viridans	S. pneumoniae	L. monocytogenes	H. influenzae	E. coli	Klebsiella spp.	Serratia spp.	Enterobacter spp.	Pseudomonas aeruginosa	Oral anaerobic flora	Gut anaerobic flora	atypicals
Colistin	0	0	0	0	0	0	0	0	0	0	2	2	0	2	2	0	0	0
Azithromycin	0	0	0	0	0	1	1	1	0	2	0	0	0	0	0	1	0	2
Clindamycin	0	2	1	1	1	2	1	1	0	0	0	0	0	0	0	2	1	1
Vancomycin	0	2	**2**	2	**2**	1	2	2	0	0	0	0	0	0	0	0	0	0
Daptomycin	**2**	2	2	2	2	2	2	2	0	0	0	0	0	0	0	0	0	0
Linezolid	**2**	2	2	2	2	2	2	2	1	0	0	0	0	0	0	0	0	0
TMP/SMX	0	0	2	2	2	0	0	0	2	1	1	2	1	2	0	0	0	0
Doxy.	1	1	1	1	1	1	1	1	0	1	1	1	0	1	0	1	1	2
Metro.	0	0	0	0	0	0	0	0	0	0	0	0	0	0	0	1	2	0

0: High rates of resistance
1: Some decreased susceptibility
2: High levels of susceptibility
Bold numbers indicate drug of choice for initial therapy

Antibiotics

General advice: If possible, know what organism is causing the infection. Balance the need for early antimicrobial therapy with the danger of inappropriate antibiotic use. Consider: What is the margin of error for delaying effective therapy in this patient? What data (history, physical, laboratory tests, radiographs, knowledge of local microbial susceptibility profiles) are needed to determine if the infection is amenable to antibiotic therapy and with which drug? Make every effort to obtain cultures of blood, urine, sputum, and any other relevant samples *before* treating with empiric antibiotics. Consider whether an antibiotic needs to be started or whether you can wait for laboratory results. *Ask:* Is surgery or device removal needed? Is the antibiotic safe for this patient (drug interaction, allergies, toxicity profile)? Will the antibiotic penetrate the site of infection? Once therapy is started, *consider:* Can the spectrum of coverage be narrowed? Is an antibiotic still required? Is the treatment course long enough? Is a less expensive, but equally safe and effective option available? In unstable and immunocompromised patients, earlier therapy with broader coverage can save lives. However, inappropriate use of antimicrobials in the general patient population and failure to control a source of infection can lead to worse outcomes, promote antibiotic resistance, and increase costs.

Penicillins

Table 14.6

Antibiotic (and its uses)	Usual adult dose	Adjustment for creatinine clearance (mL/min)
Penicillin (PCN): Most streptococci, *Meningococcus*, *Gonococcus*, syphilis, gas gangrene, anthrax, actinomycosis, and many anaerobes	**Aqueous PCN G:** 2–4 million U (MU)/4 h IV **PCN/Benzathine (Bicillin L-A)** 2.4 million U IM **PCN VK** 250–500 mg/6 h PO	**PCN-G:** Creatinine clearance (CrCl) 10–50:1–3 MU/4 h,<10:1–2 MU/4–6 h HD: 2 MU/4–6 h (give dose after HD or + 0.5 MU after HD) CrCl 10–50: q6-8h, <10: q8-12h HD: q8–12h (give dose after HD)
Ampicillin: Broader spectrum than penicillin; more active against gram-negative rods, but β-lactamase sensitive. Amoxicillin is better absorbed PO.	1–2 g/4–6 h IM/IV	
Amoxicillin: As ampicillin but better absorbed PO. For IV therapy, use ampicillin.	250–500 mg/8 h PO; can use 875 mg/12 h in urinary tract infection (UTI) or streptococcal cellulitis, 1,000 mg/8 h in penicillin (PCN) intermediate pneumococcal pneumonia	CrCl 10–30: 250–500 mg/12 h, <10: 500 mg/d HD: 500 mg/d (give dose after HD)

(Continued)

Table 14.6 (Continued)

Antibiotic (and its uses)	Usual adult dose	Adjustment for creatinine clearance (mL/min)
Amoxicillin/clavu-lanate: β-lactamase inhibitor confers a much broader spectrum than amoxicillin alone.	250–1,000 mg/8 h PO	CrCl 10–30:250–500 mg/12 h, <10 and HD: 250–500 mg/24 h
Ampicillin/sulbac-tam: Abdominal sepsis, diabetic foot infections, severe respiratory infections, head and neck infections	1.5–3 g/6 h IV	CrCl 15–30: q12h, CC <15: q24h HD: 1.5 g q12h + 2 g after HD
Dicloxacillin: For MSSA skin, soft-tissue, and respiratory tract infections	125–500 mg/6 h	No adjustment
Oxacillin, nafcillin: For serious MSSA infection	1–2 g/4–6 h. Higher doses with bacteremia	No change

Penicillin side effects The most common are hypersensitivity reactions (ranging from rash to anaphylaxis) and GI upset. With detailed questioning, many patients who report PCN hypersensitivity turn out to have had nonallergic reactions. Rashes with ampicillin do not necessarily indicate penicillin allergy, but a patient who is truly penicillin allergic likely has allergy to *all* penicillins. Large doses or intrathecal injections can cause seizures and coma. Less common side effects are *C. difficile* colitis, electrolyte imbalance with IV therapy, and interstitial nephropathy.

Cephalosporins

Spectrum Most cephalosporins are active against methicillin-sensitive staphylococci (including β-lactamase producers), streptococci (except group D, *Enterococcus faecalis* and *faecium*), pneumococci, *E. coli*, some *Proteus*, *Klebsiella*, *Haemophilus*, *Salmonella*, and *Shigella*. Second-generation drugs (cefuroxime, cefamandole) are active against *Neisseria* and *Haemophilus*. Third-generation drugs (cefotaxime, ceftazidime, ceftri-axone) have better activity against gram-negative organisms. Ceftazidime has less gram-positive activity, especially against *S. aureus*, and is used in the treatment of *Pseudomonas* infections. Cefepime is fourth-generation and has activity against both gram-positive and gram-negative aerobic bacteria (including *Pseudomonas*). Ceftaroline has activity against methicillin-resis-tant *Streptococcus aureus* MRSA, but not *Pseudomonas*.

Uses Cephalosporins (cefaclor, cefadroxil, cephradine, cephalexin, cefuroxime axetil) may be used in pneumonia, otitis media, skin and soft tissue infections, and UTIs. The oral cephalosporins are generally second-line agents or used to complete an antibiotic course started with an IV cephalosporin. The major use of cephalosporins is parenteral; e.g., as prophylaxis in surgery and in postoperative infection. Suspected life-threatening infections (e.g., severe pneumonia, meningitis, or gram-negative septicemia) may be treated empirically with a third-generation drug. Cephalosporins may also become the drugs of first choice in certain situations, such as penicillin hypersensitivity (beware of ~10% cross-sensitivity) or where aminoglycosides are better avoided.

The main **adverse effect** of the cephalosporins is hypersensitivity. This is seen in <10% of penicillin-sensitive patients. There may be GI upset, reversible changes in liver function tests, eosinophilia, rarely neutropenia, nephrotoxicity, and colitis. There are reports of clotting abnormalities, and there may be false-positive results for glycosuria or the Coombs' test. Most broad-spectrum cephalosporins potentiate warfarin.

There are over a dozen cephalosporins on the market. A representative sample is presented below:

Table 14.7 Cephalosporins

Antibiotic (and its uses)	Usual adult dose	Adjustment for creatinine clearance (mL/min)
First-generation cephalosporins		
Cefazolin: Range of infections due to MSSA, susceptible streptococci, *E. coli* and other gram-negative aerobes	1–2 g/6–8 h IV. Use higher doses with bacteremia	**CrCl** 10–35: 0.5–1 g/12 h, <10: 0.5–1 g/24 h HD:0.5–1 g/24 h + 1 g after HD
Cephalexin: Similar in spectrum to cefazolin, but in oral formulation	250–500 mg/6 h PO	**CrCl** 10–30: q8–12h, <10: q12–24h HD: Q12–24h dose after HD
Second-generation cephalosporins		
Cefuroxime: Range of infections due to susceptible streptococci and gram-negative aerobes, esp. respiratory and GU	0.75–1.5 g /6–8 h IV 250–500 mg/12 h PO	**CrCl** 10–50(IV): Q8–12h, <10 (IV) 0.75 g/24, (PO) 250 mg/24 h HD: Give dose after HD
Cefotetan: Range of infections due to susceptible gram-negative aerobes, and anaerobes, esp. GI/GU	0.5–3 g/12 h IV	**CrCl** 10–30 1–2 g/24, <10 1 g/24–48 h HD: 0.5–1 g/24 h + 1 g after HD
Third-generation cephalosporins		
Ceftriaxone: Many gram-positive and negative infections. Excellent CNS levels. Not active against *Listeria*, enterococci, and *Pseudomonas*	1–2 g/12–24 h IV	No adjustment
Cefixime: Similar in spectrum to ceftriaxone	400 mg/24 h PO	**CrCl** 10–50: 300 mg/d, <10: 200 mg/d HD: 300 mg/d, give dose after HD

(Continued)

Table 14.7 (Continued)

Antibiotic (and its uses)	Usual adult dose	Adjustment for creatinine clearance (mL/min)
Advanced-generation cephalosporins		
Cefepime: Good activity against *Pseudomonas*, *Enterobacter*, and other resistant gram-negative organisms, and *S. aureus*.	1–2 g/8 h IV	**CrCl** 30–60: 1–2 g/12–24 h, <30:0.5–2 g/24 h HD: 0.5–2 g/24 + 1 g after HD or dose after HD
Ceftaroline: Many gram-positive and -negative infections and MRSA; not active against *Pseudomonas*	600 mg/12 h IV	**CrCl** 30–50: 400 mg/12 h, 15–30:300–400 mg/12 h, <10: 200–400 mg/12 h

Aminoglycosides

These are broadly active against aerobic gram-negatives and synergistic with ampicillin in enterococcal endocarditis. Monitor levels and avoid extended therapy to reduce chance of renal and inner ear toxicities. AGs are dosed once daily or intermittently. Once daily is not recommended for meningitis and patients with renal dysfunction. In the latter, use intermittent dosing, start with standard loading dose, obtain pharmacist assistance for further dosing, follow levels closely, and consider nonaminoglycosides options. Try to avoid use in patients with myasthenia gravis, concomitant nephrotoxic drugs, and pregnancy.

Table 14.8 Aminoglycosides

Gentamicin	**Once daily:** 5–7 mg/kg/24 h. Target trough <1 (mcg/mL) **Intermittent:** 2–3 mg/kg load then 1.7–2 mg/kg/8 h. Target Peak >6–8, trough <2 (mcg/mL) **Enterococcus synergy:** 1 mg/kg/8 h, target peak 3–5 (mcg/mL)
Amikacin: Less resistance in some organisms than to gentamicin	**Once-daily dosing**: 15–20 mg/kg/24 h. Target trough <4 (mcg/mL) **Intermittent dosing**: 8–12 mg/kg load then 7–8 mg/kg/8 h or 7.5–10 mg/kg/12 h. Target peak >20–35, trough <10 (mcg/mL)

Macrolides

Active against many community respiratory tract pathogens, travelers' diarrhea, *H. pylori*, sexually transmitted infections, nontuberculous mycobacteria.

Table 14.9 Macrolides

Azithromycin: Available as IV or oral therapy, generally well tolerated. **No change for decreased glomerular filtration rate (GFR)**	Sinusitis/pharyngitis/otitis media/bronchitis/pertussis/mild community acquired pneumonia (CAP): 500 mg day 1 then 250 mg/d α 4 d Mild to moderate CAP: 500 mg/d α 5–10 d Moderate to severe CAP: Add β-lactam Non-gonococcal urethritis/cervicitis/*C. trachomatis* infection: 1 g α1 dose Non-TB mycobacterium (e.g., **M. avium intracellulare [MAI]**): 500 mg/24 h as part of combination therapy MAI prophylaxis: 1,200 mg/wk Travelers' diarrhea: 500 mg/24 h for 1–3 d
Clarithromycin: More GI upset than azithromycin, multiple drug interactions, mostly via P-450 metabolism. Decrease to q24h for CrCl <50	Sinusitis/pharyngitis/otitis media/bronchitis: 250–500 mg/12 h α 7 d Pertussis: 500 mg/12 h α 7 d Mild-moderate CAP: 250–500 mg/12 h α 7–14 d Non-TB mycobacterium (e.g., MAI): 500 mg/12 h as part of combination therapy *H. pylori* ulcer: 500 mg/12 h as part of combination therapy α 10–14 d

Quinolones

Active against many community-acquired respiratory, GU, and GI pathogens. Members of this class are available in oral and IV formulations and are the only oral option for susceptible *Pseudomonas aeruginosa*.

Table 14.10 Quinolones

Ciprofloxacin: Used in adult cystic fibrosis, typhoid, *Salmonella*, *Campylobacter*, prostatitis, and serious or resistant infections. Avoid overuse.	250–750 mg/12 h PO 200–400 mg/12 h IV Higher doses and longer courses for more complicated and severe infections	**CrCl** <30:400 mg/24 h IV, PO: 250–500 mg/12 h PO, HD: 200–400 mg/24 h IV, 250–500 mg/24 h HD: Give dose after HD
Levofloxacin: Less active against *Pseudomonas*	250–750 mg/24 h IV or PO	**CrCl** <50: 250 mg/24–48 h IV
Moxifloxacin: Less active against *Pseudomonas*, poor urine penetration	400 mg/24 h IV or PO	No adjustment

Carbapenems

Very broad-spectrum activity against gram-positive, gram-negative, and anaerobic bacteria. *Stenotrophomonas,* MRSA, and carbapenemase producing gram-negative rods not susceptible. Imipenem has better activity against *E. faecalis* than ertapenem and meropenem. Carbapenems may cause seizures, particularly imipenem.

Table 14.11 Carbapenems		
Ertapenem: Not active against *P. Aeruginosa* and *Acinetobacter.*	1 g/24 h IV	**CrCl** <10: 500 mg/24 h
		HD: 500 mg/24 h and dose post HD
Imipenem/Cilastatin: Most likely to cause seizures.	500–1,000 mg/6–8 h IV	**CrCl** 40–70:500 mg/6–8 h IV,20–40: 250 mg/6 h or 500 mg/8 h, <20 250–500 mg/12 h
		HD: 250 mg/12 h + 250 mg after HD
		Consider meropenem with lower **CrCl**
Meropenem: May be used in CNS infections	1–2 g/8 h IV	**CrCl** 25–50: 1 g/8–12 h, 10–25: 500–1,000 mg/12 h, <10: 500–1,000 mg/24 h HD: 500–1,000 mg/24 h, dose after HD

Table 14.12 Other antibiotics		
Aztreonam: Active against aerobic gram-negative rods, generally safe to use in PCN allergic patients	1–2 g/6–8 h IV	**CrCl** l30–50: Q8–12h, 10–30: Q12h, <10: Q24h
		HD: 1–2 g/24 h, dose after HD or + 250 mg after HD
Clindamycin: Active against gram-positive cocci including penicillin resistant staph, and anaerobes	150–300 mg/6 h PO; max 450 mg/6 h PO. 0.2–0.9 g/8 h IV or IM (by IV only, if >600 mg used)	No renal adjustment
Daptomycin: Broadly active against many aerobic gram positives (including VRE and MRSA, VISA), not active in lung infections. May cause myopathy	4–10 mg/kg/24 h IV	<30 q48h

(Continued)

Table 14.12 (Continued)

Doxycycline: Broadly active many organisms including intracellular bacteria and spirochetes (e.g., rickettsia, Lyme, syphilis). Can cause photosensitivity. Do not use in pregnancy.	100 mg/12 h IV or PO	No adjustment
Linezolid: Broadly active against many aerobic gram-positives; myelotoxicity and neuropathy with extended use,	600 mg/12 h PO or IV	No adjustment
Metronidazole: Drug of choice against anaerobes, *Gardnerella*, *Entamoeba histolytica*, and *Giardia lamblia*; mild to moderate *C. difficile* colitis	250–500 mg/12 h PO or 500 mg/6 h IV	No adjustment
Nitrofurantoin monohydrate macrocrystals: Broadly active against many UTI pathogens. May cause pulmonary fibrosis	UTI (uncomplicated) 100 mg/12 h PO UTI prophylaxis: 50–100 mg/24 h	**CrCl** <50: DO NOT USE, levels in urine inadequate and high serum levels may lead to toxicity
Rifampin: Key component of combination therapy in TB and in salvage of infected orthopedic devices. Associated with many drug interactions through P-450 metabolism	Dose examples: 600 mg/24 h PO for TB, 600 mg/12 h α 2 d for N. meningitis prophylaxis	No adjustment
TMP/SMX: Drug of choice for prevention and treatment of *Pneumocystis*. Active against toxoplasmosis, many *Nocardia*, *Stenotrophomonas*, *Listeria*, community-acquired *Staph aureus*, *E. coli*. Allergic reactions, myelotoxicity, jaundice may occur.	SS = 400 mg TMP/80 mg SMX, DS = 800 mg TMP/160 mg SMX GI/GU/Skin: 1–2 DS/12 h PO Serious invasive disease (e.g., PCP): 5 mg/kg (TMP component) /8 h PCP Prophylaxis: 1 SS or DS/24 h or 1 DS every other day	**CrCl** 10–30: 5 mg/kg/12 h <10: Avoid TMP/SMX if possible. If using: ½ to 1/3 standard doses. HD: Dose after HD

(Continued)

<table 14.12>

Table 14.12 (*Continued*)

Vancomycin (IV): Broadly active against many aerobic gram-positives. Histamine release syndrome with rapid infusion. Potential for nephrotoxicity	15 mg/kg/12 h IV, adjust dose by levels. Target trough: 15–20 for serious infections	**CrCl** 30–60: 15 mg/kg/24 h, <30: 15 mg/kg α 1 then adjust dose by levels
Vancomycin (oral): Moderate to severe *C. difficile* colitis	125–500 mg/6 h	No adjustment

Empiric treatment

History A detailed history will usually reveal the source of infection. Listen to the paient! Ask about respiratory, skin, GI, GU, symptoms; any travel, sexual partner, or possible immunocompromised state. Knowledge of local (including hospital) infectious diseases epidemiology and resistance patterns is essential in selecting the best empiric regimen (see Table 14.13).
Examination Evaluate the fever curve and examine for localizing signs.
Investigations Diagnostic testing should be driven by the results of the history and physical examination. Try to avoid "fishing expeditions." If possible, culture all likely sources before treating (blood, sputum, urine, feces, skin/wound swabs, cerebrospinal fluid [CSF], aspirates). As appropriate, check CBC, urine analysis (U/A), erythrocyte sedimentation rate (ESR), c-reactive protein (CRP), electrolytes, liver function tests (LFT), clotting, malaria film, respiratory and serum viral studies, save acute-phase serum, radiographic imaging, arterial blood gas (ABG; as clinically indicated).
Treatment Follow local guidelines. Change to the most appropriate drug once sensitivities are known. Treatment of most infections should not exceed 7 d. Intravenous antibiotic therapy should preferably not exceed 48–72 h; review the need and change to PO if possible. If in doubt, ask for Infectious Disease consultation.

Table 14.13 Empiric treatment

Infection	Treatment (with normal GFR)
	Urinary tract infections
UTI (uncomplicated)	TMP/SMX 160/800 mg/12 h PO α 3 d
	Nitrofurantoin monohydrate macrocrystals 100 mg/12 h PO α 5 d
	Ciprofloxacin 250 mg/12 h α 3 d
UTI (pyelonephritis): Adjust therapy once susceptibilities known	Ciprofloxacin 400 mg/12 h IV or 500/12 h mg oral, ceftriaxone 1 g/24 h IV, gentamicin 5–7 mg/kg/24 h IV
UTI with sepsis	Many options, one approach is broad spectrum β-lactam (e.g., piperacillin/tazobactam, Cefepime) + aminoglycoside

(*Continued*)

Table 14.13 (Continued)

	Skin and soft tissue
Abscess/furuncle/carbuncle (MRSA suspected)	Incision and drainage. Not all MRSA skin infections require systemic therapy
Cellulitis (nonpurulent): Length of therapy guided by response to antibiotic. Elevation of affected limb is very important.	PO: Dicloxacillin 500 mg/6 h, cephalexin 500 mg/6 h, clindamycin 300 mg–450 mg/8 h, amoxicillin/clavulanate 875 mg/12 h IV: Cefazolin 1 g/6–8 h, ampicillin/sulbactam 1.5 g/6 h, ceftriaxone 1 g/24 h, clindamycin 600 mg/8 h.
Purulent cellulitis (MRSA suspected)	PO: TMP/SMX 1–2 DS tabs/12 h, clindamycin 300–450 mg/8 h, doxycycline 100 mg/12 h, linezolid 600 mg/12 h IV: Vancomycin 15–20 mg/kg/8–12 h, daptomycin 6 mg/kg/24 h, linezolid 600 mg/24 h, clindamycin 600 mg/8 h, telavancin 10 mg/kg/d
Diabetic foot infection: Management requires multidisciplinary approach	**Mild (PO):** Dicloxacillin, cephalexin 500 mg/6 h, clindamycin 300 mg–450 mg/8 h, TMP/SMX 2 DS tabs/12 h, amoxicillin/clavulanate 875 mg/12 h, levofloxacin 500 mg/d, **Moderate (PO):** TMP/SMX 2 DS tabs/12 h, amoxicillin/875 mg/12 h, ciprofloxacin 500 mg/12 h + either metronidazole 500 mg/8 h or clindamycin 300/8 h **Moderate (IV):** Ertapenem 1 g/24 h, ampicillin/sulbactam 3 g/6 h, **Severe (IV):** Piperacillin/tazobactam 4.5 g/6 h ± vancomycin 15–20 mg/kg/8–12 h
Life- or limb-threatening soft-tissue infection: Obtain surgical evaluation	**IV:** Many options, one approach: Piperacillin/tazobactam 4.5 g/6 h + vancomycin 15–20 mg/kg/8–12 h + clindamycin 600 mg/8 h (if deep tissue infection)
Surgical wound infection: If possible, await deep swab results. Strongly consider wound exploration.	Following clean procedures: Treat as nonpurulent cellulitis. If concern for MRSA, treat with vancomycin. Following contaminated procedures: Piperacillin/tazobactam and vancomycin

Pneumonia: Pathogens differ between community-acquired (CAP), hospital-acquired (HAP) and ventilator-acquired (VAP)

Mild CAP (ambulatory), otherwise healthy	Azithromycin 500 mg/24 α 5–10 d Clarithromycin 250–500 mg/12 h α 7–14 d
Mild-moderate CAP (ambulatory)	Respiratory quinolones (e.g., moxifloxacin 400 mg/24 or levofloxacin 750 mg/24 h β-lactam (e.g., amoxicillin 1 g/8 h, amoxicillin/clavulanate 2 g/12 h) + macrolide
Moderate CAP (inpatient)	Respiratory quinolones β-lactam (e.g., ceftriaxone 1 g/24 h) + macrolide

(Continued)

Table 14.13 (Continued)

Severe CAP (inpatient)	β-lactam (e.g., ceftriaxone) + either a macrolide or respiratory quinolone. If risk for pseudomonas use cefepime or piperacillin/tazobactam as β-lactam
HAP and early onset VAP	Respiratory quinolone or β-lactam (e.g., ceftriaxone) ± macrolide. If risk for pseudomonas use cefepime or piperacillin/tazobactam as β-lactam
Late onset VAP (>72 hours of hospitalization)	Antipseudomonal β-lactam (e.g., cefepime, piperacillin/tazobactam) + vancomycin ± aminoglycoside

Bacterial meningitis: In adults with suspected or proven pneumococcal meningitis, dexamethasone (0.15 mg/kg/6 h) should be given just before or with the first dose of antibiotics and continued for 2–4 d.

Adult v 50: *S. pneumoniae*, *N. meningitidis*, *H. influenzae*, Group B strep)	Vancomycin 15–20 mg/kg/8–12 h IV + ceftriaxone 2 g/12 h IV
Adult <50 or immunocompromised: Also, *Listeria* and aerobic gram-negative rods	Vancomycin IV + ceftriaxone IV + ampicillin 2 g/4h IV
Following penetrating head trauma or neurosurgery: Aerobic gram-negative rods and staphylococci	Vancomycin IV + either cefepime 2 g/8 h IV or meropenem 2 g/8 h IV
If HSV encephalitis possible	Add acyclovir 10 mg/kg/8 h IV

Bacterial endocarditis (native valve): If at all possible, therapy should be driven by organism identified on culture.

S. viridans and *S. bovis* (MIC v 0.12)	PCN-G 3 million units/4–6 h IV or ceftriaxone 2 g/24 h IV α 4 wks
S. viridans and *S. bovis* (MIC >0.12, v 0.5)	PCN-G 4 million units/4 h or 6 MU/6 h IV or ceftriaxone 2 g/24 h IV **and** gentamicin 3 mg/kg/24 h IV for first 2 wks
S. viridans and *S. bovis* (MIC >0.5), *Enterococcus* (PCN susceptible)	Ampicillin 2 g/4 h IV or PCN-G 3–5 million units/4 h IV **and** gentamicin 1 mg/kg/8 h IV
MSSA	Oxacillin 2 g/4 IV, cefazolin 2 g/6 h IV α 6 wks
MRSA	Vancomycin 15–20 mg/kg/12 h IV
HACEK organisms: *Haemophilus parainfluenzae*, *H. aphrophilus*, *Actinobacillus actinomycetemcomitans*, *Cardiobacterium hominis*, *Eikenella corrodens*, and *Kingella kingae*	Ceftriaxone 2 g/24 h IV, ampicillin/sulbactam 3 g/6 h IV α 4 wks

38

Table 14.13 (Continued)

Culture negative: Effort should be made to establish microbiologic diagnosis	Ampicillin/sulbactam 3 g/6 h IV **and** gentamicin 1 mg/kg/8 h IV X 4–6 wks

Prosthetic valve endocarditis: Management requires a multidisciplinary approach and should be directed toward specific pathogen as soon as feasible

Initial therapy	Vancomycin 15–20 mg/kg/12 h + gentamicin 1 mg/kg/8 h + rifampin 900 mg/24 h

Intra-abdominal infections: In addition to antibiotics, patients should be evaluated for surgical management/source control.

Mild-moderate	Piperacillin/tazobactam 3.375 g/6 h IV, ertapenem 1 g/24 h IV, moxifloxacin 400 mg/24 h, or metronidazole 500 mg/6–8 h + either cephalosporin or quinolone,
Severe	Piperacillin/tazobactam IV, meropenem 2 g/8 h IV, imipenem/cilastatin 500 mg/6 h IV, **or** metronidazole + Cipro or cefepime IV

Sepsis in ICU without clear etiology: Piperacillin/tazobactam 4.5 g/6 h or Cefepime 2 g/8 h ± vancomycin 15–20 mg/kg/6–8 h, ± aminoglycoside
Osteomyelitis/septic arthritis/discitis: Make every effort to obtain microbiological diagnosis. In case of spine infections, closely evaluate for neurological injury: Vancomycin 15–20 mg/kg/6–8 h IV ± late generation cephalosporin (e.g., ceftriaxone 2 g/24 h or Cefepime 2 g/8 h IV)

Adult immunization

Active immunization usually stimulates the immune system (humoral and cellular immunity). **Passive immunization** provides preformed antibody (nonspecific or antigen-specific).

Table 14.14 Adult immunization

Vaccine	Comment
Influenza	Annually, intranasal OK for healthy, nonpregnant adults age <50. Others should receive injection.
Tetanus, diphtheria (Td) + acellular pertussis (Tdap)	Tdap once and then Td every 10 yrs
Varicella	Two doses if not immune. **Contraindicated in immunocompromised and pregnant women.**
HPV2 or HPV4	Three doses through age 26 (females), HPV4 may be given to males through age 26.
Zoster	One dose age >65. **Contraindicated in immunocompromised and pregnant women.**

(Continued)

Table 14.14 (Continued)

Vaccine	Comment
Measles, mumps, rubella (MMR)	Born before 1957: 1–2 doses, after 1957 (without evidence for immunity): 1–2 doses. **Contraindicated in immunocompromised and pregnant women.**
Pneumococcal polysaccharide	Age >65, chronic medical condition (e.g., lung, liver, sickle cell, asplenia, immunocompromised, cochlear implants, CSF leaks), tobacco use: 1 dose, 5-yr booster.
Meningococcal	Expected to have exposure (e.g., first-year college students, military recruits, microbiologists, travelers to endemic area or Hajj: 1 dose (2 doses in such patients who also have HIV).
	Asplenia, complement deficiency: 2 doses.
Hepatitis A	Men who have sex with men, injection drug use, chronic liver disease, travelers to endemic area: 2 doses.
Hepatitis B	Patients at risk for exposure (e.g., through occupation, sexual activity, injection drug use, prison), those with chronic liver, renal, and HIV disease: 3 doses.
Haemophilus influenza (HiB)	Previously unvaccinated patients with HIV, asplenia, sickle cell, leukemia.

Recommended adult immunization schedule — United States, 2011. *MMWR*. February 4, 2011;60(4).

Drug abuse and infectious diseases

Clues to substance abuse

- Request for analgesics from multiple providers
- Transient residency in the area
- Demand for analgesia/antiemetic and specific requests for medications on your institution's formulary
- Erratic behavior in the clinic or ward; unusual absences and/or visitors; mood swings
- Patient is difficult to arouse in the mornings; agitation from day 2
- Heavy smoking; strange smoke smells (cannabis, cocaine, and heroin)

Physical clues

- Acetone or glue smell on breath (solvent abuse)
- Small pupils on eye exam (opiates), reversed by naloxone
- Needle tracks on arms, groin, legs, between toes, and difficult IV access
- Abscesses and lymphadenopathy in nodes draining injection sites
- Evidence of illnesses associated with substance abuse (e.g., endocarditis, HIV, chronic viral hepatitis)

Table 14.15 Drug abuse presentation

Unconscious	Narcotics (consider naloxone), barbiturates, solvents, benzodiazepines
Psychosis or agitation	Ecstasy, LSD, amphetamine, anabolic steroids, benzodiazepines. Haloperidol may help.
Asthma or dyspnea	Consider opiate-induced pulmonary edema. Asthma may follow the smoking of heroin.
Lung abscess	Right-sided endocarditis (*S. aureus*) until proved otherwise
Fever/FUO	Is it endocarditis?
Shivering and headache	After a "bad hit" (chemical/organism contamination). Beware of myoglobinuria, DIC, renal failure. Obtain blood cultures and consider empiric antibiotics
Abscesses	If over injection site, then often of mixed organisms.
DVT	Due to injections into groin.
Pneumonia	Pneumococcus, *Haemophilus*, Tuberculosis (TB), *Pneumocystis*
Tachyarrhythmia	(If young); cocaine, amphetamines, endocarditis
Jaundice	Hepatitis B, C, or D; anabolic steroids (cholestasis)
Lymphadenopathy with fever	May be presentation of HIV seroconversion illness
Osteomyelitis	Including spinal and sternoclavicular infections. Consider *S. aureus*/gram-negative organisms
Constipation	If severe, opiate abuse may be the cause.
Blindness	Consider fungal endophthalmitis, septic emboli.
Runny nose	Opiate withdrawal (colic/diarrhea, yawns, lacrimation, dilated pupils, insomnia, myalgias, mood ↓; cocaine use)
Neuropathies	Consider solvent abuse.
Infarctions of spinal cord, brain, myocardium	Suspect cocaine use or septic emboli.

541

General management A nonjudgmental approach will produce better cooperation and may avoid the patient leaving against medical advice. Establish firm rules and, if necessary, a written contract of acceptable behavior. NSAIDs are useful for pain relief. Try to avoid prescribing benzodiazepines.

Many people trade sex for drugs. If evidence of unsafe sex behaviors, need sexually transmitted disease (STD) screen and cervical cytology (women) as carcinoma *in-situ* is common. Screen for HIV, hepatitis B, C (provide vaccination when indicated); safer sex and safer injection advice.

Fever of unknown origin

Consider the type of patient

Classical Fever of unknown origin (FUO) is defined as a prolonged fever (>3 wks), temperature ≥38.3°, undiagnosed despite 3 d of testing in the hospital, or 2 or more outpatient visits. Main causes of this type of FUO are infections, rheumatic/connective tissue disease, neoplasm, and miscellaneous. In up to 30% of patients a diagnosis is not achieved. In general, fevers that persist despite a prolonged and intense search for diagnosis are less likely to be due to infection. Bacteremia is not a common cause of FUO.

FUOs in immunocompromised patients: Typically due to infections or immune reconstitution.

Health care-associated FUO: Defined as illness that developed while in hospital with temperature ≥38.3° for 3 d. This is usually due to infections and iatrogenic (e.g., postsurgical, drug fever) complications.

Infectious: Most classical infectious FUOs are due to TB, subacute and culture-negative endocarditis, intraabdominal and pelvic abscesses, EBV, CMV, typhoid fever, and cat scratch disease. Less common causes of FUO include chronic sinusitis, relapsing fever, toxoplasmosis, Whipple's disease, visceral leishmaniasis, HIV, Q fever, brucellosis, trichinosis, trypanosomiasis, malaria, schistosomiasis, histoplasmosis, and coccidioidomycosis. Evaluation for presence of rare and unlikely infections may lead to unnecessary and useless tests. *Pitfalls:* Chest radiograph may be negative in TB and diagnosis may require culture of sputum, urine, and gastric aspirate. Blood cultures may be negative with endocarditis.

Neoplasm: Especially lymphomas (HL and NHL), myeloma, renal cell carcinoma (hypernephroma). Occasionally, fevers are due to solid tumors (especially with hepatic metastasis—breast, lung, GI). Fever with leukemia is usually due to infection.

Connective tissue disease: Rheumatoid arthritis, polymyalgia rheumatica, still's disease, giant cell arteritis, granulomatous hepatitis, systemic lupus erythematosus (SLE), polyarteritis nodosa (PAN), Kawasaki's disease.

Others: Drug fever (fever may occur months after starting but remits within days of stopping; eosinophilia is an inconsistent clue); pulmonary embolism; stroke; Crohn's; ulcerative colitis; sarcoid; amyloid; factitious fever, familial Mediterranean fever—recurrent polyserositis (peritonitis, pleurisy) + fevers, abdominal pain, and arthritis; treat with colchicines.

Fever patterns May offer some information, but are rarely diagnostic and can be altered by widespread use of antipyretics and empiric antibiotics.

- *Intermittent:* SBE; TB, filarial fever, amyloidosis, brucellosis
- *Daily fever spikes:* Abscess, malaria, schistosomiasis
- *Saddleback fever:* Fever that resolves for a few d and then returns: Colorado tick fever, borreliosis, Leptospirosis, dengue, ehrlichiosis
- *Longer periodicity:* Pel–Ebstein.
- *Remitting:* Diurnal variation, not dipping to normal. Amebiasis, malaria, salmonellosis, Kawasaki disease, CMV

History Ask about weight changes, sweats, cough, sinus congestion, mild diarrhea, rashes and itching, bites, cuts, surgery, implanted medical devices, drugs (including nonprescription); immunization, cardiac valve problems, immunosuppressive illness, sexual history, travel, former residences, hobbies, occupations, IV drug abuse, animal exposures, sick contacts, and family history. If a patient has been to an exotic locale, find an expert on that area or else you might miss diagnoses you may have never heard of.

Examination *Verify fever,* perform a thorough physical exam. Repeated exams are often required. Remember eyes, teeth, rectal/vaginal exams, skin lesions, lymphadenopathy, hepatosplenomegaly, nails, joints, and temporal arteries.

Tests

Stage 1 (the rst day): CBC, ESR, electrolytes, LFTs (especially alkaline phosphatase), CRP, white blood cell (WBC) differential, save acute-phase serum, blood cultures (several, from different veins, at various times of day; prolonged culture may be needed for *Brucella* spp.); baseline serum for virology, sputum microscopy and culture (specify for TB), urine dipstick, microscopy, and culture stool for microscopy (ova, cysts, and parasites), chest x-ray (CXR).

Stage 2: Repeat history and examination, obtain protein electrophoresis, computed tomography (CT) (chest, abdomen), rheumatoid factor, antinuclear antibodies (ANA), antistreptolysin titer, purified protein derivative (PPD) or interferon γ-release assay (IGRA), electrocardiogram (ECG), consider bone marrow biopsy and lumbar puncture. Consider prostate-specific antigen (PSA), carcino-embryonic antigen (CEA), and withholding drugs, one at a time for 48 h each. Consider temporal artery biopsy, HIV (with counseling).

Stage 3: Follow any leads uncovered. Consider echocardiography, CT, liver biopsy, bronchoscopy.

Empiric treatment Except in the case of neutropenia and otherwise very immunosuppressed patients, hold off, if possible, on antimicrobial therapy for FUO until a diagnosis is established. An empiric trial for TB or endocarditis may be attempted in selected patients. A trial of steroids should be considered early if there is suspicion for temporal arteritis.

Gastroenteritis

Ingestion of certain bacteria, viruses, and toxins (bacterial and chemical) is a common cause of diarrhea and vomiting (Table 14.16). Contaminated food and water are common sources but often no specific cause is found. Ask about details of stool characteristics, food and water taken, cooking method, time for onset of symptoms, and whether other diners were affected. Ask about travel, sexual activity, swimming, canoeing, and exposure to day-care centers.

Table 14.16 Causes of gastroenteritis

Causative agent	Incubation period	Predominant Clinical features	Food associations
Scombrotoxin ingestion	10–60 min	Diarrhea, flushing, erythema, hot mouth	Fish or Swiss cheese
Red kidney bean poisoning (phytohemagglutinin ingestion)	1–3 h	Nausea, vomiting, diarrhea	Undercooked or raw kidney beans
Ciguatera poisoning		Nausea, vomiting, diarrhea, perioral tingling/numbness, range of neurological symptoms	Warm-water fish

(Continued)

Table 14.16 (Continued)

Causative agent	Incubation period	Predominant Clinical features	Food associations
S. aureus (preformed toxin)	1–6 h	Nausea, vomiting, cramping, may cause hypotension	Range of foods, esp. meats
Bacillus cereus (pre-formed toxin)	1–6 h	Nausea, vomiting, cramps	Rice and other starchy products
Bacillus cereus (toxin produced in vivo)	8–16	Diarrhea, cramps	Range of foods
Clostridium perfringens (toxin produced in vivo)	8–24 h	Diarrhea, cramps	Meats
Clostridium botulinum (toxin)	12–36 h	Double vision, vertigo, symmetric descending paralysis	Home-canned food
Vibrio cholera (produce toxin in small intestine)	2 h–5 d	Diarrhea with "rice water" stool	Contaminated water due to poor sanitation
Vibrio parahaemolyticus (produce toxin in small intestine)	12–24 h	Vomiting, cramps, diarrhea	Seafood
Noroviruses, enteric adenovirus, parvovirus, calicivirus, enteroviruses	1–5 d	Nausea, vomiting, diarrhea, cramping	Contaminated food/water
Rotavirus	1–7 d	Vomiting, diarrhea, low-grade fever	Contaminated food
Salmonella spp.	12–48 h	Vomiting, diarrhea, abdominal pain, fever, septicemia	Meat, eggs, poultry
Yersinia entero-colitica and Y. pseudotuberculosis	24–36 h	Diarrhea, fever, abdominal pain, may mimic appendicitis	Meats, seafood, raw milk
Campylobacter spp.	2–5 d	Diarrhea (may have red blood cell [RBC] or WBC), abdominal pain, headache, myalgias, fever	Undercooked chicken, raw milk, non-chlorinated water
Shigella spp.	12–50 h	Bloody diarrhea, tenesmus, pus in stools, abdominal pain, fever	Any food

(Continued)

Table 14.16 (*Continued*)

Causative agent	Incubation period	Predominant Clinical features	Food associations
E. coli type 0157:H7	12–72 h	Bloody diarrhea, hemolytic-uremic syndrome	Undercooked hamburger meat
E. coli (enterotoxigenic)		Diarrhea, cramps, low-grade fever	Contaminated water/food in developing countries
E. coli (enteropathogenic)		Watery or bloody diarrhea,	Undercooked meat
Listeria monocytogenes	Days to weeks	Meningoencephalitis, septicemia, often preceded by influenza-like symptoms, sometimes GI symptoms	Meats, cheese, pâtés, raw milk
Clostridium difficile		Diarrhea, may be bloody, fever, leukocytosis, may lead to toxic megacolon/ perforation	Antibiotic exposure
Cryptosporidium	4–12 d	Diarrhea	Contaminated water/food, manure
Giardia lamblia[1]	1–4 wks	Diarrhea, lactose intolerance	Contaminated water
Balantidium coli	Variable, often asymptomatic	Diarrhea, abdominal pain	Contaminated water

Characteristic	Testing (stool)
Community acquired or recent travel	Salmonellosis, Shigellosis, *E. coli* 0157:H7
Nosocomial	*C. difficile*
>7 d of symptoms and/or immunosuppressed patients	*Cryptosporidium*, *Giardia*, *Cyclospora*, *Isospora*, lactoferrin, *Salmonella*, *Shigella*, *E. coli* 0157:H7. Add *Microsporidia* and MAI, CMV, lymphoma in highly immunosuppressed.

(*Continued*)

Table 14.16 (Continued)

Management is usually symptomatic. Maintain **oral fluid intake** (± oral rehydration solution). For severe symptoms (but not in dysentery), give **antiemetic** (e.g., prochlorperazine 12.5 mg/6 h IM) and an **antidiarrheal** (e.g., codeine 30 mg PO/IM or loperamide 4 mg initially then 2 mg after each loose stool). In general, routine antibiotics may cause more harm than good, and antimotility agents should be avoided in those with *C. difficile* infection. Antibiotics are generally recommended in travelers' diarrhea (often Enterotoxigenic *E. coli*) and in patients who are systemically unwell, immunosuppressed, or elderly. Treat all typhi species of *Salmonella* and non-typhi in patients who are >50, or have prosthetic devices, severe atherosclerosis, valvular heart disease, cancer, uremia.

Organism	Treatment (when electing to treat)
Vibrio cholera	Doxycycline 300 mg PO α 1, TMP/SMX DS/12 h PO α 3 d, ciprofloxacin 1 g PO α 1, Azithromycin 1 g PO α 1
Salmonella	TMP/SMX DS/12 h PO, Ciprofloxacin 500 mg/12 h PO, ceftriaxone 1–2 g/24 h IV X 5–7 d (longer if immunocompromised or extraintestinal)
Shigella	TMP/SMX DS/12 h PO, ciprofloxacin 500 mg/12 h PO, azithromycin 500 mg α 1, then 250 mg/12 h PO, ceftriaxone 1–2 g/24 h α 3–5 d (longer if immunocompromised)
Campylobacter	Erythromycin 500 mg/12 h PO α 5 d (longer if immunocompromised)
E. coli species (except enterohemorrhagic)	TMP/SMX DS/12 h PO, ciprofloxacin 500 mg/12 h PO α 3 d
C. difficile: STOP causative antibiotic if possible	Metronidazole 500 mg/8 h PO or oral vancomycin 125–250 mg/6 h α 10 d or longer
Cyclospora, Isospora	TMP/SMX DS/12 h PO α 7–10 d (consider q6h and longer in immunocompromised)
Giardia	Metronidazole 250–500 mg/8 h α 7–10 d
E. histolytica	Metronidazole 750 mg/8 h α 7–10 d + luminal agent (iodoquinol 650 mg/8 h α 20 d or paromomycin 500 mg/8 h α 7 d)
Balantidium coli	Tetracycline 500 mg/6 h α 10 d, iodoquinol 650 mg/8 h α 20 d, metronidazole 750 mg/8 h α 5 d

Bad Bug Book: Foodborne Pathogenic Microorganisms and Natural Toxins Handbook. Washington, DC: U.S. Food and Drug Administration, 2012.

Evaluating the tropical traveler

In every ill traveler, consider

Malaria: Presentation: Fever, rigors, headaches, dizziness, flu-like symptoms, diarrhea, and thrombocytopenia. *Complications:* Anemia, parasite counts >5%, renal failure, pulmonary edema, cerebral edema. *Diagnosis:* Serial thick and thin blood films. *Note:* Mosquitoes may stowaway in luggage causing malaria in nontropical areas.

Typhoid: Presents with fever, relative bradycardia, abdominal pain, dry cough, constipation, lymphadenopathy, headache, and splenomegaly ± rose spots (rare). *Complications:* GI perforation. *Diagnosis:* Blood or stool culture.

Dengue fever: Presents with fever, headache, myalgias, rash (flushing or petechial), thrombocytopenia, and leucopenia. *Diagnosis:* Serology.

Amoebic liver abscess: Presents with fever, jaundice, right upper quadrant (RUQ) pain.

Do serology and ultrasound. Blood cultures to rule out septicemia. See Table 14.17.

A visit to the tropics does not preclude the mundane fevers (e.g., flu).

Jaundice Think of viral hepatitis, cholangitis, liver abscess, leptospirosis, typhoid, malaria, dengue fever, yellow fever, and hemoglobinopathies.

Hepatosplenomegaly Viral hepatitis, malaria, *Brucella*, typhoid, leishmaniasis, schistosomiasis, toxoplasmosis.

Gross splenomegaly Malaria, visceral leishmaniasis (kala-azar).

Diarrhea and vomiting Enterotoxigenic *E. coli* (travelers' diarrhea) is most common. Consider *Salmonella, Shigella, Campylobacter, Giardia lamblia, Vibrio cholerae, Yersinia, Cryptosporidium, Isospora, E. coli 0157, Enteroinvasive E. coli, Aeromonas, Rotavirus, Noroviruses,* etc. If diarrhea prolonged, consider protozoal infection of small bowel or tropical sprue. *In HIV:* MAC, CMV, *Cryptosporidium, Microsporidium,* and *Isospora belli.*

Respiratory symptoms Common respiratory pathogens, typhoid, *Legionella,* TB, Q fever, histoplasmosis, Löffler's syndrome.

Arthritis Gonococcus; septicemia; viruses (Ross River, Chikungunya).

Erythema nodosum *Causes:* Strep, TB, leprosy, fungi, Crohn's, ulcerative colitis, sarcoidosis, pregnancy, drugs (sulfonamides).

Anemia Hookworm, malaria, kala-azar, hemolysis, and malabsorption.

Skin lesions Scabies (itchy allergic rash + burrows, e.g., in finger web-spaces), bed bugs (grouped papules), myiasis (nodules—larvae of various insects), orf (pustules), molluscum contagiosum (pearly, punctate, papules), leprosy (anesthetic, hypopigmented areas), Loa loa (calabar swellings), cercarial dermatitis (swimmer's itch), leishmaniasis (ulcers/nodules), rickettsial infections (African tick typhus, Mediterranean tick typhus, scrub typhus [painless eschar = scab]), drug reactions.

Acute abdomen Perforation of a typhoid ulcer, toxic megacolon in amoebic or bacillary dysentery, sickle-cell crisis, ruptured spleen.

Rarities to consider Use local emergency isolation policy. *Rabies* and other CNS viral infections (e.g., encephalitis). *Yellow fever :* Suspect in travelers from Africa. *Lassa fever:* Occurs in Nigeria, Sierra Leone, or Liberia. Signs: Fever; sore throat with exudates; face edema; shock. *Marburg and Ebola virus:* Seen in Sudan, Zaire, and Kenya. Signs: Fever, myalgias, diarrhea, nausea and vomiting (N&V), pleuritic pain, hepatitis, shock, and bleeding tendency. Maculopapular rash appears on day 5–7 and desquamates in <5 d. Patients may bleed from all orifices and gums. *Viruses that cause hemorrhage:* Dengue, Marburg, Lassa, Ebola, Crimea-Congo fever, hemorrhagic fever with renal syndrome, yellow fever.

Table 14.17 Incubation times for fever in the tropical traveler

The incubation times below are typical, but considerable variation occurs.

<14 d	2–6 wks	>6 wks
Undifferentiated fever		
Malaria		
Typhoid		
Leptospirosis		
Acute HIV infection		
Dengue fever		
Rickettsial		
	Acute schistosomiasis	
	Hepatitis E	
	Hepatitis A	
		Amoebic liver abscess
		Lymphatic filariasis
		Kala-azar
		Hepatitis B
Fever with CNS signs		
<14 d	2–6 wks	>6 wks
East African trypanosomiasis		
Rabies		
Viral and bacterial meningitis/ encephalitis		
Poliomyelitis		
		African trypanosomiasis
Fever with chest signs		
<2 wks	2–6 wks	>6 wks
Q fever		
Histoplasmosis		
Coccidioidomycosis		
Influenza		
Legionellosis		
SARS		
		Tuberculosis

Ryan ET. Illness after International Travel. *N Engl J Med.* 2002;347:505.

Malaria

Clinical features and diagnosis Malaria is caused by plasmodium protozoa injected by the nighttime biting female *Anopheles* mosquito. *P. falciparum* and *P. vivax* are the most common. The organisms multiply in the liver and then infect RBCs causing hemolysis, RBC sequestration, and cytokine release. Malaria is one of the most common causes of fever and illness in the tropics. There are >200 million cases of malaria each year. The infection kills nearly 800,000 people each year, mostly children in Africa. Partially protective immunity develops over time, but wanes once a person leaves an endemic area. Thus, expatriates and travelers who normally live in nonendemic areas and enter malarious regions are at high risk for severe complications.

P. falciparum malaria is the most deadly. *Incubation:* 12 d. Most travelers present within 2 months. *Symptoms:* Nonspecific flu-like prodrome: Headache, malaise, myalgias, and anorexia followed by fever and chills ± syncope. Classic periodic fever (peaking every third day, i.e., tertian), headache and rigors are unusual initially. *Signs:* Anemia, jaundice, and hepatosplenomegaly. No rash or lymphadenopathy. *Complications: Cerebral malaria:* Seizures ± confusion then coma. Focal signs unusual. May have variable tone, extensor posturing; up going plantars, dysconjugate gaze. *Mortality:* ~20%. *Metabolic (lactic) acidosis* giving labored deep (Kussmaul's) breathing also major cause of death. *Anemia* is common due to hemolysis of parasitized RBCs. Elevated transaminases levels, *hyperparasitemia* (>5% of RBCs parasitized), and *hypoglycemia* can occur in severe malaria (8% of adults) or with quinine therapy. *Acute renal failure* from acute tubular necrosis, sometimes with hemoglobinuria (*blackwater fever*), and *pulmonary edema* are important causes of death in severe malaria (*algid malaria*) from bacterial septicemia, dehydration or, rarely, splenic rupture. In pregnancy, the risk of miscarriage is up to 60% and death in the mother is up to 50%. Advise pregnant women to defer travel to malarious regions. If that is not feasible, meticulous mosquito avoidance and chemoprophylaxis should be used. Relapse occurs as parasites lie dormant in the liver (*P. vivax* and *P. ovale*) or at low levels in the blood (*P. malariae*). Nephrotic syndrome (glomerulonephritis) may occur in chronic *P. malariae* infection.

Diagnosis Serial thin and thick blood films (needs much skill, don't always believe negative reports or reports based on thin-film examination alone); if *P. falciparum*, use smears to determine level of parasitemia. Antigen detection of *P. falciparum* and *P. vivax* using rapid diagnostic tests is emerging as an option in settings lacking timely access to high quality microscopy. Serology is not useful. *Other tests:* CBC (anemia, elevated transaminases, thrombocytopenia), clotting, glucose (hypoglycemia), ABG/lactate (lactic acidosis), electrolytes (renal failure), urinalysis (hemoglobinuria, proteinuria, casts), blood culture. See Table 14.18.

549

Poor prognostic signs

Severe *P. falciparum* malaria, >5% parasitemia, hypotension, severe anemia, DIC, spontaneous bleeding, jaundice, seizures, impaired consciousness/coma, repeated seizures, respiratory distress, acidemia, renal failure, hemoglobinuria. If 20% (or $>10^4$/mcL) of parasites are mature trophozoites or schizonts, the prognosis is poor, even if few parasites seen (reflects critical mass of sequestered RBCs)

Table 14.18 Key points in diagnosis and management of malaria
Think about malaria as a possible diagnosis!
Take a full travel history, including stopovers in transit
Before excluding the diagnosis, make sure enough blood smears (three sets) have been performed and check if the patient has already received treatment, which might make the blood smear negative.
Don't delay therapy when there is a strong clinical suspicion, severe disease, or difficulty in getting timely laboratory confirmation of infection.
Use IV quinidine as part of therapy in patients with severe disease.
Make sure the drug gets to the patient promptly. Avoid potential delays due to inadequate communication between medical, nursing and pharmacy staff.
Do not delay therapy while trying to figure out if the patient should get artesunate or an exchange transfusion.
Unless certain, assume patient has *P. falciparum* and that the infection is chloroquine resistant.
Follow the patient closely for first few days.
Remember that malaria is an important cause of coma, deep jaundice, severe anemia, and renal failure in the tropics.

Treatment If species unknown or mixed infection, treat as *P. falciparum*. Nearly all *P. falciparum* is now resistant to chloroquine and in many areas is also resistant to Fansidar® (pyrimethamine + sulfadoxine). If in doubt, consider as resistant. Chloroquine is the drug of choice for nonfalciparum malarias in most parts of the world, but chloroquine-resistant *P. vivax* occurs in Papua New Guinea, Indonesia, and some areas of Brazil, Colombia, and Guyana. Never rely on chloroquine if used alone as prophylaxis. *P. falciparum* is still susceptible to chloroquine in Central America (West of the Panama Canal Zone), Haiti, Dominican Republic, and most of the Middle East. See Table 14.19.

If seriously ill, take to ICU and give quinidine IV with telemetry. Observe for QT prolongation, ventricular arrhythmias, hypotension and hypoglycemia. Consider exchange transfusion if parasitemia is >10%, patient has altered mental status, *ARDS* or renal complications. *Do not delay quinidine for exchange transfusion.* Artesunate can be obtained from *CDC* for severe malaria.

CDC Malaria Hotline: 770–488–7788, 855–856–4713 (toll free), (770–488–7100 (after hours)

Table 14.19 Malaria treatments

Organism	Modifying factor	Regimen
Uncomplicated P. falciparum (CQ susceptible), P. malariae, P. knowlesi, species not known		CQ 1,000 mg α 1, then 500 mg at 6, 24, and 48 h
		Hydroxy-CQ 800 mg α 1, then 400 mg at 6, 24, and 48 h
Uncomplicated P. falciparum (CQ resistant or unknown)		Atovaquone (250 mg)/Proguanil (100 mg) 4 tabs/24 h α 3 d **Avoid in pregnancy**
		Artemether (20 mg)/lumefantrine (120 mg) 4 tabs, Day 1 given at 0 and 8 h, d 2, 3 bid (total = 24 tabs) **Avoid in pregnancy**
		Quinine sulphate 650 mg/8 h α 3 d (7 d if malaria acquired in SE Asia) **and** doxycycline 100 mg/12 h PO α 7 d (or clindamycin 7 mg/kg/8 h PO α 7 d) **Avoid doxycycline in pregnancy**
Uncomplicated P. vivax, P. ovale		CQ 1,000 mg α 1, then 500 mg at 6,24 and 48 hours or Hydroxy-CQ 800 mg α 1, then 400 mg at 6, 24, and 48 h
		and
		Primaquine 30 mg/24 h α 14 d to treat liver stage and prevent relapse. **Avoid in** G6PD **deficiency (screen before giving) and pregnancy**
Severe (typically P. falciparum)		Quinidine gluconate: 10 mg/kg loading dose IV over 1–2 h, then 0.02 mg/kg/min continuous infusion α 24 h. After 24 h, if parasitemia is <1% and patient can tolerate orals, switch IV quinidine to PO quinine, otherwise continue IV. Total quinidine/quinine course generally 3 d (7 d if disease acquired in SE Asia)
		and
		Doxycycline 100 mg/12 h PO or IV α 7 d (or clindamycin 7 mg/kg/8 h PO. If giving IV: 10 mg/kg α 1 then 5 mg/kg/8 h α 7 d). **Avoid doxycycline in pregnancy**

CQ, chloroquine, all CQ, H-CQ, quinine and quinidine doses are for salt form of drug.

Other treatments

Acetaminophen for fever. Transfuse if severe anemia. Consider exchange transfusion if patient severely ill. Monitor bp, urine output, and blood glucose frequently. Follow daily parasite count, platelets, LFT, and electrolytes.

Antimalarial side effects

- *Artemether/lumefantrine:* Headache, anorexia, and dizziness
- *Atovaquone/Proguanil:* Abdominal pain, GI disturbances, headache
- *Chloroquine and hydroxychloroquine:* GI disturbances, dizziness, blurred vision, headache, insomnia, pruritus psychosis and retinopathy (chronic use)
- *Doxycycline:* Phototoxicity, yeast vaginitis, GI disturbances, and pill esophagitis

- *Mefloquine:* GI disturbances, headache, and neuropsychiatric symptoms ranging from sleep disturbances to psychosis. Avoid mefloquine if low risk of chloroquine-resistant malaria, past or family history of epilepsy, or need to perform complicated task (e.g., pilots). Give patient FDA mefloquine medication guide.
- *Primaquine:* Epigastric pain, hemolysis if G6PD-deficient, methemoglobinemia

Mycobacterium tuberculosis

Basic terms

Latent infection: Presence of *M. tuberculosis* in the body (detected by TST or IGRA) without disease. This person is not infectious.

Active TB: Evidence of active infection (e.g., abnormal CXR) in a person with + TST or IGRA **and/or** smear, culture or polymerase chain reaction (PCR) evidence of *M. tuberculosis.*

Clinical features

Approximately one-third of the world's population is infected with TB. The vast majority (90%) will not develop active TB. The prevalence and mortality of TB has declined in recent years, but in 2010 there were about 9 million new active TB cases and 1.4 million deaths from TB. The rates of developing active infection are much higher in those with HIV. TB is the leading cause of death in people with HIV. In the United States, great strides have been made in controlling TB. In 2009, there were about 11,000 new cases and 500 deaths. About 3.3% of new TB cases are due to MDR-TB (resistant to isoniazid and rifampin). Most of those are from Eastern Europe, Asia, and parts of Africa. There are an estimated 25,000 cases/year of XDR-TB (resistant to isoniazid [INH], rifampin, quinolones, amikacin, capreomycin, and kanamycin).

Primary TB Initial infection is usually pulmonary (by droplet spread). A lesion forms and its draining nodes are infected. There is early distant spread of the bacilli, then an immune response suspends further multiplication at all sites. Primary TB is often asymptomatic or there is fever, anorexia, productive cough, or conjunctivitis (small, multiple, yellow-gray nodules near the limbus). Acid-fast bacilli (AFB) may be found in sputum. CXR may be abnormal. The commonest nonpulmonary *primary* infection is GI, typically affecting the ileocecal junction and associated lymph nodes.

Latent TB Rates of latent TB are highest in close contacts of those with active TB, homeless, foreign-born persons, prisoners, and injection drug users. Universal screening (with TST or IGRA) is not recommended. Many people with latent TB are at low risk for reactivation, and many false-positive tests are expected in low-risk groups. Screening is most useful (with an intention to treat positive results) in people with HIV, recipients of immunosuppressive medications, the homeless, injection drug users, health care workers, and people whose test is newly positive (within 2 yrs).

Table 14.20 Tests to diagnose latent tuberculosis (TB)

Tuberculin skin test (aka Mantoux, TST, PPD) Read at 48–72 h

Patient characteristic	Positive test (induration diameter)
HIV+, TNF-β inhibitors, recent contact with person who has active TB, organ transplant recipients, corticosteroids (e.g., prednisone >15 mg/d α >1 month), fibrotic changes on CXR	" 5 mm
Recent immigrants from endemic regions, injection drug users, lived or worked in high-risk setting (e.g., homeless shelter, prison, health care facility, microbiology laboratory), high-risk clinical conditions (e.g., chronic renal disease, silicosis, diabetes, heme malignancies, gastrectomy, chronic weight loss)	" 10 mm
No known risk factor for TB	" 15 mm

BCG vaccine, may give a false positive skin test result, but results should be interpreted regardless of BCG history

Interferon γ-release assays (IGRA) requires a blood sample, does not cross-react with BCG, does not require a return visit to read skin reaction.

Treatment of latent TB: The goal is to eradicate the latent infections in patients at risk for reactivation. **First step is to rule out active infection.** In all cases, standard anti-TB therapy should be initiated once any evidence of active disease (clinical or radiographic) is found to avoid treatment failure and development of resistance.

Regimen	Comment
INH 300 mg/d α 9 months	"Classic" regimen
INH 900 mg twice weekly α 9 months	Use directly observed therapy
INH α 6 months	9 months better, but 6 months will provide some protection
Rifampin 600 mg/d α 4 months	Lower risk of hepatotoxicity compared with INH, multiple drug interactions
INH 900 mg/rifapentine 900 mg/week α 12 (doses based on weight " 60 kg)	Use directly observed therapy

If there is a known contact with a person infected with INH-resistant TB, rifampin is an alternative, but seek help.

Reactivation >80% of active TB in the United States is due to reactivation from latent infection. Reactivation rates are particularly high in the first few years after TB exposure. Any form of immunocompromised may allow reactivation (e.g., HIV, malignancy, poorly controlled diabetes, >2 wks of ≥15 mg/d prednisone, debilitation, treatment with TNF-α inhibitor, and chronic renal failure). Reactivation is significantly associated with radiographic evidence of old healed (untreated) TB.

The lung lesions, which usually are in the upper lobes, can progress and fibrose. Any other site may become the main clinical problem. Tuberculomas contain few AFB unless they erode into a bronchus, where the favorable environment ensures rapid multiplication, rendering the patient highly contagious. In the elderly or immunocompromised, dissemination of multiple tiny foci throughout the body (including back to the lungs) results in miliary TB.

Pulmonary TB This may be silent or present with cough, sputum, malaise, weight loss, night sweats, pleurisy, hemoptysis (may be massive), pleural effusion, or superimposed pulmonary infection. An aspergilloma/mycetoma may form in the cavities.

Miliary TB Occurs following hematogenous dissemination. Clinical features may be nonspecific. CXR shows characteristic reticulonodular shadowing. Look for retinal TB. Biopsy of lung, liver, lymph nodes, or marrow may yield AFB or granulomas.

Meningeal TB Subacute onset of meningitis symptoms: Fever, headache, nausea, vomiting, neck stiffness, and photophobia.

Genitourinary TB May cause frequency, dysuria, flank/back pain, hematuria, and, classically, sterile pyuria. Take three early-morning urine samples for AFB. Renal ultrasound may help. Renal TB may spread to bladder, seminal vesicles, and epididymitis or fallopian tubes.

Bone TB Look for vertebral collapse adjacent to a paravertebral abscess (Pott's vertebra). Do biopsies for AFB stains and culture.

Skin TB **(lupus vulgaris)** Jelly-like nodules; e.g., on face or neck.

Peritoneal This causes abdominal pain. Look for AFB in ascites (send a *large* volume to lab); laparotomy may be needed.

Acute TB **pericarditis** Think of this as a primary exudative lesion.

Chronic pericardial effusion and constrictive pericarditis These reflect chronic granulomas. Fibrosis and calcification may be prominent with spread to myocardium.

Additional points in all those with TB

Advise **HIV** testing. **Notify** local health department to arrange contact tracing and screening. Explain that **prolonged treatment** will be necessary. All patients should receive **directly observed therapy** (DOT). **Monitoring** of blood tests will be needed (LFTs). Explain the need for **respiratory isolation** procedures while infectious until three negative sputa for AFB. See Table 14.21.

Tuberculosis diagnosis and treatment

Diagnosis In all suspected cases, it is important to obtain the relevant clinical samples (sputum, pleural fluid, pleura, urine, pus, ascites, peritoneum, or CSF) for culture (or other testing) to establish the diagnosis. Get advice on testing contacts from health department. **Microbiology:** AFB resist acid–alcohol decolorization under auramine or Ziehl–Neelsen (ZN) staining. Sputum sample typically show few if any AFB. Send three expectorated sputum samples, preferably on different days, for AFB stain and culture. Cultures require prolonged incubation (usually 2–6 wks or longer). Sputum may be induced with aerosolized hypertonic saline. If no expectorations, bronchoalveolar lavage (BAL) fluid can be tested. Smears of BAL fluid can be negative even when there is extensive disease. Many patients develop productive sputum after bronchoscopy. This sputum should be tested for AFB. Any suspicious lesions in liver, lymph nodes, or bone marrow can be biopsied. **TB PCR:** Can be applied to AFB + sputum specimen to facilitate rapid diagnosis of TB. A negative PCR does not rule out TB. Interpretation of AFB negative smears with + PCR requires clinical judgment. PCR can also be used to test CSF, pleural and peritoneal fluid specimen. New PCR-based tests allow rapid identification of rifampicin (and likely multi-drug) resistance. **Histology:** The hallmark is the presence of **case-**

ating granulomas. *Radiological features:* CXR may show **consolidation, cavitation, fibrosis**, and **calcification** in pulmonary TB

Phases of therapy Initial phase (8 wks on four drugs) is followed by continuation phase (4 months on two drugs) with rifampicin and INH at same doses. Give pyridoxine throughout treatment. *There are multiple dosing schedules:* **Phase 1 (8 wks):**

INH/rifampin/PZA/ethambutol: 7 d/wk α 8 wks, 5 d/wk α 8 wks, 5 d or 7 d/wk α 2 wks, then 2α/wk α 6 wks, 3 d/wk α 8 wks. **Phase 2 (18 wks):** INH/rifampin: There are multiple dosing schedules including: 7 d/wk α 18 wks, 5 d/wk α 18 wks, 3 d/wk α 18 wks, 2 d/wk α 18 wks

Table 14.21 Tuberculosis and HIV/AIDS

TB is a common, serious, but treatable complication of HIV infection.

Worldwide, 10% of patients with new cases of TB also have HIV (40% in Africa).

Screening tests may be negative with CD4 <200. After initiation of anti-viral therapy, retest those with negative TB test.

Reactivation of latent TB can occur at any CD4 level

Presentation may be atypical.

Previous BCG vaccination does not prevent development of TB.

Smears may be negative for AFB in patients with pulmonary TB with or without HIV. Smears that are positive tend to contain few AFB. This makes culture all the more important and is vital to characterize drug resistance.

Atypical CXR: Lobar or bibasilar pneumonia, hilar lymphadenopathy.

Extra pulmonary and disseminated disease is much more common.

More toxicity from highly active antiretroviral therapy and anti-TB therapy due to drug interactions with rifampin.

Antiretroviral therapy reconstitutes CD4 count and immune function, which may lead to a paradoxical worsening of TB symptoms.

All persons with HIV who have evidence of latent TB should be treated.

Respiratory isolation is essential when TB patients are near other patients, including those who are HIV positive. Nosocomial (hospital-acquired) and MDR-TB are now major problems worldwide. Mortality with MDR-TB is high. Test TB cultures against first- and second-line chemotherapeutic agents; 5+ drugs may be needed in MDR-TB.

Basic principles of treatment:

1. Adherence to therapy is crucial. It helps the patient, reduces development of resistance, and inhibits further propagation of infection.

2. DOT is the preferred method of assuring adherence.

3. Treatment is long and should be coordinated with the health department.

4. Monitor for toxicity (symptoms, CBC, liver, and renal function). A small rise in LFTs is common and acceptable and often resolves without change in therapy. Ethambutol may cause ocular toxicity, so test color vision (Ishihara chart) and acuity before and during treatment if using ethambutol dose "25 mg/kg/d.

5. Seek help in patients with renal or hepatic failure, or pregnancy.

6. Steroids may be indicated in meningeal and pericardial disease.

(Continued)

Table 14.21 (Coninued)

Drug	Dose (max)	Potential side effects
First-line antitubercular agents: All are PO. All doses given as daily. Intermittent dosing options should be given as DOT		
Isoniazid	5 mg/kg/d (300 mg), 15 mg/kg (900 mg) once, twice, or thrice weekly	Hepatitis, neuropathy, pyridoxine deficit, agranulocytosis
Rifampin	10 mg/kg (600 mg) daily, twice or thrice weekly	Hepatitis, orange discoloration of urine and tears (contact lens staining), rash, many drug interactions (e.g., inactivation of birth control pills), flu-like syndrome with intermittent use.
Rifabutin	5/mg/kg (300 mg) daily, twice or thrice weekly	Heme toxicities, rash, GI intolerance, drug interactions often require dose adjustments
Ethambutol	15 mg–20 mg/kg/d, 56–75 kg: 2 g thrice/wk, 2.8 g twice/wk 76–90kg: 2.4 g thrice/wk, 4 g twice/wk	Optic neuritis, color vision is first to deteriorate
Pyrazinamide	20–25 mg/kg/d, 56–75 kg: 2.5 g thrice/wk, 3 g twice/wk 76–90 kg: 3 g thrice/wk, 4 g twice/wk	Hepatitis, non-gout polyarthritis, arthralgias (gout is a contraindication)
Second-line antitubercular agents: Associated with increased toxicity, some only available by injection		
Cycloserine	10–15 mg/kg/d (1,000 mg). Usually 500–750 mg/d in two doses	Neuropsychiatric (including psychosis and seizures). Pyridoxine (100–200 mg/d) may help
Ethionamide	10–15 mg/kg/d (1,000 mg). Usually 500–750 mg/d	Severe GI, liver, endocrine, neuropathy
Streptomycin, amikacin, kanamycin, capreomycin (injected)	15 mg/kg/d (1 g)	Nephrotoxicity and ototoxicity
p-Aminosalicylic acid	4 g/8–12 h/d	Hypothyroid, GI, liver
Quinolones	Levofloxacin: 500–1,000 mg/d Moxifloxacin: 400 mg/d	GI, liver, neuropathy, tendinopathy

(Continued)

Table 14.21 (Coninued)

Stopping the spread of MDR-TB

Early identification and isolation and full treatment: Control depends upon early isolation of suspected patients. If there is a suspicious CXR or a past history of MDR-TB, don't wait to prove the diagnosis. Isolate. Isolate if cough >2 wks and abnormal CXR. Provide negative air pressure in isolation rooms and N95 masks for staff. Obtain respiratory samples for microbiology testing in a timely fashion. Sputum induction/expectoration should be confined to isolation rooms. Only stop isolation after three sputum samples are AFB negative on culture for MDR-TB. Remove barriers for completion of therapy. Best achieved by directly observing and confirming that patients take all prescribed drugs. Frequent tuberculin skin surveillance tests for workers and contacts. Contact evaluation.

Herpes infections

Varicella zoster Chickenpox is the primary infection; after infection, virus remains dormant in dorsal root ganglia. Reactivation causes shingles. Shingles affects 20% at some time. High-risk groups: Elderly or immunosuppressed. *Clinical features:* Pain in a dermatomal distribution precedes malaise and fever by a few days. Some days later, macules, papules, and vesicles develop in the same dermatome. Thoracic dermatomes and the ophthalmic division of trigeminal nerve are most vulnerable. If the sacral nerves are affected, urinary retention may occur. Motor nerves are rarely affected. Herpes zoster oticus (Ramsey Hunt syndrome II) involves the ear, mouth, and CN VII). Zoster recurrence suggests immunosuppression. *Investigations* are rarely necessary; diagnosis can be confirmed by PCR, immunohistochemical study, and culture of suspected lesion fluid. *Indications for treatment (systemic antiviral therapy):* All immunocompromised patients, otherwise: Age " 50, moderate or severe rash/pain, nontruncal involvement. Consider therapy in all patients to reduce risk of postherpetic neuralgia. If possible, start therapy <72 h after onset. For immunocompetent patients, use PO acyclovir 800 mg/4–5 h, famciclovir 500 mg/8 h, or valacyclovir 1 g/8 h for 7–10 d. If patient severely immunocompromised, start with IV acyclovir 10 mg/kg/8 h until infection is controlled, then switch to oral therapy. For less immunosuppressed patients, try oral famciclovir or valacyclovir as initial therapy (with careful monitoring). Control pain with oral analgesic ± gabapentin, tricyclics, carbamazepine, lidocaine patch and/or narcotics (underutilized). A course of corticosteroids tapered over 3 wks (prednisone 60 mg, 30 mg, 15 mg) can be considered in patients without contraindications. Care of herpes zoster ophthalmicus should involve an ophthalmologist. Use IV acyclovir in cases of retinitis. Use topical antibacterial to protect ocular surface. Beware of iritis. Measure visual acuity often. Advise patient to report *any* visual loss at once. *SE of acyclovir:* Renal impairment (check electrolytes) vomiting, urticaria, and encephalopathy. *Complications:* Postherpetic neuralgia in the affected dermatome can persist for years and be very hard to treat. Try carbamazepine, phenytoin, amitriptyline, gabapentin, or capsaicin cream and narcotics. As a last resort, ablation of the appropriate ganglion may be tried. Refer to a pain clinic.

Herpes simplex virus (HSV) Manifestations of primary infection:
- **Systemic infection:** Fever, sore throat, and lymphadenopathy may pass unnoticed. If immunocompromised, it may be life-threatening with fever, lymphadenopathy, pneumonitis, and hepatitis.
- **Gingivostomatitis:** Ulcers filled with yellow slough appear in the mouth.
- **Herpetic whitlow:** A breach in the skin allows the virus to enter the finger, causing a vesicle to form. This often affects children's nurses.
- **Traumatic herpes (herpes gladiatorum):** Vesicles develop at any site where HSV is ground into the skin by brute force.
- **Eczema herpeticum:** HSV infection of eczematous skin; usually in children.
- **Herpes simplex meningitis:** This is uncommon and usually self-limiting (typically HSV-2 in women during a primary attack). May be recurrent. CSF PCR is test of choice.
- **Genital herpes:** At least 50 million people in America are infected. HSV-2 is most common and more likely to be recurrent. Most people do not know they have genital HSV, but still shed virus intermittently. Classic lesions are painful, may appear as ulcers or grouped vesicles and papules, develop around anus and penis (with pain, fever, and dysuria) ± palms, feet, or throat. Recurrent infection is generally less symptomatic than primary infection. *Diagnosis:* Classic lesions are frequently absent. Obtain PCR or culture of skin lesions. Negative test does not rule out infection. HSV-2 antibodies are highly sensitive and specific. Tzanck smear is not reliable. *Treatment:* Give analgesia and one of the regimens in Table 14.22 for acute, recurrent, and suppressive therapy. Suppressive therapy may improve quality of life and decrease transmission in discordant couples.
- **HSV keratitis:** Corneal dendritic ulcers. *Avoid steroids.* Trifluridine eye drops, 1 drop q2h up to 9 α/d α 21 d.
- **Herpes simplex encephalitis:** Usually HSV1. Virus spreads centripetally (e.g., from cranial nerve ganglia, to frontal and temporal lobes). Suspect this if there are fevers, seizures, headaches, odd behavior, dysphasia, hemiparesis, or coma or subacute brainstem encephalitis, meningitis, or myelitis. *Diagnosis:* Urgent PCR on CSF sample (CT/magnetic resonance imaging (MRI) and electroencephalogram (EEG) may show temporal lobe changes but are nonspecific and unreliable; brain biopsy rarely required). Seek expert help: Consider admitting to ICU; careful fluid balance is important to minimize cerebral edema. Poor predictors are age >30, delay in starting acyclovir >4 d, altered consciousness. Prompt acyclovir (e.g., 10 mg/kg/8 h IV for 14–21 d) decreases mortality to 8% (untreated mortality 70%).

Table 14.22 Genital herpes treatment			
	Acute	**Recurrent**	**Suppression**
Acyclovir	400 mg/8 h or 200 mg/4–5 h α 7–10 d	400 mg/8 h, 800 mg/12 h α 5 d, 800 mg/8 h α 2d	400 mg bid
Famciclovir	250 mg/8 h α 7–10 d	125 mg/12 h α 5 d, 500 mg α 1 then 250 mg/12 h α 2 d, 1 g/12 h α 1 d	250 mg bid
Valacyclovir	1 g/12 h α 7–10 d	500 mg/12 h α 3 d or 1 g/d α 5 d	0.5–1 g/d

Severe disease: Acyclovir 10 mg/kg q8h IV
Acyclovir resistance: Foscarnet 120–200 mg/d iv or topical cidofovir gel 1% applied daily α 5 d

- **Recurrent HSV:** HSV lying dormant in ganglion cells may be reactivated by illness, immunosuppression, menstruation, or even sunlight. Cold sores (perioral vesicles) are one manifestation. Acyclovir cream is not recommended.

Infectious mononucleosis

This is a common disease of young adults that may pass unnoticed or cause acute illness. Spread is thought to be by saliva or droplet. The incubation period is uncertain, but may be 4–5 wks. EBV is the cause of classic mononucleosis, but other viruses (e.g., HIV, CMV) can cause a similar syndrome. EBV preferentially infects B-lymphocytes. There follows a proliferation of T-cells (the "atypical" mononuclear cells), which are cytotoxic to EBV-infected cells. The latter are "immortalized" by EBV infection and can, very rarely, proliferate to form a picture indistinguishable from immunoblastic lymphoma in immunodeficient individuals (whose suppressor T-cells fail to check multiplication of these B-cells).

Symptoms and signs include sore throat, fever, anorexia, malaise, lymphadenopathy, palatal petechiae, splenomegaly, hepatitis, and hemolytic anemia. Occasionally, there is encephalitis, myocarditis, pericarditis, or neuropathy. Rashes may occur, particularly if the patient is given ampicillin.

Differential diagnosis Streptococcal sore throat (may coexist), CMV, viral hepatitis, HIV seroconversion illness, adenovirus, toxoplasmosis, leukemia, diphtheria, drug reaction (e.g., phenytoin).

Investigations Blood lm shows lymphocytosis (up to 20% of WBC) and atypical lymphocytes (large, irregular nuclei). Such cells may be seen in many viral infections (e.g., CMV, HIV, parvovirus, dengue fever), toxoplasmosis, leukemia, lymphomas, drug hypersensitivity, and lead poisoning. Serological tests are listed in Table 14.23:

Treatment Avoid alcohol and trauma to LUQ. Steroids are rarely recommended for severe symptoms. Ampicillin and amoxicillin should not be given for sore throat if mononucleosis is suspected as they may cause a severe rash in those with acute EBV infection.

Complications Depression, fatigue, and lethargy, which may persist for months. Also, mononucleosis can be associated with thrombocytopenia, ruptured spleen, splenic hemorrhage, upper airways obstruction (may need observation in ICU), secondary infection, pneumonitis, aseptic meningitis, Guillain–Barré syndrome, renal failure, lymphoma, and autoimmune hemolytic anemia. All are rare.

Table 14.23 Serological tests for mononucleosis

559

Test	Comment
Heterophil antibody (e.g., monospot)	Becomes + with acute infection and persists for 4–12 wks. False + possible in hepatitis, lymphoma, leukemia, SLE
Viral capsid antigen (VCA)	Become + with acute infection
	IgM: Persists 4–6 wks
	IgG: Persists for life
Early-antigen IgG	Become + with acute infection, persists for 3–6 months or longer (lifelong in 20%)
Antibody to EBV nuclear antigen (EBNA)	Becomes + 2–4 months after disease onset and persists for life.

Other EBV-associated diseases Burkitt's lymphoma in Africa and nasopharyngeal carcinoma in Asia. EBV positive large cell (B-cell) lymphomas occasionally appear in the immunocompromised (e.g., post-transplantation lymphoproliferative disorder). The EBV genome has also been found in the Reed–Sternberg cell of Hodgkin's lymphoma. Oral hairy leukoplakia is caused by EBV and may respond to antivirals such as acyclovir and valacyclovir.

Cytomegalovirus

CMV may be acquired by direct contact, blood transfusion, or organ transplantation. After acute infection, CMV becomes latent, but the infection may reactivate at times of stress or immunocompromise. If immunocompetent, primary infection is usually asymptomatic but acute hepatitis may occur. In solid organ transplant patients, CMV infection may be acquired from the transplanted graft as primary infection or reactivate from the recipient's own CMV. *CMV disease after solid organ or post bone marrow transplantation:* CMV syndrome (fever, myalgias, bone marrow suppression) > pneumonitis > colitis > hepatitis > retinitis. *In AIDS:* Retinitis > colitis > esophagitis > CNS disease. (Here, > means "is more common than.")

Diagnosis of acute CMV infection is occasionally difficult; growth of the virus is slow and there may be prolonged CMV excretion from a distant source of infection. For CMV disease in transplant recipients CMV PCR (including quantitative tests) of blood/CSF/bronchoalveolar lavage are becoming widely available. CMV retinitis is diagnosed by fundus exam in atypical host; no lab tests are necessary. Extensive CMV involvement of GI tract or lung can be present even with negative serum PCR. Histopathology (lung, gut, etc.) shows typical inclusions.

Treatment is stratified by scenario : Mainstay of therapy in nonimmunocompromised patients is supportive. In transplant and HIV patients, treatment is with ganciclovir IV or valganciclovir PO. In eye disease, direct antiviral injections and intraocular implants are used as well. Main toxicity of systemic therapy is leukopenia. Dose must be adjusted for renal dysfunction. Treatment is individualized. In invasive disease, try to reduce immunosuppression. If feasible, treat infection for at least 2 wks after resolution of viremia and symptoms. After completion of therapy, secondary prophylaxis for 1–3 months or longer should be considered.

Table 14.24 Cytomegalovirus treatment

Scenario	Antiviral Treatment (for normal GFR)
Acute CMV infection: Normal host	None
Asymptomatic CMV viremia: Transplant	Valganciclovir 900 mg/12 h PO
CMV syndrome: Transplant	Valganciclovir 900 mg/12 h PO or ganciclovir 5 mg/kg/12 h IV
GI: Transplant, HIV	Ganciclovir 5 mg/kg/12 IV, can switch to PO valganciclovir when stable
Lung: Transplant	Ganciclovir 5 mg/kg/12 IV, consider CMV Ig 100–150 mg/kg thrice weekly, can switch to PO valganciclovir when stable
CNS: Transplant, HIV	Ganciclovir 5 mg/kg/12 IV
Retinitis: HIV, transplant	Valganciclovir 900 mg/12 h PO or ganciclovir 5 mg/kg /12 h IV. Duration guided by eye exam. In severe disease, intraocular antiviral injection
Ganciclovir-resistant infection (test for UL97 and UL54 mutations)	Ganciclovir 7.5–10 mg/kg/12 h IV, Foscarnet 60 mg/kg/8 h or 90 mg/kg/12 h, cidofovir 5 mg/kg/wk α 2, then every other week. Consider CMV Ig.

Nonspecific upper respiratory tract infections (common cold)

>200 viruses are potentially responsible. Rhinoviruses are the main culprits (dozens of strains). Other viruses include parainfluenza, respiratory syncytial virus (RSV), adenovirus, and influenza. Illness usually includes a self-limiting nasal discharge (which becomes mucopurulent over a few days), sore throat, watery eyes, mild body aches, and headache. Symptoms last average of 7–11 d. Influenza is the most important (see below), but other viruses (e.g., RSV, parainfluenza, and adenovirus) can cause devastating illness in immunocompromised patients.

Incubation 1–4 d.

Complications Sinusitis, lower respiratory tract infection.

Treatment Avoid smoking or second-hand smoke; humidifier may help with coughing; ice chips or throat lozenges for sore throat; ibuprofen, acetaminophen for low-grade fevers and pain. First-generation antihistamines and decongestants may also help with symptoms.

Influenza

This is a very important viral respiratory infection because of its frequency and complication rate, particularly in the elderly and in those with underlying medical conditions. Influenza is responsible for ~ 20,000 deaths/year in the United States. Compared to seasonal influenza, when pandemic strains evolve, mortality may be significantly higher and/or new groups may be particularly vulnerable. The virus (RNA orthomyxovirus) has three types (A, B, C). Only types A and B cause significant morbidity in humans. Subtyping (for type A) is by hemagglutinin (H) and neuraminidase (N) characteristics. Frequent mutations give strains with new antigenic properties. Minor changes (antigenic drift) and especially major changes (antigenic shift) can place whole areas at risk. World Health Organization (WHO) classification specifies: Type/host origin/geographic origin/strain number/year of isolation/subtype (e.g., A/Swine/Taiwan/2/87/[H3, N2]).

Spread is by droplets or hands. **Incubation period:** 1–4 d. **Infectivity**: 1 d before to 7 d after symptoms start. **Immunity**: Those attacked by one strain are immune to that strain only. **Convalescence**: May be slow.

Symptoms Fever, headache, malaise, myalgias, nausea, vomiting, and conjunctivitis/eye pain (even photophobia).

Tests Only test if result will change management or infection control practices. PCR of nasopharyngeal aspirates is highly sensitive and specific. Other tests have limitations. These include rapid flu tests (<60% sensitive), immunofluorescence (requires lab expertise), and culture (results not available in timely fashion).

Complications Bronchitis 20%, pneumonia (especially *S. pneumoniae* and *S. aureus*), sinusitis, otitis media, encephalitis, pericarditis, and Reye's syndrome (coma, increased LFTs; may be associated with ASA use).

Treatment With mild disease, recommend rest at home until afebrile >24 hours. Symptom relief with acetaminophen may help. Antiviral therapy should be considered in all patients diagnosed within 48 h of symptom onset and those requiring hospitalization. Also consider therapy in those with immunosuppression, underlying illnesses (e.g., sickle cell, cancer, pulmonary, renal, heart, neurological, diabetes mellitus), residents of long-term care facilities, and age >65. If severe pneumonia, most authorities recommend rapid transfer to ICU as sepsis and hypoxia may rapidly progress to circulatory collapse and death.

Antiviral: Oseltamivir 75 mg PO bid for 5 d eases symptoms if started within 48 h of onset of symptoms. Amantadine and rimantadine are only effective against influenza type A virus. Zanamivir (an inhaled neuraminidase

Table 14.25 Influenza treatments			
Medication	**Dose**	**Spectrum**	**Toxicity**
Oseltamivir	Treatment: 75 mg/12 h α 5 d, prophylaxis: 75 mg/d	A, B	GI, neuropsychiatric
Zanamivir	Treatment: Two 5 mg inhalations/12 h α 5d. Prophylaxis: Two inhalations/d	A, B	Bronchospasm
Rimantadine/ amantadine	Treatment or prophylaxis: 200 mg/d **or** 100 mg/12 h α 5 d	A, but resistance in H3N2	GI, neuropsychiatric

inhibitor) and oseltamivir are active against influenza types A and B. *Note:* Inhalation is not an ideal route if elderly or prone to bronchospasm. May also cause oropharyngeal edema.

Prevention *Seasonal inuenza (trivalent) vaccination:* Inactivated virus (injected) and live attenuated virus (intranasal). It is prepared from current serotypes and takes <2 wks to work. *Indications:* Inactivated virus: All persons ≥6 months. Particularly important for health care workers with patient contact, household contacts of high-risk persons, persons ≥50 yrs, pregnant women (second- and third-trimester), residents of long-term care facilities, and patients with high-risk comorbidity (e.g., neurologic disorders; morbid obesity; diabetes; chronic lung, heart, or renal disease; immunosuppression; hemoglobinopathies).

Dose: 0.5 ml SC (once). Side effects *(SE):* Mild pain or swelling (17%). Fever, headaches, and malaise are reported in 10%. *Live attenuated influenza vaccine:* Indicated for immunocompetent persons aged 5–49 yrs. Do not use in immunosuppressed patients or their close contacts; persons with asthma, chronic underlying illnesses, and pregnant women. *Antiviral prophylaxis:* Consider using in high-risk patients when influenza is circulating until vaccine becomes effective (about 2 wks).

Poliomyelitis

Poliovirus is highly contagious, although only 4–8% of patients develop any illness from the infection and <1% become paralyzed (usually lower extremities). **Spread** is by droplets or fecal–oral. Polio has been eliminated from the Americas, Europe, and the Western Pacific. Polio remains endemic in India, Pakistan, Afghanistan, and Nigeria.

The patient 7 d incubation, then a flu-like prodrome, leading to a "pre-paralytic" stage: Fever, tachycardia, headache, vomiting, neck stiffness, and unilateral tremor. In <50% of patients, this progresses to the paralytic stage: Myalgias, lower motor neuron signs, and respiratory failure. *Tests:* CSF: WBC elevation, polymorphs then lymphocytes, otherwise normal; paired sera (14 d apart); throat swab and stool culture identify virus. *Natural history:* 5–10% of those with paralysis die. There may be delayed progression of paralysis. *Risk factors for severe paralysis:* Adulthood, pregnancy, post-tonsillectomy, muscle fatigue/trauma during incubation period. *Prophylaxis:* Vaccination.

Toxoplasmosis

The protozoan *Toxoplasma gondii* infects via gut, lung, or broken skin. Cats (the primary host) excrete oocysts, but the ingestion of poorly cooked infected meat by humans may be as important as contact with cat feces. In humans, the oocysts release trophozoites, which migrate widely, with a predilection for eye, brain, and muscle. Toxoplasmosis occurs worldwide, but is common in the tropics. Infection is life-long. HIV may reactivate it. *Note:* Rats are also sources of infection.

The patient In any patient with granulomatous uveitis or necrotizing retinitis, think of toxoplasmosis. Most infections are asymptomatic. Symptomatic acquired toxoplasmosis resembles infectious mononucleosis and is usually self-limiting. *Eye infection,* usually congenital, presents with posterior uveitis, often in the second-decade of life, and may cause cataract. *In the immunocompromised (e.g., aids):* Encephalitis with CD4 <100, ring enhancing lesion(s) on MRI, and positive IgG serology; clinical symptoms include focal neurological signs, stroke, or seizures.

Tests Acute infection is confirmed by a fourfold rise in antibody titer over 4 wks or specific IgM. Parasite isolation is difficult but easily seen on histopathology; lymph node or CNS biopsy may be diagnostic. Cerebral CT may show characteristic multiple ring-shaped contrast-enhancing lesions in compromised hosts, especially those with AIDS.

Treatment Often none is needed: Seek expert advice. If the eye is involved, or in the immunocompromised, pyrimethamine 200 mg PO α 1, then 50–75 mg PO qd plus sulfadiazine 1–1.5 g PO q6h plus leucovorin 10–25 mg po qd α " 6wks, then pyrimethamine 25–50 mg PO qd + sulfadiazine 500–1,000 mg PO qid + leucovorin 10–25 mg PO qd. If pregnant, get expert help. Alternatives: Pyrimethamine + leucovorin + either clindamycin or atovaquone or TMP/SMX.

Viral hepatitis

Hepatitis A virus (HAV) RNA virus. **Spread:** Fecal–oral, often in travelers or institutions. Most infections occur in childhood. **Incubation:** 2–6 wks. **Symptoms:** Prodrome symptoms include fever, malaise, anorexia, nausea, and arthralgias. Jaundice develops ± hepatomegaly, splenomegaly, and adenopathy. **Tests:** Serum transaminases rise 21–42 d after exposure. IgM rises from day 25 and signifies recent infection. IgG remains detectable for life. **Treatment:** Supportive. Avoid alcohol. **Prevention:** Immunization with HAV vaccine is a pillar of prevention. It is indicated for travelers to endemic areas, anyone exposed to hepatitis A, close contacts of adoptees from endemic areas, men who have sex with men (MSM), illicit drug users, and patients with chronic liver disease. Passive immunization with normal human immunoglobulin (0.02 ml/kg IM) gives <3 months' immunity to those at risk. Use passive immunization in unvaccinated persons >40 who were exposed to hepatitis A (as soon as possible) or who must travel in next 2 wks and are at risk for severe disease (older, chronic liver disease). **Prognosis:** Usually self-limiting. Fulminant hepatitis occurs rarely. Chronic liver disease does not occur, but 10–15% develop relapse of symptoms in first 6 months after acute illness.

Hepatitis B virus (HBV) DNA virus. **Spread:** Blood products, injection drug use, sexual intercourse, and vertical transmission. **Risk groups:** Health workers, hemophiliacs, hemodialysis, unprotected sex, MSM, and IV drug users (IVDU). HBV is Endemic in the Far East, Africa, and Mediterranean. **Incubation:** 6 wks to 6 months. **Clinical features:** Resemble hepatitis A, but extrahepatic manifestations are more common (e.g., arthralgias, urticaria). **Tests:** Serological markers (see Table 14.26). HBsAg (surface antigen) is present from 1 to 6 months after exposure. HBsAg (e antigen) is present for 1½–3 months after the acute illness and implies high infectivity. The persistence of HBsAg for >6 months defines carrier status and occurs in 5–10% of infections (chronic infection). Antibodies to HBcAg (anti-HBc) imply past infection; antibodies to HBSAG (ANTI-HBS) alone imply vaccination. HBV PCR allows monitoring of response to therapy. See Table 14.26. **Vaccination** is recommended for all unvaccinated adolescents, adults who wish to prevent hep B infection, and especially in adults at high risk for infection (e.g., health care workers, those in correctional facilities, MSM, persons at risk for STDs and those with HIV). Passive immunization (specific anti-HBV immunoglobulin) may be given to nonimmune contacts after high-risk exposure. **Treatment:** Supportive. Avoid alcohol. About 5–6% with acute HBV infection develop chronic HBV, define by persistence of HBsAg >6 months. Chronic HBV may respond to interferon-γ or antivirals (e.g., adefovir, tenofovir, lamivudine or entecavir). Unlike HCV, cure is rare, so the goal of therapy is conversion to e Ag negativity (most likely with viral interferon) or reduction in viral load and rates of disease progression. Immunize sexual contacts. **Complications:** Fulminant hepatic failure (rare); relapse; prolonged cholestasis; chronic hepatitis (5–10%); cirrhosis; hepatocellular carcinoma (HCC: 10-fold increased risk if

Table 14.26 Hepatitis B serology

HBsAg	Anti-HBc (IgG + IgM)	Anti-HBc (IgM)	Anti-HBs	Comment
-	-	-	+	Vaccination or past infection
-	+	-	+	Recovered from past infection
+	+	+	-	Acute infection
-	+	+	-	Resolving infection
+	+	-	-	Chronic infection
-	+	-	-	False-positive, acute, chronic or past infection

Sexually Transmitted Diseases Treatment Guidelines, 2010. *MMWR* December 17, 2010;59(RR–12).

HBsAg positive, 60-fold increased risk if both HBsAg and HBsAg positive); glomerulonephritis; cryoglobulinemia.

Hepatitis C virus (HCV) RNA virus. **Spread:** Blood, IVDU, sexual (not an efficient mode of transfer), unknown (40%). Early infection is often mild or asymptomatic. **Incubation:** HCV RNA is detectable at 1–3 wks, anti-HCV at 8–9 wks. **Clinical features:** Most (70–85%) develop chronic infection; 60–70% of patients have evidence of chronic liver disease, LFT (typically AST: ALT <1 until cirrhosis, 15–20% get cirrhosis within 20 yrs; a few also get hepatocellular cancer. **Tests:** Anti-HCV by enzyme immunoassay (EIA), enzyme-linked immunosorbent assay (ELISA), enhanced chemiluminescence assay, and recombinant immunoblot assay; PCR for diagnosis and monitoring disease progression; genotype and liver biopsy for prognosis and to guide therapeutic decisions. See Table 14.27.

Treatment: This is a rapidly evolving field. *Treatment considerations:* Treat adults with all of the following criteria: Age >18, + HCV RNA, liver biopsy that shows chronic hepatitis and significant fibrosis, compensated liver disease and no contraindications (see below). Consider treatment in those with acute infection, biopsy that shows mild or no fibrosis, renal disease, liver transplant, decompensated cirrhosis, and HIV co-infection.

Regimens: Pegylated interferon-β + ribavirin are used in chronic infection. For genotype 1, chronic HCV, the addition of a protease inhibitor (boceprevir or telaprevir) has been supported by recent studies and is now

Table 14.27 Hepatitis C serology

Anti-HCV	PCR	Interpretation
-	-	No infection
-	+	Early infection, chronic infection in immunosuppressed state
+	-	Acute or resolved infection
+	+	Chronic infection

Diagnosis, Management, and Treatment of Hepatitis C: An Update. *Hepatology.* 2009:49(4): 1335–1374.

the standard. IL28B genotype testing of patients can provide important pre-treatment information regarding response to antiviral therapy. The goal of treatment, unlike in HBV, is cure as indicated by sustained viral suppression defined as no detectable HCV at 6 months after treatment. Factors associated with favorable response to IFN/ribavirin: HCV genotype other than 1, lower viral load, white race, female sex, and age <40, weight <85 kg, HIV negative, and IL28B genotype

Contraindications: Major depression (not controlled), solid organ transplant (except liver), severe concomitant medical illness, autoimmune hepatitis, untreated thyroid disease, pregnancy, age <2, inability to comply with long-treatment course, women of childbearing potential unwilling to use contraception.

Hepatitis D virus (HDV) Incomplete RNA virus exists only with HBV. **Spread:** Coinfection or superinfection with HBV. **Clinical features:** Increased risk of acute hepatic failure and cirrhosis. **Tests:** Anti-HDV antibody. **Treatment:** Interferon-γ has limited success in treatment of HDV infection.

Hepatitis E virus (HEV) RNA virus similar to HAV. Commonly occurs in areas with poor sanitation (e.g., parts of India) and associated with high mortality in pregnancy. **Diagnosis:** Serology.

Differential diagnosis Acute hepatitis: Alcohol, drugs, toxins, EBV, CMV, leptospirosis, malaria, Q fever, syphilis, yellow fever. **Chronic hepatitis:** Alcohol, drugs, autoimmune hepatitis, Wilson's disease.

Human immunodeficiency virus/AIDS

Worldwide, there are ~ 34 million people living with HIV. In 2010, there were 2.7 million new infections and 1.8 million deaths. Two-thirds of cases and deaths are in sub-Saharan Africa. In the United States, there are ~ 1.8 million people living with HIV (about 20% undiagnosed) and 50,000 new cases each year. Most are in MSM. African Americans are disproportionately affected. HIV–1 (a retrovirus) is responsible for most cases worldwide. HIV–2 is a related virus and produces a similar illness, perhaps with a longer latent period.

Transmission The global experience is primarily by sexual contact (84%), and infected blood or blood products, IV drug abuse, or perinatally. In the United States, about 60% of new infections are in MSM and 10% in IVDU. Aggressive screening of pregnant women and modern blood banking processes has all but eliminated perinatal and blood product transmission of HIV in developed countries.

Immunology HIV binds, via its gp120 envelope glycoprotein, to CD4 receptors on helper T-lymphocytes, monocytes, macrophages, and neural cells. CD4 cells migrate to the lymphoid tissue, where the virus replicates producing billions of new virions. These are released, and, in turn, infect new CD4 cells. As the infection progresses, depletion or impaired function of CD4 cells predisposes to the development of immune dysfunction.

Virology HIV is a double-stranded RNA retrovirus. After entry into the cell, the viral reverse transcriptase enzyme (hence retrovirus) makes a DNA copy of the RNA genome. The viral integrase enzyme then integrates this into the host DNA. The core viral proteins are initially synthesized as large polypeptides that are cleaved by the viral protease enzyme into the enzymes and building blocks of the virus. The completed virions are then released from the cell by characteristic budding. The number of circulating viruses (viral load) predicts progression to AIDS.

Stages of HIV infection Acute infection is often asymptomatic. **Seroconversion** may be accompanied by a 1–2 wk illness 2–6 wks after

HIV infection: Fever, malaise, myalgias, pharyngitis, maculopapular rash, or meningoencephalitis (rare). Patients in these early stages of HIV are very contagious due to high levels of virus in serum and genital fluids.

A period of **asymptomatic infection** follows, although one-third of patients will have **persistent generalized lymphadenopathy (PGL)**, defined as nodes >1cm diameter at multiple extrainguinal sites, persisting for ≥3 months. There may be opportunistic infections prior to AIDS, such as tuberculosis, pneumococcal pneumonia, oral *Candida*, oral hairy leukoplakia, herpes zoster. **AIDS** is a stage in HIV infection characterized by the presence of an indicator disease or a CD4 count <200/mm^3.

AIDS prognosis If untreated, death in ~20 months, longer by an average of 15 yrs (or more) if treated with current regimens.

Diagnosis is based on detecting anti-HIV antibodies in serum. A positive screening test (e.g., EIA/ELISA, chemiluminescent immunoassays, rapid assays) must be confirmed with a Western blot, indirect immunofluorescent assay, or a nucleic acid test (e.g., HIV-1 RNA). Rapid assays are point-of-care tests that can detect antibodies to HIV in <1 h. Negative tests are generally definitive, except in cases of acute infection. Acute infection can be difficult to diagnose. When suspected, check an HIV antibody screening assay **and** HIV RNA-1. In cases where there is virological evidence of infection, serology should be checked in a few weeks to confirm infection. Efforts should be made to remove hurdles to testing.

Prevention About 40% of transmissions occur during early acute infection, prior to seroconversion. This makes detection of acute infection for counseling and consideration of early treatment a high priority. Partner notification, safer sex practices, and avoidance of sharing needles are important. Postexposure prophylaxis with combination antiretroviral therapy for occupational and sexual exposure should be offered. Screening of blood products, transplanted organs, universal precautions, and use of disposable equipment are important infection control measures. Antiretroviral therapy for mother and infant (± caesarean section) and bottle-feeding are a means of preventing vertical transmission. Antiretroviral therapy may also have a role in reducing horizontal transmission.

Complications of HIV infection All patients with a new diagnosis of HIV should be screened for TB and be tested for *Toxoplasma*, CMV, hepatitis B/C, and syphilis serology, to identify past or current infections that may develop as immunosuppression progresses. All AIDS-defining diagnoses are seen almost exclusively with a CD4 count <200/mm^3 and some (disseminated MAC and CMV) are seen only with a CD4 count of <50.

Pulmonary: Pneumocystis jiroveci pneumonia (PCP) remains an important life-threatening opportunistic infection in AIDS. The disease evolves over days to weeks with dyspnea, dry cough, fever, and chest pain. Diagnosis: Stains of respiratory specimen for *P. jiroveci*. Treatment: High-dose TMP/SMX IV or PO, trimethoprim-dapsone PO, primaquine-clindamycin PO, atovaquone PO, or pentamidine by slow IV for 3 wks. Steroids are beneficial if severe hypoxemia (pO$_2$ <70). Primary prophylaxis (e.g., TMP/SMX or dapsone PO) is indicated while CD4 count <200. Secondary prophylaxis is the same and continued after first attack until CD4 count >200 for >3 months. Other pathogens include *M. tuberculosis*; *M. avium intracellulare* (MAI); fungi (*Aspergillus, Cryptococcus, Histoplasma*); parasites (toxoplasmosis, cryptosporidiosis, *Isospora*), viruses (HSV, CMV, JC virus). Also: Kaposi's sarcoma, lymphoma, lymphoid interstitial pneumonitis, and non-specific pneumonitis. Community-acquired pneumonia, especially due to *S. pneumoniae*, is a major problem in HIV/AIDS patients.

GI tract: Candidiasis, HSV or aphthous ulcers, or tumors may cause oral pain. *Oral candida* is treated with nystatin suspension/pastilles or clotrimazole lozenges. *Esophageal* involvement causes dysphagia ± retrosternal discomfort. Fluconazole is the mainstay of therapy. For resistant cases, other azoles (e.g., itraconazole, voriconazole, posaconazole), the echinocandins (e.g., micafungin, caspofungin, anidulafungin) can be useful. *HSV* and *CMV* also cause esophageal ulceration, which may be difficult to differentiate from *Candida* by barium studies. EGD with biopsy facilitates diagnosis. *Anorexia and weight loss* are common in HIV infection. *Elevated LFT and hepatomegaly* are common; causes include drugs, viral hepatitis, AIDS sclerosing cholangitis, or *mai*. Disseminated mai causes fever, night sweats, malaise, anorexia, weight loss, abdominal pain, diarrhea, hepatomegaly, and anemia. *Diagnosis:* Blood cultures, but requires 7–14 d for growth; biopsies (lymph node, liver, colon, bone marrow). Treatment is with ethambutol + clarithromycin ± rifabutin/rifampin (see Table 14.28). **Primary prophylaxis:** E.g., azithromycin 1,200 mg weekly, while CD4 <100. *Salmonella, C. difficile,* and viruses often cause acute diarrhea. *Chronic diarrhea* may be caused by bacteria (MAI), protozoa (*Cryptosporidium, Microsporidium, Isospora belli, Cyclospora*), viruses (CMV, adenovirus), or meds esp. LPV/r and NFV. *Perianal disease* may be due to recurrent HSV ulceration, GC, *Chlamydia* (including LGV in MSM), perianal warts, and squamous cell carcinoma (rare). Kaposi's sarcoma and lymphomas can also affect the gut.

Neurological: Acute HIV is associated with transient meningoencephalitis, myelopathy, and peripheral neuropathy. *Chronic HIV* is associated with several CNS syndromes: Most common are HIV-associated dementia (HAD) attributed to HIV, toxoplasmosis encephalitis, cryptococcal meningitis, TB meningitis, CNS lymphoma, HIV-related meningitis, CMV encephalitis, progressive multifocal leukoencephalopathy (PML), neurosyphilis, listeriosis, vacuolar myelopathy, and peripheral neuropathy. T. gondii is an important CNS pathogen in AIDS, presenting with focal symptoms/signs. CT/MRI shows ring-shaped contrast enhancing lesions. Treatment is pyrimethamine (and folinic acid) + sulfadiazine or clindamycin for 6 months. Treatment should continue until CD4 >100 α 3–6 months. Primary prophylaxis (e.g., TMP/SMX PO) is indicated in patients with serum antitoxoplasma IgG and CD4 <100. Cryptococcus neoformans is a major cause of meningitis in HIV. It causes insidious meningitis, often without neck stiffness. Diagnosis: CSF cryptococcal antigen. Treatment is initially with amphotericin IV + flucytosine, then fluconazole for long-term treatment. Careful monitoring and management of CSF pressure is crucial in cryptococcosis. Secondary prophylaxis with fluconazole is needed until CD4 is >100–200 for ≥6 months. **Tumors** affecting the CNS include primary cerebral lymphoma, B-cell non-Hodgkin's lymphoma. CSF EBV PCR can assist with diagnosis. JC virus PCR may be useful in distinguishing lymphoma from PML.

Eye: CMV retinitis may present with floaters, scotoma, and visual field defects or decreased acuity. Funduscopy shows characteristic appearance. Treatment is with valganciclovir PO, ganciclovir IV, ganciclovir intraocular device + valganciclovir PO. Alternatives are foscarnet, cidofovir. Treatment has traditionally been lifelong, but trials suggest that therapy may be stopped in some patients when CD4 >150 after HAART. Other HIV-associated eye diseases include VZV-associated progressive outer retinal necrosis (PORN), ocular syphilis, dry eyes, and uveitis due to immune reconstitution or medications (e.g., rifabutin).

What every doctor should know about HIV

An expert should manage patients with HIV infection. HIV in developed countries is primary management of antiretroviral drugs and their toxicities and controlling HIV viral load—not opportunistic infections.

Preventing HIV spread

Screen patients for high-risk behavior and reduce barriers to safer sex: Promote *lifelong* safer sex, barrier contraception, and reduction in the number of partners. Videos followed by interactive discussions are one way to double the use of condoms. Another way is the *100% condom program* involving distribution of condoms to brothels, with enforcement programs enabling monitoring and encouraging condom use at any sex establishment. Such programs are estimated to have prevented 2 million HIV infections in Thailand. Testing enhances counseling, partner notification, and early treatment. Warn everyone about the dangers of sexual tourism/promiscuity. *Tell drug users* not to share needles. Use needle exchange programs. Vigorous control of other STIs can reduce HIV incidence. Strengthen awareness of clinics for STIs. Encourage pregnant women to have HIV tests. (Caesarean sections and HAART during pregnancy can prevent vertical transmission). All HIV-infected persons should have partner notification.

Think about acute seroconversion: The clinical features are similar to infectious mononucleosis; perform tests if there are unusual signs; e.g., oral candidiasis, recurrent shingles, leucopenia, or CNS signs (antibody tests may be negative, but HIV RNA levels are elevated in early infection). As always, take a thorough history. If you *do* identify acute seroconversion illness, get expert help promptly. Counseling to prevent HIV transmission is critical.

Occupational exposure and needle-stick injury Seroconversion rates are ~0.4% for HIV, 30% for hepatitis B, if HBeAg positive and recipient is unvaccinated, and 1.9% for hepatitis C. Wash wound well; do not suck or immerse in bleach. Note name, address, and clinical details of source patient. Report incident to Occupational Health and fill out an accident form.

Rapid HIV test should be performed on source if HIV status is unknown. Informed consent in a source patient is sometimes required for HIV serology. Also test source for HBV (HBsAg) and HCV (anti-HCV). Immunize (active and passive) against hepatitis B at once, if needed. Counsel injured person that HIV risk <0.5% if source is HIV positive and test recipient at baseline 3, 6, ±12 months (seroconversion may take this long).

Weigh risks, which are based on the viral load in the source patient and the severity of injury to the health care worker, volume of blood on instrument, and depth of injury. *Higher risk exposures include* source patients with symptomatic HIV, acute seroconversion, and viral load >1,500 and deeper injuries with needles that have hollow bores, were used in an artery or vein and/or have visible blood. Higher risk exposures should be treated with three or more antiretroviral drugs. *Lower risk exposures include* source patients who are asymptomatic and have a viral load <1,500 and superficial injuries with solid needles/instruments. These may be treated with a two-drug regimen. Mucus membrane or nonintact skin exposure carries a lower risk. If fluid volume is high and source patient is high risk, use three or more drugs. Otherwise consider two drugs, or none in the case of low-risk source patient and low fluid volume exposure.

HIV test counseling:

If in doubt, get help from an HIV care center. Routine tests in the recipient are HIV serology at baseline, 6 wks, 3 months, and 6 months. Viral load to detect acute infection should not be done unless symptomatic. Routine tests in the donor are rapid HIV serology, anti-HCV, and HBsAg if these have not been done previously. For assistance in testing and selection of therapy, health care workers can call PEPline at 888–448–4911.

Table 14.28 Prophylaxis and treatment of opportunistic infections

Infection	Prophylaxis	Indication
Pneumocystis jiroveci (PCP)	TMP/SMX DS/d, TMP/SMX SS/d, TMP/SMX DS/thrice weekly	Start: CD4<200, oropharyngeal candidiasis, h/o PCP
	Dapsone 100 mg/d, Dapsone 50 mg/12 h, Dapsone 50 mg/d + pyrimethamine 50 mg/d + folinic acid 25 mg/d, atovaquone 1,500 mg/d, atovaquone 1,500 mg/d + pyrimethamine 25 mg/d + folinic acid 10 mg/d, aerosolized pentamidine 300 mg/month.	Stop: CD4 count >200 for >3 months
	Screen for G6PD deficiency before giving dapsone	
Mycobacterium avium (MAI)	Azithromycin 1,200 mg/w, Azithromycin 600 mg/ twice weekly, clarithromycin 500 mg/12 h	Start: CD4<50 Stop: CD4>100 for " 3 months
Toxoplasmosis	TMP/SMX DS/d, TMP/SMX SS/d, dapsone 50 mg/d + pyrimethamine 50 mg/d + folinic acid 25 mg/d, atovaquone 1,500 mg/d (± pyrimethamine 25 mg/d + folinic acid 10 mg/d	Start: Toxo IgG + and CD4 <100 Stop: CD4 count >200 for >3 months
	Screen for G6PD deficiency before giving dapsone	
Tuberculosis	See TB section	Screen for and treat latent TB
Coccidioidomycosis	Fluconazole 400 mg/d Itraconazole 300 mg/12 h	CD4<250 **and** + IgM or IgG to cocci **and** from and endemic area

Infection	Treatment
PCP	**Moderate to Severe**: TMP (5 mg–kg)/SMX (25 mg/kg)/6–8 h, pentamidine 3–4 mg/kg/24 h, primaquine 15–30 mg/24 h + clindamycin 600–900 mg/8 h IV (or 300–450 mg/6–8 h PO) α **21 d**
	Hypoxemia: Room air PaO_2 <70 or Aa gradient >35: Add prednisone 40 mg/12 h α 5 d then 40 mg/d α 5 d then 20 mg/d α 11 d
	Mild to moderate: TMP/SMX as above or TMP/SMX DS 2 tab tid, Dapsone 100 mg/d + TMP 5 mg/kg/8 h, primaquine 15–30 mg/d + clindamycin 300–450/6–8 h PO, atovaquone 750 mg/12 h α **21 d**
	Check G6PD before giving Primaquine

Table 14.28 (Continued)

Disseminated MAI	Clarithromycin 500 mg/12 h (or azithromycin 500–600 mg/d) + ethambutol 15 mg/kg/d ± rifabutin 300 mg/d. Treatment is continued until sustained immune recovery
Toxoplasmosis	**Induction:** <60 kg: Pyrimethamine 200 mg α 1 then 50 mg/d + sulfadiazine 1,000 mg/6 h + folinic acid 10–50 mg/d α **6 wks**
	>60 kg: Pyrimethamine 200 mg α 1 then 75 mg/d + sulfadiazine 1,500 mg/6 h + folinic acid 10–50 mg/d α **6 wks**
	Maintenance: Pyrimethamine 25–50 mg/d + sulfa-diazine 1,000 mg/6–12 h + folinic acid 10–25 mg/d. Treatment is continued until sustained immune recovery. Clindamycin 600 mg/6 h can be used in place of sulfadiazine. Adjunctive steroids may be needed to control CNS edema.
Oropharyngeal candidiasis	Fluconazole 100 mg/d, clotrimazole 10 mg troches/4–5 h, nystatin suspension 4–6 m**L**/6 h α 7–14 d
Esophageal candidiasis	Fluconazole 100–400 mg/d IV or PO, itraconazole 200 mg/d PO, voriconazole 200 mg/12 h IV or PO, posaconazole 400 mg/12 h PO, echinocandin (e.g., caspofungin, micafungin, anidulafungin) IV
Cryptococcosis	**Induction:** Deoxycholate amphotericin B 0.7 mg/kg/d IV or lipid amphotericin B 4–6 mg/kg/d IV + flucyto-sine 25 mg/kg/6 h α **2 wks or longer**
	Consolidation: Fluconazole 400 mg/d α 8 wks
	Maintenance: Fluconazole 200 mg/d. Treatment is continued until sustained immune recovery.
	Follow flucytosine levels
Tuberculosis	See TB section
CMV retinitis	**Induction:** Ganciclovir implant + valganciclovir 900 mg/12 h PO, ganciclovir 5 mg/kg/12 h IV, foscarnet 60 mg/8 h IV or 90 mg/12 h IV α 14–21 d, cidofovir 5 mg/kg/wk α 2 then every other week (give with saline and probenecid) **Maintenance:** Valganciclovir 900 mg/d, ganciclovir 5 mg/kg/d, foscarnet 90–120 mg/kg/d, cidofovir 5 mg/kg/every other week (give with saline and probenecid)

Treatment and monitoring of patients with HIV infection

Extensive, long-term studies involving clinical end points such as death consistently show extraordinary benefit with antiretroviral therapy (ART). Mortality, AIDS rates, and hospitalization rates are reduced by 60–80%.

Goals of therapy: Reduce morbidity, prolong survival, improve immune function, suppress viral load, and prevent transmission.

Indications to start ART: Able to commit to taking medications for life *and* any of the below:

- AIDS-defining illness (especially with opportunistic infection and viral load >100,000 copies/m**L**)
- CD4 count <500 (particularly important in <200 rapidly declining CD4 counts)
- HIV-associated nephropathy
- Hepatitis B co-infection (when treatment of hepatitis B is indicated)
- Pregnant women (to prevent perinatal transmission)

Consider ART in patients with CD4 count >500

Consider a brief delay in initiating ART in cases of cryptococcosis and non-tuberculous mycobacteria infections (to reduce chance of immune reconstitution syndrome).

Check viral load at initiation or modification of ART and 2–8 wks later. If still detectable, recheck every 4–8 wks until <200 copies/m**L** Virological failure is an inability to achieve or maintain viral load <200.

Baseline tests: HIV serology, viral load and genotype CBC, CD4 count, chemistry profile, liver function tests, lipids, CXR, U/A, toxoplasmosis serology, G6PD (in appropriate risk groups), PPD or IGRA, Pap smear, HAV (total Ab), HBV (HBsAg, and antibody to HBs or HBc), HCV (anti-HCV), syphilis and other STIs, consider CMV IgG.

Special tests: HLA-B*5701 (prior to giving abacavir) and co-receptor tropism assay (prior to giving CCR5 entry inhibitor)

Monitoring: Every 3–6 months: CBC, CD4 count and viral load. Every 6–12 months: Basic chemistries, liver function tests

HIV **treatment**

The major concerns with HAART are:

- *Virologic failure*, which may be due to multiple factors including poor adherence, antiviral resistance and suboptimal antiviral potency
- *Adverse effects* of the drugs, both short- and long-term

What to start (initial regimen):

- Efavirenz /tenofovir /emtricitabine (EFV/TDF/FTC)
- Ritonavir-boosted atazanavir + tenofovir/emtricitabine (ATV/r + TDF/FTC)
- Ritonavir-boosted darunavir + tenofovir/emtricitabine (DRV/r + TDF/FTC)
- Raltegravir + tenofovir/emtricitabine (RAL + TDF/FTC)

Note: Choice of regimen should be individualized based on patient preference, side-effect profile, patient's comorbid conditions and other medications, and baseline antiviral resistance profile. Ritonavir is used to boost levels of protease inhibitors. (See DHHS Guidelines: www.aidsinfo.nih. gov.)

Antiviral agents

An HIV expert should supervise *all* HIV treatment. Classes of drugs are nucleoside reverse transcriptase inhibitors (NRTI), non-nucleoside reverse transcriptase inhibitor (NNRTI), protease inhibitors (PI), integrase inhibitors, and viral entry inhibitors.

General principle of initial therapy is to combine two NRTIs with an NNRTI, a boosted PI, or integrase inhibitor.

Nucleoside analogue reverse transcriptase inhibitors (NRTI)

- **Zidovudine (Azidothymidine, AZT)** was the first anti-HIV drug. *Dose:* 300 mg/12 h or 200 mg/8 h PO. *SE:* Anemia, leucopenia, gastrointestinal disturbance, lactic acidosis. AZT requires dosage adjustment in renal dysfunction.

- **Didanosine (DDI;Videx ec®)** *Dose:* 250 mg/24 h PO if wt <60kg; 400 mg/24 h if >60 kg. *SE:* Pancreatitis, lactic acidosis, peripheral neuropathy, GI disturbance. Stop treatment if significant rise in amylase. Take on empty stomach. DDI requires dosage adjustment with concomitant TDF use, renal dysfunction.
- **Lamivudine (3TC)** is probably the best-tolerated antiretroviral. *Dose:* 150 mg/12 h or 300 mg QD PO. *SE:* With HBV co-infection there may be flare in hepatitis with HBV resistance, immune reconstitution or flare if 3TC is stopped. 3TC requires dosage adjustment with renal dysfunction.
- **Stavudine (D4T)** *Dose:* 40 mg/12 h PO if >60 kg; 30 mg/12 h PO if <60 kg. Need to stop treatment if peripheral neuropathy, lipoatrophy, hypertriglyceridemia, pancreatitis, lactic acidosis. D4T requires dosage adjustment in renal dysfunction.
- **Tenofovir (TDF)** *Dose:* 300 mg/24 h PO. *SE:* Rare causes of renal failure including Fanconi syndrome and ABV flare if TDF stopped. Give with care in renal dysfunction and requires adjustment.
- **Abacavir (ABC)** *Dose:* 300 mg/12 h or 600 mg qd PO. *SE:* Hepatitis, hypersensitivity syndrome (5–8%): Rash, fever, vomiting; may be fatal if rechallenged; highest risk in those with HLA-B*5701, so screen before giving drug.
- **Emtricitabine (FTC)** *Dose:* 200 mg/24 h PO. *SE:* Same as lamivudine. FTC can cause hyperpigmentation/skin discoloration and requires adjustment with renal dysfunction.

Protease inhibitors (PI): PIS are often given with low-dose ritonavir (200–400 mg/d PO), which enhance drug levels except with nelfinavir (NFV). All PIs are metabolized by the cytochrome P-450 enzyme system. They may therefore increase the concentrations of certain drugs by competitive inhibition of their metabolism if administered concomitantly. Also, PI levels can be altered by other medications that impact CYP metabolism. PIs associated with body fat redistribution: Increased abdominal fat, breast enlargement, and a buffalo hump. *Other class specific SE:* Hyperlipidemia, hyperglycemia, insulin resistance, and gastrointestinal disturbance. ATV does not alter lipids or cause insulin resistance.

- Indinavir (IND) *Dose:* 800 mg/8 h or IND/r 800/100–200 mg/12 h PO, 1 h before or 2 h after a meal. *SE:* Dry mouth, taste disturbance, pruritus, alopecia, increased LFT and nephrolithiasis
- Saquinavir (SQV) *Dose:* SQV/r—1,000/100 mg bid PO. SE: GI intolerances, rash, hepatitis, lipodystrophy, and paresthesiae
- Nelfinavir (NFV) *Dose:* 1,250 mg/12 h or 750 mg/8 h PO. SE: Hepatitis, diarrhea, increased CK
- Lopinavir/Ritonavir (LPV) (Kaletra®) *Dose:* 400 mg (+ 100 mg ritonavir)/ bid PO. LPV can be used as 800 mg/200 mg/d in some patients. SE: GI intolerances, rash, hepatitis, and lipodystrophy
- Atazanavir (ATV) *Dose:* 400 mg qd with food or with RTV 300 mg/100 mg qd with food. SE: Hyperbilirubinemia (benign), GI intolerance, and nephrolithiasis (Note: Does not cause hyperlipidemia or insulin resistance.) Dose adjustment needed in patients taking efavirenz, H_2 antagonists, and proton pump inhibitors
- Tipranavir (TPV) *Dose:* With RTV 500/200 mg bid only for salvage. SE: Hepatotoxicity, rash, GI intolerances, CNS bleed (rare)
- Fosamprenavir (FPV) *Dose:* 1,400 mg/12 h PO, FPV/r, 1,400/100–200 mg/d or 700 mg/100 bid. SE: Rash, lipodystrophy, GI intolerance
- Darunavir *Dose:* With RTV 800/100/d or 600/100 mg bid. SE: GI intolerance, hepatitis, and lipodystrophy, rash with Stevens-Johnson

Non-nucleoside reverse transcriptase inhibitors (NNRTI): These may interact with drugs metabolized by the cytochrome P-450 enzyme system, which they either induce or inhibit depending on the concomitantly administered drug.

- Nevirapine (NVP) *Dose:* 200 mg/24 h for 2 wks, then 200 mg/12 h or 400 mg-XR/24 h PO. Resistant mutants emerge readily. SE: Stevens–Johnson syndrome, toxic epidermal necrolysis, hepatitis including fatal hepatic necrosis
- *Efavirenz* (EFV) *Dose:* 600 mg/24 h PO. SE: Rash, sleep disturbance, hepatotoxicity, neuropsychiatric symptoms, dizziness in first 2–3 wks. Avoid in pregnancy due to teratogenicity (category D)
- Etravirine (ETR) *Dose:* 200 mg/12 h PO. SE: Rash, Stevens-Johnson syndrome, hepatotoxicity
- Rilpivirine (RPV) *Dose:* 25 mg/24 h PO. SE: Rash, insomnia, depression, headache

Others:

- Raltegravir (RAL)Integrase inhibitor. *Dose:* 400 mg/12 h PO (increase to 800 mg/12 h if taken with rifampin). SE: GI intolerance, CPK elevation
- Enfuvirtide (T20) Fusion inhibitor. *Dose:* 90 mg (1 mL) SQ/12 h. SE: Local injection site reactions seen in almost all patients
- Maraviroc (MVC) Entry inhibitor. *Dose:* 150–600 mg/bid(depending on concomitant medications). SE: GI intolerance, hepatotoxicity

Golden rules for HAART

- Start HAART early, ideally before opportunistic infection or malignancy and with CD4 count well above 200.
- Establish a trusting relationship with the patient.
- Explain to patients that regimens are complex and stress the importance of strict adherence.
- Use a multidisciplinary team to identify and address barriers to adherence (e.g., social, psychiatric, economic, and substance abuse-related).
- Use multiple anti-HIV drugs (minimizes replication and resistance) together (see above for recommended regimens).
- Monitor plasma viral load and CD4 count. Aim for undetectable viral loads (<50 copies/mL) within 4–6 months of starting HAART. Suspect poor adherence or transmitted resistance if viral load rebounds.
- Assess adherence to regimen at every clinic visit.
- If virologic goals are not achieved, the cause is resistance or failure of drug to reach target (usually due to nonadherence, but possibly due to drug interactions, food effect, etc.). The usual reasons to change therapy are toxicity or virologic failure.
  1 If toxicity: Substitute for the implicated drug.
  2 If viral failure: Review adherence and drug interactions, etc. Changes in regimen are then made based on genotypic resistance tests.
- HIV therapy continues to evolve rapidly.
- Keep up with published guidelines and advisories.

Sexually transmitted infections

Incidence Although great progress has been made in the past decade in treating STIs, they still remains a major health problem. *Chlamydia* remains the most commonly reported infectious disease in the United States, with nearly 1.3 million cases in 2010. Additionally, there are >310,000 cases of gonorrhea and nearly 14,000 cases of syphilis reported annually. African Americans, especially women, are disproportionately affected by *Chlamydia* and gonorrhea. MSM and African Americans are most affected by primary and secondary syphilis.

Presentation Many are asymptomatic, which facilitates transmission. Therefore, screening is critical. When symptomatic, presentations include vaginal or urethral discharge, genital lesions, pelvic infection, cervical neoplasia, HIV disease, and ectopic parasites.

History Ask about *partners* (number, gender), *practice* (vaginal, oral, anal), *protection* (condoms), and *past* history of STI.

Examination Detailed examination of genitalia including inguinal nodes and pubic hair, scrotum and male urethra, rectal examination, pelvic and speculum examination.

Overview of tests Refer to STD clinic. *Urine:* Dipstick and culture for GC and *C. trachomatis*. *Ulcers:* Take swabs for HSV culture (viral transport medium). Dark field microscopy for syphilis (*T. pallidum*) requires expertise. *Men:* Urethral smear for Gram stain and culture for *N. gonorrhoeae* (send quickly to lab in Stuart's medium); urethral swab for *Chlamydia*. *Women:* High vaginal swab in Stuart's medium for microscopy and stain for *Candida*, *Gardnerella vaginalis*, anaerobes, *Lactobacillus*, *Trichomonas vaginalis*; endocervical swab for *Chlamydia trachomatis*. *Chlamydia* (an obligate intracellular bacterium) is usually asymptomatic but easy to detect with urinary nucleic acid amplification tests (NAAT) test. *Blood tests:* Syphilis, herpes type-specific antibodies, hepatitis B and C, and HIV serology.

Follow-up Arrange to see patients at 1 wk and 3 months, with repeat smears, cultures, and syphilis serology. Patients should avoid sex until treatment is completed. Partners should be referred for screening and treatment. If the partner is unlikely to present for treatment, consider giving the treatment course for the partner to deliver to the patient. *Note:* This may be prohibited in some states.

Screening programs in asymptomatic patients can reduce complications (e.g., infertility, PID) and reduce transmission. Patients seeking treatment for STD, commercial sex workers, drug users, and sexual contacts of persons with STD require aggressive and frequent screening for multiple infections. See Table 14.29.

Ectoparasites *Scabies (Sarcoptes scabiei):* Spread is common in families. *Presentation:* Papular rash (on abdomen or medial thigh; itchy at night) + burrows (in digital web spaces and flexor wrist surfaces). *Incubation:* ~6 wks (during which time sensitization to the mite's feces and/or saliva occurs). Penile lesions produce red nodules. *Diagnosis:* Tease a mite out of its burrow with a needle for microscopy. This may fail, but if a drop of oil is placed

Table 14.29 Routine screening recommendations

Population	Infection
Men who have sex with men	**Annually: G**C, *Chlamydia*, HIV, syphilis, consider anal Pap screening
Pregnant women	**First trimester: G**C, *Chlamydia*, HIV, hepatitis B surface antigen, and syphilis
Sexually active women < 25	**Annually: G**C and *Chlamydia* HIV at least once
HIV-positive	**Annually: G**C, *Chlamydia*, syphilis; in women also check trichomoniasis
Women >25 and heterosexual men	Routine screening not recommended, but testing should be considered in higher risk situations (e.g., multiple partners, African American women up to age 30, and prior STD)

on the lesion, a few scrapes with a scalpel may provide feces or eggs. Treat the entire household. Give written advice. Apply permethrin 5% cream to entire body (from neck down) and wash off in 8–14 h. Oral therapy with ivermectin 200 mcg/kg α 1 and repeated in 2 wks is another option. *Pediculosis pubis:* Often spread via sexual transmission. *Presentation:* Itching, visible lice or nits. *Treatment:* Permethrin 1% cream or pyrethrins applied to affected area; wash off after 10 minutes.

Lymphogranuloma *Presentation:* Inguinal lymphadenopathy and ulceration. *Causes:* Lymphogranuloma venereum, chancroid (*Haemophilus ducreyi*), or granuloma inguinale (*Calymmatobacterium granulomatis* [i.e., donovanosis]). The latter causes extensive, painless, red genital ulcers and pseudobuboes (i.e., abscesses near inguinal nodes), with possible elephantiasis ± malignant change. *Diagnosis:* "Closed safety-pin" inclusion bodies in cytoplasm of histiocytes. *Treatment:* Doxycycline 100 mg/12 h PO until all lesions epithelialized (at least 3 wks); alternatives include azithromycin, erythromycin, ciprofloxacin, or TMP/SMX.

Genital, anal or perianal ulcer disease Usual cause is HSV, syphilis, or both. *History and physical* exam must be backed up with laboratory confirmation. In the United States, there are ~ 50 million people with genital herpes. Most are due to HSV-2 and are asymptomatic. In young women and MSM, HSV-1 is increasingly associated with anogenital ulcers. HSV-2 is more likely to recur than HSV-1. When symptomatic, HSV infection can present as painful vesicles or ulcers. *Diagnosis* is with culture, PCR, serum HSV2 serology. See HSV section for treatment.

Syphilis is a systemic infection with potentially overlapping stages. *Primary:* A macule at site of sexual contact becomes a very infectious, painless, hard ulcer (primary chancre). *Secondary:* Occurs 4–8 wks after the chancre. Manifestations include fever, malaise, lymphadenopathy, rash (trunk, face, palms, soles), alopecia, mucocutaneous lesions, buccal snail-track ulcers; rarely hepatitis, meningitis, nephritis, uveitis. *Tertiary syphilis* follows 2–20 yrs latency (when patients are noninfectious). There are gummas (granulomas occurring in skin, mucosa, bone, joints, rarely viscera, e.g., lung, testis). *Quaternary syphilis:* Ascending aortic aneurysm ± aortic regurgitation; cranial nerve palsies; stroke; dementia; psychoses; sensory ataxia; numb legs, chest, and bridge of nose; lightning pains; gastric crises; reflex loss; extensor plantars; Charcot's joints; and Argyll Robertson pupil. *Latent infection* refers to serological evidence of syphilis without symptoms. Note that *neurological infection*, which can occur throughout the course of untreated syphilis, can present as meningitis, strokes, visual and hearing loss, and a range of potentially devastating neuropsychiatric abnormalities.

Syphilis serology (Two types):

Cardiolipin antibody: Not treponeme-specific. Indicates active disease and becomes negative after treatment. These are useful for screening and to determine response to therapy. For initial diagnosis, a positive test should be followed up by a confirmatory treponeme test. *False positives* (with negative treponemal antibody) can occur with pregnancy, immunization, pneumonia, malaria, SLE, TB, leprosy, HIV. *Examples:* Venereal disease research laboratory (VDRL) slide test, rapid plasma reagin (RPR), Wassermann reaction (WR). *Treponeme-specic antibody:* Positive in primary disease, remains so despite treatment. *Examples:* Fluorescent treponemal antibody (FTA–ABS), EIA, T. pallidum hemagglutination assay (TPHA), T. pallidum immobilization (TPI) test.

Other tests: In primary syphilis, treponemes may be seen by *dark field microscopy* of genital chancre fluid; serology at this stage is often negative. Interpretation of dark field microscopy requires expertise. In secondary syphilis, treponemes are seen in the lesions, and both types of antibody

Table 14.30 Treatment of syphilis

Scenario	Treatment
Primary or secondary:	Benzathine PCN-G 2.4 million units IM α 1 dose
	PCN allergic: Doxycycline 100 mg/12 h or tetracycline 500 mg/6 h α 14 d
Latent (<12 months from exposure)	Benzathine PCN-G 2.4 million units IM α 1 dose
Latent (>12 months or unknown time from exposure)	Benzathine PCN-G 2.4 million units IM weekly α 3 wks
	PCN allergy: Doxycycline 100 mg/12 h or tetracycline 500 mg/6 h α 28 d
Neurosyphilis and tertiary syphilis	PCN-G 3–4 million u/4 h or continuous IV α 10–14 d
	PCN allergy: Consider desensitization to PCN or ceftriaxone 2 g/d IV or IM α 10–14 d, but beware of cross-reactions

Beware of **Jarisch–Herxheimer reaction:** Fever, tachycardia, and vasodilatation hours after the first dose of antibiotic. Commonest in secondary disease; most dangerous in tertiary disease. Consider steroids.

tests are positive. In late syphilis, organisms may no longer be seen, but both types of antibody test usually remain positive (cardiolipin antibody tests may wane). In neurosyphilis, CSF VDRL may be positive, but false negatives are common.

Consider chancroid in settings where *H. ducreyi* is prevalent (e.g., sporadic outbreaks, and in parts of Africa and the Caribbean). **Presentation:** Painful ulcer, suppurative inguinal adenopathy. **Diagnosis:** Culture. **Treatment:** Azithromycin 1 g α 1, ceftriaxone 250 mg IM α 1, ciprofloxacin 500 mg/12 h α 3 d, erythromycin 500 mg/8 h α 7 d. See Table 14.30.

Vaginal discharge and urethritis

Some vaginal discharge may be physiologic. Most discharges associated with foul odor and itching are due to infection. A very foul discharge may be due to a foreign body (e.g., forgotten tampons). Discharges rarely resemble their classical descriptions.

Vaginal yeast infection (Candida albicans) This is the most common cause of pathological discharge and is classically described as white curds. The vulva and vagina may be red, fissured, and sore. This is not an STD, so partner treatment is unnecessary. **Risk factors:** Pregnancy, immunodeficiency, diabetes, birth control pills, and antibiotics. **Diagnosis:** Microscopy: Strings of mycelium or oval spores. Culture on Sabouraud's medium is rarely indicated except to test in vitro sensitivity in refractory cases. *Treatment:* Multiple topical azoles are available and (e.g., miconazole, butoconazole, and clotrimazole) can be obtained without a prescription. A single dose of fluconazole 150 mg PO is an alternative. Reassure that vulvovaginal candidiasis is not sexually transmitted.

Trichomonas vaginalis (TV) Produces vaginitis and a thin, bubbly, fish-smelling discharge. It is sexually transmitted. Exclude gonorrhea (which may coexist). The motile flagellate may be seen on wet film microscopy or cultured. *Treatment:* Metronidazole or tinidazole 2 g PO α 1 or metronidazole 500 mg/12 h PO for 7 d. Treat the partner.

Bacterial vaginosis presents with fish-smelling discharge. The vagina is not inflamed, and itch is common. Vaginal PH is >5.5, resulting in alteration of bacterial flora ± overgrowth (e.g., of *Gardnerella vaginalis*, *Mycoplasma hominis*, *Mobiluncus*, and anaerobes, such as *Bacteroides* spp.) with too few lactobacilli. There is increased risk of preterm labor and amniotic infection if pregnant. *Diagnosis:* Stippled vaginal epithelial "clue cells" may be seen on wet microscopy. *Treatment:* Metronidazole 500 mg/12 h PO for 7 d, metronidazole or clindamycin cream.

Gonorrhea (*Neisseria gonorrhea*; gonococcus, GC) can infect any columnar epithelium (e.g., urethra, cervix, rectum, pharynx and conjunctiva). *Incubation:* 2–10 d. *Symptoms:* Purulent urethral discharge, dysuria, proctitis, tenesmus, pharyngitis, vaginal discharge; many patients are asymptomatic. *Complications—Local:* Prostatitis, cystitis, epididymitis, salpingitis, bartholinitis. *Systemic:* Septicemia; e.g., with petechiae, hand/foot pustules, arthritis; Reiter's syndrome; endocarditis (rare). *Long-term:* Urethral stricture, infertility. *Diagnosis:* Gram stain, culture of relevant specimen, nucleic acid amplification test. *Treatment:* Uncomplicated infection: Ceftriaxone 250 mg IM α 1. Cefixime 400 mg α 1 is another option but does not cover pharyngeal disease well. Treat for *Chlamydia* too (e.g., doxycycline 100 mg/12 h PO for 7 d, or a single dose of azithromycin 1 g PO) as 50% of patients with urethritis or cervicitis will have concomitant *C. trachomatis* infection. Trace contacts. No intercourse or alcohol until cured. **Nongonococcal urethritis** is commoner than GC. Discharge is thinner and signs less acute, but this may not help diagnosis. Women (typically asymptomatic) may have cervicitis, urethritis, or salpingitis (pain, fever, infertility). Rectum and pharynx are not infected. *Organisms:* C. trachomatis (nucleic acid amplification tests can detect this), *Ureaplasma urealyticum*, *Mycoplasma genitalium*, *Trichomonas vaginalis*, *Gardnerella*, gram-negative and anaerobic bacteria, *Candida*. *Complications:* Similar to local complications of GC. *Chlamydia* may cause Reiter's syndrome and neonatal conjunctivitis. *Treatment:* Azithromycin 1 g α 1 or doxycycline 100 mg/12 h PO. Trace contacts. Avoid intercourse during treatment and alcohol for 4 wks.

Noninfective urethritis Traumatic, chemicals, cancer, foreign body.

Infections associated with animal contact

Bites Most common bite is from dogs (about 80%). Typical organisms in dog and cat bites are oral flora from animal (*Pasteurella*, *Capnocytophaga*, *Porphyromonas*, *Bacteroides*, and *S. aureus*) and human skin flora. *Approach:* Cleanse wound, update tetanus vaccination, and give antibiotics for all obviously infected wounds and for all human bites, all wounds that are moderate to severe, associated with edema, at hands or near a bone or joint, and in immunocompromised patients. Infected wounds should not be closed. Empiric therapy: Amoxicillin 500 mg/clavulanate 875 mg/12 h PO, ampicillin/sulbactam 1.5–3 g/6–8 h IV. *History of contact with specic animals* can be helpful: Rabbits (*Francisella tularensis*-tularemia), kittens (*Bartonella henselae*: Cat scratch disease), parturient cats (*Coxiella burnetii*: Q fever), cat litter (toxoplasmosis), sick cats and wild rodents (*Yersinia pestis*), birds (*Salmonella*, *Chlamydia psittaci*, *Cryptococcus neoformans*), reptiles (*Salmonella species*), raccoons (*Baylisascaris*), bat guano (histoplasmosis), rodents including pets (lymphocytic choriomeningitis virus,) wild mice (hantavirus), macaque monkeys (herpes B), farm animal and petting zoos (*E. coli* 0157:H7, *Campylobacter*, cryptosporidiosis), fish tanks (*Mycobacterium marinum*).

Rabies is a rhabdovirus spread by bites from any infected mammal. Most common rabid species in the United States are raccoons, skunks, bats, foxes; beware of contact with rabid dogs and cats (especially with travel outside the United States). Nearly all cases in the United States are from bat bites (beware of any exposure; bat bites may be unapparent); nearly all in developing world are dog bites. Incubation is usually 9–90 d, so give prophylaxis even several months after exposure. Prodrome symptoms include headache, malaise, abnormal behavior, agitation, fever, and itching at the site of the bite. Disease progresses to "furious rabies"; e.g., with water provoking muscle spasms and may be accompanied by profound terror (hydrophobia). In 20%, "dumb rabies" starts with flaccid paralysis in the bitten limb and spreads.

Treatment if bitten where rabies is endemic (if unvaccinated): Seek expert help. If bite is from a domestic dog, cat, or ferret, the animal can be observed for 10 d. If bite is from skunk, raccoon, fox, or bat, the animal can be euthanized and tested. If this is not possible, give *postexposure prophylaxis* (previously not vaccinated); wound cleansing, human rabies immune globulin (HRIG) 20 IU/kg, give as much as possible into wound, give rest IM + vaccine (HDCV or PCECV)1.0 mL IM (not HRIG site) on days 0,3,7,14. For those previously vaccinated, give IM vaccine at day 0 and 3 and no HRIG.

Pre-exposure prophylaxis (e.g., veterinarians, zoo-keepers, customs officials, bat handlers, and certain travelers): Give three doses of vaccine IM (days 0, 7, 21–28).

Rabies is usually fatal once symptoms begin, but survival has been documented in a handful of patients. A neuroprotective protocol is available through Children's Hospital of Wisconsin.

Miscellaneous gram-positive bacteria

Staphylococci When pathogenic, these are usually either S. aureus or coagulase-negative Staphylococci (CONS). Typically, S. aureus cause localized infection of skin, lids, or wounds, as well as invasive bloodstream and deep tissue infections. Severe infections with S. aureus include pneumonia, osteomyelitis, septic arthritis, endocarditis, and septicemia. S. aureus toxins may cause food poisoning (or the toxic shock syndrome toxin [TSST–1]). The latter presents as shock, confusion, fever, rash with desquamation of digits, diarrhea, myalgias, CPK elevation, and thrombocytopenia and is associated with colonization or infection by toxin-producing staphylococci. CONS are the most common cause of bloodstream infections in hospitalized patients and important causes of medical device-associated infections. When isolated from a culture, CONS are frequently contaminants. Up to 80% of CONS in blood cultures are contaminants. Clues to actual infection are recovery from a normally sterile site in the appropriate clinical context.

Methicillin-resistant S. aureus (MRSA) is a major issue in health care system-acquired and community-acquired infection, causing pneumonia, septicemia, wound infections, and deaths. In the United States, about 50% of nosocomial S. aureus infections are MRSA. *Management of health care system MRSA:* The usual drug is vancomycin; more recently, linezolid and daptomycin have been introduced. All three are essentially universally active against MRSA. However, daptomycin should not be used in cases of pneumonia as it is inactivated by surfactant. Community-acquired MRSA (USA 300 strain) has emerged as an important cause of skin and soft-tissue infection. Such staphylococcal infections are due to strains that are clonal, global, and harbor genes for the Panton-Valentine leukocidin that is associated with virulence. These strains usually harbor the mec IV element that confers resistance to β-lactams. Sensitivity tests usually show susceptibility to clindamycin, doxycycline, gentamicin, and TMP/SMX. The most common infections are large furuncles that require surgical drainage. Other less common infections are necrotizing fasciitis, necrotizing pneumonia, and pyomyositis. *Management:* Simple cutaneous abscess require drainage, and antibiotics are optional.

Antibiotics should be used in cases of systemic illness; cellulitis; rapid progression; deeper or extensive infection;, hand, face, or genital involvement; and in patients with immunosuppression, significant comorbid illness, septic phlebitis, and the elderly. If used, the usual recommendation is TMP/SMX or doxycycline, clindamycin, or linezolid (much more expensive). For patients requiring hospitalization vancomycin, linezolid, and daptomycin (except in lung) can be used. Ceftaroline and telavancin can be considered in skin and soft-tissue infections. *Preventive measures:* Isolate recently admitted patients with suspected MRSA. Group MRSA patients together or place in single isolation rooms. Cleanse hands (alcohol gel is good) and use gloves and gowns in patient rooms. Use dedicated stethoscope or cleanse it after contact. Ask about the need for eradication (with mupirocin). Be meticulous in looking after intravascular catheters. Perform surveillance swabs of patients and possibly staff during outbreaks. Masks may be needed during contact with MRSA pneumonia. *Management of recurrent MRSA skin infection:* Cover draining wounds to reduce spread; maintain good personal hygiene; cleanse towels, linens, and clothes that have come in contact with MRSA wound; trim long fingernails because under surfaces may be sites of colonization. Cleanse high-touch surfaces in the home. Consider personal decolonization with mupirocin twice daily to anterior nares for 5–10 d and skin antiseptic (e.g., chlorhexidine) for 5–14 d.

Streptococci Group A streptococci (e.g., *S. pyogenes*) are common pathogens, causing wound and skin infections (e.g., impetigo, erysipelas), tonsillitis, scarlet fever, necrotizing fasciitis, toxic shock, or septicemia. Late complications are rheumatic fever and poststreptococcal glomerulonephritis. *S. pneumoniae* (*Pneumococcus,* gram-positive diplococcus) causes pneumonia, otitis media, meningitis, septicemia, and peritonitis (rare). Resistance to penicillin is a problem. *S. sanguis, S. mutans,* and *S. mitis* (of the "viridans" group), *S. bovis,* and *Enterococcus faecalis* all cause SBE. *E. faecalis* also causes UTI, wound infections, and septicemia. *S. mutans* is a very common cause of dental caries. *S. milleri* forms abscesses (e.g., in CNS, lungs, and liver). Most streptococci are sensitive to the penicillins, but *E. faecalis* and *E. faecium* may present some difficulties. They usually respond to a combination of ampicillin and an aminoglycoside (e.g., gentamicin). Vancomycin-resistant enterococci (VRE) are generally sensitive to linezolid and daptomycin, although resistance is emerging.

Anthrax (Bacillus anthracis)**:** Occurs in Africa, Asia, China, Eastern Europe, and Haiti. Spread by handling infected carcasses; well-cooked meat poses no risk. In 2001, anthrax was used as a biological weapon. *Presentation:* Common form: Local cutaneous "malignant pustule." Edema may be a striking sign ± fever and hepatosplenomegaly. Anthrax may cause pulmonary or GI anthrax with breathlessness or massive GI hemorrhage (± meningoencephalitis). *Tests:* CXR may show a widened mediastinum and pleural effusion. Infiltrates are rare. Gram stain is sometimes diagnostic (gram-positive rod). *Treatment: Cutaneous disease:* Ciprofloxacin 500 mg/12 h PO or doxycycline 100 mg bid for 60 d. *Pulmonary or GI anthrax:* Ciprofloxacin 400 mg/12 h or doxycycline 100 mg bid IV with clindamycin 900 mg/8 h IV + rifampicin 300 mg/12 h IV or imipenem 1 g IV q6h. Switch to oral drugs when able; adjust based on susceptibility and treat for 60 d. *Prevention:* Immunization of animals at risk and enforcement of sound food-handling and carcass-hygiene policies. A human vaccine (AVA) is indicated for very specific groups. In bioterrorism, doxycycline or ciprofloxacin is highly effective in preventing disease among those exposed. There is also a role for postexposure vaccination with AVA. The mortality for pneumonia treated with ciprofloxacin and other agents is 40–50%. Bloody pleural effusions must be drained.

Diphtheria is caused by the toxin of *Corynebacterium diphtheriae*. Presents with tonsillitis ± a pseudomembrane over the throat and lymphadenopathy ("bull neck"). Diphtheria is extremely rare in the United States, but endemic in multiple developing countries and states of the former Soviet Union. Complications include airway obstruction, myocarditis, and polyneuropathies. *Treatment:* Equine diphtheria antitoxin (EDA) *and* erythromycin or penicillin is used to eradicate the organism. EDA can be obtained from CDC (770–488–7100). *Prevention:* Diphtheria toxoid vaccine (as part of combination with tetanus ± pertussis vaccines). Give all close contacts prophylaxis with erythromycin or penicillin.

Listeriosis is caused by *Listeria monocytogenes*, a gram-positive bacillus with an unusual ability to multiply at low temperatures. Possible sources of infection include pâtés, raw vegetables, unpasteurized milk, and soft cheeses (brie, camembert, and blue-vein types). It may cause a nonspecific flu-like illness, pneumonia, meningoencephalitis, ataxia, rash, or FUO, especially in the immunocompromised; in pregnancy, where it may cause miscarriage or stillbirth; and in neonates. *Diagnosis:* Culture blood, placenta, amniotic fluid, CSF, and any expelled products of conception. *Take blood cultures in any pregnant patient with unexplained fever for 48 h.* Serology, vaginal, and rectal swabs don't help (it may be a commensal here). *Treatment:* Ampicillin IV (TMP/SMX if allergic) ± gentamicin. *Prevention in pregnancy:* Avoid soft cheeses, pâtés, and undercooked meat. Observe "use by" dates. Ensure reheated food is piping hot; observe standing times when using microwaves; throw away any leftovers.

Nocardia species In the United States, nocardiosis is typically a disease of immunocompromised patients (e.g., steroids, transplant, advanced HIV), where it can cause pulmonary, liver, and brain abscesses. *Microscopy:* Branching gram-positive chains. *Treatment:* TMP/SMX ± amikacin is the mainstay of therapy. Imipenem, minocycline are alternatives. Check susceptibilities. In warm climates, *Nocardia* can cause subcutaneous infection (e.g., Madura foot).

Clostridia (*C. perfringens*) causes wound infections and gas gangrene ± shock or renal failure after surgery or trauma. *Treatment:* Debridement is essential; penicillin 1.2–2.4 g/6 h IV + clindamycin 900 mg/8 h IV, antitoxin, and hyperbaric oxygen may also be used. Amputation may be necessary. *Clostridia food poisoning:* See section on GI illness. *C. difcile:* Diarrhea (the cause of pseudomembranous colitis following antibiotic therapy). This has emerged as a major problem in hospitalized patients. Keys to management include discontinuation of offending antibiotics whenever feasible, metronidazole, or vancomycin. Fidaxomicin is newly approved for *C. difficile* colitis and may be associated with fewer recurrences. *C. botulinum (botulism):* *C. botulinum* toxin blocks release of acetylcholine causing descending flaccid paralysis. Botulism is not spread from one person to another. There are two adult forms of botulism: Food-borne and wound botulism, which is a problem in IV drug abusers if heroin is contaminated with *C. botulinum*. *Signs:* Afebrile, flaccid paralysis, dysarthria, dysphagia, diplopia, ptosis, weakness, respiratory failure. *Autonomic signs:* Dry mouth, fixed or dilated pupils. *Tests:* Find toxin in blood samples or, in the case of wound botulism, by the identification of *C. botulinum* in wound specimens. Samples include serum, wound pus, swabs in anaerobic transport media. *Management:* Get help and transfer to ICU. Botulinum antitoxin works if given early. Before giving antitoxin, skin testing is required to evaluate for sensitivity to serum or antitoxin. Then give one vial of IV antitoxin. Also consider in those who have ingested toxin but who have not yet developed symptoms. *C. botulinum* is sensitive to penicillin and metronidazole. If suspecting a case of botulism, contact local state health department for assistance. If not available, contact CDC at (770) 488–7100.

581

Actinomycosis is usually caused by *Actinomyces israelii*. *Presentations* include subcutaneous infections, forming chronic sinuses with sulfur granule-containing pus. It commonly affects the area of the jaw. It may cause abdominal masses (may mimic appendix mass). *Treatment:* Penicillin for many months. Consult with surgeons.

Miscellaneous gram-negative bacteria

Enterobacteriaceae Some are normal gut commensals, others environmental organisms. They are the most common cause of UTI and intra-abdominal sepsis, especially postoperatively and in the acute abdomen. They are also a common cause of septicemia due to nosocomial pneumonia and catheter-associated infection. Enterobacteriaceae are a rare cause of meningitis or endocarditis but may cause these infections when there are indwelling devices (e.g., prosthetic valves, ventricular drains). These organisms are often sensitive to ampicillin and TMP/SMX, but in serious infections, use cefuroxime or third- or fourth-generation cephalosporin, quinolones, or carbapenems ± an aminoglycoside. **Pseudomonas aeruginosa** is a serious pathogen, especially in the immunocompromised and in patients with cystic fibrosis. It causes pneumonia, septicemia, UTI, wound infection, osteomyelitis, and cutaneous infections. The main problem is its tendency to be resistant to many antibiotics. *Treatment:* Piperacillin/tazobactam, cefepime, ceftazidime, aztreonam, meropenem, imipenem, or doripenem. If using aminoglycosides (e.g., amikacin, gentamicin, tobramycin) or colistin, these should not be used alone. Ciprofloxacin and other quinolones are the only oral anti-*Pseudomonas* antibiotics. *Acinetobacter baumannii* has recently emerged as a major cause of health care system- and traumatic injury-associated infection. *A. baumannii* causes skin, soft-tissue, and bone infections in soldiers injured in Iraq and Afghanistan, as well as postoperative, bloodstream, and lung infection in hospitalized patients. These organisms are often resistant to multiple classes of antibiotics.

Multi-drug resistant Acinetobacter, Enterobacteriaceae, and pseudomonal infections are an increasingly important problem in hospitalized patients and, in some cases, therapeutic options are extremely limited.

Haemophilus influenzae type B typically affects unvaccinated children usually <4 yrs old. It causes otitis media, acute epiglottitis, pneumonia, meningitis, osteomyelitis, and septicemia. In adults, nontypeable strains may cause exacerbations of chronic bronchitis, sinusitis, and pneumonia. *Treatment:* Unreliably sensitive to ampicillin and TMP/SMX; cefotaxime, quinolones, azithromycin amox-clavulanate are more reliable. Capsulated types tend to be much more pathogenic than noncapsulated types. *Prevention:* Immunization with HIB vaccine has resulted in a dramatic fall in incidence.

Plague is caused by *Yersinia pestis*. *Spread:* Fleas of rodents or cats, or droplets from other infected humans. *Incubation:* 1–7 d. **Bubonic plague** presents with lymphadenopathy (buboes). **Pneumonic plague** may present with lymphadenopathy or a flu-like illness leading to dyspnea, cough, copious, bloody sputum, septicemia, and a hemorrhagic fatal illness. *Diagnosis:* Phage typing of bacterial culture or a fourfold rise in antibodies to F antigen. *Treatment:* Isolate suspects. Streptomycin 15 mg/kg/12 h IV or gentamicin 5 mg/kg/d or 2 mg load followed by 1.7 mg/kg/8 h for 10 d. Doxycycline and ciprofloxacin are alternatives. Patients with suspected or confirmed *Y. pestis* infection should be maintained in respiratory droplet isolations (gloves, gowns, eye protection) until at least 48 h of ABX therapy and clinical improvement. *Postexposure prophylaxis:* Doxycycline 100 mg/12 h PO for 7 d or ciprofloxacin 500 mg PO bid α 7 d and monitor for fever or cough during this time.

Brucellosis This zoonosis (carried by domestic animals) is common in multiple countries including those in the Middle East, Mediterranean basin, South and Central America, and Africa. Typically affects vets or farmers, but can be foodborne. Unpasteurized dairy products (e.g., "village cheese") are a risk to travelers. *Cause:* B. melitensis (the most virulent), B. abortus, B. suis, or B. canis. *Symptoms* may be indolent and last for years with fever, sweats, malaise, anorexia, vomiting, weight loss, hepatosplenomegaly, constipation, diarrhea, myalgias, backache, arthritis, sacroiliitis, rash, bursitis, orchitis, and depression. *Complications:* Osteomyelitis, SBE (culture negative), abscesses (liver, spleen, lung), meningoencephalitis. *Diagnosis:* Blood culture (may take many days to grow), serology: If titers equivocal (e.g., >1:40 in nonendemic zones) do ELISA ± immunoradiometric assays; pancytopenia is a clue. Notify laboratory if *Brucella* is a possibility; it is a laboratory hazard. *Treatment:* Doxycycline + rifampin α 6 wks, or doxycycline for 6 wks + streptomycin (α 2–3 wks) or gentamicin (α 1 week); some recommend doxycycline + rifampin α 6 wks + gentamicin α 2 wks.

Whooping cough is caused by Bordetella pertussis. *Presentation:* This begins with a prodromal catarrhal phase with fever and cough. After a week or so, the patient develops paroxysms of coughing. There may be the characteristic inspiratory whoops, but this is not always present in adults. Most patients recover without complication, although the cough may last some months. Some, especially the very young, may develop pneumonia (and consequent bronchiectasis) or convulsions or brain damage. *Prevention* efforts include vaccinating adults with DTaP in place of Td. *Diagnosis:* Nasopharyngeal aspirate or Dacron swab culture or PCR. *Treatment:* A macrolide given early in the course can decrease the duration, severity, and communicability of pertussis. Treatment is with azithromycin 500 mg/d α 1, then 250 mg/d α 4 d, clarithromycin 500 mg/12 h α 7 d, erythromycin 500 mg/6 h α 14 d, and TMP/SMX DS/12 h α 14 d. Administer postexposure prophylaxis with the above courses of antibiotics to close contacts.

Pasteurella multocida is acquired via domestic animals, especially cat or dog bites. *Presentation:* It can cause cutaneous infections, septicemia, pneumonia, UTI, or meningitis. *Treatment:* Susceptible to PCN, but best to treat with amoxicillin/clavulanate or ampicillin/sulbactam to cover potential co-pathogens from animal oral flora.

Yersinia enterocolitica In Scandinavia, this is a common cause of a reactive, asymmetrical polyarthritis of the weight-bearing joints, and, in America, of enteritis. It also causes uveitis, appendicitis, mesenteric lymphadenitis, pyomyositis, glomerulonephritis, thyroiditis, colonic dilatation, terminal ileitis and perforation, and septicemia. *Diagnosis:* Serology is often more helpful than culture, as there may be quite a time lag between infection and the clinical manifestations. Agglutination titers of >1:160 indicate recent infection. *Treatment:* None may be needed, or ciprofloxacin 500 mg/12 h PO for 3–5 d, TMP/SMX, gentamicin, and third-generation cephalosporin are usually effective.

Moraxella catarrhalis (gram-negative diplococcus) is a rare cause of pneumonia and occasional cause of exacerbations of COPD, otitis media, sinusitis, and septicemia. *Treatment:* Clarithromycin 500 mg/12 h PO. Azithromycin, doxycycline, amoxicillin-clavulanate, and quinolones are effective.

Tularemia is caused by *Francisella tularensis* (gram-negative bacillus), which may be acquired by multiple routes (tick bites, contact with infected animal carcasses, inhalation of contaminated dust or aerosol, ingestion of contaminated water). It causes rash, fever, malaise, tonsillitis, headache, hepatosplenomegaly, and lymphadenopathy. There may be papules at sites of inoculation (e.g., fingers). It has the potential for use as a bioweapon. *Complications:* Meningitis, osteomyelitis, SBE, pericarditis, septicemia.

Diagnosis: Contact local microbiologist for advice. Only use laboratories with safety cabinets suitable for dangerous pathogens. Swabs and aspirates must be transported in approved containers. *Treatment:* Gentamicin 1–1.7 mg/kg/8 h or streptomycin 7.5–10 mg/kg/12 h IM for 2 wks. Oral tetracycline or ciprofloxacin are suitable for chemoprophylaxis. *Prevention:* Find the animal vector; reduce human contact with it as much as possible. Vaccination may be possible for high-risk groups.

Cat scratch disease Mostly due to *Bartonella henselae* (a small, curved, pleomorphic, gram-negative rod) or *Afipia felis*. Think of this with an inoculating cat scratch + regional lymphadenopathy + negative evaluation for other causes of lymphadenopathy; *establish diagnosis* with Warthin-Starry stain of biopsy or serology; skin lesions may resemble Kaposi's sarcoma. *Treatment:* Usually resolves spontaneously within 1–2 months. One trial found that azithromycin hastened resolution of lymph nodes. Other drugs that have been used include ciprofloxacin, rifampin, and TMP/SMX.

Tetanus

Toxin of *Clostridium tetani* produces the exotoxin tetanospasmin, which causes muscle spasms and rigidity, the cardinal features of tetanus ("to stretch").

Incidence ~ 30 cases per year in the United States. **Mortality** is about 10–20%.

Pathogenesis Spores of *C. tetani* live in feces, soil, dust, and on instruments. A tiny breach in skin or mucosa (e.g., cuts, burns, ear piercing, banding of hemorrhoids) may allow entry of the spores. (Diabetics are at increased risk.) Spores may then germinate and make the exotoxin. This then travels up peripheral nerves and interferes with inhibitory synapses.

The patient *15–25% will have no evidence of recent wounds.* Signs appear from 1 day to several months from the (often forgotten) injury. There is a prodrome of fever, malaise, and headache before classical features develop: *Trismus* (lockjaw; difficulty in opening the mouth); *risus sardonicus* (a grin-like posture of hypertonic facial muscles); *opisthotonus* (arched body with hyperextended neck); *spasms* (which at first may be induced by movement, injections, noise, etc., but later are spontaneous; they may cause dysphagia and respiratory arrest); *autonomic dysfunction* (arrhythmias and wide fluctuations in BP).

Differential diagnosis includes dental abscess, rabies, phenothiazine toxicity, and strychnine poisoning. Phenothiazine toxicity typically affects facial and tongue muscles.

Poor prognostic signs are short incubation, rapid progression from trismus to spasms (<48 h), development postpartum or postinfection, and tetanus in neonates and old age.

Treatment Get expert help; use ICU, monitor electrocardiogram (ECG) + blood pressure (BP), and monitor fluid balance. Clean/debride wounds, IV metronidazole 500 mg/6 h for 7–14 d is preferred; can also use PCN. If tetanus is established, give human tetanus immune globulin (HTIG) 500 units IM or IV (WHO recommendation) or 3,000–5,000 units IM (CDC) to neutralize free toxin. Some advocate intrathecal administration of antitoxin. Early ventilation and sedation if symptoms progress. *Control spasms:* Diazepam 0.05–0.2 mg/kg/h IV or phenobarbital 1.0 mg/kg/h IM or IV + chlorpromazine 0.5 mg/kg/6 h IM (IV bolus is dangerous) starting 3 h after the phenobarbital. If this fails to control the spasms, paralyze and ventilate (get anesthetist's help).

Postinjury prophylaxis Td or Tdap: Any cut merits an extra dose of tetanus toxoid IM, unless history of three or more toxoids or a booster in last 10 yrs (5 yrs for more severe wounds).

Human tetanus immunoglobulin: This is required for those with fewer than three toxoid boosters in past and with dirty, old (>6 h), infected, devitalized, or soil-contaminated wounds. Give 250–500 units IM, using a separate syringe and site to the toxoid injection. If immune status is unknown, assume that the patient is nonimmune. Routine infant immunization started in 1961, so many adults are at risk. Hygiene education and wound debridement are of vital importance.

Enteric fever

Typhoid and paratyphoid are caused by *Salmonella typhi* and *S. paratyphi* (types A, B, and C), respectively. (Other *Salmonella* species cause diarrhea and vomiting.) *Incubation:* 3–21 d. *Spread:* Fecal-oral. 1% can become chronic carriers. *Presentation:* Usually malaise, headache, high fever with relative bradycardia, cough, and constipation (or diarrhea). CNS signs (coma, delirium, meningitis) are serious. Diarrhea is more common after the first week. Rose spots occur on the trunk of 40%, but may be very difficult to see. Epistaxis, bruising, abdominal pain, and splenomegaly may occur. *Tests:* First 10 d: Blood culture. Later: Urine/stool cultures. Bone marrow culture has highest yield (infiltration may cause decreased platelets and WBC). LFT can be elevated. Widal test is unreliable. DNA probes and PCR tests have been developed, but are not widely available. *Treatment:* Fluid replacement and good nutrition. There is good evidence that quinolones (e.g., ciprofloxacin 500 mg/12 h PO for 6 d) are the best antimicrobial treatment for typhoid. Chloramphenicol is still used in many areas, but generally avoided in the United States because of myelotoxicity. *Other alternatives:* Amoxicillin (if fully susceptible), cefixime, and azithromycin. In severe disease, give IV ciprofloxacin, cefotaxime, or ceftriaxone for 10–14 d. In encephalopathy ± shock, give dexamethasone 3 mg/kg IV stat, then 1 mg/kg/6 h for 48 h. Drug resistance is a problem, even with ciprofloxacin; e.g., due to mutations in the DNA gyrase enzyme of *S. typhi.* *Complications:* Osteomyelitis (e.g., in sickle-cell disease); DVT; GI bleed or perforation; cholecystitis; myocarditis; pyelonephritis; meningitis; abscess. *Chronic carriage* occurs in 1–5% of patients. Treat if at risk of spreading disease (e.g., food handlers). Amoxicillin 4–6 g/d + probenecid 2 g/d for 6 wks may work (*alternative:* Ciprofloxacin 500 mg/12 h PO for 6 wks), but cholecystectomy may be needed, particularly in those with cholelithiasis.

Bacillary dysentery

Shigella causes abdominal pain and bloody diarrhea ± sudden fever, headache, and occasionally neck stiffness. CSF is sterile. Dysentery may be severe (often *S. flexneri* or *S. dysenteriae*). *Incubation:* 1–7 d. *Spread:* Fecal-oral. *Diagnosis:* Stool culture. *Treatment:* TMP/SMX DS/12 h, ciprofloxacin 500 mg/12 h, azithromycin 500 mg/d α 3–5 d (or longer in immunocompromised patients). Imported shigellosis is often resistant to several antimicrobials: Sensitivity testing is important. There may be associated spondyloarthritis.

Cholera

Vibrio cholerae (gram-negative comma-shaped rod): Pandemics or epidemics may occur; e.g., 1990s epidemic in South America and Bangladesh (Bengal *Vibrio cholerae 0139*). *Incubation:* Ranges from a few hours to 5 d. *Spread:* Fecal-oral. *Presentation:* Profuse (e.g., 1 L/h) watery ("rice water") stools, fever, vomiting, and rapid dehydration (the cause of death). *Diagnosis:* Stool microscopy and culture. *Treatment:* Strict barrier nursing. Replace fluid and salt losses meticulously. A single dose of ciprofloxacin 1 g PO may reduce fluid loss. Doxycycline, erythromycin, and TMP/SMX are also effective. *Prevention:* Only drink boiled or treated water. Cook all food well; eat it hot. Avoid shellfish. Peel all vegetables. Heat-killed vaccine (serovar O1) gives limited protection and is no longer needed for international travel; newer vaccines are nonstandard.

Hansen's disease (leprosy)

It is a chronic infection due to *Mycobacterium leprae* predominantly involving skin, mucosa and peripheral nerves. Historically, victims have been ostracized, and this may still be a barrier to self-reporting and early treatment. Consider avoiding use of term "leprosy" due to stigma. Hansen's disease is rare in the United States (150–250 cases/year). Cases can be imported (e.g., immigrants from endemic countries) or locally acquired in Florida, Texas, Louisiana, and California. Armadillos may be a source of infection in the Southern United States. Worldwide, there are ~ 250,000 new cases/year. Most are from Asia and Africa.

Clinical presentation The incubation period is months to years, and the subsequent course depends on the patient's immune response. 95% of the world's population is not susceptible to infection. If the immune response is ineffective, *lepromatous* or *multibacillary* (WHO classification) disease develops, dominated by foamy histiocytes full of bacilli, but few lymphocytes. If there is a vigorous immune response, the disease is called *tuberculoid* or *paucibacillary* (WHO classification), with granulomata containing epithelioid cells and lymphocytes, but few or no demonstrable bacilli. Between these poles lie those with *borderline* disease.

Skin lesions Hypopigmented anesthetic macules, papules, or annular lesions (with raised erythematous rims). Erythema nodosum occurs in "lepromatous" disease, especially during the first year of treatment.

Nerve lesions Major peripheral nerves may be involved, leading to much disability. Sometimes a thickened sensory nerve may be felt running into the skin lesion (e.g., ulnar nerve above the elbow, median nerve at the wrist, or the great auricular nerve running up behind the ear).

Eye lesions Refer promptly to an ophthalmologist. The lower temperature of the anterior chamber favors corneal invasion (so secondary infection and cataract). *Inammatory signs:* Chronic iritis, scleritis, and episcleritis. There may be reduced corneal sensation (V nerve palsy), reduced blinking (VII nerve palsy), lagophthalmos (difficulty in closing the eyes), ± ingrowing eyelashes (trichiasis).

Diagnosis *Biopsy* a thickened nerve; *in vitro* culture is not possible. Split skin smears for AFB are positive in borderline or lepromatous disease. Classification matters as it reflects the biomass of bacilli, influencing treatment: The more organisms, the greater the chance that some will be drug resistant. *Other tests:* Neutrophilia, ESR elevation, IgG elevation.

Treatment It is useful to check with a local expert about resistance patterns (e.g., to dapsone). Treatment for limited disease (tuberculoid, borderline tuberculoid- paucibacillary using WHO classification) is with dapsone 100 mg/d and rifampin 600 mg/d α 12 months. In widespread disease (lepromatous, borderline lepromatous, mid borderline-multibacillary using WHO classification) treat patient with dapsone 100 mg/d + rifampin 600 mg/d + clofazimine 50 mg/d α 24 months. Clofazimine is obtained from National Hansen's Disease Program: 800-642-2477). Minocycline and clarithromycin are also active and may be used in place of dapsone or clofazimine. Ofloxacin can also be used instead of clofazimine. Single lesion skin paucibacillary disease is treated with a rifampin 600 mg, ofloxacin 400 mg, and minocycline 100 mg as a one-time treatment.

Beware of *inflammatory reactions* with therapy caused by infection and/or dying bacilli. *Erythema nodosum leprosum*, which may present as sudden nerve inflammation (± orchitis, lymphadenitis, nephritis, periostitis, irido-cyclitis) may be seen with treatment of widespread infection. Treat with steroids and referral to ophthalmologist for ocular disease. Thalidomide or clofazimine may be useful. The latter causes skin pigmentation. Edema and erythema of preexisting lesions (reversal reactions) may even cause skin ulceration and neuritis. Treat with corticosteroids. Neuritis can occur in the absence of a reactive episode and may respond to steroids.

Spirochetes

Lyme disease is a tick-borne infection caused by *Borrelia burgdorferi*. Although originally described in Lyme (Connecticut) it is now widespread. Not all will remember being bitten by a tick. *Presentation:* Erythema migrans ± malaise, cognitive impairment, lymphadenopathy, arthralgias, myocarditis, heart block, meningitis, ataxia, amnesia, cranial nerve palsies (Bell's palsy), neuropathy, lymphocytic meningoradiculitis (Bannwarth's syndrome). *Diagnosis:* If erythema migrans is present at evaluation, then serology is not needed. Otherwise, diagnose using clinical features + serology at 4–6 wks. Serology is a two-step process with a screening ELISA followed by confirmatory IgG and IgM immunoblot if ELISA is positive. If symptoms are present >4 months, IgG must be present to be considered positive. *Treatment:* Skin rash, isolated cranial nerve palsy: Doxycycline 100 mg/12 h PO (amoxicillin, cefuroxime also active) for 14–21 d, arthritis (21 d). CNS, peripheral nerve disease, carditis, or recurrent arthritis: Ceftriaxone 2 g/d IV (cefotaxime, PCN G also good). *Prevention:* Keep limbs covered; use insect repellent; tick collars for pets; check skin often when in risky areas. Vaccination is no longer available. A single dose of doxycycline 200 mg PO given within 72 h of a bite is effective prophylaxis; in highly endemic areas, this may be worthwhile (e.g., if risk is >1%). *Removing ticks:* Using fine-tipped tweezers, gently remove tick by grasping it as close to skin surface as possible, then pull up with steady, even pressure.

Endemic treponematoses *Yaws* is caused by *T. pertenue*, which is serologically indistinguishable from *T. pallidum*. It is a chronic granulomatous disease prevalent in children in the rural tropics. Spread is by direct contact, via skin abrasions, and is promoted by poor hygiene. The primary lesion (an ulcerating papule) appears ~4 wks after exposure. Scattered secondary lesions then appear (e.g., in moist skin, but can be anywhere). These may become exuberant. Tertiary lesions are subcutaneous gummatous ulcerating granulomata, affecting skin and bone. Cardiovascular and CNS complications do not occur. *Pinta* (*T. carateum*) affects only skin; seen in Central and S America. Endemic nonvenereal syphilis (bejel; *T. pallidum*) is seen in third-world children, when it resembles yaws. In the developed world, *T. pallidum* causes syphilis. *Diagnosis:* Clinical. *Treatment:* Procaine penicillin.

Leptospirosis Caused by bacteria in the genus *Leptospira*. Spread is by contact with soil or water contaminated by urine or body fluids of infected animals (e.g., rodents, livestock, and dogs). Typical exposures involve swimming/rafting/kayaking in fresh water, especially in tropical regions (e.g., Hawaii, Caribbean) and exposure to surface water in endemic regions. *Presentation:* Fever, jaundice, headache, red conjunctivae, tender legs (myositis), purpura, hemoptysis, hematemesis, or any bleeding. Meningitis, myocarditis, and renal failure may develop. AST rise may be small. *Diagnosis:* Rapid serological assays are replacing the old microscopic

587

agglutination test. Also take blood, urine, and CSF culture (for 4–6 wks). *Treat* symptomatically; give doxycycline 100 mg/12 h or, in serious disease, IV benzylpenicillin 600 mg/6 h for 7 d. Prophylaxis (e.g., doxycycline 200 mg/wk PO) may be useful for those at high risk for short periods.

Canicola fever is aseptic meningitis caused by *Leptospira canicola*.

Relapsing fever Tick-borne relapsing fever (TBRF) is usually caused by *Borrelia hermsii*. Transmission is via a soft tick. In the United States, most cases are in western mountainous regions. **Louse-borne relapsing fever (LBRF)** is caused by *B. recurrentis* transmitted person to person by the body louse. It typically occurs in epidemics following war or disaster. Illness may be severe (30–70% mortality) with enormous death tolls in outbreak settings. *Incubation:* 4–18 d. *Presentation:* Abrupt onset of fever, rigors, and headache. A petechial rash (which may be faint or absent), jaundice, and tender hepatosplenomegaly may develop. Serious complications include myocarditis, hepatic failure, and DIC. Crises of very high fever and tachycardia occur. When the fever abates, hypotension due to vasodilatation may occur and be fatal. Relapses occur, but are milder. *Tests:* Organisms are seen on Leishman-stained thin or thick films. *Treatment:* TBRF: Erythromycin 500 mg/6 h PO or IV, tetracycline 500 mg/6 h PO or 250 mg/6 h IV, or doxycycline 100 mg/12 h PO or IV α 7 d. LBRF can be treated with a single dose of ABX. Monitor for *Jarisch-Herxheimer reaction* (fevers chills, hypotension with lysis of organisms) in first few hours after ABX. Delouse the patient and his or her clothes. Doxycycline is useful prophylaxis in high-risk groups.

Viral hemorrhagic fevers

Yellow fever An epidemic arbovirus disease spread by *Aedes* mosquitoes (Brazil, Bolivia, Peru, and Central and West Africa). *Incubation:* 2–14 d. *Clinical presentation:* In mild forms, fever, headache, nausea, albuminuria, myalgias, and relative bradycardia. If severe: 3 d of headache, myalgias, anorexia ± nausea, followed by abrupt fever, a brief remission, then prostration, jaundice (± fatty liver), hematemesis and other bleeding, oliguria. *Mortality:* <10% (day 5–10). *Diagnosis:* ELISA. *Treatment:* Symptomatic.

Lassa fever, Ebola virus, Marburg virus, and dengue hemorrhagic fever (DHF) These diseases may start with sudden-onset headache, pleuritic pain, backache, myalgias, conjunctivitis, prostration, dehydration, facial flushing (dengue), and fever. Bleeding soon supervenes. There may be spontaneous resolution or renal failure, encephalitis, coma, and death. *Treatment:* Primarily symptomatic; ribavirin is useful in Lassa fever if given early in disease. Use special infection control measures (Lassa, Ebola, and Marburg); get expert help at once.

Dengue is the most prevalent arbovirus disease. There is a global pandemic of this RNA flavivirus, related to poor vector control (*Aedes* mosquitoes), urbanization, and rapid migrations bringing new strains (DEN–2), which become more virulent in those who have had mild dengue. About 50 million cases of dengue infection occur each year and 500,000 are hospitalized each year with DHF. Infants typically have a simple febrile illness with a maculopapular rash. Older children/adults have flushing of face, neck, and chest or a centrifugal maculopapular rash from day 3, or a late confluent petechiae with round pale areas of normal skin. Also, patients may have headache, arthralgias, jaundice, hepatosplenomegaly, and anuria. *Hemorrhagic signs:* (Unlikely if AST normal), petechiae, GI, gum or nosebleeds, hematuria, hypermenorrhea. *Monitor:* BP, urine flow, WBC, HCT, PLT. A positive tourniquet test (>20 petechiae inch^2) + rise in HCT by 20% are telling signs (rapid endothelial plasma leak is the key pathophysiology of DHF). *Differential diagnosis:* Chikungunya, measles, leptospirosis, typhoid, malaria. *Exclusion:* If symptoms start >2 wks after leaving a dengue-endemic area, or if fever lasts >2 wks, dengue can be ruled out. *Treatment:* With more severe disease (e.g., DHF or dengue shock syndrome) fluid and electrolyte resuscitation/management is critical. Blood transfusions may be required as well. If in shock mortality is high, fluid resuscitation should be aggressive: Give a bolus of 15 mL/kg; repeat as necessary until BP rises and urine flow is >30 mL/h.

Rickettsia and arthropod-borne bacteria

Rickettsial infections are carried by host arthropods and invade human mononuclear cells, neutrophils, or blood vessel endothelium (vasculotropic). All the cataclysmic events of the last century (war, revolution, flood, famine, genocide, and overcrowding) have favored lice infestation. As a result, these infections (in particular typhus) have killed untold millions.

Q fever is caused by *Coxiella burnetii*. It is so named because it was first labeled "query fever" in workers in an Australian abattoir. *Epidemiology:* Occurs worldwide and is usually rural, with its reservoir in cattle and sheep. The organism is very resistant to drying and is usually inhaled from infected dust. It can be contracted from unpasteurized milk, directly from carcasses in abattoirs, sometimes by droplet spread, and occasionally from tick bites. *Clinical features:* Q fever should be suspected in patients with FUO or atypical pneumonia. It may present with fever, myalgias, sweats, headache, cough, and hepatitis. In chronic cases, suspect endocarditis (typically "culture-negative"). This usually affects the aortic valve, but clinical signs may be absent. It also causes miscarriages and CNS infection. *Investigations:* CXR may show consolidation (e.g., multilobar or slowly resolving). Liver function tests may be hepatitic, and biopsy may show granulomata. Platelets may be low. Diagnosis is serologically, but may be negative in first 7–10 d of infection. Phase I antigens indicate chronic infection; phase II antigens indicate acute infection. A fourfold rise antibody titer is diagnostic. PCR may be used on serum and tissue samples. CSF tests may be needed. *Treatment:* Get expert microbiological help. *Acute:* Doxycycline 100 mg/12 h for 2–3 wks. *Chronic:* Doxycycline 100 mg/12 h + Chloroquine 200 mg/8 h α 18 months. Valve replacement may be needed in cases of endocarditis.

Bartonellosis is caused by *Bartonella bacilliformis*, a gram-negative, motile, bacillus-like organism that infects red blood cells. Spread is by sandflies in the Andes regions of Peru, Ecuador, and Colombia. The disease has two phases, an acute hemolytic febrile illness called *Oroya fever* and an eruptive phase with red to purple angioproliferative nodular skin lesions (verruga peruana). *Clinical features* of acute infection include fever, myalgias, headache, hepatosplenomegaly, lymphadenopathy, and anemia. *Complications* include end organ damage (e.g., CNS, liver, GI, pulmonary) due to microvascular thrombosis. *Diagnosis* is by observation of the organism on Giemsa-stained blood films or by culture. A similar acute syndrome has been described due to *B. rochalimae*, a newly described organism. With recovery from acute infection, patients are at transient risk for opportunistic infection with toxoplasmosis and salmonellosis. *Treatment:* Acute infection: Ciprofloxacin, doxycycline, ampicillin, TMP/SMX α 7–14 d. Eruptive phase: Rifampin 10 mg/kg/d (max 600 mg) α 10–14 d or streptomycin 15–20 mg/kg/d α 10 d. Steroids may be indicated if there is severe neurological involvement.

Cat scratch disease is caused by *Bartonella henselae*. *Bacillary angiomatosis/ peliosis:* May occur in immunocompromised patients (e.g., those with AIDS) and is manifested by neovascular proliferation that may involve skin, lymph nodes, liver, spleen, bone, brain, cervix, lung and bowel, caused by *B. henselae* or *B. quintana*. *Treatment* is with doxycycline for several months.

Trench fever is caused by *Bartonella quintana* inoculated from infected louse feces, not only in soldiers, but also in the homeless and in alcoholics. *Clinical features:* Fever, headache, myalgias, dizziness, back pain, macular rash, eye pain, leg pain, splenomegaly, and rarely, endocarditis. In HIV-infected patients, the skin lesions may resemble Kaposi's sarcoma. May cause culture negative endocarditis; may relapse after clinical improvement. *Investigations:* Blood culture, serology, PCR. *Treatment:* Doxycycline 100 mg/12 h PO for 15 d. Endocarditis requires long therapy.

Ehrlichiosis is caused by organisms related to *Rickettsia* that target macrophages (*Ehrlichia chaffeensis*) and granulocytes (*E. ewingii* and *Anaplasma phagocytophilum*). Ticks spread ehrlichiosis. *Symptoms:* Fever, headache, anorexia, malaise, abdominal pain, epigastric pain, conjunctivitis, lymphadenopathy, jaundice, rash, confusion, and cervical lymphadenopathy. *Investigations:* Leucopenia, thrombocytopenia, AST elevation. Serology and PCR are used for diagnosis. Intracellular inclusions may rarely be observed on buffy coat preparation of blood smear. *Treatment:* Doxycycline 100 mg/12 h PO for 7–14 d.

General comments about rickettsial infections

- *Typhus:* The archetypal disease. Organisms are transmitted between hosts by arthropods. The incubation period is 2–23 d. Do not delay therapy while waiting for laboratory confirmation.
- *Pathology:* Widespread vasculitis and endothelial proliferation may affect any organ, and thrombotic occlusion may lead to gangrene.
- *Clinical features:* Infection may be mild and asymptomatic or severe and systemic. There may be sudden onset of fever, frontal headache, confusion, and jaundice. With some species, an *eschar* (black scar at the site of the initial inoculation) may be present. A rickettsial rash may be macular, papular, petechial, or hemorrhagic.
- *Investigations* may show hemolysis, neutrophilia, thrombocytopenia, clotting abnormalities, hepatitis, and renal impairment. Patients die of shock, renal failure, DIC, or stroke.
- *Rocky Mountain spotted fever (R. rickettsii):* Tick-borne and endemic in the Rocky Mountains and the southeastern states of the United States. The rash begins as macules on the hands and feet, then spreads becoming petechial or hemorrhagic.
- *Tick typhus (R. conorii):* Endemic in Africa, the Arabian Gulf, and the Mediterranean. A black eschar may be visible at the site of the infecting bite. The rash starts in the axillae, becoming purpuric as it spreads.
- *Other features:* Conjunctival suffusion; jaundice, deranged clotting, renal impairment.
- *Epidemic typhus (R. prowazekii):* Carried by human lice (*Pediculus humanus*) whose feces are inhaled or pass through skin. Typhus may become latent, only to recrudesce later (Brill–Zinsser disease).
- *Murine (endemic) typhus (R. typhi):* Transmitted by fleas from rats to humans. It is more prevalent in warm, coastal ports.
- *Rickettsialpox (R. akari):* Mite-borne infection. Rash is macular, papular, or vesicular.
- *Scrub typhus (Orienta tsutsugamushi):* Most common in Southeast Asia.

Diagnosis: This is difficult as often the picture is nonspecific, the organisms are difficult to grow, and the traditional heterophil antibody Weil–Felix test has low sensitivity and specificity. A rise in antibody titer in paired sera is diagnostic. Latex agglutination, indirect immunofluorescence, and ELISAs are available. An accurate, rapid dot blot immunoassay is available for scrub typhus. Skin biopsy may be diagnostic in Rocky Mountain spotted fever. *Treatment:* Doxycycline 100 mg/12 h for at least 7 d or longer (2 d after fever resolves).

Giardiasis

Giardia lamblia is a flagellate protozoon that lives in the duodenum and jejunum. It is spread by the fecal–oral route. Risk factors for transmission are travel, immunosuppression, MSM, achlorhydria, playgroups, and swimming. Drinking water may become contaminated. *Presentation:* Often asymptomatic. Lassitude, bloating, flatulence, abdominal discomfort, loose stools ± explosive diarrhea are typical. Malabsorption, weight loss, and lactose intolerance may occur. *Diagnosis:* Organisms are excreted intermittently and even repeated stool microscopy for cysts or trophozoites may be negative. Fecal immunoassays are more sensitive and specific. Finally, a trial of therapy may be needed. *Differential diagnosis:* Any cause of diarrhea, tropical sprue, celiac disease. *Treatment:* Scrupulous hygiene. Metronidazole 250 mg/8 h α 5 d, tinidazole 2 g PO once, nitazoxanide 500 mg/12 h α 3 d. If treatment with metronidazole fails, treat longer or try nitazoxanide. For further recurrences, consider treating the whole family. If diarrhea persists, avoid milk, as lactose intolerance may persist for 6 wks.

Other GI protozoa *Cryptosporidium*, *Microsporidium* and *Isospora* occur in AIDS, *Balantidium coli*, and *Sarcocystis*.

Amebiasis

Entamoeba histolytica occurs worldwide. *Spread:* Fecal–oral. Boil water and infected food to destroy cysts. Trophozoites may remain in the bowel or invade extraintestinal tissues, leaving "flask-shaped" GI ulcers. *Presentation* may be asymptomatic, with mild diarrhea or with severe amoebic dysentery.

Amoebic dysentery may occur yrs after the initial infection. Diarrhea begins slowly, but becomes profuse and bloody. An acute febrile prostrating illness does occur but high fever, colic, and tenesmus are rare. May remit and relapse. *Diagnosis:* Stool microscopy shows trophozoites, red and white blood cells. Distinguish from *E. dispar*, which looks identical, is more common, and doesn't cause disease. Fecal antigen detection makes this distinction and is a preferred test. Serology indicates previous or current infection and may be unhelpful in acute infection. *Differential diagnosis:* Bacillary dysentery often has a sudden onset and may cause dehydration. Stools are more watery initially, then bloody. *E. coli* 0157 is a common cause of acute bloody diarrhea without fever. *Acute ulcerative colitis* has a more gradual onset and the stools are very bloody. **Amoebic colonic abscess** may perforate causing peritonitis. **Amoeboma** is an inflammatory mass most often found at the cecum, where it must be distinguished from other RLQ masses.

Amoebic liver abscess is usually a single mass in the right lobe and contains "anchovy-sauce" pus. There is usually a high swinging fever, sweats, RUQ pain, and tenderness. WBC elevation, LFT may be normal or elevated (cholestasis). 50% have no history of amoebic dysentery. *Diagnosis:* Ultrasound/CT ± aspiration; positive serology in almost all patients. *Treatment: Asymptomatic colonization:* Paromomycin 10 mg/kg/8 h α 5–7 d. *Colitis:* Metronidazole 750 mg/8 h PO for 5–10 d, then paromomycin to destroy gut cysts. *Liver abscess:* Metronidazole for 10 d or longer. Aspirate if no improvement within a few days of starting metronidazole and in lesions at high risk for rupture (cavity >5 cm, left lobe of liver).

Trypanosomiasis

African trypanosomiasis (sleeping sickness) In West and Central Africa, *Trypanosoma brucei gambiense* causes a slow, wasting illness with a long latent period. In East Africa, *T. brucei rhodesiense* causes a more rapidly progressive illness. Spread by tsetse flies, entering skin following an insect bite. It spreads via the blood to the lymph nodes, spleen, heart, and brain. *Prevalence:* ~ 30,000 cases in 2009. Nearly all cases are due to *T. b. gambiense.* Infections to international travelers or imported cases to the United States in immigrants are rare. *Presentation:* A tender, subcutaneous nodule (*T. chancre*) develops at the site of infection. Two stages follow: *Stage I (hemolymphatic):* Nonspecific symptoms including fever, rash, rigors, headaches, hepatosplenomegaly, lymphadenopathy, and joint pains. Winterbottom's sign (enlargement of posterior cervical nodes) is a reliable sign, particularly in *T. b. gambiense* infections. In *T. b. rhodesiense* infections, this stage may be particularly severe, with potentially fatal myocarditis. *Stage II (meningoencephalitic):* Occurs weeks (in *T. b. rhodesiense*) or months (in *T. b. gambiense*) after initial infection. Patients exhibit CNS features; e.g., convulsions, agitation, and confusion, with later apathy, depression, ataxia, dyskinesias, dementia, hypersomnolence, and coma. *Diagnosis:* T. b. rhodesiense trypomastigotes can be seen in blood films or from fluid expressed from lymph nodes or chancres. *T. b. gambiense* is more difficult to see in blood films. Repeated tests and concentration techniques (analysis of buffy coat and use of miniature anion exchange centrifugation) can improve yield. Analysis of fluid from lymph nodes may be positive in 40–80% of cases. Serology is only reliable in *T. b. gambiense* infections. *Staging:* Hemolymphatic phase (fevers, headaches, arthralgias, and pruritus) and neurological phase (change of behavior, confusion, ataxia, sensory abnormalities). CSF should be evaluated in all patients for disease staging. Presence of trypanosomes or ≥6 WBC in CSF indicate neurological phase. *Treatment:* Seek expert help. Suramin, melarsoprol, and eflornithine are available through Division of Parasitic Diseases at CDC, 410–718–4745, and E-mail parasites@cdc.gov

Treat anemia and other infections first.

Hemolymphatic phase: T. b. rhodesiense: Suramin 1 g on days 1, 3, 5, 14, 21. *T. b. gambiense:* Pentamidine 4 mg/kg/d IV or IM α 7–10 d. *Neurological phase:* T. b. rhodesiense: Melarsoprol "3 by 3" regimen. 2–3.6 mg/kg/d α 3 d, 7 d later repeat series at 3.6 mg/kg/d α 3 d, 7 d later repeat series again at 3.6 mg/kg/d α 3 d. Melarsoprol is associated with lethal encephalopathy in up to 10% (abnormal behavior, seizures, and coma). This is partly preventable with prednisolone (1 mg/kg/24 h, max 40 mg/24 h), starting the day before the first injection. T. b. gambiense: Eflornithine 100 mg/kg/6 h α 14 d.

American trypanosomiasis (Chagas disease) is caused by *T. cruzi.* It occurs in Latin America and is spread by triatomine bugs. *Presentation:* Acute disease predominantly affects children. An erythematous, indurated nodule (chagoma) forms at the site of infection, which may then scar. *Signs:* Fever, myalgias, rash, lymphadenopathy, hepatosplenomegaly. If the eye is infected, unilateral conjunctivitis and periorbital edema may occur (Romaña's sign). Occasionally death is from myocarditis or meningoencephalitis. In up to 30% of cases, progression to chronic disease occurs after a latency of about 20 yrs. Multiorgan invasion may cause megaesophagus (dysphagia, aspiration), megacolon (abdominal distension, constipation), or dilated cardiomyopathy (chest pain, heart failure, arrhythmias, syncope, thromboembolism). CNS lesions may occur in HIV-positive patients. *Diagnosis:* Acute disease: Trypomastigotes may be seen in or grown from blood, CSF, or lymph node aspirate. *Chronic disease:* Serology (Chagas' IgG ELISA). *Treatment:* Nifurtimox 2 mg/kg/6 h PO after food α 90 d, or, alternatively, benznidazole 3.7 mg/kg/12 h PO for 60 d. *Both are toxic and only available from CDC.* Decisions regarding treatment need to be individualized. Infected children, patients with acute infections or reactivated disease, and those aged 19–50 without advanced heart disease should be offered treatment.

Leishmaniasis

Leishmania protozoa are intracellular organisms that cause granulomata. They are spread by sandflies and occur in Africa, India, Latin America, the Middle East, and the Mediterranean. Clinical effects reflect the ability of each species to induce or suppress the immune response, to metastasize, and to invade cartilage, and the speed and efficiency of the patient's immune response. *L. major*, for example, is the most immunogenic and allergenic of cutaneous Old World *Leishmania* and causes necrosis. *L. tropica* is less immunogenic and causes less inflamed, slow healing sores with relapsing lesions having tuberculoid histology.

Cutaneous leishmaniasis (CL) Almost all cases occur in parts of Afghanistan, Algeria, Syria, Iran, Saudi Arabia (*L. tropica* and *L. major*) and parts of South America (*L. mexicana, L. panamensis,* and *L. braziliensis*). Lesions develop at the site of the bite, beginning as an itchy papule, from which the crust may fall off to leave an ulcer. Most heal spontaneously, typically within 3–18 months, with scarring (disfiguring if extensive). *L. mexicana* may cause destruction of the pinna. *L. braziliensis and L. panamensis* can cause mucocutaneous disease months to years after spontaneous healing of primary cutaneous lesion. Typically, this involves mucosa of the nose, pharynx, palate, and larynx. Nasopharyngeal lesions are called espundia. *Diagnosis:* Microscopy, culture, and PCR of skin scraping from the edge of the ulcer. Punch biopsy can be helpful if skin scrapings are unrevealing. *Treatment:* Get help. Not all cutaneous lesions need to be treated, but scarring will likely happen without treatment. Standard therapy is with Pentostam (sodium stibogluconate, a pentavalent antimonial) 20 mg/kg/d α 20 d. This is available through CDC. *L. major* can be treated with fluconazole 200 mg/d PO for 6 wks. *L. major, L. mexicana,* and *L. panamensis* can be treated with ketoconazole 600 mg/d α 28–30 d. Treatment is unsatisfactory once mucosae are involved, so treat all cutaneous lesions due to *L. brasiliensis* and *L. panamensis* early. Data on alternative therapies are limited. These include liposomal amphotericin B, topical paromomycin, intralesional pentavalent antimonial injections, thermotherapy, and oral miltefosine.

Visceral leishmaniasis (kala-azar) Kala-azar means "black sickness" and is characterized by dry, warty, hyperpigmented skin lesions. Almost all cases are in the Asian subcontinent, Sudan, and Brazil. It is usually caused by *L. donovani* and *L. infantum* (also called *L. chagasi*). *Incubation:* Usually 2–6 months, but may be 2 wks–2 yrs. The organisms spread via lymphatics from minor skin lesions and multiply in macrophages of the reticuloendothelial system (Leishman–Donovan bodies). There are 30 subclinical cases for every clinical case. Increased risk in HIV infection. *Presentation:* Insidious onset of fevers, malaise, wasting, splenomegaly, hepatomegaly, cytopenias, decreased albumin, hypergammaglobulinemia, immunosuppression with bacterial superinfection. *Complications:* Over months to years, emaciation and exhaustion occur, with a protuberant abdomen. Intercurrent infections are common, especially pneumococcal otitis, pneumonia and septicemia, tuberculosis, measles. *Untreated mortality:* >80%; with treatment ~ 10%. Poorer outcomes are seen in those with HIV, jaundice, and wasting, and severe anemia. *Diagnosis:* Leishman–Donovan bodies in bone marrow (80%), lymph node, or splenic aspirates (95%).Serology is useful, but may be negative in those with HIV. *Treatment:* Seek expert help. *First line:* Liposomal amphotericin B 3 mg/kg IV on days 1–5, 14, and 21. Use higher doses for longer in HIV (and post-treatment prophylaxis recommended).

Pentostam 20 mg/kg/24 h IV or IM, for 28–30 d is a widely used alternative (available from CDC). Other therapies include miltefosine, deoxycholate, amphotericin B, and parenteral paromomycin. **Post kala-azar dermal leishmaniasis** may occur months or years following successful treatment; lesions resemble leprosy.

Fungal infections

Fungi may cause disease by acting as airborne allergens, by producing toxins, or by direct infection. Fungal infection may be superficial or deep, and both are much more common in the immunocompromised. Corticosteroids increase risk dramatically.

Superficial mycoses Dermatophytes infection (*Trichophyton, Microsporum, and Epidermophyton*) causes tinea (ringworm). *Diagnosis* Skin scraping microscopy. *Treatment:* Topical clotrimazole 1%. Continue for 14 d after healing. If intractable, try itraconazole (100–200 mg/24 h PO for 7 d), terbinafine (250 mg/24 h PO for 4 wks), or griseofulvin 0.5–1 g/24 h (*SE:* Agranulocytosis; SLE). *Candida albicans* causes skin infection in moist macerated skin regions (e.g., under breasts, oral and vulvovaginal infections). *Malassezia furfur* causes pityriasis versicolor; a macular rash that appears brown on pale skin and pale on tanned skin. *Diagnosis:* Microscopy of skin scrapings under Wood's light. *Treatment:* Ketoconazole 200 mg/24 h PO with food for 7 d (also available as a cream); alternatively selenium sulfide lotion.

Some superficial mycoses penetrate the epidermis and cause chronic subcutaneous infections such as **Madura foot or sporotrichosis**. Treatment is complex and may require amputation of the affected limb.

Systemic mycoses *Aspergillus fumigatus* may precipitate asthma, allergic bronchopulmonary aspergillosis (ABPA), or cause aspergilloma. Pneumonia and invasive aspergillosis occur in the immunosuppressed, particularly with defects in neutrophil number and/or function. *Diagnosis:* Culture of organism from affected area, galactomannan (serum or BAL); CT scan with "halo sign" in neutropenic patient is suggestive of invasive aspergillosis. Successful *treatment* of invasive infection depends on host factors (immune reconstitution) and appropriate antifungal therapy. Voriconazole is first-line therapy. Amphotericin B preparations are an alternative. Echinocandins (e.g., caspofungin, micafungin, and anidulafungin) are probably less effective. Combination therapy with voriconazole and an echinocandin may have a role in selected patients.

Invasive candidiasis is a major cause of bloodstream infections in hospitalized patients. *Risk factors* include central venous catheters (especially with parenteral nutrition and hemodialysis), abdominal surgery, and cytotoxic chemotherapy with mucositis, neutropenia, and stay in ICU. Other sites of infection can include peritoneal cavity, post sternotomy wounds, and, rarely, heart valves. Candidemia may be complicated by endophthalmitis. *Treatment* is with echinocandins, fluconazole (unless *C. krusei* or many *C. glabrata* isolates). Alternatives are amphotericin B and voriconazole. Candiduria often responds to removal of urinary catheter and does not usually require antifungal therapy. *Empiric therapy* in high-risk ICU patients targeting *Candida species* may be considered. Empiric therapy in patients with neutropenia and persistent fever should target *Candida* spp. and filamentous fungi (e.g., with amphotericin B or an echinocandin).

Cryptococcus neoformans causes pneumonia and/or disseminated disease with fungemia and meningitis, or pneumonia. *Risk factors* are advanced HIV, solid organ transplantation, and other chronic immunosuppressing conditions (e.g., long-term corticosteroid use). *Presentation:* The history may be subacute and there may be features suggesting elevated intracranial pressure (e.g., confusion, papilledema, cranial nerve palsies). *Diagnosis:* Serum and CSF cryptococcal antigen; India ink CSF staining; and blood, sputum, and CSF culture. All immunocompromised patients require evaluation of CSF that includes pressure measurement. *Treatment:* Amphotericin B deoxycholate 0.7–1.0/kg/d (or liposomal 3–4 mg/kg/d) IV + flucytosine 25 mg/kg/6 h PO α 14 d or longer, then fluconazole 400–800 mg/d α 8 wks or longer, then 200 mg/d until CD4 >200 α 6 months (AIDS patients). If CSF opening pressure (OP) is >250 mm H_2O, drain CSF until OP decreases 50%. Repeat drainage daily until OP is <200. Failure to do this is an important cause of morbidity and mortality due to cryptococcal meningitis.

Fluconazole at 400 mg/d for 6–12 months can be used in patients with mild to moderate pulmonary disease only (CSF evaluation required).

Other fungi causing deep infection

Histoplasma capsulatum, Coccidioides immitis, Paracoccidioides brasiliensis, and *Blastomyces dermatitidis* may cause asymptomatic infections, acute or chronic lung disease, or disseminated infection. Acute histoplasma pneumonitis is associated with arthralgias, erythema nodosum, and erythema multiforme. Chronic disease may cause upper-zone fibrosis or radiographic "coin lesions." *Diagnosis:* CXR, serology, culture, and biopsy. When severe (usually in immunocompromised patients), treatment is with an amphotericin B formulation. After stabilization or when mild to moderate, these diseases are treated with itraconazole, except coccidioidomycosis, which may be treated with fluconazole (especially with cocci meningitis).

Preventing fungal infections

This is a goal in the immunocompromised. Fluconazole, posaconazole, voriconazole, and topical nystatin have roles in prevention of infection depending on risk factors (e.g., cytotoxic chemotherapy, solid organ transplantation, bone marrow transplant, and as secondary prophylaxis after cryptococcal meningitis in HIV patients). Decisions regarding prophylaxis depend on knowledge of risk factors.

Table 14.31 Fungal prophylaxis

Infection	Patient type
Candidiasis	Oropharyngeal: HIV, radiation therapy, cytotoxic chemotherapy, poor-fitting dentures
	Vulvovaginal: Antibiotics, DM, otherwise healthy women
	Disseminated: Central venous catheters, cytotoxic chemotherapy, neutropenia, abdominal surgery, burns, parenteral nutrition
Aspergillosis	Invasive disease in those with neutropenia, transplant, corticosteroids, chronic granulomatous disease (CGD).
Cryptococcosis	HIV, transplant, corticosteroids, lymphoma
Mucormycosis	Neutropenia, transplant, uncontrolled DM, deferoxamine
Histoplasmosis	Exposure in endemic areas (e.g., Ohio River Valley), usually a self limited disease. Disseminated disease in those with risks similar to cryptococcosis
Coccidioidomycosis	Exposure in endemic area (e.g., Southwestern United States, California's Central Valley), usually a self limited disease (valley fever). Disseminated disease in those with risks similar to cryptococcosis
Rare filamentous fungal infections	*Fusarium, Scedosporium, Ochroconis,* and many others: Risk for invasive disease similar to aspergillosis

Table 14.32 Treatment of fungal infections

Antifungal	Typical use	Typical dose (normal GFR)	Toxicity
Fluconazole	*Candida, Cryptococcosis, Coccidioides*	Loading dose: 800 mg α 1 then 400-mg/d (IV or PO). Lower doses oral candidiasis, 150 mg α 1 for vulvovaginal disease	Liver, drug interactions,
		Renal adjustment required	

(Continued)

Table 14.32 (Continued)

Antifungal	Typical use	Typical dose (normal GFR)	Toxicity
Voriconazole	*Aspergillus, candida*, other filamentous fungal infections (not mucormycosis)	IV: Loading dose of 6 mg/kg/12 h α 2 then 4 mg/kg/d PO: Loading dose: 400 mg/12 h α 2, then 200 mg/12 h. Decrease doses by 50% for patients <40 kg	Liver, CNS, skin, QT, multiple drug interactions Caution with IV solution with GFR <50; cyclodextrin vehicle may cause renal accumulate and exacerbate renal damage
Posaconazole	*Aspergillus, Candida*, mucormycosis (not first line)	200 mg/8 h PO	Liver, QT, multiple drug interactions
Itraconazole	Histoplasmosis, blastomycosis	200 mg/12 h PO. Oral solution better absorbed than tabs	Liver, GI upset, negative inotrope, QT, drug interactions
Echinocandins	*Candida, Aspergillus* (not first line)	Anidulafungin: 200 mg α 1, then 100 mg/d IV Caspofungin: 70 mg α 1, then 50 mg/d IV Micafungin 100 mg/d IV	Histamine release, liver
Amphotericin B (AmB)	*Candida, Aspergillus*, mucormycosis, Cryptococcus, *Histoplasma, Coccidioides*	Deoxycholate AmB: 0.7–1.0 mg/kg/d IV Liposomal AmB: 3–6 mg/kg/d IV (less toxic than deoxycholate)	Infusion reaction, renal and electrolyte
Flucytosine (5-FC)	Used as part of combination therapy with AmB for cryptococcosis	25 mg/kg/6 h Renal adjustment required	Myelosuppression colitis, hepatitis

Nematodes (roundworms)

Worldwide, ~1 billion people are hosts to nematodes. Ascariasis can cause GI obstruction, hookworms can stunt growth, necatoriasis can cause debilitating anemia, and trichuriasis causes dysentery and rectal prolapse. Mass population treatment (e.g., albendazole 400 mg/24 h PO for 3 d) to school children or immigrants from endemic areas *may* be beneficial.

***Necator americanus* and *Ankylostoma duodenale* (hookworms)** Occur in the Indian subcontinent, Southeast Asia, Central and North Africa, and parts of Europe. *Necator* is also found in the Americas and sub-Saharan Africa. *Presentation:* Numerous small worms attach to upper GI mucosa, causing bleeding and consequent iron-deficiency anemia. Eggs are excreted in the feces and hatch in soil. Larvae penetrate feet, thus starting new infections. Oral transmission of *Ankylostoma* may occur. *Diagnosis:* Stool microscopy. *Treatment:* Mebendazole 100 mg/12 h PO for 3 d, and iron.

Strongyloides stercoralis is endemic in the (sub) tropics. *Transmission:* Percutaneous. *Presentation:* Causes rapidly migrating urticaria over thighs and trunk (*cutaneous larva migrans*). Pneumonitis, enteritis, and malabsorption may occur. *Chronic signs:* Diarrhea, abdominal pain, and urticaria. The worms may take bacteria into the bloodstream, causing gram-negative bacterial septicemia ± meningitis. *Diagnosis:* Stool microscopy and culture, serology, or duodenal aspiration. *Treatment:* Ivermectin 200 mcg/kg/d α 2 or albendazole 400 mg/12 h PO for 7 d. Hyperinfestation is a problem if immunocompromised (e.g., on steroids, or, more rarely, in AIDS). Therapy may need to be prolonged or repeated in immunocompromised patients.

Ascaris lumbricoides occurs worldwide. It looks like (and is named after) the garden worm (*Lumbricus*). An unusual characteristic is that it has three finely toothed lips. *Transmission:* Fecal–oral. It migrates through liver and lungs, then settles in the small bowel. It is usually asymptomatic, but death may occur from GI obstruction or perforation. If a worm migrates into the biliary tract, cholangitis or pancreatitis can result. A worm may grow very long (e.g., 25 cm). *Diagnosis:* Stool microscopy shows ova (stained orange by bile); worms on barium x-rays; eosinophilia (may be absent if immunosuppressed). *Treatment:* Mebendazole 100 mg/12 h PO for 72 h or ivermectin 150–200 mcg/kg α 1.

Trichinella spiralis occurs worldwide and is *transmitted* by uncooked pork. *Presentation:* It migrates to muscle, causing myalgias, myocarditis, and periorbital edema ± fever. *Treatment:* Albendazole 400 mg/12 h PO for 8–14 d, with concomitant prednisolone 40 mg/d PO. Alternative is mebendazole 200–400 mg/8 h α 72 h, then 400–500 mg/8 h α 10 d.

***Trichuris trichiura* (whipworm)** may cause nonspecific abdominal symptoms. *Diagnosis:* Stool microscopy. *Treatment:* Mebendazole 100 mg/12 h PO or ivermectin 200 mcg/kg PO α 3 d.

***Enterobius vermicularis* (pinworm)** is common in temperate climes. *Presentation:* It causes anal itch as it leaves the bowel to lay eggs on the perineum. Apply sticky tape to the perineum and identify eggs microscopically. *Treatment:* Mebendazole 100 mg PO. Repeat at 2 wks if >2 yrs and treat the whole family. *Hygiene is more important than drugs* as adult worms die after 6 wks. Continued symptoms suggest a reinfection.

Toxocara canis Most common cause of **visceral larva migrans**. The infection presents with eye granulomas (squint, blindness, pigmentary retinopathy) or visceral involvement (fever, myalgias, hepatomegaly, asthma, cough). *Diagnosis:* Ophthalmoscopy, serology, may require histology. *Treatment:* Albendazole 400 mg/12 h α 5 d or mebendazole 100–200 mg/12 h α 5 d. In ocular disease, visible larvae can sometimes be photocoagulated by laser. Systemic or topical ocular steroids may be needed to control eye inflammation. *Toxocara* is commonly acquired by ingesting soil contaminated by animal feces so de-worm pets regularly and exclude them from play areas.

Filarial infections

Onchocerciasis is caused by *Onchocerca volvulus* and is *transmitted* by the black fly. *Presentation:* It causes river blindness in parts of Africa and South America. Worldwide, ~37 million are affected, 500,000 have visual impairment, and 270,000 are blinded by this pathogen. Initially, a nodule forms at the site of the bite, shedding microfilariae to distant skin sites, which develop altered pigmentation, lichenification, loss of elasticity, and poor healing. Disease manifestations are mainly due to the localized host response to dead/dying microfilariae. Eye manifestations include keratitis, uveitis, cataract, fixed pupil, fundal degeneration, or optic neuritis/atrophy. Lymphadenopathy and elephantiasis also occur. *Diagnosis:* Visualization of microfilaria in eye or skin snips. Remove a fine shaving of clean, unanesthetized skin with a scalpel. Put on slide with a drop of 0.9% saline and look for swimming larvae after 30 min. *Treatment:* Seek expert help. Ivermectin is the drug of choice (e.g., 1 dose of 150 mcg/kg PO repeated, e.g., every 6 months for *Onchocerca*). Ivermectin does not kill adult worms so treatment needs to be repeated every 6 months. Length of therapy depends on symptoms, eye findings, and ongoing presence of microfilaria in skin. Doxycycline 200 mg/d α 6 wks may help by killing *Wolbachia*, an endosymbiont of adult worms. Must rule out Loa loa before giving ivermectin as fatal encephalitis may ensue.

Lymphatic filarial Affects 120 million worldwide and occurs in Asia, Africa, South America, and parts of the Caribbean (Haiti, Dominican Republic). Mosquito vectors transmit the infection. Acute infections cause fever and lymphadenitis. *Wuchereria bancrofti* causes lower limb lymphedema (elephantiasis) and hydroceles. *Brugia malayi* causes elephantiasis below the elbow/knee. *Wuchereria* life cycle: A mosquito bites an infected human → ingested microfilariae develop into larvae → larvae migrate to mosquito's mouth → mosquito bites another human → Wuchereria gains access to bloodstream → adult filariae lodge in lymphatic system. Lymphedema occurs after initial infection. *Diagnosis:* Blood film (draw blood at night to coincide with organisms' nighttime periodicity), serology. A rapid immunochromatographic finger-prick test has been developed for use in the field. *Complications:* Immune hyperreactivity may cause tropical pulmonary eosinophilia (TPE) with cough, wheeze, lung fibrosis, eosinophilia, elevated IgE and IgG. *Treatment:* Diethylcarbamazine (DEC) 6 mg/kg/d α 1 day for early lymphatic disease and 14–21 d for TPE. Ivermectin is effective against *W. bancrofti* microfilaria, but not adult worms. Late disease manifestations are not amenable to antiparasitic therapy, but may improve with elevation and management by a lymphedema specialist. DEC is available from CDC. Must rule out *O. volvulus* infection, as DEC can cause blindness with this pathogen. Also DEC must be used with care in patients with Loa loa; see below.

Loiasis is caused by *Loa loa*. It occurs in West and Central Africa and is transmitted by the *Chrysops* fly. It causes painful "Calabar" swellings of the limbs and eosinophilia, and may migrate across the conjunctiva. *Diagnosis:* Blood film (draw around noontime), serology, and identification of worm in eye or from skin. *Treatment:* Seek expert help and treat symptomatic patients depending on microfilaria (MF)/mL counts. <8,000: DEC 3 mg/kg/8 h α 21 d, ≥ 8,000 albendazole 200 mg/12 h until <8,000, then complete 21 d with DEC. If available, consider apheresis for >8,000. DEC can be obtained from CDC. It must be used with caution due to risk for fatal encephalitis with high Loa loa counts. Steroids may help. Must rule out *O. volvulus* infection as DEC can cause blindness with this pathogen.

Cestodes (tapeworms)

Taenia solium (pork tapeworm) infection occurs by eating uncooked pork. **T. saginata** is contracted from uncooked beef. Both cause vague abdominal symptoms and malabsorption. Sometimes worms can become lodged in appendix or biliary or pancreatic ducts. Patients may report seeing worm parts in stool. Diagnosis is by examination of stool specimen. Treatment is with praziquantel 5–10 mg/kg α 1 or niclosamide 2 g α 1. Use praziquantel with caution in those who also have cysticercosis (see below).

Larval cysts of *T. solium* are the cause of cysticercosis. Transmission is by ingestion of food or water contaminated with eggs fecally shed from a person who is infected with *T. solium* worms. Autoinoculation by fecal–oral route is possible. In the intestine, the eggs mature, penetrate the circulation, and disseminate throughout the body, encysting in muscle, skin, heart, eye, and CNS, causing focal signs. *Subcutaneous cysticercosis* causes palpable subcutaneous nodules in the arms, legs, and chest. *Ocular cysticercosis* causes conjunctivitis, uveitis, retinitis, choroid atrophy, and blindness.

Neurocysticercosis is the most common cause of seizures in some places (e.g., Mexico). *Other features:* Focal CNS signs (e.g., hemiplegia), odd behavioral, dementia—or no symptoms. Cysticerci may cluster like bunches of grapes ("racemose" form) in the ventricles (causing hydrocephalus) and basal cisterns (causing basal meningitis, cranial nerve lesions, and raised ICP). Spinal cysticerci may cause radicular or compressive spinal symptoms. *Diagnosis:* Usually diagnosed by appearance on neuroimaging and clinical history. Stool microscopy and examination of perianal swabs is reserved for difficult cases. *Serology:* Indirect hemagglutination test. *CSF:* May show eosinophils in neurocysticercosis, and a CSF antigen test is available. X-rays of soft tissues may show calcified cysts. *Treatment:* Antihelminthic therapy will not treat dead worms (in calcified cysts). *Active parenchymal disease:* Anticonvulsants for cysticercosis associated seizure disorder, albendazole 7.5 mg/kg/12 h PO with food, or praziquantel 17 mg/kg/8 h PO for 15 d. Treatment duration may need to be longer in patients with extensive or extraparenchymal (e.g., ventricle) disease. An inflammatory response to the dying larvae may require corticosteroids. Dexamethasone 6 mg/d may be effective at reducing seizures when used with antiparasitic therapy. If CSF ventricles are involved, consult neurosurgeon to evaluate for cyst removal and shunt before starting drugs. Antiparasitic drugs may worsen the acute phase of cysticercosis encephalitis.

Diphyllobothrium latum is a fish tapeworm acquired from uncooked fish. It causes similar symptoms to *T. solium* and is treated with praziquantel 5–10 mg/kg α 1. It is a cause of vitamin B_{12} deficiency.

Hymenolepis nana and H. diminuta (dwarf tapeworms) are rarely symptomatic. Treat with praziquantel (25 mg/kg PO).

Hydatid disease Cystic hydatid disease is a zoonosis caused by ingesting eggs of the dog parasite *Echinococcus granulosus* (e.g., in rural sheep-farming regions). Hydatid is a public health problem in parts of China, Russia, Alaska, Wales, and Japan. *Presentation:* Most cysts are asymptomatic, but liver cysts may present with hepatomegaly, obstructive jaundice, cholangitis, or FUO. Lung cysts may present with dyspnea, chest pain, hemoptysis, or anaphylaxis. Parasites migrate almost anywhere (e.g., CNS or incidentally on CXR). *Diagnosis:* Plain x-ray, ultrasound, and CT of cysts. A reliable serological test has replaced the variably sensitive Casoni intradermal test. *Treatment:* Seek expert help. The drug of choice is albendazole 400 mg/12 h/d for 1–6 months. A common approach is to excise/drain symptomatic cysts, but beware spilling cyst contents (causes anaphylaxis; praziquantel may be useful presurgery of in case of spill). Chemotherapy + the PAIR approach is increasingly replacing surgery: Puncture, aspirate cyst, inject hypertonic saline, and reaspirate. Give albendazole pre- and postdrainage to prevent recurrence. *Note:* Alveolar hydatid is caused by *E. multilocularis*.)

Trematodes (flukes)

Schistosomiasis (bilharzia) is the most prevalent disease caused by flukes, affecting 200 million people worldwide. Most are in Africa. The snail vectors release cercariae that can penetrate the skin (e.g., during swimming or walking in contaminated water). This may cause an itchy papular rash ("swimmer's itch"). The cercariae shed their tails to become schistosomula and migrate via lungs to liver where they grow. ~2 wks after initial infestation, there may be fever, urticaria, diarrhea, cough, wheeze, and hepatosplenomegaly ("Katayama fever"). In ~8 wks, mature flukes couple and migrate to resting habitats; that is, vesical veins (*S. hematobium*) or mesenteric veins (*S. mansoni* and *S. japonicum*). Eggs released from these sites can cause granulomata and scarring. Clinical schistosomiasis is caused by an allergic response to the eggs.

Presentation is likely to have visited or be from Africa, the Middle East, or Brazil (*S. mansoni*) and present with abdominal pain and stomach upset, and, later, hepatic fibrosis, granulomatous inflammation, and portal hypertension (transformation into true cirrhosis has not been well-documented). *S. japonicum*, often the most serious, occurs in Southeast Asia, tends to affect the bowel and liver, and may migrate to lung and CNS ("travelers' myelitis"). Urinary schistosomiasis (*S. hematobium*) occurs in Africa, the Middle East, and the Indian Ocean. *Signs:* Frequency, dysuria, hematuria (± hematospermia), incontinence. It may progress to hydronephrosis and renal failure. There is an increased risk of squamous cell carcinoma of the bladder.

Diagnosis is based on finding eggs in the urine (*S. hematobium*) or feces (*S. mansoni* and *S. japonicum*) or rectal biopsy (all types). Radiographs may show bladder calcification in chronic *S. hematobium* infection. Renal ultrasound identifies renal obstruction, hydronephrosis, thickened bladder wall. Schistosoma ELISA is most sensitive.

Treatment: Praziquantel: 40 mg/kg PO with food divided into 2 doses separated by 4–6 h for *S. mansoni* and *S. hematobium*, and 20 mg/kg/8 h for 1 d in *S. japonicum*. Sudden transitory abdominal pain and bloody diarrhea may occur shortly after.

Fasciola hepatica (liver fluke) is spread by sheep, water, and snails. It causes hepatomegaly, then fibrosis. People usually become infected after eating raw watercress from endemic areas. *Presentation* is with fever, abdominal pain, diarrhea, weight loss, jaundice, and eosinophilia. *Tests:* Stool microscopy, serology. *Treatment:* Get help. Treat with triclabendazole 10 mg/kg PO α 1 (may repeat once). This medication is available from CDC. A possible alternative is nitazoxanide 500 mg/12 h α 7 d.

Opisthorchis and **Clonorchis** are liver flukes common in the Far East, where they cause cholangitis, cholecystitis, and cholangiocarcinoma. Eating raw or undercooked fresh water fish from endemic areas can cause this infection. *Tests:* Stool microscopy. *Treatment:* Praziquantel 25 mg/kg/8 h PO for 1 d.

Fasciolopsis buski is a big intestinal fluke, ~7 cm long, causing ulcers or abscesses at the site of attachment. Eating raw or undercooked aquatic plants from endemic areas can cause disease. *Treatment* is as for opisthorchiasis.

Paragonimus westermani (lung fluke) is contracted by eating raw freshwater crabs or crayfish. *Presentation:* Parasites migrate through gut and diaphragm to invade the lungs, causing cough, dyspnea, and hemoptysis. *Secondary complications:* Lung abscess and bronchiectasis. It occurs in the Far East,

South America, and the Congo, where it is commonly mistaken for TB (similar clinical and CXR appearances). *Tests:* Ova in sputum. MRI/CT may disclose CNS/lung lesions. *Treatment:* Praziquantel (25 mg/kg/8 h PO for 2 d) or bithionol (30–50 mg/kg on alternate days PO for 10 d). With cerebral disease, a short dose of corticosteroids may help to decrease inflammatory response to dying parasites when praziquantel is given.

Exotic infections

Exotic infections may be community-acquired or nosocomial (acquired in hospital). The increased prevalence of immunosuppression, both drug-induced and innate, international travel, human encroachment on animal habitats, and the widespread use of broad-spectrum antibiotics have led to increases in rates of exotic infections. New techniques such as PCR have enabled the identification of more putative infective agents.

History When an infection is suspected (fever, sweats, inflammation, diarrhea and vomiting, WBC elevation, or *any* unexplained symptom), ask the patient about:

- Foreign travel
- Artificial implantable material (e.g., hip prosthesis, prosthetic heart valves)
- Risk factors for HIV
- Treatment with immune modulator, steroids, transplantation
- Necrotic tissues
- Pets
- Animal exposure (including insects)
- Sick contacts

Diagnosis Take appropriate cultures (blood, urine, stool, CSF) or swabs as clinically indicated. Consult early with an infectious diseases physician. Consider CXR, ultrasound, or CT as clinically indicated. If the infection appears to be localized, consider surgical debridement ± drainage. Do not give up if you cannot culture an organism; tests may need to be repeated. Perhaps the organism is "fastidious" in its nutritional requirement or requires prolonged incubation? Even if culture *is* achieved, it may be that the organism is pathogenic, or it could be a commensal (i.e., part of the normal flora for that patient). If culture is not possible, look for antibodies or antigen in the serum or other body fluids. It is generally agreed that a fourfold increase in antibody titers in convalescence (compared with the acute sera) is indicative of recent infection, although not diagnostic. PCR is increasingly being used to make identifications; however, it is far from infallible, and contamination with DNA from the lab or elsewhere is a potential problem.

Treatment Table 14.33 suggests treatment options, but it is only a guide, as susceptibility patterns may vary be local epidemiological patterns. Consult with local microbiologist and/or Infectious Diseases specialist.

Table 14.33 Treating exotic infections

Organism	Site or type of infection	Treatment example
Acanthamoeba spp. (free living amoeba)	Keratitis	Topical chlorhexidine or polyhexamethylene biguanide ± propamidine isethionate
Acinetobacter complex	CNS disease	Pentamidine + azole + TMP/SMX ± flucytosine
Actinobacillus actinomycetemcomitans	UTI, CSF, lung, bone, bloodstream, conjunctiva	Carbapenems, aminoglycosides, colistin
	IE, CNS, UTI, bone, thyroid, lung, periodontitis, abscesses	Penicillin, third-generation ceph ± gentamicin
Actinobacillus lignieresii	CSF, IE, wounds, bone, lymph nodes	Ampicillin, third-generation ceph ± gentamicin
Actinobacillus ureae	Bronchus, CSF post-trauma, hepatitis	Ampicillin, third-generation ceph ± gentamicin
Aerococcus viridans	Empyema, UTI, CSF, bone	Penicillin ± gentamicin
Aeromonas hydrophila	IE, CSF, cornea, bone, D&V, liver abscess	Gentamicin, ciprofloxacin
Afipia broomeae	Marrow, synovium	Imipenem or ceftriaxone
Alcaligenes species	Dialysis peritonitis, ear, lung	Amox/clav, piperacillin/tazobactam, cefepime, TMP/SMX
Angiostrongylus cantonensis (rat lung worm)	Eosinophilic meningitis	Corticosteroids ± albendazole
Arcanobacterium	Throat, cellulitis, leg ulcer	Azithromycin, doxycycline, clindamycin, quinolones
Babesia microti (protozoa)	FUO ± haemolysis if old/splenectomized	Atovaquone + azithromycin
Bacillus cereus	Wounds, eye, ear, lung, UTI, IE	Vancomycin
Balamuthia mandrillaris (free living amoeba)	CNS, skin, adrenals, kidneys	Pentamidine + macrolide + sulfadiazine + flucytosine + fluconazole
Baylisascaris procyonis (raccoon roundworm)	Eosinophilic meningoencephalitis	Albendazole + corticosteroids

(Continued)

Table 14.33 (Continued)

Organism	Site or type of infection	Treatment example
Bifidobacterium	Vagina, UTI, IE, peritonitis, lung	Penicillin
Bordetella bronchiseptica	URTI, CSF (after animal contact)	Doxycycline. TMP/SMX
Burkholderia cepacia, etc (formerly Pseudomonas)	Wounds, lungs (esp. in CF), IE, CAPD, UTI, ecthyma gangrenosa, peritonitis	Ceftazidime, minocycline, meropenem
Burkholderia pseudomallei (formerly Pseudomonas)	Melioidosis: Self-reactivating septicemia + multiorgan, protean signs (e.g., in rice farmers, via water/soil in Southeast Asia)	Ceftazidime ± TMP/SMX, meropenem
Capnocytophaga canimorsus	Cellulitis, sepsis with DIC in asplenics	Ampicillin/sulbactam
Capnocytophaga ochracea and C. sputagena	Oral ulcer, stomatitis, arthritis, blood, cervical abscess	Penicillin or ciprofloxacin
Cardiobacterium hominis	IE	Penicillin + gentamicin
Chromobacterium violaceum	Nodes, eye, bone, liver, pustules	Quinolones, TMP/SMX, imipenem
Citrobacter koseri/diversus	CSF, UTI, blood, cholecystitis	Cephalosporins
Corynebacterium jeikeium	Fever/sepsis in neutropenia	Vancomycin
Corynebacterium striatum	Indwelling device infection	Vancomycin, non-PCN β-lactams
Corynebacterium ulcerans	Diphtheria-like ± CNS signs	Penicillin + diphtheria antitoxin
Cyclospora cayetanensis	Diarrhea (via raspberries)	TMP/SMX
Edwardsiella tarda	Cellulitis, abscesses, BP↓, dysentery via penetrating fish injuries	Cephalosporins + gentamicin
Eikenella corrodens	Sinus, ears, PE postjugular vein phlebitis (postanginal sepsis) via bites	Penicillin ± gentamicin, **Resistant to metronidazole and clindamycin**

Elizabethkingia meningosepticum	Lungs, epidemic neonatal meningitis, postop bacteremia	TMP/SMX, minocycline, quinolone or vancomycin + rifampin
Erysipelothrix rhusiopathiae	Erysipelas-like, IE	Penicillin
Finegoldia magna	Bone, joint, wound, teeth, face	Penicillin, imipenem
Fusobacterium necrophorum	Jugular venous septic thrombophlebitis	Clindamycin, ampicillin/sulbactam
Gemella haemolysans	IE, meningitis after neurosurgery	Penicillin + gentamicin
Gnathostoma spingerum (helminth)	Migrating subcutaneous lesions with eosinophilia, CNS disease	Ivermectin or albendazole
Helicobacter cinaedia	Proctitis in homosexual men	Ampicillin or gentamicin
Kingella kingae	Throat, larynx, eyelid, joint, skin	Third-generation cephalosporin, ± gentamicin
Lactobacillus	Teeth, chorioamnionitis, pyelitis	Penicillin ± gentamicin, clindamycin
Mobiluncus curtisii/mulieris	Vagina, uterus, septicemia in cirrhosis	Cephalosporins or ampicillin
Moraxella osloensis and M. nonliquefaciens	Conjunctiva, wound, vagina, UTI, CSF CNS, bone, hemorrhagic stomatitis	Penicillin
Naegleria fowleri (free living amoeba)	Meningoencephalitis	Amphotericin B IV ± AmB by IT, ± azole, ± rifampin
Neisseria cani	Wounds from cat bites	Amoxicillin
Neisseria cinerea/mucosa; N. subflava; N. flavescens	IE, CNS, bone, post human bites or from peritoneal dialysis	Penicillin, cephalosporin
Pasteurella multocida	Bone, lung, CSF, UTI, pericarditis epiglottitis. Post cat/dog bite	Amoxicillin/clavulanate, doxycycline
Pasteurella pneumotropica	Wounds, joints, bone, CSF	Penicillin, cephalosporins

(Continued)

Table 14.33 (Continued)

Organism	Site or type of infection	Treatment example
Plesiomonas shigelloides	D&V, eye, sepsis post fishbone injury	Ciprofloxacin, TMP/SMX
Propionibacterium acnes	Face, wounds, CSF shunts, bone, IE liver granuloma (botryomycosis)	Penicillin, vancomycin, doxycycline, clindamycin
Prototheca wickerhamii/ zopfii (achlorophyllous algae)	Subcutaneous granuloma, bursitis lymphadenitis, nodules, granuloma	Amphotericin or azoles
Providencia stuartii	UTI, burn or lung infections	Carbapenems, piperacillin/tazobactam, gentamicin
Ralstonia pickettii	CSF, lungs, blood in ICUs	Cephalosporin
Rhodococcus equi	Lung, CNS, wounds	Vancomycin, meropenem + rifampin or Cipro
Rothia dentocariosa	Appendix abscess	Penicillin, vancomycin
Serratia marcescens	Wound, burns, lung, UTI, liver, CSF, bone, IE, red diaper syndrome	Imipenem, ceftazidime, ciprofloxacin
Shewanella (Pseudomonas) putrefaciens	CSF post CNS surgery/head trauma	Advanced-generation Cephalosporins
Sphingobacterium multivorum	Peritonitis (spontaneous)	Cephalosporins, carbapenems, TMP/SMX

Stenotrophomonas maltophilia	Wounds, ear, eye, lung, UTI, IE	TMP/SMX, levofloxacin, ticarcillin/clavulanate
Staphylococcus lugdunensis	IE, skin, bone, prosthetic devices	Oxacillin, vancomycin
Streptococcus bovis	IE if colon cancer, do colonoscopy	Penicillin + gentamicin
Tropheryma whipplei	Whipple's disease (GI, CNS, lymphadenopathy, FUO, IE)	PCN, ceftriaxone
Vibrio vulnificus	Wounds, muscle, uterus, fasciitis	Doxycycline + ceftazidime

IE, infective endocarditis; D+V, diarrhea and vomiting; CNS, central nervous system; UTI, urinary tract infection; URTI, upper respiratory tract infection.

Hematology

Alison R. Moliterno, M.D.

Contents

Relevant pages elsewhere: Transfusion (p. 456)

Anemia

Anemia is defined as a low hemoglobin concentration due a decreased red cell mass. If the low Hb concentration is due to increased plasma volume, as in pregnancy, the anemia is then considered physiological. A low hemoglobin (Hb) level is <13.5 g/dL for men and <11.5 g/dL for women. Anemia may be due to reduced production or increased loss of red blood cells (RBCs) and has many causes. The cause of the anemia will be resolved by synthesis of the history, physical examination, and inspection of the blood smear.

Symptoms Fatigue, dyspnea, palpitations, headache, tinnitus, anorexia, dyspepsia, bowel disturbance and angina if there is preexisting coronary artery disease. Patients who have developed their anemia rapidly are often more symptomatic than those who have developed anemia slowly, in which case there has been time for physiologic compensations for their anemia to occur.

Signs Pallor (evident in conjunctivae) and retinal hemorrhages. In severe anemia (Hb <8 g/dL), there may be signs of a hyperdynamic circulation, with tachycardia, a systolic ejection murmur, and cardiac enlargement. Later, heart failure may occur and, in this state, rapid blood transfusion may be fatal.

Types of anemia The first step in diagnosis is to look at the mean cell volume (MCV, *normal MCV is 80-100 fL*) and the red cell distribution width (RDW, a measure of the variability of the red cell size).

Low MCV (microcytic):

• Iron-deficiency anemia (IDA, most common cause; p. 609)
• Anemia of inflammation
• Thalassemia
• Sideroblastic anemia

NB: Anemia of inflammation is distinguished from iron deficiency by iron studies: Serum iron, transferrin, and transferrin saturation will be reduced whereas ferritin will be normal or elevated. Both the anemia of inflammation and some thalassemias tend to have near normal RDWs.

Normal MCV (normocytic anemia)

• Anemia of chronic disease	• Hypothyroidism (or ↑MCV)
• Bone marrow failure	• Hemolysis (or ↑MCV)
• Chronic Kidney Disease	• Pregnancy

High MCV (macrocytic anemia)

• B_{12} or folate deficiency	• Myelodysplastic syndromes
• Alcohol	• Marrow infiltration
• Liver disease	• Hypothyroidism
• Reticulocytosis	• Antifolate drugs
• Cytotoxics, e.g., hydroxyurea	• Bone marrow failure states

Hemolytic anemias: Do not fall neatly into the above classification as the anemia may be normochromic, or, if the reticulocyte percentage is very high, macrocytic. Suspect a hemolytic anemia if there is a reticulocytosis (>2% of RBCs; or reticulocyte count >85 α 10⁹/L), mild macrocytosis, haptoglobin ↓ (p. 616), bilirubin ↑, and urobilinogen ↑. If the RDW is very elevated (>20), consider a microangiopathic process such as disseminated intravascular coagulation (DIC) or thrombotic thrombocytopenic purpura (TTP).

Blood transfusion Avoid unless Hb has fallen acutely and the patient is symptomatic. Transfusion decisions will depend on the severity, the cause, and the underlying medical status of the patient. If risk of hemorrhage (e.g., active peptic ulcer), transfuse up to 8 g/dL. In severe anemia with heart failure, transfusion is vital to restore Hb to safe levels: e.g., 8-10/dL, but must be done with great care. Give packed cells *slowly* with 10-40 mg furosemide IV/PO with alternate units (dose depends on previous exposure to diuretics). Check for rising jugular venous pressure (JVP) and basal crackles.

Iron-deficiency anemia

Iron deficiency is common (seen in up to 14% of menstruating women) and, worldwide, is the most frequent cause of nutritional anemias. The most common cause is blood loss, particularly menorrhagia or GI bleeding from esophagitis, peptic ulcer, carcinoma, colitis, or diverticulitis. In the tropics, hookworm (GI blood loss) is the most common cause. Poor diet may cause iron-deficiency anemia (IDA) in infants and children, those on special diets, strict vegetarians, or wherever there is poverty. Iron deficiency anemia due to malabsorption (gastric surgery, gastric bypass, celiac disease, Whipple's disease, inflammatory bowel disease) may be accompanied by other deficiency states, such as of folate and B$_{12}$. See Table 15.1.

Symptoms: Associated symptoms include ice craving (pagophagia), restless leg syndrome, and short-term memory loss (adolescents).

Signs: Koilonychia (p. 43), atrophic glossitis, and, rarely, postcricoid webs.

Investigations: Microcytic, hypochromic blood film showing anisocytosis and poikilocytosis (p. 612). Confirmed by showing serum iron↓ and ferritin↓ (more representative of total body iron) with TIBC↑. If MCV↓, and there is a good history of menorrhagia, oral iron may be started without further tests. Otherwise investigate: Fecal occult blood, barium enema or colonoscopy, gastroscopy, microscope stool for ova. *Iron deficiency without an obvious source of bleeding mandates a careful gi workup.*

Treatment: If the MCV is low and there is a history of menorrhagia, oral iron may be started without further diagnostic workup: Oral iron salts (e.g., ferrous sulfate 324 mg bid or tid PO). *Side effects (Se):* Constipation, black stools. Hb should rise by 1 g/dL/wk, with a modest reticulocytosis (i.e., young RBC [p. 612]). Continue until Hb is normal and for at least 3 months to replenish stores. Parenteral iron is reserved for patients who fail oral iron trials or dialysis patients and is available as iron gluconate, sucrose, or ferumoxytol (well tolerated) or iron dextran (higher side-effect profile).

Refractory anemia The usual reason that IDA fails to respond to iron replacement is failure of compliance, often because of GI disturbance. Altering the dose of elemental iron or the formulation of elemental iron may be helpful, or considere IV iron in appropriate situations. Other reasons for failure of oral iron supplementation include continued blood loss or malabsorption. Importantly, anemia of inflammation or thalassanemia will not respond to iron supplementation.

The anemia of chronic disease

This is associated with many diseases, including infection, collagen vascular disease, rheumatoid arthritis, malignancy, and chronic kidney disease. *Investigations:* Mild normocytic anemia (e.g., Hb >8 g/dL), TIBC↓ serum iron↓, ferritin normal or↑. *Treatment:* Treat the underlying disease. The anemia of chronic kidney disease is partly due to erythropoietin deficiency, and recombinant erythropoietin is effective in raising the hemoglobin level (maintenance dose example: 50–150 U/kg twice weekly; *se:* Hypertension in patients with chronic kidney disease). It is also effective in raising HB and improving quality of life in those with HIV-related anemia, chemotherapy induced-anemia, chronic bone marrow failure states, and the anemia of many chronic inflammatory states.

Sideroblastic anemia

Characterized by dyserythropoiesis and iron loading (bone marrow) and sometimes hemosiderosis (endocrine, liver, and cardiac damage), sideroblastic anemia (SA) may be congenital (rare, X-linked) or acquired (usually idiopathic, part of the spectrum of the myelodysplastic disorders), but may follow alcohol or lead excess, myeloproliferative disease, malignancy, malabsorption, or anti-tuberculosis (TB) drugs. Stippled, hypochromic RBCs are seen on the blood film with sideroblasts in the marrow (erythroid precursors with iron deposited in mitochondria in a ring around the nucleus).

Table 15.1 Interpretation of iron studies

	Iron	tibc	Ferritin
Iron deficiency	↓	↑	↓
Anemia of chronic disease	↓	↓	↑
Chronic hemolysis	↑	↓	↑
Hemochromatosis	↑	↓ (or ↔)	↑
Pregnancy	↑	↑	↔
Sideroblastic anemia	↑	↔	↑

Treatment is supportive; pyridoxine may occasionally be of benefit (e.g., 10 mg/24 h PO; higher doses may cause neuropathy); remove the cause if possible. In myelodysplasia, erythropoietin, with or without human granulocyte colony-stimulating factor (G-CSF) may be effective, although the cost benefit of this approach is controversial.

The peripheral blood film

Many primary hematological diagnoses and other systemic diagnoses can be made by careful examination of the peripheral blood film. It is also necessary for interpretation of the RBC indices.

Acanthocytes: RBCs show many spicules.

Anisocytosis: Variation in red cell size.

Basophilic stippling: Stippling of RBCs is seen in lead poisoning, thalassemia, and other dyserythropoietic anemias.

Blasts: Nucleated precursor cells; they are not normally seen in peripheral blood.

Burr cells: Irregularly shaped cells occurring in uremia or liver disease.

Dimorphic picture: A mixture of RBC sizes (e.g., partially treated iron deficiency, mixed deficiency [Fe with B_{12} or folate deficiency], post-transfusion, sideroblastic anemia).

Howell-Jolly bodies: Nuclear remnants seen in RBCs post splenectomy; rarely leukemia, megaloblastic anemia, IDA, hyposplenism (e.g., celiac disease, neonates, thalassemia, SLE, lymphoma, leukemia, amyloid).

Hypersegmentation: Hypersegmented neutrophils (>5 lobes to nucleus) seen in megaloblastic anemia, uremia, and liver disease.

Hypochromia: Less dense staining of RBCs seen in IDA, thalassemia, and sideroblastic anemia (iron stores unusable).

Left shift: Immature white cells seen in circulating blood in any marrow outpouring, such as infection or marrow infiltration.

Leukoerythroblastic anemia: Immature cells (myelocytes, nucleated red blood cells, and large platelets) seen in film. Due to extramedullary hematopoiesis associated with marrow infiltration, hypoxia, marrow fibrosis, or severe anemia.

Leukemoid reaction: A marked reactive leukocytosis. Usually granulocytic, and observed in severe infection, burns, acute hemolysis, metastatic cancer.

Myelocytes, promyelocytes, metamyelocytes, normoblasts: Immature cells seen in the blood in leukoerythroblastic anemia.

Normoblasts or nucleated red cells: Immature red cells with a nucleus. Seen in leukoerythroblastic anemia, marrow infiltration, hemolysis, hypoxia.

Pappenheimer bodies: Granules of siderocytes (e.g., lead poisoning, carcinomatosis, post splenectomy).

Poikilocytosis: Variation in red cell shape.

Polychromasia: RBCs of different ages stain unevenly, the younger erythrocytes being bluer. An indirect assessment of reticulocytosis.

Reticulocytes: (Normal: 0.8–2%; or <85 α 10^9/L) Young, larger RBCs (contain RNA) signifying active erythropoiesis. Elevated in hemolysis, hemorrhage, and if B$_{12}$, iron or folate is given to marrow that lack these.

Rouleaux formation: Red cells stack on each other (the visual "analogue" of a high erythrocyte sedimentation rate [ESR, p. 612]).

Schistocytes: Fragmented RBCs sliced by fibrin bands observed in microangiopathic hemolytic processes (DIC, TTP, malignant hypertension).

Spherocytes: Red blood cells lacking central pallor. Observed in extravascular hemolytic processes such as autoimmune hemolysis, hereditary spherocytosis, burns.

Target cells: RBCs with central staining, a ring of pallor, and an outer rim of staining seen in liver disease, thalassemia, or sickle-cell disease, and, in small numbers, in IDA.

The differential white cell count

Neutrophils 2–7.5 α 10^9/L (40–75% of the total white blood cell (WBC) count; absolute values are more meaningful than percentages).

Elevated in:
- Bacterial infections
- Trauma, surgery, burns, hemorrhage
- Inflammation, infarction, polymyalgia rheumatica, polyarteritis nodosa (PAN)
- Myeloproliferative disorders
- Steroids
- Disseminated malignancy

Reduced in:
- Viral infections, HIV, liver disease, hepatitis C, brucellosis, typhoid, kala-azar, TB
- Drugs (e.g., hydroxyurea, sulfonamides)
- Hypersplenism or neutrophil antibodies (seen in SLE and rheumatoid arthritis); increased destruction
- B$_{12}$ or folate deficiency; in bone marrow failure states, stem cell disorders; decreased production (p. 613)

Lymphocytes 1.3–3.5 α 10^9/L (20–45%).

Elevated in:

- Viral infections, toxoplasmosis; whooping cough; brucellosis
- Chronic lymphocytic leukemia

Large numbers of abnormal ("atypical") lymphocytes are characteristically seen with Epstein-Barr virus (EBV) infection: These are T-cells reacting against EBV-infected B-cells. They have a large amount of clear cytoplasm with a blue rim that flows around neighboring RBCs ("Dutch skirting"). Other causes of "atypical" lymphocytes:

Reduced in:
- Steroid therapy, systemic lupus erythematosus (SLE), uremia, legionnaire's disease, HIV infection, marrow infiltration, post chemotherapy or radiotherapy

T-lymphocyte subset reference values: CD4 count: 537–1,571/mm³ (low in HIV infection). CD8 count: 235–753/mm³; CD4/CD8 ratio: 1.2–3.8.

Eosinophils 0.04–0.44 α 10⁹/L (1–6%). *Elevated in:* Asthma/atopy, parasitic infections (especially invasive helminths), PAN, skin disease (especially pemphigus), urticaria, malignant disease (including lymphomas and eosinophilic leukemia, systemic mastocytosis), adrenal insufficiency, irradiation, Löffler's syndrome, during the convalescent phase of any infection.

The hypereosinophilic syndrome is seen when there is development of end-organ damage (restrictive cardiomyopathy, neuropathy, hepatosplenomegaly) in association with a raised eosinophil count (>1.5 α 10⁹/L) for >6 wks.

Monocytes 0.2–0.8 α 10⁹/L(2–10%).

Elevated in: Acute and chronic infections (e.g., TB, brucellosis, protozoa); malignant disease, including M4 and M5 acute myeloid leukemia (p. 627) and Hodgkin's disease; myelodysplasia.

Basophils 0–0.1 α 10⁹/L (0–1%).

Elevated in: Viral infections, urticaria, myxedema, post splenectomy, chronic myeloid leukemia (CML), ulcerative colitis (UC), malignancy, systemic mastocytosis (urticaria pigmentosa), hemolysis, chronic myeloproliferative neoplasms.

Macrocytic anemia

Macrocytosis (*MCV >100 fl*) is a common finding, often due to alcoholism (usually without any accompanying anemia).

Causes of macrocytosis (*MCV >110* fL):Vitamin B_{12} or folate deficiency; hydroxyurea.

MCV 100–110 FL:

- *Drugs:* Alcohol, azathioprine, zidovudine
- Marrow infiltration
- Hemolysis
- Liver disease
- Pregnancy
- Hypothyroidism
- Myelodysplasia

Investigations

Blood film: May show hypersegmented polymorphs (B_{12}↓) or target cells (liver disease).

Other tests: ESR (malignancy),liver function tests (LFTs) (include γ-glutamyl transpeptidase [GGT]), T4, serum B_{12}, and serum folate (or red cell folate). *Bone marrow biopsy* is indicated if the cause is not revealed by the above tests. It is likely to show one of these four states:

- *Megaloblastic:* B_{12} or folate deficiency (or cytotoxic drugs). (A megaloblast is a cell in which cytoplasmic and nuclear maturation are out-of-phase because nuclear maturation is slowed.)
- *Normoblastic marrow:* Liver damage, myxedema
- *Increased erythropoiesis:* E.g., hemolysis
- *Abnormal erythropoiesis:* Sideroblastic anemia, leukemia, aplastic anemia

If B_{12} deficiency, consider a *Schilling test* to help identify the cause. This determines whether a low B_{12} is due to malabsorption (B_{12} is absorbed from the terminal ileum) or to lack of intrinsic factor by comparing the proportion of an oral dose (1 mcg) of radioactive B_{12} excreted in urine with and without the concurrent administration of intrinsic factor. (The blood must be saturated by giving an IM dose of 1,000 mcg of B_{12} first.) If intrinsic factor enhances absorption, lack of it (e.g., pernicious anemia [p. 614]) is likely to be the cause.

Causes of a low B_{12} Pernicious anemia, post gastrectomy (no intrinsic factor to facilitate B_{12} absorption in the terminal ileum), dietary deficiency (vegans, children, and elderly living in vegetarian households); rarely, disease of terminal ileum (where B_{12} is absorbed), e.g., Crohn's disease, resection, blind loops, diverticula, worms (*Diphyllobothrium*). B_{12} is found in liver and all animal foods. *Body stores:* Sufficient for 3 yrs.

Causes of low folate Poor diet, heavy alcohol use, increased requirements (pregnancy, hemolysis, malignancy, long-term hemodialysis), malabsorption (especially celiac disease, tropical sprue), drugs (phenytoin and trimethoprim). Folate is found in green vegetables, fruit, liver. *Body stores:* Sufficient for 3 months. Maternal folate deficiency is associated with the development of fetal neural tube defects.

NB: In ill patients with megaloblastic anemia, it may be necessary to treat before the results of serum B_{12} and folate are at hand. Use large doses (e.g., hydroxocobalamin 1 mg/24 h IM, with folic acid 5 mg/24 h PO). Blood transfusions are very rarely needed (p. 456).

Folate given alone for the treatment of megaloblastic anemia when low B_{12} is the cause may precipitate, or worsen, subacute combined degeneration of the spinal cord.

Pernicious anemia

Pernicious anemia (PA) affects all cells of the body and is due to malabsorption of B_{12} resulting from atrophic gastritis and lack of gastric intrinsic factor secretion. In B_{12} deficiency, synthesis of thymidine, and hence DNA, is impaired and, consequently, red cell production is reduced. In addition, the central nervous system (CNS), peripheral nerves, gut, and tongue may be affected.

Incidence 1:1,000; increased with advancing age.

Common features
- Tiredness and weakness (90%)
- Dyspnea (70%)
- Paraesthesia (38%)
- Sore red tongue (25%)
- Diarrhea
- Mild jaundice (lemon tinge to skin)

Other features
- Retinal hemorrhages
- Prematurely gray hair
- Retrobulbar neuritis
- Mild splenomegaly
- Fever
- Neuropsychiatric (dementia)

Subacute combined degeneration of the spinal cord: This may be seen in any cause of a low B_{12}. Posterior and lateral columns are often affected, not always together. Onset is usually insidious with peripheral neuropathy. Joint position and vibration sense are often affected first (dorsal columns) followed by distal paraesthesia (neuropathy). If untreated, stiffness and weakness ensue. The classical triad is:

- Extensor plantars
- Brisk knee jerks
- Absent ankle jerks

Less common signs: Impaired cognition, reduced vision, absent knee jerks with brisk ankle jerks and flexor plantars, Lhermitte's sign (p. 373). Pain and temperature sensation may be intact even when joint position sense is severely affected. CNS signs can occur without anemia.

Associations Thyroid disease (~25%), vitiligo, Addison's disease, carcinoma of stomach (maintain a low threshold for endoscopy).

Tests
- Hb↓ (3–11 g/dL)
- MCV >~110 fL
- Hypersegmented neutrophils

- Serum B_{12} <200 pg/mL
- Reduced WCC and platelets ↓
- Megaloblasts in the marrow

Megaloblasts are abnormal red cell precursors in which nuclear maturation is slower than cytoplasmic maturation. Antibodies to parietal cells (high sensitivity but low specificity) or to intrinsic factor (higher specificity but lower sensitivity) are present in PA. The vast majority of B_{12} deficient patients will have elevations in serum homocysteine and methylmalonic acid. However, both homocysteine and methylmalonic acid are elevated in renal disease, and hyperhomocysteinemia is present in folate deficiency. A Schilling test (p. 613) may be appropriate occasionally (expect it to show that <7% of an orally administered dose of labelled B_{12} is excreted unless concurrent intrinsic factor is given).

Treatment Replenish stores with cyanocobalamin (B_{12}) 1 mg IM every day for 2 wks (or, if CNS signs, until improvement stops). *Maintenance:* 1 mg IM every month for life. Initial improvement is heralded by a marked reticulocytosis (after 4–5 d, but serum iron falls first). Watch for early hypokalemia and rebound thrombocytosis if severely B_{12} deficient.

Practical hints

- Beware of diagnosing pernicious anemia in those <40 yrs: Look for GI malabsorption (small bowel biopsy).
- Watch for hypokalemia in early days of therapy.
- Pernicious anemia with high-output congestive heart failure (CHF) may require exchange transfusion after blood for CBC, folate, B_{12}, and marrow sampling.
- As hematopoiesis accelerates on treatment, additional Fe and folate may be needed.
- WBC and platelet count should normalize in 1 wk. Hb rises ~1 g/dL per week of treatment.
- Dramatic rebound thrombocytosis is often observed, is transient, and does not appear to be harmful.

Prognosis Complete neurological recovery is possible. Most see improvement in the first 3–6 months. Patients do best if treated as soon as possible after the onset of symptoms.

An approach to hemolytic anemia

Hemolysis is the premature breakdown of RBCs. It may occur in the circulation (intravascular) or in the reticuloendothelial system (extravascular). Normal RBCs have a lifespan of ~120 d. In sickle-cell anemia, e.g., the lifespan may be as short as 5 d. If the bone marrow does not compensate sufficiently, a hemolytic anemia will result.

Causes of hemolysis These are either genetic or acquired.

Genetic:

1 Membrane: Hereditary spherocytosis or elliptocytosis
2 Hemoglobin: Sickling disorders (p. 616), thalassemia
3 Enzyme defects: G6PD and pyruvate kinase deficiency

Acquired:

1 Immune: Either isoimmune (hemolytic disease of newborn, blood transfusion reaction), autoimmune (warm or cold antibody mediated), or drug-induced
2 Nonimmune: Trauma (cardiac hemolysis, microangiopathic anemia [p. 617]), infection (malaria, septicemia), membrane disorders (paroxysmal nocturnal hemoglobinuria, liver disease)

In searching for evidence of significant hemolysis (and, if present, its cause), try to answer these four questions:

- *Is there increased red cell breakdown?* Bilirubin↑ (unconjugated), urinary urobilinogen↑, haptoglobin↓ (binds free Hb avidly, and is then removed by the liver, so it is a good marker of hemolysis).
- *Is there increased red cell production?* Demonstrated by reticulocytosis, polychromasia on the blood smear, macrocytosis, marrow hyperplasia.
- *Is the hemolysis mainly extra- or intravascular?* Extravascular hemolysis may lead to splenic hypertrophy. The features of intravascular hemolysis are methemalbuminemia, free plasma hemoglobin, hemoglobinuria, low haptoglobin, and hemosiderinuria.
- *Why is there hemolysis?* See below and p. 617.

History Ask about family history, race, jaundice, hematuria, drugs, previous anemia.

Examination Look for jaundice, hepatosplenomegaly, leg ulcers (seen in sickle-cell disease).

Investigation

- CBC, reticulocytes, bilirubin, lactate dehydrogenase (LDH), haptoglobin, urinary urobilinogen. Films may show polychromasia, macrocytosis, spherocytes, elliptocytes, fragmented cells or sickle cells, and nucleated RBCs if severe.
- Further investigations: *Direct antiglobulin test (DAT; Coombs' test).* This will identify red cells coated with antibody or complement, and a positive result usually indicates an immune cause of the hemolysis. The nonimmune group are usually identifiable by associated features.
- RBC lifespan may be determined by *chromium labeling,* and the major site of RBC breakdown may also be identified. *Urinary hemosiderin* (stains with Prussian blue) indicates chronic intravascular hemolysis.
- The cause may now be obvious, but further tests may be needed. Membrane abnormalities are identified on the film and can be confirmed by *osmotic fragility* testing. Hb *electrophoresis* will detect Hb variants. *Enzyme assays* are reserved for situations in which other causes have been excluded.

Causes of hemolytic anemia

Sickle-cell disease (see p. 617).

Hereditary spherocytosis Autosomal dominant RBC membrane defect (RBCs are osmotically fragile). Hemolysis is variable. *Signs:* Splenomegaly ± ↑ risk of gallstones. RBCs show increased fragility. *Diagnosis:* Hb 8–12 g/dL. Osmotic fragility tests. Film: Many spherocytes. *Treatment:* Folate replacement; splenectomy if warranted (there are risks with ensuing hyposplenism).

616

Hereditary elliptocytosis Usually inherited as autosomal dominant. The degree of hemolysis is variable; splenectomy may be indicated in severe cases.

Glucose-6-phosphate dehydrogenase deficiency is the commonest RBC enzyme defect. Inheritance is sex-linked with 100 million affected in Africa, the Mediterranean, and the Middle/Far East. Neonatal jaundice occurs, but most are symptomless with normal Hb and blood film. They are susceptible to oxidative crises precipitated by drugs (primaquine, sulfonamides, ciprofloxacin), exposure to fava beans (favism), or illness. Typically, there is rapid anemia and jaundice with RBC Heinz bodies (denatured Hb stained with methyl violet). *Diagnosis:* Enzyme assay. Don't do until some weeks *after* a crisis as young RBCs may have sufficient enzyme to make the results appear normal. *Treatment:* Avoid/remove precipitants; transfusion if severe.

Pyruvate kinase deficiency Usually inherited as autosomal recessive; homozygotes often have neonatal jaundice; later, chronic hemolysis with splenomegaly and jaundice. *Diagnosis:* Enzyme assay. Often well-tolerated. There is no specific therapy but splenectomy may help.

Drug-induced immune hemolysis Due to formation of new RBC membrane antigens (e.g., penicillin in prolonged, high dose), immune complex formation (many drugs, rare), or presence of autoantibodies to the RBC: α-methyldopa, mefenamic acid, L-dopa (rare, Coombs' +ve).

Autoimmune hemolytic anemia (aiha) *Causes:* Warm or cold antibodies. They may be primary (idiopathic) or secondary, usually to lymphoma or generalized autoimmune disease (e.g., SLE). *Warm aiha:* Presents as chronic or acute anemia. *Treatment:* Steroids (± splenectomy). *Cold aiha:* Chronic anemia made worse by cold, often with Raynaud's or acrocyanosis. *Treatment:* Keep warm. Blood transfusion is the main therapy, but chlorambucil may help. Mycoplasma and EBV may produce cold agglutinins, but hemolysis is rare.

Paroxysmal cold hemoglobinuria

is caused by Donath–Landsteiner antibody (seen in mumps, measles, chickenpox, syphilis) sticking to RBCs in cold, which causes complement-mediated lysis on rewarming.

Cardiac hemolysis Cell trauma in prosthetic aortic valves. It may indicate valve malfunction.

Microangiopathic hemolytic anemia (MAHA) Suspect if marked schistocytes and microspherocytes on the blood smear. Includes hemolytic-uremic syndrome, TTP (p. 260), and pre-eclampsia. Treat underlying disease; blood and fresh frozen plasma (FFP) transfusions, plasma exchange.

Paroxysmal nocturnal hemoglobinuria RBCs are unusually sensitive to complement due to loss of complement-inactivating enzymes on their surface, causing pancytopenia, abdominal pain, or thrombosis (e.g., Budd–Chiari syndrome) and hemolysis. *Diagnosis:* Test for glycosylphosphatidylinositol (GPI)-linked antigen loss (CD55 and CD59). *Treatment:* Anticoagulation; blood product replacement; consider stem cell transplant, complement inhibitors.

Factors exacerbating hemolysis

Infection often leads to increased hemolysis. Also, parvoviruses cause cessation of marrow erythropoiesis. Parvovirus infection can cause acute decompensation in patients with chronic hemolytic anemias due to reticulocytopenia associated with parvovirus B_{19}.

Sickle-cell anemia

Sickling disorders are due to the production of abnormal β-globins. An amino acid substitution in the β-globin gene (Glu → Val at position 6), results in the production of HbS rather than HbA. Hemoglobin S is prevalent in individuals descended from malaria-endemic regions (sub-Saharan Africa, Southeast Asia, and the Middle East). ~10% of African Americans have sickle-cell *trait* (HbAS), which causes no disability (and may protect from *falciparum* malaria) except in hypoxia, when veno-occlusive events may occur. Symptomatic sickling occurs in homozygotes and in compound heterozygotes with genes coding other amino acid substitutions with sickling properties (e.g., HBSC and SD diseases). Homozygotes (CC,

DD) have asymptomatic mild anemia. Individuals who are homozygous for hemoglobin S have sickle-cell anemia.

Pathogenesis HbS polymerizes when deoxygenated, causing RBCs to sickle. Sickle cells are fragile, have a shortened red cell survival, and can obstruct small vessel circulation.

Tests Hb ≈ 6–8 g/dL; reticulocytes 10–20%: (hemolysis is variable); ↑bilirubin. *Hemoglobin electrophoresis:* Distinguishes SS, AS, and other Hb variants. *Blood smear:* Polychromasia, nucleated red cells, sickle forms, targets. Aim for diagnosis *at birth* to aid prompt pneumococcal prophylaxis (vaccine [p. 158] and penicillin V).

Signs and symptoms *Early:* Anemia and jaundice, with painful swelling of hands and feet (dactylitis); also splenomegaly (rare if >10 yrs, as the spleen infarcts). Youngsters with sickle cell disease may have periods of good health with acute crises (below). *Later:* Adult complications of sickle-cell anemia include recurrent vaso-occlusive crisis, bone infarction and avascular necrosis, osteomyelitis, renal failure, leg ulcers, transfusional iron overload, pulmonary hypertension, and stroke.

Sickle-cell crises These may be from vaso-occlusive crisis, venous thrombosis, hemolysis (rare), red cell aplasia, sequestration, or stroke.

Vaso-occlusive crisis: Common, often causing severe pain. Precipitated by cold, dehydration, infection, or physical stress. May mimic an acute abdomen or pneumonia. *CNS signs:* Seizures, focal signs. Transcranial Doppler can indicate risk of impending stroke (preventable by transfusion). Priapism may occur; if >24 h, arrange prompt cavernosus-spongiosum shunting to prevent impotence; priapism also occurs in CML (p. 628).

Acute chest syndrome: Defined as fever, infiltrate on chest x-ray, and chest pain. Must be monitored very closely and red cell exchange arranged if clinical status deteriorates.

Aplastic crises: These are due to parvoviruses, characterized by sudden lethargy and pallor and absent reticulocytes. Urgent transfusion is needed.

Sequestration/hepatic crises: Spleen and liver enlarge rapidly from trapped RBCs. Signs: Right upper quadrant (RUQ) pain, International Normalized Ratio (INR)/LFT↑, Hb↓↓. Treatment includes red cell exchange transfusion.

Management of chronic disease
- Consider hydroxyurea if frequent crises.
- Chronic blood transfusion to keep HbS level <30% will prevent occurrence of stroke and chest syndrome but there is a high incidence of development of antibodies to red cell antigens and iron overload.
- Marrow transplant can be curative, but remains controversial.
- Splenic infarction leads to hyposplenism, and appropriate prophylaxis, in terms of antibiotics and immunization, should be adopted.

Prevention Genetic counseling; prenatal tests. Parental education and prompt medical attention for febrile illnesses prevents 90% of childhood deaths from infection, sequestration crises.

Management of sickle-cell crisis
Seek expert help.
- Give *prompt*, generous analgesia with opiates.
- Cross-match blood. CBC, reticulocytes, blood cultures, chest x-ray (CXR).
- Rehydrate with IV fluids and keep warm.
- Give O_2 by mask if P_aO_2 ↓.
- Empiric antibiotics for fever after culturing.
- Measure hematocrit (HCT), reticulocytes, liver, and spleen size daily.

- Give blood transfusion if HCT or reticulocytes fall sharply, or if there are CNS or lung complications (when the proportion of sickled cells should be reduced to <30%). This may require urgent exchange transfusion.

The acute chest syndrome entails pulmonary infiltrates associated with chest pain and fever. It is a serious condition. *Incidence:* ~0.1 episodes/patient/yr. 13% in the landmark Vichinsky study needed ventilation, 11% had CNS symptoms, and 9% of those >20 yrs old died. Prodromal painful crisis occur ~2.5 d before any abnormalities on CXR in 50% of patients. The chief causes of the infiltrates are fat embolism from bone marrow; infection with *Chlamydia*, *Mycoplasma* , or virus; and sickled RBCs. *Bronchodilators* have proved to be very effective in 20% with wheezing or obstructive pulmonary function at presentation. *Antibiotics* have an important role. *Red cell transfusion* improves oxygenation; red cell exchange should be emergently arranged if respiratory status deteriorates.

Thalassemia

Hemoglobin (Hb) is a tetramer consisting of 2 α- and 2 β-globin molecules. Hb is heterogeneous. Adults have 95% HbA ($\alpha_2\beta_2$) and a little HbA$_2$ ($\alpha_2\delta_2$). HbF ($\alpha_2\gamma_2$) predominates in fetal life and HbA predominates after birth. HbA$_2$ and fetal hemoglobins may be relatively elevated in β-chain disorders such as β-thalassemia and sickle cell anemia.

The thalassemias are a group of disorders resulting from reduced rate of production of one or more globin chains. This leads to an imbalance between α- and β-chains, precipitation of excess globin chains, and anemia due to ineffective erythropoiesis and hemolysis. They are common in a band stretching from the Mediterranean to the Far East. The most important are α- and β-thalassemia, in which there is reduced production of α- and β-chains, respectively. Since there are two genes for β-globin and four for α-globin in each individual, there are numerous varieties of genetic defects associated with thalassemias. It is possible to correlate clinical severity with the specific genetic defect to some extent, although many other genetic and acquired factors modify the clinical phenotype.

β-thalassemia major: This is the homozygous form in which very few β-chains are formed, and it results in a severe anemia presenting in the first year, often as failure to thrive. Death results in 1 yr without transfusion. If adequate transfusion is given, development is normal but symptoms of iron overload appear after 10 yrs as endocrine failure, liver disease, and cardiac toxicity. Death usually occurs at 20–30 yrs due to cardiac siderosis if long-term iron chelation is not provided. If transfusion is inadequate, there is chronic anemia with reduced growth and skeletal deformity due to bone marrow hyperplasia (bossing of skull). The smear shows very hypochromic, microcytic cells with target cells and nucleated RBCs. HbF↑, HbA$_2$ variable, HbA absent. *Prevalence of carriers:* Cypriot 1:7; southern Italy 1:10; Greek 1:12; Turkish 1:20; English 1:100.

619

β-Thalassemia minor: This is the heterozygous state, recognized as MCV <75 fL, HbA$_2$ >3.5%, and mild anemia (9–11 g/dL) that is usually well tolerated but may be worsened in pregnancy.

α-Thalassemia: Four varieties are defined, depending on the number of defective α genes. Absence of one or two genes is common in individuals of African descent and is either undetectable or produces a mild microcytic anemia.

Hb H disease: In patients with three α gene deletions, HbH (β_4) is present at 5–30% throughout life with moderate hemolytic anemia and splenomegaly. Prognosis: Good.

Hb Barts: Infants are stillborn or have neonatal jaundice (hydrops fetalis). They lack all α genes. Hb Barts is γ_4, and physiologically useless. Obstetric problems are common.

Thalassemia intermedia: This is a term used to describe individuals with thalassemia of intermediate severity who are not transfusion-dependent but have severe anemia. They often have substantial splenic enlargement. Usually the explanation for the mildness of the disease is a residual ability to make β-chains.

Diagnosis Family history, CBC, MCV, smear, iron, HbA_2, HbF, Hb electrophoresis.

Treatment
- Transfusion to keep Hb >9 g/dL
- Iron-chelating agent, e.g., deferoxamine. *Large doses of ascorbic acid also increase iron output but can cause cardiac failure due to sudden, rapid iron release,
- Perform splenectomy if hypersplenism exists.
- Give folate supplements. A histocompatible marrow transplant can offer the chance of a cure in childhood.[1] Genetic counseling should be offered. It may be particularly useful if abortion is an acceptable option.

Bleeding disorders

After trauma, three processes control hemorrhage: Vasoconstriction, platelet adhesion and aggregation, and fibrin deposition from activation of the coagulation cascade. Disorders of hemostasis fall into these three groups. The pattern of bleeding is important to the diagnostic approach—vascular and platelet disorders lead to prolonged bleeding from cuts, purpura, and bleeding from mucous membranes, whereas coagulation disorders produce prolonged bleeding after injury, into joints, muscle, and the GI and GU tracts.

Vascular defects Causes may be congenital (Osler–Weber–Rendu) or acquired (senile purpura, steroids, trauma, pressure, vasculitis, diabetes, connective tissue disease, scurvy).

Platelet disorders These may be due to quantitative or qualitative platelet defects. Causes of thrombocytopenia include:
- *Decreased production:* Marrow failure states, megaloblastosis, drugs (chemotherapy), liver disease, alcohol
- *Increased destruction:* Immune thrombocytopenia (ITP), infection (EBV), DIC, drugs, SLE, TTP, hypersplenism, heparin induced thrombocytopenia, pregnancy, sepsis

Qualitative platelet defects are most frequently acquired from drugs (aspirin, Plavix®), uremia, myeloproliferative disorders, or, less commonly, can be due to congenital platelet disorders (Glanzmann's thrombasthenia, Bernard–Soulier).

ITP may be acute or chronic. Acute ITP is most commonly observed in children after viral infections, with rapid onset and spontaneous resolution within a year. Chronic ITP is the rule in adults, with a fluctuating course of bleeding, purpura, or epistaxis. Treatment is indicated when symptomatic bleeding occurs or when platelet counts are <20,000/mcL. Treatment options include steroids, splenectomy, high-dose immune globulin, or anti-D (WinRho). Other treatments include rituximab and other immunosuppressive agents and thrombopoietic mimetics. Platelets transfusions are only transiently successful and should be used if serious bleeding ensues.

1 Rund D. Rachmilewitz E. Beta-thalassemia. *NEJM* 2005;**353**:1135–1146.

Coagulation disorders Coagulation defects include congenital disorders such as hemophilia and von Willebrand's disease or acquired processes including anticoagulants, liver disease, DIC (p. 626), vitamin K deficiency, or acquired factor inhibitors. *Hemophilia A:* Congenital factor VIII deficiency, sex-linked recessive in 1 of 10,000 male births. New mutations are common. The presentation depends on the severity of the deficiency and is frequently detected early in life, after surgery or trauma, or due to spontaneous bleeding into joints and muscle. Acquired hemophilia is due to factor VIII autoantibodies. These may appear in pregnancy, autoimmune diseases, or malignancy. Diagnosed by family history, bleeding history, prolongation of the activated PTT (aPTT), and factor VIII assay. *Management:* Seek expert advice. Avoid antiplatelet agents and IM injections. Major bleeding (hemarthrosis) requires factor VIII levels to be raised to 50% of normal. Life-threatening or CNS bleeding requires levels of 100% of normal. Both recombinant and plasma-derived factors are available. *Hemophilia B (Christmas disease):* Due to factor IX deficiency and behaves clinically like hemophilia A. *Liver disease* produces a complicated bleeding disorder, with decreased clotting factor synthesis, dysfibrinogenemia, and decreased clearance of circulating anticoagulants. *Malabsorption* leads to reduced absorption of vitamin K. *Treatmen:* Vitamin K 10 mg sq or FFP for acute hemorrhage.

The intrinsic and extrinsic pathways of blood coagulation

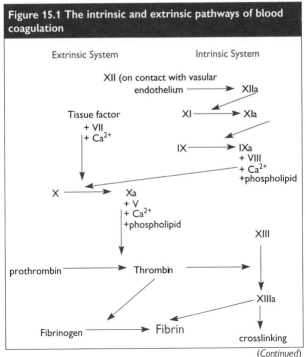

Figure 15.1 The intrinsic and extrinsic pathways of blood coagulation

621

(Continued)

Figure 15.1 (Continued)

The fibrinolytic system The coagulation cascade simultaneously activates factors that result in fibrin dissolution by the activation of plasmin from plasminogen. The process starts by the release of tissue plasminogen activator (t-PA) from endothelial cells, a process stimulated by fibrin formation. t-PA converts inactive plasminogen to plasmin, which can then cleave fibrin, as well as several other factors.

Fibrinolytic agents

1 *Alteplase* (RT-PA;Actilyse®; from recombinant DNA) is a fibrinolytic enzyme imitating t-PA, as above. Plasma $t_{1/2}$ = 5 min.
2 *Anistreplase* (anisoylated plasminogen streptokinase activator complex; APSAC®) is a complex of human plasminogen and streptokinase (so anaphylaxis is possible). Plasma $t_{1/2}$ = 90 min.
3 *Streptokinase* is a streptococcal exotoxin and forms a complex in plasma with plasminogen to form an activator complex which forms plasmin from unbound plasminogen. Initially, there is rapid plasmin formation that can cause uncontrolled fibrinolysis. However, plasminogen is rapidly consumed in the complex and then plasmin is only produced as more plasminogen is synthesized.
4 *Urokinase* is produced by the kidney and is found in urine. It also cleaves plasminogen.

Coagulation tests

Coagulation tests

If using sodium citrate tube, beware of falsely elevated results if tube is incompletely filled or insufficiently mixed. See Table 15.2.

1 *aPTT*: Activated partial thromboplastin time; measure of the intrinsic pathway. Prolonged by abnormalities in fibrinogen (I), II, VII, IX, X, XI, XII. Abnormalities can be qualitative (dysfibrinogenemia), quantitative (von Willebrand's disease, hemophilia), or acquired (heparin therapy, DIC, VIII antibodies). Also prolonged by the misnamed lupus "anticoagulant" as an artifact of cross-reaction with the lipid component of the test.
2 *Prothrombin time*: (PT) Expressed as a ratio compared to control: International Normalized Ratio (INR); normal, 0.9–1.2. Thromboplastin is added to test the extrinsic system. Prolonged by abnormalities in factors I, II, VII, X; warfarin, liver disease, or vitamin K deficiency.
3 *Thrombin time*: Thrombin is added to plasma to convert fibrinogen to fibrin. Prolonged in heparin treatment, DIC, or dysfibrinogenemia. Reptilase time is similar to the thrombin time but is not affected by heparin, which can help distinguish heparin effect from other causes.
4 *Bleeding time*: A measure of platelet and vascular function. Prolonged in von Willebrand's disease, NSAIDs, uremia, all platelet numeric or functional defects, vascular problems (diabetes).
5 *Platelet aggregation studies*: Used to evaluate defects in platelet function. Abnormal in NSAIDs, congenital defects, myeloproliferative or myelodysplastic disorders.
6 *Mixing studies* and *inhibitor screens*: Used for evaluating prolonged PT or aPTTs. If prolongation of the PT or aPTT is corrected by the addition of normal plasma, then a factor deficiency is established. If addition of normal plasma does not correct the clotting test, then inhibitors are suspected and further testing is required. Seek expert help for evaluation and treatment.

Table 15.2 Interpreting investigations into bleeding disorders						
Disorder	INR	aPTT	Thrombin time	Platelet count	Bleeding time	Notes
Heparin	↔	↑↑	↑↑	↔	↔	
DIC	↑↑	↑↑	↑↑	↓	↑	FDP↑ (p. 626)
Liver disease	↑	↑↔	↑↔	↓↔	↔↑	↑LFTs
Platelet defect	↔	↔	↔	↔↓	↑	
Vitamin K def	↑↑	↑	↔	↔	↔	
Hemophilia	↔	↑↑	↔	↔	↔	p. 570
von Willebrand's	↔	↑	↔	↔	↑	

Special tests may often be required. Consult a hematologist. FDP, fibrin degradation products.

Anticoagulants

Consider bleeding as a cause of any symptom in anyone on anticoagulants.

The main indications for anticoagulation

- Deep vein thrombosis/pulmonary emboli
- To prevent embolism in atrial fibrillation or in those with mechanical heart valves
- To prevent deep venous thrombosis/pulmonary emboli in high-risk patients (p. 446)

Types of anticoagulant Standard unfractionated(~13,000 daltons) heparin (IV or SC) is inexpensive, acts fast, and is monitored by the aPTT. Heparin inactivates thrombin by binding to antithrombin III, leading to inactivation of coagulation enzyme Xa. Plasma infusion will not reverse the effect of heparin. *Low-molecular weight-heparin preparations* (5,000 daltons, dalteparin, enoxaparin) $T_{1/2}$ are two- to fourfold longer than unfractionated heparin, and response is more predictable. They can be given once daily SC, no monitoring is needed, and can be used in the outpatient setting. Low-molecular-weight heparin inactivates factor Xa, and its activity can be monitored by Xa levels. *se:* Bleeding (at operative site, intracranial, retroperitoneal). *Contraindications (CI):* Uncontrolled bleeding/risk of bleeding (active peptic ulcer); endocarditis.

Warfarin: Warfarin inhibits the vitamin K-dependent production of the co-agulation factors II, VII, IX, and X, and the anticoagulants protein C and S. Warfarin has both a large volume of distribution and a very long $t_{1/2}$. Therapy is monitored with the INR. *CI:* Peptic ulcer, bleeding disorders, severe hypertension, liver failure, infective endocarditis, cerebral aneurysms, history of falls. Use with caution in the elderly and those with remote GI bleeds.

Beginning anticoagulation Heparin bolus (5,000–10,000 U IV over 5 min) if anticoagulation is urgent (e.g., deep vein thrombosus [DVT], pulmonary embolus (PE), unstable angina, myocardial infarction [MI]). Giving a bolus is contraindicated (by convention) for stroke. *Infusion:* Start at 800–l,400 U/h. Check aPTT 4–6 h after starting; aim for target of 1.5–2.5× the upper limit of the control (target = 60–80 sec). Adjust as follows (check with the guidelines established in your institution):

PTT (sec)	Bolus (U)	Hold (min)	Rate change (U/h)	Repeat ptt
<50	5000	0	+120	4–6 h
50–59	0	0	+120	4–6 h
60–80	0	0	0	Next day
81–110	0	30	–50	4–6 h
>110	0	60	–160	4–6 h

- Start warfarin 10 mg PO qd when aPTT is therapeutic on heparin. If the INR at 18 h after the first dose is <1.8, continue 10 mg of warfarin; if INR >1.8, reduce to 5 mg.
- Use the sliding scale below to keep INR in the target range. Do INR daily for 5 d, then alternate days until stable, then weekly or less often.

INR	<2	2	2.5	2.9	3.3	3.6	4.1
Third dose	10 mg	5 mg	4 mg	3 mg	2 mg	0.5 mg	0 mg
Maintenance	≥6 mg	5.5 mg	4.5 mg	4 mg	3.5 mg	3 mg	*

*Skip a dose; give 1–2 mg the next day (if INR >4.5, skip two doses)

- Stop heparin when INR >2. Check platelet count if on heparin >5 d.

Antidotes Consult a hematologist. Stop anticoagulation; if further steps are needed, protamine sulfate can counteract heparin: 1 mg IV neutralizes 100 U heparin given within 15 min. Maximum dose: 50 mg (if exceeded, may itself have anticoagulant effect). For warfarin reversal or overdose, use phytomenadione (vitamin K): 5–10 mg PO or SC for serious bleeding, 0.5–2 mg for simple hematuria or epistaxis; consider 0.5 mg if INR >7 without any bleeding. This takes some hours to act and may last for weeks. If serious bleeding, and INR↑, give a concentrate of activated clotting factors, activated VII, or, if unavailable, infuse fresh frozen plasma.

Thrombin inhibitors and Factor Xa inhibitors Are anticoagulants available in oral and parenteral formulations and are indicated in patients who cannot be exposed to heparins (due to the development of heparin-induced thrombocytopenia [HIT]). Oral thrombin inhibitors are approved in some instances and can replace warfarin-based anticoagulation regimens.

Warfarin: INR guidelines

The target level represents a balance between too little anticoagulation (and risk of thromboembolism) and too much anticoagulation (risk of bleeding). Since the risks of thromboembolism vary with the clinical situation, optimum INR varies. Recommendations are likely to change as further trials are done: Check with a hematologist.

Choose a target INR within the range (not the range itself). This reduces the chance that the INR will stray outside the optimum range.

The incidence of fatal bleeding due to warfarin is 0.3/100 patient years. Severe bleeding is tenfold more common.

- *Prosthetic heart valves*. The degree of anticoagulation depends on the location and type of prosthetic valve, the presence of atrial fibrillation or CHF, and the left atrial size. Aortic valves 2.5 (2–3) INR, mitral 3 (2.5–3.5). Caged-ball valves generally require higher INR.
- *Atrial fibrillation*: Important clinical parameters in determining thrombotic risk include congestive heart failure, hypertension, age >75, diabetes, and previous stroke, TIA, or systemic embolic event. For medium-risk patients (one or two risks), guidelines are an INR of 2–3; for higher risk, 2.5–3.5. An alternative for low-risk patients (0 risks) is aspirin, particularly if the

risk of bleeding is high (serious comorbidity or difficulty with monitoring INR).

- *Pulmonary embolism and above-knee DVT*: Aim for INR of 2–3, and treat for 3–6 months (depends on risk of recurrence).

Leukemia and the resident

Patients with leukemia fall ill suddenly and can deteriorate rapidly. The most important acute issues are bleeding, infection, and leukostasis. Unlike the differentiated cells in chronic lymphocytic leukemia (CLL) and myeloproliferative disorders, where elevated cell counts are not usually dangerous in themselves, leukemic blasts are large and sticky and can obstruct the small circulations in the lungs, heart, and brain. Leukemic blasts can also secrete substances that generate disseminated intravascular coagulation. Thus it is important not only to review the blood smear in patients presenting with elevated white cell counts to make the diagnosis of leukemia, it is also crucial to evaluate and treat leukemic patients who present with markedly elevated blast counts.

Neutropenic precautions and approach to febrile neutropenia If the absolute neutrophil count is <500/mcL, then neutropenic precautions are as follows:

- Strict hand washing
- No rectal temperatures or unnecessary rectal examinations
- No IM injections
- Low-bacteria diet (fresh fruit and vegetables carry risk of *Pseudomonas*)
- No fresh flowers
- Examine mouth, perineum, axillae, IV sites, and indwelling catheter sites carefully
- Vital signs q4h
- Culture urine, sputum, stool, blood (peripheral and catheter lines), CXR, computed tomography (CT) of chest and sinuses, place PPD
- Oral *Candida* prophylaxis

Antibiotic use in neutropenia: Treat known infections promptly. After cultures are drawn, start empiric antibiotics for fever >38.3°C or >38°C on separate occasions 1–2 h apart. In the absence of fever, empiric antibiotics should also be given if the patient has hypotension, tachycardia, or a new oxygen requirement. The choice of antibiotic coverage should conform to organisms common in your community and hospital. Generally, an antipseudomonal penicillin or fourth-generation cephalosporin with the addition of vancomycin (if line sepsis is suspected or if there is a high prevalence of community-onset methicillin-resistant strep [MRSA]) is acceptable. Any suggestion of a fungal infection (sinusitis, thrush) mandates early antifungal therapy. If there are chest symptoms or significant hypoxia, additionally treat presumptively for *Pneumocystis*. Continue antibiotics until afebrile and neutrophils recover. If fever persists despite antibiotics, start antifungal therapy. If the patient has a defect in cell-mediated immunity (AIDS, chronic immunosuppression for solid tumor, or bone marrow transplant) consider treatment for cytomegalovirus (CMV). Recombinant human colony-stimulating factors (G-CSF, GM-CSF) usually are not useful in the treatment of neutropenic fever, although their use in individual cases may be indicated.

Hyperviscosity If the white cell count is >70–100,000/dL, WBC thrombi may form in the brain, lung, and heart. Emergent leukapheresis with concomitant high doses of cyclophosphamide or hydroxyurea must be considered in patients with leukostasis.

Cell lysis syndrome Hyperkalemia and hyperuricemia follows the massive destruction of cells from tumor necrosis and chemotherapy. Maintain a high urine output, alkalinize the urine, and give allopurinol or rasburicase before cytotoxic therapy.

Disseminated intravascular coagulation Occurs in many leukemias and particularly in acute promyelocytic leukemia. DIC is the result of pathological thrombin formation, leading to inappropriate intravascular fibrin deposition, and platelet and clotting factor consumption. In addition to leukemia, DIC also occurs in malignancy, infection, trauma, and in obstetrical disasters. DIC results in both small vessel clotting and bleeding and is associated with extensive purpura, oozing from venipuncture sites, and bleeding in the brain, GI tract, and lungs. The blood smear may identify schistocytes (red cell fragments). Fibrinogen and platelets are reduced, whereas PT, aPTT, and fibrin degradation products are elevated. Treatment of DIC includes reversal of the underlying medical condition, platelet and plasma support. Heparin may have a place in the treatment of DIC, but it is case- and center-dependent in its use. The use of all transretinoic acid (ATRA) has significantly reduced the risk of DIC in patients with acute promyelocytic anemia.

Acute lymphoblastic leukemia

Many leukemias are associated with specific gene mutations, deletions, or translocations. Acute lymphoblastic leukemia (ALL) manifests as a neoplastic proliferation of lymphoblasts. The latest WHO classification of tumors divides ALL into precursor B lymphoblastic leukemia/lymphoblastic lymphoma and precursor T lymphoblastic leukemia/lymphoblastic lymphoma. However, the immunologic classification is still widely applied.

Immunologic classification
• *Common ALL:* 75%; defined by the presence of CD10 on the blasts. Any age may be affected; common in 2–4-yr-olds.
• *T-cell ALL:* Any age but peaks in adolescent males, who present with a mediastinal mass and a high white cell count.
• *B-cell ALL:* Burkitt or Burkitt-like leukemia. Rare, with a poor prognosis. Surface immunoglobulin is present on the blasts.
• *Null cell ALL:* Undifferentiated; lacking the markers listed above.

Morphologic classification The French American British (FAB) classification divides ALL into three types, L1, L2, L3, by microscopic appearance. It provides only limited information compared with other systems.

Signs and symptoms: Anemia, infection, bleeding, splenomegaly, lymphadenopathy, thymic enlargement, CNS involvement (cranial nerve palsies).

Common infections: Zoster, CMV, measles, candidiasis, pneumocystic pneumonia (p. 567), bacteremia. Consider immune globulin for patients in contact with measles or zoster when on chemotherapy.

Diagnosis Characteristic cells in blood and bone marrow.

Treatment
• *Supportive care:* Blood and platelet transfusions, IV antibiotics (p. 625) at first sign of infection (neutropenic regimen).
• *Chemotherapy:* As with most leukemias, patients are entered into clinical trials. A typical program is organized to achieve:
1 *Remission induction:* Vincristine, prednisone, L-asparaginase, and daunorubicin
2 *cns prophylaxis:* Intrathecal methotrexate; cranial irradiation
3 *Consolidation:* Courses of high-dose chemotherapy for 2–3 yrs. Relapse is common in blood, CNS, and testes.

Hematological remission means no evidence of leukemia in the blood, a normal or recovering blood count, and <5% blasts in a normal regenerating bone marrow, and normal cytogenetics.

Bone marrow transplant (p. 627) is considered for patients with high-risk leukemia (especially those with 9:22 translocation). Other poor prognostic indicators are adults, males, presentation with CNS signs or WBC >100,000, B-cell phenotype. Cure rates in children are 70–90% while only 35% in adults and even worse in older adults. Future therapy will more specifically target leukemic cells according to their specific genetic defect.

Acute myeloid leukemia

Acute myeloid leukemia (AML) arises from a normal marrow hematopoietic stem cell that has acquired genetic damage leading to aberrant proliferation and variable degrees of differentiation. It is a very rapidly progressive malignancy in which survival is on the order of weeks to months if untreated.

Morphological classification is now based on the WHO criteria, which is complex and requires specialist interpretation. The WHO classification recognizes important prognostic information from cytogenetics and molecular genetics and includes five main types:

1 AML with recurrent genetic abnormalities
2 AML with multilineage dysplasia
3 AML and myelodysplastic syndromes, therapy-related
4 AML not otherwise categorized
5 Acute leukemias of ambiguous lineage

Incidence is 1/10,000/yr and increases with age. AML is becoming more common as a consequence of high-dose chemotherapy for both solid tumors and lymphoma.

Signs and symptoms: Anemia; infection (often Gram negative); bleeding; DIC; hepatosplenomegaly; lymphadenopathy; bone pain (sternal tenderness); leukemic infiltration of gums, testes, and orbit; CNS involvement (cranial nerve palsies, cord compression).

Diagnosis: WBC is variable, and blasts are few in the peripheral blood of up to one-third of AML patients. Diagnosis relies therefore on bone marrow biopsy. Differentiation from ALL may be evident from microscopy, where presence of Auer rods is diagnostic for AML, but overall is secured by flow cytometric immunophenotyping and molecular methods. Molecular basis of the leukemia may dictate the specific type of treatment and helps determine prognosis.

Complications Infection, related both to the disease and complications of its therapy. Be alert to septicemia (p. 625). Oral infections are common. Both tumor lysis syndrome and leukostasis (p. 625) are common and must be treated.

Treatment *Supportive care:* Red cell and platelet support, antibiotics, neutropenic precautions. AML itself can cause fevers, common organisms can present oddly, and candida and aspergillus are not uncommon.

Chemotherapy: Courses are intensive and include cytosine arabinoside and daunorubicin. Prognosis is better for younger patients and is also linked to specific lesions.

Bone marrow transplant (BMT): Allogeneic transplants from histocompatible siblings or from unrelated donors (accessed through national and international databases) may be indicated after remissions are obtained with chemotherapy. The idea is to destroy residual leukemic cells and the patient's own immune system with high-dose cyclophosphamide and total body irradiation, then intravenously infuse the donor's marrow to replace the host's. BMT allows the most intensive chemotherapy regimens because marrow suppression is not an issue. Immunosuppressants are required to restrain the donor immune system from attacking the patient's body (graft vs. host disease). Complications of BMT include graft versus host disease (graft vs. leukemia effect is very important to the overall success of BMT in AML); infections; venoocclusive disease; leukemia relapse. *Prognosis* Allogeneic transplant survival may approach 60%. Autologous BMT in AML is intermediate between chemotherapy alone and allogeneic BMT; the role of reduced-conditioning BMT is under study.

Chronic myeloid leukemia

CML is a hematopoietic stem cell disorder in which there is uncontrolled proliferation of well-differentiated myeloid cells. It accounts for 15% of leukemias. As a myeloproliferative neoplasm (MPN) (p. 637), it has features common to other MPNs including splenomegaly. However, given its unique molecular pathogenesis and natural history, it is considered separately from the other MPNs. It commonly presents with constitutional symptoms, but may be picked up inadvertently on routine blood work. It occurs most often in the middle-aged, with a slight male predominance.

Philadelphia chromosome (Ph^1) A hybrid chromosome due to translocation between the long arms of chromosome 9 and 22 (t9:22). The translocation generates an oncogene, BCR/ABL, that constitutively signals within the cell, causing aberrant growth. The Philadelphia chromosome is present in granulocytes, platelet, and red cell precursors in >95% of those with CML. Those without the Philadelphia chromosome have a worse prognosis. Some patients have a masked translocation in which standard cytogenetics do not reveal Ph^1, but the BCR/ABL oncogene can be detected by fluorescent in situ hybridization (FISH).

Symptoms and signs Mostly chronic and insidiuous: Malaise, weight loss, gout, fever, night sweats, bleeding or abdominal pain. Splenomegaly, hepatomegaly, anemia, bruising.

Diagnosis WBC is often markedly elevated, with an orderly left shift in the differential and an increase in basophils and eosinophils. Hb can be normal or low, platelets usually are elevated. Leukocyte alkaline phosphatase (LAP) is reduced. Uric acid and alkaline phosphatase are increased.

Natural history Untreated median survival of 3–5 yrs. Three phases: Chronic, lasting months or years with few or any symptoms; accelerated phase, with increasing symptoms, spleen size, and difficulty in controlling counts; blast crisis occurs uniformly and has features of acute leukemia.

Treatment

I   *Imatinib mesylate* a specific tyrosine kinase inhibitor, has revolutionized the management of CML. It is more effective than the previous gold standard therapy for CML, α-interferon, plus or minus cytarabine, in chronic-phase patients. Imatinib therapy produced complete hematologic responses, major cytogenetic responses, and complete cytogenetic responses in the majority of patients treated in chronic phase and improved survival over interferon when compared using historical controls. The drug is also effective in patients who have failed interferon and to some extent in both accelerated phase and blast crisis. Side effects include nausea, cramps, edema, skin rash, cytopenias, and abnormal LFTs.

II   The use of *interferon* in CML has declined dramatically with the introduction of tyrosine kinase inhibitors (imatinib, desatinib), but it may still have a role in combination therapy.

III The role of *allogeneic transplantation* from a HLA matched sibling or unrelated donor must be reconsidered given the success of tyrosine kinase inhibitors. This approach should be considered as first-line therapy in patients in whom trans-plant-related mortality is estimated to be very low. Other patients should be offered a trial of a tyrosine kinase inhibitor first.

IV Treatment of transformed CML is difficult. Although patients may respond to imatinib, this is temporary. Some patients who develop a lymphoblastic transformation may respond to therapy as for ALL. Patients who develop a myeloblastic transformation rarely achieve lasting remission, and allogeneic transplant offers the only hope of long-term survival.

Chronic lymphocytic leukemia

CLL is a monoclonal proliferation of small lymphocytes that are most frequently of B-cell origin. CLL typically occurs in adults >40 yrs, with men more frequently affected than women. CLL comprises 25% of all leukemias and is the most common hematopoietic malignancy.

Staging correlates with survival:

0	Absolute lymphocytosis >15,000/mcL
I	Stage 0 + enlarged lymph nodes
II	Stage I + enlarged liver or spleen
III	Stage II + anemia
IV	Stage III + thrombocytopenia

Symptoms None in 25%; weight loss, bleeding, infection, anorexia.

Signs Enlarged nontender nodes, hepatosplenomegaly

Blood smear This is a diagnosis made by observing small, normal-appearing lymph nodes, many of which fracture on the smear and are termed "smudge cells." May also be signs of autoimmune hemolytic anemia (spherocytes) or autoimmune thrombocytopenia (large platelets).

Complications (1) Autoimmune hemolytic anemia; (2) infection, either bacterial of the respiratory tract due to low immunoglobulin levels or viral due to altered cell-mediated immunity; (3) bone marrow failure; (4) immune-mediated thrombocytopenia.

Natural history Some remain in Stage 0 for years without progressing. Usually, nodes slowly enlarge. Death is often via infection (pneumococcus, haemophilus, meningococcus, candida, aspergillosis) or transformation to aggressive lymphoma (Richter's syndrome).

Treatment Chemotherapy is often not required initially. Chlorambucil, effective in reducing WBC and node size, was the mainstay of therapy, but is now being supplanted by rituximab, fludarabine, bendamustine, other monoclonal antibody therapies, and other agents in clinical trials. Steroids are useful in controlling autoimmune processes. Radiotherapy can be used for relief of lymphadenopathy or splenomegaly.

629

Supportive care: Transfusions, prophylactic antibiotics, immune globulin.

Prognosis is often good, depending on stage, age, and molecular/immuno-logical factors such as ZAP70 or CD38.

Hodgkin's lymphoma

Hodgkin's lymphoma (HL) is a cancer characterized by the presence of clonal malignant Reed–Sternberg cells within a reactive cellular background comprised of variable numbers of granulocytes, plasma cells, and lymphocytes. Reed–Sternberg cells are transformed B lymphocytes, many of which contain Epstein–Barr genome, suggesting an association of previous infection in the pathogenesis of HL in many patients.

Classification (in order of incidence)	*Prognosis:*
Nodular sclerosing	Good
Mixed cellularity*	Good
Lymphocyte predominant	Good
Lymphocyte depleted*	Poor

* Higher incidence and worse prognosis if HIV positive.

Clinical features The usual presentation is with enlarged, painless lymph nodes, usually in the neck or axillae. Rarely, there may be alcohol-induced pain or features due to the mass effect of the nodes. 25% have constitutional symptoms such as fever, weight loss, night sweats (often drenching), pruritus, and loss of energy. If the fever alternates with long periods (15–28 d) of normal or low temperature, it is termed a Pel–Ebstein fever (other causes of this rare fever: TB, renal cell cancer). *Signs:* Lymphadenopathy (note position, consistency, mobility, size, tenderness). Look for weight loss, anemia, hepatosplenomegaly.

Tests Lymph node biopsy for diagnosis. CBC, smear, ESR, LFTs, CXR, bone marrow biopsy, abdominal or magnetic resonance imaging (MRI) scan. Lymphangiography is no longer used routinely. Staging laparotomy is performed if finding abdominal disease will change the therapy. It involves splenectomy with liver and lymph node biopsy.

Staging influences treatment and prognosis.

I Confined to single lymph node region

II Involvement of ≥2 regions on same side of diaphragm

III Involvement of nodes on both sides of diaphragm

IV Spread beyond the lymph nodes

Each stage is subdivided into A (no systemic symptoms) or B (presence of weight loss >10% in last 6 months, unexplained fever >38°C, or night sweats). These indicate more extensive disease. Pruritus is not a B symptom. Extranodal disease is indicated by a subscripted "E" (e.g., IA_e).

Treatment XRT for stages IA and (IA, chemotherapy for IIA → IVB). HA patients with very large mediastinal masses also receive chemotherapy. Chemotherapy is given with an "*ABVD"-type regimen (Adriamycin, bleomycin, vinblastine, dacarbazine). Regimens containing nitrogen mustard such as MOPP are less common because of the risk of sterility and secondary AML. Recently, more intensive regimens have been used, particularly for advanced disease. *Peripheral stem-cell transplantation:* Autologous or allogeneic transplantation of blood progenitor cells helps restore marrow function after myeloablative therapy, as do agents that stimulate progenitor cells (e.g., filgrastim).

Complications of treatment: Radiation-induced lung fibrosis and hypothyroidism. Chemotherapy—nausea, alopecia, infertility in men, infection due to myelosuppression, mucositis, and second malignancies, especially AML, breast cancer, and non-Hodgkin's lymphoma (NHL). Autologous marrow transplant may help in relapses after chemotherapy or in previously irradiated sites.

5-yr survival Depends on stage and grade, ranging from >90% in IA lymphocyte-predominant disease to <40% with IVB lymphocyte depletion.

Emergency presentations SVC obstruction presents with JVP↑, a sensation of fullness in the head, dyspnea, blackouts, and facial edema. Arrange urgent radiotherapy (XRT). High-dose corticosteroids may also be useful.

Non-Hodgkin's lymphoma

This group includes all lymphomas without the Reed–Sternberg cell and is a very diverse group. Classification is now based on cell of origin and integrates histology, immunophenotype, and molecular studies. Historically, NHL was clinically classified by grade of tumor, given the observations that low-grade lymphomas are more indolent but incurable whereas the high-grade types are more aggressive, but long-term cure is achievable.

The low-grade group includes CLL/SLL, follicular lymphoma, mantle cell, marginal zone, splenic marginal zone, and others whereas the high-grade lymphomas include centroblastic, immunoblastic, and lymphoblastic.

Incidence has doubled since 1970 (to 1:10,000), perhaps from immunosuppression in the setting of chronic viral infections (HIV, HTLV-I, and EBV) or transplant.

The patient
- Typically an adult with lymphadenopathy
- Extranodal spread occurs early, so presentation may be in skin, bone, gut, CNS, or lung. Often asymptomatic.
- Pancytopenia occurs (marrow dysplasia) ± hemolysis
- Infection is common.
- Systemic symptoms as in Hodgkin's. Examine all over. Note nodes (if any is >10 cm across, staging is advanced). Do ear-nose-throat (ENT) exam if GI lymphoma (GI and ENT lymphoma often coexist).

Tests, diagnosis, and staging As for Hodgkin's (staging is less important as 70% have widespread disease at presentation). Always do node biopsy, CXR, abdomen + pelvis CT, CBC, LFT, cytology of a pleural or peritoneal effusion, CSF cytology if CNS signs, highly aggressive phenotype or HIV positive. *NB*: Survival is worse if elderly or symptomatic.

Treatment Asymptomatic low-grade tumors may not need treatment and occasionally enter spontaneous remission; chlorambucil or cyclophosphamide may control symptoms. Radiation therapy can be used for local bulky disease. More aggressive disease requires combination chemotherapy, CHOP with Rituxan.

Lymphoblastic lymphoma; treat as for ALL. Small noncleaved lymphomas are very aggressive and require extremely intensive therapy.

Burkitt's leukemia/lymphoma Endemic in African children, also associated with HIV and sporadic forms and is associated with chromosomal translocations involving immunoglobulin loci and the myc oncogene. Jaw tumors are common, usually with GI involvement. Histology shows a "starry sky" appearance (isolated histiocytes on background of abnormal lymphoblasts). Spectacular remission may result from a single dose of a cytotoxic drug (e.g., cyclophosphamide).

Bone marrow failure

The bone marrow is responsible for hematopoiesis and, in adults, is found in the vertebrae, sternum, ribs, skull, and proximal long bones, although it may expand in anemia (e.g., thalassemia). All blood cells are thought to arise from an early, pluripotent stem cell that divides in an asymmetric fashion to provide a committed progenitor and other stem cells. Committed progenitors then undergo further differentiation before releasing formed elements into the blood. Bone marrow failure usually produces a pancytopenia, often with sparing of the lymphocyte count.

Causes of pancytopenia Aplastic anemia, hypersplenism, SLE, megaloblastic anemia, paroxysmal nocturnal hemoglobinuria, leukemia, myelodysplasia, drugs, liver disease.

Causes of marrow failure *Stem cell or erythroblast loss:* (1) Aplastic anemia; this can be toxic (e.g., drug, benzene), immunologic, congenital, viral (esp. hepatitis B and parvoviruses), or idiopathic (most common). (2) *Inltration:* From malignancy, infection (TB, *M. avium intracellulare* [MAI]). (3) *Fibrosis:* Primary myelofibrosis, HIV, SLE. (4) Abnormal differentiation of a genetically damaged clone of cells, such as myelodysplastic syndromes, acute leukemia.

Aplastic anemia This presents as pancytopenia with a hypoplastic marrow (i.e., the marrow stops producing cells). Causes are idiopathic (50%), radiation, drugs (e.g., cytotoxics, chloramphenicol, anticonvulsants and gold), viruses, congenital.

Incidence: 10–20 per million per year. Presents as bleeding, anemia, or infection. In ~50% of cases there is response to immunosuppressive therapy.

Treatment of aplastic anemia: Marrow transplantation is the best treatment for younger patients if there is a histocompatible sibling donor. In patients in whom transplantation is not feasible, immunosuppressive regimens are effective. Many patients respond to regimens incorporating cyclosporine, antithymocyte globulin, or high-dose cyclophosphamide. Responses to androgens are rare.

Bone marrow support The symptoms of bone marrow failure are due to the pancytopenia. Red cells survive for ≈120 d, platelets for an average 10 d, and neutrophils for 1–2 d, so early problems are mainly from neutropenia and thrombocytopenia.

Erythrocytes: A 1 unit transfusion should raise the Hb by about 1—2 g/dL assuming that there are no antibodies.

Platelets: Spontaneous bleeding is unlikely if platelets >20,000/dL. Platelets require irradiation or leukocyte depletion prior to transfusion. Indications for transfusion are counts <10,000/dL and bleeding. One unit of fresh platelets should raise the count to >10,000/dL unless the patient is alloimmunized or febrile.

Neutrophils: Use "neutropenic precautions" if the count is <500/dL. There is no role for neutrophil transfusions typically, although active fungal processes are exceptions.

Bone marrow biopsy Ideally, an aspirate *and* biopsy should be taken. Biopsies may be taken from the posterior iliac crest, aspirates may be taken from anterior iliac crest or sternum. Thrombocytopenia is rarely a contraindication. Severe coagulation disorders may need to be corrected. Apply pressure afterward (lie on that side for 1–2 h if platelets are low).

The myeloproliferative disorders

Polycythemia vera, essential thrombocytosis, and idiopathic myelofibrosis are bone marrow disorders characterized by excess proliferation of myeloid elements—RBC, WBC, and platelets. These disorders are clonal hematopoietic stem cell disorders in which all of the circulating cells are derived from a transformed stem cell clone. The progeny of the aberrant stem cell differentiate and function normally. The three disorders share several features, including the fact that all may present with constitutional symptoms such as fever, weight loss, night sweats, pruritus, and malaise, and have varying degrees of extramedullary hematopoiesis, myelofibrosis, and leukemic transformation. These disorders are closely related pathogenetically, many associated with a mutation in the JAK2 gene. These disorders are closely related clinically, with frequent disease evolution between different MPN subtypes over the years in a single patient.

Often these diseases are a "panmyelosis" indicating that more than one cell line is increased. This may generate diagnostic confusion, especially between essential thrombocytosis and polycythemia vera.

Erythrocytosis may be relative (plasma volume contraction) or absolute (increased red cell mass). This distinction is made by red cell mass estimation using radioactive chromium. Relative erythrocytosis is often due to dehydration (alcohol or diuretics). Absolute polycythemia may be primary (polycythemia vera) or secondary from smoking, sleep apnea, chronic lung disease, tumors (fibroids, hepatoma, renal cell cancer), altitude, or rarely from high-affinity Hb.

Polycythemia rubra vera *Incidence:* 1.5/100,000/yr, peaks at 45–60 yrs. *Signs:*

- Elevated hemoglobin, white cells, or platelets variably affected
- MCV normal or microcytic
- Splenomegaly (60%)

Presentation is determined by hyperviscosity (CNS signs [p. 636]; angina; itching—typically after a hot bath) and WBC turnover (gout). It may also present with bruising or be detected incidentally after a routine CBC. *Diagnosis:* Red cell mass >125% of predicted (^{51}Cr studies). JAK2 mutation test is positive in >95% with PV clinical phenotype. Erythropoietin levels are normal or low, O_2 saturation is normal. *Treatment:* Keep HCT <42% by phlebotomy. Iron deficiency may result from repeated phlebotomies. Myelosuppressive agents (hydroxyurea, interferon) may be required to control extramedullary disease or blood counts. *Prognosis:* Variable; many often remain well for decades, but complications include extramedullary hematopoiesis, myelofibrosis, marrow failure, or even leukemia. A particular risk is from thrombotic disorders that may derive from ↑ HCT and viscosity and/or activated white cells or platelets.

Essential thrombocytosis is defined as thrombocytosis (>600,000/mcL) in the absence of a defined stimulus, such as iron deficiency, inflammation, polycythemia vera or primary myelofibrosis. Platelet function can be abnormal, and presentation may be by bleeding or thrombosis. Microvascular occlusion may lead to erythromelalgia (painful burning and erythema in fingertips and toes).

Treatment: Hydroxyurea, interferon, or anagrelide may be needed for symptoms or in high-risk patients (age >60, previous thrombosis history, hypertension, coronary artery disease); however, platelet count correlates poorly with the risk of thrombosis. Aspirin is useful, especially if there is any evidence of a thrombotic diathesis. *Causes of a raised platelet count:* Other myeloproliferative or inflammatory disorders, bleeding, malignancy, post-splenectomy, Kawasaki disease.

Primary myelofibrosis There is marrow fibrosis with associated hematopoiesis in the spleen and liver (myeloid metaplasia, extramedullary hematopoiesis) associated with significant degrees of anemia and wasting.

Clinical features: Variable—constitutional, splenomegaly, bone marrow failure. *Smear:* Leukoerythroblastic; teardrop RBCS. *Marrow tap:* Often dry. Treatment is supportive, iron and folate supplements ± splenectomy, consideration of stem cell transplantation, interferon or JAK2 inhibitor trials.

Other causes of marrow fibrosis Any myeloproliferative disorder, lymphoma, secondary carcinoma, TB, leukemia (especially, megakaryoblastic [M7]) irradiation, SLE, HIV.

Myeloma

Myeloma is a plasma cell neoplasm that produces diffuse bone marrow infiltration and focal osteolytic lesions. An M component (M for monoclonal—not IgM) is seen on serum and/or urine electrophoresis.

Incidence 5/100,000. Peak age: 70 yrs.

Classification Based on the principal neoplastic cell product:

• IgG	55%
• IgA	25%
• Light chain disease	20%

IgD, IgE, and nonsecretory types are less common.

60% of IgG and IgA myelomas also produce free light chains that are filtered by the kidney and may be detectable as Bence Jones protein (these precipitate on heating and redissolve on boiling). They may cause renal damage or amyloidosis.

Clinical features
- Bone pain/tenderness is common, often postural (e.g., back ribs, long bones, and shoulder). Occasionally presents as pathological fracture (but 25% have no clinical or x-ray signs of bone disease at presentation).
- Fatigue (anemia, renal failure or dehydration).
- Infection (poor Ig production).
- Amyloid
- Neuropathy
- Viscosity
- Visual acuity-I ± hemorrhages/exudates on funduscopy
- Bleeding

Diagnosis Abundant, clonally restricted plasma cells in marrow. Component M or urinary light chains on serum/urine electrophoresis (Bence Jones proteins) and abnormal serum; free light chain ratios are supportive evidence. *Other tests:* CBC, ESR ↑, alk phos usually normal (unless healing fracture). Nonmyeloma immunoglobulins can be suppressed; urea, creatinine, urate + Ca^{2+} ↑ in 30–50%. *Bone x-rays:* Punched-out lesions, osteoporosis.

Treatment *Supportive:* Bone pain, anemia, and renal failure cause most symptoms. Give analgesia and transfusions PRN. Advise high fluid intake. Solitary lesions can be given XRT and may heal. Bed rest tends to exacerbate hypercalcemia, so mobilization is important—this may require surgical stabilization of lytic lesions and analgesia. Pamidronate (and other newer bisphosphonates) and erythropoietin are promising for reducing bone pain, hypercalcemia, and transfusion requirements.

Chemotherapy None may be needed (none is curative) unless: HCT ↓ or:

- Troublesome symptoms
- Many osteolytic lesions
- Impending fracture
- Creatinine >1.5 mg/dL
- Marrow >30% plasma cells
- Serum β_2 micro-globulin >4 mcg/mL.
- More light chains in urine than creatinine (mcg/mL)

Optimal therapy is evolving but includes combinations of steroids, melphalan, and thalidomide or bortezomib and other intensive chemotherapeutic regimens. Autologous bone marrow transplant may offer an advantage after induction therapy for many patients who are suitable candidates and have high-risk disease. Survival worse if blood urea nitrogen (BUN) >28 mg/dL or Hb <7.5 g/dL.

Dangers

1 *Hypercalcemia:* Use IV normal saline (NS) 4–6 L/d with careful fluid balance and furosemide. Consider steroids; e.g., hydrocortisone 100 mg IV q8h; bisphosphonates may be needed in refractory disease, calcitonin, mithramycin, and gallium nitrate also may be useful.
2 *Hyperviscosity:* May need plasmapheresis
3 Acute renal failure may be precipitated by IVP; therefore avoid IV contrast.

Paraproteinemia

Paraproteinemia refers to the presence in the circulation of immunoglobulin produced by a single clone of plasma cells or their precursors. The paraprotein is recognized as a sharp M component (M for monoclonal, not IgM) on serum electrophoresis. There are six major categories:

1 *Multiple myeloma*(p. 634)
2 *Waldenström's macroglobulinemia:* This is a lymphoplasmacytoid malignancy producing an IgM paraprotein, lymphadenopathy, and splenomegaly. CNS and ocular symptoms of hyperviscosity may occur. Chemotherapy and plasmapheresis (p. 637) may help.
3 *Primary amyloidosis:* See below.
4 *Monoclonal gammopathy* (monoclonal gammopathy of unknown significance or MGUS) is common (3% >70 yr). In contrast to myeloma, in MGUS the paraprotein level is stable, immunosuppression and urine light chains are absent and there is little plasma cell marrow infiltrate.
5 *Paraproteinemia in lymphoma or leukemia:* CLL
6 *Heavy chain disease:* Production of free heavy chains, causing malabsorption from infiltration of small bowel wall. It may terminate in lymphoma.

Amyloidosis

635

This is characterized by extracellular deposits of an abnormal protein resistant to degradation called amyloid. Various proteins, under a range of stimuli, may polymerize to form amyloid fibrils. They are shown with Congo Red staining (apple-green birefringence in polarized light).

Classification

1 *Systemic:*
- Immune dyscrasia (fibrils of immunoglobulin light chain fragments, known as "AL" amyloid)
- Reactive amyloid ("AA" amyloid; nonglycosylated protein)
- Hereditary amyloid (type I familial amyloid polyneuropathy)
2 *Localized:* Most often cutaneous; or cerebral, cardiac, endocrine

AL amyloid (primary amyloidosis) is associated with monoclonal proliferation of plasma cells (e.g., in myeloma). Clinical features include carpal tunnel syndrome, peripheral neuropathy, purpura, cardiomyopathy, and macroglossia (a large tongue).

AA amyloid (secondary amyloidosis) is associated with chronic infections (e.g., TB, bronchiectasis), inflammation (especially rheumatoid arthritis), and neoplasia. It may affect kidneys, liver, and spleen. Presents as proteinuria, nephrotic syndrome, and/or hepatosplenomegaly.

The diagnosis of amyloidosis is made after Congo Red staining of affected tissue. The rectum is a common site for biopsy.

Treatment rarely helps, but AA amyloid may improve with treatment of the underlying disease.

A rare complication of amyloid is the intravascular adsorption of factor X, resulting in a prolonged PT and a serious coagulopathy.

Inflammatory markers

The ESR is a nonspecific indicator of the presence of inflammation. It measures the rate of sedimentation of RBCs in anticoagulated blood over 1 h. If red cells are coated by proteins (such as IgG or fibrinogen), then the normal negative charge on the cell surface is masked and the cells will tend to stick to each other in columns (the same phenomenon as rouleaux on the blood smear [p. 612]),and so they will fall faster. The ESR rises with age and anemia. It is reduced in polycythemia, CHF, sickle-cell anemia, trichinosis. Patients with a markedly raised ESR (>100 mm/h) may have a serious malignancy, connective tissue diseases (e.g., giant cell arteritis), rheumatoid arthritis, renal disease, sarcoidosis, or infection.

C-reactive protein (CRP) is an acute-phase protein that is very helpful in the monitoring of inflammation. The best test is quantitative, normal <0.80 mg/L. Like the ESR, it is raised in many inflammatory conditions but is much less sluggish in its response and falls within 2–3 d of the inciting event. Therefore, it can be used to follow the response to therapy (e.g., antibiotics) or activity of disease (e.g., in Crohn's disease). If the CRP has fallen 3 d after the onset of treatment for infection then the choice of antibiotics is probably appropriate.

CRP is raised by active rheumatic disease (rheumatoid arthritis, rheumatic fever, seronegative arthritis, vasculitis), tissue injury or necrosis (acute MI, transplanted kidney or bone marrow rejection, malignancies—esp. breast, lung, GI), burns, infection (bacterial more than viral). It is very useful for diagnosis of postoperative or intercurrent infections when the ESR may still be elevated. If the CRP has not started to fall 3 d after surgery then complications must be considered (e.g., infection, PE). CRP is NOT raised by SLE, leukemia (fever, blast crisis, or cytotoxins), ulcerative colitis, osteoarthritis, anemia, polycythemia, or CHF. Its highest levels are seen in bacterial infections. Absence of an elevated CRP significantly reduces the pretest probability of other investigations for bacterial infection (e.g., bone or gallium scan) and so may be a cheaper, more comfortable alternative.

Hyperviscosity syndromes

These occur if the plasma viscosity rises to such a point that the microcirculation is impaired. Usually relative viscosity >4 (four times the viscosity of water) is necessary to produce symptoms.

Causes Myeloma (p. 634) (IgM and IgA ↑ viscosity more than the same amount of IgG because they are multimeric), Waldenström's macroglobulinemia, polycythemia. High leukocyte counts in leukemia may produce leukostasis, which differs from hyperviscosity per se.

Presentation Visual disturbance, retinal hemorrhages, headaches, coma, and GU or GI bleeding.

The visual symptoms ("slow-flow retinopathy") may be described as "looking through a watery windshield." Other causes of slow-flow retinopathy are carotid occlusive disease and Takayasu's disease.

Treatment Removal of as little as 1 L of blood may relieve symptoms. Plasmapheresis is useful in the paraproteinemias, especially IgM, since it is mostly intravascular. Plasmapheresis for hyperviscosity due to IgG is usually less effective as it is deposited extravascularly.

The spleen and splenectomy

Splenomegaly is not uncommon and the differential diagnosis can be divided on the basis of the degree of splenic enlargement.

Massive splenomegaly Myeloproliferative neoplasms (CML, PV, primary myelofibrosis), malaria (hyperreactive malarial splenomegaly), schistosomiasis, leishmaniasis, kala-azar, "tropical splenomegaly" (idiopathic, in Africa and SE Asia)

Moderate splenomegaly Infection (malaria, EBV, subacute bacterial endocarditis [SBE], TB), portal hypertension, hemolytic anemia, hematologic malignancy (leukemia, lymphoma), splenic lymphoma, connective tissue disease (rheumatoid arthritis [RA], SLE), glycogen storage diseases, common variable immunodeficiency, splenic cysts, idiopathic.

Splenomegaly can cause abdominal discomfort or more commonly pain in the left shoulder (because of the embryologic origin of the organ). It may lead to hypersplenism, defined as pancytopenia due to cells becoming trapped in the reticuloendothelial system (symptoms of anemia, infection, and bleeding). When faced with a mass in the left upper quadrant, it is important to be able to recognize the spleen. The spleen moves with inspiration, enlarges toward the umbilicus, may have a notch, and "you can't get above it" (the top margin disappears under the ribs). Ultrasound or CT may help in evaluation of the spleen. When hunting for the cause for enlargement, look for lymphadenopathy and liver disease. Appropriate tests are CBC, ESR, LFTs and liver, lymph node or marrow biopsy. Aspiration or biopsy of the spleen is not commonly performed.

Splenectomy may be indicated for splenic trauma or splenic cysts, or as therapy for autoimmune thrombocytopenia and autoimmune hemolytic anemia, or for the diagnosis and treatment of splenic lymphomas.

Post-splenectomy, there may be a prompt, dramatic, and transient rise in the platelet count, so patients should be mobilized early. All patients, especially children, remain at increased risk of infection, particularly pneumococcal septicemia. Most children are advised to take daily penicillin V until aged 20 yrs. In adults, prophylaxis of 2–5 yrs is recommended unless there is coexisting hematologic disease; broader spectrum agents such as amoxicillin may be more appropriate. Give adults and unvaccinated children pneumococcal (Pneumovax®) haemophilus (HiB), and meningococcal A & C (Mengivac®) 2 wks preoperatively. Warn asplenic travelers that they face an increased risk of tropical infections, and to adhere closely to antimalarial prophylaxis, while recognizing that this may not be effective. Counsel the patient to have standby amoxicillin to start at once if any symptoms of infection present, and to seek urgent hospital care.

637

Thrombophilia

Thrombophilia is a primary coagulopathy resulting in a propensity to thrombosis, and can be due to genetic predisposition or to acquired factors, or both. Thrombophilia is not rare and needs special precautions in surgery, pregnancy, and immobilization.

Risk factors associated with venous thrombosis include stasis, inflammation, endothelial injury, and an imbalance between activated clotting factors and anticoagulants—these types of risk factors are primarily acquired and transient. Although many genetic risk factors for thrombosis have been identified, they do not exert a strong effect in healthy individuals; in the setting of other acquired risks, however, they will strongly increase the risk of venous thrombosis.

Suspect a primary hypercoagulable state in a young patient presenting with unprovoked thrombosis. Suspicion grows if there is a personal or family history of recurrent arterial or venous thrombosis or first-trimester spontaneous abortion.

Inherited thrombophilia Activated protein C resistance (APC resistance) is the most common inherited risk for venous thrombosis. APC resistance is overwhelmingly due to a single nucleotide polymorphism in the factor V gene (Factor V Leiden) present in the carrier state in 5% of individuals of Northern European descent. Factor V Leiden renders factor Va resistant to cleavage by activated protein C and is associated with an mildly increased risk of deep venous thrombosis in the heterozygous state and a marked increase in the homozygous state. The prothrombin 20210 polymorphism is present in ~2% of the Mediterranean population (carrier state) and is less strongly associated with increased risk of DVT than is Factor V Leiden. Far less common are inherited deficiency states of antithrombin III, protein S, and protein C. *Treatment:* Those with a history of thrombosis and with inherited abnormalities should be considered for long-term anticoagulation.

Acquired thrombophilia Common risk factors include venous stasis (after knee or hip replacement surgery), endothelial injury, congestive heart failure, bed rest, obesity, the postoperative state, indwelling catheters, cancer, heparin-induced thrombocytopenia, and certain blood disorders including myeloproliferative neoplasms, sickle cell anemia, paroxysmal nocturnal hemoglobinuria (PNH), and hemolytic anemias.

Cancer: There is a high risk of occult malignancy becoming evident within a year of seemingly unprovoked thrombotic events in patients <60 yrs of age. It is not current practice, however, to investigate aggressively in a search for cancer in all patients with DVT, but rather to limit the investigation to age-appropriate cancer screening. Trousseau's syndrome—migratory thrombophlebitis associated with visceral carcinoma—classically resists treatment with warfarin and requires unfractionated or low-molecular-weight heparin.

Antiphospholipid antibody syndrome is recurrent venous and/or arterial thrombotic events in association with an antiphospholipid antibody. There are two well-recognized aPL antibodies and three common ways of measuring them: The anticardiolipin antibody (measured with an enzyme-linked immunosorbent assay [ELISA] or the dilute Russell's viper venom time [RVVT]) and the lupus anticoagulant (a misnomer, it falsely prolongs the aPTT by interfering with the assay in vitro but is a procoagulant nonetheless) measured by the aPTT. aPL syndrome can be primary or associated with autoimmune disorders such as SLE. The annual risk of recurrent thrombosis after a confirmed thrombotic event in patients with an antiphospholipid antibody is ~30%. Warfarin anticoagulation with a target INR >3 is effective in reducing thrombotic recurrences. Treatment during pregnancy includes both aspirin and heparin.

NB: Hypercoagulable studies performed at the time of a thrombosis can be misleading because of alterations of clotting factors due to acute illness or the thrombosis itself and should be avoided.

Immunosuppressive drugs

Immunosuppressive drugs are used in organ and marrow transplants, rheumatoid arthritis, psoriasis, chronic hepatitis, asthma, giant cell arteritis, polymyalgia, SLE, PAN, and inflammatory bowel disease and many other autoimmune diseases.

Prednisone Steroids can be life-saving, but a number of points should be taken into consideration before initiating treatment.

• Hypertension, osteoporosis, and diabetes may be exacerbated by steroids.
• Do not stop steroids suddenly. Adrenal insufficiency may result, as endogenous production takes time to restart (p. 312).
• Increase steroid dosing at times of illness/stress (e.g., flu or preop).
• Minimize side effects by using the lowest dose possible for the shortest amount of time. Give doses in the morning, and alternate days if possible, to minimize adrenal suppression.
• Before starting steroid treatment, extensively counsel your patient regarding the risks and benefits of steroids and the impact of steroids on their comorbidities.
• Avoid concurrent drugs bought over the counter (e.g., aspirin, ibuprofen); the danger is steroid-associated GI bleeds: If NSAIDs are essential ask the patient to come to you for advice. You might consider an NSAID combined with misoprostol, a prostaglandin analogue.
• Interactions: Antiepileptics (below) and rifampin.
• Strongly consider pneumocystic pneumonia (PCP) prophylaxis in patients who are on other chemotherapeutic regimens, who require moderate steroid dosing for long periods of time, or in patients who are otherwise immunocompromised.
• *SE:* TB reactivation, edema, osteoporosis, cataracts, euphoria, elevated glucose, *Pneumocystis*, urinary tract infection (UTI), toxoplasmosis, aspergillus, serious chicken pox/zoster, so avoid contacts (and so the need for varicella zoster immunoglobulin).
• Avoid pregnancy.

Azathioprine *SE:* Peptic ulcer, marrow suppression, reduced WBC. Do CBCs. *Interactions:* Mercaptopurine and azathioprine (which metabolized to mercaptopurine) are metabolized by xanthine oxidase (XO). Azathioprine toxicity results if XO inhibitors (allopurinol) are coadministered. Genotype testing for thiopurine methyltransferase (TPMT) should be done prior to initiating treatment. Patients with low enzyme activity have increased risk of toxicity.

639

Cyclosporine Transplant patients usually require 6 mg/kg/d; in other patients, keep the dose <4 mg/kg/d. Monitor urine (UA) and creatinine every 2 wks for the first 3 months, then monthly if dose >2.5 mg/kg/d (every 2 months if less than this). Reduce the dose if creatinine rises by >30% on two measurements even if the creatinine *is still in the normal* range. Stop if the abnormality persists. Monitor blood levels in transplant patients. *SE:* Nephrotoxicity, hepatotoxicity, edema, gum hyperplasia, tremor, paresthesia, hypertension, confusion, seizures, lymphoma, skin cancer. Interactions are legion. Cyclosporine levels are increased by ketoconazole, diltiazem, nicardipine, verapamil, oral contraceptives, erythromycin. Cyclosporine levels are reduced by barbiturates, carbamazepine, phenytoin, rifampin.

Avoid concurrent nephrotoxics: Gentamicin, amphotericin. Concurrent NSAIDs augment nephrotoxicity: Monitor LFTs.

Methotrexate Inhibits dihydrofolate reductase, which is involved in the synthesis of purines and pyrimidines. *SE:* Hepatitis, lung fibrosis, CNS signs, teratogenicity. Methotrexate's action is increased by NSAIDs, aspirin, penicillin, probenecid.

Cyclophosphamide *SE:* Carcino- and teratogenic, hemorrhagic cystitis, marrow suppression.

Geriatric medicine

Colleen Christmas, M.D.

Contents

What is special about geriatric patients?

Many aspects regarding older adults make them a challenging and rewarding patient population to work with. Most of the care of older adults consists of simultaneous management of multiple chronic diseases. The course of their medical conditions will be punctuated by episodes of exacerbation of acute illness. With each successive exacerbation, prognosticating the amount of recovery becomes increasingly difficult. Another challenge in providing care to geriatric patients is that quality of life, risks of treatment, and functional disability take on greater importance in making treatment decisions.

Geriatric patients represent an incredibly heterogeneous group demographically and physiologically. From person to person the effects of lifestyle, genetic, and environmental factors produce variable results in aging of different organ systems. While one octogenarian may be active, driving, caring for grandchildren, and have well-controlled chronic conditions, the next may be severely debilitated, dependent on others for most of his or her care needs, and profoundly cognitively impaired. Thus, the approach to geriatric patients must be highly individualized.

The final principle to be considered in caring for older adults is that of intrinsic vulnerability. Although exercise may ameliorate some of the adverse effects of aging on most organ systems, even the very healthy aged suffer from a reduced ability to withstand physiologic perturbation. Examples of this may include glucose metabolism that appears normal during usual situations but becomes abnormal with mild disturbance, such as a urinary tract infection. This dictates a requirement to "stay on your toes," treat gingerly, and frequently reassess the impact of interventions in geriatric patients.

The elderly patient in the hospital

It is only in the past 200 yrs that life-expectancy has risen much above 40 yrs. *An aging population is a sign of successful social, health, and economic policies.*

Beware of ageism. Old age is associated with disease but doesn't cause it. Any deterioration is from treatable disease *until proven otherwise*.

• Contrary to stereotype, most old people are independent. 95% of those >65 yrs and 80% of those >85 yrs old do not live in institutions; about 70% of the latter can manage stairs and can bathe without help.

- With any problem, find the cause; resist temptation to think: *This is simply aging*. Look (within reason) for treatable disease, especially medication adverse effects, ↓ fitness, and social factors.
- Do not restrict treatment simply because of age. Old people vary. Age alone is a poor predictor of outcome and should not be used as a substitute for careful assessment of each patient's potential for benefit and risk.

Characteristics of disease in old age There are differences of emphasis in the approach to old people compared with young people.

- *Multiple pathology:* Several disease processes may coincide: Find out which impinge on each complaint (e.g., senile cataract + arthritis = falls).
- *Multiple causes:* One problem may have several causes. Treating each alone may do little good; treating all may be of much benefit.
- *Nonspecific presentations:* Some presentations are common in old people: Incontinence, immobility, instability (falls), weight loss, and delirium/confusion. Any disease may present with these. Also, typical signs and symptoms may be absent (myocardial infarction [MI] without chest pain; pneumonia, but no cough, fever, or sputum).
- *Rapid worsening if treatment is delayed:* Complications are common. Often a muted presentation, such as excess sleepiness, may belie a life-threatening disease, such as acute MI.
- *More time is required for recovery:* Impairment in homeostatic mechanisms leads to loss of physiological reserve.
- *Impaired metabolism and excretion of drugs:* Doses may need lowering, both because of declines in liver and kidney function with aging and because there is often less tolerance to side effects.
- *Social factors:* These are central in aiding recovery and return to home.

Special points in caring for the elderly

In the history: Assess all disabilities, then:

- *Home details:* E.g., stairs; access to toilet?
- *Medication:* What? When? Assess understanding and concordance. How many different medications can they cope with? Which are the most important drugs? You may have to ignore other desirable remedies or enlist the help of a friend, spouse, or pharmacist (who can batch morning, noon, and night doses in compartmentalized containers so complex regimens may be reduced to "take the morning compartment when you get up, the noon compartment before lunch, etc.").
- *Social network:* Regular visitors; family and friends
- *Care details:* What services are available (meals delivered, home care nurse, community psychiatric agency, physical therapist)? Who else is involved in the care? Speak to others (relatives, loved ones, neighbors, caregivers, personal physician). See Table 16.1.

On examination:

- Do blood pressure (BP) readings lying and standing (postural hypotension may lead to falls).
- Rectal exam: Impaction may lead to overflow incontinence.
- Watch the patient walk; this is a good way to assess balance, strength and coordination simultaneously and also determine if the patient is safe to return to home independently or may benefit from a stay in rehabilitation.
- Detailed central nervous system (CNS) examination is often needed (e.g., if presentation is nonspecific).

Start planning discharge from day 1. A very common question on rounds is: "Will this patient do OK at home? We've got them as good as we can, but is discharge safe?" In answering this, take into account:

- Most patients want to go home promptly. If not, find out why.
- Is the home suitable for a frail person? Stairs? Toilet on same floor?
- If toilet access is difficult, can they transfer from chair to commode?
- Can they open a can, use the phone, turn on a microwave, cook soup?
- Does the patient live alone?
- Does the caregiver have family support? Is he or she already exhausted by other duties (e.g., young children at home)?
- Is the family supportive—in theory or in practice?
- Are the neighbors friendly?
- Are social services and community geriatric services well integrated? Proper *case management programs* with defined responsibilities, entailing integration of social and geriatric services, really can help.

Make a care plan:

- Include nutrition. Is the patient able to eat the food that is delivered?
- Involve a multidisciplinary team. Including nonphysician health care professionals. Their expertise can maximize the treatment plan.

Frailty, falls, and postural hypotension

Frailty is a syndrome that best incorporates the notion of increased vulnerability to insults and subsequent exaggerated effects of insults. A phenotype has been described[1] in which three or more of five recognized characteristics describe this syndrome:

- Unintended weight loss of ≥10 pounds over the previous 12 months
- Poor grip strength
- Self-reported poor endurance and exhaustion
- Slow walking time
- Low physical activities level

Studies demonstrate that frailty is associated with aging and is associated with higher rates of health care utilization, disability, and mortality.

The biologic mechanisms contributing to the development of frailty are just beginning to be unraveled, with the hopes that discovery of such mechanisms will lead to interventions that favorably alter the clinical course.

Falls are common (30% of those >65 who live in the community fall in a year), and this may be the start of a fatal course of events. There are many causes. 10% are related to loss of consciousness or dizziness. For most, there is no clear single cause, and many factors conspire.

History: Exact circumstances of fall. Find out about any CNS, cardiac, or musculoskeletal abnormalities. Drugs causing postural hypotension: sedation; arrhythmia, parkinsonism (e.g., tricyclics, neuroleptics, including metoclopramide and prochlorperazine, as well as alcohol).

Examination: For causes: Postural hypotension; arrhythmias; detailed neurological examination, including cerebellar signs, parkinsonism, proximal myopathy, gait; watch patient get up from chair; test for Romberg's sign; mechanical instability in knees or feet.

Consequences: Cuts; bruises; fractured ribs (± pneumonia) or limbs, especially of femur; head injury (± subdural hematoma). Often patients who fall significantly restrict activities because of intense psychological fear of falling.

Management: The patient's confidence may be shattered even if there is no serious injury. Look for causes and treat. Consider physical therapy; include learning techniques on how to get up from floor. Occupational therapists may advise on reducing household hazards and adding aids. Exercise and balance training can prevent falls.

Postural hypotension is important because it is common and a cause of falls and poor mobility. Typical times are after meals, on exercise, and on getting up at night. May be transient with illness (e.g., flu).

Causes: Leg vein insufficiency, autonomic neuropathy, drugs (diuretics, nitrates, antihypertensives, antidepressants, sedatives). Red cell mass may be low. *Management:* Reduce or stop drugs if possible. Counsel patient to stand up slowly in stages. Try compression stockings. Reserve fluid-retaining drugs (fludrocortisone 0.1 mg PO daily, ↑ as needed) in those severely affected when other measures fail.

Impairment, disability, and stroke rehabilitation

Doctors are experts at diagnosing disease and identifying impairment. But we are slow to see the patient's perspective. Considering the concepts of impairment and disability may help.

Impairment refers to systems or parts of the body that do not work. "Any loss or abnormality of psychological, physiological or anatomical structure or function." For example, following stroke, paralysis of the right arm or aphasia would be impairment.

Disability refers to things people cannot do. "Any restriction or lack (resulting from an impairment) of ability to perform an activity in the manner, or within the range, considered normal for a human being." For example, following stroke, difficulties in "activities of daily living" (e.g., with dressing, walking).

Making use of these distinctions Two people with the same impairment (e.g., right hemiparesis) may have different disabilities (e.g., one able to dress, the other unable). The disabilities are likely to determine the quality of the person's future. Treatment may usefully be directed at reducing disabilities. For example, Velcro® fasteners in place of buttons may enable a person to dress.

Three stages of management

Assessment of disability: Traditional "medical" assessment focuses on disease and impairment. Full assessment requires a thorough understanding of disability. Discuss detailed assessments with expert therapists, the patient, and relatives to help define their problems.

Who can help? Hospital doctors are part of a large team. Involve other members of the team early, including nurses, occupational and physical therapists, social workers, and the primary care physician. Also, there are self-help organizations for most chronic diseases aimed both for patients and their caregivers.

Generate solutions to problems: A list of disabilities is the key. Rehabilitation should look at each disability (e.g., unable to undress). Uncover the origin of the disability (in terms of disease and impairment). Mutual goals should be agreed upon with the patient and relatives in accordance with their wishes. At every visit, review, renew, and adapt goals.

Rehabilitation after stroke

Good care consists of attention to detail. The principles of rehabilitation are those of any chronic disease and are best carried out in specialist inpatient stroke units (they reduce morbidity and institutionalization).

Special points in early management: Watch the patient drink a glass of water: If they cough or gag, they should be kept NPO for several days.

Maintenance IV fluids should (almost) always be ordered at the same time as making someone NPO. The optimal use of nasogastric (NG) and percutaneous endoscopic gastrostomy (PEG) tubes is controversial, although a randomized clinical trial demonstrated no benefit compared to NPO in the first week after a dysphagic stroke. Consider consulting with the speech and swallowing service.

Avoid injuring the extremities of patients through careless lifting.

Ensure good bladder and bowel care through frequent toileting. Avoid early catheterization, which may prevent return to continence.

Position the patient to minimize spasticity.

Urinary incontinence

Incontinence is never normal although it occurs in up to 30% of the elderly at home and 50% in long-term care. It is transient in 30%–40% of patients, and the causes are multiple and frequently coexist.

Intrinsic urinary tract malfunction can result in *detrusor overactivity*, involuntary contractions of the bladder; *detrusor underactivity*, failure of adequate bladder contraction; *stress incontinence*, abnormally low urethral resistance; or *obstruction*, abnormally high urethral resistance.

Causes of transient incontinence are often (but not always) outside the urinary tract. Remember "*DIAPPERS*": **D**elirium; **I**nfection of the urine (not asymptomatic bacteriuria); **A**trophic urethritis and vaginitis (responds to estrogen); **P**harmaceuticals (sedatives, anticholinergics, antipsychotics, antidepressants, narcotics, α-adrenergics, diuretics, angiotensin-converting enzyme [ACE]-inhibitors), **P**sychological (severe depression), **E**xcess urine (↑ input; ↑ production—diuretics, EtOH, ↑ glucose, ↑ calcium; mobilized peripheral edema), **R**estricted mobility (arthritis, pain, gait disorders), **S**tool impaction.

Points in the history *Urgency* (the abrupt need to void or a spontaneous emptying of the bladder without warning) suggests detrusor overactivity. Leakage during stress maneuvers (e.g., coughing, laughing, sneezing) suggests reduced urethral resistance. Prostatism suggests obstruction. Ask about other medical illnesses—cancer, diabetes mellitus (DM), urinary tract infections (UTIs), H/O pelvic radiotherapy (XRT). A 2–7-d voiding diary is useful, both to understand the pattern of incontinence and as a baseline to compare treatment outcomes. The patient should record the time, volume, situation, and associated symptoms whenever urine is passed.

Physical examination A comprehensive physical examination is vital. Look for abnormal affect, functional impairment (e.g., ↓ mobility, vision, etc), congestive heart failure (CHF), orthostasis, peripheral edema, atrophic vaginitis. Test perianal sensation and reflexes (anal wink, S4–5; bulbocavernosus, S2–4). Do a rectal exam for resting and voluntary anal tone, fecal impaction, and prostate enlargement. The cough stress test is useful (especially in women). Check the postvoid residual (PVR) by in/out, "straight" catheter, or ultrasound estimation after a voluntary void (normal: <50–100 mL).

Investigations Chemistry panel, Ca^{2+}, urinalysis, and culture. In selected patients, consider renal US, urine cytology, urodynamic studies.

Treatment is aimed at the cause. Specific measures may include altered timing of medications, compression stockings during the day to reduce nocturnal mobilization of edema, and behavioral techniques such as frequent voiding (e.g., q2–3h; refer to the voiding diary for guidance) to avoid bladder overdistension and involuntary contraction. Pelvic floor or "Kegel" exercises (voluntary contraction of the external urethral sphincter for 10 sec × ~50/d) can help stress incontinence in women. Drugs with anticholinergic or α-adrenergic antagonist activity may be useful (see Table 16.2). Surgery, prostheses (e.g., penile clamps), intravaginal pessaries, external collecting devices (indwelling or condom catheters), and absorbent pads are reserved for refractory incontinence.

Complications Perineal rash, decubitus ulcers, indwelling catheters and UTIs, social stigmatization, anxiety/depression, ↓ sexual activity, institutionalization.

Drugs for urinary incontinence Start with the lowest dose, then titrate up until symptoms improve or intolerable side effects develop. The expected benefits are small.

Table 16.2 Medications For the Treatment of Urinary Incontinence

Detrusor overactivity:	
Propantheline	7.5–30 mg PO 3–4 times a day
Oxybutynin	2.5–5 mg PO 3–4 times a day
Imipramine	25–50 mg PO 1–3 times a day
Tolterodine	1–2 mg PO bid
Darifenacin	7.5–15 mg PO daily
Fesoterodine	4–8 mg PO daily
Solifenacin	5–10 mg PO daily
Trospium	20 mg PO bid
Stress incontinence:	
Phenylpropanolamine	25–50 mg PO 2–3 times a day
Outlet obstruction	
Prazosin	1–2 mg PO 2–4 times a day
Phenoxybenzamine	5–10 mg PO daily (for short-term use only)
Tamsulosin	0.4 mg PO daily
Dutasteride	0.5 mg PO daily
Doxazosin	1–8 mg PO daily
Terazosin	1–10 mg PO daily
Alfuzosin	10 mg PO daily
Silodosin	8 mg PO daily
Finasteride	5 mg PO daily

Polypharmacy

Geriatric patients disproportionately consume prescription and nonprescription medications. Additionally, geriatric patients have poorer tolerance for adverse drug effects and more commonly suffer from the harms of medications than their younger counterparts. Thus, trying to minimize the total number of drugs consumed is both a laudable and formidable goal.

Drugs that should be avoided because safer alternatives exist include cyclo-oxygenase (COX)-2 inhibitors and non-COX-specific NSAIDs and meperidine. Benzodiazepines and nonbenzodiazepine sleeping agents should be avoided for insomnia as they substantially increase the risks of falls and confusion. Drugs to treat Alzheimer's disease (AD) have demonstrated little, if any, meaningful clinical benefit; their use should be considered carefully as a trial in an individual. Atypical antipsychotics do not offer benefit over older, less expensive agents for behavioral problems in dementia. Finally, any new drug must also be very carefully considered. In seeking FDA approval for release, most drugs have not been tested on the average geriatric patient with multiple comorbidities and medications. Most certainly, they have not been tested on the frailest elderly. Only after a drug has been on the market and used in large numbers of "average" people do many of the serious toxicities become apparent. Many elderly are seriously injured as the result of new medications. Adhere to the adage, "start low, go slow" with any new medicine.

Costs, ability to take, and potential toxicity are important determinants in selecting drugs. Opportunities to get "double duty" from medications should be explored. For example, a person with neuropathic pain and depression may derive good benefit from nortriptyline at bedtime for both of these problems, rather than gabapentin three times a day and an selective serotonin reuptake inhibitor (SSRI) once a day.

Finally, the selection of medications must consider the overall treatment goals for each individual and whether or not data exist that the considered medication will reasonably further those goals.

Examination of mental state

The examination of cognitive functions is important in every patient. Much can be accomplished by careful observation during the course of the history and physical examination. For more detailed assessment of specific cognitive functions, you should have a set of questions (and tasks) with which to test the patient. Use these whenever an altered mental state is contributing to the clinical problem. A description of each of the tests performed, and the patient's response, is more useful for the clinical record than a "score" on a question set. Before starting, tell the patient that you are going to test his thinking. Reassure him that it is a standard part of the examination.

Components of the mental state examination

Level of arousal: E.g., alert, drowsy, asleep but responds to voice/touch/gentle shake/pain. Rouses for x seconds, then falls back to sleep.

Orientation: Ask the patient's name, the place where you are located, and the time (day of the week, date, month, year, season).

Attention: Recite months of the year forward and backward. If unable, try days of the week, the word "world."

Memory: Distant: Names of children, where they grew up, jobs. *Recent:* Describe news events, details of recent illness, dinner last night. *Learning:* Give three objects to remember (e.g., "glass, a duck, and a shoe"). Make sure they can repeat them without prompting after a 30 sec delay without distractions. Ask them again in 3–5 min (don't forget!).

Speech: Fluency, naming, repetition, comprehension.

Calculation: Serial 7's. How many quarters in $1.50? Nickels in $1.10? Simple addition, multiplication, etc.

Reading: Read aloud (e.g., lunch menu), then describe what they read.

Writing: Write a sentence, e.g., about the weather.

Construction: Draw the numbers inside a circle as if it were a clock. Copy intersecting pentagons. Copy a cube.

Left/right discrimination:

Praxis: Salute. Pretend to comb, roll dice, deal a pack of cards.

"Frontal" functions: Copy a sequence of three hand movements; *Go/No-go task:* "Every time I tap my hand twice, you tap once. When I tap once, you do nothing." *Word lists:* "In one minute, tell me all of the words that you can think of that begin with the letter *F.*"

Cortical sensation: Graphesthesia: Ask the patient to identify numbers, drawn in each palm. *Stereognosis:* Identify objects (e.g., comb, quarter, nickel, pen) placed in each hand without looking. *Note:* These terms refer to normal functions. "Agraphesthesia" and "astereognosis" are abnormal.

Sometimes a complex multidimensional question can be used as a screening test for cognitive dysfunction. For example:

"Pretend that you are looking at a clock. The little hand is on the 7 and the big hand is on the 3. What time will it be in 15 minutes?"

A correct response on this task ("7:30") requires many faculties, including attention, language comprehension, calculation, visual memory, and construction. In selected patients, in whom mental state is not the issue, this may be sufficient to satisfy yourself that there are no gross cognitive abnormalities. Never document that the mental status is normal unless you have tested it.

Approach to dementia

An altered mental state is due to a treatable illness until proved otherwise. Dementia is not a part of normal aging. It is a syndrome—with many causes—of progressive impairment of cognition with the preservation of clear consciousness.

Clinical features The key to diagnosis is a good history (usually requiring an informant) of progressive impairment of memory and other cognitive functioning, together with objective evidence of such impairment. The history should go back at least several months and usually years. Typically, the patient has become increasingly forgetful and has performed normal tasks (e.g., cooking, shopping, finances, work) with reduced competence. Sometimes the patient appears to have changed personality (e.g., uncharacteristically rude or aggressive).

Points in the history:
- Baseline personality, education, profession
- Duration of illness
- Onset (abrupt or insidious)
- Comorbid disease
- Past medical history: Poor nutrition, head trauma, depression or other psychiatric illness
- Medications (including PRNs)
- Toxins (occupational, EtOH)

- Risk factors for infections(HIV, syphilis)
- Family history of depression, dementia, or other degenerative disease

Epidemiology Incidence increases with age. Very rare in those <55 yrs. 5–10% prevalence >65; up to 50% >85. In the United States, there are ~4 million people with AD, at a cost of ~$90 billion/yr.

Causes Definitive diagnosis requires a pathological specimen (biopsy or autopsy). Premorbid diagnoses are often mistaken. *AD* is the most common cause of dementia (55–70% of all cases). *Vascular dementia* comprises 5–25% of all cases; essentially, multiple small strokes. Usually evidence of vasculopathy (high BP, previous strokes); sometimes of focal neurological damage. Onset sometimes sudden, and deterioration may be "stepwise." Optimize vascular risk factors to try to prevent further progression of disease. *Lewy body disease* is characterized by Lewy bodies in the brainstem and cortex. There are fluctuating but persisting cognitive deficits, parkinsonism, and hallucinations.

Less common causes HIV (*not uncommon* in those known to have HIV), progressive multifocal leukoencephalopathy, Pick's disease, progressive supranuclear palsy, Parkinson's disease, Jakob-Creutzfeldt disease, Huntington's disease, Wernicke-Korsakoff disease.

Initial assessment *For all patients with progressive dementia:* Careful history (as above); CNS exam (including mental state); CBC, erythrocyte sedimentation rate (ESR), chemistry, thyroid-stimulating hormone (TSH), B$_{12}$, syphilis serology, drug levels; computed tomography (CT) or magnetic resonance imaging (MRI) of the brain. *For selected patients:* Neuropsychology testing, psychiatric examination, electroencephalogram (EEG), HIV testing, liver profile (LP), toxic screen.

Management Treat any treatable cause. Treat concurrent illnesses (these may contribute significantly to confusion). In most people, the dementia remains and will progress. Involve relatives and social services.

Potentially treatable dementias The frequency of reversible dementias that present to memory specialists is somewhere between 0% and 30%. The reason to investigate dementia is to find one of the causes that can be fixed.

Drug toxicity: Check *all* medications.

Chronic metabolic disturbance: Organ failure (heart, kidney, liver, lungs), Wilson's disease, obstructive sleep apnea, dialysis encephalopathy (?aluminum toxicity), heavy metals (e.g., lead).

Normal pressure hydrocephalus is thought to be due to impaired cerebrospinal fluid (CSF) absorption, causing dementia, gait apraxia, and urinary incontinence. Disproportionately large ventricles on CT/MRI. Diagnosis is difficult to confirm, although *some* patients benefit from CSF shunts (e.g., ventriculoperitoneal). Good prognosticators for response to shunting include short duration of symptoms, more prominent gait disorder than dementia, known etiology (e.g., history of subarachnoid hemorrhage, head trauma), altered CSF dynamics (with invasive monitoring).

Intracranial mass: Tumors (especially meningiomas), subdural hematoma.

Infection: Syphilis, Lyme, chronic meningitis (tuberculosis [TB], fungal, parasitic).

Connective tissue disease: SLE, sarcoidosis, primary angiitis of the CNS and other vasculitides.

Endocrine: Hypo-/hyperthyroidism, parathyroid, adrenal and pituitary disease, insulinoma.

Nutritional: Deficiencies of B$_{12}$, nicotinamide (pellagra), thiamine.

Psychiatric: Pseudodementia of depression.

Alzheimer dementia

This is often considered the worst neuropsychiatric disorder of our times. Suspect AD in adults with any persistent, acquired deficit of memory and cognition; e.g., as revealed in the mental test score and other neuropsychometric tests. Onset may be from 40 yrs (or earlier; e.g., in Down's syndrome), so the notions of "senile" and "presenile" dementia are irrelevant.

Diagnosis is often haphazard. Specialist assessment with neuroimaging for all would be ideal (this would help rule out frontal lobe and Lewy body dementias, and Pick's disease).

Histology (rarely used)
- Deposition of β–amyloid protein in cortex (a few patients have mutations in the amyloid precursor protein)
- Neurofibrillary tangles and an increased number of senile plaques

Presentation Early (stage I) in AD, there is failing memory and spatial disorientation. In stage II (follows after several years), personality changes (e.g., increased aggression and focal parietal signs—dysphasia, apraxia, agnosia, and acalculia). Parkinsonism may occur. In stage III, the patient becomes apathetic, wasted, bedridden, and incontinent. Seizures and spasticity are common. **Mean survival** 7 yrs from onset.

Management *Theoretical issues:* Potential strategies:
- Preventing the breakdown of acetylcholine (e.g., donepezil; see below)
- Augmenting nerve growth factor (NGF), which is taken up at nerve endings and promotes nerve cell repair
- Stimulating nicotinic receptors that may protect nerve cells
- Inhibiting the enzymes that snip-out β–amyloid peptide from amyloid precursor protein (APP), so preventing fibrils and plaques
- Using anti-inflammatories to prevent activation of microglial cells to secrete neurotoxins (e.g., glutamate, cytokines), which stimulates formation of APP
- Regulating calcium entry (mediates the damage of neurotoxins)
- Preventing oxidative damage by free radicals

Practical issues: Treat concurrent illnesses (they contribute significantly to confusion). In most people, the dementia remains and will progress. Involve relatives and community services.

Consult with an expert; if the dementia is mild or moderate, consider increasing acetylcholine availability by inhibiting acetylcholinesterase (e.g., donepezil 5 mg PO every night at bedtime; increasing to 10 mg after 1 month). Effects may be minimal, but subtle cognitive changes can cause significant behavioral improvement even without "objective" improvement in bedside tests of cognition. The need for institutional care may be delayed.

Prevention There are no clear ways to avoid this disease. Hormone replacement therapy (HRT) and controlling vascular risk factors may offer some protection.

651

Preventive geriatrics

Although even the most fit elderly will have continued declines in most organ systems with aging, evidence clearly supports that exercise can ameliorate many of these losses substantially and help preserve function and independence. It may help improve range of movement and decrease pain associated with knee osteoarthritis. It has been shown to both treat osteoporosis and, in retrospective studies, prevent it. Exercise, particularly exercises that incorporate some aspect of balance training, have been shown to reduce falls, even in high-risk individuals. As with their younger counterparts, exercise may lower BP and favorably alter lipid profiles. Clearly, the most fit individuals tend to have the longest life expectancy and longest period of functional independence. Epidemiologic studies demonstrate that improving fitness state is associated with beneficial effects on mortality, even when this change is enacted in older age.

Although the best exercise regimen has not been firmly established, most elderly are remarkably sedentary and will gain substantially simply from reducing their inactivity by altering lifestyle. Examples of this include watching less television, taking the stairs rather than the elevator, parking farther away from the entrance of stores, and walking up and down every aisle in the grocery store. Walking is an inexpensive exercise that has functional relevance. The physician may assist in improving fitness by endorsing exercise and identifying barriers and facilitators to exercise with patients.

Most authorities endorse screening examinations for older individuals similar to those of younger individuals when the projected life expectancy is >10 yrs and when such screening (and subsequent decisions based on the results) is consistent with the overall goals of care of the individual. Although accurate prognosis is extremely difficult in patients with severe chronic conditions that exacerbate and remit, some evidence suggests that most physicians tend to underestimate life expectancy in the elderly when considering these decisions. Be particularly cautious of the risk of ageism. For example, the life expectancy of an 85-yr-old woman who is in the top quartile of functional status is nearly 10 yrs. Screening decisions about patients with cognitive impairment are particularly vexing and must take into careful consideration the ability of the patient to participate in the testing, the risks of such testing, the ability of the patient to undergo treatments if a disease is found, and, most important of all, the overarching goals of care. Prevention of injury in the elderly would include assessment for falls; discussions about firearms, particularly if a demented individual is in the home; use of seat belts in cars; evaluation for continued ability to drive; and home safety assessment.

Smoking cessation reduces the risk of lung cancer at any age. Although not proven for primary prevention of coronary artery disease (CAD), it continues to have an important role in prevention of MI in patients with established CAD. Thus, cessation of smoking is important to endorse and encourage even in the elderly.

Finally, several periodic immunizations are advised in the elderly, although their benefits for all subgroups is often debated. Pneumococcal vaccination is recommended at least once over the age of 65 yrs, with consideration of revaccination in certain subgroups. Influenza vaccination is advised annually for all elderly; although likely the most effect approach to preventing influenza in nursing homes is to aggressively immunize staff. Periodic (every 10 yrs) revaccination for tetanus is also advised. Vaccination to prevent shingles is now advised once in a lifetime >50 yrs.

Biochemistry

Paul E. Segal, D.O. and Joshua D. King, M.D.

Contents

On being normal in the society of numbers

Laboratory medicine reduces our patients to a few easy-to-handle numbers: This is the discipline's great attraction—and its greatest danger. The normal range (reference interval) is usually that which includes 95% of patients. If variation is randomly distributed, 2.5% of our results will be "too high" and 2.5% "too low" when dealing with apparently normal people using this statistical definition of normality. Other definitions may be *normative*—i.e., stating what an upper or lower limit *should* be (see Table 17.1). For example, the upper end of the reference interval for low-density lipoprotein (LDL) cholesterol may be given as 130 mg/dL because this is what preventative cardiologists state to be the *desired* maximum, although the risk of coronary heart disease (CHD) increases above 100 mg/dL (and even 70 mg/dL). The World Health Organization (WHO) definition of anemia in pregnancy is an Hgb of <11 g/dL, which makes 20% of mothers anemic. This "lax" criterion has the presumed benefit of triggering actions that result in fewer deaths by hemorrhage. So do not just ask "What is the normal range?"; also question who set the range, for what population, and for what reason.

Table 17.1 The essence of laboratory medicine

Only do a test if the result will influence management. Make sure you look at the result! Explain to the patient where this test fits into his or her overall plan of management. Do not interpret laboratory results except in the light of clinical assessment.

If there is disparity, trust clinical judgement and repeat the test.

Reference intervals (normal ranges) are usually defined as the interval, symmetrical about the mean, containing 95% of results on the population studied. The more tests you run, the greater the probability of an "abnormal" result of no clinical significance.

Artifacts Delayed analysis for plasma potassium

Anion gap (AG) Reflects unmeasured anions (e.g., lactate, uremic toxins, organic acids)

Biochemistry results: Major disease patterns ($\uparrow$ = raised, $\downarrow$ = lowered)

Hypovolemia: Urea$\uparrow$, albumin$\uparrow$ (useful to plot change in a patient's condition). Hematocrit (PCV)$\uparrow$, creatinine$\uparrow$; also urine volume$\downarrow$; skin turgor$\downarrow$

Renal failure: Creatinine$\uparrow$, urea$\uparrow$, AG$\uparrow$, $K^+\uparrow$, $PO_4^{3-}\uparrow$, $HCO_3^-\downarrow$

Diuretic use	Loop	Thiazide	K⁺-sparing
Serum Na^+	Normal, $\uparrow$	$\downarrow$	Normal, $\downarrow$
Serum K^+	$\downarrow$	$\downarrow$	$\uparrow$
Serum HCO_3^-	$\uparrow$	$\uparrow$	$\downarrow$
Serum Ca^{2+}	$\downarrow$	$\uparrow$	Normal, $\downarrow$
Serum Mg^{2+}	$\downarrow$	$\downarrow$	$\uparrow$
Serum uric acid	$\uparrow$	$\uparrow$	$\uparrow$

Bone disease	Ca^{2+}	PO_4^{3-}	Alk phos
Osteoporosis	Normal	Normal	Normal
Osteomalacia	$\downarrow$	$\downarrow$	$\uparrow$
Paget's	Normal	Normal	$\uparrow\uparrow$
Myeloma	$\uparrow$	$\uparrow$, Normal	Normal
Bone metastases	$\uparrow$	$\uparrow$,Normal	$\uparrow$
1° Hyperparathyroidism	$\uparrow$	$\downarrow$, Normal	Normal, $\uparrow$
Hypoparathyroidism	$\downarrow$	$\uparrow$	Normal
Renal failure (low glomerular filtration rate;GFR)	$\downarrow$	$\uparrow$	Normal, $\uparrow$

Hepatocellular disease Bilirubin$\uparrow$, aspartate aminotransferase (AST)$\uparrow$ (alk phos slightly $\uparrow$, albumin $\downarrow$)

Cholestasis: Bilirubin$\uparrow$, γ-glutamyl transpeptidase (GGT)$\uparrow\uparrow$, alk phos$\uparrow\uparrow$, AST$\uparrow$

Myocardial infarct (MI): AST$\uparrow$, lactate dehydrogenase (LDH)$\uparrow$, creatine kinase (CK)$\uparrow$, troponin T/I $\uparrow$

Diabetes mellitus: Glucose$\uparrow$ (bicarbonate$\downarrow$ and AG$\uparrow$ if diabetic ketoacidosis)

Addison's disease: Potassium$\uparrow$, sodium$\downarrow$

Cushing's syndrome: May show potassium$\downarrow$, bicarbonate$\uparrow$, sodium$\uparrow$

Hyperaldosteronism: May present with potassium$\downarrow$, bicarbonate$\uparrow$ (and high blood pressure [BP]); sodium normal or $\uparrow$

(Continued)

Table 17.1 (Continued)

Diabetes insipidus (DI): Sodium↑, plasma osmolality↑, urine osmolality ↓ (both hypercalcemia and hypokalemia may cause nephrogenic DI)

Inappropriate antidiuretic hormone (ADH) secretion: Na$^+$↓ with normal or low urea and creatinine, plasma osmolality↓; urine osmolality ↑ (can be > than plasma osmolality), urine Na ↑ (>20 mmol/L)

Excess alcohol intake: Evidence of hepatocellular disease. Early evidence in GGT ↑, mean cellular volume (MCV)↑, ethanol in blood before lunch

Some immunodeficiency states: Normal serum albumin but *low* total protein (low as immunoglobulins are missing—also making cross-matching difficult because expected hemagglutinins are absent)

Life-threatening biochemical derangements (See pp. 657–658).

The laboratory and ward tests

Laboratory staff like to have contact with you. Consult with a clinical pathologist for unusual or uncommon laboratory tests; their input may be invaluable.

10 tips to better laboratory results

1 Interest someone from the laboratory in your patient's problem.
2 Fill in the request form fully.
3 Give clinical details, not your preferred diagnosis.
4 Ensure that the lab knows who to contact.
5 Label specimens as well as the request form.
6 Follow the hospital labeling routine for cross-matching.
7 Find out when analyzers run, especially batched assays.
8 Talk with the lab before requesting an unusual test.
9 Be thoughtful: Don't "shoot the messenger."
10 Plot results graphically: Abnormalities show sooner (see Table 17.2).

Artifacts and pitfalls in laboratory tests

- Do not take blood sample from an arm that has IV fluid running into it.
- Repeat any unexpected result before acting on it.
- For clotting time, do not sample from a heparinized IV catheter.
- Serum K$^+$ is overestimated if sample is old or hemolyzed (this occurs if venipuncture is difficult).
- If using Vacutainers, fill *plain* tubes first; otherwise, anticoagulant contamination from previous tubes can cause errors.
- Total calcium results are affected by albumin concentration.
- International normalized ratio (INR) may be overestimated if citrate bottle is underfilled.
- Drugs may cause *analytic* errors (e.g., prednisolone cross-reacts with cortisol). Be suspicious if results are unexpected.
- Food may affect result (e.g., bananas raise urinary hydroxyindoleacetic acid [HIAA]).

656

Using urine dipsticks Store dipsticks in a closed container in a cool, unrefrigerated place. If improperly stored, or past expiration date, do not use. For urine tests, dip the dipstick briefly in urine, run edge of strip along container, and hold strip horizontally. Read at the specified time—check instructions for the type of stick.

Urine specific gravity (SG) can be measured by dipstick. It is not a good measure of osmolality. Causes of low SG (<1.003) are DI, water diuresis.

Causes of high SG (>1.025) are hypovolemia, diabetes mellitus, adrenal insufficiency, liver disease, heart failure.

Sources of error in interpreting dipstick results

Bilirubin: False positive: Phenothiazines. False negative: Urine not fresh, rifampicin.

Urobilinogen: False negative: Urine not fresh. (Normally present in urine due to metabolism of bilirubin in the gut by bacteria and subsequent absorption).

Ketones: L-dopa affects color (can give false-positive). β-hydroxybutyrate gives a false-negative result.

Blood: False-positive: Myoglobin, profuse bacterial growth. False-negative: Ascorbic acid.

Urine glucose: Depends on test. Pads with glucose oxidase are not affected by other reducing sugars (unlike Clinitest®) but can give false-positive to peroxide, chlorine; and false-negative with ascorbic acid, salicylate, L-dopa.

Protein: Highly alkaline urine can give false-positive.

Blood glucose: Sticks use enzymatic method and are glucose specific. A major source of error is applying too little blood (a large drop to cover the pad is necessary) and poor timing. Reflectance meters increase precision but introduce new sources of error.

Table 17.2 Laboratory results: When to take action NOW

- On receiving a dangerous result, first check the name and date.
- Go to the bedside. If the patient is conscious, turn off any IVF (until fluid is checked: A mistake may have been made) and ask the patient how he or she is. *Any seizures, syncope, or unexpected symptoms?*
- Be skeptical of an unexpected wildly abnormal result with a well patient. Could the specimens be mixed up? Is there an artifact? Was the sample taken from the "drip" arm? A low calcium may be due to a low albumin. Perhaps the lab is using a new analyzer with a faulty wash cycle? *When in doubt, repeat the test.*

The values chosen below are somewhat arbitrary and must be taken as a guide only. Many results less extreme than those below will be just as dangerous if the patient is elderly, immunosuppressed, or has some other pathology, such as pneumonia.

Plasma biochemistry Beware electrocardiological ± central nervous system (CNS) events (e.g., seizures)

Calcium (corrected for albumin) >13 mg/dL: If shortening QT interval on electrocardiogram (ECG) or symptoms, then dangerous hypercalcemia.

Calcium (corrected for albumin) <7.5 mg/dL + symptoms such as tetany or long QT: *Dangerous hypocalcemia.*

Magnesium <1.5 mg/dL + ventricular arrhythmia or long QT: *Dangerous hypomagnesemia.*

Phosphorus <1 mg/dL or <2 mg/dL + symptoms of muscular weakness: *Dangerous hypophosphatemia.*

Glucose <60 mg/dL: *Hypoglycemia. Glucose 50 mL 50% IV if symptoms; can give oral glucose if asymptomatic.*

Glucose >400 mg/dL: *Severe hyperglycemia. Is parenteral insulin needed?*

Potassium <2.5 mEq/L: *Dangerous hypokalemia, especially if on digoxin.*

Potassium >6.5 mEq/L: *Dangerous hyperkalemia.*

Sodium <120 mEq/L: *Dangerous hyponatremia.*

Sodium >155 mEq/L: *Dangerous hypernatremia.*

657

(Continued)

Blood gases

PaO$_2$ <60 mm Hg: Severe hypoxia. Give O$_2$.

pH <7.1: Dangerous acidemia.

pH >7.55: Dangerous alkalemia.

Hematology results

Hbg <7 g/dL with low mean cell volume (<75 fL) or history of bleeding: This patient may need urgent transfusion (no spare capacity).

Neutrophils <1,000/µL: Dangerous neutropenia. *Treat any fever as an emergency and give early antibiotic therapy.*

Platelets <40 × 10^9/L: *May need a platelet transfusion; consult a hematologist.*

Plasmodium falciparum seen: Start antimalarials now; consult infectious diseases.

CSF results

>1 neutrophil/mm^3: Consider meningitis.

Positive Gram stain: Talk to a microbiologist; urgent broad-spectrum therapy.

Conflicting, equivocal, or inexplicable results Get prompt help; repeat test.

IV fluid therapy

There are three reasons to use intravenous fluids (IVFs): To prevent volume depletion and hypotension, to maintain normal plasma osmolality, and to replace ongoing losses/match insensible losses if the patient is unable to keep up with oral fluids (see Table 17.3). There are only *two* instances to use *both* IVF therapy and diuretics: **Hypercalcemia** (*only* use loop diuretics after repletion of intravascular volume or symptomatic fluid overload) and **Rhabdomyolysis** (*only* use loop diuretics if evidence of volume overload).

Principles of IVF therapy

- Pay careful attention to intake, output, and *daily* morning weights.
- Always evaluate *daily* whether IVF should be continued:
  - *What are your goals?* Does lab data and exam support the continued need for IVF? Does the patient have evidence of extracellular fluid excess or depletion on exam? Does the patient have an inability to access oral fluids (decreased mental status or debility preventing access)?
- *Maintenance IVF therapy:* Replaces *normal* ongoing losses (see insensible losses below). It is used when a patient is unable to drink (postoperative states or ventilator use). Water losses lead to ↑ serum sodium, stimulating thirst and ↑ ADH. A patient with access to water will typically *not* become hypernatremic.
- Typical maintenance IVF regimen consists of:
  - Total fluid requirements per day = 2,000 mL/d = IVF at ~ 84 mL/h.
  - *Which fluid to use?* Total Na requirements per day = 50–150 mEq/d (77 mEq Na/L = ½ isotonic fluid = 0.45% normal saline (NS) if not volume depleted or with large ongoing fluid losses. Total K requirements per day = 20–60 mEq/d = addition of 20 mEq KCL/L of IVF. *KCL should not be added if there are concerns for acute kidney injury or worsening renal failure.* Addition of dextrose to prevent ketosis = D$_5$W. *Example of maintenance IVF: D$_5$W 0.45% NS with 20 mEq KCL/L @ 84 mL/h.*

- *The original solution may need to be modified* if there is increased GI or third-space losses (sequestration of fluid in a body compartment *not* equilibrated with the extracellular fluid [ECF]). This may require a change to 0.9% NS. If serum sodium falls, use a *more concentrated* solution (NS), or, if serum sodium rises secondary to increased insensible losses, use a *more dilute* solution (¼ NS or D_5W); see Table 17.4.
- *Daily fluid balance:* Normal intake: 2–2.9 L/d. Ingested fluids = 1–1.5 L/d. Water from food = 1 L/d. Water from oxidation (of carbohydrates) = 300–400 mL/d.

Normal output: 2–2.7 L/d. Urine output = 1–1.5 L/d. Insensible losses: Losses of fluid from skin, respiratory and GI tract. Normal insensible losses = 500–800 mL/d.

Fever, excessive sweating, burns, drains, increased GI losses and can increase insensible losses. For each degree >37°C, water loss increases by 100–150 mL/d.

- *Replacement therapy:* Corrects existing water and electrolyte deficits in excess of normal losses (e.g., nasogastric tube, vomiting, diarrhea, drains)
- The volume deficit may be estimated based on the change between pre-morbid and current weight.
- Rate of replacement depends on the degree of hypovolemia. If the patient has shock, this is best treated by bolus therapy (i.e., 200–250 mL or 3 mL/kg over 5 min of 0.9% NS (total of 1–2 L of 0.9% NS IV over 30 min to 1 h.
- Choice of replacement fluid; see Table 17.4.
- *Colloids:* Given their large size, tend to stay in the intravascular space. Albumin administration is safe *except* in traumatic brain injury. The "rule" of 3–4 mL of crystalloid to 1 mL of colloid for fluid resuscitation needs to be re-evaluated in clinical trials. Hydroxyethyl starch and dextrans may carry a risk of bleeding and acute kidney injury.

Table 17.3 Examples of fluid replacement based on total fluid requirements

For each kilogram	100:50:20 Rule (daily requirements)	4:2:1 Rule (Holliday and Segar)(hourly requirements)
1st 10 kg	100 mL	4 mL/h
2nd 10 kg	50 mL	2 mL/h
For each kg >20 kg	20 mL/kg	1 mL/h
Example: 70 kg person	1st 10 kg × 100 mL = 1,000 mL 2nd 10 kg × 50 mL = 500 mL 50 kg × 20 mL = 1,000 mL Total = 2,500 mL ÷ 24 h = 104 mL/h	1st 10 kg × 4 mL/h = 40 mL/h 2nd 10 kg × 2 mL/h = 20 mL/h 50 kg × 1 mL/h = 50 mL/h Total = 110 mL/h

Table 17.4 Replacement fluids

Soln	Glu	Na	K	CL	Ca²⁺	HCO₃⁻	Lactate	Osm
D₅W	50[a]	0	0	0	0	0	0	252
LR[b]	0	130	4	109	3	[c]	28	275
0.9%NS	0	154	0	154	0	0	0	308
3% Saline	0	513	0	513	0	0	0	1026

Glucose (g/dL), Na, K, Cl, Ca2+, HCO₃⁻ and Lactate units are mEq/L
[a] 1 g of glucose = ~4 calories
[b] LR, lactated Ringer's; NS, normal saline
[c] Lactate acts as a source of bicarbonate when normal production and utilization of lactic acid is not impaired (adjusted pH of solution = 6.6–6.75).

Acid-base balance

Arterial blood pH is closely regulated as processes necessary for life are pH sensitive and cannot occur outside a range of body fluid pH of 6.8–7.8. The carbonic acid (H_2CO_3): bicarbonate (HCO_3^-) buffer system is the most relevant clinically and is regulated by both the kidneys (which regulate HCO_3^-) and the lungs (which regulate CO_2).

How to approach an arterial blood gas (ABG)

Use the *Henderson-Hasselbalch equation* to determine the pH (and consistency) of the data. Arterial pH = $6.1 + \log [HCO_3^-] / 0.03 \times CO_2$

Evaluate the pH: *Acidemia* refers to the pH level, versus *acidosis*, which refers to the process. Simultaneously measure an ABG and electrolytes. Normal pH = 7.36–7.44. A pH <7.35 is acidemia and a pH >7.45 is alkalemia. A normal pH does *not* rule out an acid-base disorder.

Respiratory disorders: pH, HCO_3^-, and CO_2 move in *opposite directions*. Normal CO_2 = 35–45 mm Hg.

Metabolic disorders: pH, HCO_3^-, and CO_2 move in the *same direction*. Normal HCO_3^- = 22–26 mEq/L. The HCO_3^- recorded on the ABG is calculated from the Henderson-Hasselbalch equation from the ratio of CO_2/HCO_3^-. The HCO_3^- on a basic metabolic panel is measured as the total CO_2 (includes *dissolved* CO_2) and is ~1.2 mEq/L greater than calculated CO_2

Primary changes in HCO_3^- are termed *metabolic*, whereas primary changes in CO_2 are termed *respiratory*.

Calculate the *AG* and, if elevated, calculate an *osmolar gap* if toxic alcohol ingestion is suspected. Osmolar gap = measured – calculated. Calculated osmolality = $2 \times Na^+$ + blood urea nitrogen (BUN)/2.8 + glucose/18. Normal osmolar gap = (-) 10 to (+) 10 with a normal plasma osmolality = 285–295 mOsm/L. *A normal osmolar gap does not rule out toxic alcohol ingestion.* Note: *Early* in toxic alcohol ingestion, the AG will be mildly elevated and the osmolar gap will be *high*; *Late* in a toxic alcohol ingestion, the AG will be *high*, and the osmolar gap may be mildly elevated. See Table 17.5.

Differential diagnosis of an elevated AG is listed below under metabolic acidosis.

Check the degree of compensation (Table 17.6):

Determine the "delta-delta" or delta AG/delta HCO_3^- ratio (see example below). This allows you to determine if a non-AG metabolic acidosis or metabolic alkalosis is present in addition to an AG metabolic acidosis.

Table 17.5 Differential diagnosis of an elevated osmolar gap based on AG category

Low AG	Normal AG	High AG
Lithium	Isopropanol (isopropyl alcohol)	Methanol
	Glycine	Ethylene glycol
	Mannitol	Diethylene glycol
	Severe hypertriglyceridemia (TG >1,500 mg/dL)	Propylene glycol
		Ethanol (ETOH)
		End-stage renal disease
		Diabetic ketoacidosis

Table 17.6 Degree of compensation

Disorder	Compensation
Metabolic acidosis	$CO_2 = 1.5 \times HCO_3^- + 8 \pm 2$ (Winter's formula)
	$CO_2 = HCO_3^- + 15$
Metabolic alkalosis	$CO_2 = \uparrow 0.5$–0.7 mm Hg for each 1 mEq $\uparrow$ HCO_3^-
	$CO_2 = HCO_3^- + 15$
	$CO_2 = 0.7*([\text{measured } HCO_3^-]-24) + 40$

Metabolic acidosis Primary disturbance is a decreased pH and HCO_3^-. Overproduction (or ingestion) of a fixed acid or loss of base will produce a decrease in arterial pH (acidemia) and HCO_3^- will be used to *buffer* the extra fixed acid, resulting in a decrease in arterial HCO_3^-. The development of acidemia will lead to *hyperventilation*, which provides the respiratory compensation (by lowering the CO_2) to decrease the initial *fall* in pH.

Metabolic acidosis is further divided into either increased (high) AG metabolic acidosis or normal AG (hyperchloremic, due to the $\uparrow$ in CL^-) metabolic acidosis by calculating the AG:

$AG = [Na^+ - (CL^- + HCO_3^-)]$ with a normal range of 8 ± 4 (if ion selective electrodes are used). In healthy individuals, the AG is 11 ± 2.5 mEq/L[1] AG is an estimate of *unmeasured anions*. It is important to know what the patient's normal AG is prior to the development of an acidosis. Individual's *maximum AG* = (albumin × 2.5) + phos × 0.5).

Clinical pearl: Always correct the AG for albumin (major source of unmeasured anions). The AG decreases ~2.5 mEq/L for every 1.0 g/dL decrease in albumin from normal. *Example:* AG = 12 and serum albumin = 2.0 gm/dL. Normal serum albumin minus measured serum albumin = 4.0 - 2.0 = 2.0 × 2.5 = 5 mEq/L. You **add** 5 mEq/L to the current AG of 12 = 17 (corrected AG). See Table 17.7.

661

1 Kraut JA, Madias NE. Serum anion gap: Its uses and limitations in clinical medicine. *Clin J Am Soc Nephrol.* 2007;2:162–174.

Table 17.7 Differential diagnosis of an AG

Low	Normal/ Hyperchloremic Mnemonic = **HARDUP**	Elevated Mnemonic = **GOLDMARK**[*]
Lab error	**H** = Hyperventilation/ Hyperalimentation	**G** = Glycols (ethylene, propylene)
Hypoalbuminemia	**A** = Acetazolamide (carbonic anhydrase inhibitors) Addison's disease/ Amphotericin B	**O** = Oxoproline (pyroglutamic acid)
Hypercalcemia Hypermagnesemia Hyperkalemia	**R** = Renal tubular acidosis (RTA) Urine AG = Positive with distal and type 4 RTA (hyporenin-hypoaldosteronemia)	**L** = L-Lactate/Linezolid
Lithium toxicity	**D** = Diarrhea Urine AG = Negative	**D** = D-Lactate
Multiple myeloma (IgG = cationic protein)	**U** = Uretero-enteric diversion/fistula/urinary obstruction	**M** = Methanol/meds (Metformin, INH)
	P = Pancreatico- duo-denal fistula/ parenteral saline	**A** = Aspirin
		R = Renal failure **K** = Ketoacidosis (diabetic, alcoholic, or starvation)

[*]Adapted from Mehta AN, Emmett JB, Emmett M. GOLD MARK: An anion gap mnemonic for the 21st century. *Lancet*. 2008;372:892.

Example: pH = 7.2, pCO_2 = 25 mm Hg, HCO_3^- = 10 mEq/L, Na^+ = 135 mEq/L, CL^- = 100 mEq/L, glucose = 130 mg/dL, BUN = 15 mg/dL, albumin = 4.0 g/dL, measured osmolality = 290 mOsm/L.

Internal consistency via Henderson-Hasselbalch = correct (pH = 7.22).

pH <7.35 = acidemia (with *both* the pH and HCO_3^- low = Metabolic).

AG = 135 − (97 + 10) = 25 = elevated;

osmolar gap = 290 − (270 + 5 + 7) = 8 (normal).

Expected pCO_2 compensation = 1.5 × HCO_3^- + 8 ± 2 = 21–25 = Compensated.

Delta-Delta:

Typically, when a fixed acid accumulates in the extracellular fluid, the decrease in HCO_3^- is equivalent to the increase in AG (ratio 1:1).

When a non-AG (hyperchloremic) metabolic acidosis occurs with an increased AG acidosis, the decrease in HCO_3^- is greater than the increase in AG (*delta-delta <1*) = coexistent non-AG metabolic acidosis. Additionally, the chloride change equals the bicarbonate change (for every 1 mEq ↑ in chloride, the bicarbonate ↓ 1 mEq).

If the *delta-delta* is >2.0, then the decrease in HCO_3^- is less than the increase in AG = coexistent metabolic alkalosis.

From the example, delta-delta calculated by: (measured AG-8)/(normal HCO_3^- – 10) = 17/14.

Clinical pearl:

Only used when there is an already noted elevated AG metabolic acidosis.

Metabolic alkalosis

Primary disturbance is an increased pH and HCO_3^-.

Occurs either from excess base (from intake, loss of acid (H^+), or generated by kidneys) or a failure of the kidneys to excrete excess bicarbonate.

The work-up of metabolic alkalosis hinges on measurement of spot urine chloride, BP, serum potassium, plasma renin activity, and serum aldosterone. See Table 17.8.

Typically, there are two phases: *Generation* (initiation) and *maintenance*.

Respiratory acidosis

Primary disturbance is decreased **pH** and increased CO_2. Typically divided into CNS causes, neuromuscular disorders, or acute-chronic lung disease. Always consider oversedation with narcotics as a cause of respiratory acidosis. *Need to look at P_aO_2 to evaluate if oxygen therapy is needed.* See Table 17.9.

Respiratory alkalosis

Primary disturbance is increased **pH** and decreased CO_2. Typically divided into CNS causes or Other causes. *Clinical pearl:* Sepsis and salicylate intoxication can cause *both* a respiratory alkalosis and metabolic acidosis. See Table 17.9.

Table 17.8 Metabolic alkalosis

Chloride depleted saline responsive (urine chloride <15 mEq/L)	Saline unresponsive (urine chloride >15 mEq/L)
Vomiting/nasogastric tube (NGT) suction	**Current** diuretics
Prior diuretics	Primary hyperaldosteronism
Post hypercapnia	Bartter's or Gitelman's syndrome
Villous adenoma	Liddle's syndrome
Laxative abuse /chloride-rich diarrhea	Cushing's syndrome or ectopic adrenocorticotropic hormone (ACTH) production
Profound K^+ depletion	Exogenous or endogenous mineralocorticoid production (certain forms of licorice, chewing tobacco, or carbenoxolone)
Severe Mg^{++} depletion Cystic fibrosis	

Hypertension (HTN) + Metabolic Alkalosis Differential

Renin	Aldosterone	Causes
Low	Low	Glycyrrhizic acid (certain forms of licorice or chewing tobacco)
		Carbenoxolone
		Exogenous mineralocorticoids
		Liddle's syndrome
		Cushing's Syndrome
		Congenital adrenal hyperplasia
		Deoxycorticosterone (DOC) producing tumor
Low	High	Primary hyperaldosteronism
		Glucocorticoid remediable aldosteronism (GRA)
High	High	Renovascular HTN
		Malignant HTN
		Renin-secreting tumor
		Secondary Hyperaldosteronism

Table 17.9

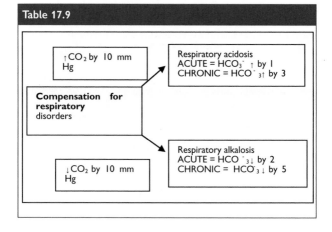

$\uparrow CO_2$ by 10 mm Hg

Compensation for respiratory disorders

Respiratory acidosis
ACUTE = HCO_3^- $\uparrow$ by 1
CHRONIC = HCO_3^- $\uparrow$ by 3

$\downarrow CO_2$ by 10 mm Hg

Respiratory alkalosis
ACUTE = HCO_3^- $\downarrow$ by 2
CHRONIC = HCO_3^- $\downarrow$ by 5

Urate and the kidney

Causes of hyperuricemia **Hyperuricemia may result from either ↑ turnover or ↓ excretion of urate. Associated conditions may include: Gout and nephrolithiasis.**

Drugs: Diuretics (both thiazide and loop diuretics), chemotherapy (cisplatin, cyclophosphamide and vincristine), alcohol, cyclosporine, low-dose salicylates, ketoconazole, ethambutol, pyrazinamide, theophylline, and levodopa.

Increased cell turnover: Lymphoma, leukemia, myeloproliferative disorders, hemolysis, rhabdomyolysis or tumor lysis syndrome (see below).

Reduced excretion: Primary hyperuricemia (± gout), chronic kidney disease (CKD), volume depletion, lead nephropathy, pre-eclampsia or toxemia of pregnancy.

Miscellaneous: G6PD deficiency, Lesch-Nyhan syndrome, metabolic syndrome.

Hyperuricemia is normally defined as a serum uric acid >7.0 mg/dL. In CKD, serum urate increases. Hyperuricemia in CKD has been defined as[3]

- >9 mg/dL for serum creatinine ≤1.5 mg/dL
- >10 mg/dL for serum creatinine of 1.5–2.0 mg/dL
- >12 mg/dL for serum creatinine of 2.1–3.0 mg/dL

There is an association between hyperuricemia and CKD. The mechanism may be inflammatory from deposition of urate crystals in the interstitium → progressive tubulointerstitial injury.

Tumor lysis syndrome (TLS) Constellation of metabolic abnormalities including hyperuricemia, hyperkalemia, hyperphosphatemia, hypocalcemia; frequently associated with acute kidney injury (AKI; see p. 277, Oncology; see p. 430; Table 17.10)

Table 17.10

Pathophysiology and risk factors
  Rapid cell breakdown post chemotherapy with release of **intracellular** contents.
  Hyperuricemia can lead to deposition of uric acid crystals within the tissues and renal tubules → AKI.
Highest risk of development: Burkitt's lymphoma, lymphoblastic lymphoma, B-cell acute lymphoblastic lymphoma, acute leukemia (especially if WBC count ≥100,000/μL)
Cairo-Bishop* definition of tumor lysis syndrome
Serum values included in the definition of laboratory TLS:
- Uric acid ≥8 mg/dL or 25% ↑ from baseline
- Potassium ≥6 mEq/L or 25% ↑ from baseline
- Phosphorus ≥4.5 mg/dL or 25% ↑ from baseline
- Calcium ≤7 mg/dL or 25% ↓ from baseline

Criteria included in the definition of clinical TLS:
- Serum creatinine ≥1.5 mg/dL greater than the value of the upper limit of the age-adjusted normal range
- Cardiac arrhythmia or sudden death
- Seizure

* **Cairo MS, Bishop M. Tumor lysis syndrome: New therapeutic strategies and classification.** *Brit J Haematol.* 2004;127(1):3–11.

665

3 Murray T and Goldberg M. Chronic Interstitial Nephritis: Etiologic Factors. *Annals of Internal Medicine.* 1975;82(4):453–459.

Treatment Prevention is the cornerstone, based on recognizing which patient population is at risk for TLS. Treatment may include:

- *Aggressive hydration* intravenously, minimum of 2–3 L/d, maintaining a urine output of 100–200 mL/h (typically started 48 h before chemotherapy).
- *Allopurinol* (a competitive inhibitor of xanthine oxidase) administered prior to the onset of chemotherapy at a dosage of 300–800 mg/d (dosage reduction if CKD or AKI).
- *Rasburicase* (recombinant urea oxidase that converts uric acid to water-soluble allantoin), IV at a dose of 0.20 mg/kg in a 30-min infusion for up to 5 d. Considered first-line therapy over allopurinol in patients at significant risk for TLS. Rasburicase typically results in a shorter time to control of uric acid than does allopurinol.
- *Urinary alkalinization* is controversial as it requires a urine pH of 7.0 to be effective, which may promote calcium-phosphate crystallization and precipitation.
  - Currently *not* recommended in the therapeutic management of TLS.
  - If progressive oliguric AKI develops, intermittent hemodialysis or continuous forms of renal replacement therapy may be required.

Gout See p. 408.

Electrolyte physiology

Sodium is pumped out of the cell in exchange for K^+ by the sodium-potassium pump, which requires energy from adenosine triphosphate (ATP). Sodium is the major extracellular cation; potassium is the major intracellular cation.

- *Osmolarity* is the number of osmoles per L of solution.
- *Osmolality* is the number of osmoles per kg of solvent (*normal:* 280–300).

To calculate plasma osmolality $2(Na^+)$ + urea/2.8 + glucose/18. If the measured osmolality >10 mmol/L higher than the calculated osmolality, an osmolar gap is present. Consider the presence of ketones, ethanol, methanol, or ethylene glycol (see page xxx).

Fluid compartments For 70 kg man: *Total fluid* = 42 L (60% body weight). *Intracellular fluid* = 28 L (67% body fluid), *extracellular fluid* = 14 L (33% body fluid). *Intravascular component* = 5 L of blood (see Figure 17.1).

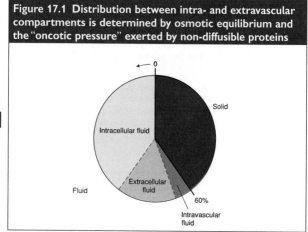

Figure 17.1 Distribution between intra- and extravascular compartments is determined by osmotic equilibrium and the "oncotic pressure" exerted by non-diffusible proteins

Control of sodium *Renin* produced by the juxtaglomerular apparatus responds to decreased renal blood flow and catalyses conversion of *angiotensinogen* to *angiotensin I*. This is then converted by angiotensin-converting enzyme (ACE), located in the lung and blood vessels, to *angiotensin II*, which increases efferent renal arteriolar constriction (↑ perfusion pressure), systemic vasoconstriction, and stimulation of the adrenal cortex to produce *aldosterone*, which activates the sodium-potassium pump and other ion channels in the collecting duct, leading to reabsorption of sodium and water from the urine in exchange for potassium and hydrogen.

High renal peritubular blood flow and hemodilution ↓ sodium reabsorption in the proximal tubule.

Control of water Controlled mainly by sodium concentration. Increased plasma osmolality stimulates thirst and the release of ADH from the posterior pituitary, which increases the water reabsorption from the collecting duct by opening water channels to allow water to flow from the hypotonic luminal fluid into the hypertonic renal interstitium. See Table 17.11.

Table 17.11 Natriuretic peptide

Brain natriuretic peptide (BNP) is a hormone originally identified from pig brain (hence the B) and is mostly secreted from ventricular myocardium. Plasma BNP is closely related to left ventricular (LV) pressure. In MI and LV dysfunction, these hormones can be released in large quantities. Secretion is also increased by tachycardia, glucocorticoids, and thyroid hormones. Vasoactive peptides (endothelin-1, angiotensin II) also influence secretion. BNP increases GFR and decreases renal Na^+ reabsorption; it also decreases preload by relaxing smooth muscle.

BNP as a biomarker of heart failure* Increased BNP distinguishes heart failure from other causes of dyspnea more accurately than does LV ejection fraction(sensitivity, >90%;specificity, 80–90%). BNP is highest in decompensated heart failure, intermediate in LV dysfunction but not acute heart failure exacerbation, and lowest in those without heart failure or LV dysfunction.

What is the BNP threshold for diagnosing heart failure? If BNP >100 ng/L, this "diagnoses" heart failure better than history, examination, and chest x-ray (CXR). BNP can be used to rule out heart failure if <50 ng/L (negative predictive value [PV] 96%). In those with heart failure, BNP is higher in systolic dysfunction than in isolated diastolic dysfunction and is highest in those with systolic *and* diastolic dysfunction.

Threshold (ng/L)	Sensitivity (%)	Specificity (%)	Positive PV	Negative PV	Accuracy (%)
50	97	62	71	96	79
100	90	76	79	89	83
150	85	83	83	85	84^2

- BNP increases in proportion to right ventricular dysfunction (e.g., in primary pulmonary hypertension, cor pulmonale, PE, and congenital heart disease, but rises are less than in LV disorders).

Prognosis in heart failure: The higher the BNP, the higher the cardiovascular and all-cause mortality (independent of age, New York Heart Association (NYHA) class, previous MI, and LV ejection fraction). Increased BNP in heart failure is also associated with sudden death. Serial testing may be important: Persistently high BNP levels despite vigorous treatment predict adverse outcomes.

(continued)

Table 17.11 (Continued)

Prognosis in angina and MI: BNP has some prognostic value here (adverse LV remodeling; LV dysfunction; death post-MI).

Prognosis in COR pulmonale/primary pulmonary hypertension: BNP is useful.

Cautions with BNP: A BNP >50 ng/L does not exclude other coexisting diseases such as pneumonia. Assays vary, so consult with your lab.

* Lemos J. B-type natriuretic peptide in cardiovascular disease. *Lancet.* 2003;**362(9380)**:316–322.

Sodium: Hyponatremia

How to think about hyponatremia Hyponatremia does not actually imply reduced total body sodium; it is a disorder of *excess water relative to total body sodium*. It results from either loss of solute (Na^+, K^+) or gain of excess water. ADH mediates water retention by concentrating the urine and is involved in most causes of hyponatremia.

Signs and symptoms depend on severity and rate of change in serum sodium; these include confusion, seizures, anorexia, nausea, muscle weakness.

Diagnosis See tree in diagram, p. 670. Key information needed is patient's volume status, serum osmolality, urine osmolality, and urinary sodium.

Causes of hyponatremia For a full list, see Figure 17.2.

- *Hypovolemic hyponatremia:* Renal or nonrenal (GI, sweat) volume loss
- *Hypervolemic hyponatremia:* Heart failure, kidney failure, cirrhosis, nephrotic syndrome
- *Euvolemic hyponatremia:* Excess water intake, syndrome of inappropriate antidiuretic hormone (SIADH) secretion, cortisol insufficiency
- *Pseudohyponatremia:* Measurement artifact as plasma water concentration is decreased from very high lipids or protein(myeloma), and the **measured** plasma Na^+ concentration measured plasma Na^+ concentration is indirectly measured, but actual Na^+ concentration and plasma osmolality is unchanged.
- *Dilutional hyponatremia:* If plasma glucose 200 mg/dL, make a correction. Add 1.6 mEq/L to plasma Na^+ concentration for every 100 that glucose is >100 mg/dL to correct for water movement from cells to the extracellular space due to excess glucose. Plasma osmolality is increased.

Management Don't base treatment on plasma Na^+ concentration alone. The presence of symptoms, duration, and volume status influence treatment. If possible, correct the underlying cause. Treat hyponatremia much more slowly if chronic, as patients can be at risk for osmotic demyelination syndrome, a condition caused by rapid shifts of fluid in the CNS potentially causing permanent neurological side effects such as paralysis, cognitive disorders, or death. *When treating patients who are asymptomatic from hyponatremia, aim for a rate of rise of serum sodium concentration of <10–12 mEq/L/24 h.* Acute hyponatremia may initially require more rapid rates of correction, but attempts should be made to keep the rise to <10–12 mEq/L/24 h. If patients have severe symptoms or if hypertonic saline is being considered, nephrology consultation is strongly advised.

Hypovolemic hyponatremia Renal or nonrenal losses (urine sodium distinguishes the two). Usually evident from exam. Treatment is volume resuscitation, but be cautious not to raise sodium too quickly. Attempt to determine whether the condition is likely to be temporary (diarrhea, diuretics) or more long-lasting (high-output ostomy, salt-wasting nephropathy).

Hypervolemic hyponatremia e.g., congestive heart failure (CHF), cirrhosis, nephrotic syndrome. Treat the underlying disorder, typically with water restriction and perhaps loop diuretics. Aim to normalize the patient's volume status.

SIADH An important but overdiagnosed cause of hyponatremia. Typically, patients will have a normal plasma volume. Urine osmolality is inappropriately high; urine sodium will usually be >20 mEq/L and can be very high, and urine osmolality is >100 mOsm/kg which is not maximally dilute. Importantly, if urine osmolality is >300 mOsm/kg, then administration of normal saline will worsen hyponatremia (the urine is more concentrated than 0.9% saline, resulting in net retention of water). *Causes:*

- *Malignancy*: E.g., small cell lung cancer, pancreas cancer, prostate cancer, lymphoma
- *CNS disorders:* Meningoencephalitis, abscess, stroke, subarachnoid hemorrhage, subdural hemorrhage, head injury, many others
- *Chest disease:* TB, pneumonia, abscess, aspergillosis
- *Metabolic disease:* Porphyria, trauma
- *Drugs:* Opiates, chlorpropamide, antipsychotics and antiemetics, selective serotonin reuptake inhibitors (SSRIs), cytotoxics

Treatment Treat the cause. Fluid restriction is one mainstay of treatment. Cases with very high urine osmolality usually require either hypertonic saline (3% NaCl) for severe symptoms such as seizures or coma. Vasopressin (V_2) receptor antagonists such as tolvaptan may be useful, but these drugs are very expensive and not recommended for severe symptoms at present. Furosemide may help lower urinary sodium acutely. Demeclocycline should be avoided due to nephrotoxicity.

Figure 17.2

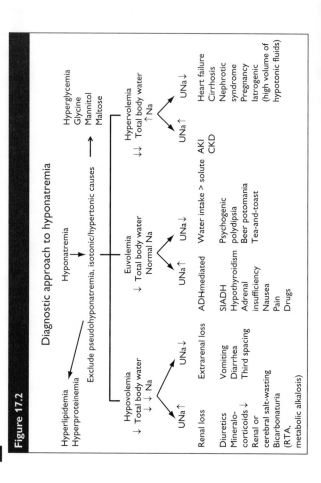

Diagnostic approach to hyponatremia

Hyperlipidemia
Hyperproteinemia

Hyponatremia

Exclude pseudohyponatremia, isotonic/hypertonic causes →

Hyperglycemia
Glycine
Mannitol
Maltose

Hypovolemia
↓ Total body water
↓ → Na

UNa↑   UNa↓

Renal loss   Extrarenal loss

Diuretics
Mineralo-
corticoids ↓
Renal or
cerebral salt-wasting
Bicarbonaturia
(RTA,
metabolic alkalosis)

Vomiting
Diarrhea
Third spacing

Euvolemia
↓ Total body water
Normal Na

UNa↑   UNa↓

ADHmediated   Water intake > solute

SIADH
Hypothyroidism
Adrenal
insufficiency
Nausea
Pain
Drugs

Psychogenic
polydipsia
Beer potomania
Tea-and-toast

Hypervolemia
↓↓ Total body water
↑ Na

UNa↑   UNa↓

AKI
CKD

Heart failure
Cirrhosis
Nephrotic
syndrome
Pregnancy
Iatrogenic
(high volume of
hypotonic fluids)

Sodium: Hypernatremia

How to think about hypernatremia Unlike hyponatremia, most causes of hypernatremia are due to dehydration with *water loss in excess of sodium loss;* typically implies impaired access to water.

Signs and symptoms Look for thirst, confusion, coma, and seizures with signs of dehydration: Dry skin, reduced skin turgor, postural hypotension, and oliguria if water deficient. Laboratory features: Hematocrit (HCT) ↑, ↑albumin, ↑urea.

Causes Mostly related to dehydration:

- *Fluid loss* without water replacement (e.g., diarrhea, vomiting, burns)
- *DI:* Caused by inability of the kidney to concentrate urine. Suspect if large urine volume. Can be central (deficiency of ADH [may follow head injury, or CNS surgery, especially pituitary]) or nephrogenic (resistance to ADH [lithium, NSAIDs, genetic diseases]).
- *Osmotic diuresis* (e.g., mannitol, very high-protein diet).
- *Incorrect iv fluid replacement* (excess hypertonic fluid); patients are hypervolemic.
- *Primary aldosteronism:* Patients not dehydrated, results from excess sodium retention. Plasma Na^+ concentration is usually only mildly elevated. Suspect if BP↑, K^+↓, alkalosis (HCO_3^- ↑). Licorice and Cushing's syndrome can cause a similar picture.

Management Give water orally if possible; if not, dextrose 5% IV guided by urine output and plasma Na^+ concentration. Giving 0.9% saline can be helpful if the patient is hypovolemic as this causes less marked fluid shifts and is hypotonic in a hypernatremic patient. Aim for a rate of sodium correction of 10 mEq/L/24 h to avoid cerebral edema from rapid overcorrection.

DI is treated differently, depending on whether it is central or nephrogenic, but free access to water is crucial to avoid dehydration (see page 325; Endocrine). Central DI can be treated with long-term arginine vasopressin (DDAVP, which is the same compound as ADH). Nephrogenic diabetes insipidus (DI) can be treated with thiazide diuretics.

Potassium

General Points

98% of potassium (K^+) is intracellular (~3,500 **meq** total with the majority found in skeletal muscle), thus the serum potassium is a poor reflection of total body potassium.

The main factors that control the internal distribution of K^+ are insulin and β_2 stimulation, which drive K^+ into cells by stimulation of the $Na^+K^+ATPase$ pump.

Mineralocorticoid activity (aldosterone) and the delivery of sodium to the cortical collecting duct (CCD) are the main regulators of K^+ secretion. Addison's disease may cause hyperkalemia due to loss of **mineralocorticoid** activity.

Hyperkalemia

The urgency of treatment depends on several factors: The cause of hyperkalemia (hemolysis or muscle/tissue breakdown), preexisting chronic hyperkalemia, the presence of oliguric/anuric renal failure, and the rate of rise (Figure 17.3). Aggressive treatment may be required even in modest degrees of hyperkalemia or associated ECG manifestations. Persistent hyperkalemia requires an associated impairment in urine potassium excretion.

Although there are no standard definitions, a K^+ ≥6.5–7.0 mEq/L requires *urgent* evaluation and treatment.

Signs and Symptoms Muscle weakness/paralysis, cardiac conduction abnormalities, and decreased ammonium excretion (NH_4^+) leading to metabolic acidosis.

Tall, peaked T waves and shortened QT interval are the earliest changes.

Clinical pearl: The ECG is *insensitive* for the diagnosis of hyperkalemia, especially if of rapid onset. The presence of hypocalcemia or metabolic acidosis may precipitate symptoms or ECG abnormalities at a lower serum K^+.

Causes

Pseudohyperkalemia: Mechanical trauma (hemolysis due to tourniquet compression), marked leukocytosis (white blood cells [WBC] >100,000/µL) or thrombocytosis (platelet count >700,000/µL). To diagnose, draw a plasma K^+ in a heparinized tube to determine the actual K^+ level.

Excessive K^+ intake: Typically seen in disorders with reduced renal function. Always consider nutritional products (noni or coconut juice) or salt substitutes.

Cell shifts: Rhabdomyolysis, TLS, drugs (digoxin, RAAS blockers, trimethoprim), diabetic ketoacidosis (DKA)/hyperosmolar states, inorganic or mineral acidosis due to buffering of excess H^+ ions with movement of K^+ out of cells.

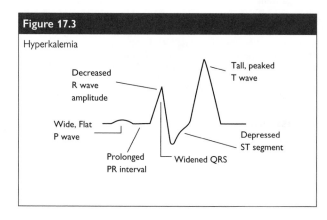

Figure 17.3

Hyperkalemia

Decreased R wave amplitude

Tall, peaked T wave

Wide, Flat P wave

Depressed ST segment

Prolonged PR interval

Widened QRS

Impaired renal excretion: Most common cause of sustained hyperkalemia. Typically *not* seen until the eGFR is <15 mL/min/1.73 m² unless other factors.

Treatment **of severe hyperkalemia** Three guiding principles:

1. *Antagonize metabolic effects of* ↑ K⁺ with calcium gluconate 1 g IV given over 5–10 min, especially if loss of P waves or QRS widening. May be repeated if ECG manifestations continue.

2. *Drive K⁺ into cells.* Insulin (given as bolus or continuous infusion, *not* subcutaneously) ± D₅₀W IV (*not* used if significantly hyperglycemic already, i.e., ≥250 mg/dL).

Inhaled albuterol (double to quadruple strength, 5–10 mg) may be synergistic with insulin therapy.

The role of *sodium bicarbonate* is controversial and may only be helpful in associated states of metabolic acidosis.

3. *Remove K⁺ from the body.* Diuretics (loop diuretics) may be *best* for patients with mild or moderate degree of kidney failure.

Cationic exchange resins (sodium polystyrene sulfonate [SPS]) may take 4–6 h to be effective; *not* helpful if post colectomy. May be dangerous with ileus (potential for intestinal ischemia and ulcerations). Typical dose is 15–60 g.

Dialysis: Indicated if the above measures are *not* successful, progressive oliguria ensues, or there is significant K⁺ release from tissue. Hemodialysis is *preferred* over continuous renal replacement therapy or peritoneal dialysis.

Eliminate reversible causes of impairment in renal function (drugs, hypovolemia, or urinary obstruction).

Hypokalemia

Typically, there are no symptoms until the serum K⁺ is <3.0 mEq/L, but a serum K⁺ <2.5 mEq/L (especially if accompanied by symptoms) requires *urgent* treatment (Figure 17.4). Symptoms may depend on the speed of development. It may be potentiated by use of digoxin or underlying cardiovascular disease.

Signs and symptoms Muscle weakness, cramps, paralysis, rhabdomyolysis, respiratory failure from respiratory muscle weakness, ileus, impaired urinary concentration (polyuria), and cardiac arrhythmias and ECG abnormalities.

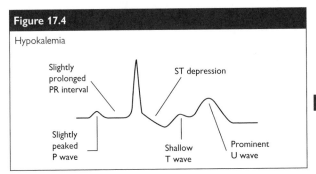

Figure 17.4

Hypokalemia

Slightly prolonged PR interval

ST depression

Slightly peaked P wave

Shallow T wave

Prominent U wave

Causes

- *Shift or redistributive process* (typically transient): Insulin or hypokalemic periodic paralysis
- *Decreased intake*: Unusual cause by itself
- *Gastrointestinal losses*: Diarrhea, villous adenoma or chronic laxative abuse
- *Renal losses*
- *Miscellaneous*: Hypothermia can lead to a decrease in K^+. Metabolic and respiratory alkalosis facilitates entry of K^+ into cells (trivial effect).

Diagnosis Urine K^+/Cr ratio <15 mmol/g of creatinine is seen with poor dietary intake, transcellular K^+ shifts, GI loss, or prior diuretic usage.

Treatment Depends on urgency and symptoms. If mild (>2.5 mEq/L and no symptoms), given oral K^+ supplements, 20–40 mEq at a time. If severe (<2.5 mEq/L and musculoskeletal or cardiac symptoms), give IV potassium *cautiously* (10 mEq/h via a peripheral IV, 20 mEq/h via a central line). Never give IV K^+ as a bolus; typically give over 1 h; *be cautious if patient is oliguric or anuric.*

Always evaluate for magnesium deficiency and replete. It will be difficult to normalize low potassium levels unless hypomagnesemia is normalized.

Calcium: Physiology

General points About 40% of plasma calcium is bound to albumin. Usually, it is total plasma calcium that is measured although it is the unbound, ionized portion that is important. Therefore, *adjust total calcium level for albumin as follows*: Add 0.8 mg/dL to the measured calcium for every 1 g/dL that albumin is below 4.0 g/dL (perform the reverse if albumin is elevated). However, many factors affect binding (e.g., other proteins in myeloma, cirrhosis, acid–base status, individual variation) so be cautious in your interpretation. If in doubt over an abnormal calcium, check the ionized calcium.

The control of calcium metabolism

- *Parathyroid hormone (PTH)*: A rise in PTH causes a rise in plasma Ca^{2+} and a ↓ in plasma PO_4^{3-}. This is due to ↑Ca^{2+} and ↑ PO_4^{3-} reabsorption from bone; and ↑Ca^{2+} but ↓ PO_4^{3-} reabsorption from the kidney. PTH secretion enhances active vitamin D formation. PTH secretion is itself controlled by ionized plasma calcium levels.
- *Parathyroid hormone-related peptide (PTHrP)*: A substance mostly secreted by tumors, it acts similarly to PTH. If elevated, a cause of hypercalcemia in malignancy.
- *Vitamin D*: Cholecalciferol (vitamin D_3) and ergocalciferol (vitamin D_2) are biologically identical in their actions. Serum vitamin D is converted in the liver to 25-hydroxy vitamin D (25[OH] vitamin D). In the kidney, a second hydroxyl group is added to form the biologically active 1,25-dihydroxy vitamin D (1,25[OH]$_2$ vitamin D), also called calcitriol. Calcitriol production is stimulated by ↓Ca^{2+}, ↓PO_4^{3-}, and PTH. Its actions include ↑Ca^{2+} and ↑PO_4 absorption from the gut; ↑Ca^{2+} and ↑PO_4^{3-} reabsorption in the kidney; enhanced bone turnover; and inhibition of PTH release.
- *Calcitonin*: Made in C-cells of the thyroid, this causes a decrease in plasma calcium and phosphate, but its physiological role is unclear. It is a marker to detect recurrence or metastasis in medullary carcinoma of the thyroid.
- *Thyroxine*: May increase plasma Ca^{2+}, although this is rare.
- *Magnesium*: ↓Mg_{2+} prevents PTH release, and may cause hypocalcemia.

Hypercalcemia

Signs and symptoms "Bones, stones, groans, and psychic moans": Abdominal pain, vomiting, constipation, polyuria, polydipsia, depression, anorexia, weight loss, tiredness, weakness, BP↑, confusion, fever, renal stones, acute kidney injury, corneal calcification, cardiac arrest. *ECG:* QT interval↓.

Causes and diagnosis See Figure 17.5. Most commonly, malignancy (myeloma, bone metastases, PTHrP↑) and primary hyperparathyroidism. Others include sarcoidosis or lymphoma (granulomas activate vitamin D to the 1,25-hydroxylated form), vitamin D intoxication, and familial benign hypocalciuric hypercalcemia (rare; defect in calcium-sensing receptor). Pointers to malignancy are ↓albumin, ↓Cl⁻, ↓K⁺, alkalosis, ↓PO₄³⁻, ↑alk phos. Other investigations (e.g., isotope bone scan, CXR, ESR) may also be of diagnostic value.

Treat the underlying cause. If Ca^{2+} >13 mg/dL, and severe abdominal pain, vomiting, fever, or confusion, aim to reduce calcium as follows:

- *Blood tests:* Measure urine and electrolytes, Mg^{2+}, creatinine, Ca^{2+}, PO_4^{3-}, alk phos.
- *Fluids:* Rehydrate with IVF 0.9% saline (e.g., 4–6 L in 24 h as needed). Correct hypokalemia/hypomagnesemia (mild metabolic acidosis needs no treatment). This will reduce symptoms, and increase renal Ca^{2+} loss. Monitor urine and electrolytes.
- *Diuretics: Controversial,* but can increase renal calcium loss. Use loop diuretics, avoid thiazides, and be careful not to volume deplete.
- *Bisphosphonates:* IV pamidronate will lower Ca^{2+} over 2–3 d. Maximum effect is at 1 wk. These drugs inhibit osteoclast activity and so bone resorption.
- *Steroids:* Useful in granulomatous disease (e.g., prednisone 40–60 mg/d for sarcoidosis).
- *Salmon calcitonin:* Used for temporization of symptomatic hypercalcemia. Less effective than bisphosphonates, but quicker onset. Inhibits osteoclasts. *Tachyphylaxis* occurs after several doses, reducing its effectiveness.
- *Other:* Chemotherapy may deplete Ca^{2+} in malignant disease (e.g., myeloma).

Hypocalcemia

Apparent hypocalcemia may be an artifact of hypoalbuminemia (above).

Signs and symptoms Tetany; depression; perioral paresthesias; carpopedal spasm (wrist flexion and fingers drawn together), especially if brachial artery is occluded with BP cuff (*Trousseau's sign*); neuromuscular excitability (e.g., tapping over parotid [facial nerve] causes facial muscles to twitch [*Chvostek's sign*]). Cataract if chronic Ca^{2+}↓. *ECG:* QT interval↑.

Causes Most commonly, hypoparathyroidism (may be a consequence of thyroid or parathyroid surgery). Check PTH and phosphate levels. *If phosphate raised,* then either chronic kidney disease (high phosphate causes ↑PTH, which ↑urinary Ca^{2+} excretion), hypoparathyroidism, pseudohypoparathyroidism, or acute rhabdomyolysis. If phosphorus normal or decreased ↓, then either osteomalacia (high alkaline phosphatase), overhydration, or pancreatitis. In respiratory alkalosis, the total Ca^{2+} may be normal, but ionized Ca^{2+}↓ due to increased binding to albumin, and the patient may have symptoms because of this. Prolonged IV fluid administration (e.g., long hospital stay) can also cause hypocalcemia.

Treatment If *symptoms are mild,* replete calcium orally (e.g., 5 mmol/6 h). Check daily plasma and periodic ionized calcium levels. If hypoparathyroidism

Figure 17.5

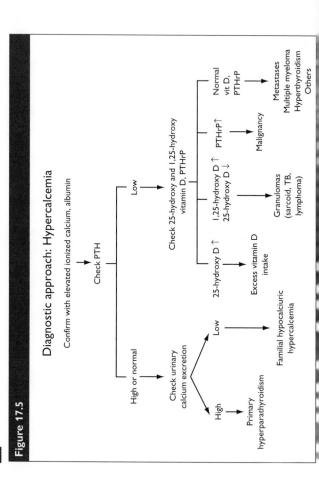

Diagnostic approach: Hypercalcemia

Confirm with elevated ionized calcium, albumin

Check PTH

High or normal

Check urinary calcium excretion

- High → Primary hyperparathyroidism
- Low → Familial hypocalciuric hypercalcemia

Low

Check 25-hydroxy and 1,25-hydroxy vitamin D, PTHrP

- 25-hydroxy D ↑ → Excess vitamin D intake
- 1,25-hydroxy D ↑
  25-hydroxy D ↓ → Granulomas (sarcoid, TB, lymphoma)
- PTHrP↑ → Malignancy
- Normal vit D, PTHrP → Metastases
  Multiple myeloma
  Hyperthyroidism
  Others

is the cause, calcitriol is often necessary to maintain a normal calcium. If *symptoms are severe*, give 10 mL of 10% calcium gluconate (2.25 mmol) IV over 30 min (bolus injections are only needed very rarely). Repeat as necessary. If due to alkalosis, correct the alkalosis and recheck values.

Magnesium

Magnesium is distributed 65% in bone and 35% in cells; plasma concentration tends to follow that of Ca^{2+} and K^+. Magnesium excess is usually caused by renal failure, but rarely requires treatment in its own right.

Hypomagnesemia causes paresthesias, seizures, tetany, and arrhythmias. Digitalis toxicity may be exacerbated. *Causes:* Severe diarrhea; ketoacidosis; alcoholism or poor diet; diuretics or other medications (e.g., tacrolimus, proton pump inhibitors), total parenteral nutrition (monitor weekly); accompanying hypocalcemia. May accompany hypokalemia (especially with diuretics) and hypophosphatemia. *Treatment:* Give magnesium salts. IV is more effective than PO.

Hypermagnesemia is usually iatrogenic or from excessive intake (e.g., antacids). *Features:* Neuromuscular depression, ↓BP, CNS depression, coma.

Trace elements

A number of trace elements are of biological importance and can cause clinical disease in deficiency or excess. Disorders of most trace elements are rare without a very unusual diet or long-standing malabsorptive process (e.g., short gut syndrome).

Zinc is important in many enzymatic processes and plays multiple roles in insulin metabolism. Zinc deficiency may occur in parenteral nutrition or, rarely, from a poor diet (too few cereals and dairy products, anorexia nervosa, alcoholism). Rarely, it is due to a genetic defect. *Signs and symptoms:* Look for red, crusted skin lesions, especially around nostrils and corners of mouth. *Diagnosis:* Therapeutic trial of zinc (plasma levels are unreliable as they may be low, e.g., in infection or trauma, without deficiency).

Zinc excess is rare, usually related to excess intake. Its major clinical effect is copper deficiency (through inhibiting copper absorption).

Copper An essential element for synthesis of heme and oxidation of metals. Copper deficiency can result from parenteral nutrition, zinc excess, malabsorption (e.g., short bowel). Deficiency can cause anemia and neutropenia. Diagnosis of copper deficiency: Check serum copper levels. Copper excess is rare outside of Wilson's disease and is caused by excess intake, often from contaminated water. Copper toxicity causes cirrhosis, kidney disease, and various neurological diseases. Treatment can involve chelation with penicillamine; consult an expert.

Selenium An essential element present in cereals, nuts, and meat. It is required for the antioxidant glutathione peroxidase (which protects against harmful free radicals). It is also antithrombogenic and is required for sperm motility proteins. Deficiency may increase the frequency of neoplasia and atheromata and may lead to a cardiomyopathy (Keshan's disease). There is interest that selenium may modulate the oxidative stress response in sepsis. Serum levels are a poor guide. Toxic symptoms may also be found with excessive supplementation or contaminated food products.

677

Plasma proteins

Serum protein electrophoresis (SPEP) distinguishes a number of bands (see Figure 17.6, p. 680).

Albumin is synthesized in the liver; $t_{\frac{1}{2}} \approx 20$ d. It binds *bilirubin, free fatty acids, calcium,* and some *drugs (penicillin and acetylsalicylic acid)*. It typically requires a fall in albumin of 30% before it shows up on an electrophoresis. *Low albumin* may result in edema from low oncotic pressure. *Causes:* Liver disease, nephrotic syndrome, burns, protein-losing enteropathy, malabsorption, malnutrition, late pregnancy, artifact (e.g., from arm with IVF), posture (5 g/L higher if upright), genetic variations, malignancy. *Causes of high albumin:* Acute dehydration; artifact (e.g., stasis).

α₁ Zone α_1-Antitrypsin, thyroid-binding globulin, α_1 glycoprotein (orosomucoid), and high-density lipoprotein (HDL). A decreased band may be seen: Cirrhosis and nephrotic syndrome.

α₂ Zone α_2-Macroglobulin, ceruloplasmin, and haptoglobin (predominant component). The $\alpha2$ zone is typically decreased in hemolytic anemia.

β Zone Transferrin (major band), low-density lipoprotein (LDL), fibrinogen, and C3 complement (C4 may be visible if increased or high-normal). Reduced in active glomerulonephritis and systemic lupus erythematosus (SLE).

γ Zone Immunoglobulins and C-reactive protein (CRP). *Diffusely raised* in chronic infections, liver cirrhosis, sarcoidosis, SLE, rheumatoid arthritis (RA), Crohn's disease, TB, bronchiectasis, primary biliary cirrhosis (PBC), hepatitis, and parasitemia. It is *low* in nephrotic syndrome, malabsorption, malnutrition, immune deficiency (severe illness, diabetes mellitus, renal failure, malignancy, or congenital).

Paraproteinemia See p. 635.

Acute-phase response The body responds to a variety of insults with, among other things, the synthesis by the liver of a number of proteins (normally present in serum in small quantities)—e.g., α_1-antitrypsin, fibrinogen, complement, haptoglobin, and CRP. An increased density of the α_1- and α_2-fractions, often with a reduced albumin level, is characteristic of conditions such as infection, malignancy (especially if the α_2-fraction is elevated), trauma, surgery, and inflammatory disease.

CRP Levels help monitor inflammation/infection. Normal <0.5 mg/dL, *but can be elevated age, race, BMI, and smoking.* Like the ESR, it is raised in many inflammatory conditions, but changes more rapidly; increases in hours and falls within 2–3 d of recovery. Therefore, it can be used to follow the response to therapy (e.g., antibiotics in osteomyelitis) or disease activity (e.g., Crohn's disease). CRP values in mild inflammation are 10–50 mg/L; active bacterial infection, 50–200 mg/L; severe infection or trauma >200 mg/L; see Table 17.12. Elevated CRP levels may suggest an increased risk in patients with cardiovascular disease if measured using a highly sensitive assay. Low risk <1 mg/dL; moderate risk 1–3; and high risk >3 mg/L.

Urinary proteins

If urinary protein loss is >0.15 g/24 h (24 h urine), then this is considered pathological.

Albuminuria Caused by kidney disease. Microalbuminuria (albumin excretion between 30–300 mg/d) is an important screening test for diabetic nephropathy. >300 mg/d of albuminuria is considered macroalbuminuria or clinical proteinuria. Microalbuminuria by spot urinary albumin to creatinine ratio is 30–300 mg/g creatinine.

Bence Jones proteinuria consists of light chains excreted in excess by some patients with myeloma. They are not detected by dipsticks and may occur with normal serum electrophoresis. Typically diagnosed with urinary electrophoresis (UPEP).

Serum free light chains Recently, a highly sensitive assay has been developed to measure κ and λ light chains (Freelite™) as an indicator of monoclonality. Serum free light chains have a greater sensitivity than SPEP, UPEP, and immunofixation electrophoresis (IFE) alone in the detection of myeloma, light chain myeloma, and nonsecretory myeloma and are important in both treatment response and prognosis.

Plasma enzymes

Reference intervals vary between laboratories.

Raised levels of specific enzymes can be a useful indicator of a disease. However, remember that most can be raised for other reasons, too. The major causes of *raised enzymes* are given below.

Alkaline phosphatase
- Liver disease (suggests cholestasis)
- Bone disease (isoenzyme distinguishable, reflects osteoblast activity) especially Paget's, growing children, healing fractures, osteomalacia, metastases, primary hyperparathyroidism, and renal failure
- Pregnancy (placenta makes its own isoenzyme)

Alanine-amino transferase (ALT; serum glutamic-pyruvic transaminase [SGPT])
- Liver disease (suggests hepatocyte damage); also raised in shock

Amylase
- Acute pancreatitis (not chronic pancreatitis as little tissue remaining)
- Severe uremia, diabetic ketoacidosis

Aspartate-amino transferase (AST; serum glutamic-oxaloacetic transaminase [SGOT])
- Liver disease (suggesting hepatocyte damage)
- MI
- Skeletal muscle damage and hemolysis

CK
- MI (isoenzyme "CK-MB." MI diagnosed if CK-MB >6% total CK, or CK-MB mass >99 percentile of normal)

Table 17.12 CRP	
Marked elevation	*Normal to slight elevation*
Bacterial infection	Viral infection
Abscess	Steroids/estrogens
Crohn's disease	Ulcerative colitis
Connective tissue diseases (± SLE)	
	Atherosclerosis
Neoplasia	
Trauma	
Necrosis (e.g., MI)	

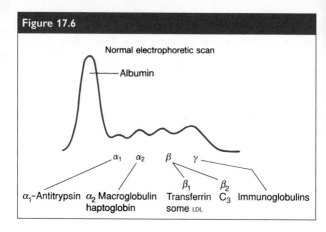

Figure 17.6

Normal electrophoretic scan

Albumin

α_1 α_2 β γ

β_1 β_2

α_1-Antitrypsin α_2 Macroglobulin haptoglobin   Transferrin some LDL C_3 Immunoglobulins

- Muscle damage (rhabdomyolysis, prolonged running, hematoma, seizures, IM injection, defibrillation, bowel ischemia, myxedema, dermatomyositis) and *drugs* (e.g., statins). A raised CK does not necessarily mean an MI.

GGT
- Liver disease (particularly alcohol-induced damage, cholestasis, drugs)

LDH
- MI(nonspecific)
- Liver disease (suggests hepatocyte damage)
- Hemolysis, pulmonary embolism, and tumor necrosis

Tumor markers

Tumor markers are rarely sufficiently specific to be of diagnostic value. Their main value is in monitoring the course of an illness and the effectiveness of treatment. Reference ranges vary between laboratories.

α-Fetoprotein Elevated in hepatocellular CA, germ cell tumors (not pure seminoma), hepatitis, cirrhosis, pregnancy, open neural tube defects.

CA 125 Elevated in carcinoma of the ovary, uterus, breast, and hepatocellular carcinoma. Also raised in pregnancy, cirrhosis, and peritonitis.

CA 15–3 Elevated in carcinoma of the breast and benign breast disease

CA 19–9 Elevated in colorectal and pancreatic carcinoma, and in cholestasis

Carcino-embryonic antigen (CEA) Elevated in gastrointestinal neoplasms, especially colorectal CA. Also cirrhosis, pancreatitis, and smoking.

Human chorionic gonadotrophin Elevated in pregnancy and germ cell tumors.

Neurone specific enolase (NSE) Elevated in small-cell carcinoma of lung and neuroblastoma.

Placental alkaline phosphatase (PLAP) Elevated in pregnancy, carcinoma of ovary, seminoma, and smoking.

Prostate-specific antigen (PSA) See Table 17.13.

Table 17.13 Prostate specific antigen (PSA)

As well as being a marker of prostate cancer, PSA is (unfortunately) Elevated in benign prostatic hypertrophy. 25% of large benign prostates emit PSA up to 10 mcg/L; levels may be higher if recent ejaculation; therefore, avoid ejaculation for 24 h prior to measurement. Other factors causing raised PSA include recent rectal examination, prostatitis, and UTI (PSA levels may not return to baseline for some months after the latter).[*] Plasma reference interval is age-specific; an example of the top end of the reference interval for total PSA is:

Healthy males of age (yrs)	PSA mcg/L
40–50	2.5
50–59	3.5
60–69	5.0
70–79	6.5
80–89	7.5

- This is a rough guide only; different labs have different reference ranges and populations vary. More specific assays, such as free PSA/total PSA index, and PSA density, are also becoming available, which may partly solve these problems. It is shown to illustrate the common problem of interpreting a PSA of ~8—and as a warning against casual requests for PSAs in the (vain) hope of simple answers. The following indicates the proportion of patients with a raised PSA and benign hypertrophy or carcinoma.

	PSA mcg/L	
Benign prostatic hypertrophy	<4 in 91%	PSA will be ~50% lower after 6 months on 5× reductase inhibitors
	4–10 in 8%	
	>10 in 1%	
Prostate carcinoma	<4 in 15%	
	4–10 in 20%	
	>10 in 65%	

[*] Up to 6 months in one study (Aus G. *Urology.* 2003;62:278).

The porphyrias

The acute porphyrias are rare genetic diseases caused by errors in the pathway of heme biosynthesis resulting in the toxic accumulation of porphobilinogen and δ-aminolevulinic acid (porphyrin precursors). Characterized by acute neurovisceral crises, due to the increased production of porphyrin precursors and their appearance in the urine. Some forms have cutaneous manifestations. Prevalence: 1–2/100,000.

Acute intermittent porphyria A low-penetrant autosomal dominant condition (porphobilinogen deaminase gene); 28% have no family history (*de novo mutations*). ~10% of those with the defective gene have neurovisceral symptoms. Attacks are intermittent, more common in women, and may be precipitated by many drugs (see below). Urine porphobilinogens are raised during attacks and often (50%) between them (the urine may go deep red on standing). Fecal porphyrin levels are normal. There are no skin manifestations.

Variegate porphyria and hereditary coproporphyria: Autosomal dominant, characterized by photosensitive blistering skin lesions, and/or acute attacks. The former is prevalent in Afrikaners in South Africa. Porphobilinogen is high only in an attack, and other metabolites may be detected in feces.

Features of an acute attack Colic ± vomiting ± fever ± WBC↑—so mimicking an acute abdomen (anesthesia can be disastrous here). Also:

- Hypotension
- Hyponatremia
- Hypokalemia
- Hypotonia
- Proteinuria
- Psychosis/odd behavior
- Peripheral neuritis
- Paralysis
- Seizures
- Sensory impairment
- Sight may be affected
- Shock (± collapse).

Drugs to avoid in acute intermittent porphyria are legion (they may precipitate above symptoms ± quadriplegia); they include: Alcohol, several anesthetic agents (barbiturates, halothane), antibiotics (chloramphenicol, sulfonamides, tetracyclines), painkillers (pentazocine), oral hypoglycemics, contraceptive pill.

Treatment of an acute attack
- Remove precipitants, then:
- Give IV fluids to correct electrolyte imbalance.
- Institute high carbohydrate intake (e.g., Hycal®) by NG tube if necessary.
- IV hematin to replenish heme stores is the treatment of choice when available.
- Nausea is controlled with prochlorperazine 12.5 mg IM.
- Sedation, if necessary, is with chlorpromazine 50–100 mg PO/IM.
- Pain control is usually with opioids.
- Seizures can be controlled with benzodiazepines.
- Treat tachycardia and hypertension with propranolol.

Nonacute porphyrias

Porphyria cutanea tarda, erythropoietic protoporphyria, and *congenital erythropoietic porphyria* are characterized by cutaneous photosensitivity alone, as there is no overproduction of porphyrin precursors, only porphyrins.

Alcohol, lead, and iron deficiency cause abnormal porphyrin metabolism.

Offer genetic counseling to all patients and their families.

Radiology

Sumera Ali, M.D. and Clifford R. Weiss, M.D.

Contents

General principles

Help the radiologist help you!

Radiology is a powerful diagnostic and therapeutic tool that has become indispensable to modern-day medical practice. Not only have new, cutting-edge diagnostic techniques been introduced, but almost all existing modalities have been revolutionized. This has made available a wide array of imaging studies from which to choose. When faced with a diagnostic inquiry, one must choose the most appropriate imaging study. In choosing, there are many aspects to consider, including invasiveness, cost, radiation exposure, sensitivity and specificity, and local expertise. The challenge of ordering imaging tests deepens because most imaging tests can be tailored to maximize sensitivity and specificity depending on the patient's underlying disease process and suspected diagnosis (e.g., obtaining multiphasic liver computed tomography [CT] scan [unenhanced, arterial, and portal venous phases] of a patient with suspected liver lesions can help differentiate cysts, hemangiomas, and hypervascular or avascular tumors). These considerations fall well within the scope of a radiologist, and involving them at an early stage in decision making can greatly speed up the diagnostic process, saving clinician and patient time and money.

When communicating with a radiologist, it is important to realize that many imaging findings are nonspecific and can be interpreted differently depending on the clinical history. Hence, it is of utmost importance to provide relevant and specific clinical information to the radiologist when ordering the imaging study. This information may mean the difference between a broad differential diagnosis and a single definitive diagnosis, or may even allow the radiologist to detect subtle findings. For example, describing the mechanism of injury in a trauma patient can improve the detection and location of fractures or soft-tissue damage.

For any radiologic study ask yourself: How can I help the radiologist help me? Before ordering a test

Before ordering a test, ask yourself relevant questions:

- What do I need to know? How will this imaging test alter the management or change the outcome of the patient?
- What conditions will I be able to rule in or rule out with this investigation?
- Is the patient fit to have the examination?
- What is the urgency of the study?

This last question is essential to nighttime/off-hours radiology, in order to help the radiologist triage studies. Nonessential studies performed when a radiology department is understaffed can make it very difficult to provide essential care to critically ill patients.

At the time of ordering the investigation After you have decided that a patient will benefit from a certain exam, it is time to request the investigation:

Provide the radiologist with relevant clinical history:

Clear and concise clinical information allows the radiologist to perform the appropriate test, modify the imaging procedure to increase specificity in the characterization of pathology, advise an alternative test that may be more appropriate, and interpret the findings properly in the context of the clinical information at hand. The first portion of a clinical history is what is normally put in the first line of a good internal medicine presentation: The patient's age, sex, significant underlying diseases, relevant past surgical history, current symptoms prompting the examination (with as much spatial/anatomic localization as possible), and the suspected diagnosis or differential diagnosis. For example: "65-year-old woman with a past medical history of pancreatic cancer, now with calf pain followed by acute onset shortness of breath and tachycardia, suspect pulmonary embolism."

Prepare the patient before the procedure: The following questions should be considered:

- Is the patient aware that she is going to have the study, and is she willing? Is the patient able to undergo the procedure? Can the patient be moved? One key question is: Is the patient too heavy to fit on the imaging table?
- Is the study contraindicated for any reason? Contraindications will vary based on imaging modality and organ system under consideration.
- Is the patient properly prepared for the procedure? Does he need to be NPO? Does he need to have a full bladder or a Foley catheter in place? Does he need to receive oral contrast before coming down for his procedure (and if so, how much and for how long beforehand)? Is he going to receive IV contrast, and, if so, does he have appropriate IV access? Does the patient need consent for the procedure (always for interventional radiology procedures)? If so, can the patient give consent? Does the patient need to be well hydrated for the procedure? Do any medications need to be given before the procedure, either as premedication or as part of procedure, or do medications need to be stopped?

After the investigation has been performed

Does patient need observation? Many investigations may require observing the patient for a certain time. For example, creatinine needs to be monitored in patients with poor renal function who have undergone contrast-enhanced studies.

Interpreting the image: The interpretation can be very modality-, system-, and pathology-specific, but general rules are to have a systematic approach, compare it to previous examinations, and keep the patient's clinical condition in mind.

Ask the radiologist for advice: Radiologists are imaging specialists and should always be consulted for image findings post study.

Radiation exposure

Justifying the exposure Although medical imaging is an invaluable diagnostic tool, it is crucial to know that it accounts for almost half of the radiation exposure experienced by the population in the United States. Exposure from a single procedure is likely to be very small and clinically irrelevant. However, cumulative doses in a patient population undergoing frequent and repeated imaging significantly increases the risk of radiation-induced malignancies and has become a public health concern.[1]

Effective dose is the calculated measure most commonly used to compare the detrimental effects such as cancer and hereditary effects due to ionizing radiation. It is the weighted average of doses to the organs that have been exposed, taking into account the radiosensitivity of the organs. It is measured in sieverts (Sv) or rems (100 rem = 1 Sv). The average effective doses for the most common radiologic and nuclear medicine procedures in the United States for the adult population have been determined and are shown in Table 18.1.[2]

What can you do? There are guiding principles that one should keep in mind when ordering an investigation.[3] *Justification:* Make sure that there is an appropriate indication for the procedure, and it is not being repeated for no reason. *Optimization:* Following the protocols designed to obtain images at as low as reasonably achievable dose (ALARA principle) while still achieving a diagnostic study. *Limitation* : Setting a maximum aggregate dose a patient can receive in a specified time period. *Restriction:* Limit the region scanned to the smallest area necessary.

Furthermore, the American College of Radiology (ACR) has developed appropriateness criteria of imaging for specific clinical conditions to reduce the number of unnecessary scans for inappropriate indications. These can be found at http://www.acr.org/ac

Contrast agents

Intravenous contrast for imaging procedures involving ionizing radiation is iodine-based, whereas almost all magnetic resonance imaging (MRI) and magnetic resonance angiography (MRA) procedures that are contrast-based use gadolinium compounds. Iodinated radiocontrast agents can either be ionic or nonionic and are available in various concentrations as compared to plasma. These are high-osmolal (HO), low-osmolal (LO), and iso-osmolal (IO) contrast material in descending order of osmolality. Low and iso-osmolal and nonionic agents are associated with decreased incidence of immediate hypersensitivity reactions and contrast-induced nephropathy. Low osmolal nonionic agents have replaced HO contrast in clinical practice. If a contrast is required, specific indications should be present, and the patient should be assessed for potential risk factors for adverse reactions.

1 Brenner DJ, EJ Hall. Computed tomography: An increasing source of radiation exposure. *N Engl J Med.* 2007;357(22):2277–2284.
2 Mettler FA Jr., et al. Effective doses in radiology and diagnostic nuclear medicine: A catalog. *Radiology.* 2008;248(1):254–263.
3 McCollough CH, et al. Strategies for reducing radiation dose in CT. *Radiol Clin North Am.* 2009;47(1):27–40.

Examination	Average effective dose (mSv)	Values reported in literature (mSv)	Equivalent chest x-ray*
Various diagnostic radiology procedures			
Skull	0.1	0.03–0.22	1
Cervical spine	0.2	0.07–0.3	2
Thoracic spine	1.0	0.6–1.4	10
Lumbar spine	1.5	0.5–1.8	15
Posteroanterior and lateral study of chest	0.1	0.05–0.24	1
Posteroanterior study of chest	0.02	0.007–0.050	0.2
Mammography	0.4	0.10–0.60	4
Abdomen	0.7	0.04–1.1	7
Pelvis	0.6	0.2–1.2	6
Hip	0.7	0.18–2.71	7
Shoulder	0.01	–	0.1
Knee	0.005	–	0.05
Other extremities	0.001	0.0002–0.1	0.01
Dual x-ray absorptiometry (without CT)	0.001	0.001–0.035	0.01
Dual x-ray absorptiometry (with CT)	0.04	0.003–0.06	0.4
Intravenous urography	3	0.7–3.7	30
Upper gastrointestinal series	6	1.5–12	60
Small-bowel series	5	3.0–7.8	50
Barium enema	8	2.0–18.0	80
Various CT Procedures			
Head	2	0.9–4.0	20
Neck	3	–	30
Chest	7	4.0–18.0	70
Chest for pulmonary embolism	15	13–40	150
Abdomen	8	3.5–25	80
Pelvis	6	3.3–10	60
Three-phase liver study	15	–	150
Spine	6	1.5–10	60
Coronary angiography	16	5.0–32	160
Calcium scoring	3	1.0–12	30
Virtual colonoscopy	10	4.0–13.2	100

(Continued)

Examination	Average effective dose (mSv)	Values reported in literature (mSv)	Equivalent chest x-ray*
Various Interventional Radiology Procedures			
Head and/or neck angiography	5	0.8–19.6	50
Coronary angiography (diagnostic)	7	2.0–15.8	70
Coronary percutaneous transluminal angioplasty stent placement or radiofrequency ablation	15	6.9–57	150
Thoracic angiography of pulmonary artery or aorta	5	4.1–9.0	50
Abdominal angiography or aortography	12	4.0–48.0	120
Transjugular intrahepatic portosystemic shunt placement	70	20–180	700
Pelvic vein embolization	60	44–78	600

* One chest x-ray: 0.1 mSv
Adapted from Mettler FA, et al. Effective doses in radiology and diagnostic nuclear medicine: A catalog. *Radiology*. 2008; 248(1):254–263.

Immediate hypersensitivity reactions (IHR) Any contrast agent administered intravenously can cause adverse reactions. These reactions are idiosyncratic and are not related to the dose. IHR can be classified based on its severity and may range from mild flushing, pruritus, and urticaria to more severe angioedema, laryngospasm, bronchospasm, and hypotension. Adverse reactions occur in ~ 1/1,000 patients and death by anaphylaxis in 1/40,000. The osmolality of the agent is strongly associated with IHR.[4] Risk factors for contrast reaction should always be reviewed prior to imaging. The most significant risk factor for IHR is a previous IHR. Other risk factors include asthma, atopic diseases, and possibly the use of β-blockers or NSAIDs. With a previous history of IHR, the patient may require premedication with steroids. A common regimen includes prednisone 40 mg PO, 24 h, 12 h, and 1 h before and 12 h after the procedure, with or without a dose of diphenhydramine (50 mg PO or IV 1 h) before the procedure. When the patient has a history of severe anaphylactic reaction to IV contrast, iodine-based contrast is absolutely contraindicated. It is important to note that there is no proven link between seafood and contrast allergies.

Contrast-mediated nephrotoxicity Risk factors include congestive heart failure, diabetes, preexisting renal insufficiency, age >70, concurrent nephrotoxic medications, high-dose hyperosmolar IV contrast, diuretic

4 Greenberger PA, Patterson R. The prevention of immediate generalized reactions to radiocontrast media in high-risk patients. *J Allergy Clin Immunol*. 1991;87(4):867–872.

medications, or dehydration. IV 0.9% saline 1 mL/kg/h, 4–6 h before contrast administration and 12–24 h after exposure, significantly reduces the risk of contrast nephrotoxicity in patients with mild renal insufficiency. The use of sodium bicarbonate drip instead of NS is shown to be superior in some studies, but other studies have shown conflicting results. The efficacy of N-acetylcysteine, an antioxidant, to reduce the occurrence of contrast-induced nephrotoxicity (CIN) is also undetermined but is often used. It is dosed at 600 mg PO bid for 24 h before contrast administration and on the day of contrast, along with hydration. When possible, it is beneficial to discontinue nephrotoxic medications (e.g., metformin and diuretics) for at least 24 h after contrast administration. Low-osmolar contrast media are less nephrotoxic than high-osmolar contrasts in patients with renal insufficiency. Alternative imaging modalities such as magnetic resonance, ultrasound (US), and nuclear scintigraphy should be considered in patients at high risk of developing contrast nephropathy.

Gadolinium contrast Gadolinium is a very safe contrast agent used in MR imaging in patients with normal renal function. It is completely unrelated to CT/angiographic iodinated contrast, and gadolinium allergies are extremely rare. Gadolinium should be avoided in pregnant patients and in patients with renal insufficiency / failure.

Nephrogenic systemic fibrosis/Nephrogenic fibrosing dermopathy (NSF/NFD) was first described in 2000 and is a relatively newer described complication of gadolinium in patients with renal failure.

NSF/NFD is seen in patients who have noticeably advanced chronic renal failure corresponding to estimated glomerular filtration rate (eGFR) values of <29 mL/min/1.73 m^2 and acute kidney injury. The reported incidence of developing NSF ranges from 1% to 7% after exposure to gadolinium in patients with chronic renal disease. The disease causes fibrosis of the skin and connective tissues throughout the body. Patients develop skin thickening that may prevent bending and extending joints, resulting in decreased mobility of joints. In addition, patients may experience fibrosis that spreads to other parts of the body such as the diaphragm, muscles in the thigh and lower abdomen, and the interior areas of lung vessels. The clinical course of NSF/NFD is progressive and may be fatal.

In general, due to NSF/NFD, the administration of gadolinium-based contrast agents in patients with renal failure or renal insufficiency is contraindicated. However, your institution's policy regarding NSF/NFD should be consulted.

The basics of radiography

General concepts

Images are obtained by transmitting x-rays (ionizing radiation) through the body to a detector (film or a photosensitive plate in digital image systems). The image obtained represents a "shadowgram" as the body absorbs different amounts of radiation depending on the density of the tissue. Denser tissues, such as bone, absorb more radiation and appear white, and less dense tissues, such as lung, absorb less radiation and appear dark as more x-rays reach the film and expose the photosensitive cells.

Although this modality does use ionizing radiation, doses are fairly low, and, other than early pregnancy, there is essentially no contraindication to obtaining a radiograph. Radiographs also have the advantage of being portable and have no weight limitations, although heavier patients require more radiation and create noisier films.

Basic considerations

- *"One view is no view."* Because these are two-dimensional images of three-dimensional structures, two orthogonal views should always be obtained, if possible.
- *Not all radiographs are equal.* Radiographs done on fixed equipment within a radiology department are generally of higher quality than are radiographs acquired portably. This is due to the presence of a better grid system and the ability to better position the patient on the stationary system. Thus, if the patient can be safely moved to radiology department, he or she should be.
- *Order coned (region-specific) radiographs.* Radiographs are most diagnostic in the center of the x-ray beam, where the photons are parallel. Thus, if the area of interest is the wrist, order a wrist series and not a forearm series. This will place the wrist in the center of the field of view.
- *Do not skip the radiograph.* Radiographs are excellent screening tools, are often diagnostic, and usually should be obtained before other more expensive and time-consuming imaging modalities. (One glaring exception to this rule is skull radiographs—which are obsolete and have been replaced by CT.)

Basic steps in interpreting any radiograph

1 *Check the technical accuracy of the film:* Is the film named, dated, right/left orientated, and marked as to whether AP (anteroposterior), PA (posteroanterior), erect, or supine. X-ray beam penetration is important; ideally, vertebral bodies are visible through heart on a chest x-ray (CXR). If the film is underpenetrated, diffuse "whitening" effect and poor anatomical detail is present. Check for rotation (e.g., check for asymmetry of clavicles on a CXR) as this may affect the appearances of normal structures, such as the hila.

2 *Describe the abnormalities seen:* This may be a change in the appearance of normally visualized structures or an area of increased opacity or translucency.

Plain radiographs identify the interfaces between different densities. These interfaces occur, and are visible on the film, only when two different tissue densities are immediately adjacent to each other. These densities are:

- Gas
- Fat (normal adipose tissue, lipomas, oily deposits, etc.)
- Soft tissue (like muscle, tendon, ligament, water, visceral organs, blood vessels, nerves, etc.)
- Calcified structures (bone, calcified granulomas, tumoral calcinosis, etc.)
- Metallic structures (surgical clips, radiodense markers in central lines, bullet fragments)

A border is seen at an interface of two densities; e.g., heart (water) and lung (air). This "silhouette" is lost if air in the lung is replaced by consolidation (water). This is called the silhouette sign and can be used to localize pathology (e.g., right middle lobe pneumonia or collapse causing loss of distinction of the right heart border). See p. 153 (pulmonary medicine), which describes the methods for localizing collapse/consolidation in the lungs; see Figure 6.1.

3 *Translate the abnormalities into gross pathology* (e.g., pleural fluid, lung consolidation, free air in the abdomen).

4 *Suggest a differential diagnosis:* Develop a structured approach so as not to miss any major abnormality. Try not to jump immediately to one diagnosis, and develop your differential based both on radiologic findings and patient history/physical findings.

5 *Treat the patient, not the film.*

The chest film

See Figures 18.1–18.7, and PLATES 1–8

Before you start

Order the best possible exam: Upright PA and lateral views are the standard initial imaging of choice for almost all cardiopulmonary disease. These complementary views are particularly important when localization of a lesion/pathology is required.

An ideal PA view is taken with the patient in an upright position with full inspiration, and it demonstrates no rotation or motion and minimal overlying osseous structures. However, this ideal is rarely seen in chest x-rays taken in ICU and emergency settings.

The interpretation

- *Double-check the name on the film.*
- *Comment on the quality of the film ("RIPE"):*

  Rotation: The spinous process of T3 should be midway between the clavicles.

  Inspiration: 5–7 ribs anteriorly or 9–10 ribs posteriorly are visible in full inspiration.

  Position of the patient: Entire thorax from larynx to costophrenic angles should be visible.

  Exposure: Pulmonary vessels and thoracic vertebra should be visible through the heart.

- *Look thoroughly and systematically.* Examine all the structures, including visible portions of the abdomen, bones, mediastinum, lungs together (to judge symmetry), and lungs separately.
- *Compare to old examinations when possible.* Age and progression of findings can be crucial to diagnosis and treatment. For example, a calcified nodule that has remained unchanged over years may merely be a calcified granuloma.

Lines and hardware: All lines and hardware need to be identified and examined for correct location and potential complications. Remember, all the hardware visible on CXR may not be inside the patient (e.g., electrocardiogram [ECG] leads, oxygen lines, etc.). Examples of common hardware include central venous catheters (check for tip location and for pneumothorax), endotracheal tubes (typically, the tip should be above the carina to avoid endobronchial intubation), chest tubes, feeding tubes (nasogastric or naso-duodenal—tip locations are key), sternal wires (are these intact?), prosthetic valves, implantable cardioversion devices (ICDs/pacers), vagus nerve stimulators, Swan–Ganz catheters, etc.

The diaphragm: The right hemidiaphragm is higher than the left by up to 3 cm in 95% of cases. The lateral costophrenic angles should be sharp and acute. They may be ill-defined in hyperinflation or with effusion. On a lateral view, the right hemidiaphragm passes through the heart to the anterior chest wall, whereas the left ends at the posterior heart border. Causes of raised hemidiaphragm include eventration of diaphragm, enlarged liver or spleen, phrenic nerve paralysis, or lobar collapse.

Trachea: The trachea is central or maybe slightly to the right. Trachea may be deviated toward the lesion (collapse), away from the lesion (tension pneumothorax) or deviated from patient rotation. Paratracheal line is commonly <5 mm; its thickening and nodularity suggest paratracheal lymphadenopathy/mass.

Heart: Look for the landmarks. The cardiothoracic ratio is the ratio of the heart width to the chest width. It should be <50% (essential to have a PA film as the heart is magnified on AP or supine films). Ratios larger than this suggest cardiomegaly due to any number of causes.

Mediastinum: Mediastinal widening may be due to aortic aneurysm or dissection, mediastinal fluid, enlarged lymph nodes, thymus, thyroid, or tumor.

The hila: Composed of pulmonary arteries, pulmonary veins, lymph nodes, and airways. Left is higher than right (~1 cm) 95% of the time. Look for change in density and/or rounded configuration. This could be due to tumor, enlarged lymph nodes, hypoinflation, or just a rotated film.

The lungs

"Too black":

- Pneumothorax: Absent vascular markings and visceral pleura/lung edge visible
- Bullous change: I.e., emphysema
- Chronic pulmonary embolus: Localized oligemia (regional lack of visualization of pulmonary blood vessels)
- Hyperinflation in chronic obstructive pulmonary disease (COPD)
- Absent anterior chest wall structures: I.e., mastectomy or Poland's syndrome

"Too White":

- Consolidation: Lobar or segmental opacity, plus air bronchogram if airways remain air-filled but little volume change (unlike collapse)
- Collapse/atelectasis: Volume loss causes shift of the normal landmarks (hila, fissures, diaphragm, etc.)
- Pulmonary nodules ("coin" lesions <3 cm in diameter): These are often "incidentalomas" and need to be differentiated into either benign or malignant lesions based on their characteristics—but most importantly in comparison to older films.
- "Ring" shadows: Either airways with peribronchial "cuffing" (pulmonary edema, bronchiectasis), or cavitating lesions (e.g., abscess [bacterial, fungal]) or tumor
- Interstitial pattern: Pulmonary interstitium is normally not seen on CXR. Abnormal interstitial patterns maybe seen as linear opacities (*Kerley's B lines,* interlobular lymphatics seen in low-pressure pulmonary edema or lymphangitic spread of tumor); *discoid atelectasis,* linear band of atelectasis; *reticulonodular pattern,* multiple intersecting irregular lines interspersed with small 1–2 mm nodules, seen in pulmonary fibrosis or interstitial pneumonitis.

Acute conditions not to miss

- *Pneumothorax* is commonly associated with trauma or can be iatrogenic. It may occur spontaneously in emphysema. In tension pneumothorax, the lung may be severely collapsed with mediastinal shift to the opposite side, with scooping of the ipsilateral hemidiaphragm. There may also be subcutaneous air/subcutaneous emphysema. This is a medical emergency and requires immediate decompression followed by placement of a chest tube.
- *Widened mediastinum* in a patient with chest pain and/or history of trauma may represent aortic aneurysm or dissection, traumatic transection, or mediastinal hematoma.
- *Free air in the abdomen* seen under the right hemidiaphragm; this represents free intraperitoneal air and may suggest a bowel perforation.

Don't

- *Succumb to "satisfaction of search":* After identifying one example of pathology on the image, don't give up your search until you have thoroughly examined the whole film, including all the corners; there may be two or more important findings!

Figure 18.1 Posteroanterior chest radiograph of a female showing basic anatomical structures

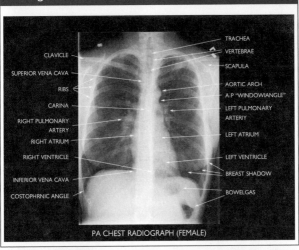

PA CHEST RADIOGRAPH (FEMALE)

Figure 18.2 Lateral chest radiograph of a female showing basic anatomical structures

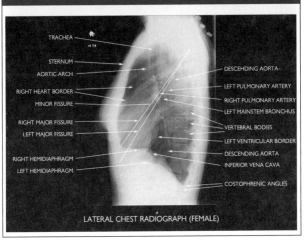

LATERAL CHEST RADIOGRAPH (FEMALE)

Figure 18.3 3D coronal CT of the chest demonstrating heart and vascular structures

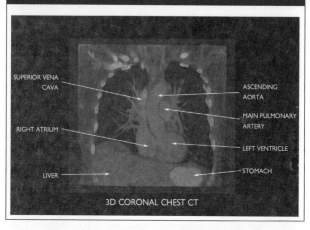

SUPERIOR VENA CAVA

ASCENDING AORTA

MAIN PULMONARY ARTERY

RIGHT ATRIUM

LEFT VENTRICLE

LIVER

STOMACH

3D CORONAL CHEST CT

Figure 18.4 3D coronal CT of the chest demonstrating heart and vascular structures

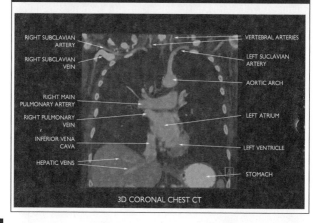

RIGHT SUBCLAVIAN ARTERY

VERTEBRAL ARTERIES

RIGHT SUBCLAVIAN VEIN

LEFT SUCLAVIAN ARTERY

AORTIC ARCH

RIGHT MAIN PULMONARY ARTERY

RIGHT PULMONARY VEIN

LEFT ATRIUM

INFERIOR VENA CAVA

LEFT VENTRICLE

HEPATIC VEINS

STOMACH

3D CORONAL CHEST CT

Figure 18.5 3D sagittal CT of the chest demonstrating midline structures of the chest and vertebral column

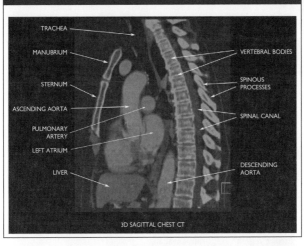

Figure 18.6 3D sagittal CT of the chest demonstrating structures on the left side of the chest

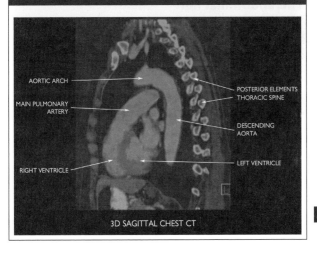

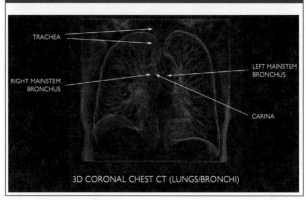

Figure 18.7 3D coronal CT of the chest demonstrating bronchial and pulmonary vascular tree

TRACHEA

LEFT MAINSTEM BRONCHUS

RIGHT MAINSTEM BRONCHUS

CARINA

3D CORONAL CHEST CT (LUNGS/BRONCHI)

- *Forget to recheck danger areas*: Apices, aortopulmonary (AP) angle, retrocardiac region, and paratracheal area
- *Fail to give an adequate history* to the radiologist and to check the radiologist's final interpretation. Basic image interpretation can be easy, but subtle abnormalities require the trained eye of a radiologist.

The abdominal film

See Figures 18.8–18.13.

Before you start

- *Order the best possible exam*: A true abdominal series of radiographs includes three films:
  1. Upright PA chest (to look for free air under the diaphragms)
  2. Upright abdomen after at least 5 min of upright positioning to allow air to percolate superiorly and appear
  3. Supine abdomen
- *Double-check the name, date and time on the film*: Make sure the patient's name matches and that you are looking at the appropriate time point.
- *Radiographs (plain films) only identify the interfaces between tissues of different densities*: Interfaces made by adjacent tissues that are of the same density cannot be seen. For example, you cannot see the interface between two adjacent loops of fluid-filled small bowel. What you can identify are abnormal contours and mass effects created by the underlying pathology (e.g., loops of small bowel displaced by a large pelvic mass).
- *Look thoroughly and systematically*: Develop a repeatable method by which you look at all abdominal films; review by organ system.
- *Compare new versus old findings*: Compare to prior films whenever possible, as age and progression of findings can be crucial to diagnosis and treatment.
- *Don't forget the patient*: Although abdominal radiographs can offer valuable clues to diagnosis, it is possible for a very sick patient to have a normal-appearing abdominal series of radiographs.

Figure 18.8 Abnormal gas patterns on plain abdominal radiography

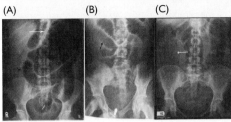

(A) Cecal volvulus: Erect abdominal radiograph demonstrating a grossly dilated loop of bowel (cecum) projected in the upper abdomen (*white arrow*). Note the lack of gas in the rest of the large bowel and dilated small bowel loops (*black arrow*). (B) Small bowel obstruction: Multiple loops of distended small bowel. Note the valvulae conniventes stretching across the bowel circumferentially (*arrow*). (C) Large bowel obstruction: Plain radiograph showing distended large bowel loops. Note grossly dilated cecum (*white arrow*).

From Musson RE, et al. *Postgrad Med J.* 2011;87:274–287. Adapted with permission from *PMJ, The Fellowship of Postgraduate Medicine.*

Observe the gas pattern and position See Figure 18.13. Small bowel is recognized by its central position and valvulae conniventes (the mucosal folds) that transverse the full width of the bowel lumen. Large bowel is more peripheral and the haustrae, colonic folds, extend only partially across the lumen. Abnormal position may point to pathology (e.g., centrally displaced loops in ascites; bowel displaced to the left lower quadrant by splenomegaly). Look for dilated bowel loops, defined as >3 cm diameter for the small bowel and as >6 cm diameter for the large bowel. Also look for air–fluid levels in the bowel on upright film.

• If the dilated loops are small bowel only, it is probably a small bowel obstruction.
• If the dilated loops are large bowel only, it may be a large bowel obstruction or a cecal or sigmoid volvulus. A volvulus appears as a large bean-shaped loop of large bowel arising from pelvis.
• If the dilated loops are seen in the small and large bowel, it may be an adynamic ileus, a large bowel obstruction with an incompetent ileocecal valve, gastroenteritis, or excessive aerophagia.

Localized peritoneal inflammation can cause a localized dilatation of bowel in response to inflammatory irritation (focal ileus). This may be seen on the plain film as a "sentinel loop" of intraluminal gas and can provide a clue to the site of pathology.

Look for extraluminal/extraintestinal gas Look for gas in the peritoneal cavity, especially air under the hemidiaphragm, which can indicate a perforated viscus. Look in the portal vein territory (peripheral liver) or biliary system (central liver and gallbladder), where air may be seen after passing a stone, after ERCP, or with gas-forming biliary infection or with bowel necrosis. Look at the GU system (enterovesical fistula,

697

pyelonephritis), in the peritoneum (*double wall sign:* Visualization of the outer wall of bowel loops caused by gas outside the bowel loop and normal intraluminal gas), *triangle sign* (represents a triangular pocket of air between two loops of bowel and the abdominal wall), *football sign* (a large collection of air that seems to outline the entire abdominal cavity; air surrounding the falciform ligament, may have the appearance of the laces of the football), the colonic wall (pneumatosis coli, infective colitis), or a subphrenic abscess. Sometimes, free air in the abdomen can be normal post surgery or after certain procedures, such as ERCP, laparoscopy, etc. Free air can be detected on the left lateral decubitus radiograph because free air collects around the inferior edge of the liver, which forms the least dependent part of the abdomen in that position.

Look for calcification in the abdomen or pelvis

Calcification in an abdominal film maybe normal or may indicate pathology. Normal structures that calcify include costal cartilage, mesenteric lymph nodes, pelvic veins (phlebolith), and prostate gland. Pathological calcification can be approached systematically:

• *Vascular:* Arteries (atherosclerosis, the eggshell calcification of an aneurysm)

• *GU:* Renal calcification or ureteric stones (usually jagged; look along the line of the ureter), bladder (stone, tumor, tuberculosis [TB], schistosomiasis), uterine fibroids, dermoid cyst of the ovary (which may contain teeth)

• *GI:* Adrenal (TB), pancreatic (chronic pancreatitis), liver, or spleen granulomas; gallstones (only 10% radiopaque), appendicoliths and incision or injection sites; may all calcify.

Bones of spine Look for metastases, which may be osteolytic (low density, black), osteoblastic (higher density, white), or mixed. Malignancies that have predominant osteoblastic lesions include prostate, carcinoid, gastrinoma, small cell lung cancer, and Hodgkin's lymphoma. Osteolytic lesions can indicate renal cell and thyroid cancer, melanoma, multiple myeloma, non-small cell lung cancer and non-Hodgkin's lymphoma. Mixed lesions are most commonly secondary to breast cancer, but osteosarcoma, Ewing's sarcoma, as well as others, can also present as mixed lesions. Paget's disease maybe identified as a "picture frame vertebral body." Other conditions visible on spine include osteomalacia, collapse, osteoarthritis, hyperparathyroidism ("rugger jersey" spine), or ankylosing spondylitis ("bamboo spine").

Bones of pelvis Look at the hip joint for any signs of fracture. Advanced osteonecrosis may be seen as loss of spherical margin and collapse of the femoral head. Osteoarthritis may present as joint-space narrowing with degenerative changes such as osteophytes.

Soft tissues These can be evaluated by the fatty rim (preperitoneal fat lines) surrounding the organs. The loss of the normal fat planes may suggest the presence of pathology; for example, the psoas lines may be obliterated in retroperitoneal processes such as inflammation, hemorrhage, or peritonitis. Note kidney size and shape (normally 2–3 vertebral bodies' length and parallel to the psoas line).

Iatrogenic or incidental objects You will be surprised to find that the abdominal cavity can be a hiding place for a wide array of objects, left both intentionally (e.g., inferior vena cava [IVC] filters, stents, surgical pins, screws, clips, etc.) and unintentionally (surgical sponges, clamps, etc.) For intentionally placed objects, make sure that they are located where they should be (e.g., an IVC filter should not be located in chest). Presence of such objects can reveal a lot about a patient's history.

Acute conditions not to miss

- *Pneumoperitoneum:* This usually means perforation unless recent instrumentation.
- *Portal venous air (peripheral liver) and/or pneumatosis coli (air in the wall of bowel, usually colon):* This often means necrotic bowel.

Don't

- Forget to look for lower lung pathology on the upright abdominal film.
- Forget to check the "corners" of any plain films as these can hide subtle and often missed pathology.

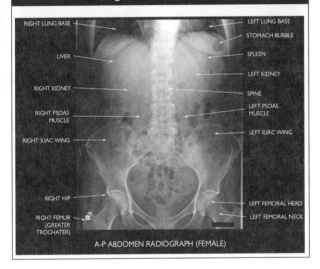

Figure 18.9 Anterio-posterior abdominal radiograph of a female demonstrating structures in the abdomen and pelvis

RIGHT LUNG BASE

LEFT LUNG BASE

STOMACH BUBBLE

LIVER

SPLEEN

LEFT KIDNEY

RIGHT KIDNEY

SPINE

RIGHT PSOAS MUSCLE

LEFT PSOAS MUSCLE

LEFT ILIAC WING

RIGHT ILIAC WING

RIGHT HIP

LEFT FEMORAL HEAD

RIGHT FEMUR (GREATER TROCHATER)

LEFT FEMORAL NECK

A-P ABDOMEN RADIOGRAPH (FEMALE)

Figure 18.10 Supine abdominal radiograph

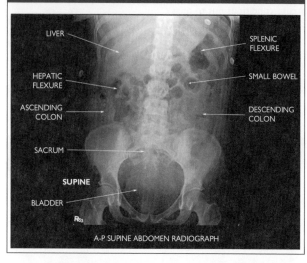

LIVER

SPLENIC FLEXURE

HEPATIC FLEXURE

SMALL BOWEL

ASCENDING COLON

DESCENDING COLON

SACRUM

SUPINE

BLADDER

R₆₃

A-P SUPINE ABDOMEN RADIOGRAPH

Figure 18.11 3D coronal CT of the abdomen—I

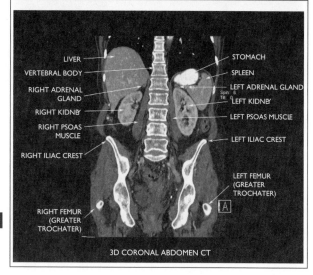

LIVER

STOMACH

VERTEBRAL BODY

SPLEEN

RIGHT ADRENAL GLAND

LEFT ADRENAL GLAND

LEFT KIDNEY

RIGHT KIDNEY

LEFT PSOAS MUSCLE

RIGHT PSOAS MUSCLE

LEFT ILIAC CREST

RIGHT ILIAC CREST

LEFT FEMUR (GREATER TROCHATER)

RIGHT FEMUR (GREATER TROCHATER)

3D CORONAL ABDOMEN CT

Figure 18.12 3D coronal CT of the abdomen—II

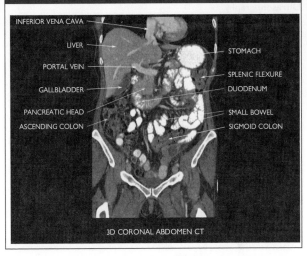

INFERIOR VENA CAVA
LIVER
PORTAL VEIN
GALLBLADDER
PANCREATIC HEAD
ASCENDING COLON

STOMACH
SPLENIC FLEXURE
DUODENUM
SMALL BOWEL
SIGMOID COLON

3D CORONAL ABDOMEN CT

Figure 18.13 3D coronal CT of the abdomen—III

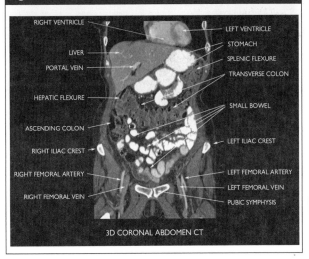

RIGHT VENTRICLE
LIVER
PORTAL VEIN
HEPATIC FLEXURE
ASCENDING COLON
RIGHT ILIAC CREST
RIGHT FEMORAL ARTERY
RIGHT FEMORAL VEIN

LEFT VENTRICLE
STOMACH
SPLENIC FLEXURE
TRANSVERSE COLON
SMALL BOWEL
LEFT ILIAC CREST
LEFT FEMORAL ARTERY
LEFT FEMORAL VEIN
PUBIC SYMPHYSIS

3D CORONAL ABDOMEN CT

Modalities

Ultrasonography

"Ultrasound" refers to the sound waves with frequency greater than the upper limit of human hearing. In ultrasonography, a sound wave that passes through a tissue interface is reflected back to the US transducer, and these reflected waves are used to construct an image of an organ or structure. Keys to US image formation are attenuation (i.e., when the signal strength is progressively reduced as waves penetrate deeper into the tissues due to its conversion to heat) and reflection (i.e., when the US wave hits a tissue boundary and is partially or completely reflected back to the transducer). These key properties help to create the US image. Beyond seeing organs and tissues, other key features can help in making a diagnosis using US. Two of these are *acoustic shadowing* (Figure 18.14A), which is a band of markedly reduced echogenicity (black) behind a strongly reflecting structure. Fibrous tissue, calcified structures, such as bones and stones, lead to this kind of acoustic shadowing. US is also unable to penetrate air-containing structures, which also leads to shadowing. In contrast, *acoustic enhancement* (Figure 18.14B) is a bright band (white) behind an anechoic structure that does not reflect any sound waves (e.g., bladder or a cyst). This phenomenon can help us differentiate an anechoic simple cyst showing distal acoustic enhancement from a hypoechoic solid breast lesion.

US is an extremely powerful tool that can be tailored to any number of diagnostic and interventional uses. It does not use ionizing radiation to produce images; hence, it is safe even in early stages of pregnancy. Furthermore, US is portable and can be used at the bedside of critically ill patients. There are essentially no contraindications to US. However, it may be of limited value in obese people because of poor tissue penetration. Bone, gas, and calcifications reflect US waves and can interfere with the ability to image subjacent structures. Of all the modalities, US is the most operator-dependent, and reliability of results may vary.

US is the imaging modality of choice in obstetrics and is often the first line of investigation for abdominal pathologies and pelvic lesions. US is often used to guide needle aspiration, biopsies, sclerotherapies, and thermal ablations.

Doppler US allows for the assessment of the direction and velocities of blood flow within blood vessels. It is based on the principal of *Doppler shift*, which is defined as the change in the frequency of a sound wave when the source and observer are in relative motion. When incident sound waves encounter the red blood cells in the circulating blood, they undergo a frequency shift proportional to the speed of red cell movement. This change in frequency helps determine the blood flow velocity. There are various modalities of Doppler US, such as color flow imaging, in which the velocities are displayed on a color scale. The transducer detects the flowing blood and arbitrarily assigns a red and blue color depending on whether the flow is toward or away from the transducer. It is most commonly used in assessment of regurgitant flow and intracardiac shunts.

Duplex US combines the Doppler flow information and conventional imaging information, sometimes called B-mode. It gives both structural and functional information and is used extensively.

Figure 18.14

Radiology

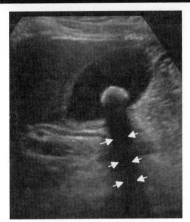

(A) US of gallbladder demonstrates a single echogenic focus (gallstone) with acoustic shadowing (*arrowheads*)

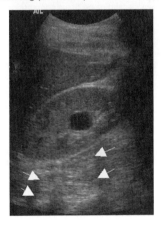

(B) US of the kidney demonstrates a cyst with acoustic enhancement (*arrowheads*)

Computed tomography

The advent of CT (also called CAT) has revolutionized medical imaging. The principal component of CT scanning is an x-ray tube that rotates around the patient and generates an x-ray beam. The opposed array of detectors record the radiation that passes through the tissues and is used to construct the images. Since its introduction, there have been several generations of scanners. In first-generation conventional "step and shoot" CT, the patient is moved into a desired position and x-ray tube rotates around the patient to acquire individual slices. Conventional CT scans are still used for some applications such as high-resolution CT (HRCT) of lungs. Conventional CTs have almost entirely been replaced by spiral or helical CT scanners. In helical CT, the x-ray beam rotates continuously around the patient in a spiral manner so that a volume of tissue is scanned rather than individual slices. The large amount of raw three-dimensional (3-D) data are then reformatted into axial, coronal, sagittal, or oblique planes. These datasets can also be used for 3-D and maximum intensity projections (MIP) postprocessing. All modern CT scanners are designed as multidetector (MDCT) or multislice scanners, in which multiple active rows of detectors acquire information as tubes rotate around patients. Multidetector imaging allows for faster scanning, thinner slices, higher imaging resolution, and better 3-D reconstruction from the entire volume of a scanned body part.

CT uses point attenuation for density measurements, which are expressed as Hounsfield units (HU). It can be used to differentiate between tissue types (air, fat, muscle, blood, fluid, bone). In Hounsfield units, bone has attenuation of +1,000, water is 0, air is –1,000, fat is <0, and the remaining tissues fall in between, depending on tissue composition (see Figure 18.15).

Contrast use in CT CT can be performed with or without IV or oral contrast. Tissue structures can be viewed in arterial, venous, and delayed phases after the injection of IV contrast. IV contrast is used to differentiate enhancing vascular structures and lesions (e.g., infections or neoplasia) from nonenhancing structures (e.g., cysts, free fluid). The contrast used for CT is similar to that used in angiographic procedures; therefore, standard precautions and consent are recommended. Oral contrast (or water for 3-D reconstructions) should be given prior to abdominal or pelvic scanning to help delineate the bowel (the exception are protocols for renal stone studies and CT angiography). To fill as much of the bowel as possible, the general rule is to give oral contrast early and often.

CT angiography High-resolution, contrast-enhanced MDCT is able to produce 3-D reconstructed images of nearly every arterial territory. CT has already begun to replace much diagnostic angiography in both emergent and nonemergent settings.

All the advances in CT have created some difficulties, including increased cost and increased computer workload and data storage. Compared to conventional radiography (plain x-rays), radiation doses from CT scanning are considerably higher. The ever-increasing use of CT scanning has

Figure 18.15 Figure demonstrates the Hounsfield unit scale on a linear grayscale diagram.

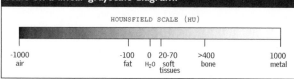

HOUNSFIELD SCALE (HU)

| -1000 air | | -100 fat | 0 H₂O | 20-70 soft tissues | >400 bone | 1000 metal |

increased the overall population radiation exposure. The long-term effects of this increased exposure are still being examined.

Magnetic resonance imaging

MRI is a powerful imaging modality that does not use ionizing radiation. Instead, it uses a powerful magnetic field to image protons within the soft tissues of the body. When a patient is placed in the magnetic field (0.2–7 Tesla), the body's nuclei align themselves in the direction of the external magnetic field. A radiofrequency (RF) pulse is then generated that excites the protons in the soft tissue, causing them to attain a higher energy level. When the RF pulse stops, the protons relax back into their equilibrium position, releasing the energy. This radiofrequency signal or echo emitted by the protons while relaxing is detected and used to create an image. The time elapsed between a RF pulse and to the peak of the echo is called the echo time (TE). The elapsed time between successive RF pulses is called the repetition time (TR). The two types of relaxation times—T1 or longitudinal relaxation and T2 or transverse relaxation—differ for various tissues and are the basis for varying contrasts seen on MRIs. The emission and reception of the RF waves are carried out by the coils that are placed over the body structure that is being imaged.

MR images are described in terms of signal intensity. Tissues that are whiter are *hyperintense* and those with low signals or black are *hypointense*. A pulse sequence with a short TR and a short TE accentuates the T1 differences between tissues (T1-weighted). A *T1-weighted image* provides excellent anatomic detail and produces increased signal intensity over baseline when a contrast agent is given (showing more vascularity). A sequence with a long TR and long TE are *T2-weighted*, which is good for visualizing pathology. A mixture of both reflects proton density weighting, which reflects the water content of the structure.

Advantages and disadvantages MRI takes advantage of multiple parameters (T1, T2, proton density) and has many imaging protocols or sequences (spin echo, inversion recovery, gradient echo), which provides an excellent soft-tissue contrast. Various sequences are available and can be tailored to ask very specific clinical questions. The exposure to magnetic fields of the strength used in clinical MRI is considered to be harmless. Because MR's safety in pregnant patients has yet to be determined, it should be used cautiously, especially in the first trimester. Although MRI is an extremely powerful and evolving technique, it is limited by a lack of portability and its relatively slow speed of imaging. MRI machines can be noisy and claustrophobic, although newer machines with open or wide bores are available.

Contraindications to MRI The specific contraindications to MRI will vary from institution to institution.

Absolute contraindications:
- Non-MRI compliant aneurysm clips or other surgical clips placed in the last 6 wks
- Neurostimulator device
- Pacemaker or defibrillator (this may vary)
- Cochlear implant
- Metallic ocular foreign body (suspect this in patients with a welding history—evaluate with orbit x-ray)
- Other metallic implanted devices such as insulin pumps
- Metallic shrapnel
- Obesity over the maximum table allowance (will vary, usually <350 lb).

Relative contraindications:
- Claustrophobia
- Unstable patients (only MR-compatible life support equipment can be used in the scanning area)
- Dependence on infusion pumps

MRI development is currently one of the most active areas of research within radiology, and its indications and uses continue to expand.

Nuclear medicine (radionuclide scanning)

Radioisotope scanning involves administration of a small amount of radioactive tracer that localizes to a specific organ or cellular receptor. The organ is subsequently imaged to study the disease process. The radioactive tracer consists of a ligand (nonradioactive) that is combined with a radionuclide. The commonly used radionuclides include technetium-99m (^{99}Tcm), indium-111 (^{111}In), iodine-123 (^{123}I), and gallium-67 (^{67}Ga). All these isotopes emit γ-rays, which are captured by a γ-camera and subsequently transformed into analog and/or digital information. Imaging performed by a rotating γ-camera is termed single photon emission computed tomography or SPECT.

Anatomic modalities such as CT or MRI are considered anatomic imaging modalities that, in general, provide exquisite anatomical detail. Radioisotope studies fill this gap by providing physiological or functional information. Using CT and MRI in conjunction with radioisotope imaging provides complementary information that is often of greater clinical relevance than either type of test individually. Because of this, most SPECT cameras have been combined with CT scanners to provide fusion images that display both function and anatomy simultaneously.

Bone scan ^{99}Tcm-MDP (methylene diphosphonate) is the commonly used radiotracer; it is retained in areas with increased osteoblastic activity. *Common indications:* Assessment of metastatic disease from a known primary, assessment of extent of Paget's disease, diagnosis of occult or stress fractures, Identification of osteoid osteoma, characterization of metabolic bone disease. Note that bone scanning it typically negative in cases of multiple myeloma.

Cardiac scan Myocardial perfusion imaging is used mainly to evaluate atypical chest pain, assess the extent of ischemic heart disease, and assess viable myocardium prior to revascularization. Dipyridamole, adenosine, or dobutamine are used as stressors if arthritis or abnormal ECG (left bundle branch block, or on digoxin with changes to the ECG) preclude exercise, or in those in whom the exercise test is inconclusive. SPECT imaging is performed after injection of ^{201}Tl (thallium-201), or ^{99}Tcm-MIBI (methoxy isobutyl isonitrile).

Radionuclide ventriculography/ Multigated acquisition scan (MUGA) ECG gated imaging is performed after radiolabeling red blood cells with radiotracer and measuring the radioactivity. It provides objective and reproducible data on ventricular ejection fractions, regional wall motion abnormalities, and information on ventricular aneurysms.

Lung scan (V̇/Q̇) ^{99}Tcm -MAA (macroaggregates of albumin) is commonly used to assess perfusion (Q) and ^{133}Xe is used to assess ventilation (V). V/Q scanning relies on the physiological principle of reduction in segmental perfusion with maintained normal ventilation in pulmonary embolism. Matched reduction in perfusion and ventilation can be seen in parenchymal lung disorders. Scans should be interpreted in conjunction with a current CXR, and reports are in the form of probabilities: High probability (>80% likelihood of pulmonary embolism [PE]), low probability (<20% likelihood of PE), intermediate probability (~20–80% likelihood of PE), or very low probability (<5% likelihood of PE). Note that CT pulmonary angiography is both sensitive and specific technique for the assessment of acute pulmonary embolism and is more commonly used.

Hepatobiliary scan (HIDA) ^{99}Tcm-mebrofenin is taken up by the hepatocytes, secreted into the bile, then disperses with the bile into the bile ducts, gallbladder, and intestine. This test is used mainly to diagnose acute cholecystitis, for biliary leaks, and for quantitative information on gallbladder kinetics (i.e., assessment of chronic cholecystitis) when used in conjunction with an IV infusion of cholecystokinin (CCK).

Thyroid scan ^{99}Tcm-pertechnetate or ^{123}I-Iodide may be used for assessment of solitary thyroid nodule, assessment of congenital hypothyroidism and localization of ectopic thyroid tissue, diagnosis of autonomous functioning thyroid adenomas, and for the differentiation of Graves' from multinodular goiter. Radioactive iodine is also used to treat hyperthyroid patients with Graves' disease, toxic adenoma, or multinodular goiter. Therapeutic sodium ^{131}I is given orally and is rapidly taken up by the thyroid gland, where it emits high-energy β rays that locally destroys the gland. It is also used as an adjuvant therapy after thyroidectomy (to destroy residual tumor or metastatic disease) in patients with well-differentiated thyroid cancer.

Parathyroid scan ^{99}Tcm -MIBI is used to localize a parathyroid adenoma once a biochemical diagnosis of primary hyperparathyroidism is made.

Adrenal scan Pheochromocytomas and other tumors of neuroectodermal origin can be localized using ^{123}I-MIBG (metaiodobenzylguanidine).

Renal scan Radioisotope scanning and computer-assisted analysis of the images of the kidneys (renography) provide vital functional information. Standard renography with ^{99}Tcm-DTPA or ^{99}Tcm-MAG3 (Mertiatide) provides data on split renal function and uptake and excretory patterns of each kidney. Diuretic renography performed by injecting furosemide at the end of a standard renogram helps to distinguish physiological dilatation of the renal pelvis from obstructive nephropathy. Captopril renography performed by repeating the standard renogram after administration of PO captopril (25–50 mg) helps to confirm renovascular disorder (unilateral better than bilateral). ^{99}Tcm -DMSA (dimethyl succinic acid), a renal cortical imaging agent, is useful in assessing chronic pyelonephritis, renal scarring, cortical cysts, and tumors.

Inflammation/infection scan (tagged white blood cell scan) ^{111}In-oxine labeled leukocytes are typically used to evaluate osteomyelitis (in conjunction with either a phase bone scan using ^{99}Tcm-MDP or a marrow scan using ^{99}Tcm-sulfur colloid). However, leukocytes radiolabeled with ^{111}In-oxine or ^{99}Tcm-HMPAO can also be used for the evaluation of fever of unknown origin, localization of abscesses (5–10 d old), evaluation of chronic inflammation, and assessment of mediastinal lymphomas, prosthetic infection (especially hip), and in patients with inflammatory bowel disease.

Radiolabeled red blood cell scans (tagged red blood cell scans) are useful in the localization of an unexplained active GI bleeding that is occurring at a rate of 0.1–0.5 mL/min. It is more sensitive than angiography in localizing a GI bleed. It can be a key to localizing bleeding—and can help direct therapeutic angiography, endoscopy, or surgery.

Positron emission tomography

Molecules labeled with positron-emitting radionuclides are injected and postannihilation event photon paths are analyzed by crystal detectors to produce 3-D images. 18F-FDG (fluorodeoxyglucose), an analogue of glucose, is the agent most commonly used. Currently, positron emission tomography (PET) is used primarily for the evaluation of recurrent or metastatic tumors, for assessing tumor response to chemo-/radiotherapy, and for assessing an unknown lesion's metabolic activity or neoplastic potential (e.g., a newly appearing lung nodule). Studies are frequently performed in a hybrid PET/CT scanner for accurate physiologic/anatomic correlation.

In the brain, 18F-FDG PET can also be used to determine the site of epileptogenic foci when there is no anatomic lesion seen on MRI or CT. PET can also be used to diagnose dementia (even before symptoms start) and to distinguish Alzheimer's from other dementias (e.g., symmetrical hypo-metabolism in parietal and temporal lobes not the frontal lobes, which are affected in Pick's dementia).

PET development is currently one of the most active areas of research within radiology, and its indications and uses continue to expand.

Organ systems

Gastrointestinal radiology

Abdominal US Abdominal US has found its major use in suspected hepatobiliary disease. It is the choice of imaging for patients who present with acute right upper quadrant pain. It can detect >95% of gallstones and can characterize the gall bladder wall along with localized tenderness (Murphy's sign) in the case of acute cholecystitis. Note that right upper quadrant and abdominal US require that the patient remain NPO 4–8 h prior to the examination in order to allow the gallbladder to expand and to minimize abdominal gas. Other clinical indications for hepatobiliary US include evaluating obstructive jaundice (dilation in obstructive jaundice; although the cause, i.e., stone vs. tumor, is less reliably seen), screening for hepatocellular carcinoma in cirrhotic patients (live size, texture [e.g., fatty or shrunken cirrhotic liver and solid or cystic masses within it]), evaluating patients before and after liver transplantation (patency and size of the portal vein, spontaneous or surgically created portosystemic shunts), and evaluating shunt patency with TIPS. Doppler of the portal and splanchnic veins is used to rule out thrombosis and assess direction of flow in the portal veins in cirrhosis, screen for vascular complications after orthotopic liver transplant, and check the patency of the stents.

Abdominal CT CT is the modality of choice for the evaluation of nearly all abdominal pathology in both solid and luminal organs. With few exceptions (such as renal stone protocols), abdominal CT should be performed with both oral and IV contrast. This provides the most contrast between abdominal structures, allows for evaluation of post-traumatic injuries (e.g., active hemorrhage, parenchymal organ and hollow organ injuries), infections/abscess, masses, adenopathy, and vascular disease throughout the abdomen. CT can be used to assess for bowel disease such as obstruction, cancer, perforation/pneumoperitoneum, and inflammatory/infectious disease. Figure 18.16 shows CT scans of some acute abdomen pathologies seen commonly in the emergency room. CTA of the abdomen is used for the evaluation of the aorta, renal arteries, celiac trunk, and superior and inferior mesenteric arteries, and can be used to assess for aneurysm, dissection, stenosis, and atherosclerotic disease.

Abdominal MRI MRI of the abdomen can be used for the evaluation of masses or infection within any of the solid abdominal and, to a lesser degree, luminal organs. MRI is most often used for the evaluation of lesions that are poorly seen on CT (e.g., metastatic disease to the liver), for the characterization of lesions that are indeterminate with other modalities (e.g. "complex" renal cysts or "indeterminate" liver or adrenal lesions), and for patients who are unable to be evaluated with CT (e.g., allergy to iodinated contrast). MRI is often used to assess the biliary tree (MRCP) to evaluate pancreatic ductal anomalies (e.g., divisum) or for the diagnosis of biliary obstruction. MRA of the abdomen is used for the evaluation of the renal arteries, celiac trunk, and superior and inferior mesenteric arteries, and of stenosis and atherosclerotic disease. MRA is also used to assess for arterial dissection or aneurysm.

GI fluoroscopy In all of these studies, radiopaque contrast (either barium or water-soluble contrast, depending on perforation and aspiration risks)

Figure 18.16

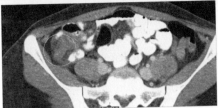

(A) Axial CT with IV and oral contrast demonstrating thickened and dilated appendix (*circle*) with mild periappendiceal fat stranding.

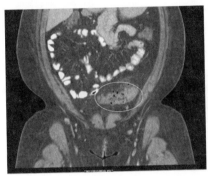

(B) Coronal CT scan with oral and IV contrast demonstrates multiple diverticula in sigmoid colon. There is bowel wall thickening and moderate fat stranding consistent with diverticulitis (*circle*).

Images courtesy of Dr. Karen Horton, MD, Johns Hopkins Hospital.

is introduced by mouth, feeding tube, or enema in order to evaluate the GI tract.

Upper GI series is performed to evaluate the esophagus, stomach, and duodenum. The upper GI series with small bowel follow-through continues to follow the contrast through the entire small bowel. Indications for these studies include perforation of the esophagus or stomach, gastric outlet obstruction, bowel obstruction, GI bleeding, Crohn's disease (when endoscopy is normal), malabsorption syndromes, and small bowel motility, and for evaluation of surgical anastomosis in a postoperative patient.

Barium swallow is a method for investigating dysphagia when motility and pharyngeal coordination need to be observed. The patient is asked to swallow barium containing solids and liquids of various consistencies under direct fluoroscopic visualization. It identifies anatomic abnormalities and aspiration.

Barium enema is commonly performed with the "double-contrast" (barium and air) technique that provides a more detailed examination of surface mucosal pattern. Cleansing the colon using a standard bowel prep is the single most important determinant of quality with barium enemas. Indications include demonstration of structural lesions (e.g., tumor, diverticula, polyps, ulcers, fistulae, perforation), evaluation of colonic obstruction and as a screening tool for colorectal cancer (CRC) especially in failed colonoscopy.

Genitourinary radiology

Renal US US is the modality of choice to look for urinary tract obstruction (hydronephrosis). It is also useful in detecting chronic kidney disease (echogenic and small) and in differentiating a benign cyst from a complex cyst or tumor. Renal Doppler can be used to evaluate vascular flow and help characterize renal vein thrombosis, infarction, and renal artery stenosis.

Renal CT A noncontrast helical CT scan is the gold standard for renal calculi (nearly 100% sensitivity; indinavir stones are not seen) (Figure 18.17). It can detect those stones that are missed on radiographs as well as on IVP. CT scan can also detect signs of obstruction (ureteric and collecting system dilation, perinephric fat stranding). Another major use of CT scan in renal pathology is to diagnose and stage renal cell carcinoma and to characterize renal cysts. *Note*: A cyst that is simple on US (round, sharp boundaries, anechoic, and strong posterior wall echo) doesn't need further imaging. CT and MRI are being increasingly used for the diagnosis of renal vein thrombosis.

Renal nuclear scans A 99mTc-mercaptotriglycylglycine (MAG-3) renal scan can be used to differentiate between obstructive and nonobstructive causes of hydronephrosis. 99mTc-DMSA is used to detect scarring in patients with reflux nephropathy. It also detects ectopic renal tissue or renal dysplasia.

Pelvic US may be used to assess (1) obstetric pathology—US is the standard imaging technique for monitoring normal and abnormal pregnancy, fetal growth and organ development, localization of the placenta, and ectopic pregnancy; (2) ovaries (masses—tumors, cysts, torsion); and (3) uterus (masses—fibroids, cysts, endometrial polyps, hyperplasia). Pelvic US in female patients may require transabdominal scan (TA) and transvaginal scan (TV). For a transabdominal scan, a full bladder either from oral intake of water or from filling of the bladder via a Foley catheter is needed.

A quantitative serum β-HCG should be obtained before all pelvic US performed in young women in order to evaluate for ectopic pregnancy because the interpretation of this examination varies widely depending on the levels of β-HCG. CT is usually not the modality of choice for the evaluation of purely pelvic pathology, especially in female patients (i.e., GU origin). Both US and MRI are more sensitive and specific, have higher resolution within the pelvis, and do not irradiate the gonads.

Testicular US Useful for the evaluation of testicular masses, infections (epididymitis, orchitis), torsion, and varicocele.

Pelvic MRI MRI is a sensitive and specific modality for the evaluation of both the male and female pelvis. In both men and women, MRI can be used to evaluate for abscess, lymphadenopathy, carcinomas of the colon and rectum, carcinomas of the bladder, and pelvic soft-tissue masses. In the postoperative setting, MRI can be used to distinguish between postoperative changes and tumor recurrence, and to monitor response to therapy. In the female pelvis, MRI is the modality of choice for the evaluation of uterine anomalies (e.g., Müllerian duct anomalies, adenomyosis), for the assessment of adnexal masses, and for the radiologic staging of cervical and endometrial cancer. It can also be used to evaluate pelvic organ prolapse. In the male pelvis, endorectal MRI is used for staging prostate cancer.

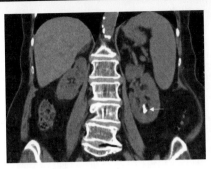

Figure 18.17 Coronal unenhanced abdominal CT demonstrating a left calyceal calculus (*arrow*)

Note there is no perinephric fat stranding or hydronephrosis. This maybe an incidental finding in many patients.

Thoracic radiology

Chest CT CT is the modality of choice for the evaluation of thoracic abnormalities. Noncontrast chest CT is able to demonstrate small pathologies such as focal pneumonias, pleural lesions, and pulmonary nodules that may not be visible using plain radiography. High-resolution chest CT is used to assess and diagnose lung parenchymal disease (e.g., emphysema, interstitial lung disease). Contrast-enhanced chest CT is used to evaluate lung and pleural masses, as well as mediastinal masses and thoracic adenopathy. CT angiography is the modality of choice for the assessment of pulmonary embolism, aortic aneurysm, and aortic dissection, as well as for post-traumatic assessment when aortic injury is suspected. ECG-gated, multidetector CT is also being used to perform coronary angiography and to assess cardiac function.

Chest MRI MRI is less sensitive in the evaluation of lung parenchyma when compared to CT. However, MRI can be used to assess mediastinal masses, chest wall tumors, and breast masses. MRI and MRA (MR angiography) is frequently used in the evaluation of the thoracic aorta for aneurysm and/ or dissection. ECG-gated cardiac MRI is also indicated for the evaluation of myocardial function, structural/congenital anomalies of the heart (e.g., atrial or septal defects), and cardiac tumors (e.g., myxoma). Furthermore, MRI's abilities to distinguish healthy myocardium from diseased or scarred myocardium allows for the evaluation of right ventricular dysplasia and hypertrophic cardiomyopathy, and for the detection of infarcted, stunned, and normal myocardium.

71

Coronary CTA (CCTA) and MRI (CMRI) are rapidly evolving technologies for the noninvasive evaluation of the native coronary arteries and coronary artery bypass grafts. These noninvasive methods have been found to be most clinically applicable in patients with symptoms who are at intermediate risk for coronary artery disease. Currently, CCTA has a better diagnostic accuracy than CMRI, and CCTA is used clinically on a routine basis. It should be noted that artifacts created by severe coronary calcification and by coronary stents affect CCTA's accuracy. CCTA and CMRI can also be used to image congenital anomalies of the coronary artery.

Neuroradiology

Head CT CT is the first-line diagnostic procedure for intracranial processes. CT can diagnose hydrocephalus, intracranial hemorrhage, masses/intracerebral edema, and cerebral atrophy. Intracranial hemorrhage can be subdural, epidural, subarachnoid, or intraparenchymal and appear differently, as described in Figures 18.18A-E. CT is indicated in the setting of moderate to severe head trauma to assess intracranial structures as well as the cranial bones, and it provides an excellent assessment of the extent and location of intracranial hemorrhage. Fresh blood has higher attenuation and therefore is brighter than the brain parenchyma but, as the hemoglobin breaks down, attenuation of hematomas decline. For example, subacute subdural hematoma at 2 wks will have the same attenuation as the adjacent brain. If injury to the face is suspected, a separate facial CT should be ordered to evaluate for facial fractures and intraorbital pathology.

A noncontrast CT is the first choice of imaging when a patient is suspected of having a stroke. Although unenhanced head CT is often normal within the first 6 h after ischemic infarction, it should still be ordered on all patients suspected of presenting with ischemic stroke to assess for the presence of hemorrhage (a contraindication to the administration of thrombolytic agents), alternative diagnoses (such as intracranial mass), and mass effect and edema that may alter the treatment plan. Contrast-enhanced multidetector CT perfusion and cerebral/cervical angiography is an exquisitely sensitive modality for assessment of acute infarction, as well as for assessing cerebrovascular embolic sources. The combination of unenhanced and contrast-enhanced CT may soon become the modality of choice for the assessment of ischemic infarction due to its widespread availability and speed.

Neck CT

Contrast-enhanced CT of the neck is useful to assess for traumatic damage to either soft tissue or the cervical spine, abscess, neoplasm, and vascular disease (CT angiography).

Head and neck MRI

MRI is the modality of choice for the evaluation of tumors and infections of the head (both intra- and extracranially), face, and neck. MRI is also indicated in the evaluation of demyelinating disease (e.g., multiple sclerosis). MRI with diffusion-weighted and perfusion imaging is an exquisitely sensitive modality for assessment of acute infarction and can demonstrate a region of infarction within minutes of symptom onset. MR angiography (MRA) can be performed to evaluate the carotid and vertebral arteries as well as the circle of Willis for atherosclerotic disease, stenosis, and aneurysm. MR venography is used for the assessment of venous sinus thrombosis.

Spine MRI

If neurologic findings related to the spine are present, or if demyelination, infection, or neoplasm involving the spinal canal is suspected, MRI is the modality of choice for the evaluation of the spinal cord and the surrounding CSF spaces. If MRI is unavailable or contraindicated, CT myelography can be considered.

Figures 18.18A–E

Types of Intracranial hemorrhage

Epidural

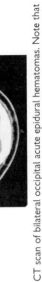

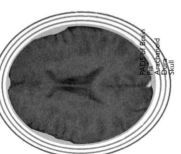

CT scan of bilateral occipital acute epidural hematomas. Note that there are two lens-shaped hematomas. They arise in the potential space between the dura and the skull. Epidural hematomas do not cross the suture lines.

Location

PADS of Brain
Pia
Arachnoid
Dura
Skull

Most common etiology

Trauma resulting in tearing of the meningeal arteries

713

(Continued)

Subdural

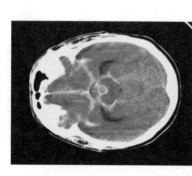

Subarachnoid

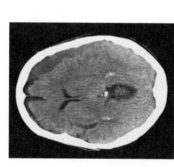

CT scan of a chronic subdural hematoma. Subdural hematomas form between the dura and the arachnoid membrane.

Note that the attenuation of the hematoma is lower than the adjacent brain allowing it to be characterized as a chronic hematoma.

Trauma resulting in tears of the bridging veins which cross the subdural space.

CT scan of an acute subarachnoid bleed. Bleeding occurs in the area between the arachnoid membrane and the pia mater.

Ruptured aneurysms

Intracerebral

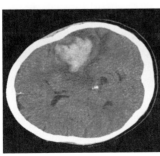

CT scan demonstrating an acute intraparenchymal hemorrhage within the brain tissue itself. Intraventricular is another subtype of intracerebral bleed that involves the ventricles (not shown here)

Hypertensive vasculopathy

Images courtesy of Dr. Nafi Aygun, MD, Johns Hopkins Hospital

Musculoskeletal radiology

Skeletal radiography Radiographic evaluation is often the first method of examination of the extremities and demonstrates fractures, joint effusions, radiodense foreign matter, and lytic or sclerotic bone lesions. Even if MR and CT are requested for further evaluation, comparison to plain films is often essential for accurate diagnosis of skeletal abnormalities and will be needed by the radiologist.

Spine radiography Although often obtained in acute trauma to assess for acute fracture, multidetector CT has largely replaced spine radiography in this area as it is far more sensitive and specific than radiography, and multiplanar reconstructions can be performed. If traumatic spinal injury is strongly suspected, CT should be the first imaging test obtained, followed by MRI as needed.

Musculoskeletal CT CT examination is generally reserved for operative planning for complex fractures or to further evaluate or characterize osseous lesions. As in other areas of the body, contrast-enhanced CT is excellent for evaluating possible soft-tissue abscess in these regions.

Spine CT If equivocal plain film findings or severe pain are present, CT scan to assess the osseous structure of the spinal column should be considered. In most major trauma centers, cervical spine CT has nearly completely replaced radiography when cervical spine trauma is strongly suspected.

Musculoskeletal MRI MRI is commonly used for the evaluation of joints for ligamentous injury, cartilaginous injury, meniscal tears, or arthritic changes. It is also the best means for examining bone marrow and soft-tissue masses. MRI is most often ordered for the evaluation of the knees to evaluate meniscal tears, anterior and posterior cruciate ligament (ACL and PCL) tears, and cartilaginous injury and for degenerative changes. MRI is also the modality of choice for the evaluation of the shoulder joints and is typically ordered for the evaluation of rotator cuff tears or for other traumatic or degenerative changes in the shoulder. MR arthrography of the shoulder is most useful for the evaluation of labral tears. MRI is used for the evaluation of suspected radiographically occult fractures, palpable soft-tissue masses, and in the staging of primary neoplasms of the bone and soft tissue. MR angiography of the extremities can be performed with or without the use of IV gadolinium for the evaluation of peripheral vascular disease.

Practical procedures

Rosalyn W. Stewart, M.D., M.S., M.B.A. and Mathew Stewart, M.D., Ph.D.

Contents

There is no substitute for learning by experience. It is better to wait for someone to assist you with nonurgent procedures when you are not fully confident in your skills than to try on your own.

Primum non nocere.

General considerations

• Always obtain informed consent; explain the procedure, the indications, risks, and alternatives.
• Getting consent for life-saving emergency procedures is not necessary.
• Universal precautions should be practiced, and proper sterile technique is essential.
• Sedation and analgesia, when required, should be planned in advance.
• Assess for presence of coagulopathy or need to modify medications (e.g., heparin drip).

Suturing

Assess for foreign body (consider x-ray), deep tissue damage, or injury to nerve, blood vessels, or tendons.

Anesthetize wound with topical, local, or regional anesthetic.

Clean wound with copious sterile normal saline irrigation.

Select suture type, staples, liquid stitches (if using glue or placing one staple, no need to anesthetize wound).

Size is indicated by a 0, the more 0's the smaller (4–0 is <3–0).

Apply topical antibiotic (if not using liquid stitches) and sterile dressing; if near joint, immobilize with a splint.

Consider need for tetanus prophylaxis.

Body region	Size of suture	Removal (days)
Scalp	Staple, or 4, 5–0	5–7
Face	6–0	3–5
Trunk	4, 5–0	5–7
Extremities	4, 5–0	7
Joints	4–0	10–14
Hand	5–0	7
Foot	3, 4–0	7–10

Nasogastric tube insertion

Indication

Aspirate stomach contents for diagnosis (e.g., assess for GI bleeding) or treatment (e.g., treatment of ileus, obstruction), or for feeding/medication.

Contraindications Facial or basilar skull fractures, esophageal stricture, history of caustic ingestion, penetrating cervical spine wounds, choanal atresia, recent surgery to upper GI tract, status post esophagectomy, Zenker's diverticulum.

Complications Pain, tracheal intubation, esophagitis, retro- or nasopharyngeal necrosis, stomach perforation.

Equipment Towel or chuck for covering patient's clothes, emesis basin, nasogastric tube, cup of water and straw, lubricating gel, vasoconstrictor spray, catheter-tip syringe, stethoscope.

Technique

1 Place patient in sitting position, have towels or chuck over chest and an emesis basin in lap in case it is needed.
2 For unconscious patient, put the patient in left lateral decubitus position with head turned downward. This position helps prevent aspiration.
3 Apply topical anesthetic to nares and pharynx.
4 Select tube by French gauge (F): 16F = large, 12F = medium, 10F = small.
5 Estimate length: Put tip at nose, loop tube over ear lobe and then down to xiphoid as well as umbilicus. Mark the latter spot with tape before insertion.
6 Spray topical vasoconstrictor.
7 Give patient water with a straw to drink and support the patient's head to prevent him from pulling away.
8 Insert lubricated tube along floor of nose with the natural curve pointing down, at a 60–90-degree angle to plane of face, and advance toward occiput.
9 Have patient swallow some water and flex head slightly, when patient swallows, advance tube into esophagus and then into stomach.
10 The patients should be able to speak, if unable, you may have just intubated the trachea inadvertently. Coughing and gagging may also indicate there may be tracheal intubation.
11 Advance to the predetermined distance.
12 Connect a 60 cc catheter-tip syringe to lumen and while auscultating over left upper quadrant, push air into tube. A bubble of air should be heard immediately.
13 Secure tube.

Placing an IV catheter

Ask for help until you are experienced.

Equipment IV catheters; gauze to stop bleeding from unsuccessful attempts; tape and sterile barrier to secure the catheter; flush.

1 *Set up* the first bag of fluid/medication.
2 *Explain* procedure to patient. Place the tourniquet around the arm.
3 *Search hard for the best vein* (palpable, not just visible). Don't be in a hurry. Rest the arm below the level of the heart to aid venous filling. Ask the patient to clench and unclench their fist.
4 *Sit comfortably,* with the patient lying (helps prevent syncope).
5 *Tap the vein* to make it prominent. Avoid sites spanning joints.
6 *Swab with iodine to clean skin*. You may use local anesthetic (or EMLA® cream). Use a fine needle to raise a bleb of lidocaine. Wait 15 sec.

After IV is placed

1 Connect fluid tube; check flow.
2 Fix catheter firmly with tape.
3 Bandage a loop of the tube to the arm.
4 Check the flow rate of the infusion. You may need to explain that no needle is left in the arm.

If you fail after three attempts or are having trouble putting in an IV—get help.

Hypotensive patients need fluid quickly

If the patient needs blood quickly, use a large size catheter.

• *"The IV is no longer working"*: Ask yourself: Is the IV still needed? Is there fluid in bag and tubing? Is the infusion pump working? Inspect the tubing. Are there kinks in the tube?
• *Inspect the IV*: Take bandage off.

Erythematous IV sites need prompt attention. The catheter should be removed and another placed at a different site.

Catheterizing bladders

Catheters *Size* (in French gauge): 12F = small; 16F = large. Usually a 12- or 14F is appropriate. Use the smallest possible. *Type:* Foley is most commonly used, a flexible tube; *coudé (elbow) catheters* have an angled tip to ease around enlarged prostates but insertion is more risky. *Condom catheters* have no in-dwelling parts and therefore cause less pain, less restriction of movement, but they may leak and fall off.

Catheter complications: Bladder infection (don't use antibiotics unless systemically ill). Consider bladder irrigation (e.g., 0.9% saline or chlorhexidine 0.02%). *Bladder spasm* may be painful. Try reducing the volume of water in the balloon.

Methods of catheterizing bladders

Per urethrae: This route is used to relieve urinary retention, monitor urine output in critically ill patients, or collect urine for diagnosis uncontaminated by urethral flora. It is contraindicated in urethral injury (e.g., pelvic fracture) and acute prostatitis. Catheterization introduces bacteria into the bladder, so aseptic technique is essential.

1 *Check the catheter's balloon capacity:* Have your equipment set up in easy reach. Place the patient supine in a well-lit area: Women with knees flexed and hips abducted with heels together. Use a gloved hand to prep urethral meatus in a pubis-to-anus direction, holding the labia apart with the other hand. With uncircumcised men, retract the foreskin; use a gloved hand to hold the penis still and off the scrotum. The hand used to hold

the penis or labia should not touch the catheter (use forceps to pick-up the catheter if needed).

2 Put sterile lidocaine 2% gel on the catheter tip and 10 mL into the urethra. In men, stretch the penis perpendicular to the body to eliminate any urethral folds that may lead to false passage.

3 Use steady gentle pressure to advance the catheter. Significant obstructions encountered should prompt withdrawal and reinsertion. With prostatic hypertrophy, a coudé tip catheter may be required to advance past the prostate.

4 Once inserted fully, wait until urine emerges before inflating the balloon. Pull the catheter back so that the balloon comes to rest at the bladder neck.

5 Remember to reposition the foreskin in uncircumcised men to prevent edema of the glans after the catheter is inserted.

Central venous catheter cannulation

Indications
- Emergency access
- Central venous pressure monitoring
- Large-volume parenteral fluid administration
- Delivery of parenteral fluids (nutrition, hyperosmolar)
- Delivery of medications (chemotherapy)
- Alternative for repetitive venous cannulations
- Procedures (hemodialysis, plasmapheresis)
- Cardiac catheterization, temporary transvenous pacemaker

Contraindications
- Abnormal or distorted anatomy
- Bleeding diathesis
- Burns over insertion site
- Cellulitis over insertion site
- If subclavian or internal jugular vein insertion, pneumothorax/hemothorax on contralateral side
- Uncooperative patient

Complications Infection, bleeding, arterial perforation, pneumothorax, hemothorax, thrombosis, catheter fracture, air embolism, injury to surrounding structures.

Equipment
- Central line kit
- Sterile gloves, sterile gown, hair cover, mask, eye protection
- Sterile drape
- Sterile gauze pads
- Needle driver
- Suture scissors
- Suture on a cutting needle
- Occlusive dressing
- Completed x-ray request form if subclavian or internal jugular vein insertion
- Bedside US, such as the Site-Rite system, if available

Access locations
- Internal jugular
- Subclavian
- Femoral

Technique (Seldinger technique)
6 Position patient, clean and prep site, drape in sterile fashion; don mask, eye protection, hair cover, sterile gown and gloves.

7 Flush central venous catheter with sterile saline; flush all ports.

8 Insert finder needle while applying negative pressure and locate vessel.

9 Using bedside ultrasound (US), such as Site-Rite system, follow the needle tip indicator to the target vein using the US display.

10 Once blood return is obtained, insert guide wire through needle into the vein.

11 Remove needle while holding onto the guide wire.

12 Enlarge entry site with dilator.

13 Pass catheter over guide wire and into vessel.

14 Remove guide wire.

15 Secure catheter with suture.

16 Apply sterile dressing.

17 Obtain a postprocedure central line placement x-ray if subclavian or internal jugular vein insertion.

Approaches

Internal jugular:

1 Position patient in 15–20-degree Trendelenburg position.

2 Turn head to contralateral side and hyperextend the neck to tense the sternocleidomastoid muscle. The internal jugular vein is anterior and lateral to the carotid. It travels under the apex of the triangle formed by the sternal and clavicular heads of sternocleidomastoid muscle and the clavicle.

3 Anesthetize with needle directed toward the ipsilateral nipple and the junction of the medial third and middle third of the clavicle.

4 Puncture skin at this site and direct needle caudally toward the ipsilateral nipple.

5 When blood flow is obtained, continue with the Seldinger technique.

6 The right side is preferred because there is no thoracic duct, there is a straight course to the right atrium, and the dome of the lung's pleura is usually lower.

Subclavian:

1 Position patient in Trendelenburg position with a towel roll under the thoracic spine, between the scapulae to hyperextend the back.

2 Anesthetize at the distal third of the clavicle.

3 Aim needle under the clavicle toward the sternal notch (see Figure 19.1).

4 When blood flow is obtained, continue with the Seldinger technique.

Femoral:

1 Palpate the femoral artery pulse at the midpoint between the anterior superior iliac spine and the symphysis pubis. The vein is parallel and immediately medial to the artery.

2 Anesthetize the skin and subcutaneous tissue.

3 Puncture needle at this site.

4 When blood flow is obtained, continue with the Seldinger technique.

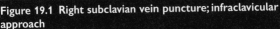

Figure 19.1 Right subclavian vein puncture; infraclavicular approach

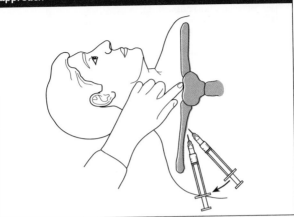

Paracentesis

Indications
- Diagnosis (cytology for neoplasia, culture for spontaneous bacterial peritonitis)
- Therapeutic relief from ascites, including relief of pain or respiratory compromise

Contraindications
- Coagulopathy
- Pregnancy
- Evidence of abdominal wall skin infection or bowel obstruction

Complications
- *Bleeding* Rare complication caused by injury to large vessels of abdominal wall, the inferior epigastric vessels, or to mesenteric vessels. Avoid injury to epigastric vessels by staying midline or lateral to the rectus abdominus. Hemodynamic instability after paracentesis requires emergency investigation and may require an exploratory laparotomy.
- *Infection* ascitic fluid leak may lead to peritonitis.
- *Injury to nearby structures including liver or spleen* Bowel and bladder injuries most likely. Bowel injuries are minimized by careful technique and patient positioning. Bowel injuries lead to delayed peritonitis and sepsis. Risk of bowel injury during procedures is increased near abdominal scars due to possible adhesion of bowel to previous abdominal incision. Bladder injuries are minimized by having the patient void or by placing a Foley catheter prior to procedure.
- *Hypotension* from rapid changes in pressure and fluid of abdominal cavity; rarely, by intravascular shift to abdominal compartment.

Equipment
- Paracentesis kit
- Specimen collection tubes and/or vacuum bottles

- Intravenous albumin for large volume paracentesis.

Technique

1 Place patient in supine position.
2 Preferably, the target site for procedure may be determined by US and marked on the patient's skin. If not available, percuss the ascites, marking a point where fluid level was identified but avoiding scars or vessels.
3 Clean the skin with iodine.
4 Anesthetize skin at the insertion site. The ideal site is midline, 1–2 cm below the umbilicus. Do not use a midline site if a previous midline incision is present (due to risk of bowel adhesion to abdominal wall). The lateral site is between the anterior-superior iliac crest and the lateral border of the rectus abdominus, at the level of the umbilicus.
5 Insert a 21F needle on a 20 mL syringe into the skin and advance while aspirating until ascitic fluid is withdrawn. Remove desired amount of fluid.
6 Remove the needle and apply a sterile dressing.
7 If indicated, send fluid for chemistry, microscopy, culture, and cytology.
8 Replace ascitic fluid with albumin if large volume paracentesis (>4–5 L) is planned. Replace 6–8 g (25%) for every liter removed. Can consider replacement for lower volumes removed as well

Transudate occurs when a patient's serum-ascites albumin gap (SAAG) level is ≥1.1 g/dL. Exudative ascites occurs when patients have SAAG levels <1.1 g/dL.

Thoracentesis

Indications

- Diagnosis (malignancy, infection, inflammation)
- Therapeutic

Contraindications

- Local skin infection,
- Uncooperative patient

Complications Bleeding; infection; pneumothorax; hemothorax; pulmonary contusion or laceration; diaphragm, spleen, or liver puncture; bronchopleural fistula; reexpansion of pulmonary edema.

Equipment

- Thoracentesis kit
- Sterile gauze pad
- Iodine
- Fenestrated drape
- Oxygen by nasal cannula
- Specimen collection tubes and/or vacuum bottles

Technique

1 Position patient sitting on edge of bed resting head and extended arms on a bedside table. If the patient is unable to sit, place the patient in the lateral decubitus position.
2 Preferably, the target site for the procedure may be determined by US and marked on the patient's skin.
3 If US marking is not available, confirm location of fluid by percussion, auscultation, and chest x-ray. Mark site with a marker.
4 Locate needle insertion site, 1–2 interspaces below the fluid level, but not below the eighth rib.
5 Prep and drape area with proper sterile technique.
6 Anesthetize skin and then insert needle until it touches the superior border of a rib while aspirating and advancing. Move needle over

the superior margin of the rib and anesthetize the intercostal muscle layers.

7 Insert the thoracentesis needle in the same tract as the anesthesia needle.

8 Draw off 10–30 mL of pleural fluid.

9 Send fluid to the lab for *chemistry* (protein, glucose, pH, lactate dehydrogenase [LDH], amylase); *bacteriology* (microscopy and culture, acid-fast bacillus [AFB] stain, tuberculosis [TB] culture); *cytology*.

10 If large-volume removal is needed, use the Seldinger technique and insert catheter through the needle and into the chest.

11 Obtain a postprocedure chest x-ray.

A pleural effusion is likely exudative if at least one of the following exists (Light's criteria):

• Pleural protein-to-serum protein ratio >0.5
• pleural LDH-to-serum LDH ratio >0.6
• Pleural LDH >0.6 or two-thirds the upper limit for serum LDH

Inserting a chest tube

NB: This is a sterile procedure.

Indications
• Hemothorax, trauma
• Chylothorax
• Empyema
• Effusion
• Pneumothorax

Contraindications
• Previous thoracic surgery
• Pulmonary blebs
• Oscillator ventilation
• Prior pleural adhesions

Complications
• Scar formation
• Injury to lung or surrounding organs
• Bleeding
• Pain
• Pneumothorax

Equipment
• Chest tube kit
• Sterile gloves, sterile gown, hair cover mask, eye protection
• Sterile drape
• Sterile gauze pads
• Needle driver
• Suture scissors
• Iodine
• 1% lidocaine
• Scalpel
• Suture
• Chest tube: 10–14F usually; 28–30F if trauma or hemothorax
• Pleuri-Vac container with water seal
• Connection tubes
• Petroleum gauze
• Occlusive dressing
• Completed x-ray request form

Technique
1. Obtain preprocedure x-ray to confirm location for chest tube insertion.
2. Choose insertion site: 4th–6th intercostal space, anterior to mid-axillary line, in the "safe triangle," see Figure 19.2.
   • A more posterior approach (e.g., the seventh space posterior), may be required to drain a loculated effusion
   • The second intercostal space in the mid-clavicular line may be used for apical pneumothoraces.
   • The posterior and anterior approaches are more uncomfortable.

725

3. Infiltrate down to the pleura with 10–20 cc of 1% lidocaine.
   - Verify that either air or fluid can be aspirated from the proposed insertion site; if not do not proceed.
   - Wait 3 min for the anesthetic to have an effect.
4. Make a 2-cm incision above anesthetized rib to avoid the neurovascular bundle under rib.
   - Blunt dissect with forceps down to the pleura.
   - Puncture pleura with scissors or forceps.
   - If inserting a large-bore tube (>24F), then sweep a finger inside chest to clear adherent lung and exclude obstructing structures (e.g., in blunt abdominal trauma, stomach in the chest).
5. Before inserting the chest tube, remove the metal trochar completely and introduce the tube atraumatically using forceps to advance it.
6. Advance the tip upward to the apex of lung (or base of lung if draining an effusion). Stop when you meet resistance.
7. Attach the chest tube to the drainage container with water seal.
   - Ensure that the chest tube is bubbling with respiration.
8. With large-/medium-bore tubes, the incision should be closed with a mattress suture or suture across the incision.
   - Purse string sutures are not recommended as they may lead to scarring and increased wound pain.
9. Fix the chest tube with a second suture tied around the chest tube.
10. Cover with petroleum gauze and occlusive dressing.
11. Secure the tube with tape to prevent slippage.
12. Obtain a postplacement x-ray to observe the position of the tube.
13. Give PO/IV/IM analgesia.

Tension pneumothorax

In a tension pneumothorax air is drawn into the intrapleural space with each breath but cannot escape due to a valve-like effect of the tiny flap in the parietal pleura. The increased pressure progressively compresses the heart and the other lung.

1. Give the patient 100% oxygen.

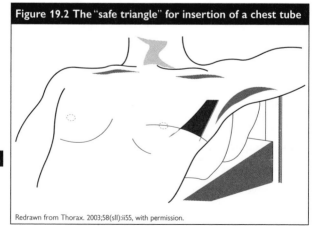

Figure 19.2 The "safe triangle" for insertion of a chest tube

Redrawn from Thorax. 2003;58(sII):ii55, with permission.

2. Insert a large-bore IV cannula through an intercostal space anywhere on the affected side (usually second intercostal space in the midclavicular line).
   - Remove the stylet, which will allow the trapped air to escape, usually with an audible hiss.
3. Secure IV cannula with tape.
4. Insert chest tube as above.
   - Chest tube is to continue to release air from the pleural space until lung rift can seal.

Lumbar puncture

Indication

- Suspected central nervous system (CNS) infection
- Suspected subarachnoid hemorrhage
- Disease diagnosis: Pseudotumor cerebri, Guillain-Barré syndrome, multiple sclerosis, systemic lupus erythematosus, meningeal carcinomatosis
- Infusion: Antibiotics, chemotherapy, contrast (myelography/cisternography)

Contraindications

- Local skin infection
- intracranial pressure (except pseudotumor cerebri)
- Supratentorial mass lesions (computed tomography [CT] first)
- Platelet count <50,000/severe bleeding diathesis
- Hemodynamically unstable patient

Complications Shooting pains in the lower extremities, infection, bleeding, spinal fluid leak, hematoma, spinal headache (10–20%), brain herniation from supratentorial mass or extreme pressure.

Spinal headache usually occurs 24–48 h after LP with resolution over hours to 2 wks:

- Constant, dull, bilateral ache more frontal than occipital; it is positional—worse with upright positioning.
- Blood patch (injection of 20 cc of autologous venous blood into the epidural space) causes immediate relief in 95%.

Equipment

- Spinal tray
- Sterile gloves
- Fenestrated drape
- Topical anesthetic cream
- 1% lidocaine

Technique

1 Apply local anaesthetic cream if sufficient time is available.
2 Position patient near edge of bed/table in the lateral decubitus or sitting position. Flex spine anteriorly (flex hips, knees, and neck).
3 Locate L3–L4 interspace at the level of the iliac crests. See Figure 19.3.
4 Open spinal tray in a sterile manner, prepare skin at the selected interspace with antiseptic solution, and cover with a fenestrated drape.
5 Anesthetize skin with 1% lidocaine.
6 Using the spinal needle, puncture the skin in the midline just caudal to the palpated spinous process; angle needle about 15 degrees cephalad toward the umbilicus.
7 Advance needle about 3–4 cm then withdraw stylet to check for cerebral spinal fluid (CSF) flow. If no fluid, replace stylus and advance a fraction then repeat.

8 Usually, a slight "pop" is felt as the needle penetrates the dura; advance 1–2 mm further.

9 If resistance is felt (bone), withdraw needle slightly and change its angle.

10 Once fluid is obtained, place end of stopcock with the attached manometer onto the needle hub to measure the opening pressure.

11 In a supine patient, normal opening pressure is 50–200 mm H_2O; elevated >250 mm H_2O.

12 Note color of fluid as well as opening pressure.

13 Opening pressure can only reliably be measured while patient is lying quietly on his side in an unflexed position (have patient straighten legs and relax; this will help prevent an artificially elevated pressure).

14 Turn stopcock to allow the CSF to flow into the test tubes; label tubes in the order collected.

15 Collect 1–3 cc of CSF in each of 3–4 tubes.

16 Send tubes for appropriate studies.

Tube 1	Tube 2	Tube 3	Tube 4
Bacteriology	Biochemistry	Hematology	Optional
Culture and Gram stain	Glucose Protein	Cell count and differential	Viral studies PCR Metabolic studies VDRL Fungus TB Electrophoresis Cytology

17 Replace stylus and withdraw the needle.

18 Cover with sterile dressing and have patient lay supine for next 2 h.

NB: CSF normal values

Lymphocytes <5/mm^3

Glucose 60–70% blood glucose

Protein 15–45 mg/dL

Bloody tap This is an artifact due to piercing a blood vessel, which is indicated by fewer red cells in successive tubes and no yellowing of CSF (xanthochromia).

If the patient's blood count is normal, the rule of thumb is to subtract from the total CSF white blood cells (WBCs) (per mcL) one white cell for every 1,000 red blood cells (RBCs). To estimate the true protein level, subtract 1 mg/dL for every 1,000 RBCs/mm^3 (be sure to do the count and protein estimation on the same tube). *Note* High protein levels in CSF make it appear yellow.

Subarachnoid hemorrhage Xanthochromia (yellow supernatant on spun CSF). Red cells in equal numbers in all tubes. RBCs can provoke an inflammatory response most marked after 48 h.

Elevated protein Meningitis; multiple sclerosis (MS); Guillain–Barré syndrome.

Very elevated CSF protein Spinal block; TB; or severe bacterial meningitis.

Figure 19.3 Method of defining the interspace between the third and fourth lumbar vertebrae

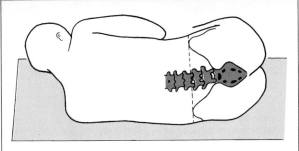

After Vakil RJV, Udwadia FEU. Diagnosis and Management of Medical Emergencies 2nd ed. Delhi: Oxford University Press, 1988.

Cricothyroidotomy

This is an emergency procedure to overcome upper airway obstruction above the level of the larynx.

Indications Upper airway obstruction when endotracheal intubation is not possible; e.g., irretrievable foreign body; facial edema (burns, angioedema); maxillofacial trauma; infection (epiglottitis).

Procedure Position the patient supine with neck extended (e.g., pillow under shoulders). Run your index finger down the neck anteriorly in the midline to find the notch in the upper border of the thyroid cartilage: Just below this, between the thyroid and cricoid cartilages, is a depression—the cricothyroid membrane (see Figure 19.4).

Needle cricothyroidotomy: Pierce the membrane with a large-bore cannula (14F) attached to syringe: Withdrawal of air confirms position. Lidocaine may or may not be required). Slide cannula over needle at 45 degrees to skin in sagittal plane. Use a Y-connector or improvise connection to O_2 supply and give 15 L/min: Use thumb on Y-connector to allow O_2 in over 1 sec and CO_2 out over 4 sec ("transtracheal jet insufflation"). See Figure 19.5.

Figure 19.4

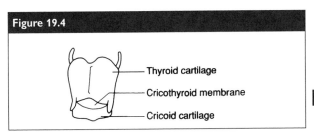

Thyroid cartilage

Cricothyroid membrane

Cricoid cartilage

Figure 19.5

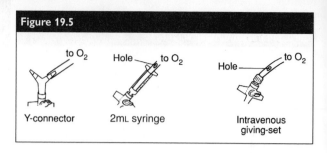

to O₂ — Y-connector

Hole — to O₂ — 2mL syringe

Hole — to O₂ — Intravenous giving-set

Surgical cricothyrotomy: Smallest tube for prolonged ventilation is 6 mm. Introduce high-volume, low-pressure cuff tracheostomy tube through horizontal incision in membrane.

Complications Local hemorrhage, posterior perforation of trachea ± esophagus, laryngeal stenosis, tube blockage, subcutaneous tunneling.

Pericardiocentesis

Figure 19.6 Emergency needle pericardiocentesis

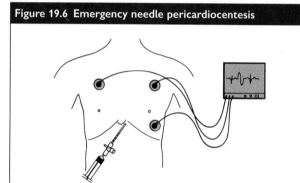

Equipment 20 mL syringe, long 18F cannula, 3-way tap, electrocardiogram (ECG) monitor, skin cleanser

Technique

1 If time allows, use aseptic technique, and, if conscious, local anesthesia technique and sedation, e.g., with midazolam: Titrate up to 0.07 mg/kg IV—start with 2 mg over 1 min, 1 mg in elderly.

2 Ensure you have IV access and full resuscitation equipment at hand.

3 Introduce needle at 45 degrees to skin just below and to left of xiphisternum, aiming for tip of left scapula. (See Figure 19.4.) Aspirate continuously and watch ECG. Frequent ventricular ectopics or an injury pattern (ST segment falls) on ECG implies myocardial penetration: Withdraw slightly.

(Continued)

Figure 19.6 *(Continued)*

4 Evacuate pericardial contents through the syringe and 3-way tap. Removal of only a small amount of fluid (e.g., 20 mL) can produce marked clinical improvement. If you are not sure whether the fluid you are aspirating is pure blood (e.g., on entering a ventricle), see if it clots (heavily bloodstained pericardial fluid does not clot).

5 You can leave the cannula *in situ* temporarily, for repeated aspiration. If there is reaccumulation, pericardiectomy may be needed. Send fluid for microscopy and culture, as needed, including tests for TB.

Complications Laceration of ventricle or coronary artery (± subsequent hemopericardium); aspiration of ventricular blood; arrhythmias (ventricular fibrillation); pneumothorax; puncture of aorta, esophagus (± mediastinitis), or pericarditis.

Cardioversion/defibrillation

Indications Ventricular fibrillation or tachycardia, fast atrial fibrillation (AF, p. 123), supraventricular tachycardias if other treatments (p. 121) have failed or there is hemodynamic compromise.

The aim is to completely depolarize the heart using a direct current.

Unless critically ill, conscious patients require sedating medication.

Procedure (for monophasic defibrillators)

Do not wait for a crisis before familiarizing yourself with the defibrillator.

1 Set the energy level (e.g., 200 J for ventricular fibrillation or ventricular tachycardia; 100 J for atrial fibrillation; 50 J for atrial flutter).

2 Place pads on chest, one over apex and one below right clavicle (less chance of skin arc than jelly).

3 Make sure no one else is touching the patient or the bed.

4 Disconnect oxygen circuit tubing during shock delivery.

5 Press the button(s) on the electrode(s) to give the shock.

6 Watch ECG. Repeat the shock at a higher energy if necessary.

NB: For AF and supraventricular tachycardia (SVT), it is necessary to synchronize the shock on the R-wave of the ECG (by pressing the "SYNC" button on the machine). This ensures that the shock does not initiate a ventricular arrhythmia. *If the SYNC mode is engaged in ventricular fibrillation (VF), the defibrillator will not discharge!*

- It is only necessary to anesthetize the patient if he or she is conscious.
- After giving the shock, monitor ECG rhythm. Consider anticoagulation, as the risk of emboli is increased. Get a postprocedure 12-lead ECG.

Inserting a temporary cardiac pacemaker

Possible indications in the setting of acute myocardial infarction

- *Complete arteriovenous (AV) block:* With inferior MI (right coronary artery occlusion), pacing may only be needed if symptomatic; spontaneous recovery may occur.
- With anterior myocardial infarction (MI) (representing massive septal infarction)
- *Second-degree block:* Wenckebach (p. 116) implies decremental AV node con-duction; may respond to atropine in inferior MI; pace if anterior MI. Type 2 block is usually associated with distal fascicular disease and carries high risk of complete heart block, so pace in both types of MI.
- *First-degree block:* Observe carefully: 40% develop higher degrees of block.
- *Bundle branch block:* Pace prophylactically if evidence of trifascicular disease (p. 96) or nonadjacent bifascicular disease.
- *Sinoatrial disease + serious symptoms:* Pace unless patient responds to atropine.

Other indications in which temporary pacing may be needed

- Drug poisoning (e.g., with β-blockers, digoxin, or verapamil)
- Symptomatic bradycardia, unresponsive to atropine
- Suppression of drug-resistant VT and SVT (overdrive pacing; do in ICU)
- Asystolic cardiac arrest with P-wave activity (ventricular standstill)
- During or after cardiac surgery (e.g., around the AV node or bundle of His)

Method and technique for temporary pacing Learn from an expert.

1 *Preparation:* Monitor ECG; have a defibrillator at hand. Create a sterile field and ensure that the pacing wire fits down the cannula easily. Insert a peripheral cannula.

2 *Insertion:* Place the cannula into the subclavian or internal jugular vein (p. 721). Pass the pacing wire through the cannula into the right atrium. It will either pass easily through the tricuspid valve or loop within the atrium. If the latter occurs, it is usually possible to flip the wire across the valve with a combined twisting and withdrawing movement. Advance the wire slightly. At this stage, the wire may try to exit the ventricle through the pulmonary outflow tract. A further withdrawing and rotation of the wire will aim the tip at the apex of the right ventricle. Advance slightly again to place the wire in contact with the endocardium. Remove any slack to decrease risk of subsequent displacement. (See Figure 19.5)

3 *Checking the threshold:* Connect the wire to the pacing box and set the "demand" rate slightly higher than the patient's own heart rate and the output to 3 V. A paced rhythm should be seen. Find the pacing threshold by slowly reducing the voltage until the pacemaker fails to stimulate the tissue (pacing spikes are no longer followed by paced beats). The threshold should be less than 1 V, but a slightly higher value may be acceptable if it is stable (e.g., after a large infarction).

4 *Setting the pacemaker :* Set the output to 3 V or >3 times the threshold value (whichever is higher) in "demand" mode. Set the rate as required. Suture the wire to the skin and fix with a sterile dressing.

5 Check the position of the wire (and exclude pneumothorax) with a CXR.

Recurrent checks of the pacing threshold are required over the next few days. The formation of endocardial edema can be expected to raise the threshold by a factor of 2–3. See Figure 19.7.

Figure 19.7

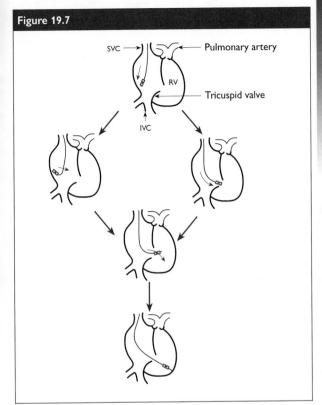

Emergency medicine

Rodney Omron, M.D., M.P.H. and Arjun S. Chanmugam, M.D.

Contents

Emergency presentations

Cardiovascular emergencies

Respiratory emergencies

Gastrointestinal emergencies

Neurological emergencies

Endocrinological emergencies

Acute poisoning: General measures 787

To manage an emergency condition, you must be prepared to treat and diagnose at virtually the same time.

Patients who present with an emergency condition generally fall into two categories: They either have a life-threatening condition or an organ-threatening condition. Knowledge of some basic disease processes and an understanding of how to approach patients who may be critically ill is important in managing their care. Recognizing that an emergent condition is present is the key first step; the second step is to activate the appropriate resources as quickly as possible. Remember, if you suspect an emergent condition, call for help as soon as possible, even if you are not sure whether there is an emergency.

Introduction to emergencies

Patients who have an emergent condition require immediate intervention. As stated earlier, recognition is the critical first step. Any patient who has a problem with his airway, who has any trouble breathing, or who has difficulty maintaining his blood pressure (ABCs) should be considered as having a potential medical emergency. The next step is to activate the appropriate resources to support the patient, which means asking for help and applying the acronym "**O**h **MI**': **O**xygen, cardiac **M**onitoring, and an **I**V catheter. While providing the patient with as much support as possible, consider the potential threats to life and the potential threats to any organ system. This list must be considered as soon as possible in order to provide the patient with the correct medical interventions. By continuing to consider the potential life and organ threats, the well-prepared provider will be in a better position to craft the all-important management plan—the plan of action.

When developing your management plan, two data sources must be used. The subjective data, which includes all the historical elements, including the patient's version of the events leading to presentation, the medical record, and comments from other people (eye witnesses, paramedics, family). The second dataset is the objective data, the physical findings, as well as any laboratory, radiological, or other studies. Very often, the heart of the diagnosis lies in the subjective data and the objective data confirms the diagnostic suspicion.

The key to good management is to identify any abnormality, any source of concern—or, to put it another way—any red flag. Every red flag must be appropriately addressed. Whenever new data are acquired, regardless of the source, the treatment plan must be modified to incorporate these new data and the evolving condition of your patient.

Continuous reevaluation is critically important because, by definition, an emergent condition is a state that can change dramatically and quickly. To that end, remember to dynamically review the temperature, pulse rate and quality, respiratory rate and pattern, blood pressure, and oxygen saturation, as well as the most important vital sign of all—the patient's mental status. All this should be done in the context of the preliminary assessment shown in Table 20.1.

Table 20.1 Preliminary assessment (primary survey)

Airway	*Assessment:* Any signs of airway obstruction? Ascertain patency.
	Management: Establish a patent airway
	Key: Avoid manipulation of and protect the cervical spine if injury is possible, especially in the presence of a change in mental status
Breathing	*Assessment:* Determine respiratory rate, check bilateral chest movement, percuss, and auscultate.
	Management: If no respiratory effort, treat as arrest, intubate, and ventilate. If breathing is compromised, give high-concentration O_2, manage according to findings, e.g., relieve tension pneumothorax.
Circulation	*Assessment:* Check pulse and blood pressure; check capillary refill; look for evidence of hypoperfusion
	Management: Peripheral or central IV catheters, fluids (crystalloids or blood products), measure urine output; consider central venous pressure measurement, ultrasound inferior vena cava measurement; consider pressors.
	If no cardiac output, treat as arrest
Disability	Assess level of consciousness with AVPU score (**A**lert? Responds to **V**oice? To **P**ain? **U**nresponsive?); check pupils: Size, equality, reactions. *Glasgow Coma scale* (GCS) if time allows.
Exposure	Undress patient, but cover to avoid hypothermia.

Quick history from relatives or significant others may assist with diagnosis: *Events* surrounding onset of illness, contributing issues, evidence of overdose/suicide attempt, any suggestion of trauma? *Past medical history:* Especially diabetes; asthma; chronic obstructive pulmonary disease (COPD); alcohol, opiate, or street drug abuse; epilepsy or recent head injury; recent travel. *Medication:* Current drugs. *Allergies*.

Once appropriate ventilation and circulation support are adequate, a more complete history and examination, along with more thorough investigations, should be undertaken as part of the appropriate management.

Cardiorespiratory arrest

Confirm absence of pulse, blood pressure, and/or respirations.

Causes Myocardial infarction (MI), pulmonary embolism (PE), trauma, tension pneumothorax, electrocution, shock (septic, cardiogenic, neurogenic, hypovolemic, and anaphylactic), hypoxia, hypercapnia, hypothermia, electrolyte/acid/base imbalance, drugs (e.g., digoxin).

Basic life support Request help immediately. Check for responsiveness. Check breathing. Ask someone to call the arrest team and bring the automatic external defibrillator. Note the time. Check the pulse for no longer than 10 seconds. Place patient in a supine position. Begin cardiopulmonary resuscitation (CPR) as follows:

Chest compressions: Give 30 compressions to 2 breaths (30:2) in adults. CPR should not be interrupted except to give shocks. Use the heel of hand with straight elbows. Center over the lower half of the sternum. Aim for 4–5 cm compression at 100/min. Allow the chest to return to normal position. Push hard and push fast.

Airway: Open airway. If no contraindications, use head tilt ± chin lift. Clear the mouth.

Breathing: Assess breathing, if inadequate, give two breaths, each inflation ~1 sec long. Use specialized bag-and-mask system (e.g., Ambu® system) if available and two resuscitators are present. Otherwise, mouth-to-mouth breathing.

Advanced life support For algorithm and details, see Figure 20.1.

- *Notes:* Place defibrillator paddles on chest as soon as possible and set monitor to read through the paddles if there is a delay in attaching leads.
- *Assess rhythm:* Is this ventricular fibrillation (VF)/pulseless VT?
- In VF/ventricular tachycardia (VT), defibrillation must occur without delay: Monophasic 360 J (biphasic maximum dose 120–200 J).
- Asystole and electromechanical dissociation (synonymous with pulse-less electrical activity) are rhythms with a worse prognosis compared to VF/VT, but potentially remediable (see Figure 20.1). Treatment may be life-saving.
- Obtain IV/IO access and intubation if possible.
- Look for reversible causes of cardiac arrest and treat accordingly.
- Check for pulse if ECG rhythm is compatible with a profusible rhythm.
- Reassess ECG rhythm. All shocks now Monophasic 360 J (biphasic 200). CPR for 2 min, epinephrine every 3–5 min; consider advanced airway/capnography. If there is a shockable rhythm, then shock and, while you perform CPR for another 2 min, start amiodarone. Repeat these steps while there is a shockable rhythm.
- Send someone to find the patient's chart and the patient's usual doctor. These may give clues as to the cause of the arrest.
- If IV access fails, **n**aloxone, **a**tropine, diazepam (**V**alium), **e**pinephrine, and **l**idocaine (**NAVEL**) may be given down the tracheal tube but absorption is unpredictable. Give 2–3 times the IV dose diluted in 10 mL 0.9% saline followed by five ventilations to assist absorption. Intracardiac injection is not recommended. Consider intraosseous line (all meds, blood, and crystalloid can be given).

When to stop resuscitation: This is one of the most difficult decisions to make, and there are no definitive recommendations. Consider stopping re-suscitation after 20 min if there is refractory asystole or electromechanical dissociation. In general, in those patients without myocardial disease, resuscitations are often continued until core temperatures are >33°C and pH and potassium are normal.

After successful resuscitation:

- 12-lead electrocardiogram (ECG); chest x-ray (CXR), comprehensive metabolic panel, glucose, blood gases, CBC, creatine kinase (CK), CK MB/troponin.
- Transfer to appropriate unit, such as a CCU/ICU.
- Monitor vital signs.
- Whatever the outcome, explain to relatives what has happened.

When "do not resuscitate" may be a valid decision

- If a patient's condition is such that resuscitation is unlikely to succeed.
- If a mentally competent patient has consistently stated or recorded the fact that he or she does not want to be resuscitated.
- If the patient has signed an advanced directive forbidding resuscitation.
- Ideally, involve patients and relatives in the decision **before** the emergency. When in doubt, resuscitate.

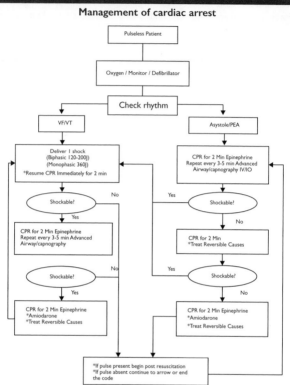

Figure 20.1 Cardiac arrest: 2010 guidelines for advanced life support

Management of cardiac arrest

Pulseless Patient

Oxygen / Monitor / Defibrillator

Check rhythm

VF/VT — Asystole/PEA

VF/VT branch:

Deliver 1 shock
(Biphasic 120-200J)
(Monophasic 360J)
*Resume CPR Immediately for 2 min

Shockable? — No

Yes

CPR for 2 Min Epinephrine
Repeat every 3-5 min Advanced
Airway/capnography

Shockable? — No

Yes

CPR for 2 Min Epinephrine
*Amiodarone
*Treat Reversible Causes

Asystole/PEA branch:

CPR for 2 Min Epinephrine
Repeat every 3-5 min Advanced
Airway/capnography IV/IO

Shockable? — Yes

No

CPR for 2 Min
*Treat Reversible Causes

Shockable? — Yes

No

CPR for 2 Min Epinephrine
*Amiodarone
*Treat Reversible Causes

*If pulse present begin post resuscitation
*If pulse absent continue to arrow or end
the code

Avoid interruption in CPR, except to defibrillate. Push hard (>2 in [5 cm]) and fast (100/min). Avoid excessive ventilation. Rotate compressions every 2 min. Consider capnography (if $PetCo_2$ is <10 mm Hg, then improve CPR quality). Consider intra-arterial line (if diastolic blood pressure [BP] is <20 mm Hg, then improve CPR quality). Return of pulse associated with sudden increase in $PetCo_2$ to >40 mm Hg and arterial waveform. (Consider the reversible causes: 5H's; 5T's: Hypovolemia, Hypoxia, Hydrogen ion (acidosis), Hypo-/Hyperkalemia, Hypothermia; Tension pneumothorax, Tamponade (Cardiac), Toxins, Thrombosis (cardiac, pulmonary). May replace first or second dose of epi with vasopressin 40 U IV/IO.

From 2010 American Heart Association Guidelines for CPR and ECC. *Circulation.* 2010;122 (suppl):729–767.

Headache

Life-threatening considerations

- Meningitis
- Encephalopathy
- Intracranial bleed

Organ-threatening causes

- Narrow angle glaucoma
- Temporal arteritis (elevated erythrocyte sedimentation rate [ESR], jaw claudication, platelet count >400)
- Severe anemia

Other potential causes

- Tension headache
- Migraine
- Cluster headache
- Post-traumatic
- Drugs (nitrates, calcium-channel blocker)
- Carbon monoxide poisoning or anoxia

Signs of meningismus?

- Meningitis (may not have fever or rash)
- Subarachnoid hemorrhage

Decreased conscious level or localizing signs?

- Encephalitis/meningitis
- Stroke
- Cerebral abscess
- Subarachnoid hemorrhage
- Tumor
- Subdural hematoma

Papilledema?

- Tumor
- Severe hypertension
- Benign intracranial hypertension
- Any central nervous system (CNS) infection, if prolonged (e.g., >2 wks); e.g., tuberculosis (TB) meningitis

Others

- Paget's disease (elevated alk phos)
- Sinusitis
- Altitude sickness
- Cervical spondylosis

Worrying headache features or "red flags"

- First headache or worst headache; *consider subarachnoid hemorrhage*
- Thunderclap headache; *consider subarachnoid hemorrhage*
- Unilateral headache and eye pain; *cluster headache*
- Unilateral headache and ipsilateral symptoms; *migraine, tumor, vascular*
- Cough-initiated headache; *raised ICP/venous thrombosis*
- Persisting headache ± scalp tenderness in those >50; *temporal arteritis*
- Headache with fever or neck stiffness; *meningitis*
- Change in the pattern of "usual headaches"
- Decreased level of consciousness

Two other vital questions:

- Where have you been? (Malaria)
- Might you be pregnant? (Eclampsia; especially if proteinuria and elevated BP)

Shortness of breath

Wheezing?

- Asthma
- COPD
- Heart failure
- Anaphylaxis

Stridor? (Upper airway obstruction)

- Foreign body or tumor
- Acute epiglottitis
- Anaphylaxis
- Trauma (e.g., laryngeal fracture)
- Angioedema

Crackles?

- Heart failure
- Pneumonia
- Bronchiectasis
- Fibrosis

Chest clear?

- Pulmonary embolism (PE)
- Hyperventilation
- Metabolic acidosis (e.g., diabetic ketoacidosis [DKA])
- Anemia
- Drugs (e.g., salicylates)
- Shock (may cause air hunger)
- Central causes

Others

- Pneumothorax; pain, increased resonance
- Pleural effusion

Chest pain: Differential diagnosis

First exclude any potentially life-threatening causes by virtue of history, brief examination, and limited investigations. Then consider other potential causes.

Immediately life-threatening

- Acute MI
- Angina/acute coronary syndrome
- Aortic dissection
- Tension pneumothorax
- Pulmonary embolism
- Esophageal rupture

Others

- Pneumonia
- Empyema
- Chest wall pain:
  - Muscular
  - Rib fractures
  - Bony metastases
  - Costochondritis
- Pleurisy
- Gastroesophageal reflux
- Pericarditis
- Esophageal spasm

- Herpes zoster
- Cervical spondylosis
- Intra-abdominal:
  - Cholecystitis
  - Peptic ulceration
  - Pancreatitis
- Sickle-cell crisis

Although cardiac pain is usually described as a dull pressure or a substernal pressure that radiates to jaw, neck, or arm, and is usually associated with exertion, not all cardiac chest pain presents classically. It is worthwhile to consider obtaining CXR, ECG, CBC, comprehensive metabolic panel (CMP), and cardiac enzymes (including troponin) on all patients who are at risk. Cardiac chest pain can, and does at times, present atypically, so please consider options such as short-stay units or observation units for low-risk patients. Cardiac monitoring in appropriate inpatient units is indicated for higher risk patients.

Discuss options with the patient. Remember, just because the patient's chest wall is tender to palpation doesn't mean the cause of the chest pain is musculoskeletal. Make sure you have excluded all potential life-threatening causes.

Coma

Definition Unarousable unresponsiveness.
Causes

Metabolic:	Drugs, poisoning (e.g., carbon monoxide, alcohol, tricyclics)
	Hypoglycemia, hyperglycemia (ketoacidotic, or hyperosmolar coma)
	Hypoxia, CO_2 narcosis (COPD)
	Sepsis
	Hypothermia
	Myxedema, Addisonian crisis
	Hepatic/uremic encephalopathy
Neurological:	Trauma
	Infection meningitis; encephalitis, e.g., herpes simplex—give IV acyclovir if the slightest suspicion; tropical: Malaria (do thick films), typhoid, rabies, trypanosomiasis
	Tumor: Cerebral/meningeal tumor
	Vascular, subdural/subarachnoid hemorrhage, stroke, hypertensive encephalopathy
	Epilepsy: Nonconvulsive status or postictal state

Immediate management See Table 20.2.
- Assess airway, breathing, and circulation. Consider intubation if GCS <8. Support the circulation if required (i.e., IV fluids). Give O_2 and treat any seizures. Protect the cervical spine.
- **Check blood glucose in all patients**. Give 50 mL 50% dextrose IV (or 1 mg of glucagon intramuscularly if no IV) immediately if presumed hypoglycemia.
- IV thiamine if any suggestion of Wernicke's encephalopathy (consider giving glucose first).

- IV naloxone for opiate intoxication (may also be given IM or via endotracheal [ET] tube); IV flumazenil for may be considered benzodiazepine intoxication *if* airway compromised and patient is not known to be chronically dependent on benzodiazepines. Caution must be exercised when administering flumazenil to a patient who has benzodiazepine dependency as it may precipitate seizures.

Examination (see Table 20.3)

- *Vital signs are vital:* Obtain full set, including rectal temperature.
- *Signs of trauma:* Hematoma, laceration, bruising, cerebrospinal fluid (CSF)/blood in nose or ears, fracture "step" deformity of skull, subcutaneous emphysema, "raccoon eyes"
- *Stigmata of other illnesses:* Liver disease, alcoholism, diabetes, myxedema
- *Skin* for needle marks, cyanosis, pallor, rashes, poor turgor
- *Smell the breath* (alcohol, hepatic fetor, ketosis, uremia)
- *Meningismus* but do *not* move neck unless cervical spine is cleared
- *Heart/lung exam* for murmurs, rubs, wheeze, consolidation, collapse
- *Abdomen/rectal exam* for organomegaly, ascites, bruising, peritoneal signs, melena
- *Are there any foci of infection?* Abscesses, bites, middle ear infection
- *Any features of meningitis?:* Neck stiffness, rash, focal neurology
- *Note the absence of signs:* E.g.,*no* pin-point pupils in a known heroin addict or a diabetic patient whose breath does *not* smell of acetone.

Quick history from family, ambulance staff, bystanders: Abrupt or gradual onset? Suicide note present? Was there any seizure activity? Be highly suspicious of cervical spinal injury and consider spinal immobilization if there is uncertainty. Recent complaints—headache, fever, vertigo, depression? Recent medical history—sinusitis, otitis, neurosurgery, ENT procedure? Past medical history—diabetes, asthma, ↑BP, cancer, epilepsy, psychiatric illness? Drug or toxin exposure (especially alcohol or other recreational drugs)? Any recent travel?

Critical considerations: In all undiagnosed coma patients or in those with focal neurological signs, a computed tomography (CT) scan is very helpful. A lumbar puncture (LP) may be needed for meningitis or subarachnoid hemorrhage.

Table 20.2 Management of coma[a]

ABC of life support

↓

O_2, IV access

↓

Stabilize cervical spine

↓

Blood glucose

↓

Control seizures

↓

Consider IV glucose, thiamine, naloxone, or flumazenil

↓

Brief examination, obtain history

↓

Investigations

Arterial blood gases (ABG), CBC, CMP, liver function tests (LFTs), ESR,
c-reactive protein (CRP), total CK

Ethanol, toxic screen, drug levels

Blood cultures, urine culture, CXR

↓

Reassess the situation and plan further investigations.

[a]*Check pupils every few minutes during the early stages*, particularly if trauma is the likely cause. Doing so is the quickest way to find a localizing sign (very helpful in diagnosis, but remember that false localizing signs *do* occur), and observing *changes* in pupil behavior (e.g., becoming fixed and dilated) is the quickest way to find out just how bad things are.

The Glasgow Coma Scale

The GCS was first developed to assess consciousness in trauma patients. This scale is now often used in a variety of situations to quantify in a reliable, objective way the conscious state of a person. It can be used by medical and nursing staff for initial and continuing assessment. Three areas are examined when obtaining a GCS score: motor response, verbal response, and eye response.

Best motor response This has six grades:

6 Follows command: The patient obeys a command to complete a simple task on your request.

5 Localizing response to pain: The patient responds to pain by reaching toward the painful stimuli.

4 Withdraws to pain: The patient retreats from the painful stimuli in some fashion, without attempting to localize the response.

3 Flexor response to pain: The patient responds to painful stimuli by abnormally flexing the upper limbs.

2 Extensor posturing to pain: The painful stimulus causes limb extension (adduction, internal rotation of shoulder, pronation of forearm); decerebrate posture.

1 No response to pain.

Note that it is the best response of any limb that should be recorded.

Best verbal response This has five grades:

5 Oriented: The patient knows who he is, where he is, and why he is where he is, the year, season, and month.

4 Confused conversation: The patient responds to questions in a conversational manner but there is some disorientation and confusion.

3 Inappropriate speech: Random or exclamatory articulated speech but no conversational exchange.

2 Incomprehensible speech: Moaning but no words.

1 None. Record level of best speech.

Eye opening This has four grades:

4 Spontaneous eye opening.

3 Eye opening in response to speech: Any speech or shout, not necessarily request to open eyes.

2 Eye opening in response to pain: Painful stimuli results in eye opening.

1 No eye opening.

An overall score is made by adding the individual scores from the three areas assessed. For example: A person who is dead has no response to pain + no verbalization + no eye opening and would have a GCS = 3. A severely ill patient would have a GCS of ≤8; a moderate injury, GCS 9–12; minor injury, 13. In general, "less than or equal to 8, intubate."

NB: An abbreviated coma scale, the AVPU, is sometimes used in the initial assessment (primary survey) of the critically ill:

- A = alert
- V = responds to vocal stimuli
- P = responds to pain
- U = unresponsive

Table 20.3 The neurological examination in coma

A patient who appears to have an altered level of consciousness has a problem in one of two areas (1) a diffuse, bilateral, cortical dysfunction (usually producing loss of awareness with normal arousal) or (2) damage to the ascending reticular activating system (ARAS) located throughout the brainstem from the medulla to the thalami (usually producing loss of arousal with unassessable awareness). The brainstem can be affected directly (e.g., pontine hemorrhage) or indirectly (e.g., compression from trans-tentorial or cerebellar herniation secondary to a mass or edema). The following are areas to be examined in these patients.

Level of consciousness: Describe using *objective* words such as *unarousable, responds to questions,* or *responds to pain.*

- *Respiratory pattern:* Cheyne–Stokes, hyperventilation (acidosis, hypoxia, or, rarely, neurogenic), ataxic or apneustic (breath-holding) breathing (brainstem damage with grave prognosis).
- *Eyes:* Almost all patients with ARAS pathology will have eye findings.

Visual fields Test fields with visual threat. No blink in one field suggests hemianopsia and contralateral hemisphere lesion.

Pupils

Normal, direct, and consensual = intact midbrain. *Midposition (3-5 mm) nonreactive ± irregular* = midbrain lesion.

Unilateral dilated and unreactive ("fixed") = third-nerve compression.

Small, reactive = pontine lesion ("pinpoint pontine pupils") or drugs.

Horner's syndrome = ipsilateral lateral medulla or hypothalamus lesion; may precede uncal herniation.

(Continued)

Table 20.3 (*Continued*)

Be aware of patients with false eyes or who use eye drops for glaucoma.

Extraocular movements (EOMs) Observe resting position and spontaneous movement, then test the vestibulo-ocular reflex (VOR) with either the *Doll's-head maneuver* (normal if the eyes keep looking at the same point in space when the head is quickly moved laterally or vertically) or *ice water calorics* (normal if eyes deviate toward the cold ear with nystagmus to the other side). If present, the VOR exonerates *most* of the brainstem from the CN VII nerve nucleus (medulla) to the CN III (midbrain). *Don't move the head unless the cervical spine is cleared.*

Fundi Papilledema, subhyaloid hemorrhage, hypertensive retinopathy, other disease (diabetic retinopathy)

• Examine for CNS asymmetry (tone, spontaneous movements, reflexes).

Shock

Definition Circulatory insufficiency resulting in inadequate tissue perfusion. Shock can be classified into four categories (1) hypovolemic (caused by inadequate circulating volume), (2) cardiogenic (caused by inadequate cardiac pump function), (3) distributive (caused by peripheral vasodilatation and maldistribution of blood flow (i.e., sepsis), and (4) obstructive (caused by extracardiac obstruction to blood flow). *Shock is often manifested by SBP <90 mm Hg; a weak pulse; evidence of end-organ dysfunction, such as cool or mottled skin; oliguria; hepatic insufficiency; or altered mental status. However, the signs of shock can be subtle depending on the cause.*

• **Hypovolemia:** *Bleeding:* Trauma, ruptured aortic aneurysm, ruptured ectopic pregnancy. *Fluid loss:* Vomiting (e.g., GI obstruction), diarrhea (e.g., cholera), burns, pools of sequestered (unavailable) fluids (third spacing; e.g., in pancreatitis). *Heat exhaustion* may cause hypovolemic shock (also hyperpyrexia, oliguria, rhabdomyolysis, unconsciousness, hyperventilation, hallucination, incontinence, collapse, coma, pin-point pupils, LFTs↑, and disseminated intravascular coagulation [DIC, p. 626]).

• **Cardiogenic:** *Heart dysfunction* that includes dysrhythmias, tachyarrhythmias, or bradyarrhythmias. Overt pump failure is another cause of cardiogenic shock and can result from acute coronary syndromes, myocarditis, or cardiomyopathy, as well as from acute valvular dysfunction (especially regurgitant lesions) or rupture of ventricular septum or ventricular wall.

• **Obstructive shock:** Pathology that prevents blood from flowing from the heart; includes pericardial disease (tamponade), tension pneumothorax, pulmonary emboli, pulmonary hypertension, or other cardiac tumor, as well as obstructive valvular disease (aortic or mitral stenosis).

• **Distributive shock:** Blood is maldistributed throughout the body; includes septic shock, anaphylactic shock, and neurogenic shock, as well as effects from vasodilator drugs and acute adrenal insufficiency.

• **Sepsis:** Gram –ve (or +ve) septic shock from endotoxin-induced vasodilatation may be sudden and severe, with shock and coma but no signs of infection (fever, white blood cells [WBCs]↑).

• **Neurogenic:** E.g.,post spinal surgery

• **Endocrine failure:** Addison's disease or hypothyroidism

• **Iatrogenic:** Drugs (e.g., anesthetics, antihypertensives)

Assessment ABC.

- *ECG:* Rate, rhythm, ischemia?
- *General:* Cold and clammy: Cardiogenic shock or fluid loss. Look for signs of anemia or dehydration: Skin turgor, postural hypotension? Warm and well-perfused with bounding pulse: Septic shock. Any features suggestive of anaphylaxis—history, urticaria, angioedema, wheeze?
- *Cardiovascular system (CVS):* Usually tachycardic (unless on β-blocker or in spinal shock) and hypotensive. But in the young and fit or pregnant women, the systolic BP may remain normal, although the *pulse pressure* will narrow, with up to 30% blood volume depletion. Difference between arms: Aortic dissection
- *JVP or central venous pressure:* If raised, cardiogenic shock is likely.
- *Check abdomen:* Any signs of trauma or aneurysm? Any evidence of GI bleeding? Check for melena.

Management If BP is unrecordable, call the cardiac arrest team.

See Table 20.4 for general management. Specific measures:

- **Anaphylaxis (covered in own section)**
- **Cardiogenic shock (covered in own section)**
- **Septic shock:** If no clue to source: Piperacillin-tazobactam 3.375–4.5 g IV q6h + vancomycin 15 mg/kg q12h ± gentamicin. Give colloid or crystalloid by IV. Consider transfer to ICU if possible for monitoring ± inotropes (norepinephrine). Goal-directed therapy now includes measurement of lactic acid, central venous pressure (CVP), inferior venous cava (IVC) measurement, urine output, and hematocrit. See Table 20.5.
- **Hypovolemic shock:**
  Fluid replacement: 20 mg/kg bolus of saline or lactated Ringer's solution initially; if bleeding use blood; assess risks and benefits. Titrate against blood pressure, CVP, and urine output. Treat the underlying cause. If severe hemorrhage, exsanguinating, or >1 L of fluid required to maintain blood pressure, consider using group-specific blood, or O Rh negative blood. Correct electrolyte abnormalities. Acidosis often responds to fluid replacement.
- **Heat exposure (heat exhaustion):** Sponge bath + fanning; avoid ice and immersion. Resuscitate with high-sodium IV fluids, such as 0.9% saline ± hydrocortisone 100 mg IV. Dantrolene seems ineffective. Chlorpromazine 25 mg IM may be used to stop shivering. Stop cooling when core temperature <39°C.

Table 20.4 Management of shock

If BP is unrecordable, call the cardiac arrest team
↓
ABC(including high-flow O₂)
↓
Raise foot of the bed
↓
IV access: Two (wide-bore; get help if this takes >2 min)
↓
Identify and treat underlying cause
↓
Infuse crystalloid *fast* to raise BP (unless cardiogenic shock)
↓
Seek expert help early
↓
Investigations
CBC, CMP, ABG, glucose, CRP
Cross-match and check clotting
Blood cultures, urine culture, ECG, CXR
Others: Lactate, echo, abdominal CT, US
↓
Consider arterial line, central venous line, and bladder catheter (aim for a urine flow >30 mL/h) 0.5–1 cc/kg/hr
↓
Further management:
Treat underlying cause if possible
Fluid replacement as dictated by BP, CVP, Ultrasound IVC measurement, urine output

Don't overload with fluids if cardiogenic shock If persistently hypotensive, consider inotropes

NB: *Remember that higher flow rates can be achieved better through peripheral lines than through standard -gauge central lines.*
If cause is unclear: Treat as hypovolemia—most common cause and reversible.
Ruptured abdominal aortic aneurysm: Aim for a systolic BP of ~90 mm Hg.

Table 20.5 SIRS, sepsis, and related syndromes

The pathogenesis of sepsis and septic shock is becoming increasingly understood. The systemic inflammatory response syndrome (SIRS) is the early phase of septic shock and is thought to involve cytokine cascades, free radical production, and the release of vasoactive mediators. SIRS is defined as the presence of ≥2 of the following features:

• Temperature >38°C or <36°C
• Tachycardia >90 bpm
• Respiratory rate >20 breaths/min
• WBC >12×10⁹/L or <4×10⁹ /L, or >10% immature (band) forms

Related syndromes include:
Sepsis: SIRS occurring in the presence of infection. If SIRS continues, then severe sepsis can result.
Severe sepsis: Sepsis with evidence of organ hypoperfusion (e.g., hypoxemia, oliguria, lactic acidosis, or altered cerebral function)

747

(Continued)

Table 20.5 (*Continued*)

Septic shock: Severe sepsis with hypotension (systolic BP <90 mm Hg) despite adequate fluid resuscitation or the requirement for vasopressors/inotropes to maintain BP. If sepsis progresses, the patient may end up with multiorgan dysfunction syndrome.

Septicemia was used to denote the presence of multiplying bacteria in the circulation, but the term has been replaced with the definitions above.

Anaphylactic shock

Type I IgE-mediated hypersensitivity reaction. Release of histamine and other agents causes capillary leak, wheeze, cyanosis, edema (larynx, lids, tongue, lips), urticaria. More common in atopic individuals. An *anaphylactoid reaction* results from direct release of mediators from inflammatory cells without involving antibodies, usually in response to a drug (e.g., *N*-acetylcysteine).

Common precipitants
• Drugs (e.g., penicillin), contrast media in radiology
• Latex
• Stings, eggs, fish, peanuts, strawberries

Signs and symptoms
• Itching, erythema, urticaria, edema
• Wheeze, laryngeal obstruction, cyanosis
• Tachycardia, hypotension

Management of anaphylaxis
Secure the airway; give 100% O_2
Intubate if respiratory obstruction imminent

↓

Remove the cause; raising the feet may help restore the circulation

↓

Give epinephrine IM
0.3 mg (i.e., 0.3 mL of 1:1000)
Repeat every 5 min if needed, as guided by BP, pulse, and respiratory function, until better

↓

Secure large-bore IV access

↓

Diphenhydramine 25–50 mg IV and methylprednisolone 125 mg IV

↓

IV (0.9% saline bolus 20 mg/kg; may repeat once)
Titrate against BP

↓

If wheezing, treat for asthma
May require ventilatory support

↓

If still hypotensive, admission to ICU and an epinephrine (adrenaline) drip may be needed ± nebulized albuterol. Get expert help.

Further management

- Admit to ward; monitor ECG.
- Continue Benadryl 25–50 mg/4–6 h PO/IV if itching.
- H$_2$ blocker, such as cimetidine 300 mg or ranitidine 100 mg (orally, IV, IM)
- Suggest a "Medic-alert" bracelet naming the culprit allergen.
- Teach about self-injected epinephrine (e.g., 0.3 mg, EpiPen®) to prevent a fatal attack.
- Skin-prick tests showing specific IgE help identify which allergens to avoid.
- Consider glucagon 1–2 mg every 5 min IM/IV if on a β-blocker (β-blockers blunt tachycardic response and worsen low BPs in this type of shock). Beware of causing nausea with glucagon in the obtunded patient without a definitive airway.

Note: Epinephrine IV should be reserved for life threatening situations or when the patient is hypotensive. The IV dose is **different: (1:10,000 solution) 0.1 mg slowly over 5 min**. Stop as soon as a response has been obtained.

Acute myocardial infarction

A common medical emergency; prompt, appropriate treatment saves lives and myocardium. If in doubt, seek immediate help.

Prehospital management

Arrange an emergency ambulance. Aspirin 325 mg PO (unless clear contraindication). Analgesia, e.g., morphine 5–10 mg IV (avoid IM injections, as risk of bleeding increases if thrombolysis ultimately given). Sublingual nitroglycerin unless hypotensive.

Management See Table 20.6 for acute measures.

Percutaneous coronary angioplasty (PCA) is preferred to thrombolysis. If PCA is not available within 1 h, then thrombolysis is also effective in reducing mortality if given early. Greatest benefit is seen if given <12 h after the onset of chest pain, but some benefit is possible up to 24 h. The door-to-needle/balloon time for thrombolysis and PCA should be <90 min.

Indications for thrombolysis: Presentation within *12 h* of chest pain with:

- ST elevation >2 mm in ≥2 chest leads *or*
- ST elevation >1 mm in ≥2 limb leads *or*
- Posterior infarction (dominant R waves and ST depression in V$_1$–V$_3$)
- New-onset left bundle branch block

Presentation within *12-24 h* if continuing chest pain and/or ST elevation.

Thrombolysis contraindications (CI): Consider urgent angioplasty instead.

• Internal bleeding	• Suspected aortic dissection
• Prolonged or traumatic CPR	• Previous allergic reaction
• Heavy vaginal bleeding	• Pregnancy or <18 wks postnatal
• Acute pancreatitis	• Severe liver disease
• Active lung disease with cavitation	• Esophageal varices
• Recent trauma or surgery (<2 wks)	• Recent head trauma
• Cerebral neoplasm	• Recent hemorrhagic stroke.
• Severe hypertension (>200/120 mm Hg)	

Relative CI: History of severe hypertension, peptic ulcer, history of CVA, bleeding diathesis, anticoagulants.

Streptokinase (SK) is the usual thrombolytic agent. *Dose:* 1.5 million units in 100 mL 0.9% saline IV over 1 h. side effects: Nausea, vomiting, hemorrhage, stroke (1%), dysrhythmias. Any hypotension usually responds to slowing down or stopping the infusion. Also watch for allergic reactions and anaphylaxis (rare). Do not repeat unless it is within 4 d of the first administration.

Alteplase (rt-PA) may be indicated if the patient has previously received SK (>4 d) or reacted to SK. *Dose:* 15 mg IV bolus, then 0.75 mg/kg (max 50 mg) over 30 min, then 0.5 mg/kg (max 35 mg) over 60 min. Accelerated rt-PA has benefit if given within 6 h, especially in younger patients with anterior MI. Standard rt-PA is given to patients presenting at 6–12 h.

Tenecteplase is given by bolus injection (over 10 sec), which in some cases may be an advantage. *Dose:* 30 mg IV (max 50 mg) if weight is <60 kg; 35 mg IV (max 50 mg) if weight is 60–69 kg; 40 mg IV (max 50 mg) if weight is 70–79 kg; 45 mg IV (max 50 mg) if weight is 80–89 kg; 50 mg IV (max 50 mg) if weight is >90 kg.

Complications

- Recurrent ischemia or failure to reperfuse (usually detected as persisting pain and ST-segment elevation in the immediate aftermath of thrombolysis): Additional analgesia, nitroglycerin, β-blocker; consider rethromboblysis or do angioplasty if persistent or new ST-segment elevation.
- Stroke
- Pericarditis: Analgesics (try to avoid NSAIDs)
- Cardiogenic shock and heart failure

Right ventricular infarction

- Confirm by demonstrating ST elevation in RV3, RV4 and/or echo. **NB:** RV4 means that V_4 is placed in the right fifth intercostal space in the midclavicular line.
- Treat hypotension and oliguria with fluids.
- Avoid nitrates and diuretics.
- Intensive monitoring and inotropes may be useful in some patients.

Table 20.6 Management of an acute MI

Attach ECG monitor and record a 12-lead ECG

↓

High-flow O$_2$ by face mask (caution, if COPD)

↓

IV access

Bloods for CBC, CMP, glucose, lipids, cardiac enzymes ↓

Brief assessment

History of cardiovascular disease; risk factors for heart disease

Contraindications to thrombolysis?

Examination: Pulse, BP, JVP, cardiac murmurs, signs of heart failure, peripheral pulses, scars from previous cardiac surgery

↓

Aspirin 325 mg if not given previously that day and no contraindications; heparin (follow weight-based nomogram); clopidogrel 300 mg PO; consider eptifibatide (Integrilin) with cardiology consult before going to percutaneous coronary angioplasty (PTCA)

↓

Nitroglycerin 0.4 mg sublingually unless hypotensive

↓

If chest pain persists, consider morphine unless hypotensive

↓

β-Blocker, e.g., metoprolol 5 mg IV (unless asthma or left ventricular failure)

↓

PTCA or thrombolysis (see chart in text)

↓

CXR

Do not delay thrombolysis while waiting unless aneurysm is suspected

↓

Consider deep vein thrombosis (DVT) prophylaxis

↓

Continue medication except calcium-channel antagonists (unless specific indication)

If pain is uncontrolled, especially if continuing ST elevation, consider rethrombolysis with rt-PA (no bolus), tenecteplase, or rescue angioplasty.

Acute coronary syndrome

Acute coronary syndrome (ACS) (without ST-elevation) includes unstable angina, evolving MI, and non-Q wave or subendocardial MI. Although the underlying pathology is similar, management differs, and, therefore, ACS is usually divided into two classes:

- *ACS with ST segment elevation* or new left bundle branch block (LBBB) (see acute MI earlier)
- *ACS without ST segment elevation* (unstable angina or non-q wave MI)

ACS is associated with a greatly increased risk of MI(up to 30% in the first month). Patients should be managed medically until symptoms settle. They are then investigated by angiography with a view to possible angioplasty or surgery (coronary artery bypass graft [CABG]).

Assessment

Brief history: Previous angina, relief with rest/nitrates, history of cardiovascular disease, risk factors for ischemic heart disease (IHD).

Examination: Pulse, BP, JVP, cardiac murmurs, signs of heart failure, peripheral pulses, scars from previous cardiac surgery.

Investigations ECG: ST depression flat, inverted t waves, or normal. CBC, CMP, glucose, lipids, cardiac enzymes, CXR.

Measurement of cardiac troponins helps predict which patients are at risk of a cardiac event, and who can be safely discharged early.

Management

See Table 20.7 for acute management.

The aim of drug therapy is twofold:

1 Anti-ischemic (e.g., β-blocker, nitrate, calcium-channel antagonist)
2 Antithrombotics (e.g., aspirin, low-molecular-weight heparin, eptifibatide), which interfere with platelet activation and so reduce thrombus formation

Further measures:

- Wean off nitroglycerin (NTG) infusion when stabilized on oral drugs.
- Stop heparin when pain-free for 24 h, but give at least 3–5 d therapy.
- Check serial ECGs and cardiac enzymes for 9 h.
- Address modifiable risk factors: Smoking, hypertension, hyperlipidemia, diabetes.
- Begin gentle mobilization.

If symptoms recur, refer to a cardiologist for urgent angiography and angioplasty or CABG.

Prognosis Overall risk of death ~1–2%, but ~15% for refractory angina despite medical therapy. Risk stratification can help predict those most at risk and allow intervention to be targeted at those individuals. The following are associated with an increased risk:

- Hemodynamic instability: Hypotension, pulmonary edema
- T-wave inversion or ST segment depression on resting ECG
- Previous MI
- Prolonged rest pain
- Older age
- Diabetes mellitus

Indications for consideration of invasive intervention:

- Poor prognosis (e.g., pulmonary edema)
- Refractory symptoms
- Positive exercise tolerance tests (ETT)at low workload
- Non-Q wave MI.

Table 20.7 Acute management of ACS without ST-segment elevation

Admit to a monitored setting

↓

High-flow O_2 by face mask

↓

Nitrates: NTG spray or sublingual tablets as required

↓

Analgesia: E.g., morphine mg IV + ondansetron 4 mg IV

↓

Aspirin: 160–325 mg if not given previously that day and no contraindications *reduces risk of mi and death*

↓

β-blocker: E.g., metoprolol 50–100 mg/8 h orally
If β-blocker is contraindicated (asthma, COPD, left ventricular function (LVF), bradycardia, coronary artery spasm), give rate-limiting calcium antagonist (e.g., diltiazem 60–120 mg/8 h PO)

↓

Low-molecular-weight heparin
e.g., enoxaparin 1 mg/kg/12 h
Alternatively: Unfractionated heparin 5,000 U IV bolus then iv infusion
Check aPTT q6h. Alter IV rate to maintain aPTT at 1.5–2.5 × control

↓

IV nitrate if pain continues
titrate to pain, and maintain SBP at >100 mm Hg

↓

Record ECG while in pain

↓

High-risk patients
(persistent or recurrent ischemia, st-depression, diabetes, ↑troponin)
Infusion of a GPIIb/IIIa antagonist (e.g., tirofiban) and, ideally, urgent angiography. Addition of clopidogrel may also be useful

↓

Optimize drugs: β-blocker; Ca^{2+} channel antagonist; angiotensin-converting enzyme (ACE)-inhibitor; nitrate
Intensive statin regimens, *starting at top dosages*, may decrease long- *and* short-term mortality/adverse events, e.g., by stabilizing plaques

↓

If symptoms fail to improve, refer to a cardiologist for urgent angioplasty ± angioplasty or CABG

Low-risk patients
(no further pain, flat or inverted t-waves, or normal ecg, **and** *negative troponin)*
May be discharged if a repeat troponin (3, 6, and 9 h) is negative. Treat medically and arrange further investigation(e.g., stress test, angiogram)

Severe pulmonary edema

Causes

- Cardiovascular: Usually left ventricular (LV) failure—post-MI—or ischemic heart disease. Also mitral stenosis, arrhythmias, and malignant hypertension
- Acute respiratory distress syndrome (ARDS) (Any cause (e.g., trauma, malaria, drugs); look for predisposing factors (e.g., trauma, postop, sepsis). *Is aspirin overdose or glue-sniffing/drug abuse likely?* Ask friends/relatives.
- Fluid overload
- Neurogenic (e.g., head injury)
- See X-RAY PLATE 2

Differential diagnosis Asthma/COPD, pneumonia, and pulmonary edema are often hard to distinguish, especially in the elderly, in whom these may coexist. Do not hesitate to treat all three simultaneously (e.g., with albuterol nebulizer, furosemide IV, morphine, fluoroquinolone).

Symptoms Dyspnea, orthopnea (e.g., paroxysmal), pink frothy sputum. **NB:** Drugs; other illnesses (recent MI/COPD) or pneumonia).

Signs

Distressed, pale, sweaty, pulse↑, tachypnea, pink frothy sputum, pulsus alternans, elevated JVP, fine lung crackles, triple/gallop rhythm, wheeze (cardiac asthma). Usually sitting up and leaning forward. Quickly examine for possible causes.

Investigations

- CXR(X-RAY PLATE 2: Cardiomegaly, signs of pulmonary edema. Look for shadowing (usually bilateral), small effusions at costophrenic angles, fluid in the lung fissures, and Kerley B lines (linear opacities).
- ECG: Signs of MI
- CMP; cardiac enzymes, arterial blood gases (ABG)
- Consider echo

Management

Begin treatment before investigations. See Table 20.8.

Monitoring progress: BP, heart rate, cyanosis, respiratory rate, JVP, urine output, ABG.

Once stable and improving:

- Daily weights; BP and pulse q6h. Repeat CXR.
- Change to oral furosemide or bumetanide.
- If on large doses of loop diuretic, consider the addition of a thiazide or metolazone 2.5–5 mg/d PO.
- ACE-inhibitor if LV failure; also consider echo. If ACE-inhibitor is contraindicated, consider hydralazine and nitrate.
- Also consider β-blocker and spironolactone.
- Is the patient suitable for cardiac transplantation?
- Consider digoxin ± warfarin, especially if AF.

Table 20.8 Management of heart failure

Sit the patient upright

↓

Oxygen
100% if no preexisting lung disease

↓

IV access and monitor ECG
Treat any arrhythmias (e.g., atrial fib)

↓

Investigations while continuing treatment

↓

Furosemide 40–80 mg IV slowly
Larger doses required in renal failure

↓

Nitroglycerin spray two puffs SL or 2 × 0.3 mg tablets SL
Don't give if systolic BP <90 mm Hg
Necessary investigations, examination, and history

↓

If systolic BP>100 mm Hg, start a nitrate infusion (*e.g., isosorbide dinitrate 2-10 mg/h IV*)
keep systolic BP >90 mm Hg

↓

If the patient is worsening: Further dose of furosemide 40–80 mg
Consider ventilation (invasive or noninvasive; e.g., CPAP; get help)or increase nitrate infusion

↓

If systolic BP <100 mm Hg, treat as cardiogenic shock; i.e., *consider a Swan-Ganz catheter and inotropic support*

↓

If systolic BP is >180 mm Hg, consider treating for hypertensive LVF

Cardiogenic shock

This has a high mortality. Ask a senior physician's help both in formulating an *exact* diagnosis and in guiding treatment. Cardiogenic shock is caused primarily by the failure of the heart to maintain the circulation. It may occur suddenly or after progressively worsening heart failure.

Causes
- Arrhythmias
- Cardiac tamponade
- Tension pneumothorax
- MI
- Myocarditis; myocardial depression (drugs, hypoxia, acidosis, sepsis)
- Valve destruction (endocarditis)
- Pulmonary embolism
- Aortic dissection

Management

If the cause is MI, prompt revascularization (thrombolysis or acute angio-plasty) is vital; see MI section for indications and contraindications.

- Manage in coronary care unit, if possible.
- Investigation and treatment may need to be done concurrently.
- See Table 20.9 for details of management.
- *Investigations:* ECG, CMP, CBC, CK, CK-MB, troponin, ABG, CXR, echo. If indicated, CT thorax (aortic dissection) and ventilation/profusion scan or pulmonary angiogram for PE.
- *Monitor* CVP, BP, ABG, ECG, urine output. Do a 12-lead ECG every hour until the diagnosis is made. Consider a Swan–Ganz catheter to assess pulmonary wedge pressure and cardiac output and an arterial line to monitor pressure. Catheterize for accurate urine output.

Cardiac tamponade

Pericardial fluid collects → intrapericardial pressure rises → heart cannot fill → pumping stops

Causes: Trauma, lung/breast cancer, pericarditis, myocardial infarct, bacteria (e.g., TB). *Rarely:* Urea↑, radiation, myxedema, dissecting aorta, systemic lupus erythematosus (SLE).

Signs: Falling BP, a rising JVP, and muffled heart sounds = Beck's triad; JVP↑ on inspiration (Kussmaul sign); pulsus paradoxus (pulse fades on inspiration). Echocardiography may be diagnostic. CXR: Globular heart; left heart border convex or straight; right cardiophrenic angle <90 degrees. ECG: Electrical alternans.

Management: Severe cases can be difficult to manage. Early recognition is important. Ensure that proper backup is available including either cardiology or cardiac surgery. With luck, prompt pericardiocentesis brings swift relief. While awaiting this, give O_2, monitor ECG, and set up IV. Draw blood.

<hr>

Table 20.9 Management of cardiogenic shock

Oxygen
Titrate to maintain adequate arterial saturations

↓

Investigations and close monitoring

↓

*Correct arrhythmias, electrolyte abnormality,
or acid-base imbalance*

↓

*Optimize filling pressure;
if available measure pulmonary capillary wedge pressure (PCWP)
If PCWP <15 mm Hg fluid load (100mg every 15 min IV to PCWP 15-20)
If PCWP >15 mm Hg Inotropic support (e.g., dobutamine 2.5-10mcg/kg/min
IV for a SBP >80 mm Hg*

↓

*Consider intra-aortic balloon pump if you expect the underlying condition to
improve or you need time awaiting surgery*

↓

*Look for and treat any reversible cause (e.g., MI or PE; consider throm-
bolysis; surgery for: Acute ventriculo-septal defect (VSD), mitral, or aortic
regurgitation)*

<hr>

Wide complex tachycardia

ECG shows rate of >100 bpm and QRS complexes >120 ms.

Principles of management

If in doubt, treat as ventricular tachycardia (the most common cause).
Identify the underlying rhythm and treat accordingly.

Differential

- Ventricular tachycardia (VT) including torsade de pointes
- SVT with aberrant conduction (e.g., AF, atrial flutter)
- Preexcited tachycardias (e.g., AF, atrial flutter, or AV reentry tachycardia with accessory pathways such as underlying Wolff–Parkinson–White [WPW] syndrome).

NB: Ventricular ectopics should not cause confusion when occurring singly; but if >3 together at a rate of >120, this constitutes VT.

Identification of the underlying rhythm may be difficult; seek expert help. Diagnosis is based on the history: If heart disease/MI, the likelihood of a ventricular arrhythmia is >95%. A 12-lead ECG and the lack of response to IV adenosine also helps to discover the underlying rhythm.

ECG findings in favor of VT:

- Fusion beats or capture beats
- Positive QRS concordance in chest leads
- Marked left-axis deviation or rightward axis
- AV dissociation (occurs in 25%) or 2:1 or 3:1 AV block
- QRS complex >160 ms
- Any atypical bundle branch block pattern

Management Give high-flow O_2 by mask and monitor O_2 saturations.

- Connect patient to a cardiac monitor and have a defibrillator at hand.
- Assess CVS: Decreased consciousness, BP <90, oliguria, angina, pulmonary edema
- Obtain 12-lead ECG(request CXR) and obtain IV access

If hemodynamically unstable:

- Synchronized DC shock
- Correct any hypokalemia and hypomagnesemia: 20–40 mEq/h IV with cardiac monitoring, 1–2 g IV magnesium sulfate over 30 min.
- Follow with amiodarone 150 mg IV over 10 min.
- For refractory cases, procainamide or sotalol may be considered.

If hemodynamically stable:

- Correct hypokalemia and hypomagnesemia, as above.
- Amiodarone 150 mg IV over 10 min
- If this fails, consider procainamide or sotalol or synchronized DC shock

After correction of VT:

- Establish the cause (via the history and tests above).
- Maintenance antiarrhythmic therapy may be required. If VT occurs after MI, give IV amiodarone; if 24 h after MI also start oral antiarrhythmic: e.g., amiodarone.
- Prevention of recurrent VT: Surgical isolation of the arrhythmogenic area or implantation of tiny automatic defibrillators may help.

Ventricular Fibrillation Use nonsynchronized DC shock (there is no R wave to trigger defibrillation).

Ventricular extrasystoles (ectopics) are the most common post-MI arrhythmias, but they are also seen in healthy people (often >10/h). Patients with frequent ectopics post-MI have a worse prognosis, but there is no evidence that antidysrhythmic drugs improve outcome; indeed they may increase mortality.

Torsade de pointes: A form of VT with a constantly varying axis, often in the setting of long-QT syndromes. This can be congenital or acquired (e.g., from drugs, such as some antidysrhythmics, tricyclics, antimalarials, newer antipsychotics, and terfenadine). Give magnesium 1–2 g IV. Torsade in the setting of congenital long-QT syndromes can be treated with high doses of β-blockers.

In acquired long-QT syndromes, stop all predisposing drugs, correct hypokalemia, and give magnesium 1–2 g IV. An alternative is overdrive pacing.

Figure 20.2 AHA 2010 guidelines for advanced life support

Management of tachycardia with a pulse

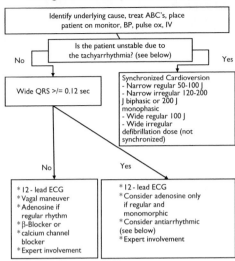

Identify underlying cause, treat ABC's, place patient on monitor, BP, pulse ox, IV

Is the patient unstable due to the tachyarrhythmia? (see below)

No / Yes

Wide QRS >/= 0.12 sec

Synchronized Cardioversion
- Narrow regular 50-100 J
- Narrow irregular 120-200 J biphasic or 200 J monophasic
- Wide regular 100 J
- Wide irregular defibrillation dose (not synchronized)

No / Yes

* 12 - lead ECG
* Vagal maneuver
* Adenosine if regular rhythm
* β-Blocker or
* calcium channel blocker
* Expert involvement

* 12 - lead ECG
* Consider adenosine only if regular and monomorphic
* Consider antiarrhythmic (see below)
* Expert involvement

Unstable is defined as: (1) hypotension, (2) acute altered mental status, (3) signs of shock, (4) ischemic chest discomfort, or (5) acute heart failure.

Antiarrhythmic infusions for stable wide complex tachycardia include:

Procainamide IV 20–50 mg/min until arrhythmia suppressed, hypotension, QRS duration increases >50%, or max of 17 mg/kg given. Infuse at 1–4 mg/min. Avoid if prolonged QT or congestive heart failure (CHF).

Amiodarone IV dose is 150 mg over 10 min. Repeat as need if VT recurs. Infuse at 1 mg/min for first 6 h.

Sotalol IV 100 mg (1.5 mg/kg) over 5 min. Avoid if prolonged QT.

From 2010 American Heart Association Guidelines for CPR and ECC. *Circulation.* 2010;122 (suppl):729–767.

Narrow complex tachycardia

ECG shows rate of >100 bpm and QRS complex duration of <120 ms.

Differential diagnosis
- Sinus tachycardia: Normal p-wave followed by normal QRS.
- *Atrial tachyarrhythmias:* Rhythm arises in atria;
  - Atrial fibrillation (AF): Absent P-wave, irregular QRS complexes
  - Atrial flutter: Atrial rate ~260–340 bpm. Saw-tooth baseline due to continuous atrial electrical activity; ventricular rate is often 150 bpm (2:1 block)
  - Atrial tachycardia: Abnormally shaped P-waves; may outnumber QRS
  - Multifocal atrial tachycardia: ≥3 P-wave morphologies; irregular QRS complexes
- *Junctional tachycardia:* AV-node is part of the pathway; P-wave either buried in QRS complex or occurring after QRS complex
  - AV nodal reentry tachycardia
  - AV reentry tachycardia, includes an accessory pathway (e.g., WPW).

Principles of management See Figure 20.2.
- If the patient is compromised, use DC cardioversion.
- Otherwise, identify the underlying rhythm and treat accordingly.
- Vagal maneuvers (carotid sinus massage, Valsalva maneuver) transiently increase AV block and may unmask an underlying atrial rhythm.
- If unsuccessful, give adenosine, which causes transient AV block. It has a short half-life (10–15 sec) and works in two ways:
  - By transiently slowing ventricles to show the underlying atrial rhythm
  - By cardioverting a junctional tachycardia into sinus rhythm

Give Adenosine 6 mg IV bolus into a large vein, followed by saline flush, while recording a rhythm strip. If unsuccessful, give 12 mg, then 12 mg again 2 min later if no response. *Warn about:* Transient chest tightness, dyspnea, headache, flushing. *CI:* Asthma, second-/third-degree AV block, or sinoatrial disease (unless pacemaker). *Interactions:* Potentiated by dipyridamole, antagonized by theophylline.

Specifics

Sinus tachycardia: Identify and treat underlying cause.

Supraventricular tachycardia: If adenosine fails, consider diltiazem (0.25 mg/kg or about 20 mg IV over 2 min. **NB:** When on a β-blocker, diltiazem should either be avoided or used with caution. *Alternatives:* Metoprolol 5 mg IV or amiodarone. If unsuccessful, use DC cardioversion.

Atrial Fibrillation/utter: Manage along standard lines (see afib section).

Atrial tachycardia: Rare; may be due to digoxin toxicity: Withdraw digoxin, consider digoxin-specific antibody fragments. Maintain K⁺ at 4–5 mmol/L.

Multifocal atrial tachycardia: Most commonly occurs in COPD. Correct hypoxia and hypercapnia. Consider Metoprolol or diltiazem if rate remains >110 bpm.

Junctional tachycardia: Where antegrade conduction through the AV node occurs, vagal maneuvers are worth trying. Adenosine will usually cardiovert a junctional rhythm into sinus rhythm. If it fails or recurs, β-blockers, diltiazem (**not** with β-blockers),or digoxin. If this does not control symptoms, consider radiofrequency ablation.

Wolff–Parkinson–White (WPW) syndrome Caused by congenital accessory conduction pathway between atria and ventricles. Resting ECG shows short P-R interval and widened QRS complex due to slurred upstroke or "delta wave." Two types: WPW type A(+ve QRS vector in V1), WPW type B(–ve QRS vector in V1). Patients present with SVT, which may be due to an AVRT preexcited AF, or preexcited atrial flutter. Risk of degeneration to VF and sudden death. Consider Procainamide or amiodarone. Refer to cardiologist for electrophysiology and ablation of the accessory pathway.

Acute severe asthma

The severity of an attack is easily underestimated. An atmosphere of calm helps.

Presentation Acute breathlessness and wheeze.

History Ask about usual and recent treatment, previous acute episodes and their severity, and best peak expiratory flow rate (PEFR). Has patient ever been admitted to ICU? or intubated, if so when?

Differential diagnosis Acute infective exacerbation of COPD, pulmonary edema, upper respiratory tract obstruction, pulmonary embolus, anaphylaxis.

Investigations PEF—but may be too ill, ABG, CXR (to exclude pneumothorax, infection), CBC, CMP.

Assessing the severity of an acute asthmatic attack

Severe attack:

- Unable to complete sentences
- Respiratory rate >25/min
- Pulse rate >110 bpm
- PEF <50% of predicted or best

Life-threatening attack:

- PEF <33% of predicted or best
- Silent chest, cyanosis, feeble respiratory effort
- Bradycardia or hypotension
- Exhaustion, confusion, or coma
- ABG: Normal/high P_aCO_2 >36 mm Hg; P_aO_2 <60 mm Hg, low pH, e.g., <7.35.

Treatment Life-threatening or severe asthma, see Table 20.10.

- Albuterol 5 mg nebulized, ipratropium bromide 500 mcg nebulized, with oxygen.
- If PEF remains <75%, repeat albuterol and give prednisone 60 mg PO.
- Monitor oxygen saturation, heart rate, and respiratory rate.

Discharge Before discharge patients must have:

- Had inhaler technique checked
- Peak flow rate >75% predicted or best with diurnal variability <25%
- Steroid and bronchodilator therapy
- Instructed on use of PEF meter and management plan
- Follow-up appointment within 1 wk
- Respiratory clinic appointment within 4 wks

Drugs used in acute asthma

Albuterol: β-agonist. *SE:* Tachycardia, arrhythmias, tremor, K+↓.

Ipratropium bromide: Anticholinergic *SE:* Dry Mouth and Sedation

Magnesium: Smooth muscle relaxant *SE:* Hypotension with rapid infusion, in high doses muscle weakness, absent reflexes, abnormal cardiac conduction, respiratory depression

Methylprednisolone/prednisone: Steroid

Table 20.10 Immediate management of acute severe asthma

Assess severity of attack (see above). Warn ICU if attack is severe. Start treatment immediately (prior to investigations).

- Sit patient up and give high-dose O_2 100% via non-rebreathing bag.
- Albuterol 5 mg every 20 min × 3 doses + ipratropium bromide 0.5 mg nebulized with O_2.
- Methylprednisolone 40–80 mg/d IV (If unable to tolerate PO) or prednisone 40–80 mg/d PO.
- CXR to exclude pneumothorax.

If life-threatening features (above) present:

- Inform ICU.
- Add magnesium sulphate ($MgSO_4$) 1.2–2 g IV over 20 min.
- Give albuterol nebulizers every 15 min, or 10 mg continuously per hour.

Further management
If improving

- 40–60% O_2
- Consider oral prednisone 10–60 mg with taper.
- Nebulized albuterol q4h
- Monitor peak flow and oxygen saturations.

If patient not improving after 15–30 min

- Continue 100% O_2 and steroids.
- Methylprednisolone 125 mg IV or prednisone 60 mg PO if not already given.
- Give albuterol nebulizers every 15 min or 10 mg continuously per hour.
- Continue ipratropium 0.5 mg q4–6h.

If patient still not improving

- Discuss with ICU staff.
- Repeat albuterol nebulizer every 15 min.
- $MgSO_4$ 1.2–2g IV over 20 min, unless already given.
- If no improvement or life-threatening features are present, consider transfer to ICU, accompanied by a doctor prepared to intubate; consider noninvasive ventilation (BIPAP).

Monitoring the effects of treatment

- Repeat PEF 15–30 min after initiating treatment.
- Pulse oximeter monitoring: Maintain S_aO_2 >92%.
- Check blood gases within 2 h if: Initial P_aCO_2 was normal/raised or initial P_aO_2 <60 mm Hg or patient is deteriorating.
- Record PEF pre- and post-β-agonist in hospital.

Once patient is improving

- Reduce nebulized albuterol and switch to inhaled β-agonist.
- Initiate inhaled steroids and stop oral steroids if possible.
- Continue to monitor PEF. Look for deterioration on reduced treatment and beware early morning dips in PEF.
- Look for the cause of the acute exacerbation and admission.

Acute exacerbations of COPD

Common medical emergency, especially in winter. May be triggered by viral or bacterial infections.

Presentation Increased cough, breathlessness, or wheeze. Decreased exercise capacity.

History Ask about usual/recent treatments (especially home oxygen), smoking status, and exercise capacity (may influence a decision to ventilate the patient).

Differential diagnosis Asthma, pulmonary edema, upper respiratory tract obstruction, pulmonary embolus, anaphylaxis.

Investigations
- PEF but patient may be too symptomatic to use)
- ABG
- CXR to exclude pneumothorax and infection
- CBC, CMP, blood cultures (if febrile)
- ECG
- Sending sputum for culture.

Management
- Look for a cause (e.g., infection, pneumothorax)
- See Table 20.11 and 20.12 for acute management.
- Prior to discharge, coordinate steroid reduction, home oxygen, smoking, pneumococcal and flu vaccinations.

Treatment of stable COPD.

Nonpharmacological:	Stop smoking, encourage exercise, treat poor nutrition or obesity, influenza vaccination

Pharmacological:

- **Mild** — Short-acting β_2-agonist or ipratropium PRN.
- **Moderate** — Regular short-acting β_2-agonist and/or ipratropium. Consider corticosteroid trial. Either po or inhaled or both
- **Severe** — Combination therapy with regular short-acting β_2-agonist and ipratropium

  Consider corticosteroid trial. Either po or inhaled or both

  Assess for home nebulizers.

  +/– macrolide antibiotic if evidence of infection

More advanced disease:

- Consider pulmonary rehabilitation in moderate/severe disease.
- Consider long-term oxygen therapy if P_aO_2 <55 mm Hg.
- Indications for surgery: Recurrent pneumothoraces, isolated bullous disease, lung volume reduction surgery (selected patients).
- Assess social circumstances and support required. Identify and treat depression.

Table 20.11 Management of acute copd

Controlled oxygen therapy
Start at 24–28%; vary according to ABG
Aim for a P_aO_2 >60 mm Hg with a rise in P_aCO_2 <12 mm Hg

↓

Nebulized bronchodilators:
Albuterol 5 mg/20 min and ipratropium 500 mcg as first two doses

↓

Steroids
IV methylprednisolone 125 mg/d or
oral prednisone 40–80 mg/d

↓

Antibiotics:
Use if evidence of infection, e.g., macrolide

↓

If no response:
Repeat nebulizers

↓

If no response:
1. Consider biphasic positive airway pressure *(BIPAP) if respiratory rate*
>30 or pH <7.35.

↓

2. Consider intubation[a] & ventilation if pH <7.26 and P_aCO_2 is rising

[a]A decision to ventilate will depend on the patient's premorbid state: Exercise capacity, home oxygen, and comorbidity. Ask about this information before you need to make this decision.

Table 20.12 Oxygen therapy

- The greatest danger is hypoxia, which probably accounts for more deaths than hypercapnia. *Don't leave patients severely hypoxic.*
- Therefore, care is required with O_2, especially if there is evidence of CO_2 retention. Start with 24–28% O_2 in such patients. Reassess after 30 min.
- In patients without evidence of retention at baseline, use 28–40% O_2 but still monitor and repeat ABG.

Pneumothorax

See **X-RAY** PLATE 6.

Tension pneumothorax requires immediate relief (see below). Do not delay management by obtaining a CXR.

Causes Often spontaneous (especially in young thin men) due to rupture of a subpleural bulla. *Other causes:* Asthma, COPD, TB, pneumonia, lung abscess, carcinoma, cystic fibrosis, lung fibrosis, sarcoidosis, connective tissue disorders (Marfan's syndrome, Ehlers–Danlos syndrome), trauma, iatrogenic (subclavian CVP line insertion, pleural aspiration or biopsy, percutaneous liver biopsy, positive pressure ventilation).

Clinical features *Symptoms:* There may be no symptoms (especially in fit young people with small pneumothoraces) or there may be sudden onset of dyspnea and/or pleuritic chest pain. Patients with asthma or COPD may present with a sudden deterioration. Mechanically ventilated patients may present with hypoxia or an increase in ventilation pressures. *Signs:* Reduced expansion, hyperresonance to percussion, and diminished breath sounds on the affected side. *With a tension pneumothorax, the trachea can be deviated away from the affected side, and the patient may be very symptomatic.*

Investigations *Immediate necessary treatment should not be delayed by a CXR.* Otherwise, request an expiratory film and look for an area devoid of lung markings, peripheral to the edge of the collapsed lung (X-RAY PLATE 6). *Ensure the suspected pneumothorax is not a large emphysematous bulla.* Check ABG/VBG in dyspneic patients and those with chronic lung disease.

Management Depends on whether it is a primary or secondary (underlying lung disease) pneumothorax, size and symptoms.

- Pneumothorax due to trauma or mechanical ventilation requires a chest tube.
- Aspiration of a pneumothorax (see below)
- Insertion and management of a chest tube

Surgical backup should be arranged anytime a chest tube is being considered.

Tension pneumothorax

See X-RAY PLATE 6. **This is a medical emergency**.

Essence: Air drawn into the pleural space with each inspiration has no route of escape during expiration. The mediastinum is pushed over into the contra-lateral hemithorax, kinking and compressing the great veins. Unless the air is rapidly removed, cardiorespiratory arrest will occur.

Signs: Respiratory distress, tachycardia, hypotension, distended neck veins, trachea deviated away from side of pneumothorax. Increased percussion note, reduced air entry/breath sounds on the affected side.

Treatment: To remove the air, insert a large-bore (14–16F) needle into the second intercostal interspace in the midclavicular line on the side of the suspected pneumothorax.

If the patient is in extremis, this procedure may be done before obtaining a chest x-ray.

Then insert a chest tube.

Chest tube drainage

- Use a small tube (10–14F) unless blood/pus is also present.
- Never clamp a bubbling tube.

- Tubes may be removed 24 h after the lung has reexpanded and air leak has stopped (i.e., the tube stops bubbling). This is done during expiration or a Valsalva maneuver.
- If the lung fails to reexpand within 48 h or if there is a persistent air leak, specialist advice should be obtained, as surgical intervention may be required.
- If suction is required, high-volume, low-pressure (–10 to –20 cm H_2O) systems are required.

Pneumonia

See X-RAY PLATES 5 and 8.

An infection of the lung parenchyma. Incidence of community-acquired pneumonia is 12:1,000 adults. Of these, one will require hospitalization, and mortality in these patients is still 10%.

Common organisms
- *Streptococcus pneumoniae* is the most common cause (60–75%).
- *Mycoplasma pneumoniae* (5–18%)
- *Staphylococcus aureus*
- *Haemophilus influenzae*
- *Legionella* sp. and *Chlamydia psittaci*
- Gram-negative bacilli, often hospital-acquired or in the immunocompromised (e.g., *Pseudomonas*, especially in those with COPD).
- Viruses including influenza account for up to 15%.

Symptoms
- Fever, rigors, malaise, anorexia, dyspnea, cough, purulent sputum (classically "rusty" with pneumococcus), hemoptysis, and pleuritic chest pain.

Signs
- Fever, cyanosis, herpes labialis (pneumococcus), confusion, tachypnea, tachycardia, hypotension, signs of consolidation (diminished expansion, dull percussion note, ↑ tactile vocal fremitus/vocal resonance, bronchial breathing), and a pleural rub.

Investigations
- CXR (see X-RAY PLATES 5 and 8).
- Oxygen saturation, ABG if S_aO_2 <92% or severe pneumonia
- CBC, CMP, LFT, CRP atypical serology
- Blood and sputum cultures
- Pleural fluid may be aspirated for culture
- Bronchoscopy and bronchoalveolar lavage if the patient is immunocompromised or in ICU.

Severity
Core adverse features "CURB" score:
- **C**onfusion
- B**U**N >20 mg/dL;
- **R**espiratory rate ≥30/min
- **B**P <90/60 mm Hg)

A score >2 indicates severe pneumonia. Other features that increase the risk of death are age >50 yrs, coexisting disease, bilateral/multilobar involvement, P_aO_2 <60 mm Hg or S_aO_2 <92%.

Management See Table 20.13

Complications

Pleural effusion, empyema, lung abscess, respiratory failure, septicemia, pericarditis, myocarditis, cholestatic jaundice, renal failure.

Table 20.13 Management of pneumonia

Oxygen to maintain P_aO_2 >60 mm Hg
Caution if history of COPD

↓

Treat hypotension and shock (p. 687)

↓

Investigations

↓

Antibiotics
see Table 20.14

↓

IV fluids may be required *(anorexia, dehydration, shock)*

↓

Analgesia for pleuritic chest pain *(e.g., acetaminophen 1 g/6 h or NSAID)*

↓

Some patients may need intubation and a period of ventilatory support

Table 20.14 Antibiotics

Community-acquired		
Mild	*Streptococcus pneumoniaeHaemophilus influenzaeMycoplasma pneumoniae*	Doxycycline 100 mg/d PO, or Azithromycin 500 mg/d × 3 d, 1 g then 500 mg/d × 2 d or 2 g one time (all above preferred) *or* clarithromycin 1 g/d or 500 bid × 7 d *or* levofloxacin 750 mg/d × 7 d *or* moxifloxacin 400 mg/d × 7 d
Severe	As above	Levofloxacin 750 mg IV/PO *or* moxifloxacin 400 mg IV/PO q24h × 7–10 days *or* (ceftriaxone 1 g IV q24h or cefotaxime 1 g IV q8h each with azithromycin 500 mg/d IV/PO × 3 days)
Atypical	*Legionella pneumophila*	Azithromycin 3–5 d or levofloxacin or moxifloxacin 7days
	Chlamydia species	Azithromycin or doxycycline 7 doxy 100 mg bid x
	Pneumocystis pneumoniae	High-dose co-trimoxazole
Hospital-acquired		
	Gram +ve bacilli *Pseudomonas* Anaerobes	If hospitalized >4 d, nursing home, ABX in last 90 d, immunosuppression then vanc/linezolid for MRSA + antipseudomonal β-lactam + either (levoflox or Cipro) *or* (gent or tobra or amikacin). If none of the above features, then ceftriaxone 2 g/d IV *or* fluoroquinolone *or* amp-sulbactam *or* ertapenem

(Continued)

| Table 20.14 | (Continued) |

Aspiration		
	Strep. pneumoniae	Clindamycin q8h IV ± fluoroqui-
	Anaerobes	nolone × 10 d

Massive pulmonary embolism

Always suspect PE in sudden collapse 1–2 wks after surgery. Mortality ranges from 0.7 to 6.0 per 100,000 persons.

Mechanism Venous thrombi, usually from DVT, pass into the pulmonary circulation and block blood flow to lungs. The source is often occult.

Risk factors

- Malignancy
- Surgery, especially pelvic
- Immobility
- Birth control pills (there is also a slight risk attached to HRT)
- Previous thromboembolism and inherited thrombophilia

Prevention Early postop mobilization is the simplest method; consider:

- Antithromboembolic stockings
- Low-molecular-weight heparin prophylaxis SC
- Avoid contraceptive pill if at risk (e.g., major or orthopedic surgery).
- Recurrent PES may be prevented by anticoagulation; vena caval filters are of limited use and should be combined with anticoagulation.

Signs and symptoms

- Acute dyspnea, pleuritic chest pain, hemoptysis, and syncope
- Hypotension, tachycardia, gallop rhythm, JVP↑, loud P_2, right ventricular heave, pleural rub, tachypnea, and cyanosis, AF

Classically, PE presents 10 d postop with collapse and sudden breathlessness while straining at stool, but PE may occur after any period of immobility or with no predisposing factors. Breathlessness may be the only sign. Multiple small emboli may present less dramatically with pleuritic pain, hemoptysis, and gradually increasing breathlessness.

Look for a source of emboli, especially DVT (is a leg swollen?).

Investigations

- CBC, CMP, baseline clotting
- ECG(commonly normal or sinus tachycardia); right ventricular strain pattern V1–3 (p. 95), right-axis deviation, RBBB, AF; may be deep S-waves in I, Q-waves in III, inverted T-waves in III ("S1 Q3 T3")
- CXR is often normal; increased vascular markings, small pleural effusion. Wedge-shaped area of infarction.
- *ABG*: Hyperventilation + gas exchange↓: P_aO_2↓, P_aCO_2↓, pH often↑
- CT pulmonary angiography is sensitive and specific in determining if emboli are in pulmonary arteries. If helical CT is unavailable, a *ventilation-perfusion (V/Q) scan* can aid diagnosis. If V/Q scan is equivocal, pulmonary angiography or bilateral lower ext ultrasound may help.
- D-dimer blood test, if low thrombosis absent. May help in excluding a PE.

Table 20.15 Management of massive pulmonary embolism

Oxygen, 100%
↓
If critically ill, consider immediate surgery
↓
IV access and start heparin *either* unfractionated heparin 80 U/kg bolus then 18 U/kg/h IV as guided by aPTT *or* low-molecular-weight heparin (e.g., enoxaparin 1 mg/kg SC q12h)
↓

What is the systolic BP?

<90 mm Hg
Start rapid fluid resuscitation
If BP still↓ after 500 mL colloid, dobutamine 2.5–10 mcg/kg/min IV; aim for systolic BP >90 mm Hg
If BP still low, consider norepinephrine
If the systolic BP <90 mm Hg after 30–60 min of standard treatment and signs of right ventricular dilation on echo, clinically definite PE and no CI, consider thrombolysis.

>90 mm Hg
Start warfarin 10 mg/24 h PO
Confirm diagnosis

Management See Table 20.15 for immediate management.

- Try to prevent further thrombosis with compression stockings.
- Heparin should be given for 3 d and until International Normalized Ratio (INR) >2. Then transition to warfarin.
- If obvious remedial cause, 6 wks treatment with warfarin may be sufficient. Otherwise, continue for at least 3–6 months (long-term if recurrent emboli or underlying malignancy).
- Is there an underlying cause (e.g., thrombophilic tendency), malignancy [especially prostate, breast, or pelvic cancer], SLE, or polycythemia)?

If good story and signs, make the diagnosis. Start treatment before definitive investigations.

Acute upper GI bleeding

Causes *Common:* Gastric/duodenal ulcer, gastritis, Mallory–Weiss tear (esophageal tear due to vomiting), esophageal varices, portal hypertensive gastropathy, drugs (NSAIDS, aspirin, thrombolytics, anticoagulants).

Rarer: Hemobilia, nose bleeds (swallowed blood), esophageal/gastric malignancy, esophagitis, angiodysplasia, hemangiomas, Ehlers–Danlos or Peutz–Jeghers syndrome, bleeding disorders, aorto-enteric fistula (in those with an aortic graft).

Signs and symptoms Hematemesis or melena, dizziness (especially postural), fainting, abdominal pain, dysphagia? Postural hypotension, hypotension, tachycardia (not if on β-blocker), ↓urine output, cool and clammy, signs of chronic liver disease; telangiectasia or purpura; jaundice (biliary colic + jaundice + melena suggests hemobilia). **NB:** Ask about previous GI problems, drug use, and alcohol intake.

Management *Assess whether patient is in shock:*

- Cool and clammy to touch (especially nose, toes, fingers); ↓capillary refill
- Pulse >100 bpm
- Systolic BP <100 mm Hg
- Postural drop
- Urine output <30 mL/h

If not in shock: Insert two big cannulae; start slow saline IV to keep lines patent; check bloods and monitor vital signs + urine output. Aim to keep hemoglobin (HG) >8 g/dL. **NB:** HG may not fall until circulating volume is restored.

If in shock: See Table 20.16 for management

Variceal bleeding: Resuscitate, then proceed to urgent endoscopy for banding or sclerotherapy. Give octreotide 50 mcg/h IV infusion for 2–5 d. If massive bleed or bleeding continues, pass a Sengstaken–Blakemore tube. Pantoprazole 40 mg IV may also be helpful in preventing stress ulceration.

Endoscopy Within 4 h, if you suspect variceal bleeding; within 12–24 h if hypotensive on admission or significant comorbidity. Endoscopy can identify the site of bleeding, estimate the risk of rebleeding (rebleeding doubles mortality), and can be used to administer treatment. *Risk of rebleeding:* Active arterial bleeding seen (90% risk); visible vessel (70% risk); adherent clot/black dots (30% risk). *No site of bleeding identied:* Bleeding site missed on endoscopy; bleeding site has healed (Mallory–Weiss tear); nose bleed (swallowed blood); site distal to third part of the duodenum (Meckel diverticulum, colonic site).

Rebleeds *Serious event:* 40% of patients who rebleed will die. If at-risk, maintain a high index of suspicion. If a rebleed occurs, check vital signs every 15 min and call senior cover. To prevent rebleeding in endoscopically proven high-risk cases, IV pantoprazole has been tried (e.g., 80 mg followed by an infusion of 8 mg/h for 72 h).

Signs of a rebleed:

- Rising pulse rate
- Falling JVP ± ↓ hourly urine output
- Hematemesis or melena
- Fall in BP (a late and sinister finding) and reduced consciousness level

Acute drug therapy Following successful endoscopic therapy in patients with **major** ulcer bleeding, IV pantoprazole (80 mg stat followed by 8 mg/h for 72 h) is recommended. There is no firm evidence to support the use of somatostatin or antifibrinolytic therapy in the majority of patients.

Table 20.16 Immediate management if hypotensive with GI bleed

Protect airway and keep NPO

↓

Insert two large-bore cannulae *14–16 g*

↓

Draw bloods
CBC, CMP, LFT, glucose, clotting screen
Cross-match 6 units

↓

Give high-flow O_2

↓

Rapid IV crystalloid infusion
Up to 1 L

↓

If remains hypotensive, give blood
Group specific or O Rh -ve until cross-match done

↓

Otherwise slow saline/lactated Ringer's infusion[a]
to keep lines open

↓

Transfuse as dictated by hemodynamics

↓

Correct clotting abnormalities
Vitamin K, fresh frozen plasma (FFP), platelet concentrate

↓

Set up CVP line to guide fluid replacement
Aim for >5 cm H_2O; CVP may mislead if there is ascites or CHF

↓

Catheterize and monitor urine output
Aim for >30 ml/h

↓

Monitor vital signs every 15 min until stable, then hourly

↓

Consider GI and/or surgery consult for all serious bleeds

↓

Urgent endoscopy for diagnosis ± control of bleeding

Poor prognostic signs:

- Age >60
- Systolic BP <100 mm Hg
- Bradycardia or rate >100 bpm
- Bleeding diathesis
- Chronic liver disease
- Consciousness level ↓
- Significant comorbidity

[a] Avoid saline in patients with decompensated liver disease (ascites, peripheral edema) as it worsens ascites, and, despite a low serum sodium, patients have a high body sodium. Use whole blood or salt-poor albumin for resuscitation and 5% dextrose for maintenance.

Acute liver failure

Fulminant liver failure is assumed to be potentially reversible. Therefore, treatment is supportive and designed to buy time for the patient's liver to regenerate.

Management

- Seek expert help. Is transfer to a ICU appropriate? Consider 20-degree head-up tilt in ICU.
- Treat the cause if known (e.g., acetaminophen overdose).
- Use caution with secretions and blood if is hepatitis suspected.
- Check blood glucose q1–4h and give 50 mL 50% dextrose IV if <3.5 mmol/L. Give 10% dextrose IV, 1 L/12 h to avoid hypoglycemia.
- NGT to avoid aspiration and remove any blood (bleeding varices) from stomach. Protect the airway with an endotracheal tube.
- Monitor temperature, pulse, respiratory rate (RR), BP, pupils, urine output.
- Daily lab blood glucose, INR, CMP, LFT, ammonia, blood cultures, and EEG. The INR (or prothrombin time [PT]) is the best measure of liver synthetic function.
- Avoid FFP unless bleeding or undergoing a surgical procedure. Some centers give vitamin K daily. Platelet transfusions may be required if thrombocytopenic and bleeding.
- Daily weights (ascites)
- Minimize absorption of nitrogenous substances and worsening of coma by restricting protein and emptying the bowel with lactulose and magnesium sulfate enemas. Aim for two soft stools per day.
- Consider neomycin 1 g/6 h PO to reduce numbers of bowel organisms.
- Consider N-acetylcysteine. Even in nonacetaminophen liver failure, this can improve oxygenation and clotting profiles.
- Watch renal function carefully. Consider hemodialysis if water overload or acute renal failure develops.
- Reduce acid secretion and risk of gastric stress ulcers; e.g., with cimetidine, ranitidine IV or a proton pump inhibitor (e.g., pantoprazole).
- Avoid sedatives (but diazepam is used for seizures) or other drugs with hepatic metabolism.
- Treat sepsis aggressively and don't forget the risk of spontaneous bacterial peritonitis.

NB: Caution should be used when attempting to correct acid–base imbalance as interventions can sometimes be more harmful than anticipated.

Meningitis

Do not delay treatment; it may save a life.

Make sure the referring physician gives a dose of antibiotic before sending the patient to you if possible.

Presentation

- Headache
- Meningismus: Neck stiffness, photophobia, Kerning's sign, Brudzinski's sign, headache, Jolt test positive (move the head quickly from side to side causing worse headache)
- Conscious level decreased; coma
- Petechial (nonblanching) rash; may only be one or two spots
- Seizures (~20%)
- Focal neurological signs (~20%)

Common organisms

- *Meningococcus*
- *Pneumococcus*

- *Haemophilus influenzae* (especially children)
- *Listeria monocytogenes*.

Management
- *Careful examination:* Pay attention to the neurological exam; look for rashes; assess GCS.
- If hypotensive, resuscitate with fluids and oxygen.
- If intracranial pressure (ICP) is raised, summon help immediately and inform neurosurgeons.
- Start antibiotics (below) immediately.

Investigations
- CMP, CBC, LFT, glucose, coagulation screen
- Blood culture, throat swabs (one for bacteria, one for virology), stool culture for viruses
- Lumbar puncture if safe. Don't forget to measure the opening pressure! **Contraindications** are suspected intracranial mass lesion, focal signs, papilledema, trauma, or middle-ear pathology; major coagulopathy. Send samples for cell count and differential, C+S, Gram stain, protein estimation, glucose, and to virology. See Table 20.17.
- CT head before LP if mass lesion or raised ICP is suspected.
- CXR

Antibiotics
Local policies vary. If in doubt, ask. The following are suggestions only, when the organism is unknown:
- <50 yrs: Vancomycin 1 g IV/12 h + ceftriaxone 2 g IV over >2 min as 1 daily dose.
- >50 yrs: Vancomycin 1 g IV/12 h + ceftriaxone 2 g IV over >2 min daily + ampicillin 2 g IV/4 h (for *Listeria*).
- Acyclovir if herpes encephalitis is suspected.
- Once organism is isolated, seek urgent microbiological advice.

Further measures
- There is some evidence that high-dose steroids may reduce neurological complications. Therefore, some centers recommend the administration of dexamethasone 10 mg IV before or with the first dose of antibiotics (but do not delay giving antibiotics), then q6h for 4 d. Avoid in patients with shock.
- General supportive measures
- Remember, meningitis is a notifiable disease.
- Inform local public health officer for contact tracing.
- Antibiotic prophylaxis for family and close contacts (depends on the organism: Ask a microbiologist)

Table 20.17 Typical CSF in meningitis

	Pyogenic	Tuberculous	Viral ("aseptic")
Appearance	Often turbid	Often fibrin web	Usually clear
Predominant cell	Polymorphs	Mononuclear	Mononuclear
White Cell count/mm³	e.g., 90–1,000+	10–1,000/mm³	50–1,000/mm³
Glucose	<½ plasma	<½ plasma	>½ plasma
Protein (g/l)	>1.5	1–5	<1
Organisms	In smear and culture	Often absent in smear	Not in smear or culture
		(There are no hard-and-fast rules)	

Cerebral abscess

Suspect this in any patient with elevated ICP, especially if there is fever or elevated WBC. It may follow ear, sinus, dental, or periodontal infection; skull fracture; congenital heart disease; endocarditis; bronchiectasis.

Signs: Seizures, fever, localizing signs, or signs of elevated ICP. Coma. Signs of sepsis elsewhere (e.g., teeth, ears, lungs, and endocarditis).

Investigations: CT/MRI (e.g., "ring-enhancing" lesion), ↑WBC, ↑ESR, biopsy.

Treatment: Urgent neurosurgical referral; treat ↑ICP. If frontal sinuses or teeth are the source, the likely organism will be *Strep. milleri* (microaerophilic) or oropharyngeal anaerobes. In ear abscesses, *B. fragilis* or other anaerobes are most common. Bacterial abscesses are often peripheral; *Toxoplasma* lesions are deeper (e.g., basal ganglia). Consider the possibility of underlying immunosuppression.

Status epilepticus

Seizures lasting for >30 min or repeated seizures without intervening consciousness. Mortality and the risk of permanent brain damage increases with the length of attack. Aim to terminate seizures lasting more than a few minutes as soon as possible (<20 min).

Status usually occurs in known epileptics. If it is the first presentation of epilepsy, the chance of a structural brain lesion is high (>50%). Diagnosis of tonic–clonic status is usually clear. Nonconvulsive status (e.g., absence status or continuous partial seizures with preservation of consciousness) may be more difficult: Look for subtle eye or lid movement. An EEG can be very helpful. *Could the patient be pregnant* (any pelvic mass)? If so, eclampsia is the likely diagnosis; check the urine and BP: Call a senior obstetrician—immediate delivery may be needed.

Investigations

- Bedside glucose; the following tests can be done once treatment has started: Glucose, blood gases, CMP, Ca^{2+}, CBC, ECG
- Consider anticonvulsant levels, toxicology screen, LP, culture blood and urine, EEG, CT, carbon monoxide level
- Pulse oximetry, cardiac monitor

Treatment

See Table 20.18. Basic life support and these agents:

Lorazepam ~2 mg as a slow bolus (over 2 min) into a large vein. Beware respiratory arrest during the last part of the injection. Have full resuscitation facilities at hand for all IV benzodiazepine use. (*Alternative:* Diazepam, but it is less long-lasting; give 10 mg IV over 2 min; if needed, repeat at 5 mg/min, until seizures stop, or 20 mg given, or significant respiratory depression occurs.) The rectal route is an alternative for diazepam if IV access is difficult.

While waiting for this to work, prepare other drugs. If seizures continue:

fosphenytoin infusion: 15–20 mg PE/kg IV, at a max rate of 150 mg/min. (Don't put diazepam in same line: They don't mix.) Beware BP↓ and do not use if bradycardic or heart block. Requires BP and ECG monitoring. 100 mg/q6–8h is a maintenance dose (check levels). If seizures continue: Dexamethasone 10 mg IV if vasculitis/cerebral edema (tumor) is possible. General anesthesia expert guidance on ICU.

As soon as seizures are controlled, start oral drugs. Ask what the cause was (e.g., hypoglycemia, pregnancy, alcohol, drugs, CNS lesion or infection, hypertensive encephalopathy, inadequate anticonvulsant dose).

Table 20.18 Management of status epilepticus

Open and maintain the airway, put patient in recovery position
Remove false teeth if poorly fitting, insert oral/nasal airway, intubate if necessary

↓

Oxygen, 100% + suction (as required)

↓

IV access and take blood
CMP, LFT, CBC, glucose, calcium, Toxicology screen if indicated, anticonvulsant levels

↓

Thiamine 100 mg IV over 10 min if alcoholism or malnourishment suspected. Unless glucose known to be normal IV glucose 50 mL 50%

↓

Correct hypotension with fluids

↓

Slow IV bolus phase to stop seizures: E.g., lorazepam 2–4 mg, or Diazepam 10mg with 5mg/min repeat to total of 20mg

↓

IV infusion phase: If seizures continue, start phenytoin, 15 mg/kg IV, at a rate of 50 mg/min or fosphenytoin at 15–20 mg PE/kg at rate of 150 mg PE/min. Monitor ECG and BPP. 100 mg/q6–8h is a maintenance dose (check levels).

↓

General anesthesia phase: Continuing seizures require propofol drip versus expert help with paralysis and ventilation with continuous EEG monitoring in ICU
Never spend >20 min on someone with status epilepticus without admission to the neurointensive critical care unit or similar type unit.

Head injury

If the pupils are unequal, diagnose rising ICP(e.g., from extradural hemorrhage) and summon urgent neurosurgical help. Retinal vein pulsation at funduscopy helps exclude ICP↑.

Initial management (See Table 20.19.) Write full notes. Record times.

- Involve neurosurgeons at an early stage, especially with comatose patients or if elevated ICP suspected.
- Examine the CNS. Chart pulse, BP, temperature, respirations + pupils every 15 min.
- Maintain c-spine immobilization until an adequate exam can be done.
- Assess antegrade amnesia (loss from the time of injury; i.e. post-traumatic) and retrograde amnesia—its extent correlates with the severity of the injury, and it never occurs without antegrade amnesia.
- Provide meticulous care to bladder and airway.

Who needs a CT head scan?

If any of the following are present, a CT is required immediately:

- GCS <13 at any time, or GCS 13 or 14 at 2 h following injury
- Focal neurological deficit
- Suspected open or depressed skull fracture or signs of basal skull fracture
- Post-traumatic seizure

Suspicion of Alcohol or drug use
- Vomiting more than once
- Loss of consciousness *or* any of the following:
  - Age 65
  - Coagulopathy
  - "Dangerous mechanism of injury" (e.g., fall from great height)
  - Confusion

When to ventilate immediately:
- Coma 8 on GCS
- P_aO_2 <70 mm Hg in air (<100 mm Hg with O_2) or P_aCO_2 >45 mm Hg
- Spontaneous hyperventilation (P_aCO_2 <26 mm Hg)
- Respiratory irregularity.

Ventilate before neurosurgical transfer if:
- Deteriorating level of consciousness
- Bilateral fractured mandible
- Bleeding into mouth (e.g., skull base fracture)
- Seizures

Risk of intracranial hematoma in adults
- Fully conscious, no skull fracture = <1:1,000
- Confused, no skull fracture = 1:100
- Fully conscious, skull fracture = 1:30
- Confused, skull fracture = 1:4

Criteria for admission
- Difficult to assess (child, postictal, alcohol intoxication)
- CNS signs, severe headache or vomiting, fracture
- Loss of consciousness does **not** require admission if patient is otherwise well and a responsible adult is in attendance.

Drowsy trauma patients (GCS <15 to >8) smelling of alcohol: Alcohol is an unlikely cause of coma if plasma alcohol <50 mg/dL. If unavailable, estimate blood alcohol level from the osmolar gap. **Never assume signs are just alcohol.**

Complications *Early:* Extradural/subdural hemorrhage, seizures.

Late: Subdural; seizures, diabetes insipidus, parkinsonism, dementia.

Indicators of a poor prognosis Increased age, decerebrate rigidity or any posturing, extensor spasms, prolonged coma, hypertension, hypoxemia, temperature >39°C. 60% of those with loss of consciousness of >1 month will survive 3–25 yrs, but may need daily nursing care.

Table 20.19 Immediate management plan for head injury

ABC's

↓

Oxygen, 100%
Intubate and hyperventilate if necessary
NB: *Beware of a cervical spine injury*

↓

Stop blood loss and support circulation
Treat for shock if required

↓

Treat seizures with benzodiazepine

↓

Assess level of consciousness (GCS)
Antegrade and retrograde amnesia

↓

Rapid examination survey

↓

Investigations
glucose, CMP, CBC, blood alcohol, toxicology screen, ABG and clotting

↓

Neurological examination

↓

Brief history
When? Where? How? Had a fit? Lucid interval? Alcohol?

↓

Evaluate lacerations of face or scalp
Palpate deep wounds with sterile glove to check for step deformity. Note obvious skull/facial fractures[a]

↓

Check for CSF leak from nose or ear
Any blood behind the ear drum?
If either is present, suspect basilar skull fracture: Do CT
Give tetanus toxoid and refer at once to neurosurgeons

↓

Palpate the neck posteriorly for tenderness and deformity. *If detected, or if the patient has obvious head injury or injury above the clavicle with loss of consciousness, immobilize the neck and get cervical spine radiographs*

↓

Radiology
As indicated: Cervical spine, CXR, CT of head

[a] Periorbital "raccoon sign" or postauricular Battle's sign ecchymoses.

Raised intracranial pressure

There are three types of cerebral edema:
- *Vasogenic:* Increased capillary permeability—tumor, trauma, ischemia, infection
- *Cytotoxic:* Cell death from hypoxia
- *Interstitial* (e.g., obstructive hydrocephalus)

Because the cranium defines a fixed volume, brain swelling quickly results in ↑ICP, which may produce a sudden clinical deterioration. Normal ICP is 0–10 mm Hg. The edema from severe brain injury is probably both cytotoxic and vasogenic.

Causes
- Primary or metastatic tumors
- Head injury
- Hemorrhage (subdural, extradural, subarachnoid; intracerebral, intraventricular)
- Meningoencephalitis, brain abscess
- Hydrocephalus, cerebral edema, status epilepticus

Signs and symptoms
- Headache, drowsiness, vomiting, seizures. History of trauma.
- Listlessness, irritability, drowsiness, falling pulse and rising BP (Cushing's response), coma, Cheyne–Stokes respiration, pupil changes (constriction at first, later dilatation—do not mask these signs by using agents such as tropicamide to dilate the pupil to aid funduscopy).
- Papilledema is an unreliable sign, but venous pulsation at the disc may be absent (absent in ~50% of normal people, but *loss* of it is a useful sign).

Investigations
- CMP, CBC, LFT, glucose, serum osmolality, clotting, blood culture, CXR
- CT head
- Then consider lumbar puncture, if safe. Measure the opening pressure!

Treatment
The goal is to lower ICP and avert secondary injury. Urgent neurosurgery is required for the definitive treatment of ↑ICP from focal causes (e.g., hematomas). This is achieved via a craniotomy or burr hole. Also, an ICP monitor (or bolt) may be placed to monitor pressure. Surgery is generally not helpful following ischemic or anoxic injury.

Holding measures are listed in Table 20.20.

Herniation syndromes *Uncal herniation* is caused by a lateral supratentorial mass that pushes the ipsilateral inferomedial temporal lobe (uncus) through the temporal incisura and against the midbrain. The third nerve, traveling in this space, is compressed, causing a dilated ipsilateral pupil, then ophthalmoplegia (a fixed pupil localizes a lesion poorly but is "ipsi-lateralizing"). This may be followed (quickly) by contralateral hemiparesis (pressure on the cerebral peduncle) and coma from pressure on the ARAS in the midbrain.

Cerebellar tonsil herniation is caused by increased pressure in the posterior fossa forcing the cerebellar tonsils through the foramen magnum. Ataxia, VI nerve palsies, and +ve Babinski (upgoing plantars) occur first, then loss of consciousness, irregular breathing, and apnea. This syndrome may proceed very rapidly given the small size of and poor compliance in the posterior fossa.

Subfalcine (cingulate) herniation is caused by a frontal mass. The cingulate gyrus (medial frontal lobe) is forced under the rigid falx cerebri. It may be silent unless the anterior cerebral artery is compressed and causes a stroke; e.g., contralateral leg weakness ± abulia (lack of decision-making).

Table 20.20 Immediate ICP management plan

ABC's
↓
Correct hypotension and treat seizures
↓
Brief examination, history if available
Any clues (e.g., meningococcal rash, previous carcinoma)
↓
Elevate the head of the bed to 30–40 degrees
↓
If intubated, hyperventilate to ↓P_aCO_2 (e.g., to 26 mm Hg)
This causes cerebral vasoconstriction and reduces ICP almost immediately
↓
Osmotic agents (e.g., mannitol) can be useful but may lead to rebound
↑ICP after prolonged use (~12–24 h) *Give 20% solution 1-2 g/kg IV over
10-20 min (e.g., 5 ml/kg). Clinical effect is seen after ~20 min and lasts for
2-6 h. Follow serum osmolality—aim for ~300 mosmol/kg but don't
exceed 310*
↓
Corticosteroids are *not* effective in reducing ICP
except for edema surrounding tumors
(e.g., dexamethasone 10 mg iv and follow with 4 mg/6 h IV/PO)
↓
Restrict fluid to <1.5 L/d
↓
Monitor the patient closely, consider monitoring ICP
↓
Aim to make a diagnosis
↓
Treat cause or exacerbating factors (e.g., hyperglycemia, hyponatremia)
↓
Definitive treatment if possible

Diabetic ketoacidosis

Hyperglycemic ketoacidotic (DKA) coma occurs mainly in type 1 diabetes:
It may be the initial presentation for a newly diagnosed diabetic patients.
Precipitants include infection, surgery, MI, noncompliance, or wrong insulin dose. The diagnosis requires the presence of ketosis and metabolic
acidosis.

Signs and symptoms
• Polyuria, polydipsia, lethargy, anorexia, hyperventilation, ketotic breath,
  dehydration, vomiting, abdominal pain, coma

Investigations
• Lab glucose, CMP, HCO_3^-, amylase, osmolality, ABG, CBC, urine and
  blood cultures, serum ketones
• Urine tests: Ketones, CXR
• To estimate plasma osmolarity: 2[Na^+] + [(urea) mg/dL]/2.8 + [(glucose)
  mg/dL]/18

Key points in the treatment of diabetic ketoacidosis
Treat dehydration aggressively with IVF.

- *Plasma glucose* is usually high, but not always, especially when insulin therapy is instituted.
- *High WBC* may be seen in the absence of infection.
- *Infection:* Often there is no fever. Do urine and blood cultures and CXR. Start broad-spectrum antibiotics early if infection is suspected.
- *Hyponatremia: Pseudohyponatremia* is common due to osmolar compensation for the hyperglycemia. Corrected plasma $[Na^+]$ = measured Na + 1.6 (Glucose − 100)
- *Ketoacidosis:* Blood glucose may return to normal long before ketones are cleared from the bloodstream. A rapid reduction in the amount of insulin administered in response to a decrease in serum glucose may lead to lack of clearance and return to DKA. This may be avoided by maintaining a constant rate of insulin (e.g., 0.1 U/kg/h IV) and co-infusing D5W to when plasma glucose falls below 250–300 mg/dL during the extended insulin regimen.
- *Acidosis* can be present without gross elevation of glucose; when this occurs, consider other causes as well (e.g., salicylates, lactic acidosis).
- *Serum amylase* is often elevated, and nonspecific abdominal pain is common, even in the absence of pancreatitis.

Management See Table 20.21. Dehydration is more life-threatening than hyperglycemia, so its correction takes precedence. See Table 20.22.

- Monitor electrolytes carefully, especially potassium levels (which may fall during therapy), glucose, creatinine, HCO_3, hourly initially. Aim for a fall in glucose of 90 mg/dL/h and correction of the acidosis. The use of venous HCO_3 can be used as a guide to progress and may prevent the need for repeated ABG sampling. K^+ disturbance may cause dysrhythmias. See Table 20.23.
- Flow chart vital signs, fluids inputs and output (urine output), and ketones; insert Foley catheter if no urine is passed for >4 h. Monitoring CVP OR ultrasound IVC measurement may sometimes be helpful in guiding fluid replacement.
- Find and treat infection (lung, skin, perineum, urine after cultures).

NB: If acidosis is severe (pH <7), some give IV bicarbonate. This remains controversial because of effects on the HG-dissociation curve and cerebral circulation—discuss with your senior resident.

Complications Cerebral edema, aspiration pneumonia, hypokalemia, hypomagnesemia, hypophosphatemia, thromboembolism.

Talk with the patient: Ensure that there are no further preventable episodes or other complicating issues.

Other emergencies: Hyperosmolar nonketotic coma and hypoglycemia

Table 20.21 DKA Management plan

IV access and start fluid (0.9% saline or lactated Ringer's)
replacement immediately

↓

Check plasma glucose: Usually >200 mg/dL
if so give 4–8 U (0.1 U/kg) regular insulin IV

↓

Investigate precipitating cause

↓

Labs electrolytes, glucose, CMP, osmolality, blood gases, CBC, serum
ketones, blood culture, mg, phos, Ca, CXR, ECG
Urine tests: Ketones, urine C+S

↓

Insulin sliding scale (below)

↓

Continue fluid replacement, K⁺ replacement

↓

Check glucose and CMP regularly (hourly initially)

↓

Continue the investigation of causes

Table 20.22 Fluid replacement

- Give 1 L of 0.9% saline immediately. Then, typically, 1 L over the next hour, 1 L over 2 h, 1 L over 4 h, then 1 L over 6 h.
- Use dextrose saline or 5% dextrose when blood glucose is <259–300 mg/dL.
- Those >65 yrs or with CHF need less saline and more cautious fluid delivery.

Table 20.23 Potassium replacement

- Total body potassium is invariably low, and plasma K⁺ falls as K⁺ enters cells with treatment.
- Don't add K⁺ to the first bag. Less will be required in renal failure or oliguria. Determine Urine output prior to K replacement. Check CMP every 2 h initially and replace K⁺ as needed.

Other diabetic emergencies

Hypoglycemic coma Usually *rapid* onset; may be preceded by odd behavior (e.g., aggression), sweating, pulse↑, seizures.

Management: Give 20–30 g dextrose IV (e.g., 200–300 mL of 10% dextrose). This is preferable to 50–100 mL 50% dextrose, which may harms veins. Expect prompt recovery. Glucagon 1 mg IV/IM is nearly as rapid as dextrose but will not work in intoxicated patients. Dextrose IV may be needed for severe prolonged hypoglycemia. Once conscious, give sugary drinks and a meal.

Hyperglycemic hyperosmolar nonketotic state Those with type 2 diabetes are at risk of this. The history is longer (e.g., 1 wk), with marked dehydration and glucose >800 mg/dL. Acidosis is absent as there has been no switch to ketone metabolism—the patient is often older and presenting for the first time. The osmolality is >340 mosmol/kg. Focal CNS signs may occur. The risk of DVT is high, so consider anticoagulation.

Rehydrate over 48 h with 0.9% saline IV (e.g., at half the rate used in ketoacidosis). Wait an hour before giving any insulin (it may not be needed, and you want to avoid rapid changes). If it is needed, 1 U/h is a typical initial dose. Look for the cause (e.g., MI, or bowel infarct).

Hyperlactatemia is a rare but serious complication of DM(e.g., after septicemia or biguanide use). *Blood lactate:* >5 mmol/L. Seek expert help. Give O_2. Treat any sepsis vigorously.

Thyroid emergencies

Myxedema coma *Signs and symptoms:* Patient looks hypothyroid; >65 yrs, hypothermia, hyporeflexia, glucose↓, bradycardia, coma, seizures.

History: Prior surgery or radioiodine for hyperthyroidism.

Precipitants: Infection, MI, stroke, trauma.

Examination: Goiter, cyanosis, heart failure, precipitants.

Treatment: Preferably in intensive care.

- Take venous blood for T3, T4, thyroid-stimulating hormone (TSH), CBC, CMP, cultures, cortisol.
- Take arterial blood for P_aO_2.
- Give high-flow O_2 if cyanosed. Correct any hypoglycemia.
- Give T3 (triiodothyronine) 5–20 mcg IV slowly. Be cautious: This may precipitate manifestations of undiagnosed ischemic heart disease.
- Give hydrocortisone 100 mg/8 h IV—vital if pituitary hypothyroidism is suspected (i.e., no goiter, no previous radioiodine, no thyroid surgery).
- IV 0.9% saline. Be sure to avoid precipitating LVF.
- If infection suspected, give antibiotic (e.g., cefuroxime 1.5 g/8 h IVI).
- Treat *heart failure* as appropriate.
- Treat *hypothermia* with warm blankets in warm room. Beware complications (hypoglycemia, pancreatitis, arrhythmias).

Further therapy: T3 5–20 mcg/4–12 h IV until sustained improvement (e.g., ~2–3 d), then thyroxine (T4 = levothyroxine) 50 mcg/24 h PO. Continue hydrocortisone. Give IV fluids as appropriate (hyponatremia is dilutional).

Hyperthyroid crisis (thyrotoxic storm) *Signs and symptoms:* Severe hyperthyroidism: Fever, agitation, confusion, coma, tachycardia, AF, vomiting and diarrhea, goiter, thyroid bruit, "acute abdomen" picture.

Precipitants: Recent thyroid surgery or radioiodine, infection, MI, trauma.

Diagnosis: Confirm with technetium uptake if possible, but do not wait for this if urgent treatment is needed.

Treatment: Enlist expert help from an endocrinologist. See Table 20.24.

Table 20.24 Management plan for thyrotoxic storm

IV 0.9% saline, 500 mL/4 h; NG tube if vomiting.

↓

Take blood for: T3, T4, cultures (if infection suspected)

↓

Sedate if necessary (e.g., midazolam 2 mg IV)

↓

If no contraindication, give propranolol 40 mg/8 h PO (maximum IV dose: 1 mg over 1 min, repeated up to 9 times at ≥2 min intervals)

↓

High-dose digoxin may be needed to slow the heart (e.g., 1 mg over 2 h IV)

↓

Antithyroid drugs: Propylthiouracil (PTU 50–200 mg q4h)

↓

Hydrocortisone 100 mg/6 h IV or
dexamethasone 4 mg/6 h PO

↓

Treat suspected infection with, e.g., cefuroxime 1.5 g/8 h IV

↓

Adjust IV fluids as necessary; cool with sponging ± acetaminophen

Addisonian crisis

Signs and symptoms: May present in shock (tachycardia, peripheral vaso-constriction, postural hypotension, oliguria, weak, confused, comatose). Typically (but not always!) seen in a patient with known Addison's disease or in someone on long-term steroids who has forgotten to take tablets. An alternative presentation is with hypoglycemia.

Precipitating factors: Infection, trauma, surgery.

Management: If suspected, treat before biochemical results.

- Take blood for cortisol (10 mL heparin or clotted) and adrenocortico-tropic hormone (ACTH) if possible (10 mL heparin, to go straight to laboratory).
- Hydrocortisone sodium succinate 100 mg IV stat.
- IV: Use 0.9% saline or lactated Ringer's solution for resuscitation.
- Monitor blood glucose: The danger is hypoglycemia.
- Take blood, urine, sputum for culture.
- Give antibiotics (e.g., cefuroxime 1.5 g/8 h IV).

Continuing treatment:

- Glucose IV may be needed if hypoglycemic.
- Continue IV fluids, more slowly. Be guided by clinical state.
- Continue hydrocortisone sodium succinate 100 mg IV/IM q6h.
- Change to oral steroids after 72 h if patient's condition is good. The ACTH stimulation test (cosyntropin) is impossible while on hydrocortisone.
- Fludrocortisone is needed only if hydrocortisone dose is <50 mg/d and the condition is due to adrenal disease.
- Search for the cause once the crisis is over.

Hypopituitary coma

Usually develops gradually in a person with known hypopituitarism. Rarely, the onset is rapid due to infarction of a pituitary tumor (pituitary apoplexy); because symptoms include headache and meningismus, subarachnoid hemorrhage is often misdiagnosed.

Presentation: Headache, ophthalmoplegia, consciousness↓, hypotension, hypothermia, hypoglycemia, signs of hypopituitarism.

Tests: T4, cortisol, TSH, ACTH, glucose; pituitary fossa CT/MRI.

Treatment:

- Hydrocortisone sodium succinate 100 mg IV/6 h
- Only after hydrocortisone begun: T3 10 mcg/12 h PO
- Prompt surgery is needed if the cause is pituitary apoplexy.

Pheochromocytoma emergencies

Stress, abdominal palpation, parturition, general anesthetic, or contrast media used in radiography may produce dangerous hypertensive crises (pallor, pulsating headache, hypertension, feels "about to die").

Treatment Get help.

- Phentolamine 2–5 mg IV; repeat to maintain safe BP.
- Labetalol is an alternative agent.
- When BP is controlled, give phenoxybenzamine 10 mg/24 h PO(↑ by 10 mg/d as needed, up to 0.5–1 mg/kg/12 h PO); *SE:* Postural hypotension, dizziness, tachycardia, nasal congestion, miosis, idiosyncratic marked BP drop soon after exposure. The idea is to increase the dose until the BP is controlled and there is no significant postural hypotension. A β-blocker may also be given at this stage.
- Surgery is usually done electively after a period of 4–6 wks, to allow full α-blockade and volume expansion. When admitted for surgery, the phenoxybenzamine dose is increased until significant postural hypotension occurs.

Acute renal failure (ARF)

Seek expert help promptly: BP, urinary sediment, serum K^+, creatinine, and US must be rapidly known. Have them at hand.

Definition Acute (over hours or days) deterioration in renal function, characterized by a rise in serum creatinine and urea, often with oliguria or anuria.

Causes

- Hypovolemia
- Low cardiac output
- Sepsis
- Drugs
- Obstruction
- Other (e.g., hepatorenal syndrome, vasculitis)

Investigations

- CMP, Ca^{2+}, PO_4^{3-}, CBC, ESR, CRP, INR, LFT, CK, lactose dehydrogenase (LDH), protein electrophoresis, hepatitis serology, autoantibodies, blood cultures.
- Urgent urine microscopy and cultures. White cell casts suggest infection, but are seen in interstitial nephritis, and red cell casts are seen in inflammatory glomerular conditions.
- US of the renal tract
- ECG, CXR

Management See Table 20.25 for acute measures. Underlying principles are:

Treat precipitating cause: Treat acute blood loss with blood transfusion, and treat sepsis with antibiotics. ARF is often associated with other diseases that need more urgent treatment. For example, someone in respiratory failure *and* renal failure may need to be managed in the ICU, not in a renal unit, to ensure optimal management of the respiratory failure.

Treat life-threatening hyperkalemia: See Table 20.26.

Treat pulmonary edema, pericarditis, and tamponade: Urgent dialysis may be needed. If in pulmonary edema and no diuresis, consider removing a unit of blood before dialysis commences.

Treat volume depletion if necessary: Resuscitate quickly; then match input to output. Use a large-bore line in a large vein (central vein access can be risky in obvious volume depletion).

Treat sepsis

Further care

- Has obstruction been excluded? Examine for rectal and vaginal masses; arrange urgent US. Is the bladder palpable? Bilateral nephrostomies relieve obstruction, provide urine for culture, and allow pyelography to determine the site of obstruction.
- If worsening renal function but dialysis-independent, consider renal biopsy.
- *Diet:* High in calories (2,000–4,000 kcal/d) with adequate high-quality protein. Consider nasogastric feeding or parenteral route if too ill.

Prognosis Depends on cause (*ATN mortality*: Surgery or trauma, 60%; medical illness, 30%; pregnancy, 10%). Oliguric ARF is worse than nonoliguric with more GI bleeds, sepsis, acidosis, and higher mortality.

Urgent dialysis if:

- K_+ persistently high (>6.0 meq/L)
- Acidosis (pH <7.2)
- Pulmonary edema and no substantial diuresis
- Pericarditis (In tamponade, only dialyze *after* pressure on the heart is relieved.)
- High catabolic state with rapidly progressive renal failure

Table 20.25 Management of ARF

Catheterize to assess hourly urine output, and establish fluid charts

↓

Assess intravascular volume BP, JVP, skin turgor, fluid balance sheet, weight, CVP, attach to cardiac monitor. *Consider inserting a central venous cannula*

↓

Investigations

↓

Identify and treat hyperkalemia—see below
Use a cardiac monitor

↓

If dehydrated
Fluid challenge: 250–500 mL of colloid or saline over 30 min

↓

Reassess
Repeat if still fluid depleted. Aim for a CVP of 5–10 cm H_2O

↓

Once fluid replete, continue fluids at 20 mL + previous hour's urine output per hour

↓

If volume overloaded, consider urgent dialysis
A nitrate infusion, or furosemide may help in the short term, especially to make space for blood transfusion etc. but does not alter outcome

↓

If clinical suspicion of sepsis, take cultures, then treat vigorously
Do not leave possible sources of sepsis (e.g., iv lines) in situ unless unavoidable

↓

Avoid nephrotoxic drugs (e.g., NSAIDs, ACE-inhibitors, gentamicin)
Check Medication Sheet for all drugs given.

Table 20.26 Hyperkalemia

The danger is ventricular fibrillation. A K^+ of >6.5 mEq/L will usually require urgent treatment, as will those with ECG changes:
- Tall "tented" T-waves ± flat P-waves ± ↑ PR interval.
- Widening of the QRS complex leads eventually, and dangerously, to a sinusoidal pattern and VF/VT.

Treatment:
- 10 mL calcium gluconate (10%)IV over 2 min, repeated as necessary if severe ECG changes. This provides cardioprotection. It does not change serum potassium levels.
- Insulin + glucose (e.g., 10 units regular insulin + 50 mL of glucose 50% IV). Insulin moves K^+ into cells.
- Nebulized albuterol (2.5 mg) also makes K^+ enter cells.
- Polystyrene sulfonate resin (e.g., Kayexalate, 15 g/8h in water) orally or, if vomiting makes the PO route problematic, as a 30 g enema (followed by colonic irrigation after 9 h, to remove K^+ from the colon).
- Dialysis

Acute poisoning: General measures

Diagnosis comes mainly from history. The patient may be reluctant or unwilling to tell the truth about what has been taken. Pill identification is occasionally helpful, and texts such as the *Physician's Desk Reference (PDR)* may useful. Multiple ingestions are common. While awaiting the results of the serum and urine toxicological screen, certain physical findings may help to narrow the potential drugs ingested.

- *Fast or irregular pulse:* Albuterol, antimuscarinics, tricyclics, quinine, or phenothiazine poisoning
- *Respiratory depression:* Opiate or benzodiazepine toxicity
- *Hypothermia:* Phenothiazines, barbiturates
- *Hyperthermia:* Amphetamines, monoamine oxidase inhibitors (MAOIs), cocaine, or ecstasy
- *Coma:* Benzodiazepines, alcohol, opiates, tricyclics, or barbiturates
- *Seizures:* Recreational drugs, hypoglycemic agents, tricyclics, phenothiazines, or theophyllines
- *Constricted pupils:* Opiates or insecticides
- *Dilated pupils:* Amphetamines, cocaine, quinine, or tricyclics
- *Hyperglycemia:* Organophosphates, theophyllines, or MAOIs
- *Hypoglycemia:* Insulin, oral hypoglycemics, alcohol, or salicylates
- *Renal failure:* Salicylate, acetaminophen, or ethylene glycol
- *Metabolic acidosis:* Alcohol, ethylene glycol, methanol, acetaminophen, or carbon monoxide poisoning
- ↑*Osmolality:* Alcohols (ethyl or methyl), ethylene glycol

Management See Table 20.27 for a general guide to management.
- *Take blood* as appropriate. Always check acetaminophen and salicylate levels.
- *Empty stomach* if appropriate.
- *Consider specific antidote* or oral activated charcoal.
- *If you are not familiar with the poison,* get more information. Call your local Poison Control Center.

Continuing care Measure temperature, pulse, BP, and blood glucose regularly. Use a continuous ECG monitor. If unconscious, turn regularly, keep eyelids closed. A urinary catheter will be needed if the bladder is distended, renal failure is suspected, or forced diuresis is undertaken. Take to ICU, e.g., if respiration decreases.

Psychiatric assessment Be sympathetic despite the hour! Interview relatives and friends if possible. Aim to establish:
- *Intentions at time:* Was the act planned? What precautions against being found? Did the patient seek help afterward? Does the patient think the method was dangerous? Was there a final act (e.g., suicide note)?
- *Present intentions*
- *What problems* led to the act: Do they still exist?
- *Was the act* aimed at someone?
- Is there a *psychiatric disorder* (depression, alcoholism, personality disorder, schizophrenia, dementia)?
- What are his *resources* (friends, family, work, personality)?

The assessment of suicide risk: The following increase the chance of future suicide: Original intention was to die, present intention is to die, presence of psychiatric disorder, poor resources, previous suicide attempts, socially isolated, unemployed, male, >50 yrs old.

Referral to psychiatrist: This depends partly on local resources. Ask advice if presence of psychiatric disorder or high suicide risk.

Table 20.27 Emergency care for poisoining

ABC's, clear airway

↓

Consider ventilation (if the respiratory rate is <8/min, or P_aO_2 <60 mm Hg, when breathing 60% O_2, or the airway is at risk, e.g., GCS <8)

↓

Treat shock

Further management

↓

Assess the patient

↓

History from patient, friends, or family is vital

↓

Features from the examination may help

↓

Investigations

Glucose, CMP, CBC, LFT, INR, ABG, ECG, lactate, acetaminophen, and salicylate levels,
urine/serum toxicology, specific assays as appropriate

↓

Monitor

T°(rectal), pulse, and respiratory rate, BP, O_2 saturations, urine output ± ECG

↓

Treatment

Supportive measures: May need catheterization
↓Absorption: Consider gastric lavage ± activated charcoal
Consider naloxone if unconscious and pin-point pupils

Acute poisoning: Specific points

Plasma toxicology For all unconscious patients, acetaminophen and aspirin levels and blood glucose are required. The necessity of other assays depends on the drug taken and the index of suspicion. Be guided by the poison information service. More common assays include digoxin, methanol, lithium, iron, theophylline. Toxicological screening of urine, especially for recreational drugs, may be of use in some cases.

Gastric lavage In general, only of use if presentation is within 40 min of ingestion and if a potentially toxic dose of a drug has been taken. Lavage beyond this time frame may make matters worse. *Do not empty the stomach* if petroleum products or corrosives such as acids, alkalis, bleach, have been ingested (*exception*: Paraquat) or if the patient is unconscious or unable to protect his airway (unless intubated). Never induce vomiting.

Gastric emptying and lavage Gastric emptying and lavage is contraindicated in patients who have a change in mental status, who are comatose, or have an absent gag reflex. These patients may require endotracheal intubation prior to insertion of a nasogastric tube. If conscious, get verbal consent.

- Monitor O_2 by pulse oximetry.
- Have suction apparatus at hand and working.
- Position the patient in left lateral position.
- Raise the foot of the bed by 20 cm.
- Pass a lubricated tube (14 mm external diameter) via the nares, asking the patient to swallow.
- Confirm position in stomach: Blow air down and auscultate over the stomach.
- Siphon the gastric contents. Check pH with litmus paper.
- Perform gastric lavage using 300–600 mL tepid water at a time.
- Repeat until no tablets in siphoned fluid.
- Leave activated charcoal (50 g in 200 mL water) in the stomach unless alcohol, iron, Li^+, or ethylene glycol was ingested.
- When pulling out tube, occlude its end (prevents aspiration of fluid remaining in the tube).

Activated charcoal reduces the absorption of many drugs from the gut when given as a single dose of 50 g with water (e.g., salicylates, acetaminophen). It is given in repeated doses (50 g q4h) to increase the elimination of some drugs from the blood (e.g., carbamazepine, dapsone, theophyllines, quinine, digoxin, phenytoin, phenobarbitone (phenobarbital), and paraquat). Lower doses are used in children.

Some specific poisons and their antidotes

Benzodiazepines Flumazenil rarely used (for respiratory arrest) 200 mcg over 15 sec; then 100 mcg at 60 sec intervals if needed. Usual dose range: 300–600 mcg IV over 3–6 min (up to 1 mg; 2 mg if on ITU). May provoke seizures.

β-Blockers Severe bradycardia or hypotension. Try atropine up to 3 mg IV. Give glucagon 2–10 mg IV bolus + 5% dextrose if atropine fails (± an atropine infusion of 50 mcg/kg/h). consider prophylactic antiemetic since glucagon provokes nausea and vomiting. If unresponsive, consider pacing or an aortic balloon pump.

Cyanide This fast-killing poison has affinity for Fe^{3+} and inhibits the cytochrome system, reducing aerobic respiration.

Three phases:
1. Anxiety ± confusion
2. Pulse↑ or ↓
3. Seizures ± shock ± coma.

Treatment: 100% O_2, GI decontamination; if reduced consciousness, give ampule of amyl nitrate for inhalation (if no IV established), 10 cc of 3% solution sodium nitrate IV, and 50 cc of 25% solution of sodium thiosulfate. Alternatively consider hydroxocobalamin 5gm IV over 15 min. *Get expert help*

Carbon monoxide Despite hypoxemia, skin is pink (or pale), not blue, as carboxyhemoglobin (COHb) displaces O2 from Hb binding sites.

Symptoms: Headache, vomiting, pulse↑, tachypnea, and, if COHb >50%, fits, coma, and cardiac arrest. Remove the source. Give 100% O2. Metabolic acidosis usually responds to correction of hypoxia. If severe, anticipate cerebral edema. Give mannitol IV. Confirm diagnosis with a heparinized blood sample (COHb >10%) quickly as levels may soon return to normal. Monitor ECG. *Hyperbaric O_2 may help: Discuss with the poison service if patient is or has been unconscious, pregnant, COHb >20%, or failing to respond.*

Digoxin *Symptoms:* Cognition↓, yellow-green visual halos, arrhythmias, nausea, and anorexia. If serious arrhythmias are present, correct hypokalemia and inactivate with digoxin-specific antibody fragments (Digibind®). If load or level is unknown, give 20 vials (800 mg) for adult or child >20 kg. Consult

Poison Control. Dilute in water for injections (4 mL/38 mg vial) and 0.9% saline (to make a convenient volume); give IV over half hour, via a 0.22 mcm-pore filter. If the amount of digoxin ingested is known, Poison Control will tell you how many vials of Digibind® to give (e.g., if 25 tabs of 0.25 mg ingested, give 10 vials; if 50 tabs, give 20 vials; if 100 tabs, give 40 vials).

Heavy metals Enlist expert help.

Iron Deferoxamine 15 mg/kg/h IV; max 80 mg/kg/d. **NB:** Gastric lavage if iron ingestion in last hour; consider whole bowel irrigation.

Oral anticoagulants If major bleed, treat with vitamin K, 5 mg slow IV; give prothrombin complex concentrate 50 U/kg IV(or, if unavailable, fresh frozen plasma 15 mL/kg IV). If it is vital that anticoagulation continues, enlist expert help. Warfarin can normally be restarted within 2–3 d.

NB: Coagulation defects may be delayed for 2–3 d following ingestion.

Opiates Many analgesics contain opiates. Give naloxone (e.g., 0.8–2 mg IV); repeat every 2 min until breathing adequate (it has a short $t_{1/2}$, so it may need to be given often or IM; max 10 mg). Naloxone may precipitate features of opiate withdrawal: Diarrhea and cramps will normally respond to diphenoxylate and atropine (Lomotil®; e.g., 2 tablets/6 h PO). Sedate as needed.

Phenothiazine poisoning (e.g., chlorpromazine) No specific antidote. *Dystonia* (torticollis, retrocollis, glossopharyngeal dystonia, opisthotonus): Try benztropine 1–2 mg IV/IM. Treat *shock* by raising the legs (± plasma expander IV or norepinephrine IV if shocked). Restore body temperature. *Monitor ECG.* Avoid lidocaine in dysrhythmias. Use diazepam IV for prolonged seizures. *Neuroleptic malignant syndrome:* Hyperthermia, rigidity, extrapyramidal signs, autonomic dysfunction (labile BP, pulse↑, sweating, urinary incontinence), mutism, confusion, coma, WBC↑, CPK↑; it may be treated with cooling. Dantrolene has been tried.

Carbon tetrachloride poisoning This solvent, used in many industrial processes, causes vomiting, abdominal pain, diarrhea, seizures, coma, renal failure, and tender hepatomegaly with jaundice and liver failure. IV acetylcysteine may improve prognosis. Seek expert help.

Organophosphate insecticides inactivate cholinesterase; the resulting increase in acetylcholine causes the SLUD response: **S**alivation, lacrimation, urination, and diarrhea. Also look for sweating, small pupils, muscle fasciculation, coma, respiratory distress, and bradycardia. *Treatment:* Wear gloves; remove soiled clothes. Wash skin. Take blood (CBC and serum cholinesterase activity). Give atropine IV = 2 mg every 10 min until full atropinization (skin dry, pulse >70, pupils dilated). Up to 3 d treatment may be needed. Also give pralidoxime 30 mg/kg slowly. Repeat as needed every 30 min; max 12 g in 24 h. Even if seizures are not occurring, diazepam 5–10 mg IV seems to help.

Paraquat poisoning Found in weed-killers. This causes painful oral and esophageal ulcers, alveolitis, and renal failure. Diagnose by urine test. Give activated charcoal *at once* (100 g followed by a laxative, then 50 g/3–4 h, ± antiemetic). *Get expert help.* Avoid O_2 early on (promotes lung damage).

Ecstasy poisoning Ecstasy is a semisynthetic hallucinogenic substance (MDMA, 3,4-methylenedioxymethamphetamine). Its effects range from nausea, muscle pain, blurred vision, amnesia, fever, confusion, and ataxia to tachyarrhythmias, hyperthermia, hyper/hypotension, water intoxication, DIC, K^+↑, acute renal failure, hepatocellular and muscle necrosis, cardiovascular collapse, and ARDS. There is no antidote, and treatment is supportive.

Management depends on clinical and lab ndings, but may include:

- Administration of activated charcoal and monitoring of BP, ECG, and temperature for at least 12 h (rapid cooling may be needed).
- Monitor urine output and CMP, LFT, creatinine kinase, platelets, and coagulation. Metabolic acidosis may benefit from treatment with sodium bicarbonate.
- Anxiety: Diazepam 0.1–0.3 mg/kg PO. Max IV does over 2 min
- Narrow complex tachycardias in adults: Consider metoprolol 5–10 mg IV.
- Hypertension can be treated with nifedipine 5–10 mg PO or phentolamine 2–5 mg IV. Treat hypotension conventionally.
- Hyperthermia: Attempt to cool, if rectal T° >39°C. Consider dantrolene 1 mg/kg IV (may need repeating: Discuss with your senior and a poison unit). Hyperthermia with ecstasy is akin to serotonin syndrome, and propranolol, muscle relaxation, and ventilation may be needed.

Snakes and Snake envenomation : *There are two types of poisonous snakes in the United States, the pit viper (rattlesnake) and the elapid (coral snake)* For suspected envenomations, consider giving 1–2 vials of specific antivenom as soon as possible. To locate antisera for exotic snakes, call a regional poison control center (800–222–1222). CroFab is now available for pit viper bites, and 4–6 vials should be given if there is evidence of local or systemic reaction *Management:* Avoid active movement of affected limb (use splints/slings). *Avoid incisions and tourniquets.* Get help.

Salicylate poisoning

Aspirin is a weak acid with poor water solubility. It is present in many over-the-counter preparations. Anaerobic metabolism and the production of lactate and heat are stimulated by the uncoupling of oxidative phosphorylation. Effects are dose-related and potentially fatal:

- 150 mg/kg: Mild toxicity
- 250 mg/kg: Moderate
- >500 mg/kg: Severe toxicity

Signs and symptoms Unlike acetaminophen, many early features. Vomiting, dehydration, hyperventilation, tinnitus, vertigo, sweating. Rarely, lethargy or coma, seizures, vomiting, ↓BP and heart block, pulmonary edema, hyperthermia. Patients present initially with respiratory alkalosis due to a direct stimulation of the central respiratory centers and then develop a metabolic acidosis. Hyper- or hypoglycemia may occur.

Management Correct dehydration. Gastric lavage if within 1 h, activated charcoal (may be repeated, but is of unproven value).

- Acetaminophen and salicylate level, glucose, CMP, LFT, INR, ABG, ,CBC. Salicylate level may need to be repeated after 2 h due to continuing absorption if a potentially toxic dose has been taken.
- Levels over 700 mg/L are potentially fatal.
- Monitor urine output and blood glucose. If severe poisoning: Salicylate levels, blood pH, and CMP. Consider urinary catheter and monitoring urine pH. Beware hypoglycemia.
- If plasma level >500 mg/L (3.6 mmol/L), consider alkalinization of the urine, with IV sodium bicarbonate. Aim to make the *urine* pH 7.5–8.5. **NB:** Monitor serum K^+ because hypokalemia may occur.
- Consider dialysis if plasma level >700 mg/L, and if patient has renal or heart failure, seizures, severe acidosis, or persistently ↑plasma salicylate. ECG monitor.
- Discuss any serious cases with the local toxicological service or national poison information service.

Acetaminophen poisoning

140 mg/kg (or 12 g) in adults may be fatal. However, prompt treatment can prevent liver failure and death.

Signs and symptoms None initially, or vomiting ± RUQ pain. Later: Jaundice and encephalopathy from liver damage (the main danger) ± renal failure.

Management *General measures*: Lavage if >12 g (or >140 mg/kg) taken within 1 h. Give activated charcoal if <8 h since ingestion. Specific measures:

- Glucose, CMP, LFT, INR, ABG, PT/PTT/INR, HCO_3^-, FBC; blood level at 4 h postingestion
- If <8 h since overdose and plasma acetaminophen is above the line on the graph in Figure 20.3, start *N*-acetylcysteine.
- If >8 h and suspicion of large overdose (>7.5 g) err on the side of caution and start acetylcysteine, stopping it if acetaminophen level is below the treatment line and INR and ALT are normal.
- Acetylcysteine is given by IV: 140 mg/kg in 200 mL of 5% dextrose over 15 min. Then 50 mg/kg in 500 mL of 5% dextrose over 4 h. Then 100 mg per kg/16 h in 1 L of 5% dextrose. Rash is a common SE: Treat with diphenhydramine and observe; do not stop unless anaphylaxis (i.e., shock, vomiting, wheeze occurs [<10%]).
- If ingestion time is unknown, it is staggered, or presentation is >15 h from ingestion, treatment *may* help. Get advice.
- The graph may mislead if HIV positive(hepatic glutathione↓), if long-acting acetaminophen has been taken, in the presence of preexisting liver disease, or if induction of liver enzymes has occurred. Beware glucose↓; bedside glucose/1hr; INR/12 h.
- Next day, do PT, PTT, INR, CMP, LFT. If INR rising, continue acetylcysteine until <1.4.
- If continued deterioration, discuss with the liver team.

Do not hesitate to get expert advice. *Criteria for transfer to ICU:*

- *Encephalopathy* or ICP↑. Signs of CNS edema: BP >160/90 (sustained) or brief rises (systolic >200 mm Hg), bradycardia, decerebrate posture, extensor spasms, poor pupil responses. ICP monitoring can help.
- INR>2.0 at <48 h *or* >3.5 at <72 h (so measure INR q12h). Peak elevation: 72–96 h. LFTs are *not* good markers of hepatocyte death. If INR is *normal* at 48 h, the patient may go home.
- *Renal impairment* (creatinine >2.2 mg/dL). Monitor urine flow. Daily CMP and serum creatinine (use hemodialysis if >2.4 mg/dL).
- *Blood pH <7.3* (lactic acidosis → tissue hypoxia)
- *Systolic BP <80 mm Hg*

Figure 20.3

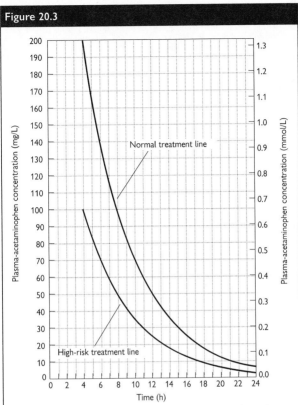

Patients whose plasma-acetaminophen concentrations are above the normal treatment line should be treated with acetylcysteine by IV infusion (or, provided the overdose has been taken within 10 – 12 h, with methionine by mouth). Patients on enzyme-including drugs (e.g., carbamazepine, phenobarbital, phenytoin, rifampicin, alcohol) or who are malnourished (e.g., in anorexia, in alcoholism, or those who are HIV-positive) should be treated if their plasma-acetaminophen concentrations are above the high-risk treatment line (We thank Dr. Alun Hutchings for permission to reproduce this graph.)

Burns

Resuscitate and arrange transfer for all major burns. (>25% partial thickness in adult and >20% in children). Assess site, size, and depth of the burn. Referral is still warranted in cases of full thickness burns >5%, partial thickness burns >10% in adults or >5% in children or the elderly, burns of special sites, chemical and electrical burns, and burns with inhalational injury.

Assessment *Burn size* is important to assess (see Figure 20.4) as it influences the magnitude of the inflammatory response (vasodilatation, ↑ vascular permeability) and thus the fluid shift from the intravascular volume. The size must be estimated to calculate fluid requirements. Ignore erythema.

Burn depth determines healing time/scarring; assessing this may be difficult, even when experienced. The big distinction is whether the burn is partial thickness (painful, red, and blistered) or full thickness (insensate/painless and white/gray). **NB:** Burns can evolve, particularly over the first 48 h.

Resuscitation

Airway: Beware of upper airway obstruction developing if hot gases inhaled. See Table 20.28. Suspect if history of fire in enclosed space, soot in oral/nasal cavity, singed nasal hairs, or hoarse voice. A flexible laryngeo/bronchoscopy is useful. Involve anesthesiologist early and consider early intubation.

Breathing: Exclude life-threatening chest injuries (e.g., tension pneumothorax) and constricting burns. Give 100% O_2 if carbon monoxide poisoning is suspected (mostly from history; may have cherry-red skin. Measure carboxyhemoglobin (COHb) and compare to nomograms. With 100% O_2, $t_{1/2}$ of COHb falls from 250 min to 40 min (consider hyperbaric oxygen if pregnant; CNS signs; >20% COHb). SpO2 measured by pulse oximeter is unreliable. Do escharotomy if thoracic burns impair chest excursion.

Circulation: Partial thickness burns >10% in a child and >15% in adults require IV fluid resuscitation. Insert two large-bore (14 or 16 g) IV lines. Do not worry if you have to put these through burned skin; intraosseous access is valuable in infants. Secure them well: They are literally lifelines.

Use a *burns calculator* flow chart or a formula, such as the *Parkland formula* (popular): 4 × weight (kg) × % burn = mL lactated Ringer's in 24 h, half given in first 8 h.

Modied Brooke formula: 2 mL/kg for each % burn = ml lactated Ringer's in 24 h.

Either formula is acceptable and the modified Brooke has been shown to require less fluids without increasing harm. Replace fluid from the time of burn, not from the time first seen in hospital. See Figure 20.4.

Formulae are only guides: Adjust IV infusion according to clinical response and urine output; aim for >0.5 mL/kg/h (>1 mL/kg/h in children), ~50% more in electrical burns and inhalation injury. Monitor temperature (core and surface); catheterize the bladder.

Treatment Do *not* apply cold water to extensive burns: This may intensify shock. If transferring to a burn unit, do not burst blisters or apply any special creams as this can hinder assessment. Simple saline gauze or Vaseline® gauze is suitable; cling film is useful as a temporary measure and relieves pain. Use morphine in IV aliquots and titrate for good analgesia. Ensure tetanus immunity. Antibiotic prophylaxis is not routine.

Definitive dressings There are many dressings for partial thickness burns, including biological (pigskin, cadaveric skin), synthetic (Mepitel® DuoDERM®), and silver sulfadiazine cream (Flamazine®). Major full thickness burns benefit from early tangential excision and split-skin grafting as the burn wound is a major source of inflammatory cytokines causing SIRS (systemic inflammatory response syndrome) and are an ideal medium for bacterial growth.

Table 20.28 Smoke inhalation

Initially, laryngospasm leads to hypoxia and straining (leading to petechiae), then hypoxic cord relaxation leads to true inhalation injury. Free radicals, cyanide compounds, and carbon monoxide accompany thermal injury. Cyanide compounds (generated from burning plastic in particular) bind reversibly with ferric ions in enzymes, thus stopping oxidative phosphorylation and causing dizziness, headaches, and seizures. Tachycardia and dyspnea soon give way to bradycardia and apnea. Carbon monoxide is generated later in the fire as oxygen is depleted; the COHb level does not correlate well with the severity of poisoning.

- 100% O_2 is given to elute both cyanide and CO.
- Involve ICU/anesthesiologist early: Early ventilation may be useful; consider repeated bronchoscopic lavage.
- Enroll expert help in cyanide poisoning. There is no single regimen suitable for all situations. Clinically mild poisoning may be treated by rest, O_2, and amyl nitrite 0.2–0.4 mL via an Ambu® bag. IV antidotes may be used for moderate poisoning: Sodium thiosulphate is a common first choice. More severe poisoning may require hydroxocobalamin, sodium nitrite, and dimethylaminophenol.

Figure 20.4 Lund & Browder charts

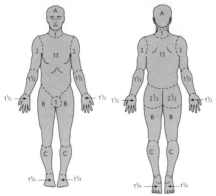

Relative percentage of body surface area affected by growth

Area	Age	0	1	5	10	15	Adult
A: half of head		$9\frac{1}{2}$	$8\frac{1}{2}$	$6\frac{1}{2}$	$5\frac{1}{2}$	$4\frac{1}{2}$	$3\frac{1}{2}$
B: half of thigh		$2\frac{3}{4}$	$3\frac{1}{4}$	4	$4\frac{1}{4}$	$4\frac{1}{2}$	$4\frac{3}{4}$
C: half of leg		$2\frac{1}{2}$	$2\frac{1}{2}$	$2\frac{3}{4}$	3	$3\frac{1}{4}$	$3\frac{1}{2}$

Hypothermia

Have a high index of suspicion and a low-reading thermometer. Most patients are elderly and do not complain of being or feel cold, so they have not tried to warm themselves up. In the young, hypothermia is usually either from cold exposure (e.g., near-drowning), or it is secondary to impaired level of consciousness (e.g., following excess alcohol or drug overdose).

Definition Hypothermia implies a core (rectal) temperature <35°C.

Causes In the elderly, hypothermia is often caused by a combination of:
- Impaired homeostatic mechanisms: Usually age-related
- Low room temperature: Poverty, poor housing
- Disease: Impaired thermoregulation (pneumonia, MI, heart failure)
- Reduced metabolism (immobility, hypothyroidism, diabetes mellitus)
- Autonomic neuropathy (e.g., diabetes mellitus, Parkinson's)
- Excess heat loss (psoriasis)
- Decreased cold awareness (dementia, confusion)
- Increased exposure to cold (falls, especially at night when cold)
- Drugs (major tranquilizers, antidepressants, diuretics), alcohol

The patient Don't assume that if vital signs seem to be absent, the patient must be dead: Rewarm (see below) and reexamine. If temperature <32°C, this sequence may occur: Drop in BP → coma → bradycardia → AF → VT → VF. If >32°C, there may simply be pallor ± apathy.

Diagnosis Check oral or axillary temperatures. If ordinary thermometer shows <36.5°C, use a low-reading one rectally. Is the rectal temperature <35°C?

Tests Urgent CMP, plasma glucose, and amylase. Thyroid function tests, CBC, blood cultures. Consider blood gases. The ECG may show J-waves or Osborn waves. See Figure 20.5.

Treatment
- Ventilate if comatose or respiratory insufficiency.
- Warm IV (for access or to correct electrolyte disturbance)
- Cardiac monitor (both VF and AF can occur during warming)
- Consider antibiotics for the prevention of pneumonia. Give these routinely in patients >65 with a temperature <32°C.
- Consider urinary catheter (to assess renal function).
- *Slowly rewarm.* Do not reheat too quickly, which causes peripheral vasodilatation, shock, and death. Aim for a rise of ½°C/h. Elderly conscious patients should sit in a warm room taking hot drinks. Thermal blankets may cause too rapid warming in older patients. The first sign of too rapid warming is falling BP.
- Rectal temperature, BP, pulse, and respiratory rate every half hour.

NB: Advice is different for victims of sudden hypothermia from immersion. Here, if there has been a cardiac arrest and T° <30°C, mediastinal warm lavage, peritoneal or hemodialysis, and cardiopulmonary bypass (no heparin if trauma) may be needed.

Complications Arrhythmias (if there is a cardiac arrest, continue resuscitating until temperature is >33°C, as cold brains are less damaged by hypoxia); pneumonia, pancreatitis, acute renal failure, intravascular coagulation.

Prognosis Depends on age and degree of hypothermia. If age >70 and temperature <32°C then mortality >50%.

Before hospital discharge Anticipate problems. *Will it happen again? What is her network of support?* Review medication (*could you stop tranquilizers?*)? *How is progress to be monitored?* Coordinate with physician/social worker.

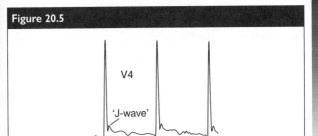

Figure 20.5

V4

'J-wave'

Kindly supplied by Drs. Richard Luke and EM McLachlan.

Major disasters

Planning All hospitals should have a detailed *disaster plan*.

At the scene Call the police and activate EMS.

Safety is paramount: Your own and others. Be visible (luminous monogrammed jacket) and wear protective clothing where appropriate (safety helmet, waterproofs, boots, respirator in chemical environment).

Triage: Label RED if victim will die in a few minutes with no treatment. Label YELLOW if victim will die in ~2 h with no treatment; label GREEN if victim can wait for treatment. (BLACK = dead).

Communications are essential: Each emergency service will dispatch a control vehicle and have a designated officer for liaison. Support medical staff from hospital report to the medical safety officer: He is usually the first doctor on the scene. His job is to assess then communicate to the receiving hospital the number and severity of casualties, organize resupply of equipment, and replace fatigued staff. He must resist the temptation to treat casualties as this compromises his role.

Equipment: Must be portable and include intubation and cricothyrotomy set, IV fluids (colloid), bandages and dressings, chest drain (+ flutter valve), amputation kit (when used, ideally two doctors should concur), drugs (*analgesic:* Morphine; *anesthetic:* Ketamine 2 mg/kg IV over >60 sec [0.5 mg/kg is a powerful analgesic without respiratory depression]), limb splints (may be inflatable), defibrillator/monitor ± pulse oximeter.

Evacuation: Remember: With immediate treatment on scene, the priority for evacuation may be reduced (e.g., a tension pneumothorax [patient labeled RED], if relieved [now patient labeled YELLOW], can wait for evacuation), but those who may suffer by delay at the scene must go first. Send any severed limbs to the same hospital as the patient, ideally chilled, but not frozen.

At the hospital a "major incident" is declared. The *first receiving* hospital will take most of the casualties; the *support* hospital(s) will cope with overflow and may provide mobile teams so that staff is not depleted from the first hospital. A control room is established, and the medical coordinator ensures that staff have been summoned, nominates a triage officer, and supervises the best use of inpatient beds and ICU/operating room resources.

Blast injury may be caused by domestic (e.g., gas explosion) or industrial (e.g., mining) accidents or by terrorist bombs. Death may occur without any obvious external injury (air emboli). Injury occurs in six ways:

Blast wave

1 A transient (milliseconds) wave of overpressure expands, rapidly producing cellular disruption, shearing forces along tissue planes (submucosal/subserosal hemorrhage) and reexpansion of compressed trapped gas: Bowel perforation, fatal air embolism.

2 **Blast wind** This can totally disrupt a body or cause avulsive amputations. Bodies can be thrown and sustain injuries on landing.

3 **Fragments** Penetration or laceration from blast fragments are by far the most common injuries. These arise from the source of explosion (e.g., bomb) or are secondary (e.g., flying glass).

4 **Flash burns** These are usually superficial and occur on exposed skin.

5 **Crush** Injuries: Beware of sudden death or renal failure after release.

6 **Psychological injury** E.g.,post-traumatic stress disorder

Treatment Approach the same as any major trauma. Have patient rest; observe others for any suspected exposure to significant blast but without other injury.

Index

Page numbers followed by *t* and *f* indicate tables and figures, respectively

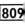